Spinal Anatomy

Jean Marc Vital • Derek Thomas Cawley
Editors

Spinal Anatomy

Modern Concepts

Springer

Editors
Jean Marc Vital
Spinal Unit
Centre Hospitalier
Universitaire de Bordeaux
Bordeaux
France

Derek Thomas Cawley
Spinal Unit
Centre Hospitalier
Universitaire de Bordeaux
Bordeaux
France

Translation from the French language edition 'Anatomie de la colonne vertébrale, Nouveaux concepts' by Jean-Marc Vital © Sauramps Medical, Montpellier, 2016; ISBN 979-10-303-0064-2

Translated by Derek Thomas Cawley

Publishing rights for the English language edition will be returned to the editor.
ISBN 978-3-030-20924-7 ISBN 978-3-030-20925-4 (eBook)
https://doi.org/10.1007/978-3-030-20925-4

This Springer imprint is published by the registered company Springer Nature Switzerland AG
The registered company address is: Gewerbestrasse 11, 6330 Cham, Switzerland

Foreword

It is difficult for the layman to understand anatomical research and discoveries, because anatomy is considered as a science of the dead, so long known without new phenomena. This book on the anatomy of the spine with its new concepts is a clear proof of this common mistake. Studying the dynamic anatomy of the living subject and using the most up-to-date technical means can open up new perspectives to elucidate the pathology of the spine and perfect its surgery!

The comparative anatomy of the spine through the vertebrate chain illustrates the Darwinian evolution of the spine to finally adapt to bipedal walking. Embryology, which is a repetition of phylogeny, shows this adaptation. Studies in erect standing have identified parameters, including "pelvic incidence," which quantifies the pelvic tilt relative to the lumbar curvature. Thus, from these parameters, it has been possible to identify four types of "vertebral equilibrium." It has appeared that a "reserve of the extension of the hips" must be considered in the operative state of sagittal imbalances.

The 3D study of vertebral movements, thanks to the "EOS system," made it possible to define an "articular chain of equilibrium" and a "cone of economy." To simplify this concept, the authors included the skull and pelvis in the spine as cephalic and pelvic vertebrae. This may seem logical and simplistic, but I doubt that anatomists agree. The new histological and chemical knowledge of the intervertebral disk enriches the chapter on this element. The posterior vertebral joints have general features specific to the cervical, dorsal, and lumbar vertebrae, which explain their dynamics and their role in the spinal balance; facet orientation variations are common. The study of ligaments and spinal muscles widens our conceptions on their structure and dynamics. In the muscles are isolated "sarcomeres" and fascicles whose angular orientation regulates their power. The tensegrity model helps in understanding the musculoskeletal system. It is necessary to emphasize the originality of the chapter on aponeuroses and fascia so little studied in classical works. The chapter on the vertebral canal makes it possible, in other interests, to discover the descriptions of the "lateral recess" and the "transverse canal." The spinal cord is the subject of an exhaustive review of our current knowledge. The spinal nerves and meninges happily complete this spinal anatomy!

It is obvious that this book deserves to be recommended to all those who are interested in the spine, including physiotherapists, rehabilitators, rheumatologists, and spinal surgeons. Congratulations to all the authors who participated in its realization!

Marseille, France

René Louis

Preface

It is interesting to know that this book *Anatomy of the Spine: New Concepts* was born naturally, following our long experience concerning spinal surgical pathologies shared with Jacques Sénégas, founder of the school of spine surgery in Bordeaux, and to the interest we have in the anatomy of the vertebral column that we have long taught to medical students.

Thanks to this double cap, anatomist and surgeon of the spine, we have been able to develop an anatomy applied to physiology, degeneration, and surgical pathology.

We also collaborated with our friends in Montpellier, François Bonnel, who opened his collection of images of the School of Anatomy, and Alain Dimeglio, with his expertise on spinal growth.

All articles are from French anatomists and clinicians. These clinicians are spinal surgeons (orthopedic surgeons (pediatricians or adult surgeons) or neurosurgeons), rehabilitation specialists, physiotherapists, and biomechanists.

These French authors have all been able to develop rather original concepts concerning the growth of the vertebral column and its aging and functioning.

We thank them very much for their active participation.

All this has led to a book that we hope will allow readers to progress in terms of diagnostic and therapeutic knowledge of the spine.

Bordeaux, France

Jean Marc Vital
Derek Thomas Cawley

Contents

Part I

Phylogenesis and Ontogenesis

Comparative Anatomy of the Axial Skeleton of Vertebrates

J. Sénégas

Introduction

Vertebrates (e.g. fish, amphibians, reptiles, birds and mammals, including primates) form a branch of the phylum chordata. They are distinguished from other animals by the existence of a bone or cartilaginous endoskeleton comprising two basic structures: the skull (hence the name Craniata) and the vertebral column which protect the central nervous system (encephalon and spinal cord). The oldest vertebrate fossils to date—*Mylokumingia fengjiaoa* and *Haikouichthys ercianunensis*—were discovered in China in 2003 in the Maotianshan Shales and date back to the early Cambrian period (535 million years ago).

It was above all, the physical constraints linked to the aquatic or terrestrial way of life that led to the selection of specific morphofunctional adaptations in these animals. They relate more specifically to the modes of respiration, locomotion, management of water loss and reproduction, and also behavioural constraints of survival (attack/defence, mating).

The Organization Plan for the Vertebrates

All vertebrates, without exception, present a bilateral symmetry which determines three axes of polarity (Fig. 1):

1. The anteroposterior axis (or craniocaudal axis) corresponds to the sequence: (1) of the head/neck complex which carries the sensory organs, the brain and the mouth; (2) the trunk complex that carries the appendicular system and (3) the tail.

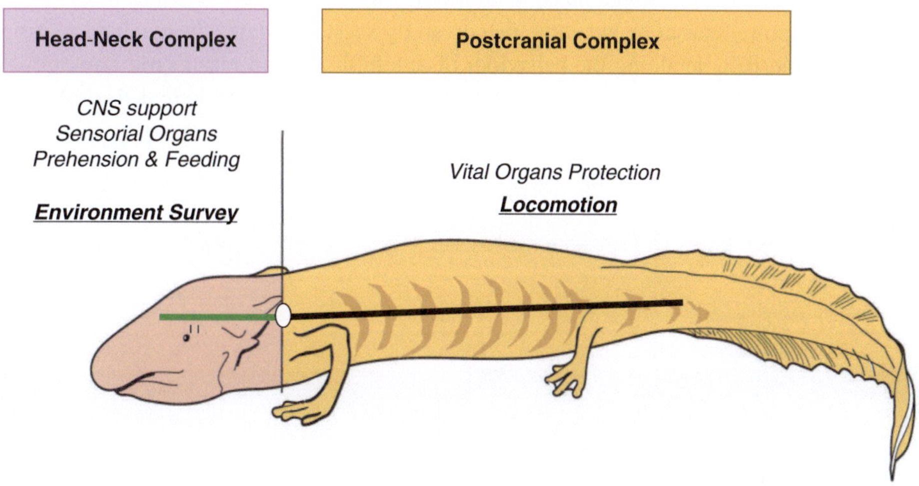

Fig. 1 The body of the vertebrates is characterized by the existence of an anteroposterior corporeal axis and a cephalocaudal bipolarization. Head and neck complex—support of the CNS and sensory organs for the analysis of environment and nutrition. Postcranial complex—protection of vital organs and locomotion

J. Sénégas (✉)
Spinal Unit, University Hospital, Bordeaux, France

J. M. Vital, D. T. Cawley (eds.), *Spinal Anatomy*, https://doi.org/10.1007/978-3-030-20925-4_1

The craniocaudal axis changes orientation during the transition from quadruped to biped with multiple angular variations between the horizontal and the vertical.
2. The dorsoventral axis with the vertebral column in dorsal position, the thorax and the abdomen in ventral position.
3. The left–right axis of symmetry in the coronal plane.

Adaptive Constraints of the Living Environment

Constraints of the Aquatic Environment

It is thought that the aquatic environment is the original environment. Oxygen is relatively rare (7.2 ml/l vs 209.5 ml/l in air) and diffuses more slowly. Oxygen is extracted by gills, extensions of the splanchnocranium. In the branchial system of fish, the partial pressure difference of oxygen between water and blood remains constant.

In the aquatic environment, postures and displacements constantly depend on Archimedes principles—the ratio of gravity/hydrostatic thrust which defines buoyancy. The force exerted on the water which determines the magnitude of the acceleration during the propulsion is a function of the displacement velocity and the viscosity of the liquid. In water, it is the axial structure (vertebral column periaxial musculature) that is the motor of locomotion, the fins (pterygium limbs) having in most fish only a directional or stabilizing role. The body, without a neck, moves as one, on itself around the three Cartesian axes, and advances in water by translation along the same axes. In attack/defence behaviours, the cephalic end of the fish is projected forward by the rest of the body [6]. Unlike amphibians, fish do not project the tongue to capture their prey, but some fish do so by suction such as anglerfish, heralding the behaviour of amphibians (sit and wait predators) (Fig. 2).

Constraints of the Terrestrial Air Environment

The terrestrialisation of tetrapods involves the extraction of oxygen from the air using lungs developed from the digestive tract. This active extraction requires the individualisation of a specific respiratory musculature whose action is reinforced by that of the appendicular musculature when the consumption of oxygen increases, especially in rapid displacements.

For the support of the body and terrestrial locomotion, the primordial adaptive stress is gravity (9.81 m/s^{-2}). It must be balanced by the resistance of the locomotor apparatus to ensure body retention. On land, it is the limbs which take on most propulsion forces. The axial system loses its flexibility, especially in large mammals, but it nevertheless contributes significantly to rapid propulsion through deformations in the sagittal plane which modify the orientation of the pelvis and thus the axis of thrust of the limbs. This intervention of the axial skeleton is essential in fast paces. The vertebral column also plays a pivotal role in postural flexibility through rotation.

Finally, to survive, an animal must be able to attack and defend itself. For this purpose, the axial skeleton of the tetrapod allows the rapid projection and retraction of the mouth, armed with teeth, towards the prey or the aggressor.

Fish

(Approximately 25,000 Species)

The axial skeleton of primitive fish such as cyclostomes (e.g. lamprey) is a flexible rod, the notochord which is formed of vacuolated chondrocytes, surrounded by a fibrous sheath. The stiffness of this hydrostatic skeleton depends on the osmotic pressure of the colloid in the vacuoles of the chondrocytes. Its mechanical properties can be compared to those of an elastic rod combining longitudinal compressive stiffness and lateral flexibility. With this configuration, the pro-

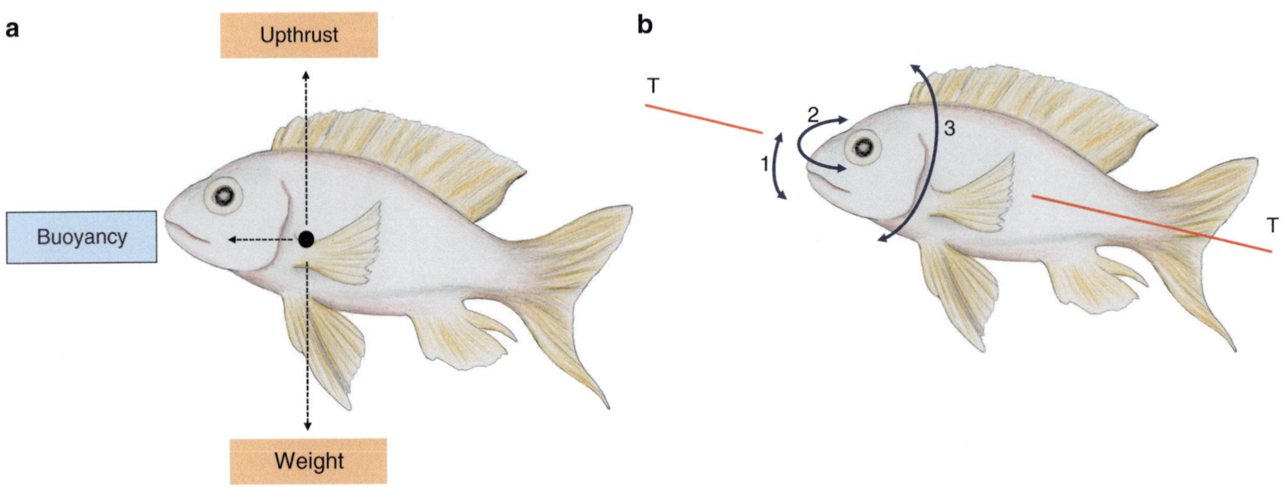

Fig. 2 (**a**) In the aquatic environment, the buoyancy depends on the hydrostatic weight/pressure ratio (Archimedes' thrust). (**b**) In fish the body uses six degrees of freedom. The linear displacements are carried out by axial translation. Buoyancy—Hydrostatic thrust—Gravity

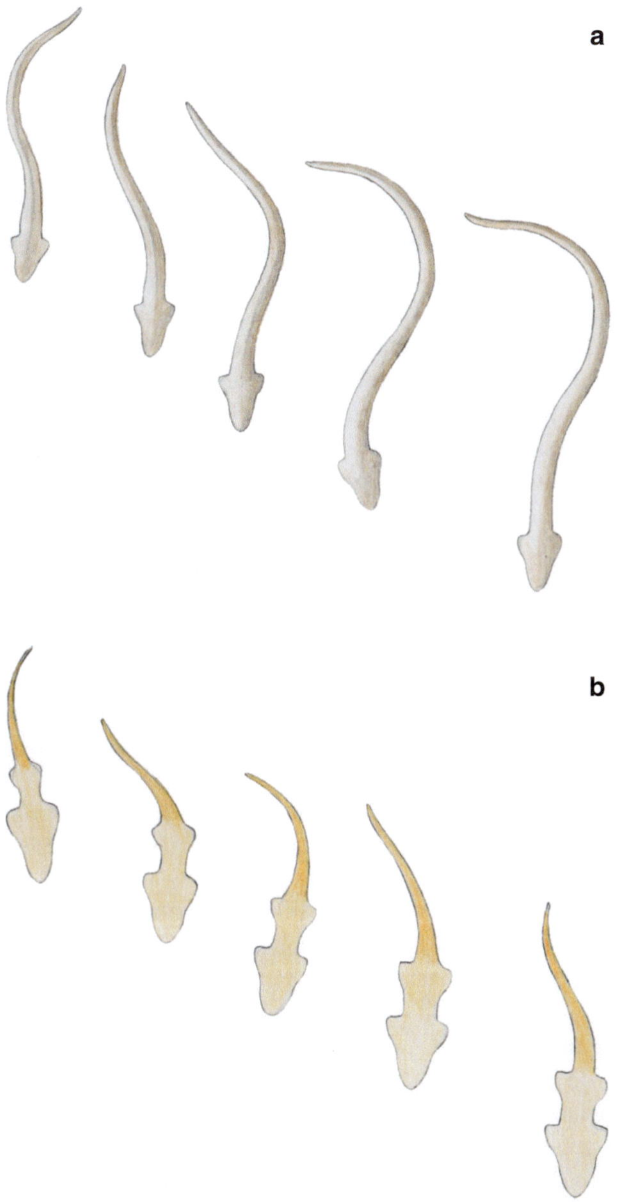

Fig. 3 The displacements of anguilliform fish (**a**) occur in an axial wave mode (the whole body is flexible and undulating). Most pelagic fish (**b**) move in an axial oscillatory mode (the propelling force originates mainly from the caudal fin). Certain fish with rigid bodies (e.g. balistidae, mormyridae and electric fish) move in a caudal oscillatory mode (the tail alone allows the propulsion)

pulsion of these species is the axial wave mode contraction of muscles composed of periaxial myotomes in sequence which generate a succession of undulating waves propagating from the head to the tail, while the animal moves forward [10].

Teleostean fish have a skeleton formed of identical cartilaginous or bony vertebrae, without zygapophyses. Although fish have no neck, there is a beginning of vertebral regionalisation, which distinguishes between a trunk segment and a more flexible caudal segment (Fig. 3).

In fish, the perivertebral musculature is organized into two groups, the dorsal epiaxial and ventral hypoaxial, separated by a horizontal septum. The myofibrils do not, however, attach directly into the vertebral parts. For pelagic fish (living neither close to the shore nor to the bottom), many myomeres regroup as large longitudinal fibre endings that resemble the organization of long muscles of tetrapods [15]. Propulsion of these species then takes place in the axial oscillatory mode, the lateral deformation of the body intensifying towards the caudal segment carrying a rigid fin.

The feeding of the fish is done either by suction/aspiration or by predators, by rapid acceleration of the mouth towards the prey. This gesture of rapid protraction of the head by impulse of the body involves the whole axial skeleton. This "push-forward-with-the-head" ability is evident with all tetrapods.

Tetrapodomorphic fish (actinistians such as coelacanth and rhipidistians like lungfish) have fleshy fins that participate in locomotion. Their pectorals have well-defined bony pieces prefiguring the anterior well-defined chiridian limbs. Tetrapod fish are characterized by the appearance of a cervical vertebra at the craniovertebral junction and chiridian limbs with three distinctly individual segments: stylopod, zeugopod and autopod. Thus, contrary to popular belief, the chiridian limbs first appeared in aquatic and non-terrestrial organisms. This is the principle of exaptation. At this stage, the functional coupling of the vertebral column of the appendicular skeleton for open-air locomotion is already in place.

In summary, fish are characterized by:

- A flexible cartilaginous or bony axial skeleton without vertebral differentiation but with truncal and caudal regionalization
- The presence of an epiaxial and hypoaxial musculature
- Only a lateral (in a horizontal plane) deformation of the column that ensures all locomotion with attack/defence behaviours.

Terrestrial Vertebrates

During life in the open air, the weight of the body is no longer balanced by hydrostatic thrust. It is the appendicular skeleton which counteracts gravity for the maintenance of the body and its displacements.

There are two spatial reference systems of terrestrial vertebrates:

At a minimum, two coordinate reference frames are needed to account for both the position and movements of the body in the environment and changes in the position of skeletal segments and organs within the body itself (Figs. 4 and 5).

1. The external (exocentric) reference frame is fixed, locked on the gravitational vertical force from which the coordinates of the centre of mass of the animal are defined.

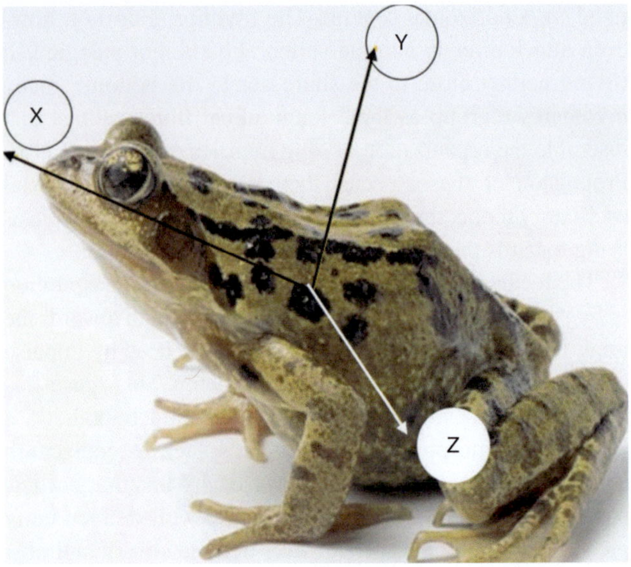

Fig. 4 Representation of the orthonormal reference formed by the three axes of polarity of the animal from the cephalocaudal axis of symmetry

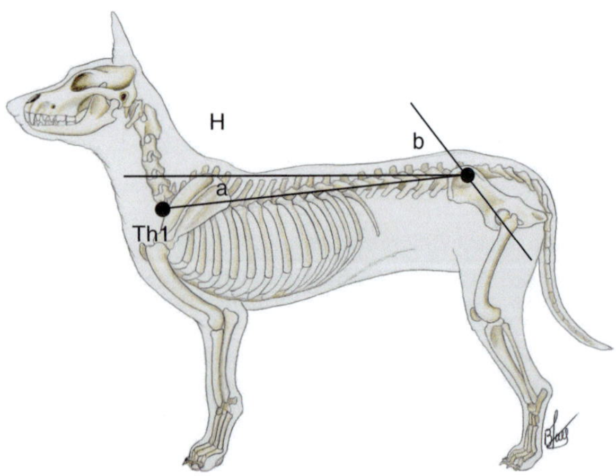

Fig. 5 In quadrupeds, the angular variations coupled between the thoracolumbar column and ilium can be measured by the spinopelvic angle. It is formed by the intersection of a line from T1 and the sacroiliac joint (the upper edge of the sacrum is very hard to visualize in animals) and the centre line between both the femoral heads (the bicoxo-femoral axis) and the sacroiliac joint. This is an adaptation of the spinopelvic angle described in humans

2. The general internal frame of reference (egocentric) corresponding to the three axes of polarity, which is an expression of the animal's body pattern (topological properties of the species).

To analyse the relative movements of the thoracolumbar spine and pelvic girdle, we propose to use the angle formed by the spinopelvic line from T1 to the centre of the sacroiliac joint (easier to locate in tetrapods than the sacral end plate), and the axis of the ilium represented by the line from the acetabulum to the same point of the sacroiliac joint.

The angle of incidence formed by the axis of the ilium and that of the sacrum is not a reliable topological data in animals because, contrary to popular belief, the sacroiliac joint is mobile, varying within and between individual cases. In man also this mobility can vary from one subject to another.

The external and internal reference systems coincide only under certain conditions (as in the strict vertical position in human bipedalism). In all other cases, data switching is required to change the repository. In animals, this switching is performed automatically by the central nervous system, which reconstructs a global pattern of data from the two references, so that the animal knows the position, speed and acceleration of the elements, its environment, its body and its own components.

Amphibians (About 7000 Species)

In amphibians, the final regionalization of the vertebral column is in place. Although reduced to a single vertebra, the cervical segment articulates with two trochoid surfaces homologous to the occiput. This is the individualized subcranial junction.

In anurans (frogs), the trunk segment is limited to 4–8 elongated vertebrae connected to the pelvis by a longitudinal urostyle. Frogs have no ribs. The truncocaudal junction is the most mobile of the column. At rest, the column is flexed at this joint, while it extends during jumping.

In the urodeles (salamanders), the elongated truncal segment comprises 12–63 vertebrae with ribs connected to the sternum.

In amphibians, the posterior vertebral arch is complemented by three types of apophyses: diaphysis (transverse), zygapophysis (articular) and neurapophysis (spinous). The first segment of the upper limb (stylopod) is horizontal, characteristic of the transverse chiridium (buttressed limbs). In amphibians, the scapular girdle is independent of the vertebral column while the pelvic girdle is secured to the sacrum through the transverse sacral processes. The ilium houses the proximal end of the femur. The pubic and ischial parts play the role of levers for the proximal muscles of posterior limbs. The axial skeleton of amphibians shows no curvature in the sagittal plane (the functional sagittal curvature of the anurans corresponds to the truncopelvic junction). The axis of the ilium is vertical (sacropelvic angle = 90°). The lumbosacral angle is approximately 0°.

On land, the anurans move by alternate advances of the limbs, but choose the jump for fast displacements in the open air. There is then a great mobility of the short thoracic column, around the lumbosacral junction. In the urodeles, walking is affected by lateral oscillations of the column, which causes an inverse rotation of the pelvis. The main role of the limbs is to lift the body off the ground, while deformation of

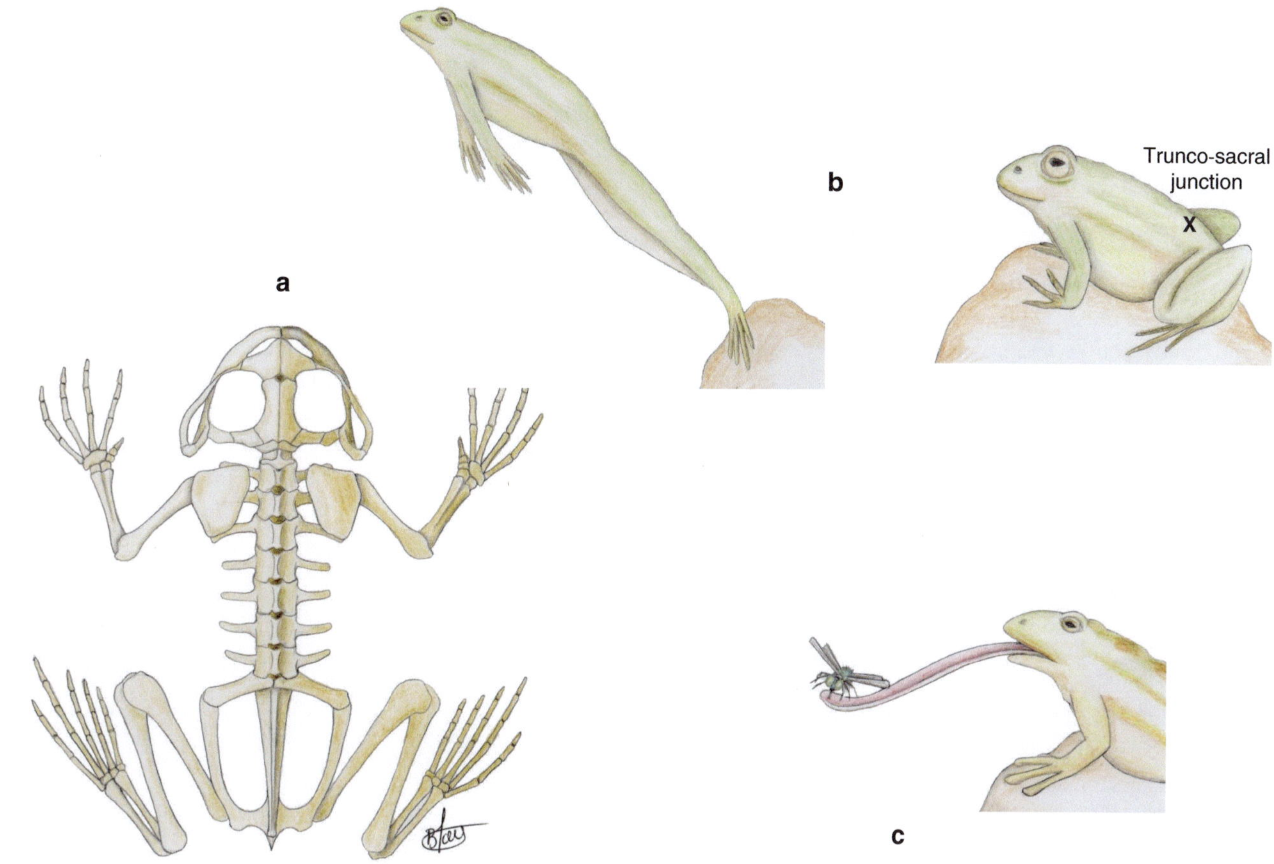

Fig. 6 (**a**) In Anurans (frogs) the craniovertebral junction is functional. The truncal segment is short and prolonged by the urostyle. (**b**) In the jump, the column is extended to the level of the truncosacral junction. (**c**) For amphibians and certain reptiles (geckos, iguanas, and chameleons), the projection of the tongue is more economical than that of the whole body for the capture of prey (sit-and-wait predators)

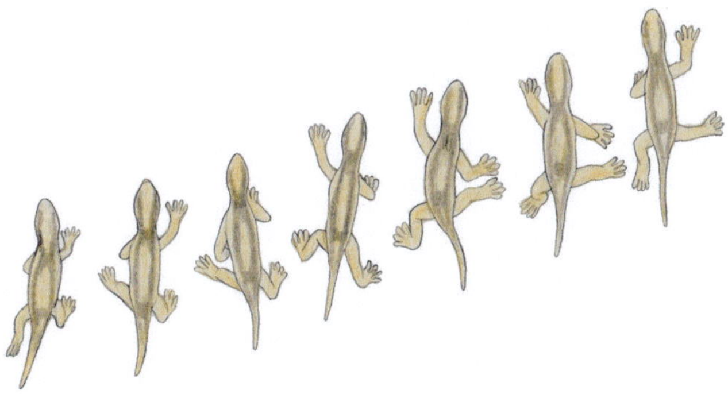

Fig. 7 Walking in Urodeles (salamanders) is done by side-to-side oscillations of the column causing an inverse rotation of the pelvis. The essential role of the limbs consists of lifting the body, while lateral deformations of the column pull the limbs forward

the vertebral column pulls the limbs forward. Different muscles ensure elevation and displacement [12] (Figs. 6 and 7).

The reduction of the cervical segment to a single vertebra does not make it possible to carry out a rapid protraction/retraction of the cephalic end of the animal for the capture of prey. The low mobility of the occipitocervical junction allows it only to bite and swallow. For reasons of saving energy that propulsion of the whole body would require, most of these species are "sit-and-wait predators" [6]. The solution of an extensible tongue projected rapidly and powerfully towards the prey was selected by evolution in many amphibians.

Respiration of amphibians is ensured by the contraction of the buccal floor, without any involvement of the appendicular musculature as seen in reptiles and mammals.

Reptiles (Approximately 8950 Species)

This class of terrestrial tetrapods remains heterogeneous and unclear in its definition. At the level of the axial skeleton, it is characterized by three major innovations:

1. a semi-independent craniocervical junction with significant mobility;
2. an epiaxial musculature differentiated into independent muscle groups;
3. and the strengthening of ties between the sacrum and the pelvis.

The Cervical Spine

The atlas articulates with a single occipital condyle. The testudines (turtles) have up to eight cervical vertebrae, the caudal aspect of which articulates with the first truncal vertebra which itself is fixed to the shell.

In reptiles, epiaxial cervical muscles become inserted on the occiput, differentiating into three groups (*vertebrocapitis superficialis* and *profundus*, and *intertransversalis capitis*). These extensor muscles of the craniocervical junction have an antigravity action which is essential for maintaining the head, which is sometimes very heavy (e.g. crocodiles).

The movements of protraction/retraction are particularly pronounced in turtles, whereas in crocodiles and most squamates (snakes), it is still the propulsion of the body that ensures the projection of the head forward. In geckos, iguanas and chameleons, the "sit-and-wait attitude" prevails, with the projection of the tongue towards the prey.

The thoracic column of the crocodiles comprises 10–11 vertebrae, 5 lumbar and 2 sacral, the transverse processes of which have a close connection with the ilium.

Like the cervical system, the muscular masses are segregated into organized bundles (*m. longissimus*, *m transverseo-spinalis* and *ilio costalis*), which generate the lateral movements of the column when they contract asymmetrically, but induce an extension of the column during a symmetrical contraction [15]. Crocodilian limbs have a first horizontal segment (buttressed limbs). It is the muscles of the pelvis that raise the body of the animal (sprawling posture).

The amplitude of mobility of the hip joint is low (less than 45°). The axis of the ilium is vertical, perpendicular to the vertebral axis at rest (pelvic version = 90°). The spinopelvic angle varies from 80 to 100° in crocodiles.

Slow locomotion in crocodiles is achieved by alternating oscillations of the column causing the front left leg and the rear right leg to move forward simultaneously with a caudal propulsion force. When the animal accelerates, as in catching prey, the entire column can participate in propelling the body forward. This new type of locomotion using a deformation of the column in the sagittal plane of flexion/extension induces backward (retroversion) and forward (anteversion) tilting of the pelvis leading to an increase in the amplitude of the stride, which increases the effect of the thrust of the posterior limbs. This new type of displacement is observed preferentially in young crocodilians, then disappears in adults as they become heavier [15] (Figs. 8 and 9).

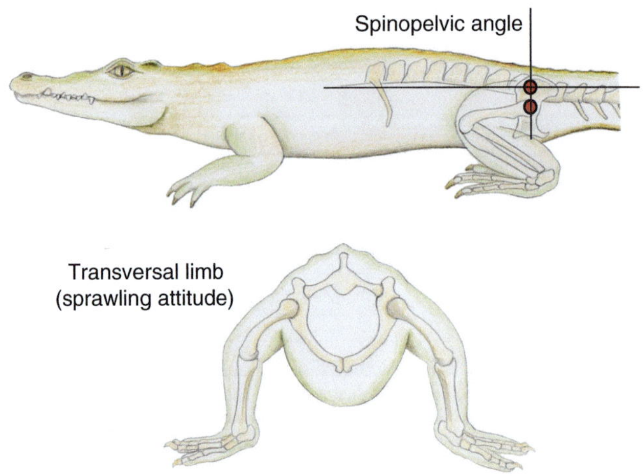

Fig. 8 In crocodiles, the axis of the ilium is perpendicular to the column. The posterior spinopelvic angle and the pelvic version approximate 90°

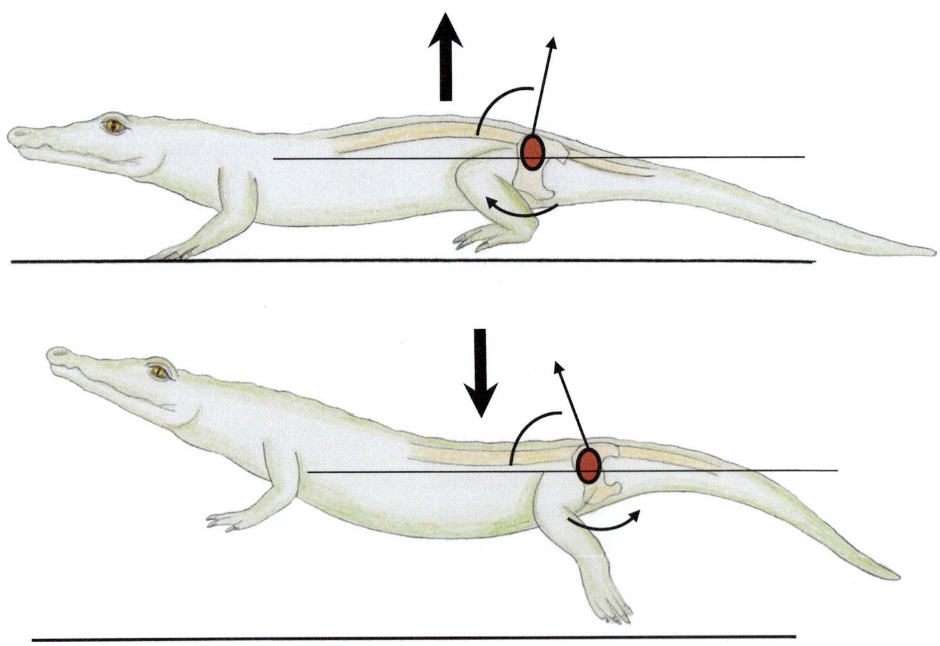

Fig. 9 Young crocodiles can mobilize their column in the sagittal plane which changes the orientation of the pelvis and thus improves the thrust of the posterior limbs. The weight of the adult makes this impossible

It is interesting to note that it is in reptiles that the coupling respiration/locomotion appears. However, the two functions cannot be carried out concomitantly. In locomotion, the appendicular musculature contracts asymmetrically, in the respiration symmetrically. This strict alternation is possible only because of the low energy expenditure of these ectothermal species.

In summary, amphibians and reptiles are characterized by:

- defining the final regionalization of the column, an SP angle varying from 80 to 120°
- locomotion by lateral oscillations or by sagittal deformation of the column for rapid displacements
- protraction/retraction of the isolated head or with the whole body creating the "push-forward-with-the-head" characteristic or the capture of prey by the tongue—"sit-and-wait predators".

Birds (Approximately 10,000 Species)

Birds have the most flexible neck of vertebrates with a rigid thorax to allow for flight. This is the most extreme example of the substitution of limbs for the axial skeleton for all movements. They are bipeds.

Birds emerge from the lineage of the middle Jurassic theropod dinosaurs that survived the Triassic-Cretaceous extinction, 65 million years ago. This line is characterized by a long moving neck that stabilizes the posture of the head during running and flight, and by its rapid projection (protraction/retraction) for the capture of prey (Fig. 10).

The vertebrae of the thoracic, lumbar and the sacral spine are fused to form the synsacrum. The truncated column only intervenes in flight and walking as a fulcrum of the muscles of the pelvis. In contrast, the S-shaped cervical segment includes many vertebrae (up to 25 in swans). The axis of the cervical spine is vertical, perpendicular to the trunk.

Mammals (About 5500 Species)

Adaptation to open-air lifestyles is fully expressed in mammals, the most widely spread and most morphologically diverse vertebrate group. This great ecological independence is the result of many evolutionary innovations [12]:

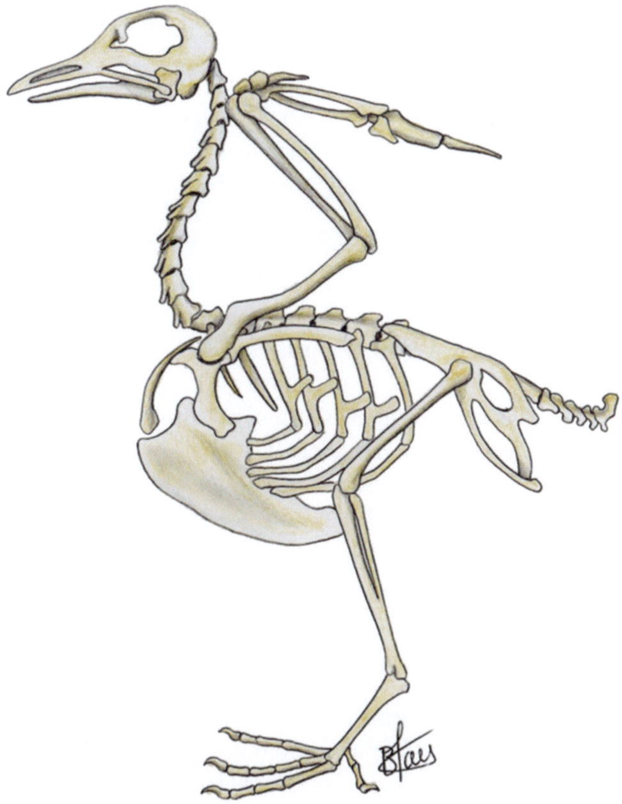

Fig. 10 In birds, the long and flexible neck allows it to project or retract the head quickly. The posterior vertebrae of the trunk are fused to form the synsacrum. The trunk is sufficiently rigid to allow flight

- Firstly, they benefit from permanent homeothermia from the embryonic stage (unlike birds).
- They also exhibit an exceptional neopallium development of the brain which allows them to perform complex behaviours "culminating in man, with language, conceptualization and symbolic thought" [12].
- Finally, their musculoskeletal system is optimized for an important metabolic energy conservation thanks to the nature and organization of the elastic connective structures of the musculature of the column and the limbs [9]; thus referred to as a spring mechanism. Indeed, the potential (slow-paced) and kinetic (fast-paced) energy released during stride is temporarily stored in the stretched muscles in the form of "elastic energy" which will be restored immediately to the same muscle group for the next phase of the locomotor cycle without metabolic cost. One of the most characteristic examples of this phenomenon is the high jump. Whatever the technique, the jumper starts by stretching the propulsion muscular chain by lowering its centre of gravity, which has the effect of passively storing

the elastic energy and thus considerably reinforcing the vertical thrust force.

At high speeds, some mammals, and man more than quadrupeds, can thus save more than half the metabolic energy that their movements would otherwise require without this mechanism.

The protein macromolecule, Titin, which is incorporated into the sarcomeres, plays a major role in this mechanism by giving its deformation to the frequency of the locomotive cycle, which reduces the dissipation of energy in the form of heat [13].

This phenomenon applies as much to the musculature of the limbs as to that of the spine. It is therefore preferable to compare the column with a bowstring or retaining bridge (by Arcy Thompson 1917).

The Cervical Spine

Functionally, the cervical column is coupled to the head and ensures its spatial orientation. The survival of terrestrial animals depends on information from one's external frame of reference. The information is captured by the visual, vestibular and somatosensory organs and then directed to the brain, whose interpretation of the data allows navigation through a complex environment without falling or failing. The vestibular system contributes to postural balance and locomotion by vestibulocollic reflexes and vestibuloocular reflexes. With the acquisition of bipedalism, the role of vision becomes predominant thanks to the high definition of macular perception and the acquisition of stereoscopic vision. This multisensory information supplies the middle and anterior brain as well as the hippocampus. The simultaneous cerebral integration of the data from the two repositories makes it possible to reconstitute and constantly update an internal map of the environment for navigation.

This central navigation function devolved mainly to the head/neck complex implies in sthenic tasks (exploration, alert, racing, combat) the possibility of horizontalizing the cephalic end which corresponds to the plane of terrestrial activity. This results in a de facto empowerment of the spatial frame of reference of the head relative to that of the rest of the body. Thus, irrespective of the inclination of the body or the type of locomotion, quadruped or biped, the plane of the base of the skull, parallel to the lateral (or horizontal) semicircular canals, presents only a slight angulation with respect to the skull [5, 8]. The neck is thus the instrument for adjusting the position of the head.

This neurological constraint is not without consequence in terms of energy. Indeed, the head/neck assembly presents itself as an inverted pendulum which poses problems of equilibrium, especially in quadrupeds. The weight of the head represents approximately 10% of body weight in large herbivores, 8% in humans and chimpanzees [16], and 6% in lemur prosimians [5]. This difference of 2–4% may seem small in absolute value, but becomes significant in relative value, given the total mass of large quadrupeds (about 500 kg for the horse). Proportionally, bending moments are 10–11 times greater than in humans and chimpanzees. Bipedalism also results in a considerable reduction in the bending moment of the head.

In aquatic mammals (whales, dolphins) secondarily adapted to life in water 50 million years ago, the cervical vertebrae became fused, with only a mobile cranial junction. Similarly, the fusion of the vertebrae of the lower cervical segment is observed in the armadillo and in some rodents such as the kangaroo rat and the jerboa, which has the effect of reducing the inertia of the weight of the head when jumping. The same applies to burrowing species such as the mole rat [11], where fusion of the vertebrae of the lower cervical spine increases its resistance to axial stresses (Fig. 11).

The centre of gravity of the head in quadrupeds is located very forward of the craniovertebral junction due to the development of the splanchnocranium, the horizontality of the base of the skull (platybasia) and the very posterior position of the occipital condyles, so that the occipitoatloid line is almost vertical. In primates and even more markedly in humans, basicranial flexion is observed in the sphenoid, with the clivus then forming an angle with the anterior part of the base of the skull. This process, probably related to the development of the cerebral hemispheres and the reduction of facial mass, coincides with the forward migration of the occipital condyles, which has the effect of considerably reducing the bending moment of the centre of mass of the head. In humans, the occipitoatloid articulation is horizontal and the head gravity line passes right in front of the dens (Fig. 12).

Structure

The cervical spine of terrestrial mammals has 7 vertebrae, except the Folivora (sloth) which has 6–9 and Sirenia (manatee) which has 6 [11].

The upper cervical spine consists of the atlas and axis; morphology varies little from one species to another, except the dens (C-shaped in herbivores and vertical in carnivores and primates). The length of the spinous processes and the width of the transverse processes are much more prominent in quadrupeds and large primates than humans. Similarly, the superior articular surfaces of the atlas corresponding to the

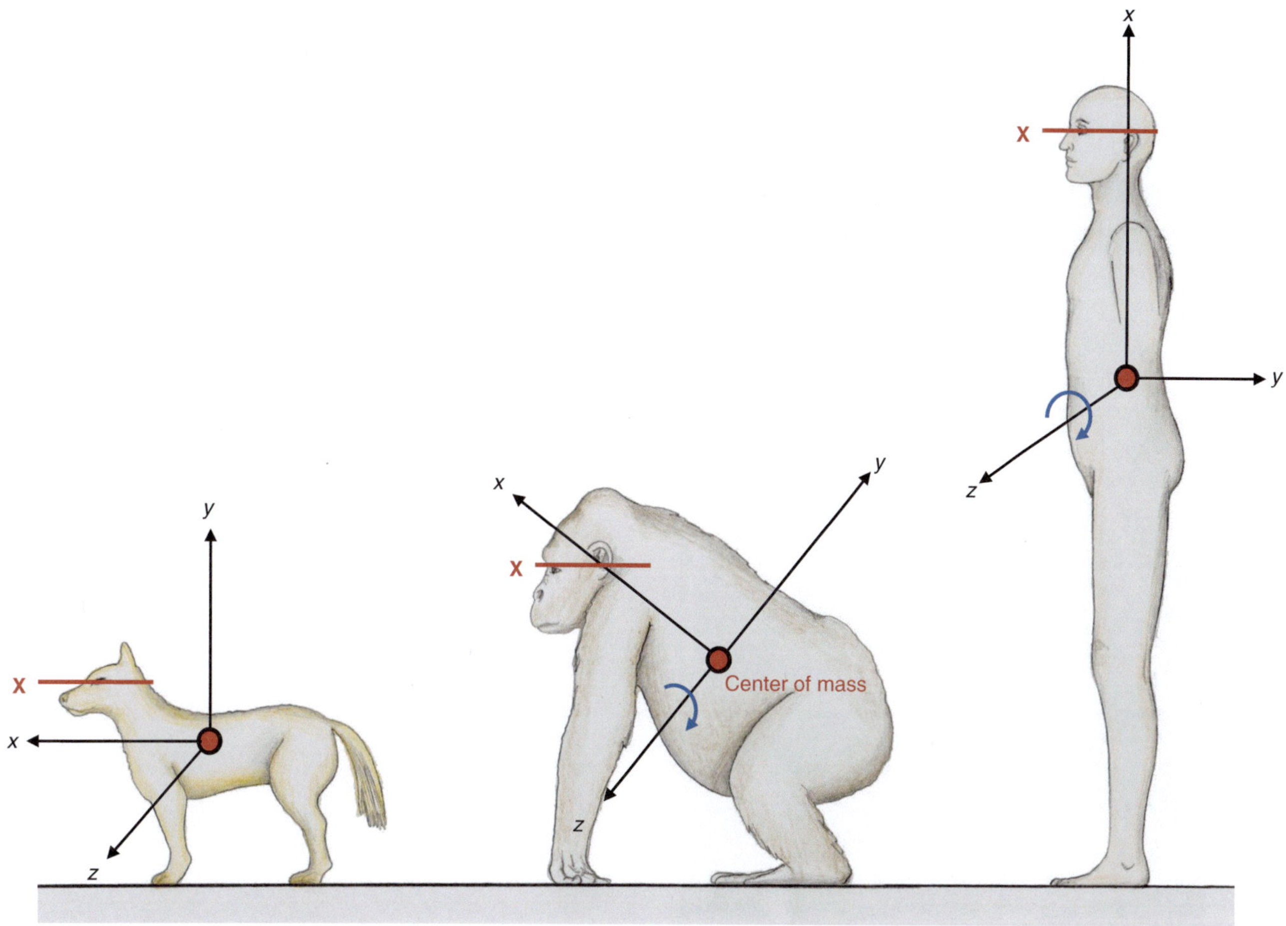

Fig. 11 In the internal frame of reference, the coordinate axes of the head are kept approximately fixed relative to the external reference frame by changes in the orientation of the cervical column, irrespective of the position of the trunk, horizontal (quadrupeds) or vertical (bipeds). This autonomy of the cephalic coordinates facilitates the switching of data between the two reference frames and allows the brain to permanently recreate a new global pattern of navigation

occipital condyles occupy in quadrupeds about 75% of the atlas ring but only 40% in humans [7].

The lower cervical spine includes the lower 5 cervical vertebrae whose configuration minimally varies. The total volume of the vertebral bodies is relatively greater among bipeds.

Movements

Mobility of the occipitocervical junction is important in the sagittal plane in quadrupeds (flexion/extension range of motion of 90–105°), whereas it is much lower in primates, including humans (13° in monkeys and 25° in man) [8]. Rotations take place in the atlantoaxial joint (Tables 1 and 2).

The mechanical coupling of both OC1 and C1C2 joints generate a toggle effect which allows more lateral tilting movements of the head (induced rotation).

It is worth noting that in quadrupeds, mobility between the vertebrae of the lower cervical spine is very small (unlike humans). It is also interesting to note that the cervicothoracic articulation encompasses more than the C7T1 anatomical junction. It encompasses C6 to T2 in small quadrupeds [8], and as far as T3 in humans. The range of motion of the cervicothoracic junction ranges from 6 to 80° in all mammals [8].

In the neck, as well as the very important intrinsic ligament mechanism, there is an extrinsic ligament (septum nuchae) specifically developed for large herbivores. This system plays a vital role in the passive stabilization of the craniocervical kinetic chain (which is not provided by the

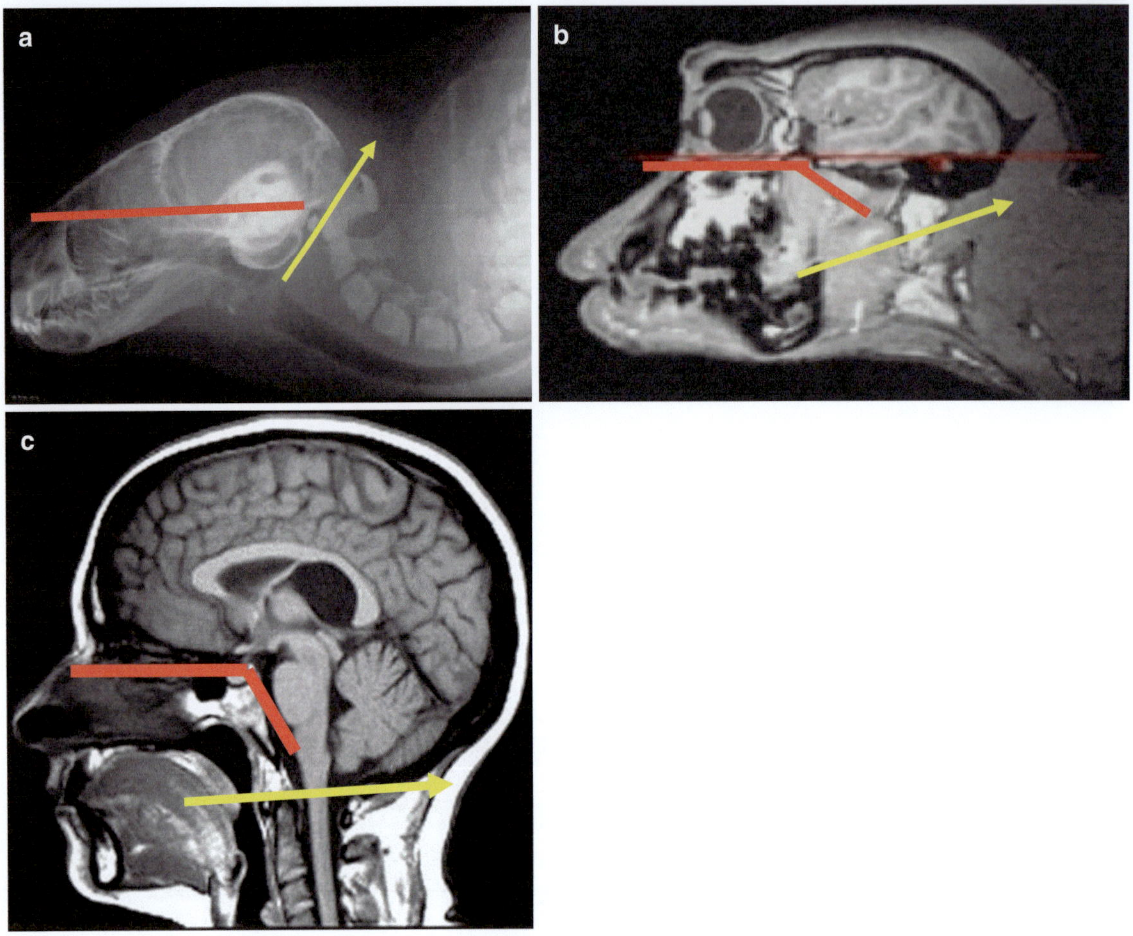

Fig. 12 In quadrupeds (**a**) the skull base is horizontal (platybasia), the occipital condyles are located at the back of the skull and the foramen magnum is tilted back and top. In monkeys (**b**) there is a basicranial bending at the sphenoid bone, the occipital condyles are located further forward. The foramen magnum tends to horizontalize. In humans (**c**) basicranial flexion is more important between the anterior floor of the skull base and clivus, the occipital condyles are almost under the skull and the foramen magnum is horizontal

Table 1 Amplitude of mobility in the sagittal plane of the atlantooccipital articulation (OC1) in various mammals [7]

Rabbit	104.6° (±15.7)
Guinea pig	106.6° (±5.9)
Cat	88.6° (±11.2)
Rhesus	13° (±14.8)
Man	25°

Table 2 Range of mobility in the sagittal plane at the cervicothoracic junction (C6T3) [8]

Rabbit	96°
Cat	82°
Rhesus	68°
Man	33°

bone passive locking cam effect, as applied to most musculoskeletal joints). This elastic passive locking allows optimum use of the inertia of the head and neck in running.

The Craniovertebral Musculature

There is a large musculature variation in mammals related to the complexity of stabilization and precise mobilization of head/neck system. One can distinguish schematically:

(1) the short muscles of the craniocervical junction (*m. recti* and *obliqui capitis anterior* and *posterior*)
(2) short intervertebral muscles, including intermetameric (*m. intertransversalis* and *m. interspinalis*) and long spinal muscles (*m. longus capitis* and *cervicis, m. longissimus and m. semispinalis*) which mainly act as stabilizers cervical flexible
(3) finally, cephalothoracoscapular muscles (*m. splenius capitis, m. levator scapulae, m. scalenius, m. trapezius* and *m. sternocleidomastoid*) that are specifically dedicated to the active mobilization of the neck and secondarily, respiration during effort. Cats have a muscle (*m.*

occipitoscapularis) that is absent in humans. The cervical muscle volume is comparatively much higher in quadrupeds than in primates, including humans.

Postures

At rest, the cervical spine of small mammals (rabbits, guinea pigs, cats) resembles an "S" shape whose average orientation is vertical. In this configuration, the craniocervical junction is maximally flexed and the cervicothoracic junction is stabilized at full extension [8]. This attitude, according to these authors, is totally passive, only assured by the tensioning of the pervertebral tissues (resting posture). In this position, the plane of the lateral semicircular canals is inclined to the horizontal at approximately 5–10° upwards. The same authors describe, next to the posture of rest, the alert or active posture, in which the head is raised by extending the occipitocervical hinge. The cervicothoracic junction is then flexed in this posture and the plane of the lateral semicircular canals moves upward [8].

However, extending the generalization of this functional dichotomy to all terrestrial mammals of the complex head/neck seems too simplistic. It is enough to be persuaded to observe the diversity of the postures of the head and the neck of large ungulates (e.g. cattle, deer and sheep) (Fig. 13).

The mechanical model of the head/neck is that of an inverted pendulum whose rod represents the cervical spine and the sphere, the head. Schematically, the rod moves around the cervicothoracic joint, while the sphere is mobilizing around the occipitocervical junction. However, it is not exactly centred on the end of the cervical rod. In quadrupeds, it is forward due to the very posterior position of the occipital condyles, which induces a significant bending moment at OC1. In primates and even humans, that moment is greatly reduced by adopting the biped posture.

In quadrupeds, verticalisation of the neck reduces the bending moment of the head. This attitude of retraction is analogous to the term used in humans. It involves an extension of the cervicothoracic junction. This posture cannot be completely passive, as in this position, the perivertebral tissues are not stretched sufficiently. Contraction is combined with two different positions of the head. When in this position the OC1 joint remains flexed, the posterior tendinoligamentous structures are likely to develop an effective passive muscle moment so that the energy cost is low (standing alert position). When the OC1 joint is actively maintained in extension, the tension moment of the passive structures decreases. The maintenance of this position necessitates contraction of the occipitocervicothoracic muscles as seen in trotting or parrying (sthenic retraction).

When the neck is flexed around the cervicothoracic joint, the bending moment increases horizontally and then decreases. This protraction movement stops when the elastic tension of ligament and muscle (whose deformation is nonlinear) reaches the value required to cancel the bending moment of the head/neck. When the protraction is combined with a bending of the OC1 joint, posture is mainly passive, energy-saving (like grazing, watering or extreme tiredness states). By contrast, when protraction is combined with an active extension of the OC1 and/or a straightening of the neck above the horizontal, it is then a sthenic posture (as in the gallop). This position optimizes the moment of inertia of the head and neck in fast running (Fig. 14).

We find these same two basic stereotypes (retraction-protraction) in primates including humans. Protraction corresponds to a passive rest position when the OC1 joint is flexed (as in reading or sleeping in a sitting position), or to an active position when the OC1C2 joint is extended under the effect of the posterior musculature. This is in fact a "push-forward-with-the-head" attitude which one observes in particular through efforts of pushing (as in the collision sports). According to Ordway et al. [14], it is in this posture that the

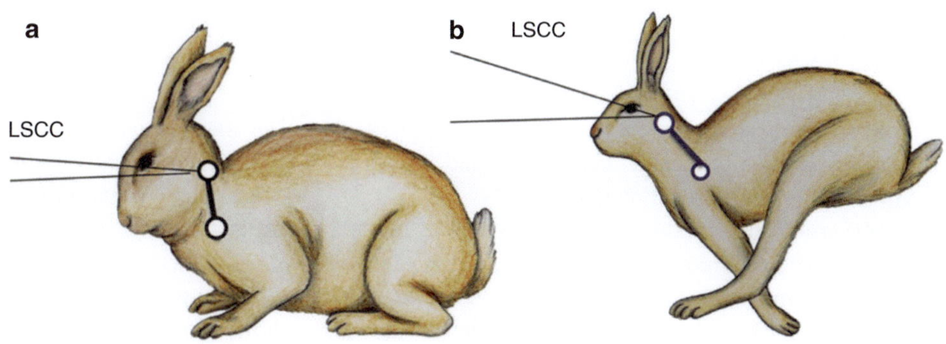

Fig. 13 In small mammals: In the rest position (**a**) the cervical spine is vertical, the craniovertebral junction is maintained in full flexion and the cervicothoracic junction in extension [4]. The plan of the lateral semicircular canals (LSCC) is slightly inclined to the horizontal (5–10°). In the alert position (**b**) the positions of the two joints are reversed. The plan of the lateral semicircular canals is shifted upwards

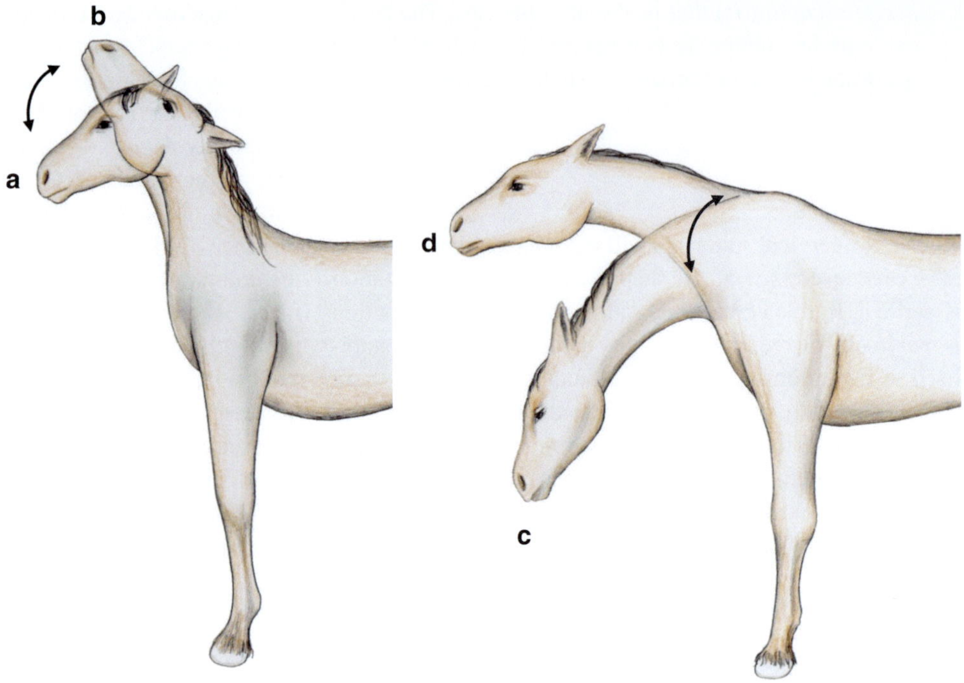

Fig. 14 Reverse coupling of the craniovertebral and cervicothoracic joints: (**a**) when the craniovertebral junction is flexed (static posture without large energy expenditure), the other (**b**) is extended (sthenic posture). Displacements at the craniovertebral junction, flexion (**c**) or extension (**d**)

craniocervical junction reaches its maximum amplitude in extension.

Retraction behaves in the same way through flexion of the OC1 joint (OC1 position where it reaches its maximum amplitude in flexion) and active extension (e.g. to charge with the head or to wear a headlight). Each of these attitudes implies a new choice of orientation of the field of view depending on the position of the eyes of the animal, the side of the head in quadrupeds and front of the head in humans and primates [5] (Fig. 15).

In running, the cervical spine plays, in quadrupeds, a significant role in breathing (respiratory locomotion coupling). Inspiration occurs when the neck is in ventral flexion, expiration when dorsi-flexing.

Thoracic Spine and Lumbosacral

The trunk of quadrupeds is almost horizontal and approximately cylindrical shaped. Its centre of mass is positioned approximately centrally. Its forward displacement, as in ungulates, promotes running, whereas the most posterior position is observed in small mammals [2].

Limbs articulate with the trunk by the shoulder and pelvic girdles. The shoulder girdle is independent of the axial skeleton and maintains a single connection to the trunk through the clavicle (collarbone). The upper limbs are involved in locomotion more as carriers and for steering than that as propellants. In many small mammals, the upper limbs acquire the faculties of grasping and manipulating objects within the field of view, which will become their primary role in bipeds. One notes by contrast, at the pelvis, increased strengthening ties between the ilium and sacrum without the loss of sacroiliac joints whose mobility in locomotion persists in many animals and also in man. In humans, it is 3–17° in adults, and up to 30° in gymnasts. In certain athletes one can even observe an opposite displacement of each iliac bone in the sagittal plane.

The proximal segments of the limbs are, in mammals, situated in a parasagittal plane, which has the effect of symmetrically supporting the body and raising the centre of gravity. This configuration reduces ground frictional force, improves manoeuvrability and allows the use of the elastic potential energy (spring effect). At the point of rapid reaction, manoeuvrability and acceleration capabilities outweigh stability however, especially in humans.

Structures

The mammalian thoracic region comprises 12–15 vertebrae. The thoracic vertebrae of large herbivores have very long spinous processes. At the transition between the thoracic and lumbar vertebrae is at the anticlinal vertebra (diaphragmatic vertebra, to which all other vertebrae are inclined) where the spinous process is short. On both sides, chest spinous processes are inclined caudally, the lumbar cephalad.

There are usually from four to seven lumbar vertebrae (the latter figure is typical of the cat and rabbit). The body of

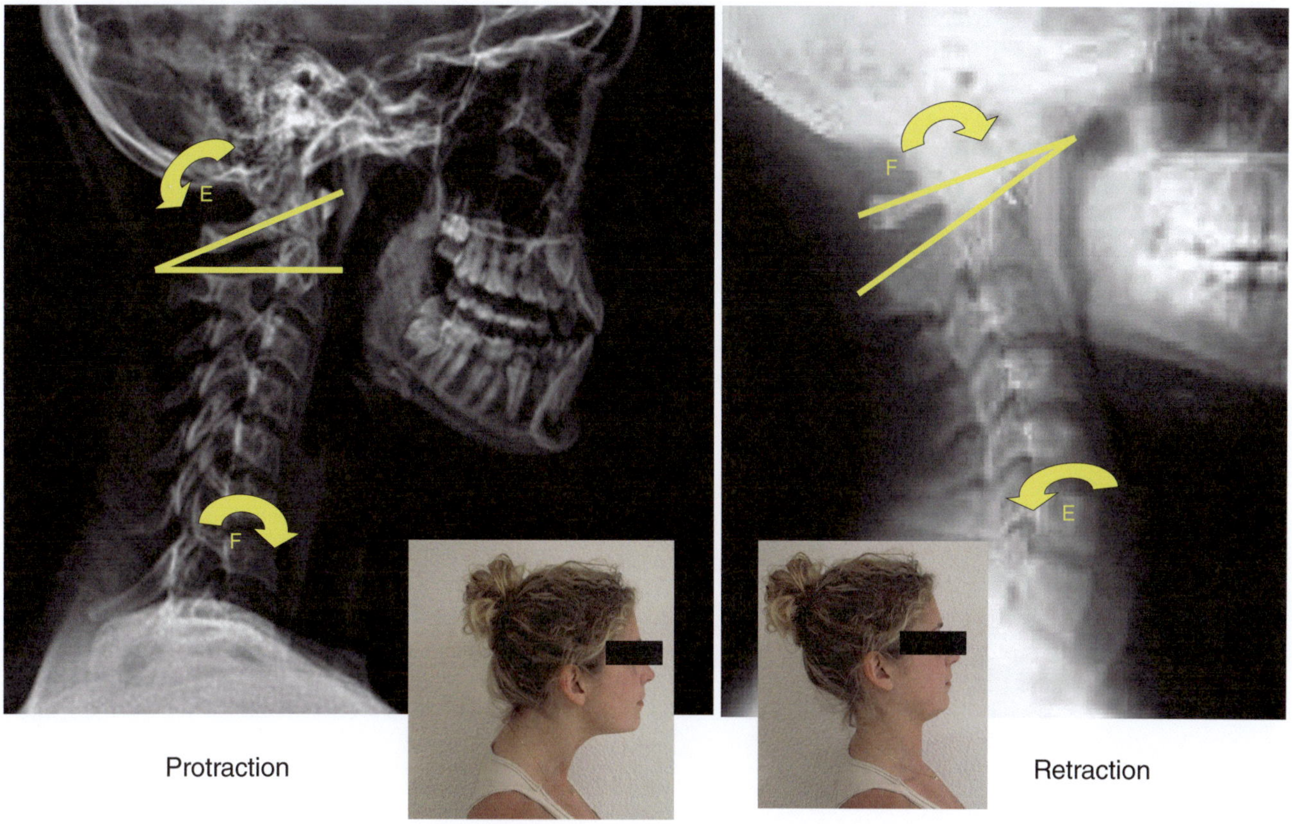

Fig. 15 Primates, including humans, use like quadrupeds, the reverse coupling of the two extreme neck positions for protraction and retraction of the neck and head

the lumbar vertebrae is proportionally larger in men and increases down to L5.

The sacrum is composed of a varying number of fused vertebrae (three in cats, four in rabbits and usually five in humans). This number can reach six to eight in perissodactyla (odd-toed ungulates—e.g. horse, zebra and rhino) and up to thirteen in edentulous (e.g. anteater and sloth). The first sacral vertebrae articulates with the ilium through its transverse processes.

The coccygeal vertebrae also vary in number, depending on the tail length (up to fifty, but usually three to five); Merged, they form the coccyx in humans [11].

Musculature

Both the body of quadrupeds and that of the bipeds present a "bowstring construction" represented by tight dorsal musculature bow and the chord of the ventral muscles, especially the *recti*. As in the neck, in terrestrial mammals there is a regression of epiaxial muscles concomitant with the trans-girdle musculature (*mm. trapezius, rhomboid, latissimus dorsi* and *glutei*) [12]. The local system of intervertebral short muscles (*m. interspinalis, m. intertranversalis*) is distinguished from a global system (*m. erector spinae*, *m. quadratus lumborum* and *m. rectus* and *obliqui abdominalis* and *m. psoas)* [3].

Postures

The quadruped truncal column is generally horizontal or kyphotic. The diaphragmatic vertebrae represents in quadrupeds, the flexion/extension hinge of the trunk.

- In all quadrupeds the lumbosacral angle (LSA) is minimal while it becomes important especially in primates and hominids. Abitbol [1] has in particular studied variations of this angle: in dogs, it varies from 4 to 14° (average 9.3°); rhesus monkeys, 20 to 35° (mean 26.7°); chimpanzee 22 to 44° (average 32°) and in humans 71 to 83° (average 77°). This angle is related to the acquisition of erect posture and the ontogeny of biped locomotion.
- The pelvic tilt that expresses the orientation of the ilium relative to the horizontal for quadrupeds and to the vertical for bipeds varies in quadrupeds from 30 to 60°. In chimpanzees, which are alternately quadru-

ped and biped, it varies from 25 to 60° (average 42°). In humans, the angle of pelvic tilt varies from 7 to 25°.

- The spinopelvic angle (SP) (Fig. 5) varies from 60 to 75° in quadrupeds, from 30 to 60° in chimpanzees and from 15 to 45° in humans.

The thoracolumbar spine helps to maintain posture and locomotion in quadrupeds as well as bipeds. In extension there is a relative shortening of the column that has the effect of pulling the sacroiliac junction forward in quadrupeds and upward among bipeds.

Contrary to what one might think, it is not the posterior limbs that guide the pelvis, but the vertebral column. This rocker promotes forward momentum when pushing off from the rear. Conversely, the bending of the thoracolumbar spine causes the pelvis to retrovert, increasing the amplitude of pushing off from the front (Fig. 16).

Primates generally move in quadrupedalism, especially in fast running, but adopt bipedal posture in either static or in slow movements or jumps (lemurs).

The physical problem of verticalisation of the body is that of balance on a considerably reduced support surface, in addition to maintenance of balance through effective musculature. In primates, the centre of mass is located at the base of the thorax which is relatively high compared to the hips. Moreover, the absence of lordosis does not allow easy adjustment of the line of gravity on the support polygon if the femurs are not bent over the pelvis. This posture is difficult to maintain in large part because of weak *glutei maximi* muscles in these animals, and instead use the *g. medius* and *g. minimus* for hip extension.

It is likely that bipedalism evolved as an adaptive process in the three-dimensional arboreal environment (Rose 1991; Preuschoft 1991). In this situation, the body weight is often supported only by the posterior limbs so that the anterior limbs are liberated for their gripping function (Fig. 17).

In humans, during walking and running, the deformation of the lumbar spine allows pelvic tilt. Pelvic retroversion increases hip flexion amplitude and extends the stride. Anteversion favours the rear step thrust by increasing the extension of the hip beyond the vertical (Fig. 18).

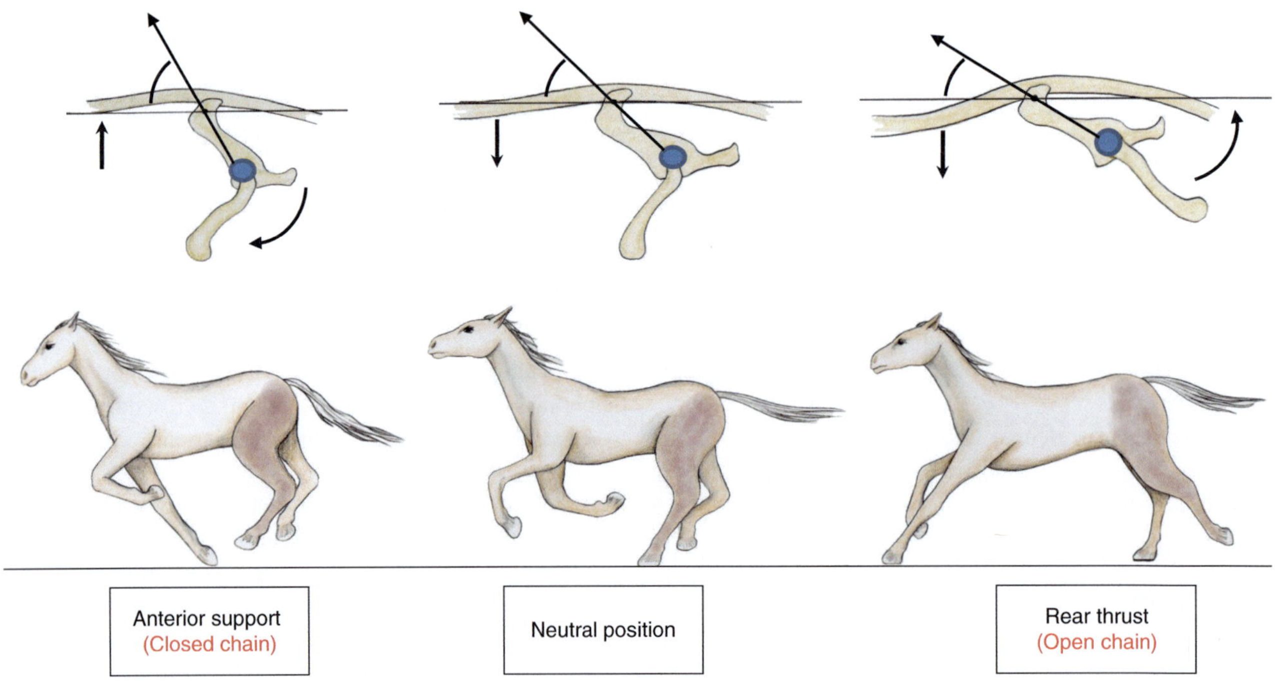

Fig. 16 In mammalian runners, the bending of the thoracolumbar spine induces pelvic retroversion which increases the amplitude of the previous step. The extension brings the pelvis in anteversion which has the effect of increasing the extension of the femur and the thrust of the posterior pitch

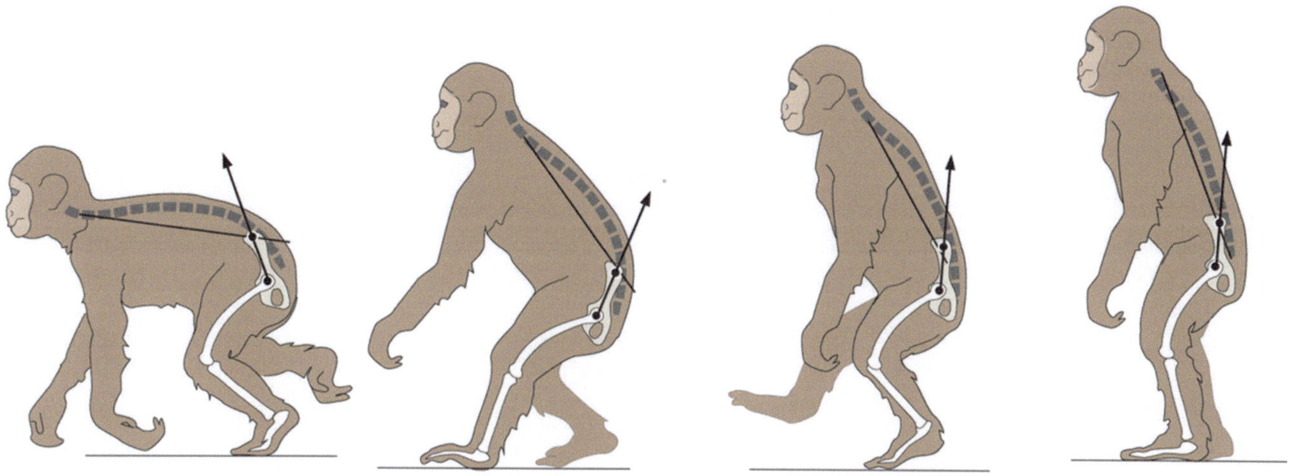

Fig. 17 Chimpanzees adopt quadrupedalism for quick trips (semibrachiateurs). They can maintain a stable bipedal posture but the lack of lumbar lordosis forces flexion of the femur on the pelvis to bring the projection of the centre of mass into the area of elevation. This position requires a significant effort from the glutei muscles

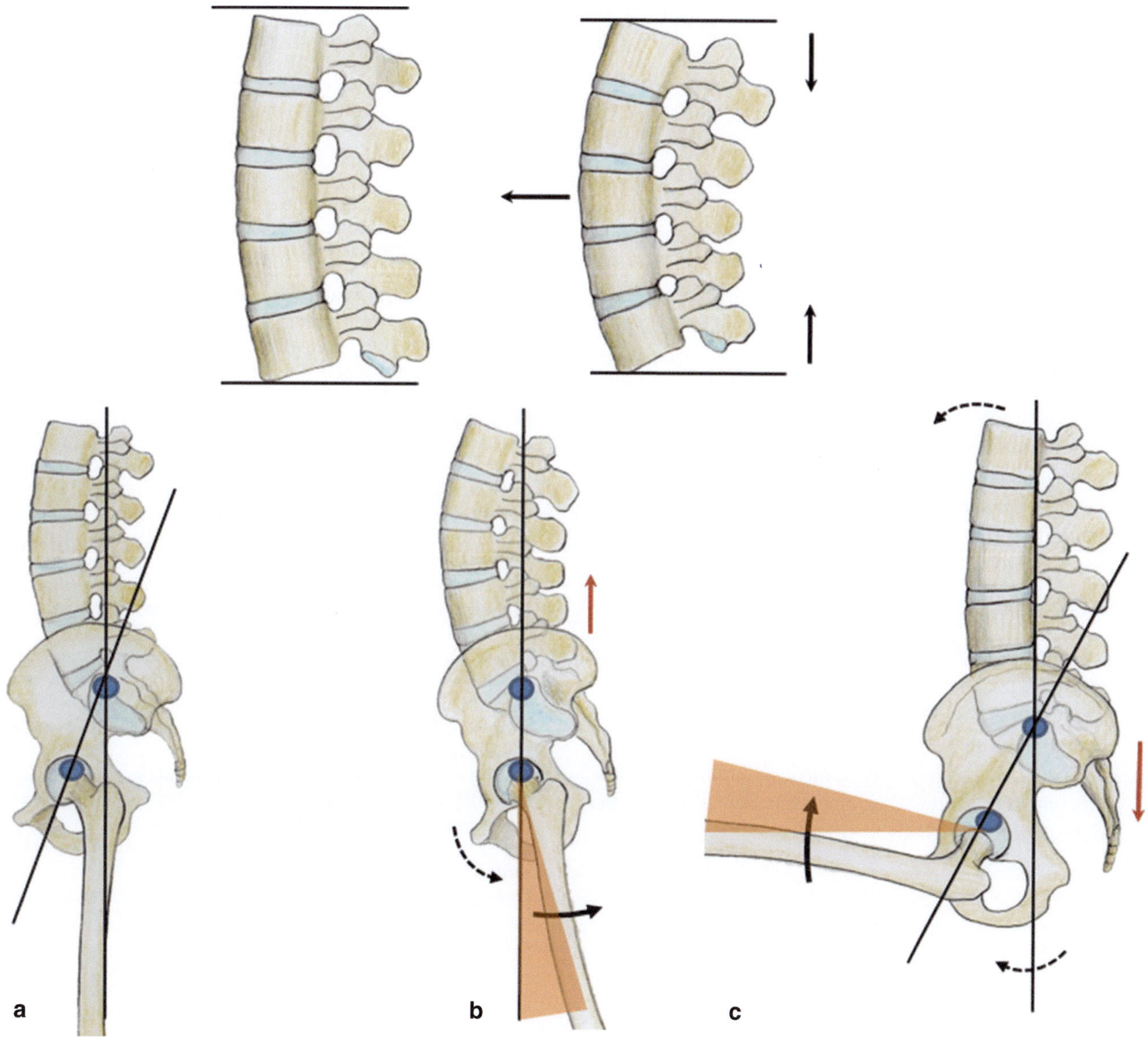

Fig. 18 The extension of the lumbar spine (**a**) pulls the pelvis in anteversion, which has the effect of granting a supplementary extension to the femur relative to the vertical (**b**) (without gain in amplitude of the hip joint). Conversely, lumbar flexion (**c**) causes pelvic retroversion and, consequently, an equivalent gain in femur flexion

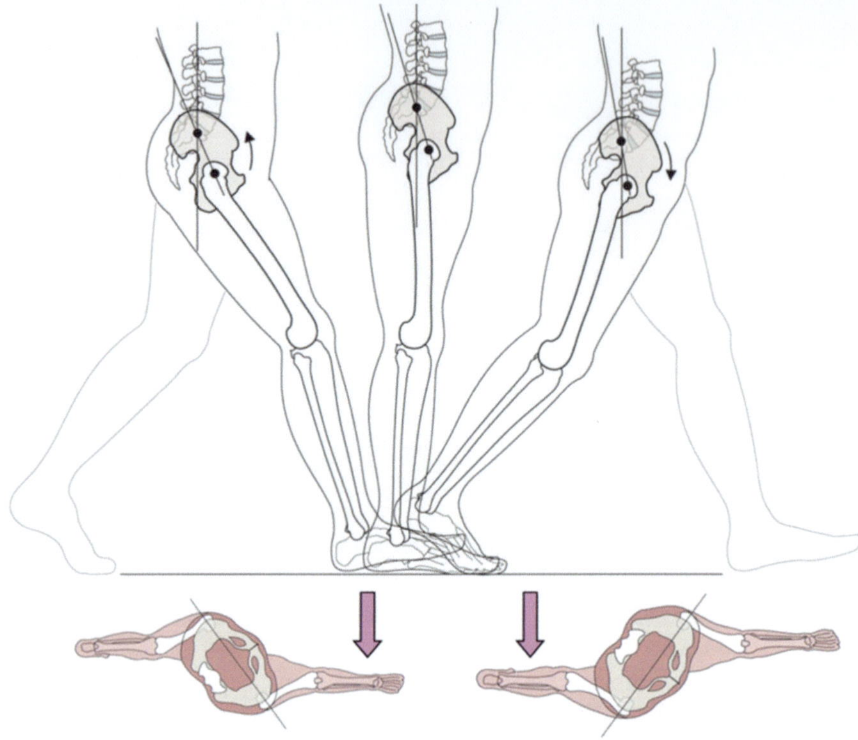

Fig. 19 In humans when walking and running, the shoulders and pelvis rotate in opposite direction with a tipping point approximately at the thoracolumbar junction

In mammals, the vertebral column plays an essential role both in posture and in movement by the axial rotational movements which are usually coupled to displacements in the coronal and sagittal planes. When walking and running the shoulders and pelvis move in opposite directions. The thoracolumbar spine is thus "twisted" from either side of the thoracolumbar junction. Rotations are expressed as the background kinematics of the spinal kinematics. This contributes to a better understanding of their role in the genesis of spinal degenerative process (Fig. 19).

In summary, the mammals are characterized by:

- A very mobile cervical spine capable of powerful and rapid protraction and retraction movements
- A thoracolumbar spine that permits the awareness and stability of postures. It is also involved in locomotion by a "spring effect" in flexion/extension which changes the orientation of the pelvis
- In bipeds exclusively, the lumbar column intervenes in locomotion. Moreover, it plays an essential role in the axial rotation of the body.

References

1. Abitbol MM. Evolution of the lumbosacral angle. Am J Phys Anthropol. 1987;72:36172.
2. Alexander RMN. Animal mechanics. Oxford: Blackwell; 1983.
3. Bergmark A. Stability of the lumbar spine. Acta Orthop Scand Suppl. 1989;60:230.
4. Berthoz A, Graf W, Vidal PP. The head-neck sensory motor system. Oxford: Oxford University Press; 1992.
5. Dunbar DC, et al. Stabilization and mobility of the head, neck and trunk in horses during overground locomotion: comparisons with humans and other primates. J Exp Biol. 2008;211(24):3889–907.
6. Gans C. Biomechanics: an approach to vertebrate biology. Philadelphia: Lippincott; 1974.
7. Goel A, et al. Comparative quantitative analysis of osseous anatomy of the craniovertebral junction of tiger, horse, deer and humans. J Craniovertebr Junction Spine. 2011;2(1):327.
8. Graf W, De Waele C, Vidal PP. Functional anatomy of the head-neck movement system of quadrupedal and bipedal mammals. J Anat. 1995;186:5574.
9. Heglund NC. Energetics and mechanics of terrestrial locomotion III. Energy changes of the centre of mass as a function of speed and body size in birds and mammals. J Exp Biol. 1982;97:4156.
10. Hilledebrand M. Walking, running, digging of the quadrupeds. In: Functional vertebrate morphology. Cambridge: Harvard University Press; 1985. p. 3857.
11. Wake MH. Hyman. Comparative vertebral anatomy. Chicago: The University of Chicago Press; 1979.
12. Jouffroy FK. Evolution of the dorsal muscles of the spine in light of their adaptation to gravity effects. In: The head and neck sensory motor system. Oxford: Oxford University Press; 1992.
13. Lindstedt S, et al. Do muscles function as adaptable locomotor springs? J Exp Biol. 2002;205:22116.
14. Ordway NR, et al. Cervical flexion, extension, protrusion and retraction: a radiographic segmental analysis. Spine. 1999;24(3):2407.
15. Renous S. Locomotion. Paris: Dunod; 1994.
16. Vital JM, Senegas J. Anatomical basis of the study of the constraints to which the cervical spine is subject in the sagittal plane. A study of the center of gravity of the head. Surg Radiol Anat. 1986;8(3):16973.

Embryology of the Vertebral Column

Sebastien Pesenti, Nicole Philip, and Gerard Bollini

Genetic and Biochemical Considerations

The fertilized egg (or first embryonic cell) is described as totipotent because it is capable of giving birth to an entire embryo. Embryonic development is the consequence of the gene activity within the cells and the interactions received by this cell from its environment. The result is changes in shape, movement, proliferation and death, differentiation, and specialization of cells. During these processes, embryonic cells receive local signals allowing their differentiation into particular cell types. Signaling molecules or ligands (morphogenetic molecules) bind to specific receptors causing a cascade of biochemical reactions within the cell leading to the target molecule. Morphogens diffuse through the tissues of the embryo during the early phase of development, establishing concentration gradients.

In vertebrates, the mesoderm is divided into axial mesoderm (prechordal plate and notochord), paraxial mesoderm (presomitic mesoderm lying on either side of the notochord and giving birth to the somites), intermediate mesoderm, and lateral plate mesoderm.

BMP4, belonging to the TGF beta superfamily, secreted by the dorsal portion of the notochord, [1] defines the dorsoventral axis of the embryo and acts as a "lateralisater" of the somitic mesoderm characteristics. The somites are formed successively from the presomitic mesoderm, from the cephalic extremity to the caudal extremity. This migration of a group of epithelial cells to the caudal end of the presomitic mesoderm is what forms the somites. The segmentation of the somites is regulated by a "clock and wavefront model" [2]. This model includes an intracellular oscillator interacting with a cephalocaudal gradient of morphogenic proteins in the presomitic mesoderm. The wavefront is a cephalocaudal gradient of FGF8 which is a major determinant of longitudinal organization [3]. In the caudal and middle part of the presomitic mesoderm, high levels of FGF8 maintain the cells in an immature and undifferentiated state. At the cephalic part, the low concentration of FGF8 allows the formation of somites. The boundary separating the two regions where the concentration of FGF8 is different is known as the determination front.

Several genes, such as CHAIRY1 and IFNG, are expressed dynamically in the presomitic mesoderm (Fig. 1). The "segmentation clock" molecular oscillator acting inside the cells of the presomitic mesoderm has also been shown to determine vertebral segmentation. This involves, in mice, the cyclic expression of 50–100 genes.

For example, expression of CHAIRY1 spreads along the presomitic mesoderm during the formation of each somite [4]. DeltaNotch is a key cascade pathway in somatogenesis and in the regulation of the "segmentation clock." This complex process can be simplified as follows: Notch active *Lunatic Fringe* which in turn inhibits the Notch receptor. Activation of Notch also stimulates activation of the HES gene which inhibits Lunatic Fringe, releasing the Notch receptor. This genetic feedback allows the cyclic expression of these genes. In humans, mutations of LFNG genes (Lunatic Fringe), HES7 (Hairyenhancer of split7), DLL3 (encoding for the Notch ligand), and MESP2 (activated Notch) are responsible for recessive forms of spondylocostal dysostoses (Fig. 2).

The positional identity of somites according to the cephalocaudal axis is defined by a combined expression of genes encoding transcription factors and belongs to the family of HOX (homeotic) genes. This specification occurs in the presomitic mesoderm prior to somitogenesis. The HOX genes are grouped into several complexes on the chromosomes. The genes of each complex are expressed sequentially in a spatial and temporal order defined by their position along the chromosome. In Drosophila, there is only one HOX gene

S. Pesenti · G. Bollini (✉)
Department of Pediatric Orthopedics, Timone Enfants, Marseille, France
e-mail: sebastien.pesenti@ap-hm.fr; Gerard.BOLLINI@ap-hm.fr

N. Philip
Department of Genetics, Timone Enfants, Marseille, France
e-mail: Nicole.philip@ap-hm.fr

J. M. Vital, D. T. Cawley (eds.), *Spinal Anatomy*, https://doi.org/10.1007/978-3-030-20925-4_2

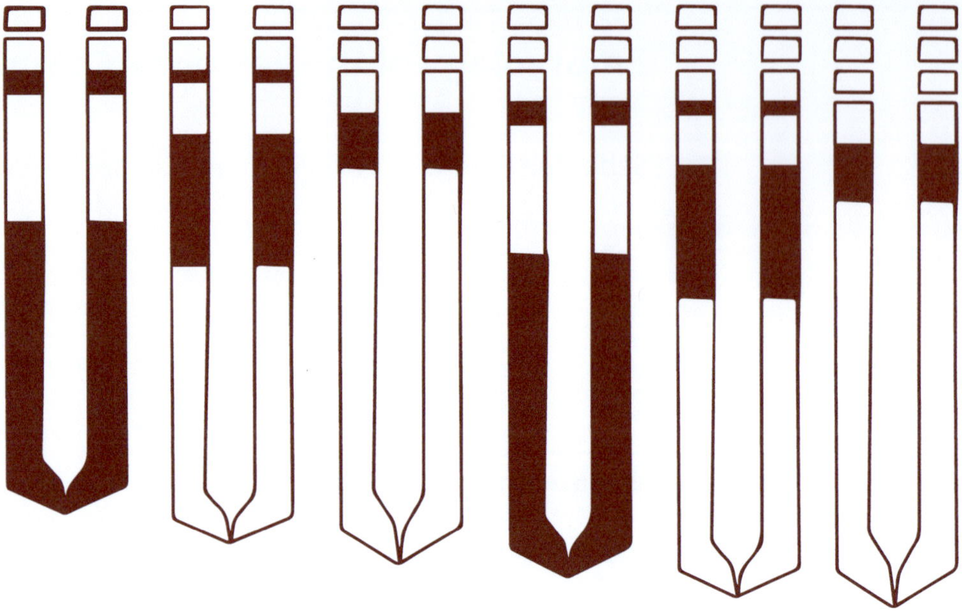

Fig. 1 Expression of the chairy1 gene in the presomitic mesoderm

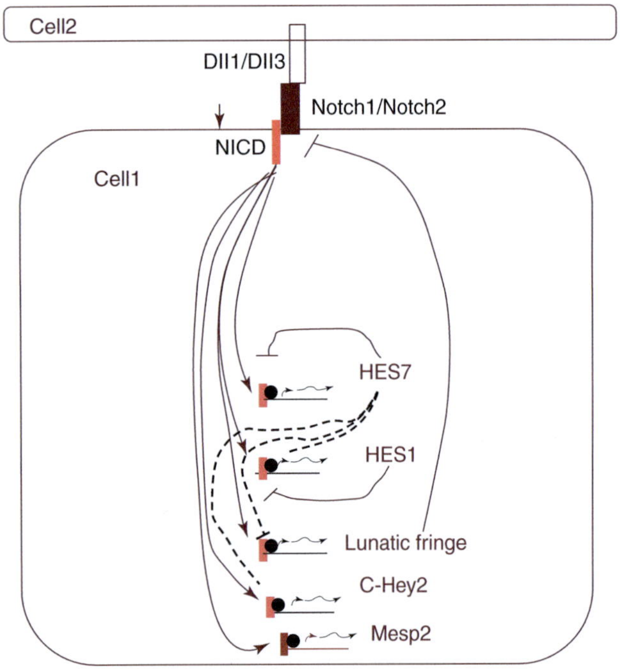

Fig. 2 DeltaNotch signaling

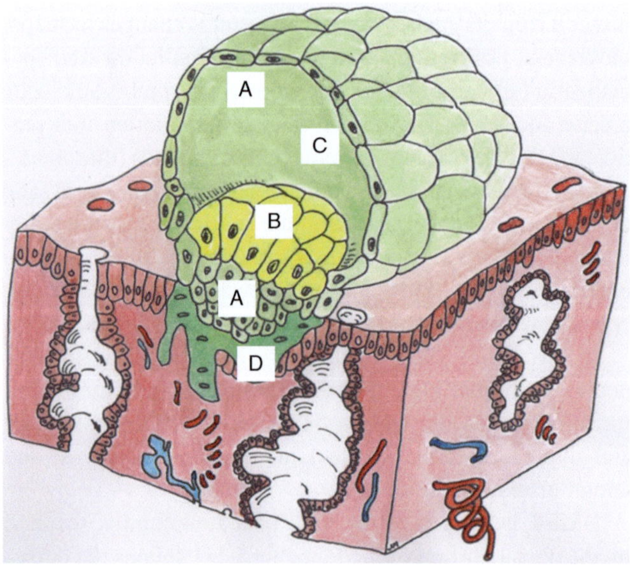

Fig. 3 (A) Cytotrophoblast; (B) Embryo; (C) Blastocele; (D) Syncytiotrophoblast

complex (initially called the HOM complex). Thus, the loss of function of one of these genes leads to a homeotic transformation in the adult insect, transforming an entire part of the body into another. In mammals, there are four HOX gene complexes on four different chromosomes. In mice, experiments have shown that inactivation of different HOX gene complexes resulted in the appearance of different phenotypes, frequently comprising vertebral malformations. In humans, no vertebral malformations have been linked to mutations in HOX gene complexes [5].

Embryology of the Vertebromedullary Axis

Early Development

The embryonic period is defined as the first 8 weeks after fertilization. During the first week after fertilization, the morula migrates along the fallopian tube. At the end of the first week, the morula became a blastocyst following the appearance of a cavity, the blastocele (Fig. 3). It is at this time that implantation takes place in the maternal uterine mucosa (Fig. 4). At this stage, the embryonic disc is trans-

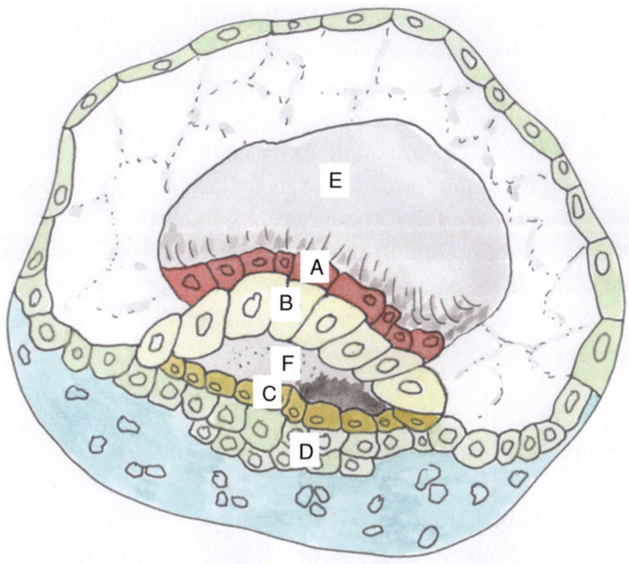

Fig. 4 Day 8: (A) Entoblast; (B) Ectoblast; (C) Amnios; (D) Cytotrophoblast; (E) Lecithocele; (F) Amniotic cavity

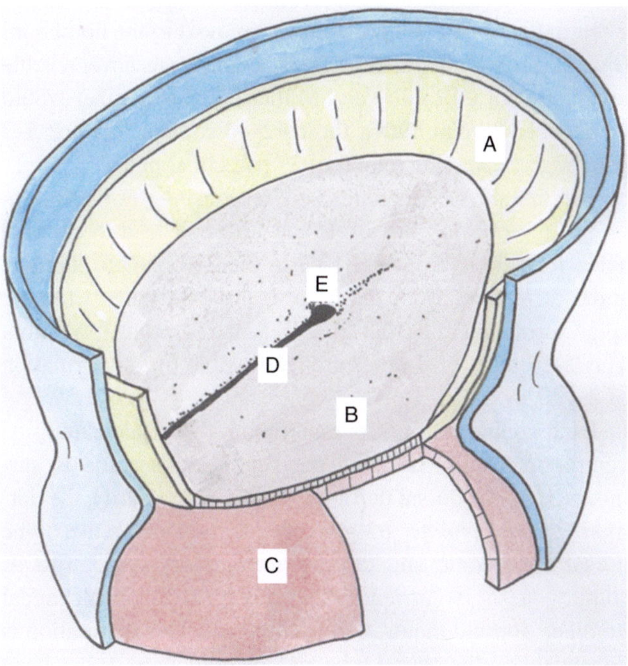

Fig. 5 Day 15: (A) Amniotic sac; (B) Ectoblast; (C) Entoblast; (D) Primary line; (E) Hensen's primitive knot

formed into a bilaminar structure, comprising two layers, the epiblast and the hypoblast. At the beginning of the third week, a primitive streak appears in the middle of the epiblast and gradually lengthens. The craniocaudal axis of the embryo that forms during the primitive streak extends from the primitive node which determines the cranial end of the embryo (Fig. 5).

Trilaminar Embryo

The third week is marked by gastrulation. The epiblastic cells migrate from the deep side of the primitive streak and the hypoblast is laterally displaced to contribute to the formation of the extraembryonic endoderm. The migration of the epiblastic cells through the primitive streak and the node leads to the formation of the three primordial germ layers: the definitive endoderm which takes the place of the hypoblast, the ectoderm that remains on the surface, and the mesoderm which lies in between.

The axial mesoderm consists of two median structures: the prechordal plate and the notochordal process. The prechordal plate, situated at the cranial extremity, is adherent to the ectoderm, whereas the notochordal process is situated more caudally and is transformed into a tubular structure, causing the yolk sac (this structure gives rise exclusively to extraembryonic structures) and the amniotic sac to communicate transiently. This communication is called the notochordal (or chordal) canal (of Lieberkühn).

Three lateral structures appear on either side of the embryo: the paraaxial mesoderm (Fig. 6), the intermediate

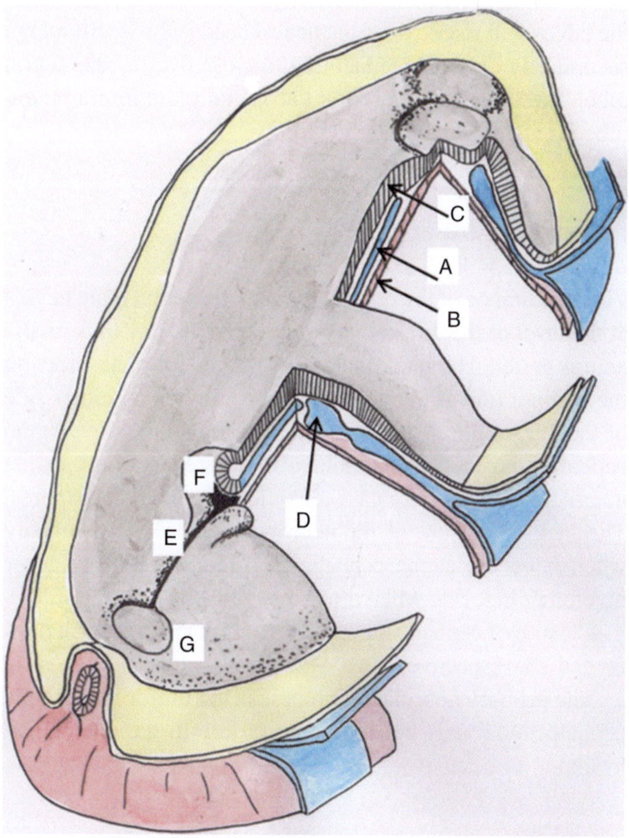

Fig. 6 (A) Notochord; (B) Endoblast; (C) Ectoblast; (D) Paraaxial mesoderm; (E) Primitive line; (F) Hensen's primitive knot; (G) Cloacal membrane

mesoderm, and the lateral mesoderm. The paraaxial mesoderm gives rise to cell lines that differentiate into an axial skeleton, paravertebral muscles, dermis, and subcutaneous tissue and muscles of the ventral wall and limbs. The intermediate mesoderm will be the origin of the urogenital tract. The ventral part of the lateral mesoderm will form the walls of the digestive tract and of the bronchopulmonary tree, while its dorsal part will form the lateral and ventral walls of the embryo.

The Notochord

The notochordal process is a mesodermal hollow tube structure that extends from the primitive node, which elongates, as primitive node cells migrate to the proximal end of the tube. The notochordal plate remains adherent to the surface ectoderm thus preventing anterior migration of the notochordal process. The notochordal process develops into the notochord and represents an early version of the future vertebrae and bony skeleton.

By the secretion of growth factors, neural induction, or planar induction, which is no longer come from the notochord but from the primitive node, will lead, from the neuroectoderm, to the initial formation of the neural plate of which the edges will rise to form the neural beads which will merge secondarily on their median line to close over as the neural tube. The transformation of a flat neural plate into a neural tube is called primary neurulation.

Primary Neurulation

The appearance of the neural crests on the neural plate begins at the level of the 4th somite around the 20th day to form the neural gutter. The lateral edges of the neural plate meet on the median line to merge. The fusion extends on either side of the 4th somite in the cephalic and caudal direction. At the cephalic and caudal extremities there are openings in the neural tube which are called cephalic and caudal neuropores. The lack of closure of the neuropores causes anencephaly when it occurs at the cephalic end and a meningocele or myelomeningocele when it occurs at the distal end.

Closure of cephalic and caudal neuropores occurs on days 26 and 28, respectively.

The primary neurulation process is not uniform along the cephalocaudal axis but differs according to the anatomical levels.

Secondary Neurulation

At the caudal neuropore, the tissue of the caudal bud contributes to the formation of the medullary cord. Subsequently, the medullary cord condenses, individualizes, and forms vacuoles. The union of these vacuoles results in the formation of a second neural tube communicating with the first neural tube formed during the primary neurulation.

A junctional neurulation has recently been described, accounting for the formation of medullary segments located between primary and secondary neurulations [6].

The dorsal portion of the neural tube produces cells that migrate into the embryo. They constitute the cells of the neural crest which form the pigment cells of the skin and the cells of the peripheral nervous system.

Formation and Differentiation of Somites

The segmental structures of mesodermal origin or somites appear on both sides of the neural tube. The first pairs of somites appear around day 20. The somites originate from the paraaxial mesoderm and develop from the cephalic end to the caudal end at the rate of 3–4 somites per day, under the action of the neural tube and the notochord.

Initially, 42–44 pairs of somites are next to the notochord (this number is disputed as these somites are never visible together). For O'Rahilly and Müller [7], this number would be between 38 and 39. Of these 42–44 somites, the last 5–7 pairs regress, leaving a total of 37 pairs of somites.

The first 4 pairs of somites are responsible for the formation of the occiput, the 5th to the 12th pair lead to cervical spine formation, from the 13th to the 24th pair to thoracic spine formation, from the 25th to the 29th pair to lumbar spine formation and 30th to 34th pair to sacrum formation. The last 3 pairs of somites are responsible for the formation of the coccyx.

Each somite, during its maturation, dissociates along its ventrodorsal axis. Initially, the ventral sclerotome is surmounted by the dorsal dermomyotome. Secondarily, the dermomyotome evolves to generate its two derivatives: the dorsal dermatome and the intermediate myotome. Just as somitogenesis is carried out according to a cephalocaudal gradient, somitic maturation follows suit. This maturation is dependent on the neural tube and the notochord. It has been shown that the morphogen Sonic hedgehog acts on the ventralization of the somite. This molecule is produced by the notochord and the neural tube floor.

It is the sclerotome that will give rise to the spine, to the set of spinal meningeal tissues (pia mater, arachnoid layer, and dura mater) and to the intervertebral ligaments. During the 4th week of development within each sclerotome, the cells migrate around the notochord and the neural tube.

The cells of the sclerotome are influenced by Sonic hedgehog. The most ventral regions of the future vertebra depend on the molecule Gli2, while the more lateral regions are in the dependence of Gli3. It is important to note that the most dorsal region of the sclerotome will give rise to the spinous process, is independent of Sonic hedgehog but responds to BMP4. This molecular peculiarity could account for malformations preferentially located in one of the three vertebral territories defined above.

Each somite is divided into two hemisomites along the cephalocaudal axis. This is the theory of resegmentation proposed by Remak in the nineteenth century. This process of resegmentation is now perfectly established experimentally. Curiously, a vertebra does not derive from a somite but from two hemisomites from different structures. The caudal end of each somite then merges with the cephalic end of the underlying somite forming the precursor of the vertebra. Thus, 8 cervical somites with 8 corresponding nerve roots will give rise to 7 cervical vertebrae, each vertebral body consisting of 2 hemisomites. This polarization, along the cephalocaudal axis, is explained by the differential expression of genes by each of the hemisomites. More than the genes and the molecules synthesized, it is necessary to specify that only the rostral hemisomite is permeable for the migration of the cells coming from the neural crest and for the axons of the motor neurons. It follows that the peripheral nervous system, initially produced by the neural tube in an unsegmented fashion, is organized according to a radicular topography due to the intrinsic properties of the somites. This explains the metamerism of the spinal ganglia and the motor roots.

The cells of the sclerotome will give rise to the annulus fibrosus of the intervertebral disc. The notochord will disappear gradually, with the exception of its remnants which will form the nucleus pulposus.

With this new organization, the segmental nerve roots become visible at the level of the disc space, whereas the segmental blood vessels appear at the height of the vertebral body.

The pairs of sclerotomes subsequently fuse in front of the median line. At the 6th week of development, chondrification occurs of vertebral precursors, thus forming the cartilaginous outline of the vertebra. These chondrification centers will evolve secondarily. Within each vertebral precursor, three nuclei of chondrification form: one anteriorly which will give rise to the vertebral body and two posteriorly, on either side of the vertebral canal, which will each give rise to a pedicle and a hemi-arch. The 2 posterior chondrification centers will remain separated from the center of chondrification prior to birth by neurocentral synchondrosis.

Five secondary ossification centers will appear after birth, each of which is apophyseal center of ossification. One will give rise to the spinous process, another two to the transverse processes, and two others located on either side of the vertebral body will give rise to the apophyseal ring.

The primary ossification centers first appear at the cervicothoracic junction at 9 weeks in utero and are followed by upper cervical then thoracolumbar vertebrae with the primary ossification centers of the lumbar neural arches the last to appear at approximately 14 weeks in utero. It progresses more rapidly at the level of the vertebral body in caudal vertebrae and at the level of the posterior arch for the cranial vertebrae.

At birth, the position of the conus medullaris (end of the spinal cord) is considered abnormal if it is below L3. The position of the conus of 84 postmortem fetuses (mean gestation: 26.3 weeks, 14–41 weeks) was studied using 3D MRI. The earlier the gestation, the higher the location of the conus. At 20 weeks gestation, 84% of the fetuses had a conus located at L4/L5 or higher. At 26 weeks, it had reached L3 in 50% of the cases and in 94% of cases at the 40th week of gestation. This means that there is a gradual ascent of the conus throughout fetal life. Although growth is not linear, most fetuses have a conus at the same level as the adult from the 33rd week of gestation [8].

It is interesting to compare this study with another analyzing a population of 231 men and 273 women of average age of 46 years. In this cohort, the position of the conus was on average at the level of the lower third of L1. There was no significant difference by sex or age [9].

The progressive rise of the conus medullaris relative to the spinal canal during fetal life is due to the difference in growth velocity between the neural tube and the spine. This phenomenon explains why the nerve roots are directed upwards and downwards from the spinal canal.

It is commonly accepted that the fetal spine forms only a single kyphotic curvature and that lumbar lordosis appears with the acquisition of erect posture. This adage was contradicted by Choufani et al. [10] in a study analyzing 45 fetal MRIs aged 23–40 weeks of gestation. The measurements made on these 3D MRIs were relevant to the radius of curvature of the lumbosacral junction. Although lumbosacral lordosis was only visible in 60% of cases, computer analysis showed that it was present in 100% of cases. Statistical analysis showed no significant correlation between gestational age and lumbosacral lordosis, which means that the existence of this curvature could be genetically determined rather than related to the acquisition of erect posture.

References

1. Tonegawa A, Funayama N, Ueno N, Takahashi Y. Mesodermal subdivision along the mediolateral axis in chicken controlled by different concentrations of BMP4. Development. 1997;124:197584.
2. Dubrulle J, Pourquié O. From head to tail: links between the segmentation clock and anteroposterior patterning of the embryo. Curr Opin Genet Dev. 2002;5:51923.
3. Dubrulle J, Pourquié O. FGF8 mRNA decay establishes a gradient that couples axial elongation to patterning in the vertebrate embryo. Nature. 2004;427:419–22.

4. Palmeirim I, Henrique D, Ish-Horowicz D, Pourquié O. Avian hairy gene expression identifies a molecular clock linked to vertebrate segmentation and somitogenesis. Cell. 1997;91:639–48.
5. Quinonez SC, Innis JW. Human HOX gene disorders. Mol Genet Metab. 2014;111(1):4–15.
6. Dady A, Havis E, Escriou V, Catala M, Duband JL. Junctional neurulation: a unique developmental program shaping a discrete region of the spinal cord highly susceptible to neural tube defects. J Neurosci. 2014;34(39):13208–21.
7. O'Rahilly R, Müller F. Human embryology and teratology. 2nd ed. New York: Wiley-Liss; 1996. 468 pp
8. Arthurs OJ, Thayyil S, Wade A, Chong WK, Sebire NJ, Taylor AM, and the Magnetic Resonance Imaging Autopsy Study Collaborative Group. Normal ascent of the conus medullaris: a post-mortem foetal MRI study. J Matern Fetal Neonatal Med. 2013;26(7):697–702.
9. Saifuddin A, Burnett SJ, White J. The variation of position of the conus medullaris in an adult population. A magnetic resonance imaging study. Spine. 1998;23:1452–6.
10. Choufani E, Jouve JL, Pomero V, Adalian P, Chaumoitre K, Panuel M. Lumbosacral lordosis in fetal spine: genetic or mechanic parameter. Eur Spine J. 2009;18:1342–8.

The Growing Spine

A. Dimeglio, F. Bonnel, and F. Canavese

A Mosaic of Growth Cartilage

130 growth cartilages are implicated in the formation of the spine. Their roles are well defined. The programme is hierarchical.

Spine growth is complex, different from one level to another. Each component has its own growth rate, but all are synchronized and fit into a well-coordinated schedule. The first two months of life are defined: the migration of somites and the differentiation of sclerotomes, which are organized around the notochord, the true axis of reference. The slightest slip in this well-organized scenario… and everything changes.

Three major periods mark the growth of the spine:

- *The embryonic period* in which all the elements are set up, i.e., the vertebral envelope and the cord;
- *The fetal period* that corresponds to the beginning of vertebral ossification;
- *The postnatal period* is characterized by progression in ossification and decisive phases, such as the first 5 years of life or the pubertal growth spurt.

A. Dimeglio (✉)
Department of Pediatric Orthopedic Surgery, Polyclinique Saint Roch, Montpellier, France

F. Bonnel
Orthopedic Surgery, Clinique Beau Soleil, Montpellier, France

F. Canavese
Department of Pediatric Orthopedic Surgery, University Hospital Estaing, Clermont Ferrand, France

Vertebral Growth Is Growth by Endochondral Ossification

This is characterized by a first mesenchymal step, followed by a cartilaginous step that serves as a matrix for the third step, ossification. Ossification begins early in the third month of uterine life and will last for 15 years.

The growth is distinct for the posterior arc whose closure is linked to the presence of the neural tube and for the vertebral body which behaves like a long bone. The rate of growth is different not only at each stage of the spine but also at each vertebra. Morphology at the end of growth is the product of the synchronized work of more than 130 growth cartilages. Any spinal pathology is allied to the dynamics of these cartilages.

The growth of the spine is therefore a complex and hierarchical growth.

Embryology Holds First Truths

The embryonic period extends from Day 0 to Day 60: 60 decisive days during which the two essential players, that is to say the cord and its roots on one side and the vertebra on the other, are placed (Figs. 1, 2, 3, and 4).

The growth cartilage roles are well distributed; the programming is hierarchical.

Without going back to the main embryonic stages, we note (Fig. 5) the following:

- the decisive role of the future notochord
- the redistribution of sclerotomes… crucial time
- the closing of the posterior arc which is linked to the closure of the tube.

The sequences are linked to an immutable rhythm.

J. M. Vital, D. T. Cawley (eds.), *Spinal Anatomy*, https://doi.org/10.1007/978-3-030-20925-4_3

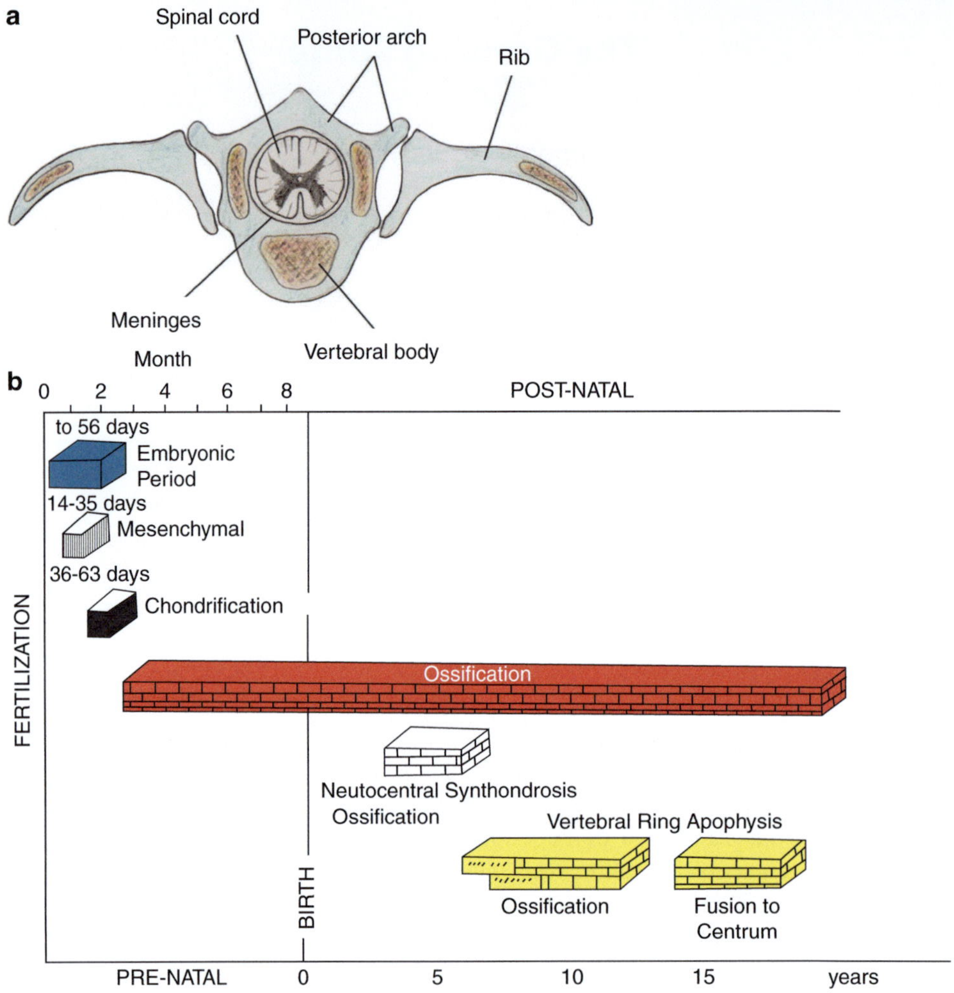

Fig. 1 (**a**) Thoracic vertebra. Transverse section. Fourth month of intrauterine life. The ossification centers are now in place in the future vertebral body and in the posterior arcs. (**b**) Three successive and overlapping phases: Mesenchyme, Cartilage, and Ossification. According to Tsou. Embryology of congenital kyphosis. Clin Orthop 1977, 128, 18–25 (with his permission)

The failed closure of the neural stem (which normally closes around the 4th week of intrauterine life) determines the persistent opening of the posterior arch. All of these multiple, complex processes are contemporary and can be associated. *This explains why a vertebral malformation can be a polymalformation (eg, spina bifida).*

The vertebral body is a vascular sponge.

The Fetal Period: The Strongest of All Growth Is the Intra-Uterine Period

The fetal period extends from Day 60 to birth. It corresponds to the very beginning of the ossification of the vertebral body. Cartilage is gradually replaced by the mesenchyme (Figs. 6 and 7).

The appearance of cartilage is rapidly followed by ossification fronts that progress in the posterior arcs as well as the center of the vertebra.

During the fetal period, the proportions change. In the 2nd month of intrauterine life, the spine is about 2/3 of the length of the body. This proportion gradually changes as the lower extremities develop (Fig. 8).

In the 5th month of intrauterine life, the length of the spine represents only 3/5 of the total length of the fetus. It represents only 2/5 at birth toward adulthood (Fig. 9).

Annual growth rate vertex–coccyx: 44 cm!

The vertex–coccyx distance.

The neurocentral cartilage has a bidirectional activity.

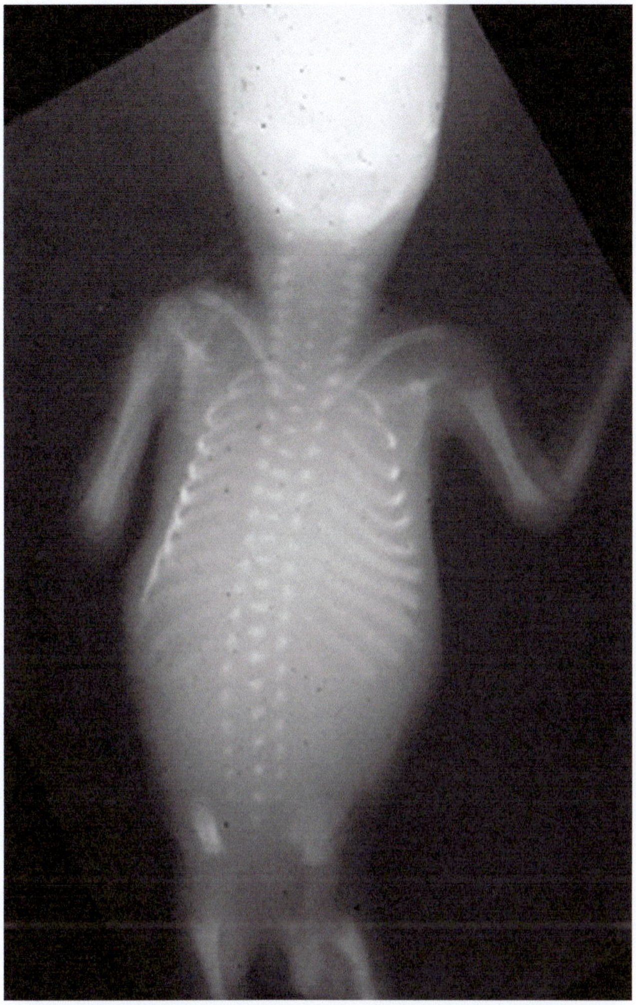

Fig. 2 Ossification of the spine in the third month of intrauterine life

Vertebral ossification does not occur simultaneously or in parallel across the bony parts of the vertebral column. It begins in the cervical region and then progresses smoothly up and down to the coccyx, at the level of the vertebral body. It first appears in the thoracic region, and then from this thoracic region, it progresses to the lumbar region and to the cervical region. The ossification nucleus of the vertebral body morphology changes. It is at first ovoid and becomes rectangular with time (Fig. 10).

The ossification of the odontoid and the apex of the odontoid is very late, as are those of the sacral pieces (Fig. 11).

The work of ossification progresses extremely slowly. It begins in the 2nd month of intrauterine life but only ends around the 18th year, and for some, at the 25th year!

Vertebral Curves Are Not Primitive But Acquired

During the first period of intrauterine life, the vertebral column is substantially rectilinear or with a slight anterior concave curve (Figs. 12 and 13). In the 5th month occurs a slight sacro-vertebral angle, establishing the respective limit of the lumbar region and the sacral region. But even at birth, there is virtually no trace of the inflections that characterize the cervical or lumbar regions.

In the fetus *the vertex–coccyx distance* is 10 cm at 3 months and 25 cm at 4 months— the growth is very important between the 3rd and 4th months. At the 5th month, the vertex–coccyx distance is 30 cm and it will be 35 cm at birth (Fig. 6).

At Birth, 30% of the Spine Is Ossified

At birth, two elements will play a key role (Fig. 13):

- neurological maturation
- sitting height whose evolution directly reflects vertebral growth.

At birth, the vertebrae have three centers of ossification: one for the central anterior part, one for each posterior arc. The length at the end of growth will have almost tripled.

About 30% of the spine is ossified at birth. There is no significant difference between the vertebrae. The vertebral body of a thoracic vertebra is about 7 mm in height. The sitting size measures 35 cm.

Evolution of spinal curvatures

Growth is a change of proportions

The First Five Years of Life Are Decisive: Living Growth

The first year of life is dominated by two events (Figs. 14, 15, 16, and 17):

- the establishment of the osseous medulla, which is adjusted relative to its container (cortex);
- the constitution of cervical, thoracic, and lumbar curvatures which are dependent on verticalization.

Once erect, around the age of 1 year, the cervical curvature and lumbar curvature settle, they are dependent on neuromotor development and neurological maturation which is cephalocaudal.

> After 5 years, the lower limbs grow 3.5 cm per year.

During the first year of life, the vertebral body may present as two ossification nuclei, but these small occurrences in ossification will unify rapidly. On the other hand, the coronal cleft, which is visible sometimes at birth, will disappear during the first year. This radiographic image can be

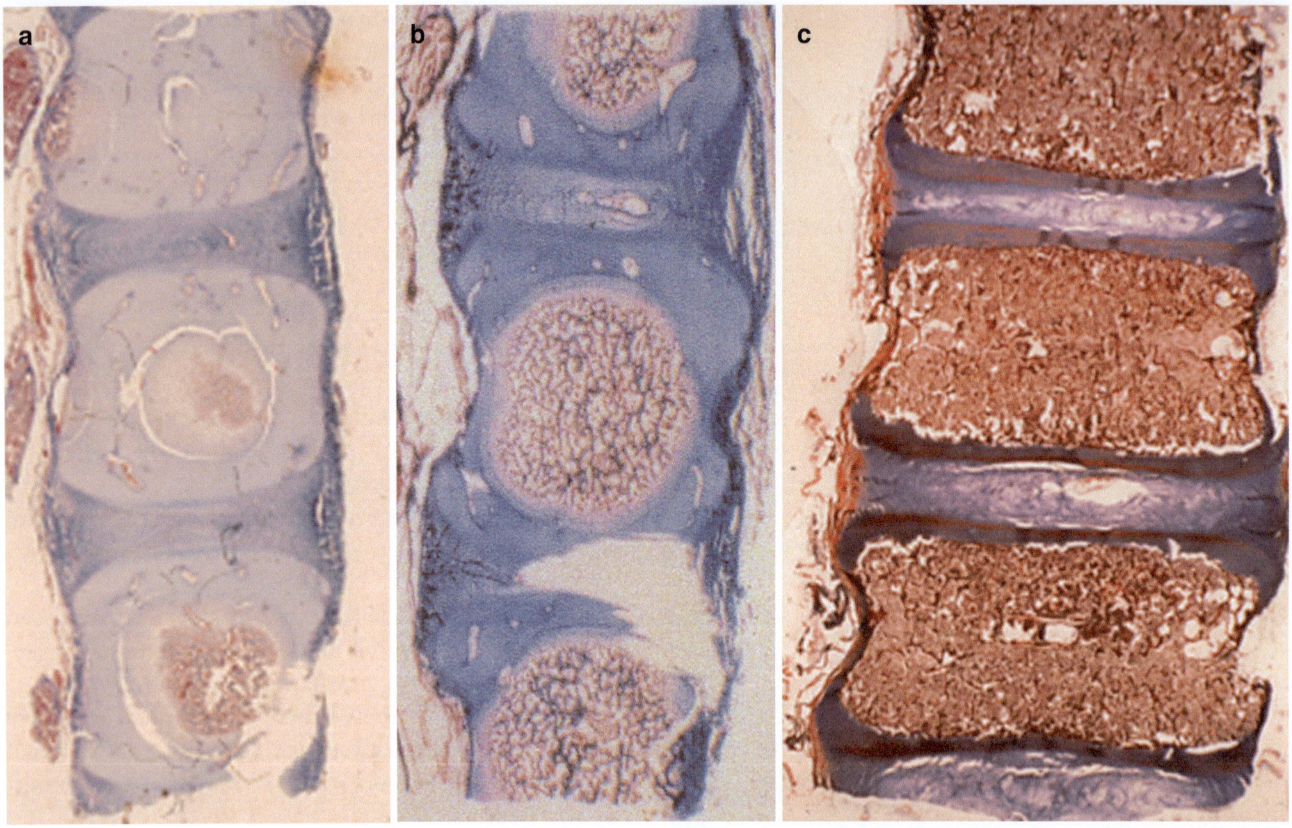

Fig. 3 The morphology of the vertebral body evolves: (**a**) at 3 months of intrauterine life, (**b**) at 4 months of intrauterine life, and (**c**) at 8 years. The osseous nucleus changes its morphology, it has the shape of a lens at 3 months, then it is ovoid at 4 months of intrauterine life, and quadrangular at 8 years

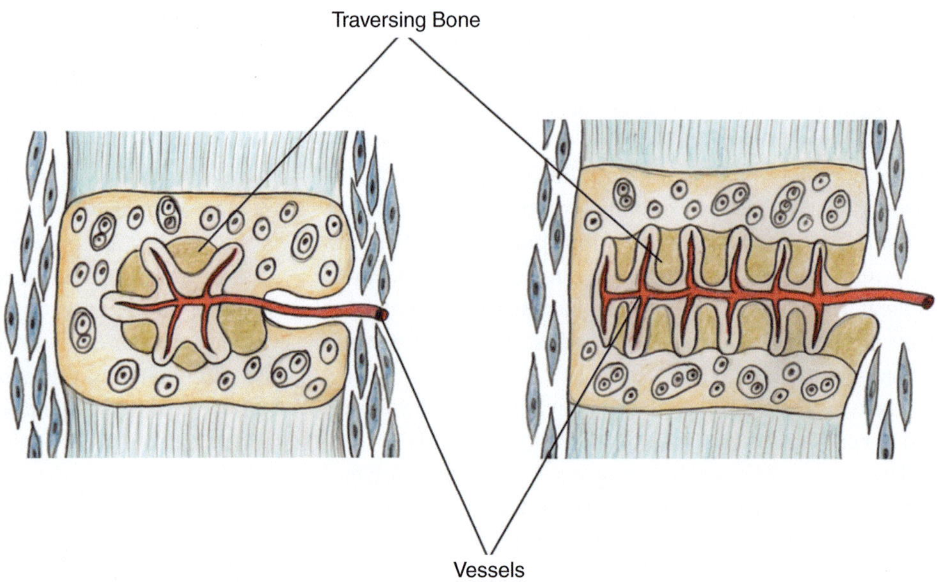

Fig. 4 Cellular organization of the vertebral body around the vessels: (**a**) 2 months of intrauterine life and (**b**) 4 months of intrauterine life. The upper and lower parts of the vertebral body are marked by growth cartilage (Baldet)

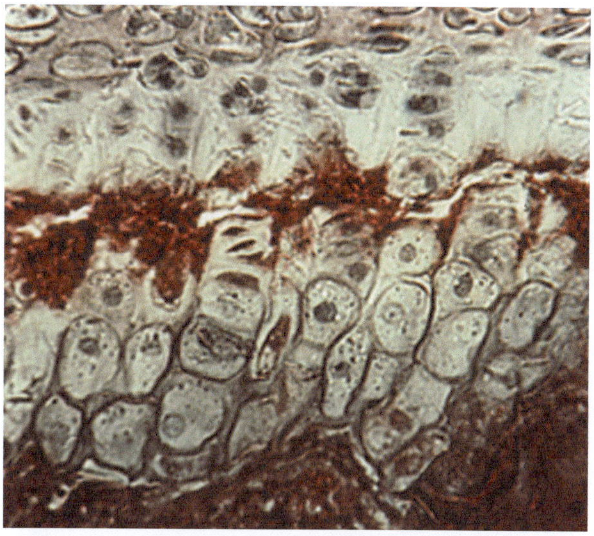

Fig. 5 Cartilage growth. Histological structure: with its germ cells, its column cells, its chondrocytes, and its ossification front

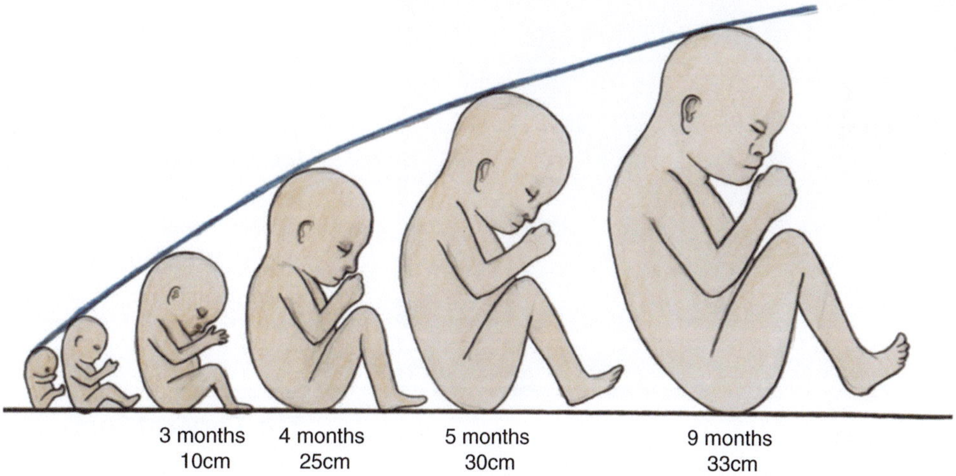

Fig. 6 The vertex–coccyx distance. In the fetus, at 3 months, it is about 10 cm and reaches 25 cm at 4 months. Thus, between the 3rd and the 4th month, growth is very important. In the 5th month, the vertex–coccyx distance is 30 cm, and will be 34 to 35 cm at birth

visualized until the age of 4, and it must be considered as a variation of endochondral ossification.

From 1 to 5 years, the medullary systemization is refined.

Once the closure of neurocentral synchondrosis is completed, then commences the closure of the posterior arc, then only one can really speak of the posterior arc and vertebral body, whereas the denomination which precedes these actions is the following one: neural arc for the posterior part and central point for the future vertebral body.

Growth during this period remains very strong. The sitting height gain is 12 cm in the first year of life; the sitting height then increases from 35 to 47 cm. From 1 to 5 years the sitting height gain is 15 cm; sitting height increases from 47 to 62 cm.

The sitting height at the end of growth represents 52% of the standing height.

Sitting height has increased by 27 cm in 5 years! The remaining growth of sitting height after 5 years is 30 cm. In other words, within a few centimeters the spine grows as much during the first 5 years of life as during all of the rest of growth. It is necessary to put in perspective this increase of growth of the first 5 years of the life (+27 cm) compared to the puberty period where the sitting height grows 12–14 cm.

This growth spurt in the first 5 years of life is even stronger than during the pubertal period.

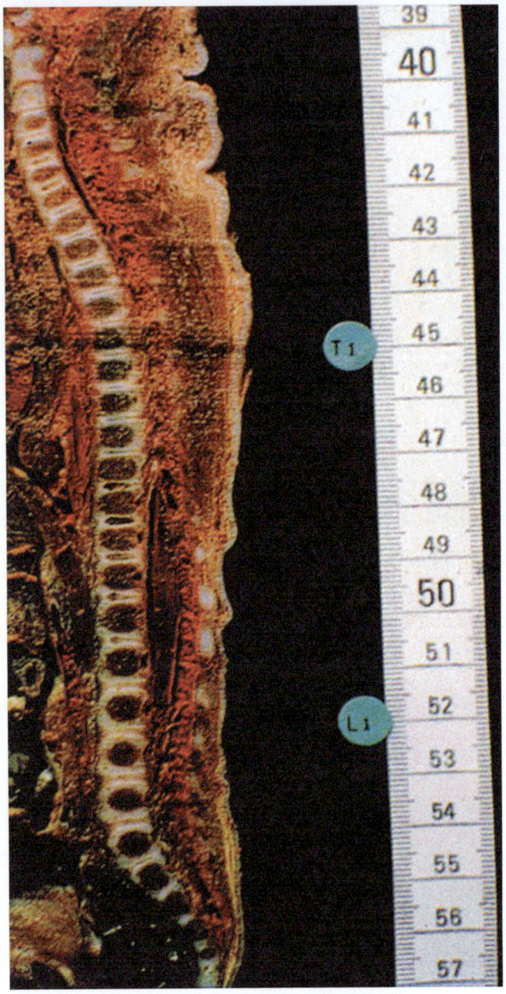

Fig. 7 Sagittal section of the spine at 8 months. Ossification is first posterior; it extends radiating upwards and downwards

Growth Between 5 Years and the Beginning of the Puberty

From 5 to 10 years, the growth of the trunk, and therefore of the spine, slows down as the sitting height will increase by about 10 cm. The annual growth rate of the trunk is 2 cm. The T1-LS segment grows 1.2 cm per year. *The annual elongation of the T1-L5 spine should theoretically not exceed 1.2 cm per year.* We must exploit this soft growth, especially when we manage an infantile scoliosis.

Puberty, a Decisive Turn: New Acceleration

The pubertal peak begins at 11 years of bone age in the girl. The remaining growth in sitting height is about 12 cm, including 2 years of strong growth where the sitting height will increase by 7 cm and 3 years of soft growth where the sitting height will increase by only 5 cm. Growth slows down after the closing of the elbow growth cartilages.

The pubertal peak in the boy starts later, at 13 years of bone age. The remaining growth on the sitting size is 13 cm: a sharp growth for 2 years, 13–15 years of bone age, with a sitting height gain of 8 cm and a gentle growth at 15–18 years, where the sitting height gain is 5 cm.

Growth slows down significantly after the closure of the elbow growth cartilages.

All these figures are valuable because sitting height is a reflection of macrocrine growth, and this macrocrine growth is the product of microcurrents that occur mainly in the spine.

Between the ages of 10 and 17, the vertebra has almost doubled in size. It is at the time of puberty that the secondary ossification nuclei appear (especially at the level of the posterior arc) and the marginal vertebral apophysis that comes to sit above and below the vertebral body (Fig. 8).

Each Level of the Spine: A Different Growth

The spine has almost tripled in length from birth to adulthood. It measures in adulthood of 70 cm in the boy, 65 cm in the girl. The cervical spine measures approximately 12 cm; thoracic spine of about 28 cm; the lumbar spine of approximately 18 cm; the sacrum of approximately 12 cm. The medullary canal reaches at 5 years 95% of its final size (Figs. 18 and 19).

The Cervical Spine

The cervical spine represents 22% of C1-S1 segments. The volume of the cervical spine is 9 cm^3 at birth. It is 110 cm^3 at the end of growth. It has been multiplied by 12.

It measures 3.7 cm at birth and 12–13 cm at the end of growth. It has almost quadrupled in length. It represents approximately 15% of the sitting height at the end of growth and as mentioned, 22% of the C1S1 segment. The cervical cord is comfortable in the medullary canal. It occupies in the adult a surface of 80 mm^2, while the average surface of the vertebral canal is of the order of 376 mm^2.

It is necessary to differentiate the high cervical spine C1-C2 and the low cervical spine.

Central Spinal Canal at the End of Growth

Two entities must be distinguished:

- the superior cervical spine: C1–C2.
- the inferior (subaxial) cervical spine: C3–C4–C5–C6–C7.

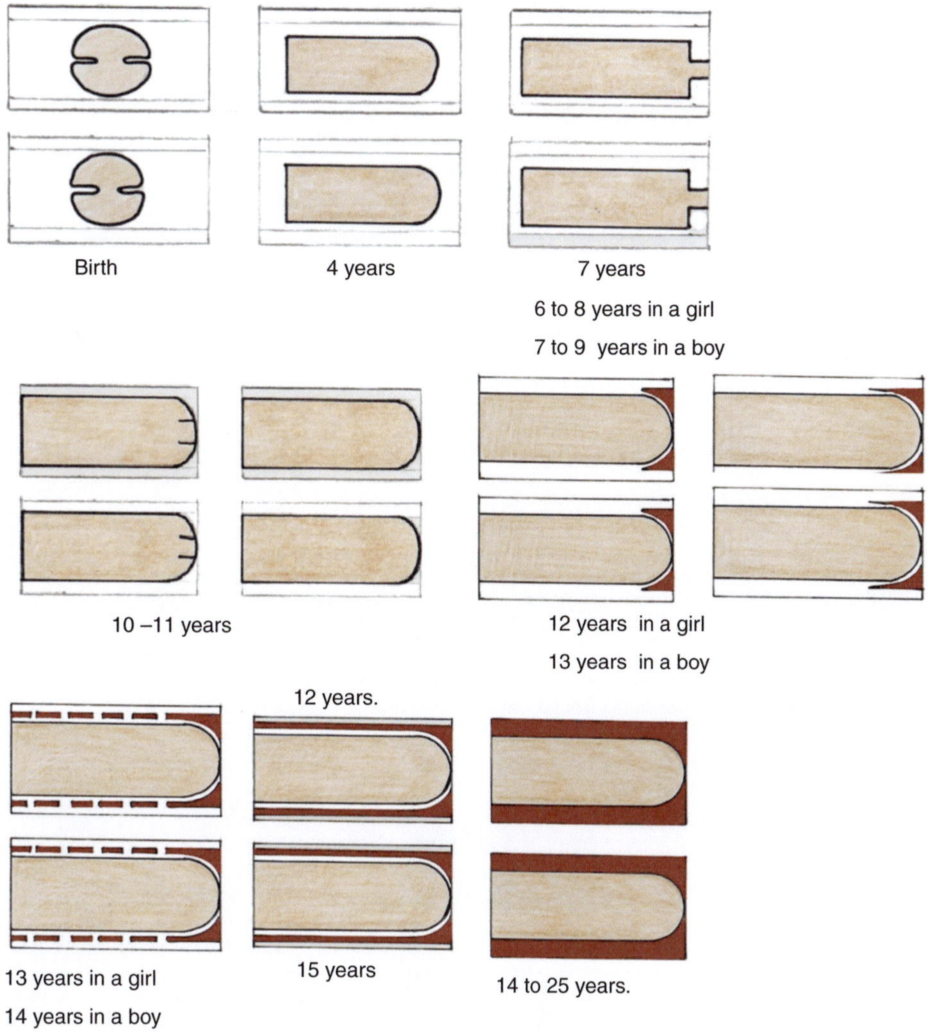

Fig. 8 The morphology of the vertebral body evolves. The marginal listel appears at the beginning of puberty; the complete integration of all the listels can occur until the age of 25 years

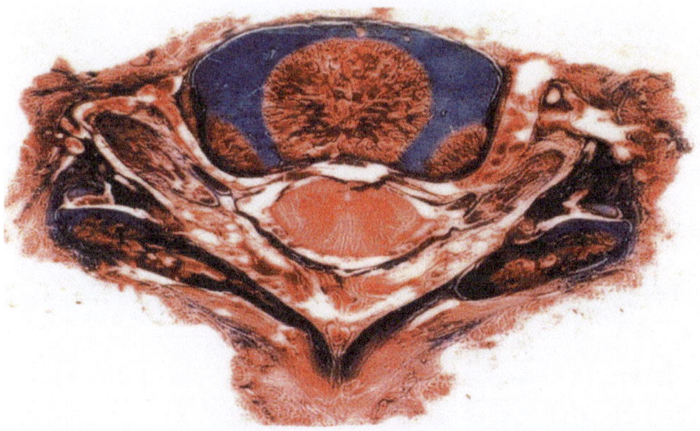

Fig. 9 Neurocentral cartilage has bidirectional activity. It contributes posteriorly to the ossification of the posterior arc and anteriorly to a third of the ossification of the vertebral body

Cervical Spine Height

Dimensions			
Newborn	6 years	10 years	15 years
3.7 cm	7.5 cm	10 cm	13 cm

From the age of 5 years the medullary canal reaches 95% of its area.

The Superior Cervical Spine

Characterized by its embryological singularity. The lower part of the 4th occipital sclerotome and the upper part of the 1st cervical sclerotome form the top of the odontoid (Figs. 20, 21, 22, 23, and 24). The lower part of the first cervical sclerotome and the upper part of the 2nd sclerotome form the atlas and the base of the odontoid (Fig. 25).

The lower part of the 2nd sclerotome and the upper part of the 3rd sclerotome form the body of the atlas (Fig. 26).

The Growth of the Atlas (Figs. 27, 28, and 29)

The body of the odontoid practically represents the body of the atlas, but they merge and fit into the vertebral body of the axis.

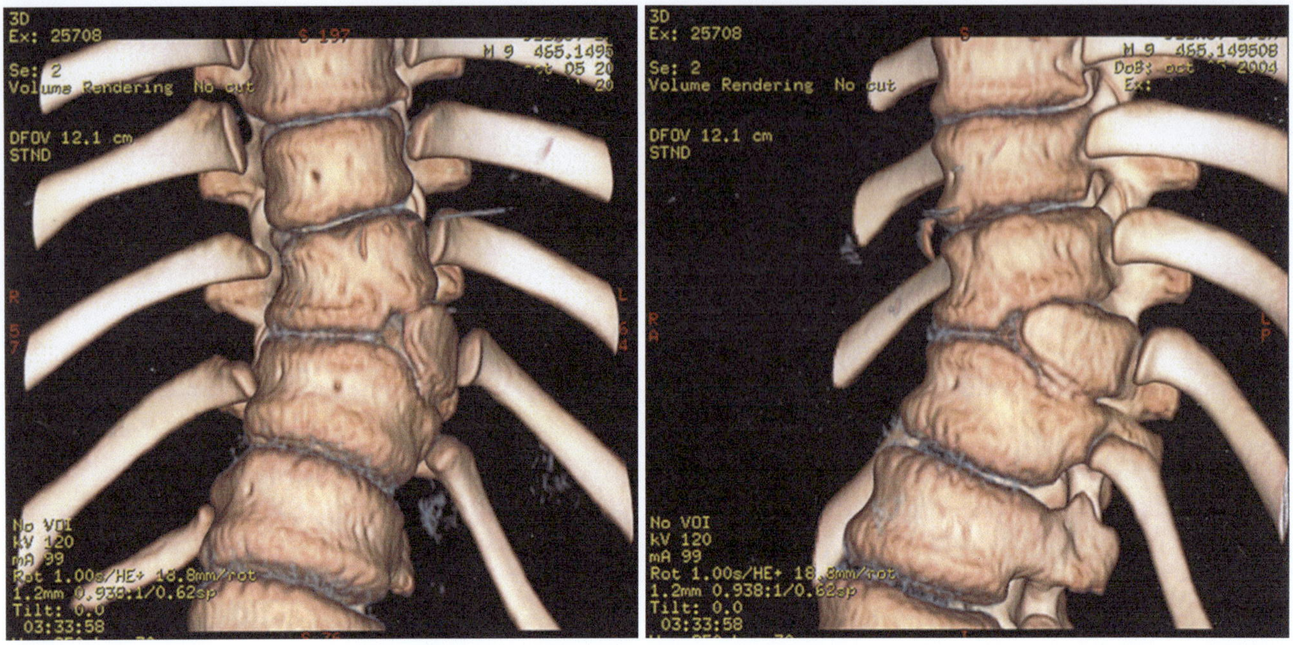

Fig. 10 Congenital scoliosis. The slightest aggression during embryonic life may be responsible for a malformation of the spine. The hemivertebra deforms the growing spine in the frontal and sagittal plane

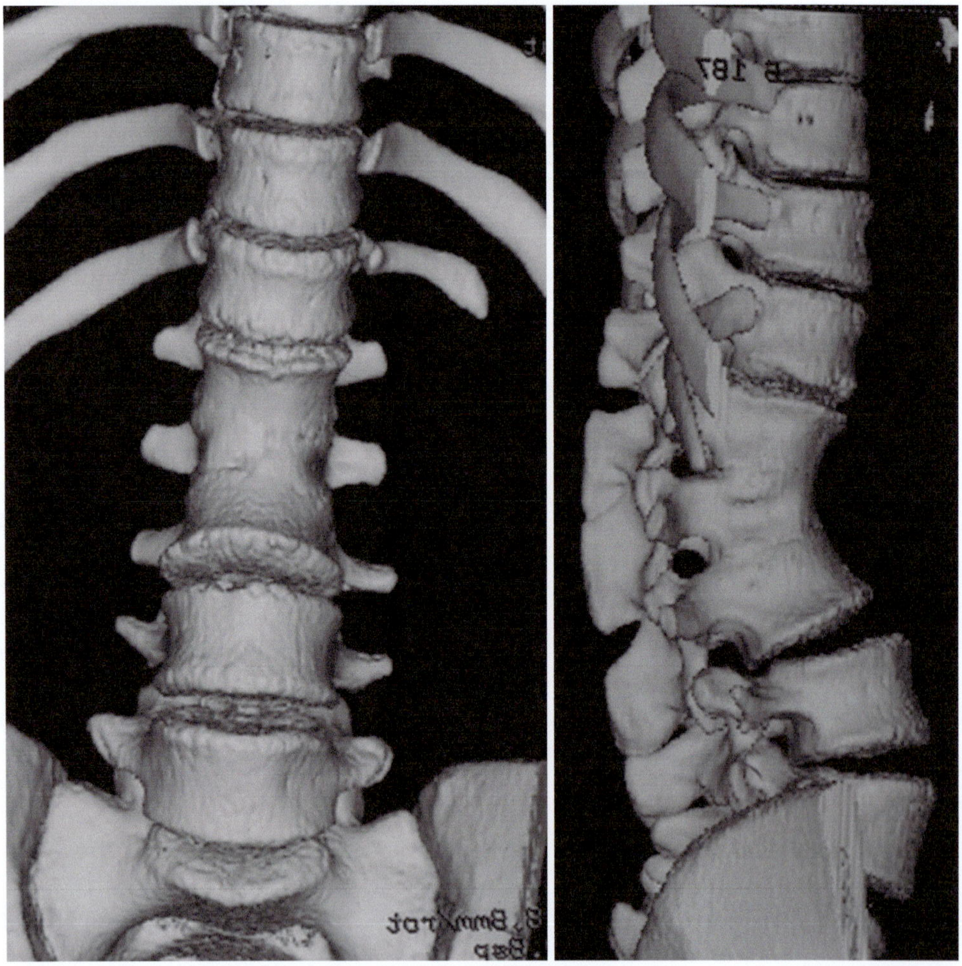

Fig. 11 Congenital kyphosis by failure of segmentation

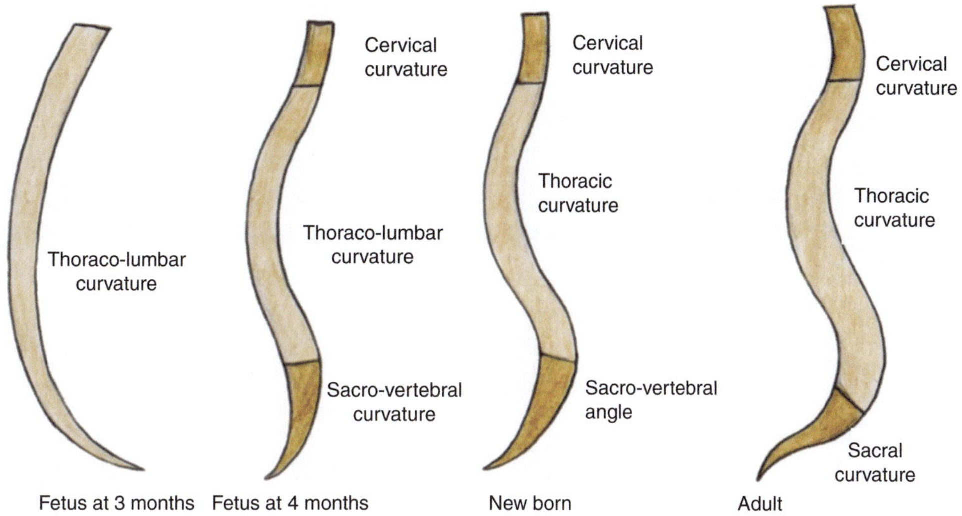

Fig. 12 Evolution of spinal curvatures. Fetus at 3 months: large "C" curvature. Fetus at 4 months: note the appearance of the sacro-vertebral angle. From birth to 1 year: spinal curvatures depending on the neurological calendar. The holding of the head heralds the cervical lordosis, the holding of the trunk, the thoracic kyphosis and the postural verticalization is accompanied by the lumbar curvature

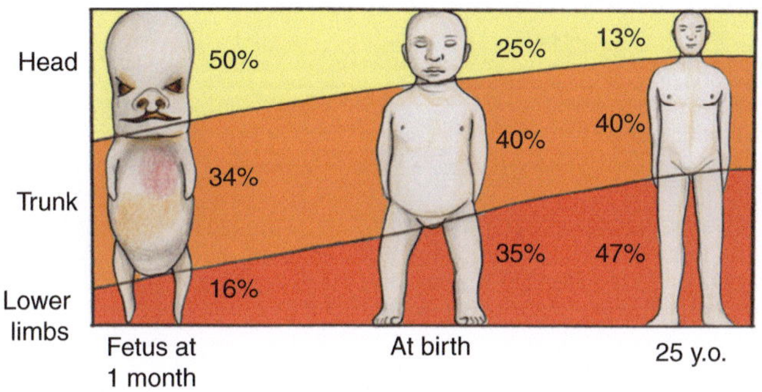

Fig. 13 Growth is a change of proportions. The lower limbs grow larger than the trunk, the cephalic sphere diminishes in proportion. At birth, the lower limbs measure 15 cm; sitting height 35 cm; at the end of growth, the sitting height represents 52–53% of the standing height

The atlas has two lateral ossification nuclei that become the lateral masses.

> After the age of 8, there is no visible growth cartilage.

There is a third nucleus of ossification which is anterior and which also contributes to the formation of the posterior arc. This ossification nucleus does not appear sometimes before the age of 1 year. It can be bifid but it is not pathological.

The ossification of the atlas may be incomplete resulting from a pseudo spina bifida. It should not be confused with a fracture.

The Growth of the Axis Is Even More Complex

Ossification of the odontoid appears very early in the 5th month of intrauterine life. Two ossification centers appear and merge at birth. The top of the odontoid ossifies around the age of 6 years.

This terminal ossification fuses with the rest of the body of the odontoid at the age of 12 years.

The non-fusion of this center of ossification with the body of the odontoid creates the conditions of the odontoid bone whose pathogenesis is not very precise. Perhaps congenital? Traumatic?

The body of the odontoid is separated from the body of the axis by a growth cartilage. But this growth cartilage does not have a very elaborate structure. The body of the odontoid fuses with the body of the axis around the age of 6. In children, before the age of 6, an injury of the odontoid can therefore lead to detachment of this growth cartilage.

The Lower Cervical Spine

The lower part of the cervical spine C3–C4–C5–C6–C7 is characterized by two elements (Fig. 30):

The synchondrosis between the vertebral body and the vertebral arch disappears at the age of 6 years. Posterior arc fusion occurs around the age of 4 years.

The neurocentral cartilage has a double activity. It contributes anteriorly to 30% of the volume of the vertebral body and posteriorly to the growth of the posterior arc.

The medullary canal is wide. It can fit the thumb. The anteroposterior diameter reaches its maximum around the age of 8 years.

It is 9 mm at birth, 16 mm at 5 years, and 19 mm at adulthood.

An anteroposterior diameter at adulthood less than 15 mm indicates a narrow canal at C5.

The transverse diameter is wider than the anteroposterior diameter:

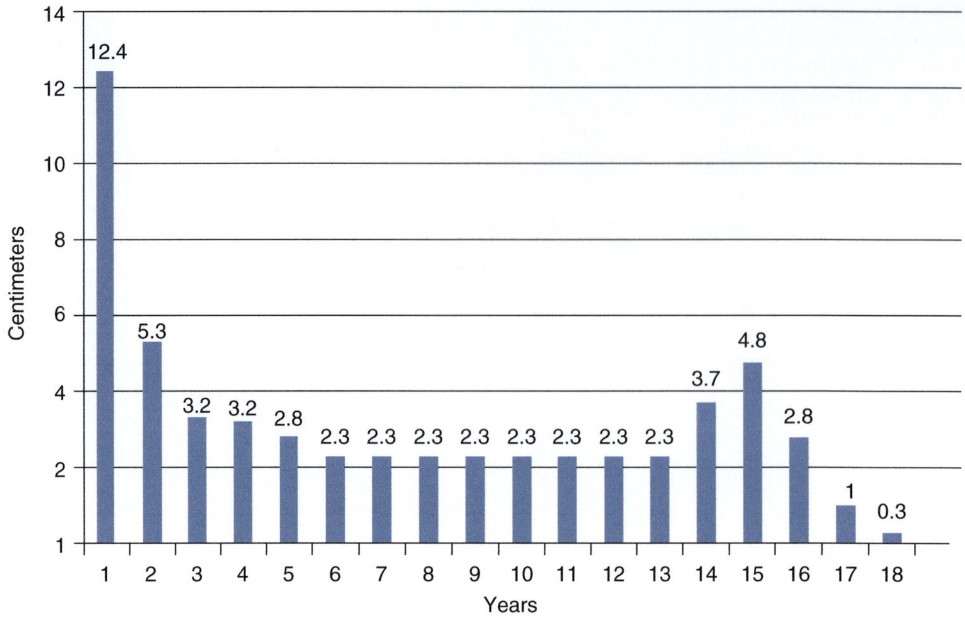

Fig. 14 Annual speed of male sitting height—12.4 cm gain in the first year of life; note the slowdown after the age of 5. From 0 to 5 years, sitting height increases as much as the lower limb. After 5 years and until puberty, the lower limb increases more than the trunk. After puberty, the trunk grows larger than the lower limb

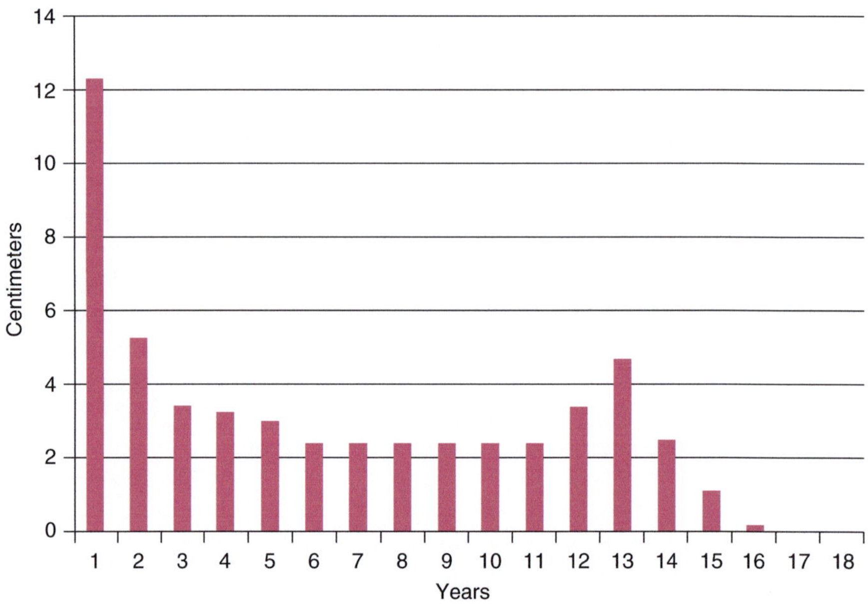

Fig. 15 Annual growth rate of sitting waist in the girl. The sitting height gain is 12 cm in the first year of life; after the age of 5 and until puberty: annual gain is about 2.4 cm

13 mm at birth, 22 mm at 10 years, and 27 mm at 16 years. The cervical cord is comfortable in the medullary canal. In adulthood its surface is 80 mm^2, while the surface of the spinal canal is 376 mm^2 (Table 1).

The T1-S1 Segment (Figs. 31a, b, 32, and 33)

It represents almost 50% of the sitting height. It is on this segment that presents all of the most common spinal affections such as scoliosis or kyphosis. It measures about 19 cm at birth, 45 cm at the end of growth in the boy and 42–43 cm in the girl.

The Thoracic Spine T1-T12 (Figs. 34 and 35)

The thoracic spine represents 2/3 of the T1-S1 segment. It measures schematically 11 cm at the birth and 26 cm at the end of growth in the girl, 28 cm in the boy. It grows from 15 to 17 cm during all of the growth. It is more than doubling its birth size.

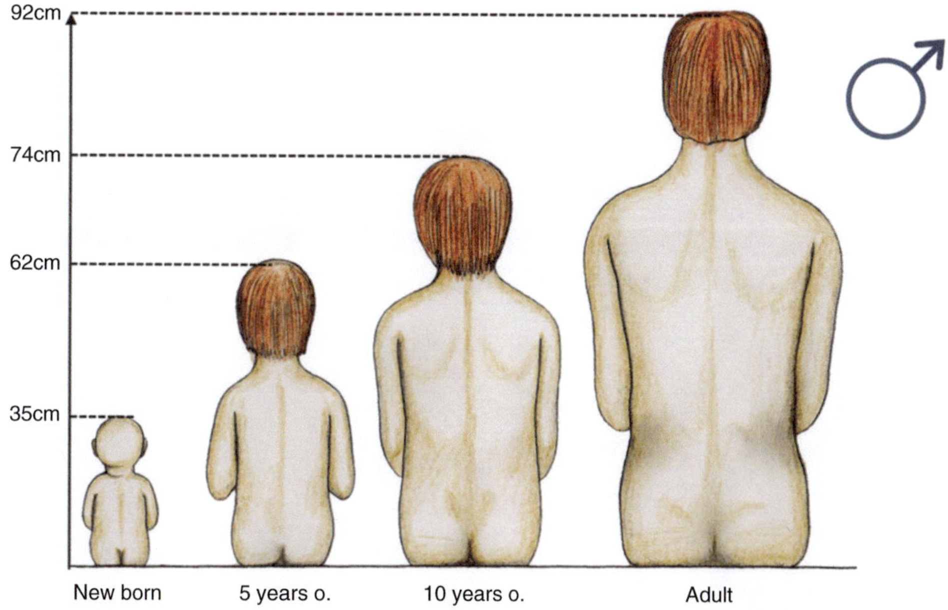

Fig. 16 Average sitting height in the boy. At the end of growth, the average sitting height of a boy measuring 1.75 m is 92 cm

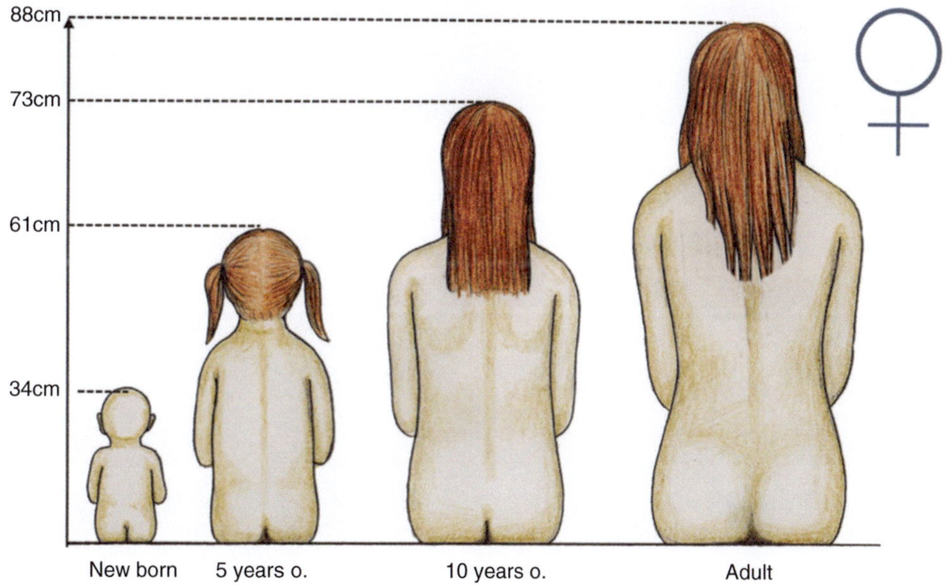

Fig. 17 Average sitting height in the girl. At the end of growth, the average sitting height of a girl who measures 1.67 m is 88 cm

The T1T12 segment represents 30% of the sitting height: in other words, a thoracic vertebra represents 2.5% of the sitting height, which means that a perivertebral epiphysiodesis will result in a statural deficit of 2.5% of the sitting height. Posterior arthrodesis results in only one-third of this deficit, i.e., 0.8% per thoracic vertebra, i.e., less than 1%. The medulla occupies an area of 0.4 mm^2, that is to say about 25% of the area of the vertebral canal (Table 2).

The Lumbar Spine L1-L5 (Figs. 36 and 37)

It represents 1/3 of the T1-S1 segment. Around 7 cm at birth: 16 cm at the end of growth in the boy and 15.5 cm in the girl.

The L1-L5 segment represents 18% of the sitting height: a lumbar vertebra is 3.5% of the sitting height, which means that a total perivertebral epiphysiodesis sterilizing all the growth cartilages would result in a deficit of 3.5% of the final sitting size. On the other hand, posterior vertebral epiphysiodesis would result in only one-third of this deficit, or just over 1% (Table 3) (Figs. 38 and 39).

The Sacrum

Its ossification is complex. It measures 3 cm at birth and 12 cm at the end of growth. Like the cervical spine, it represents about 15% of sitting height. It is composed of a large number of growth cartilages (see pelvic vertebra).

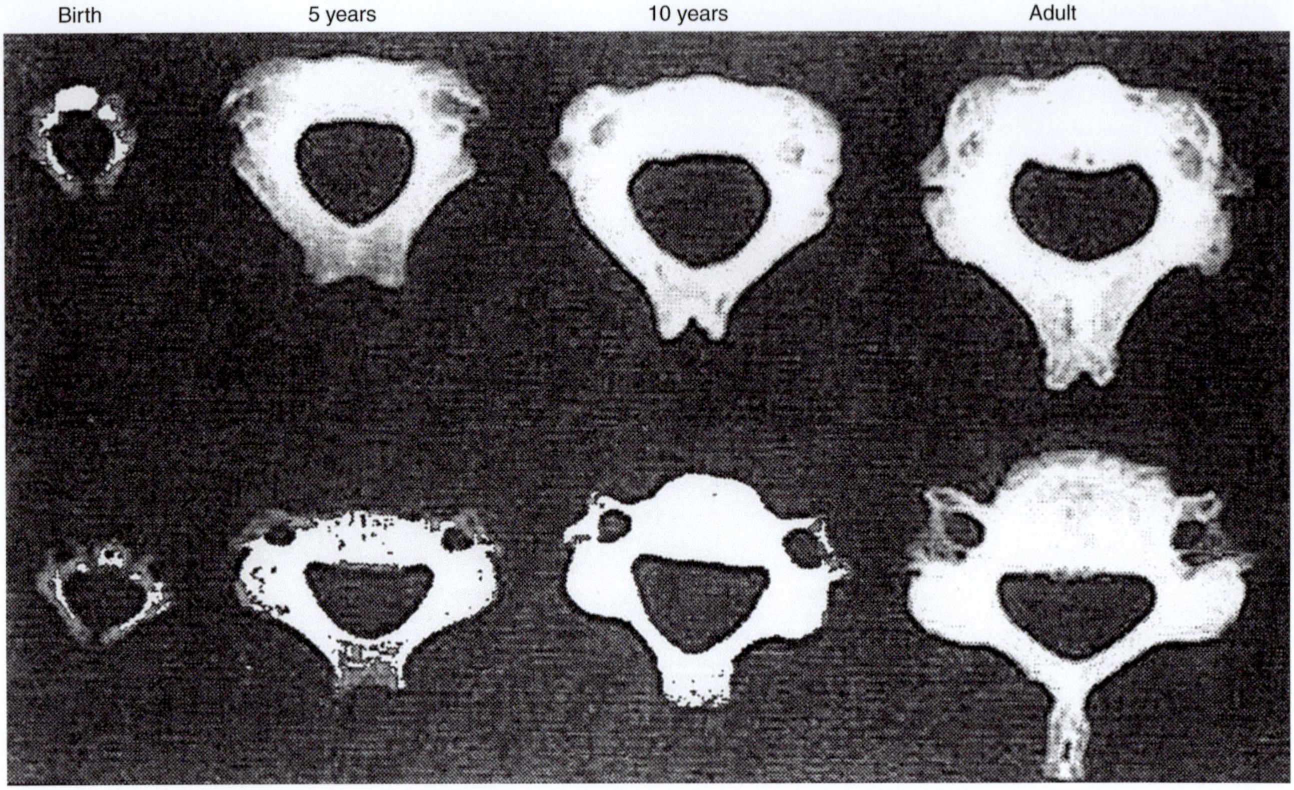

Fig. 18 From left to right. Cervical spine 2nd vertebra at birth, 5 years old, 10 years old, adulthood. From the age of 5, the cervical spine is fully grown. Inferior cervical spine, C4 at birth, 5 years old, 10 years old, and as an adult

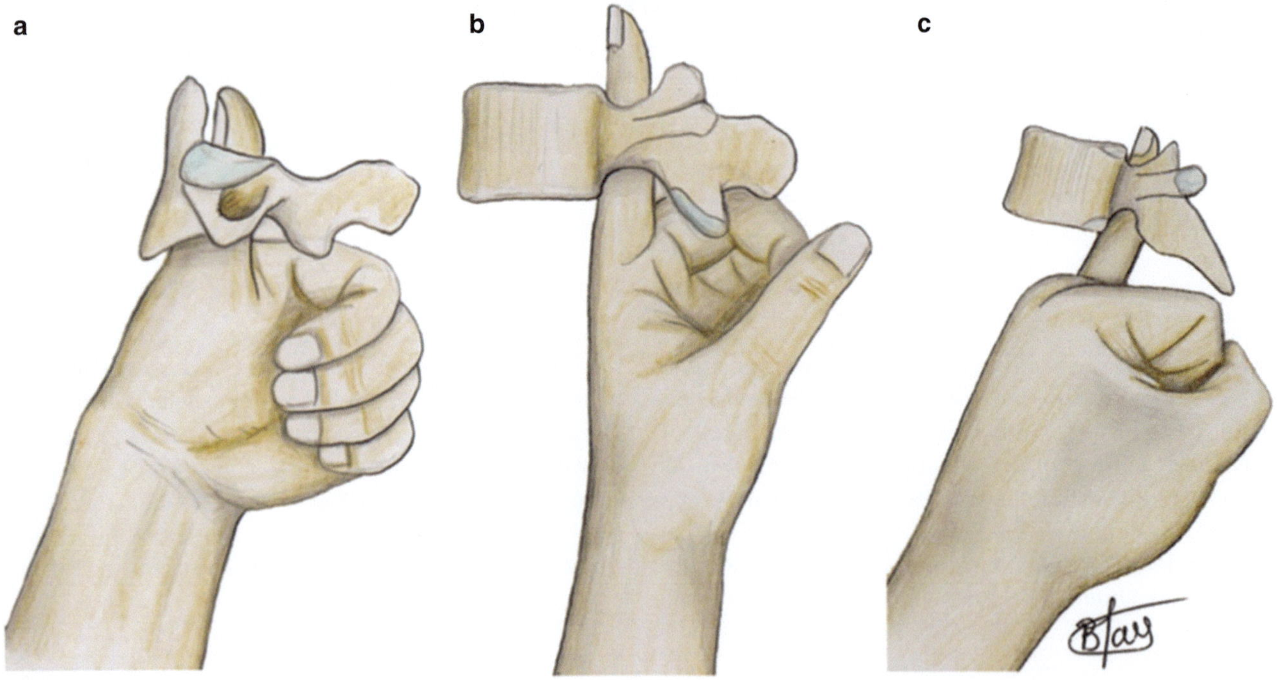

Fig. 19 Central spinal canal at the end of growth. (**a**) The cervical vertebra admits the thumb. (**b**) The lumbar vertebra admits the index. (**c**) The thoracic vertebra admits the 5th finger

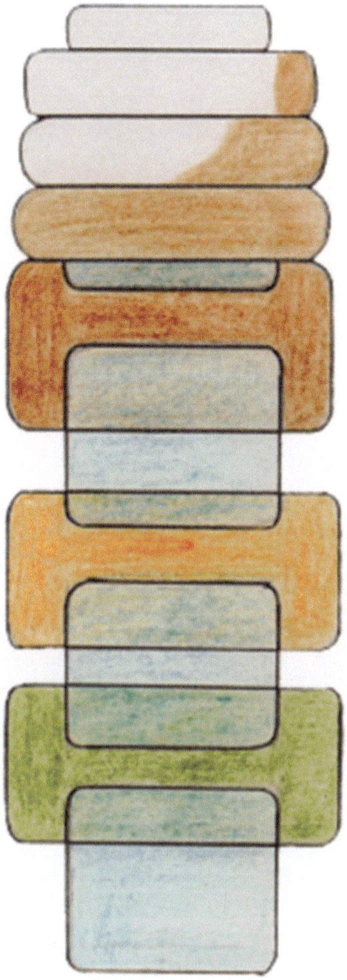

Fig. 20 Evolution of the 4 occipital somites and the first 3 cervical somites. The darker areas represent the 2nd to the 4th occipital somites, which contribute to the formation of the superior cervical spine

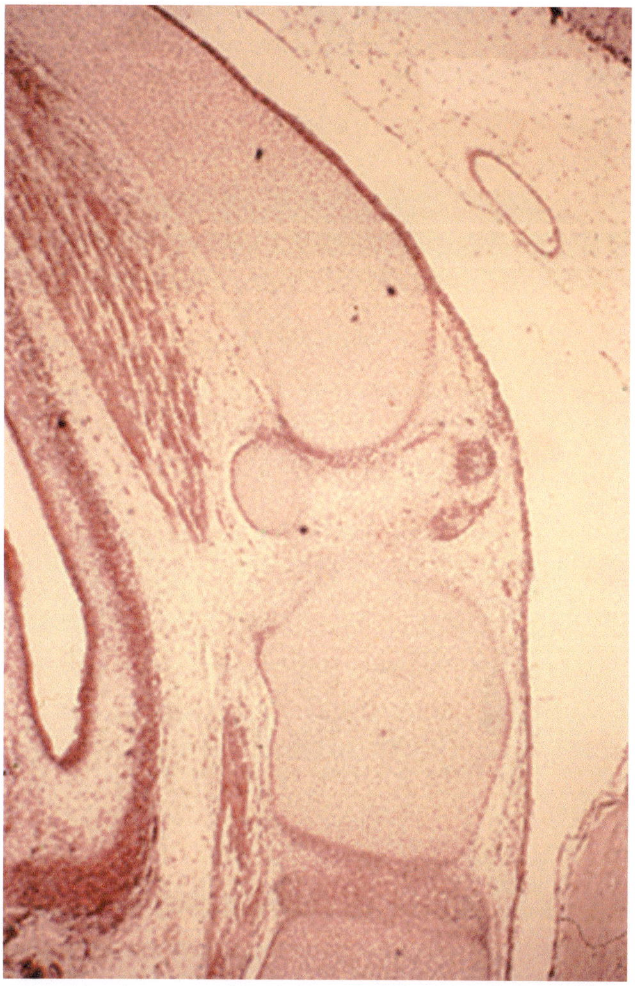

Fig. 21 Embryology: formation of the odontoid within the mesenchymal tissue

When comparing the sitting height to the chest perimeter, it turns out that at 10 years old, the child reaches 80% of his final sitting size, while the chest perimeter reaches 73–74%. He thus has an asynchronous growth between the sitting height and the thoracic size.

The Intervertebral Disc

Its height varies from cervical spine to lumbar spine. Overall, the intervertebral discs represent 24% of the spine.

The thoracic perimeter grows much faster than the upper segment or sitting height of 0 to 1 year, much less quickly between 1 and 10 years, and much faster from 10 years.

The Growth of the Thorax: 4th Dimension of the Spine

The growth of the thorax (Figs. 40, 41, and 42) is part of the growth of the spine. The reasoning on scoliosis is theoretically three-dimensional reasoning. This reflection was done in successive stages. At first, deformations of the vertebra on the horizontal plane were noted; secondly, it was understood that balancing the spinal profile was perhaps more important than correcting the frontal plane; Today, it remains an additional step to make that of the 4th dimension: to control a scoliosis, it is also to balance the thorax and to take account of its growth. *Scoliosis is a four-dimensional disease.*

The thoracic perimeter is a crude and valuable indicator of chest growth. Growth evolves on a ternary rhythm: active during the first 5 years of life, slower from 5 years to puberty, then very strong at puberty.

The thoracic perimeter is about 32 cm at birth; it will later measure about 89 cm. It grows about 56 cm, measuring almost 2.8 times its birth size. It has more than doubled, almost tripled.

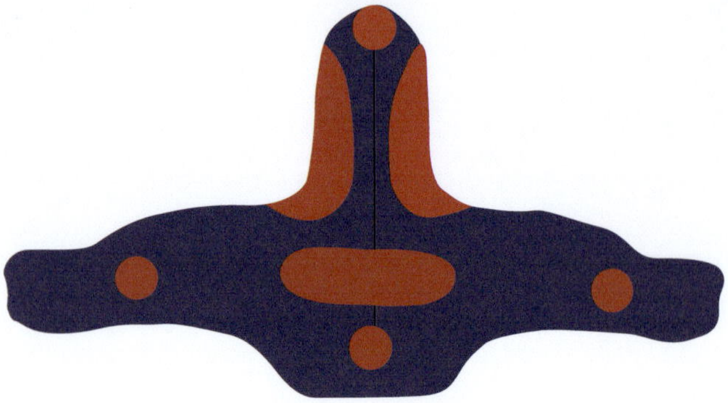

Fig. 22 The growth cartilages of the first cervical vertebra. The 2 lateral nuclei of the body of the odontoid merge before birth

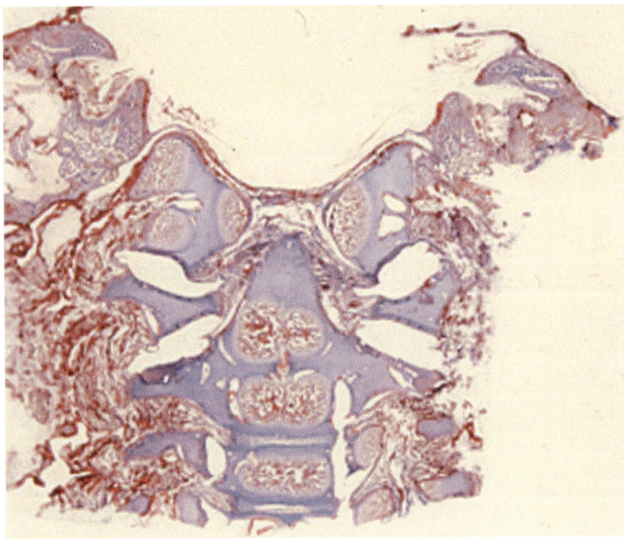

Fig. 23 Odontoid in the 8th month of intrauterine life. The 2 body cores of the odontoid are about to merge

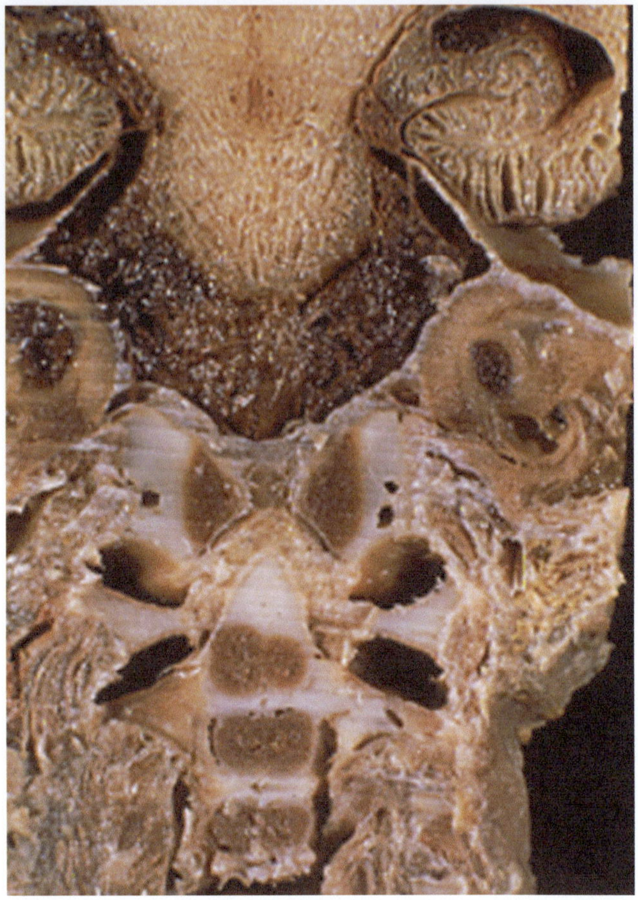

Fig. 24 Odontoid at birth. Frontal cut

At birth, the chest perimeter represents 97% of the sitting height: it measures 32 cm while the sitting size measures 35 cm.

At 1 year, the sitting height is almost the same value as the chest perimeter.

At the end of growth, the chest perimeter represents 95% of the sitting height.

The growth of the thoracic perimeter is active from 0 to 5 years. It increases by 24 cm.

From 5 to 10 years, growth is slower. The chest perimeter measures 66 cm at 10 years, so it increases by 9.9 cm. At 10, it represents 73% of its final value.

At 18: new acceleration. The thoracic perimeter measures 89 cm in the boy; it has increased by 23 cm between 10 and 18 years.

From 10 years to 18 years the thoracic perimeter increases as much as between birth and 5 years.

The anteroposterior diameter in boys is about 11 cm at birth, which is about 53% of the anteroposterior diameter of the adult; at the end of growth it measures about 21 cm so a boy can grow about 10 cm and double his birth measurement.

Growths are interdependent but not all grow at the same pace.

In the girl, the values are almost superimposable.

The transverse thoracic diameter is approximately 14 cm at birth, i.e., approximately 50% of the thoracic and transverse diameter; at the end of growth it measures 28 cm, so it doubles its birth size. The transverse diameter grows much more than the anteroposterior diameter. Between the transverse diameter and the anteroposterior diameter, the difference is about 2.5 cm at birth, it is about 7 cm at the end of growth. The ratio of the transverse diameter to the thoracic diameter is relatively stable. It is stable from the age of 4 years.

Volumetric growth of the thorax.

All growths do not evolve at the same rate.

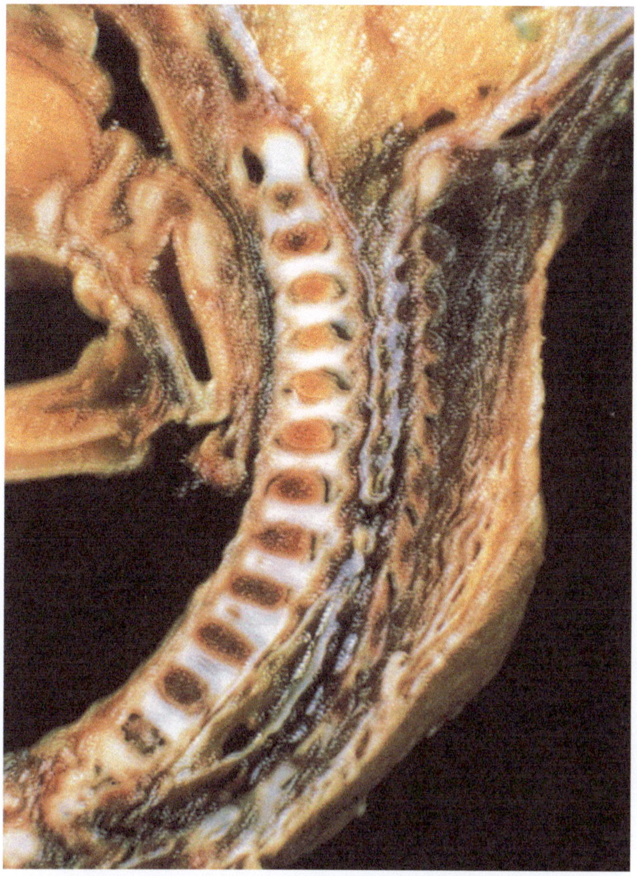

Fig. 25 Cervical spine, sagittal cut. Ossification is initially dorsal and extends radiating upwards and downwards. Note that the odontoid process is still completely cartilaginous on an 8-month-old fetus

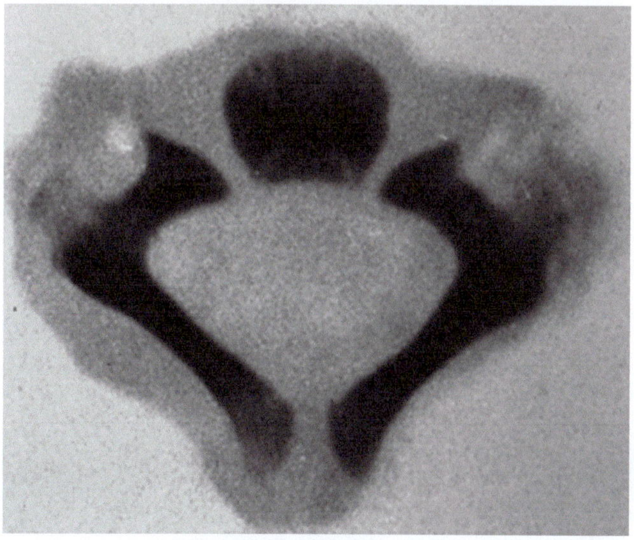

Fig. 26 Cervical vertebra at birth. X-ray horizontal section. Note the importance of the cartilaginous mass; the vertebral body can appear only at the age of 1 year. The neurocentral cartilage merges. The 2 posterior arcs merge posteriorly toward 6 years

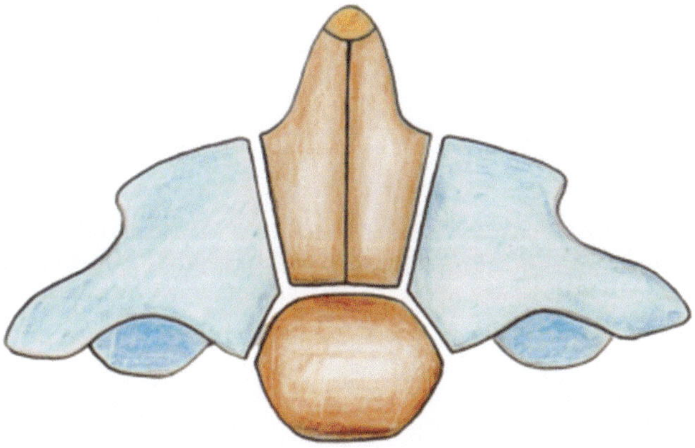

Fig. 27 Odontoid calendar. Development of the second cervical vertebra. Two centers of ossification appear "in the heart of the odontoid" at the 4th month of the fetal life; they merge before birth. The fusion between the body of the odontoid and the neurocentral cartilages occurs around the age of 6 years. A nucleus of higher polar ossification appears around the age of 3. The odontoid bone fuses at the top of the odontoid with the body of the odontoid around the age of 12 years. The two neural arches fuse posteriorly around the age of 4, it persists at about 6 years, a much reduced growth sequence between the body of the odontoid and the body of the atlas

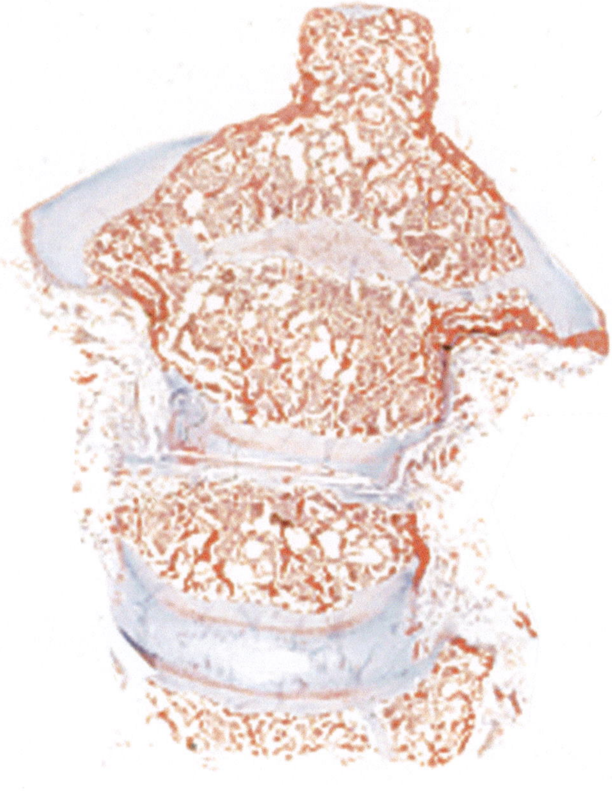

Fig. 28 The odontoid process at age 8 is completely ossified

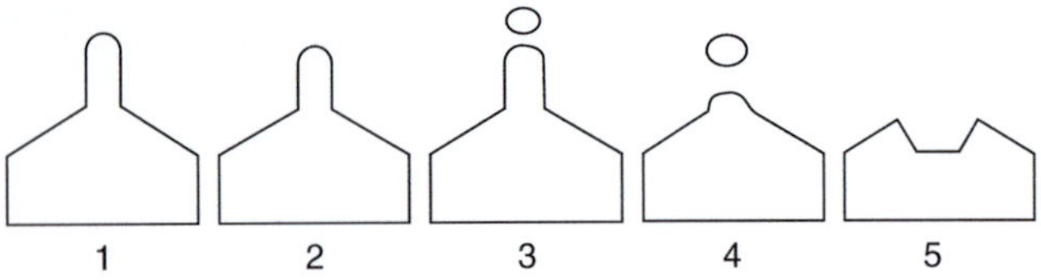

Fig. 29 Morphological abnormalities of the odontoid. 1. Normal odontoid apophysis; 2. Atrophic odontoid apophysis; 3. Os odontoideum; 4. More severe os odontoideum malformation; 5. Absence of odontoid process

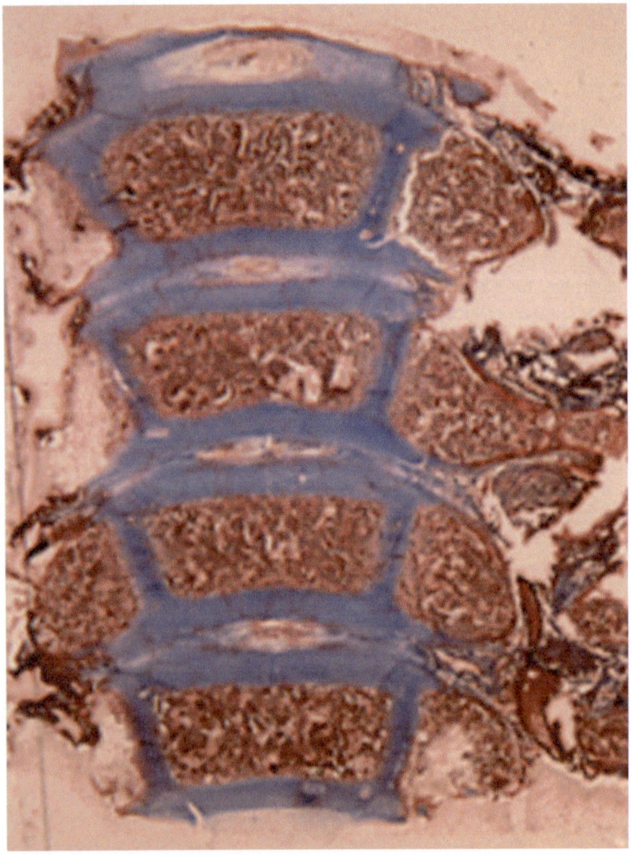

Fig. 30 Lower cervical spine. Frontal cut at 8 years old

Table 1 The cervical spine

	Anteroposterior diameter	Transverse diameter	Surface
Canal	17 mm	27 mm	376 mm^2
Cord	8 mm	13 mm	80 mm^2
Cord	Anteroposterior diameter	Transverse diameter	Surface
Cervical	8 mm	13 mm	8 mm^2
Thoracic	6 mm	8 mm	4 mm^2

Bodyweight

The anteroposterior diameter represents 75% of the transverse diameter from the age of 5 years. The anteroposterior diameter represents on average 21% of the sitting height.

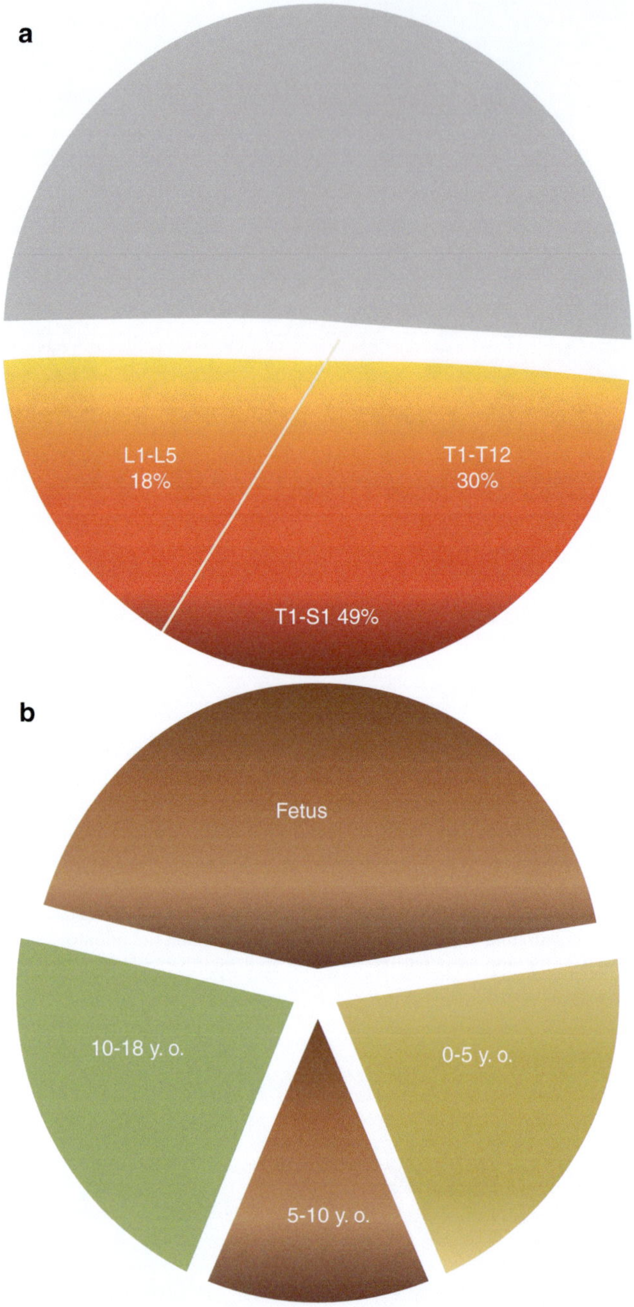

Fig. 31 (**a**) The T1-S1 segment represents approximately 49–50% of the sitting height, the thoracic spine 30%, and the lumbar spine 18%. (**b**) The T1-S1 segment represents at birth 44% of its final size; high growth is recorded in the first 5 years of life and at puberty

The transverse diameter represents on average 30% of the sitting height.

There are two types of thorax to differentiate:

- *a balanced thorax*: the anteroposterior diameter and the frontal diameter represent more than 50% of the sitting size. The chest perimeter represents 95% of the sitting height.

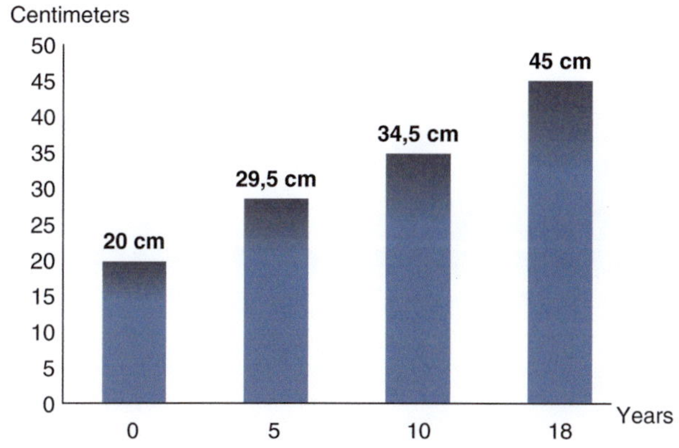

Fig. 32 Segment T1-S1 in the boy. T1-S1 is about 45 cm in adulthood. The increase is about 25 cm during entire growth. Between 5 and 10 years the speed of growth collapses (1 cm/year). In the 10-year-old boy, there is 9.5 cm left to run on the thoraco-lumbar spine

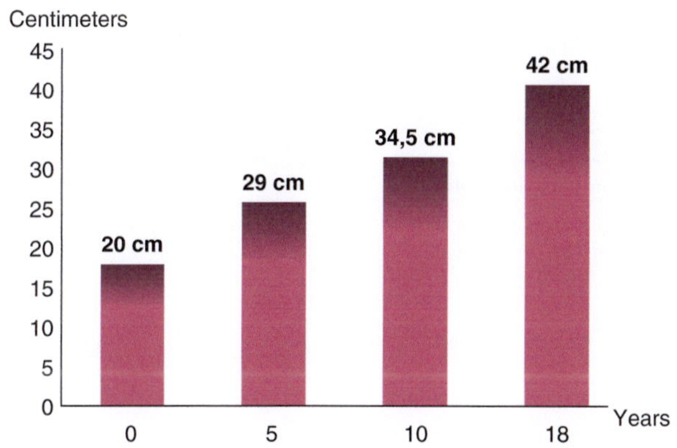

Fig. 33 Segment T1-S1 in the girl. T1-S1 is about 42 cm in adulthood. The increase is about 22 cm during entire growth. Between 5 and 10 years, the growth rate is only 1 cm per year. In the girl, at 10 years, there is 6.5 cm left to grow in the thoraco-lumbar spine (T1-S1)

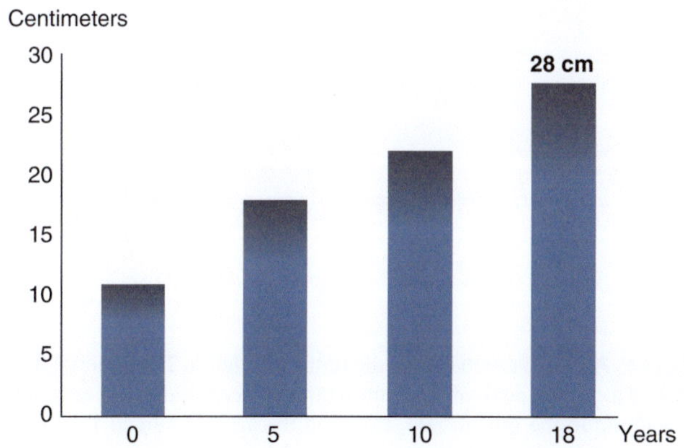

Fig. 34 T1-T12 segment in the boy. The thoracic segment of the boy is a little larger (28 cm versus 26.5) than that of the girl at the end of growth. It is multiplied by 2.5 cm between birth and adulthood. It has almost doubled to 10 years. Of all growth, the most important is that which occurs from 0 to 5 years. In the boy, at 10 years, there is 6 cm left to grow on the thoracic spine

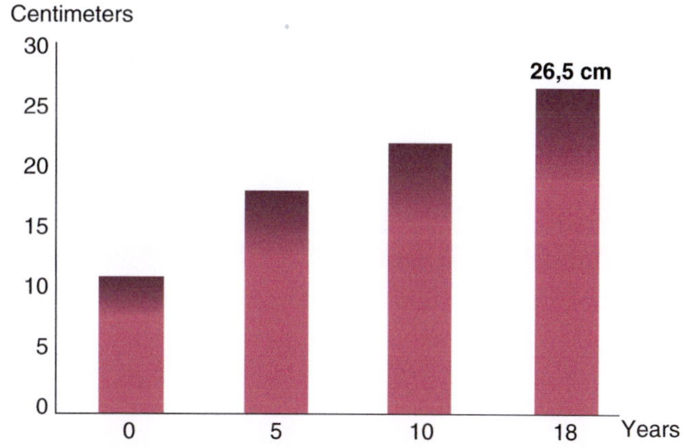

Fig. 35 Segment T1-T12 in the girl. At birth, the T1-T12 segment is 11 cm, there is actually about 4 cm of disc, or more than 30%. Up to 10 years, there is less significant difference between boy and girl. The T1-T12 segment of the girl is a little smaller than that of the boy at the end of growth. In the girl, at 10 years, there is 4 cm left to grow on the thoracic spine. The thoracic vertebra represents 2.5% of the sitting height

Table 2 Thoracic vertebra

Age (years)	Size	Volume
New born	0.6 cm	1.2 cm^3
2 years	1.1 cm	8.6 cm^3
4 years	1.3 cm	12.8 cm^3
10 years	1.6 cm	18.7 cm^3
18 years old	2.2 cm	39.4 cm^3

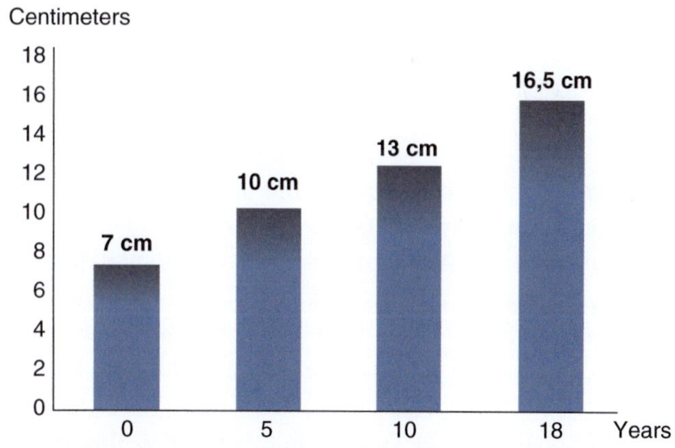

Fig. 36 L1-L5 segment in the boy. At birth, the L1-L5 segment is 7 cm. It is approximately identical to that of the girl until adulthood, or greater by 0.5 cm. In the boy, at 10 years, there remains 3.5 cm left to grow on the lumbar spine

- *an unbalanced thorax*: the anteroposterior diameter and the frontal diameter represent less than 45% of the sitting size. The chest perimeter is less than 90% of the sitting height.

In both boys and girls, the thoracic volume at birth represents 6–7% of the final thoracic volume. It increases about

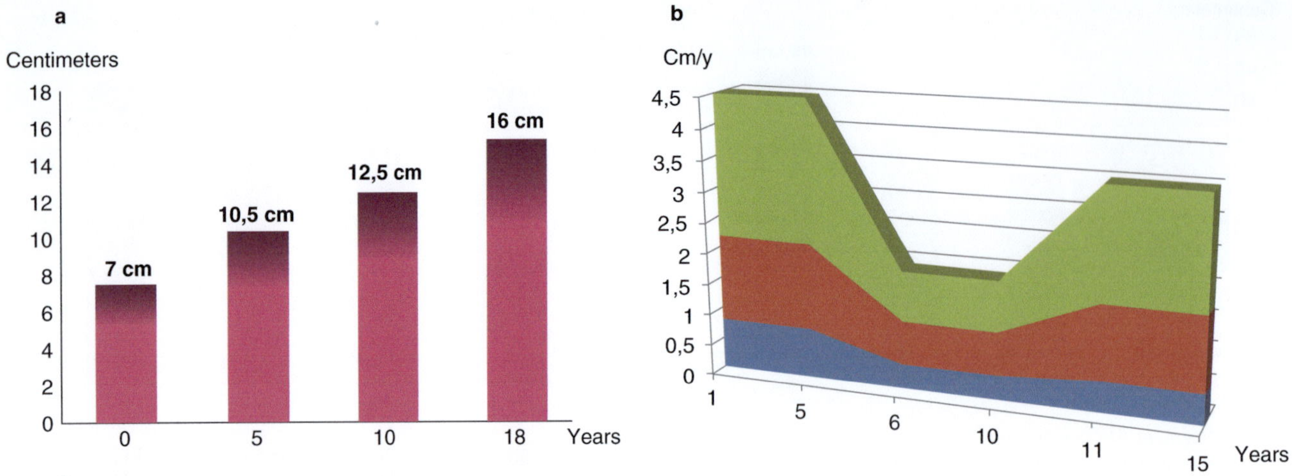

c

Spinal segment	Birth–5 years	5–10 years	10–16 years
T1-S1	2.2	0.9	1.8
T1-T12	1.4	0.6	1.2
L1-S1	0.8	0.3	0.6

Fig. 37 (**a**) L1-L5 segment in the girl. At birth, the L1-L5 segment is 7 cm. The L1-L5 segment is constantly about 0.5 cm greater than the boy, up to 10 years. At the end of growth, it is about 0.5 cm less than in the boy. (**b**) Segment growth rate curve (average between girl and boy). The fastest growth is between 0 and 5 years old. The peak of pubertal growth shows a strong recovery. (**c**) Speed of growth expressed in centimeters in infantile scoliosis

Table 3 Lumbar vertebra

Age (years)	Height	Volume
New born	0.83 cm	2.0 cm^3
2 years	1.6 cm	18.4 cm^3
4 years	2.0 cm	24.0 cm^3
10 years	2.4 cm	43.0 cm^3
18 years old	3.3 cm	87.0 cm^3

25% during the first 5 years of life and especially it will increase by 50% between 10 and 15 years.

Campbell (San Antonio) (Fig. 43) has shown that in severe scoliosis (the first five years of life), it is preferable to "open the thorax" rather than strive to reduce a spine deformed by major kyphosis or progressive scoliosis. He has therefore devised an instrumentation which makes it possible to create distraction or compression; similar to that of an Ilizarof apparatus, a circular external fixator, likely to open the ribcage when the thorax is too retracted.

He understood that the fundamental objective in any scoliotic or kyphotic curvature was to protect the spinal cord and also to give the space necessary for pulmonary development, avoiding the retraction of the thoracic cage. This new conception of scoliosis surgery has opened up many perspectives, particularly in the treatment of severe paralytic scoliosis, severe congenital scoliosis, and severe juvenile scoliosis.

The opening and the maintenance of the thorax are similar to the opening of an umbrella or a parasol. The study of severe infantile scoliosis revealed the interaction of growths:

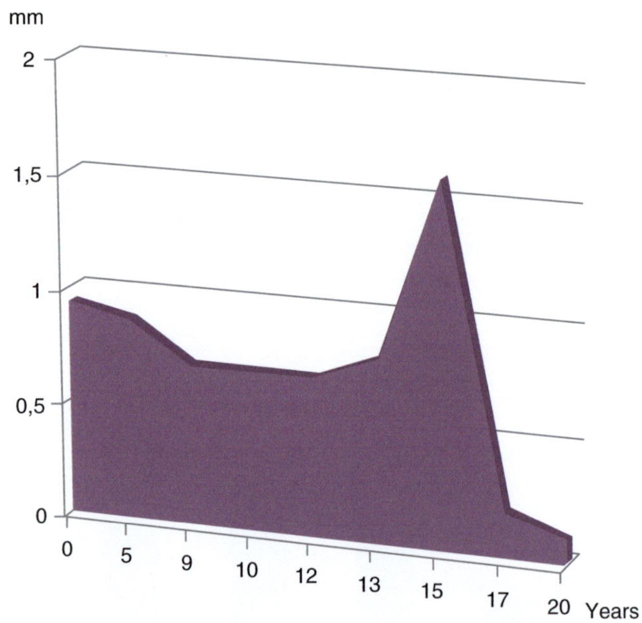

Fig. 38 Annual growth rate of the lumbar vertebra. The pubertal thrust creates a growth peak of 1.6 mm, while between 5 and 10 years, there is a slump in the growth rate. Between the ages of 13 and 15 years in boys, there is a marked increase in growth rate

growth of the spine, growth of the thorax and sternum, cardiopulmonary growth. *The vertebral-costo-sternal frame under the effect of scoliosis deformity and loses its elasticity (Figs. 44 and 45).*

Parasol Effect

Early vertebral graft blocks thoracic growth and lung development:

- The spinal canal is predominately that of early growth, around the age of 5. As a result, early perivertebral arthrodesis (around the age of 5 years) is not likely to lead to stenosis of the spinal canal;
- Only perivertebral arthrodesis can control all anterior and posterior growth cartilages, especially in severe scoliosis. *Theoretically*, the best way to control an evolutionary curvature is to lock all the growth cartilages involved in the curvature—to avoid the crankshaft effect;
- Posterior vertebral graft slows the growth of the vertebral body by 23% anteriorly. The vertebral bodies are therefore partly influenced by the posterior graft. Winter showed that posterior arthrodesis was able to correct a congenital kyphosis;
- Hemi-arthrodesis can be performed in congenital scoliosis; they relate to the convex side of the spinal deviation, thus fixating the physis for half of the vertebral body and thus half of the vertebra. In addition, Winter has shown that anterior and posterior hemi-arthrodeses are effective only to the extent that it is performed before the age of 5 years.
- Roaf has shown that an epiphysiodesis of the vertebral body is likely to cause at each vertebral segment an angular gain of the order of 10–15°. Hence the interest in vertebral staples previously, or more conventionally, that of tethering.
- Canavese and Karol showed that *early arthrodesis of the thoracic spine before the age of 5 blocks the growth* of the anteroposterior diameter of the thorax, vertebral body growth, thoracic growth, and lung development. This fundamental work led to a strategic reversal. The distraction of the spine, the opening of the thorax to facilitate the development of the lung has replaced early vertebral fixation (Table 4).

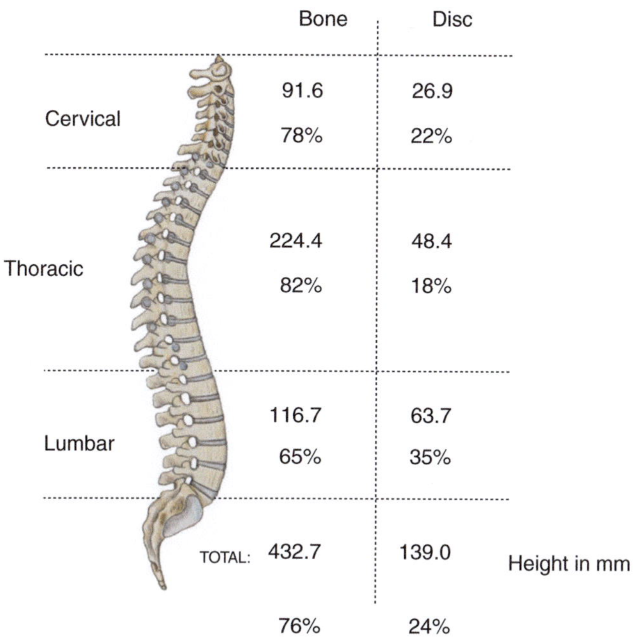

Fig. 39 Respective percentages of bone and disc in the total height of the spine. In the cervico-thoracic spine, the discs represent about 1/4 of the total height, the vertebrae 3/4. At the lumbar level, the discs represent about 1/3 of the height, whereas the lumbar vertebrae represent only 2/3 of the height

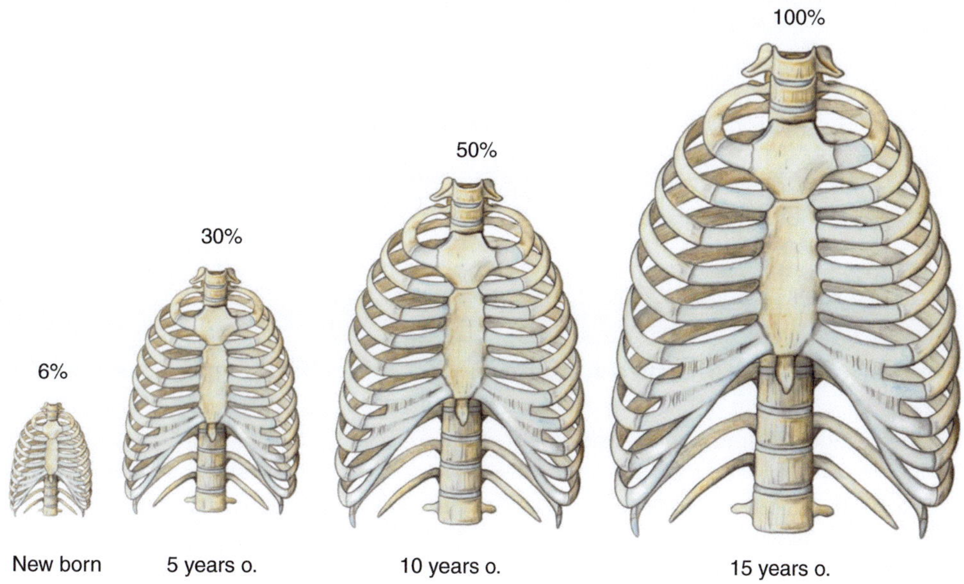

Fig. 40 At 5 years, the thoracic volume reaches 30% of its final size; the volume of the thorax doubles from 10 years to skeletal maturation

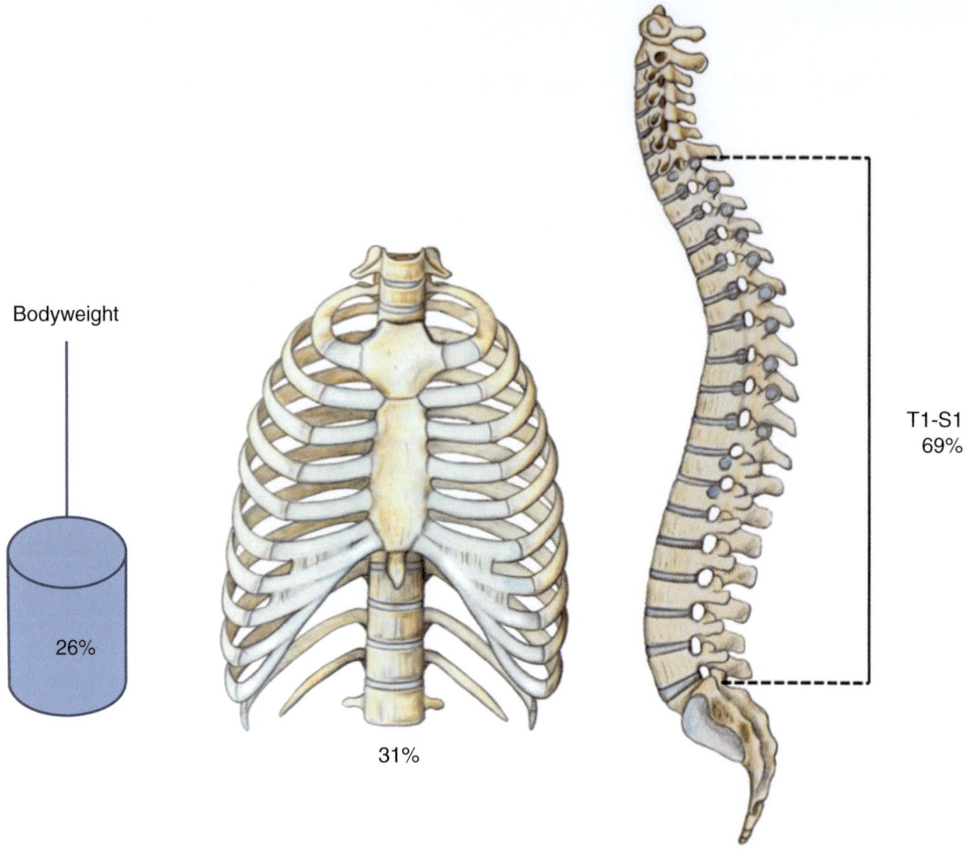

Fig. 41 At the age of 5, the weight reaches 26% of its final size; the chest is 31% while the T1-S1 segment is 69% of its final size

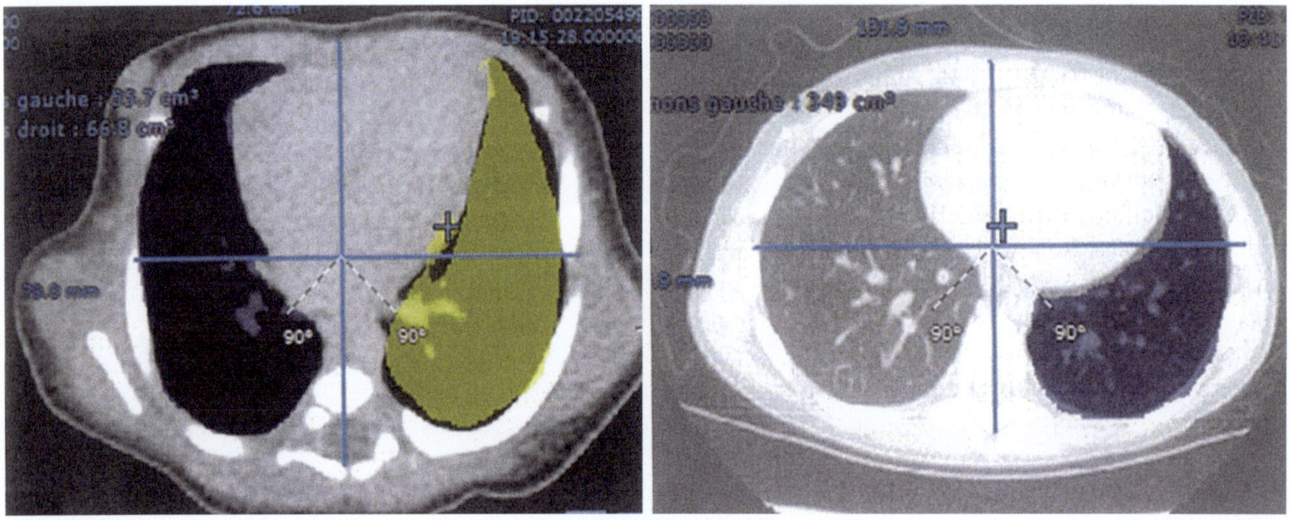

Fig. 42 The shape of the thorax evolves with growth. The thorax is spherical at birth, it becomes ovoid with growth, the anteroposterior diameter grows less rapidly than the transverse diameter. The volume of the thorax is multiplied by five from birth to 5 years

What Size Deficit for Which Arthrodesis?

Three questions must first be answered:

- specify the bone age. Bone age is in phase with chronological age in only 50% of cases;
- measure sitting height;
- evaluate on the growth curves the remaining sitting size (Figs. 46, 47, 48, and 49).

First Scenario: Arthrodesis of the Thoracic Spine

The thoracic spine represents 30% of the sitting height. This ratio is constant from the age of 5 years. Each thoracic vertebra represents approximately 2.5% of the sitting height.

When puberty begins, there remains 13% of growth both in the boy and in the girl for sitting height. When the elbow fuses, there remains at 13 years of bone age in the

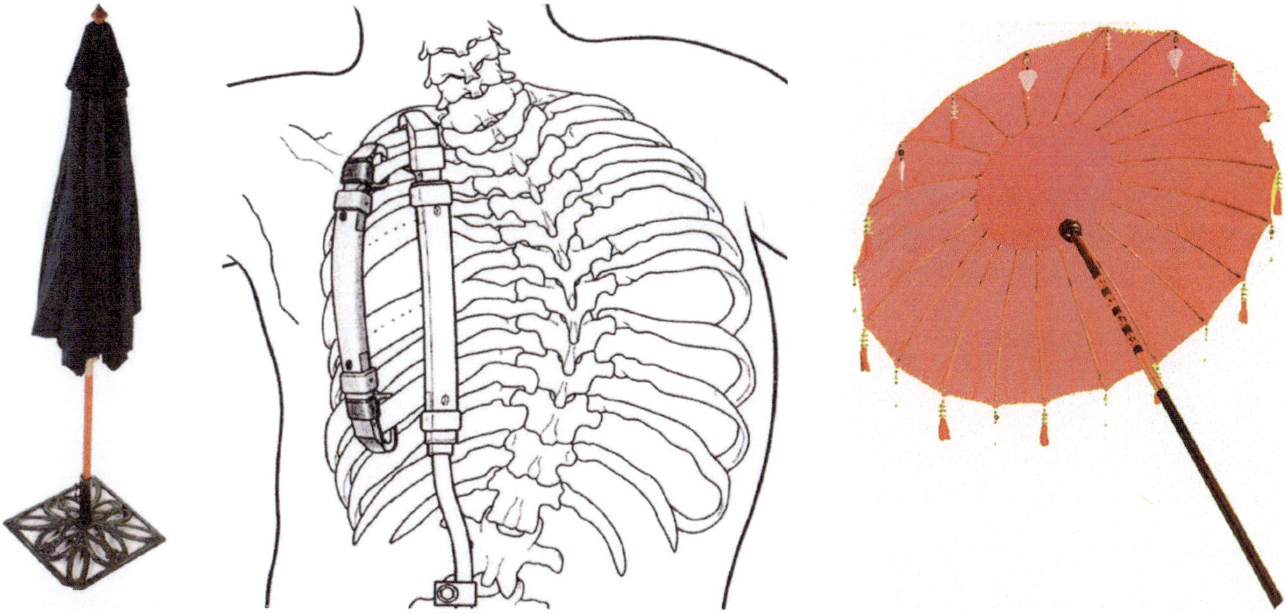

Fig. 43 In severe scoliosis before the age of 5, the retraction of the thorax compromises cardiopulmonary growth. Campbell et al. (San Antonio) has proposed correcting this retraction and opening the thoracic parasol

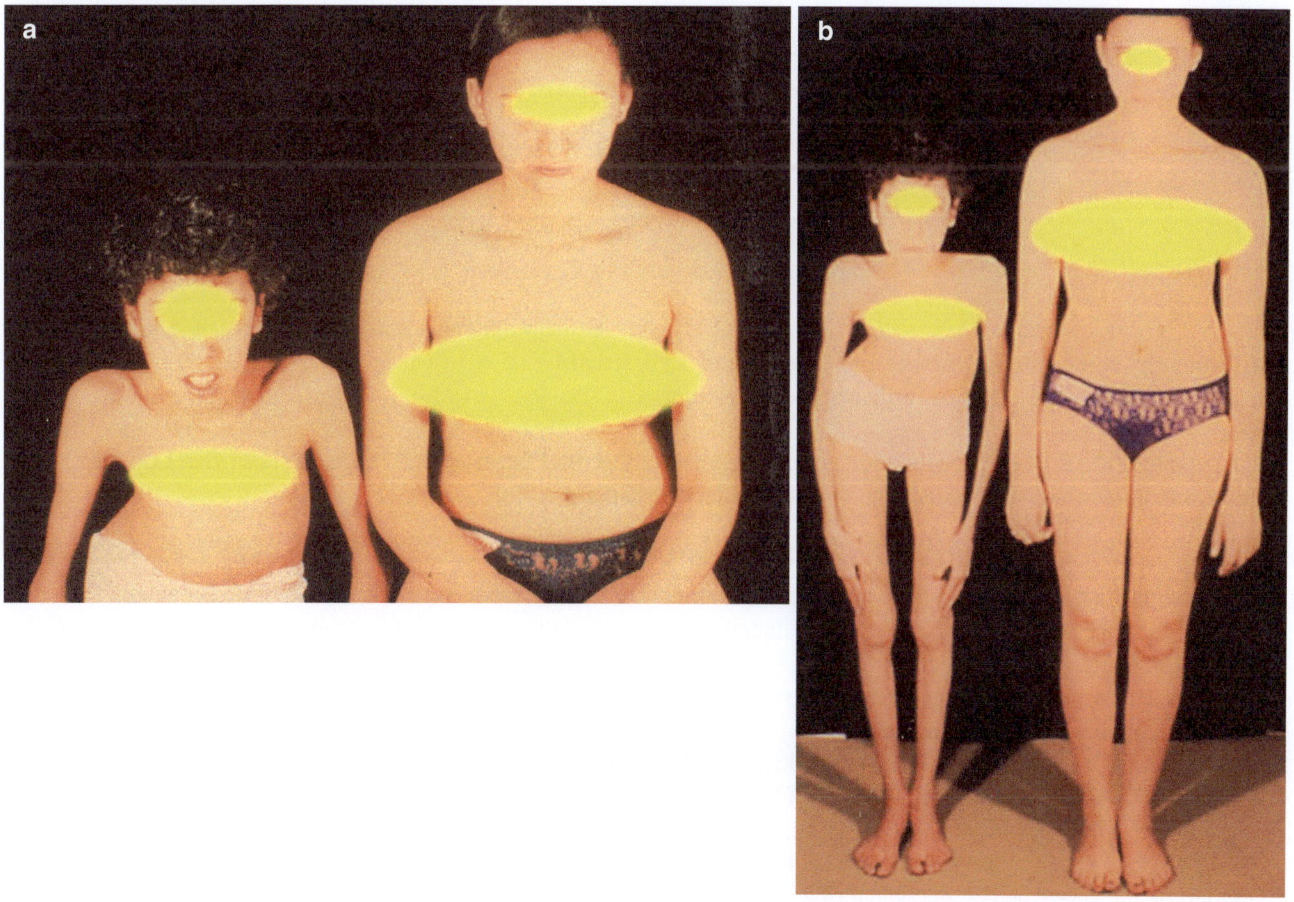

Fig. 44 (**a** and **b**) Infantile scoliosis causes a severe deficit in sitting height. Infantile scoliosis at 16 years old. Deficit on sitting height, 25 cm. Weight, 22 kg (weight of a child of 6 years). Abnormal growth of the lower limbs

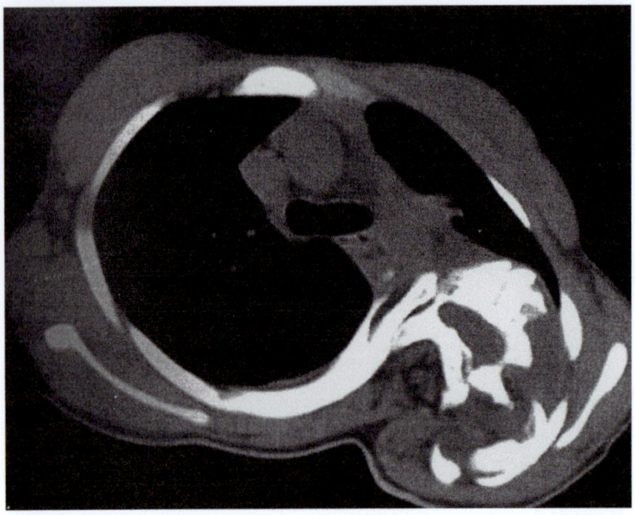

Fig. 45 Infantile scoliosis causes penetration of the vertebral body into the thorax

Table 4 Spine growth in percentage

Age (years)	% sitting height (girls)	% sitting height (boys)
2	58%	57%
5	70%	67%
10	84%	80%
11	87%	82%
12	91%	84%
13	95%	87%
14	97%	91%
15	100%	95%
16	100%	97%
17	100%	100%
18	100%	100%

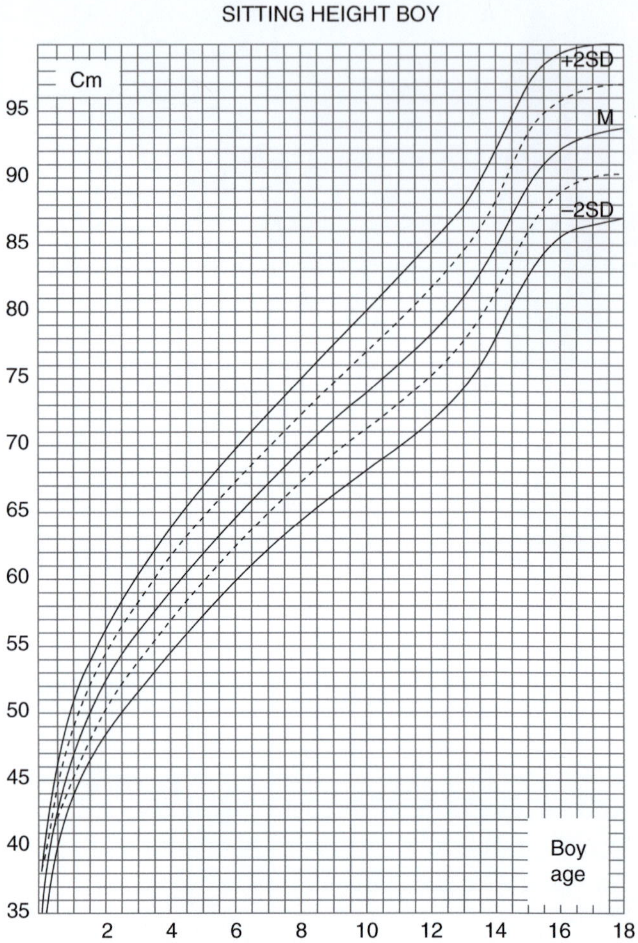

Fig. 46 Evolution of sitting height in boys

girl (6 months before the appearance of Risser I) and 15 years of bone age in the boy, 5% further growth in sitting height.

The epiphysiodesis of all growth cartilages of a thoracic vertebra therefore results in a "remaining" sitting size deficit of 2.5%.

The epiphysiodesis of the thoracic spine at the age of 5 years in the boy is analyzed as follows: remaining sitting height of 31 cm; neutralization of 30% of the remaining sitting size. The deficit of sitting height of 9.3 cm.

For girls: 5 years, sitting height 28 cm: neutralization of 30% of the remaining sitting size is 7.8 cm.

At the age of 10 years, the remaining sitting height in the boy is about 20 cm. Blocking growth of the T1-T12 segment will result in a deficit of 5 cm.

When the boy's puberty begins at age 13, there is about 13 cm left on the sitting height; the deficit of a perivertebral arthrodesis T1-T12 will be of the order of 3.9 cm.

Growth diagrams make it easily possible to evaluate the deficit.

Second Scenario: Arthrodesis of the Lumbar Spine

The lumbar spine represents 18% of the sitting height. Each lumbar vertebra contributes 3.5% of sitting height.

An arthrodesis of the entire lumbar spine in the boy at 5 years will result in a deficit of 5.6 cm, at 10 years of 3.6 cm, to 13 years of 2.3 cm, at 15 years of 0.9 cm.

In the girl a perivertebral arthrodesis of the complete lumbar spine will result in a deficit of 5 years of 4.7 cm, at 11 years of 2.1 cm, at 13 years of 0.9 cm.

The detailed analysis of these deficits shows that a periventricular arthrodesis performed at the onset of puberty finally leads to a relatively small sitting height deficit.

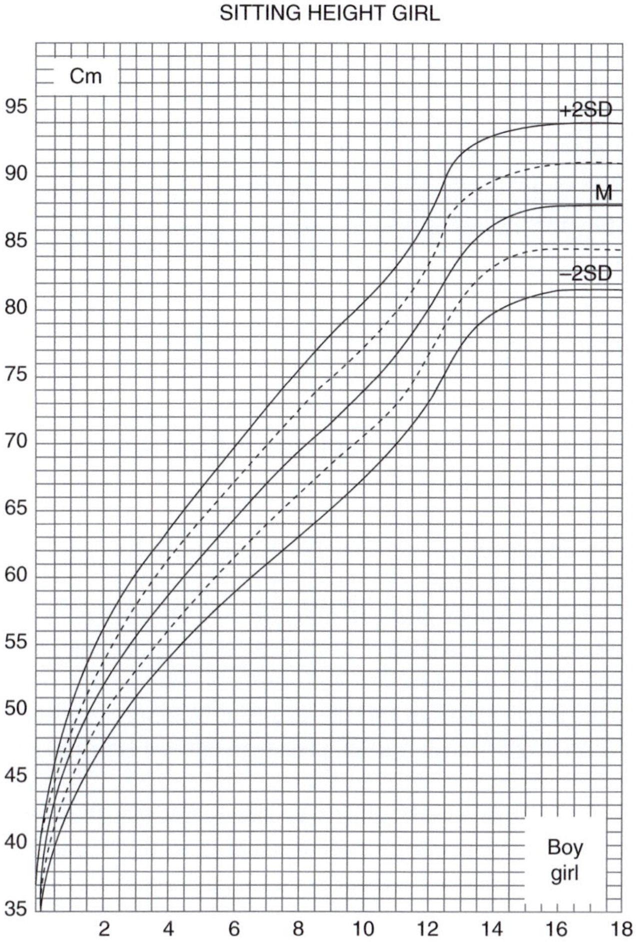

Fig. 47 Evolution of sitting height in girls

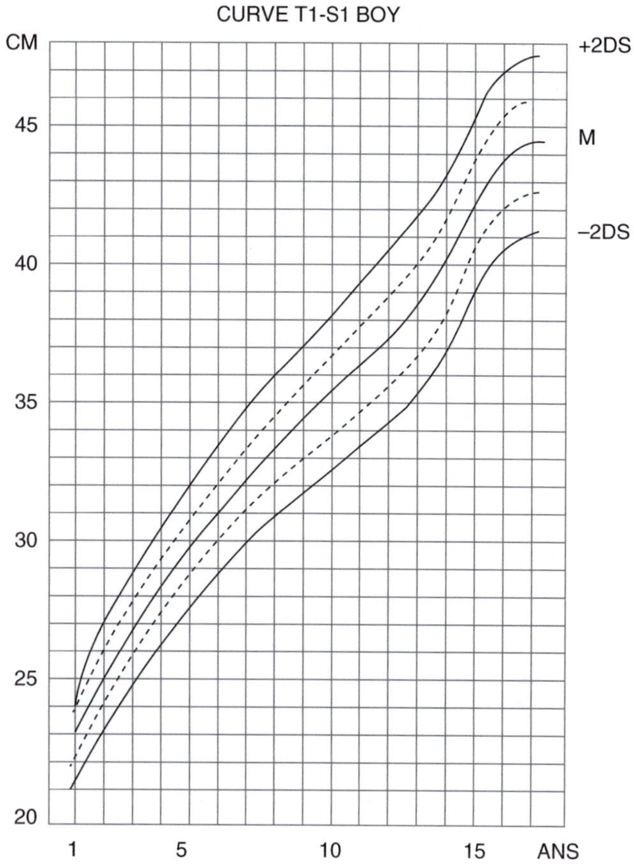

Fig. 48 Standard deviations of T1-S1 in the boy

These figures relate to periventricular arthrodesis. When arthrodesis is only posterior, the deficit to be considered is only 1/3 compared to a deficit of periventricular arthrodesis (Figs. 50 and 51).

All Scoliosis Will in Time Become Identified as a Growth Cartilage Disease

Disturbing a single cartilage challenges the morphology of the whole vertebra. Any aggression on a growth cartilage that is mechanical, malformative, or metabolic resonates on the whole vertebral column.

The growth disorder can strike indiscriminately at all the cartilages of the same vertebra, it can be more selective and touch the posterior cartilages or the anterior cartilages. In this case, it determines an asynchronous growth that will result in a deviation. The involvement of the posterior structures leads to a sagittal imbalance. Disturbance of one side of the vertebral body can lead to vertebral deviation. Scoliosis exerts greater pressure in the concave zone and weaker in the convex zone. It compresses some cartilages and limits other cartilages. It is responsible for a curvature that is self-sustaining. Kyphosis is due to a malformation of the anterior growth cartilages; it creates a difference of growth potential in favor of the posterior arc. Vertebral ossification is progressive, which explains why radiographically a segmentation defect due to a congenital malformation does not always appear clearly at birth.

It is necessary to wait several years for example, before identifying on radiograph, a defect of vertebral ossification caused by Klippel-Feil syndrome.

These vertebrae are sensitive to pressure, so the vertebral bodies have an abnormally high height in bedridden children, often seen in cerebral palsy, due to a lack of stress on the vertebral body (Fig. 52).

The Growth of the Spine: From Normal to Pathological

Normality makes it possible to better assess deficits. To grasp the complexity of growth, it is necessary to regularly measure the sitting height, the chest perimeter, the T1-S1 segment and especially the annual growth rate of the sitting height (Figs. 53 and 54).

In severe infantile scoliosis, the loss of sitting height for a curvature of 100° can be 15 cm!

The interdependence of growth is at the heart of the problem. The growths are synchronized but do not evolve at the same pace. For example, at age 5, the growth of the thorax is very late compared to the growth of the spine. But at puberty, there is a catch-up. The thorax grows larger than the sitting size.

The risk of infantile scoliosis is primarily cardiorespiratory! It is necessary to act quickly during the first 5 years of life (Campbell). The lung abnormalities are irreversible. Abnormal growth tends to spread. This is a domino effect: abnormal growth of the spine, then the chest, then the lung.

Infantile scoliosis with growth changes in nature. It becomes a pediatric condition with cardio-respiratory and nutritional problems.

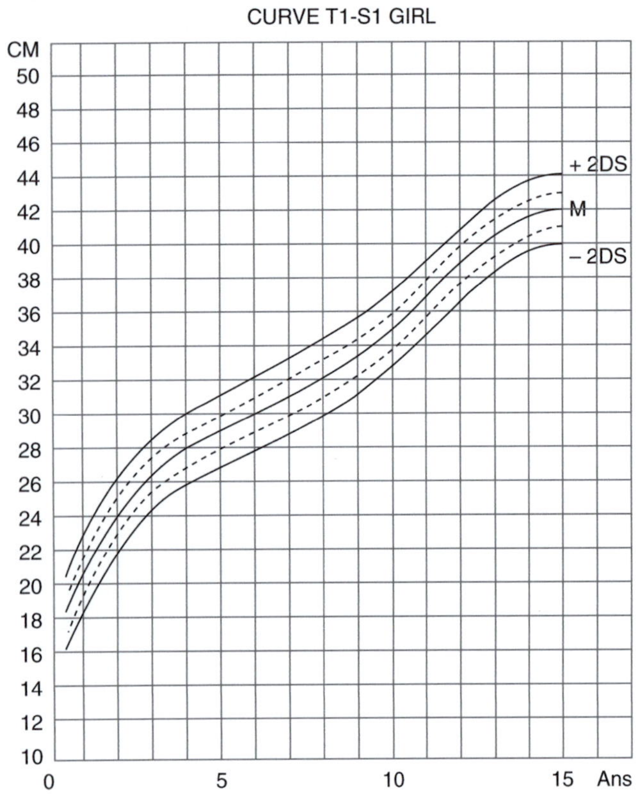

Fig. 49 Standard deviations of T1-S1 in the girl. Expression of the average in percentage. At birth T1-S1 represents 36%, at 10 years 83.3%, at 11 years (beginning of puberty), it represents 87.6%

Managing Infantile Scoliosis Is Controlling the Vilebrequin Effect

It means approximating a course of normality. It is to marry the growth rhythms.

The crankshaft effect is omnipresent. There is no ideal instrumentation to control it. Its expression is multiple. It is expressed on the apical curvature, on the frontal, sagittal, horizontal plane, upstream, and downstream! Nothing can contain it (except unfortunately a complete perivertebral arthrodesis).

1. *The first five years of life*: do not forget that the spine grows more than during all the other years (by 5 years the sitting height increases to 27 cm and the weight to 17 kg).
2. *Between 5 years and the beginning of puberty*, the sitting height increases by about 2.5 cm per year, the weight by 2.5 kg per year. To stay on course is to respect those numbers.
3. *At puberty*, one has to prepare for acceleration. Knowing that a scoliosis of 30° at the beginning has a 100% risk of being surgical. One must anticipate this.

Fig. 50 Remaining growth on the T1-S1 segment in the boy

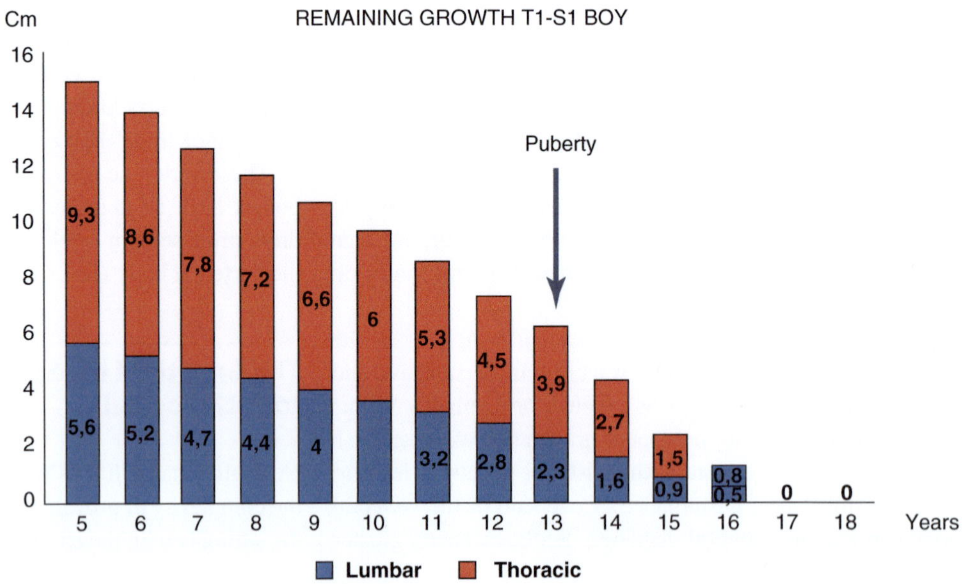

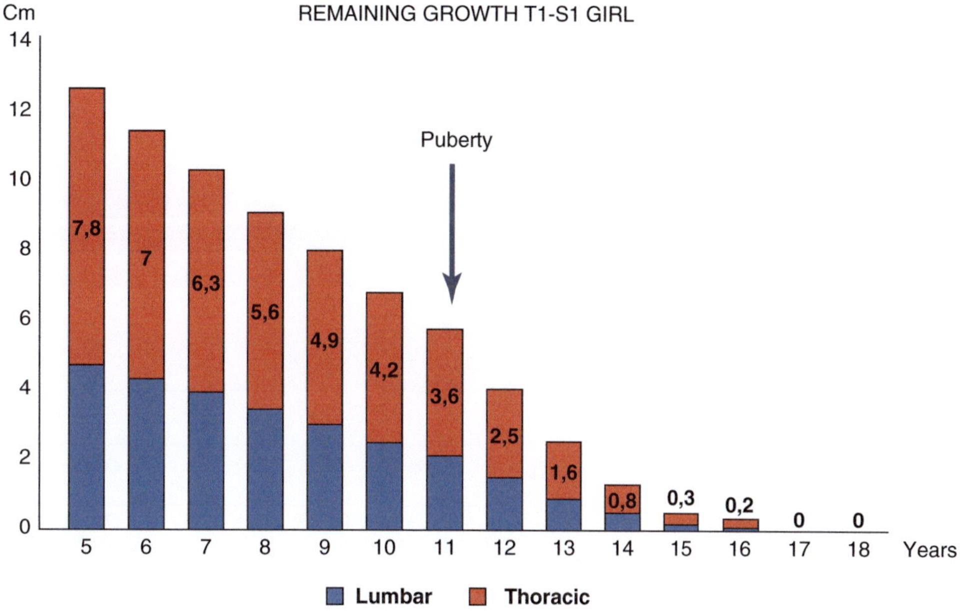

Fig. 51 Remaining growth on the T1-S1 segment in the girl

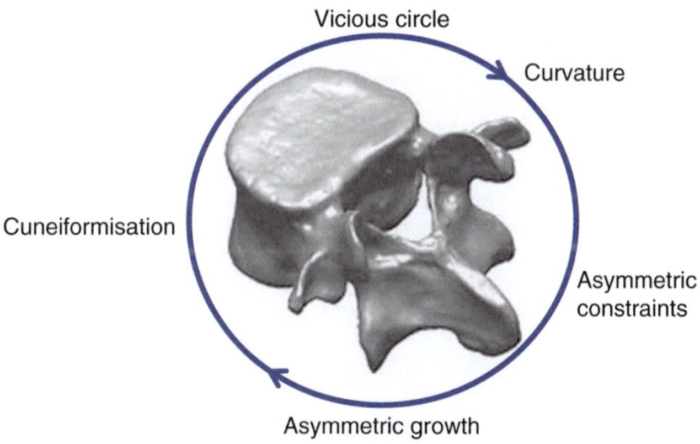

Fig. 52 Spinal curvature leads to asymmetric growth cartilage constraint that leads to cuneiformisation (wedge-shaped)

One must not forget that the volume of the thorax doubles and the weight doubles. It goes from 30 kg at 10 years to 60 kg at 15 years. The centimeters that are lost from fixation during puberty are minute. To keep control of the events, it is necessary to anticipate the accelerations.

The aim for infantile scoliosis at the end of growth is as follows: a weight greater than 40 kg, a vital capacity of at least 50%, a length of the thoracic spine of 22 cm, a length of T1-S1 of 30 cm (Table 5).

> To know a little more: all the growth curves are in the book "La croissance du rachis" (A. DImeglio - F. Bonnel) SpringlerVerlag 1990.

Fig. 53 Ascending and descending phases of puberty relative to Risser stages and physeal closures

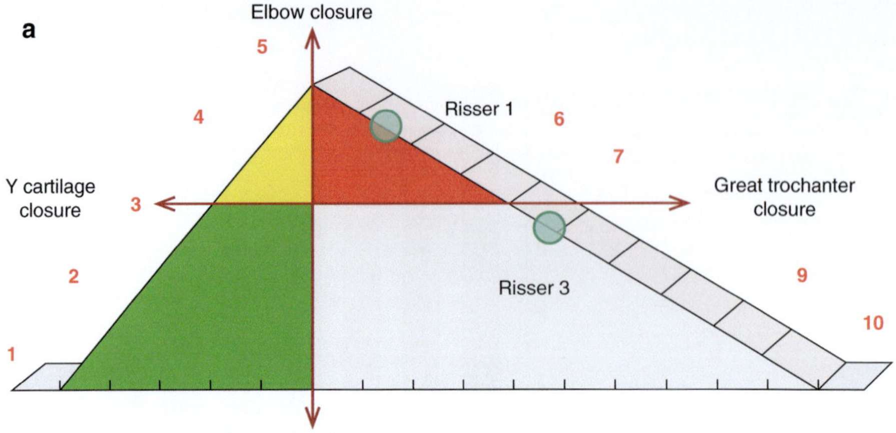

b

	Hand	Olecranon	Triradiate certilage	Risser
1	Sesamoid of the thumb	Double ossification	Open	0
2	Sesamoid of the thumb	Ovoid	Open	0
3	Sesamoid of thumb	Quadrangular	Closed	0
4	Sesamoid of thumb	Start of fusion	Closed	0
5	Distal fusion of the thumb	Fused	Closed	0
6	Distal phalanx fusion	Fused	Closed	1
7	Metacarpophalangeal fusion	Fused	Closed	2
8	Interphalangeal fusion	Fused	Closed	3
9	Fusion ulna	Fused	Closed	4
10	Fusion radius	Fused	Closed	5

Sequences 1 to 5, the ascending growth phase of puberty (from 11 years to 13 years of age in the girl, from 13 to 15 years of age in the boy), sequences 6 to 10, descending phase of puberty (13 to 15 years and 6 month in the gil, 15 to 17 years and 6 month in the boy).

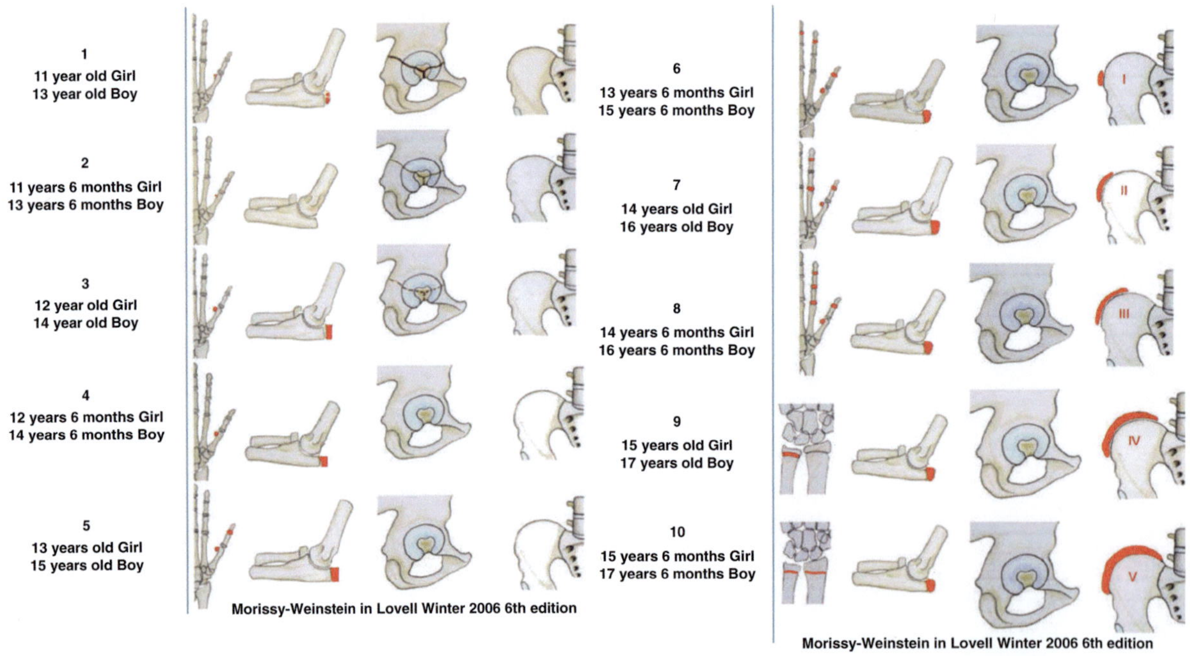

Fig. 54 Wrist, Elbow, Acetabular and Pelvic Ossification staging, from Morissy-Weinstein in Lovell Winter 2006 6th Edition

Table 5 Reference figures worth knowing

Birth	Standing height: 50 cm Sitting height: 35 cm
5 years	Standing height: 1.04 m–1.10 m Sitting height: 62 cm (approximately) Remaining sitting height: 33% for boys: about 30 cm 30% for girls: about 25 cm
11 years old bone age Girls	Early puberty in girls Remaining standing height: 18 cm Remaining sitting size: 12 cm Remaining sitting height: 13%
13 years old bone age Boys	Early puberty in boys Remaining standing height: 20–22 cm Remaining sitting size: 13 cm Remaining sitting height: 13%
Sitting size End of growth	End of growth 52% of the standing height Average: 90 cm/1.70 m standing height in boys 85 cm/1.65 m standing height in girls
Vertebral column	2nd month of intrauterine life: 2/3 of body length 5th month of intrauterine life: 3/5 of body length Birth: 2/5 of body length End of growth: 70 cm in boys (approximately) 65 cm in girls (approximately)
Spinal discs	24% of the spine
T1 S1	50% of the sitting height (exactly 49%) At birth: 19 cm At the end of growth: 45 cm/1.70 m of standing height in boys 42 cm/a sitting height of 85 cm in girls
T1 T2	2/3 of T1-S1 30% of sitting height Birth: 11 cm in length End of growth: length Girls: 26 cm Boys: 28 cm
L1 L5	1/3 of the T1-S1 segment Birth: length 7 cm End of growth: 16 cm 18% of sitting height 3.5% of sitting height per vertebra
Thoracic perimeter	Birth: 32 cm/97% of sitting height End of growth: 95% of sitting height
Anteroposterior diameter of the thorax	75% of the transverse diameter Birth: 11 cm End of growth: 22 cm 21% of the sitting height
Transverse diameter of the thorax	Birth: 12 cm End of growth: 28 cm 30% of sitting height
Balanced chest	Beginning of puberty: Front diameter + anteroposterior diameter = 50% of the sitting height Thoracic Perimeter: 95% of the sitting height
Unbalanced chest	Start of puberty: Front diameter + anteroposterior diameter = 45% of sitting height Thoracic perimeter: 90% of sitting height
Thoracic	Birth: 6% 5 years: 30% 10 years: 50% 17 years: 100%
Risser I	Fusion of distal phalanges "In general" Bone age: 13 years 6 months in girls 15 years 6 months in boys Remaining growth: 4–4.5 cm End of growth of the lower limbs
Risser II	Fusion of metacarpophalangeal growth cartilages Bone age: 14 years in girls; 16 years in boys Remaining growth on the spine: 3 cm
Risser III	Fusion of the interphalangeal cartilages Bone age: 14 years 6 months in girls; 16 years 6 months in boys Growth remaining on the spine: 2 cm
Risser IV	Fusion of the distal elbow Bone age: 15 years in girls 17 years in the boy Growth remaining on the spine: 1 cm
Risser V	Fusion of the radial epiphysis Bone age: 15 years 6 months in the girl; 17 years 6 months in boys Growth remaining on the spine: 0 cm

T1-S1 segment = 50% of the sitting height
T1-T12 thoracic segment = 2/3 of the T1-S1 segment
L1-L5 lumbar segment = 1/3 of the T1-S1 segment

Suggested Readings

Dimeglio A. Growth in pediatric orthopedics. In: Morrissy R, Weinstein S, editors. Lovell and winters pediatric orthopedics, vol. 1. Philadelphia: Lippincott Williams and Wilkins; 2006.

Dimeglio A. Growth of the spine before age 5 years. J Pediatr Orthop B. 1993;1:102–7.

Dimeglio A, Bonnel F. In: Al R, Choux M, Di Rocco C, editors. Principles of pediatric neurosurgery, the pediatric spine, vol. 9. New York: Springer; 1989. p. 39.

Dimeglio A, Bonnel F. Le Rachis en Croissance. Paris: Springer; 1990.

Dimeglio A, Bonnel F, Canavese F. In: Arkbania BA, et al., editors. The normal growing spine in the "growing spine": Springer; 2014. p. 47–81.

Dimeglio A, Canavese F. In: Nnadi C, editor. Development of the spine in early onset: Ed Thieme; 2015. p. 13–22.

Dimeglio A, Canavese F. The growing spine: how do spinal deformities influence normal spine and thoracic spine growth. Eur Spine J. 2012;21:64–70.

Dimeglio A, Canavese F, Charles YP. Growth and adolescent idiopathic scoliosis: when and how much? J Pediatr Orthop. 2011;31(Suppl):S28–6.

Canavese F, Dimeglio A. In: Nnadi C, editor. Frontier of the impossible in early onset scoliosis: Ed Thieme; 2015. p. 1–12.

Canavese A, Dimeglio A, Granier M, et al. Arthrosis of the first six dorsal vertebrae in prepubertal New Zealand white rabbits and dorsal growth to skeletal maturity: the role of the rib-vertebral-sternal complex. Minerva Ortop Traumatol. 2007a;58:369–78.

Canavese F, Dimeglio A, Volpatti D, et al. Dorsal arthrodesis of thoracic spine and effects on thorax growth in prepubertal New Zealand white rabbits. Spine. 2007b;32:E443–5.

Campbell RM Jr, Smith MD, Mayes TC, et al. The effect of open wedge thorascotomy on thoracic insufficiency syndrome associated with fused ribs and congenital scoliosis. J Bone Joint Surg Am. 2004;86A:1659–74.

Karol LA, Johnston C, Mladenov K, Schochet P, Walters P, Browne RH. Pulmonary function following early thoracic fusion in non-neuromuscular scoliosis. J Bone Joint Surg Am. 2008;90: 1272–81.

Dubousset J. The crankshaft phenomenon. J Pediatr Orthop. 1989;9:541–50.

Arkbania BA, Campbell RM, Dimeglio A, et al. Fusionless procedures for the management of early-onset spine deformities in 2011: what do we know? J Child Orthop. 2011;5:159–72.

The Growth Cartilages of the Spine and Pelvic Vertebra

Jean Marc Vital, A. Dimeglio, M. Petit, and L. Boissière

Growth cartilages forge the morphological identity of the spine and pelvis. The pelvic vertebra is considered part of this ensemble.

The radiological images of these growth cartilages reliably document the maturation of the spine. They constitute a true calendar on which the clinician can define their strategies and make their decisions.

Frequent questions:

> From what age can a screw be inserted to the growing pedicle without compromising the dimensions of the spinal canal?

> Does unilateral screw fixation of the neurocentral cartilage induce scoliosis?

> How early can one radiologically detect an abnormal ring apophysis in a Scheuermann's disease before vertebral body wedging?

> Should timing of surgery be based on the closing of the triradiate cartilage to limit the risk of a crankshaft effect?

> What value should be attributed to Risser staging?

> How can one plan the surgical strategy for a Risser 0 despite knowing that Risser 0 represents two thirds of puberty?

> Can we decide on the timing or removal of a spinal brace based only on Risser's staging?

We will describe in this chapter aspects of secondary ossification of the spine and pelvis as described by Jean Dubousset (see Chapter "Sacrum Anatomy: New Concepts"). We will describe the neurocentral cartilage (NCC) and the ring apophysis of the spinal vertebra, the triradiate (or Y) cartilage and the epiphyseal nucleus of the iliac wing (as applied to the Risser staging) for the pelvic vertebra regarding monitoring growth and their involvement in scoliosis or kyphosis of Scheuermann's disease.

Neurocentral Cartilage (NCC)

The NCC (or intermediate cartilage or synchondrosis of Schmorl and Junghanns [1]) (Fig. 1) is located at the junction of the body (or centrum) and the neural arch. Histologically, it is bipolar with an alignment of cell columns facing each other, as it is located at the junction between the two primary ossification nuclei of the vertebral body and the neural arch (Fig. 2). It has a histological structure quite like that of the Y cartilage, which will be described later. Its maximum activity is in the first 5–6 years and its closure date has been approximated to 5–6 years by Knutsson [2], 5 years by Nicoladoni

J. M. Vital (✉) · M. Petit · L. Boissière
Spinal Unit, University Hospital, Bordeaux, France

A. Dimeglio
Department of Pediatric Orthopedic Surgery, Polyclinique Saint Roch, Montpellier, France

J. M. Vital, D. T. Cawley (eds.), *Spinal Anatomy*, https://doi.org/10.1007/978-3-030-20925-4_4

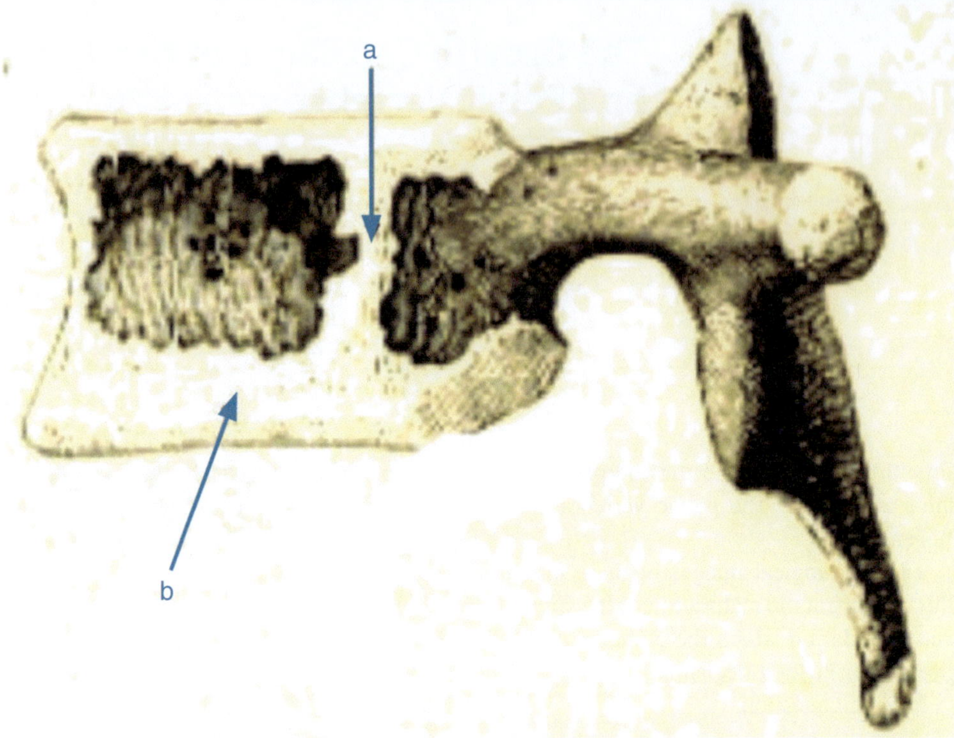

Fig. 1 Schmorl's original drawing of a thoracic vertebra showing (**a**) the NCC and (**b**) the ring apophysis

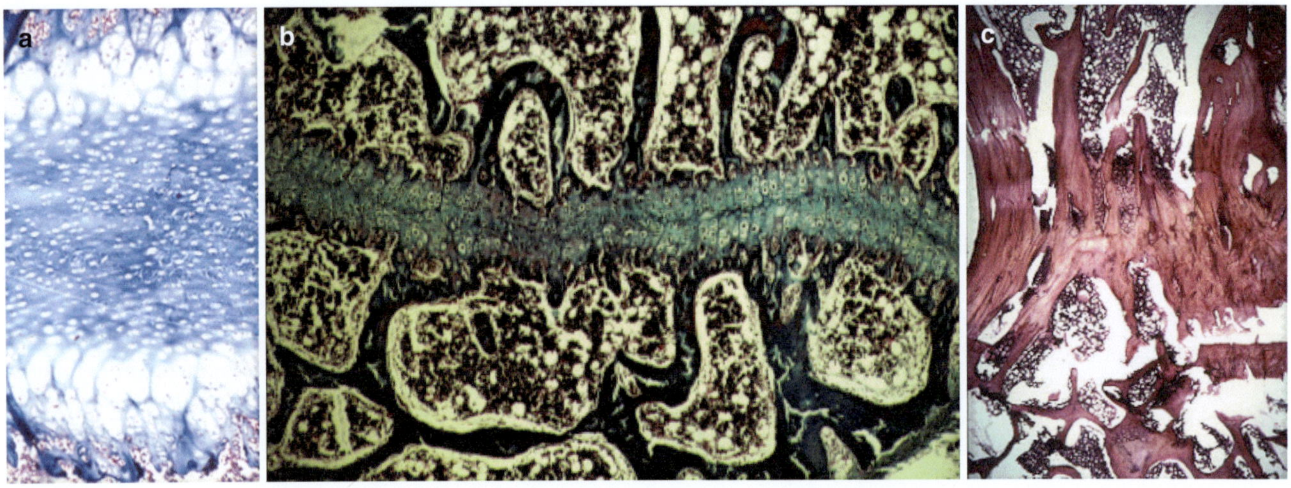

Fig. 2 Histology of the NCC: (**a**) active bipolar cartilage, (**b**) cartilage at a later age, (**c**) closed cartilage

[3], 10 years by Ottander [4], 14 years by Bouillet [5], 15 years by Mineiro [6] and 16 years by Canadell [7]. The authors concur that the cervical and lumbar NCCs close before the thoracic NCCs (Figs. 3 and 4).

We studied the anatomy of 20 children from under 1 year to 16 years and CT scans of 30 children from 3 to 18 years (10 healthy children with axial images at T8 and 20 pathological cases including 15 congenital scoliosis, 2 lordoscoliosis and 3 severe kyphoses) [8].

Table 1 shows the series of anatomical specimens studied by Beguiristain (Fig. 5). On these vertebrae of different ages, there was a natural progressive narrowing of the NCC towards closure, a relative decrease in the antero-posterior direction (study of the ratio (AC/AB)) due to the continued growth of the vertebral body while the posterior arc no longer increases (Figs. 6 and 7) and a relative horizontalization of the NCC in the axial plane (Fig. 8). For the CT scan, general anaesthesia had to be performed in those under 3 years of age and positioned in the lateral decubitus with a small bolster in the cases of scoliosis to horizontally align the inclined vertebrae and avoid a false image plane (pre-digital imaging) (Figs. 9 and 10). The constants selected for the CT were 800–1600 Hounsfield units. The sections studied were sagittal and coronal (Fig. 11). This examination, more precise in the study of the NCC than MRI, made it possible to recognize its shape, and thus its complete closure, occurring very late (Fig. 12). We have also shown the asymmetrical closure of concave and convex NCCs in scoliosis, as discussed later. MRI was used by Yamazaki et al. [9] to study the age of NCC closure in the thoracic spine: between 11 and 16 years for girls and 12 and 16 years for boys.

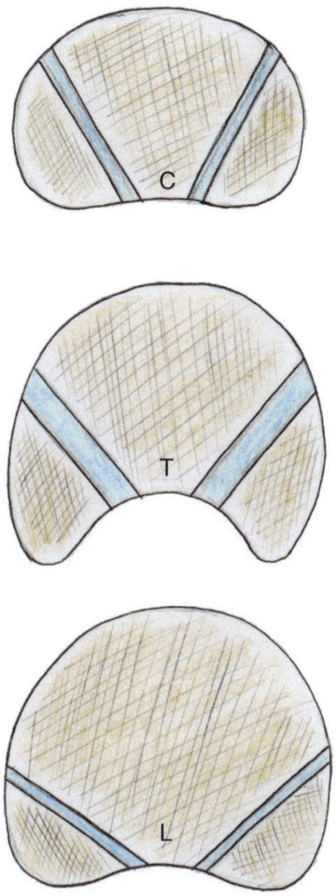

Fig. 3 Chronology of closure of the NCC initially in cervical and lumbar, then in the thoracic spine

> The NCC has a dynamism of growth: it changes spatial orientation as it self horizontalises over time.

> The NCC has another polarity: it ossifies the vertebral body and the posterior arch

Table 1 Anatomical specimens

Number	Age	Gender
1	Foetus	M
3	New born	1M 2F
1	3 months	M
1	11 months	M
2	2 years	1M 1F
2	3 years	2M
1	4 years	F
2	5 years	2F
1	6 years	M
1	7 years	M
1	9 years	F
1	11 years	M
1	12 years	M
1	14 years	F
1	16 years	M
20		12M 8F

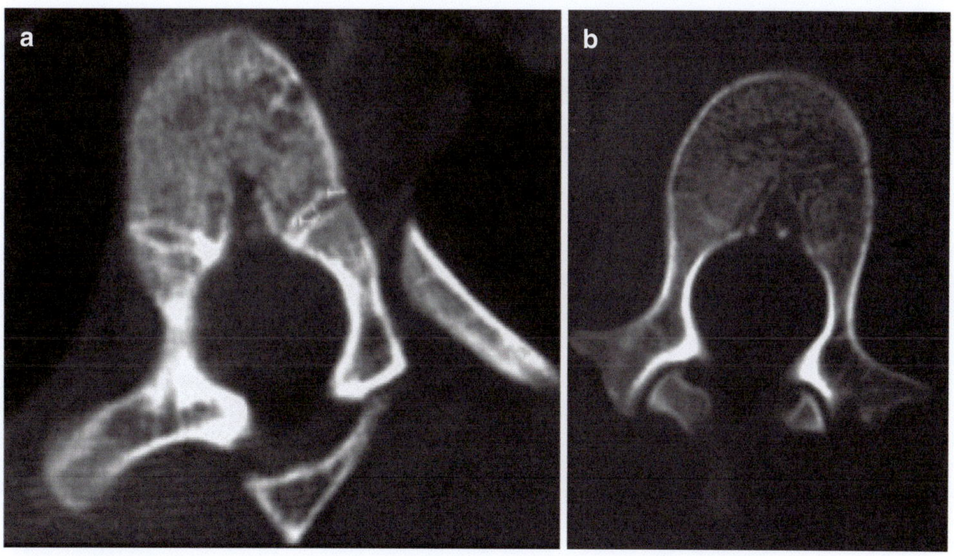

Fig. 4 Chronology of closure of the NCC in the same child with a double curvature: (**a**) right thoracic, (**b**) left lumbar. The closure is earlier in lumbar than in the thoracic

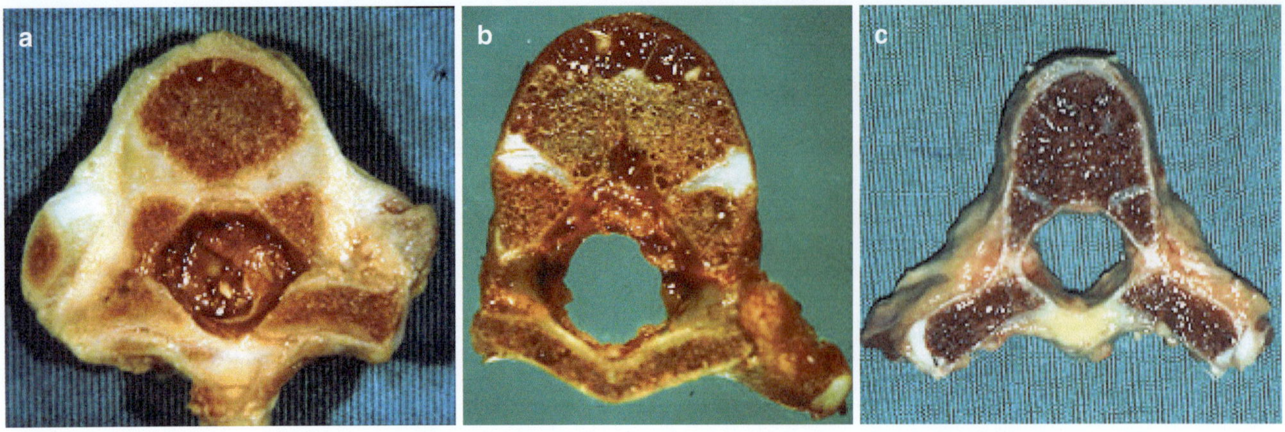

Fig. 5 Anatomy of the NCC on 3 thoracic vertebrae of different ages, **a** = newborn, **b** = 6 years, **c** = 12 years

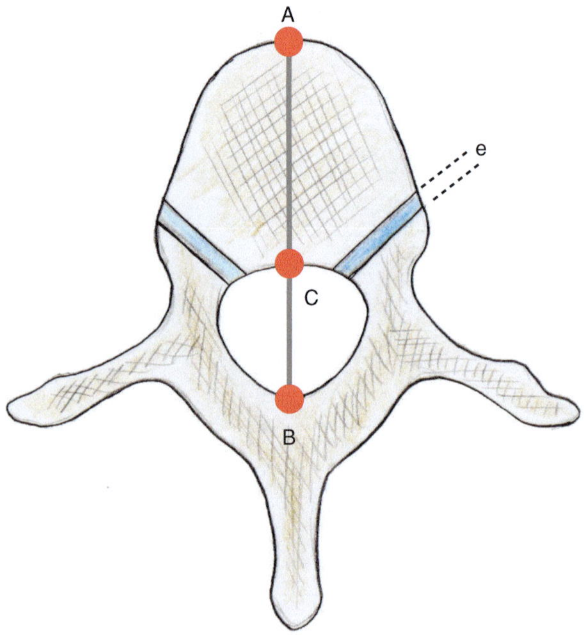

Fig. 6 NCC anatomy: e = thickness, AC/AB = anteroposterior position of the NCC

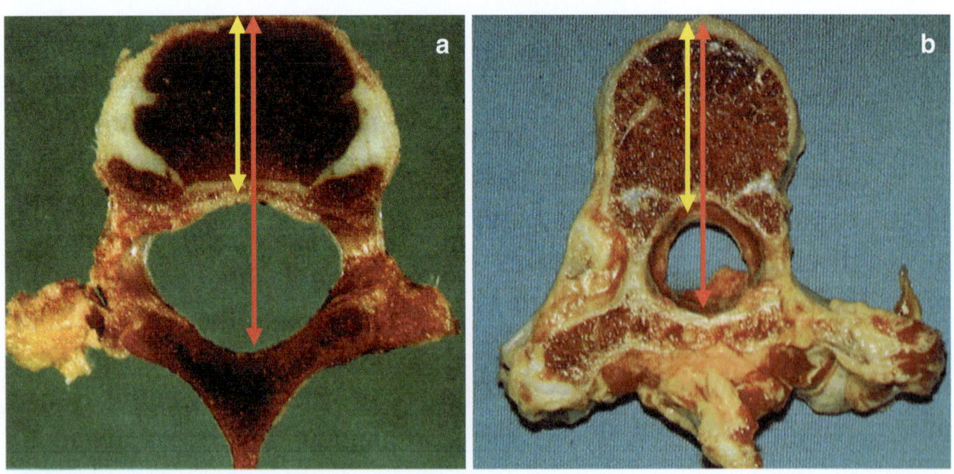

Fig. 7 NCC anatomy evolution of the AC/AB ratio: **a** = vertebra of 10 years, **b** = vertebra of 16 years

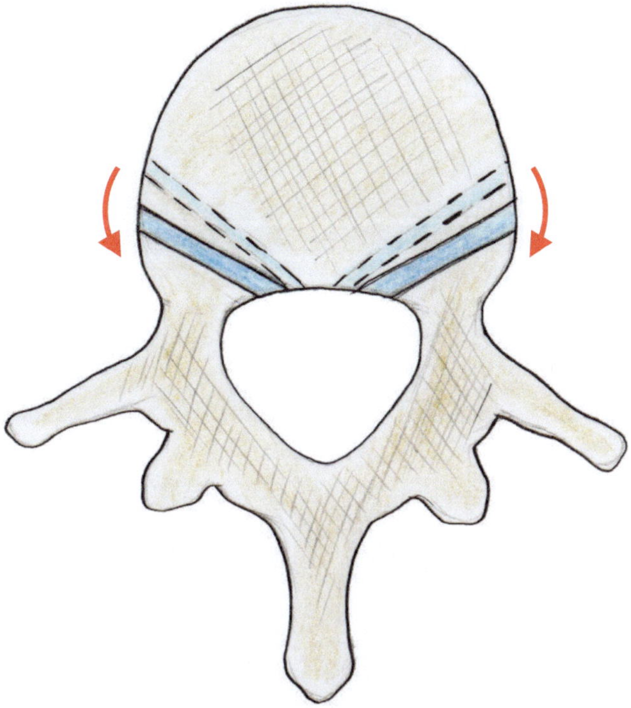

Fig. 8 Anatomy of the NCC: Horizontalisation over time

The NCC has a double action (Figs. 13, 14): control of the anteroposterior dimension of the central spinal canal, which is therefore fixed early, as shown by Knutsson [2] (Fig. 15), and height of the posterior 1/3 of the vertebral body.

Nicoladoni [3] has shown, on histological sections of scoliotic vertebrae, the earlier closure of the convex NCC (Fig. 16). Beguiristain et al. [10] showed on the growing pig that unilateral screw fixation of the NCC caused a scoliosis with rotation of the convex side corresponding to the side of the NCC interupted by the screw fixation (Fig. 17). The same result was obtained more recently by Zhang and Sucato [11]. In our study, the scanners performed early in the case of early scolioses allowed us to recognize this early closure of the NCC on the convex side (Fig. 18); The concave part of the neural arc is longer, since the NCC acts longer on this side, which goes in the direction of the rotation of the body towards the convexity (Fig. 19). We can compare this dysfunction of the NCCs in the axial plane of the hyperlordotic spine observed in the most severe scoliosis because of the action of the NCC in the growth of the posterior part of the vertebral body (Fig. 20). This corresponds to Dickson's scheme [12], which has shown that the thoracic scoliotic segment where there is rotation is in hypokyphosis or even in lordosis (Fig. 21).

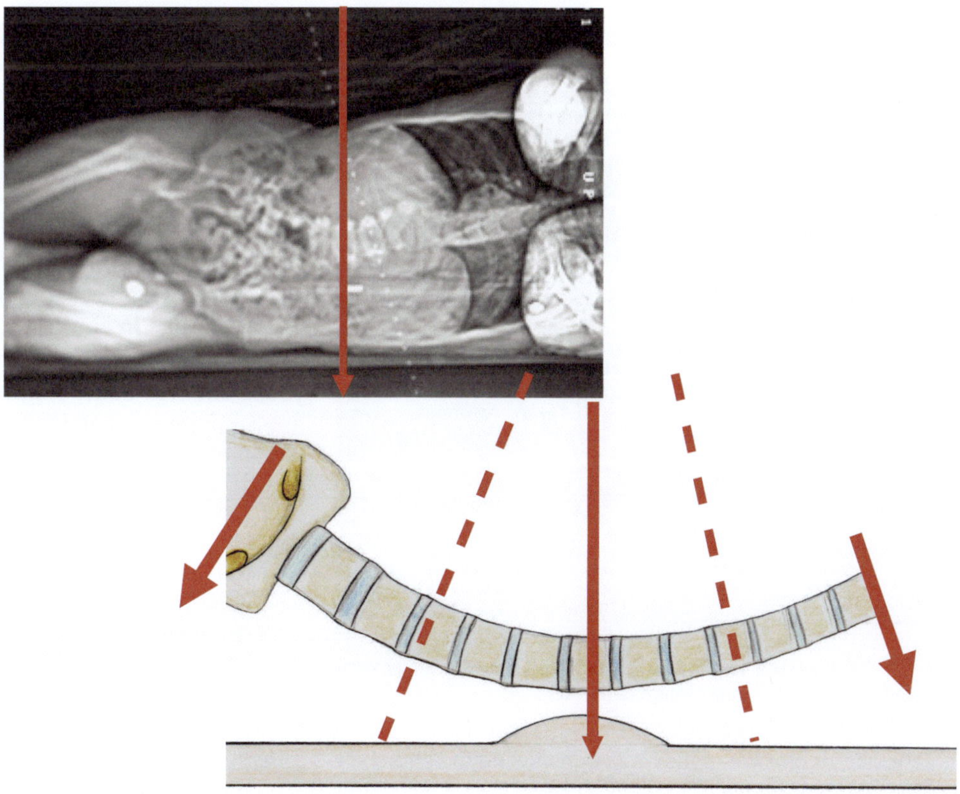

Fig. 9 Positioning in lateral decubitus to minimize scoliosis, with an image taken at the level of the apical vertebra

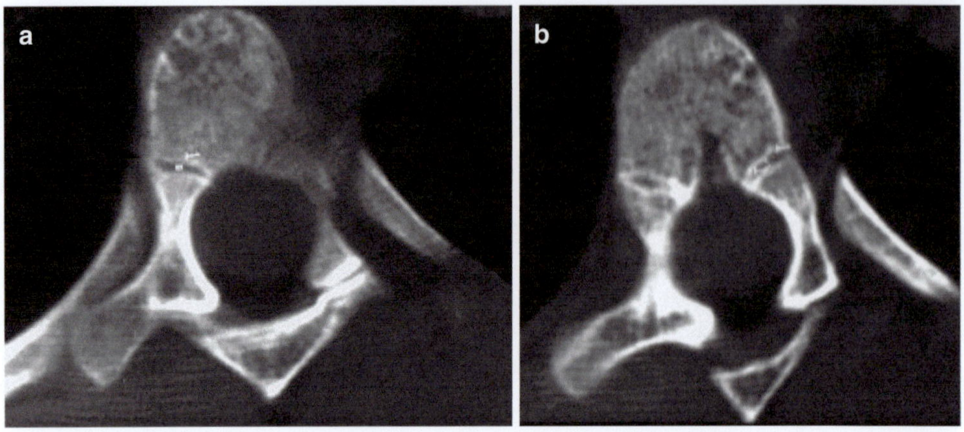

Fig. 10 Comparison of two images: (**a**) non-horizontal and uninterpretable, (**b**) correct

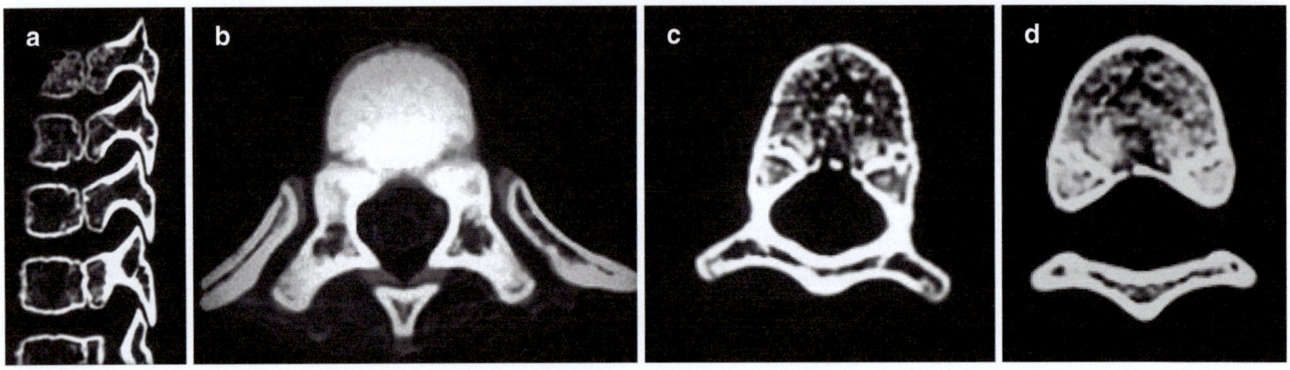

Fig. 11 CT Scan of a thoracic vertebra in a 6-year-old child; sagittal cut (**a**) and axial at different levels (**b**, **c**, **d**)

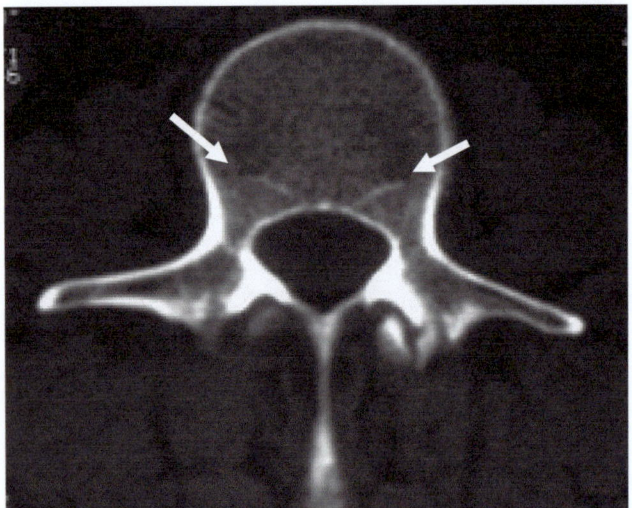

Fig. 12 CT Scan of a vertebra in a young adult showing the physeal scar and therefore the recent closure of the NCC

The age of closure of the NCC depends on the choice of investigation used; we have mainly used CT data, probably the most sensitive examination that recognizes very faint remnants of the NCC. Zhang et al. [13] with MRI estimate that in 95% of cases the cartilage is closed at 5 years. This end of very early activity explains that unilateral pedicle screw insertion in children does not cause the same scoliosis as observed in immature animals. This is in theory an attractive method of scoliosis correction that has not yielded results in clinical practice. Olgun et al. [14] could control the size of the pedicles and the spinal canal in 15 young children under 5 who had undergone pedicle screw insertion: they noted no abnormality following this perforation of NCCs, thus assuming that it was still a little active in this series.

This bipolar cartilage has maximum activity before 5 years; it seems to close late, but only on the CT scan, sometimes after the end of growth. It controls the growth of the spinal canal thus its dimensions are fixed early in life. It provides 1/3 of the ossification of the vertebral body.

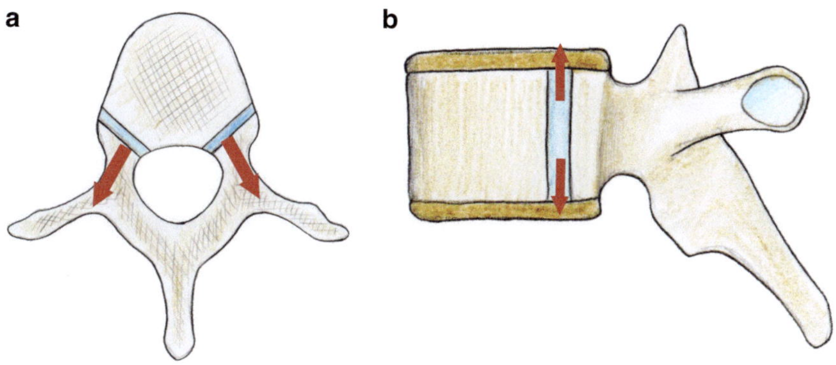

Fig. 13 Action of the NCC: control of the size of the central spinal canal (**a**) and control of the height growth of the posterior part of the vertebral body (**b**)

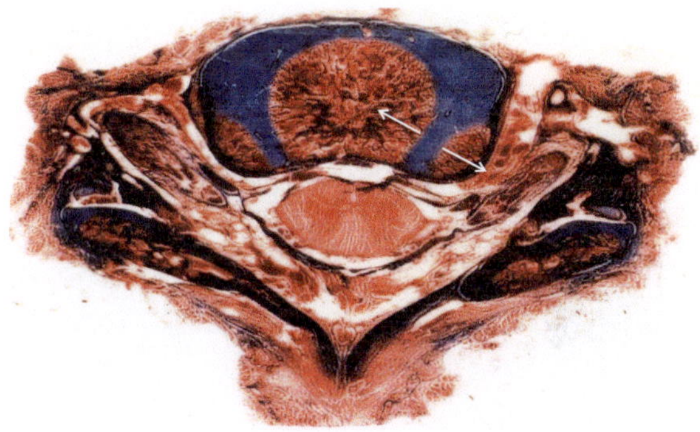

Fig. 14 Neurocentral cartilage has a bidirectional activity. It contributes posteriorly to the ossification of the posterior arch and anteriorly to a third of the ossification of the vertebral body

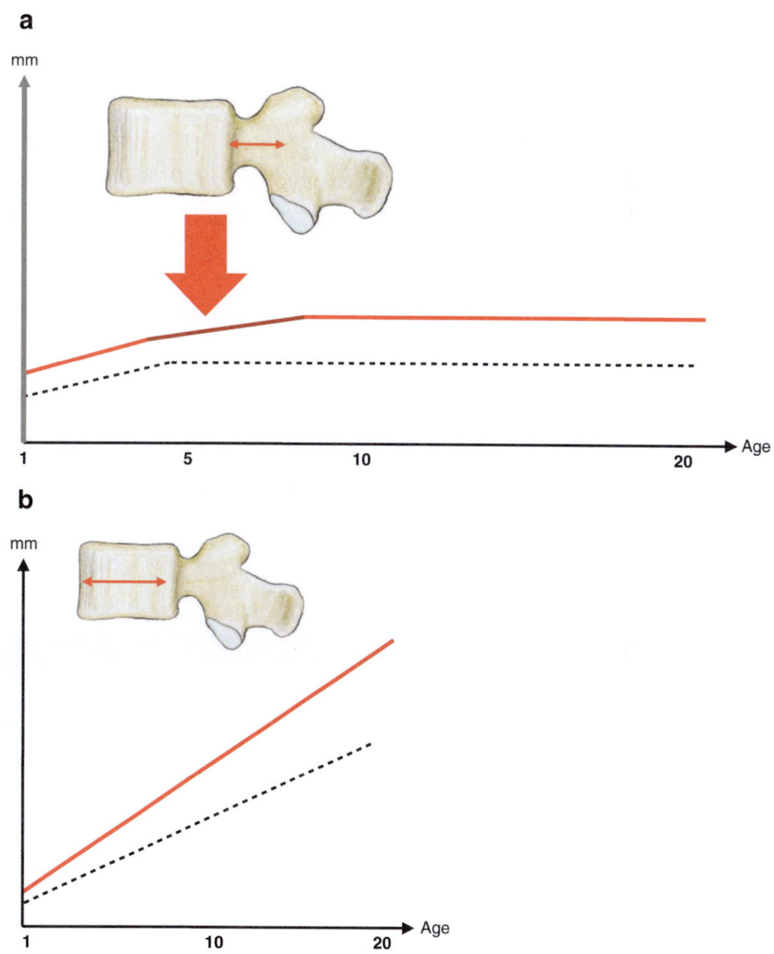

Fig. 15 Evolution of the dimensions of the spinal canal (**a**) and the anteroposterior diameter of the vertebral body (**b**), according to Knutsson [2]

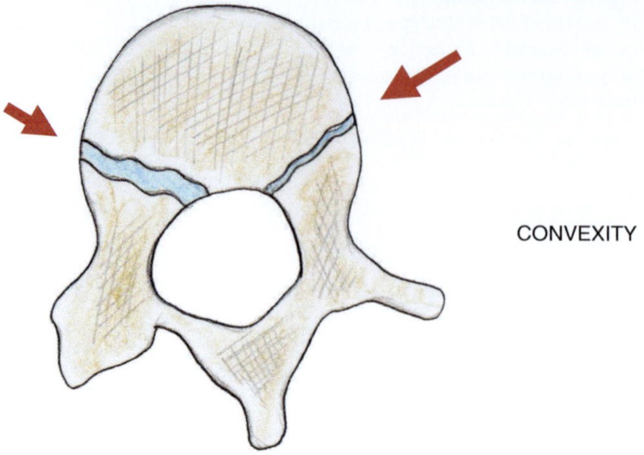

Fig. 16 Scoliotic vertebra as described by Nicoladoni [3] noting the asymmetry of concave and convex NCCs

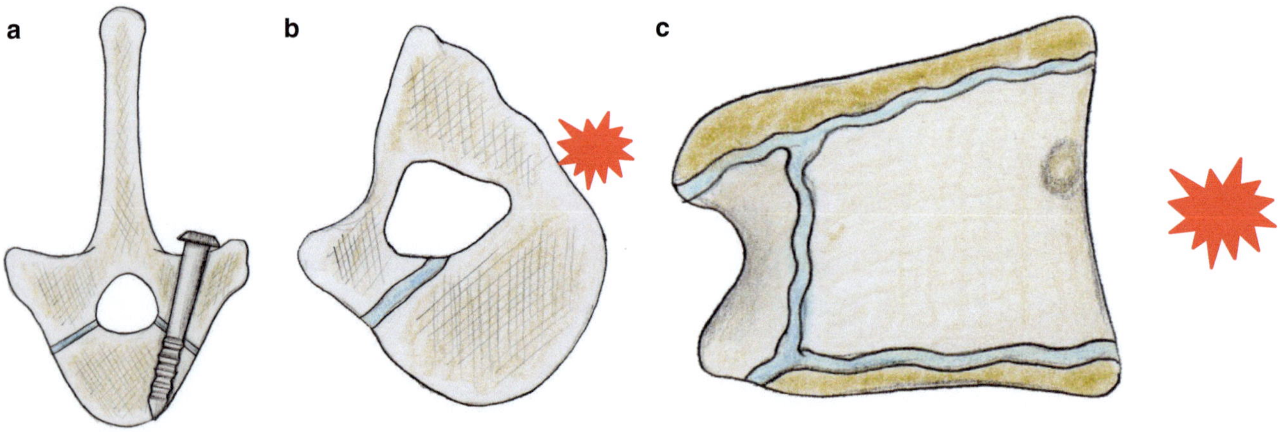

Fig. 17 (a) Pedicle screw epiphysiodesis (fixation of the NCC) with (b) consequential growth inhibition and deformity towards the affected side and (c) inhibition of the posterior vertebral height creating a segmental lordosis

Studies of the vertebrae of scoliotic youths and the experiments of unilateral screw fixation of the NCC conclude an early closure of the convex side compared to the concave to perhaps explain the scoliotic rotation on convex side. The question is whether this phenomenon is the cause or consequence of early structural scoliosis.

Recent clinical studies suggest that after 5 years of age, pedicle screw insertion does not create a risk of premature NCC closure (especially after what Zhang et al. [13] calls the early juvenile period (4–7 years)) and especially since the vertebra outside this cartilage remains very cartilaginous and therefore malleable.

Growth cartilage works in three dimensions.

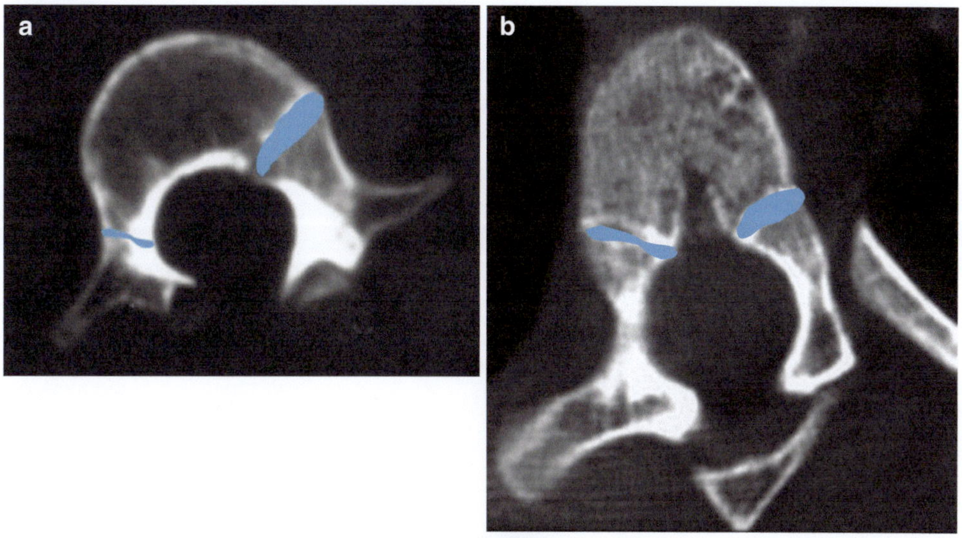

Fig. 18 Lumbar (**a**) and thoracic (**b**) scoliotic vertebrae

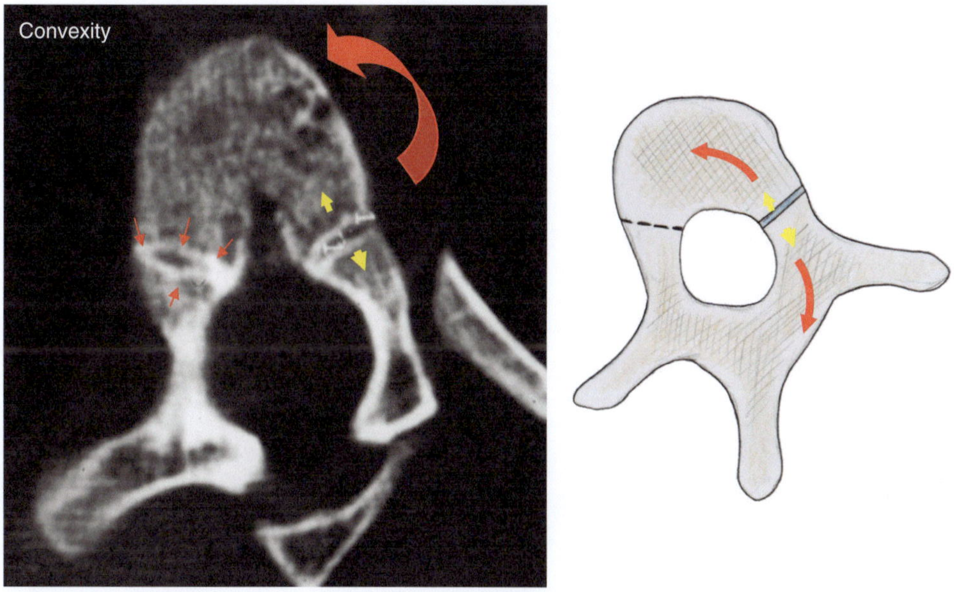

Fig. 19 Asymmetric closure of NCC in thoracic idiopathic scoliosis with convexity to the patient's right side (left side of CT scan); The convex right NCC closes earlier than the left NCC; The pedicle on the convex side is therefore shorter in the anteroposterior direction which goes in the direction of the rotation of the body towards the convexity, and wider than on the concave side

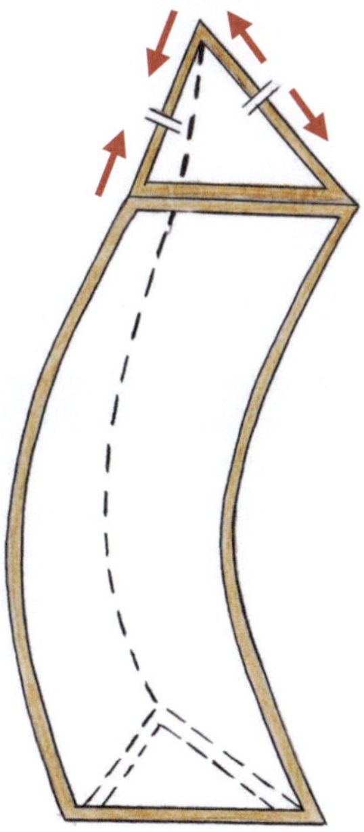

Fig. 20 Posterior view of a schematic scoliotic column; The growth progression of the NCC (according S Eguiraun) explains the rotation towards the convexity and hyperlordotic shape

The Ring Apophysis

It appears at 2 years, ossifies back and forth in a "comet tail" fashion and merges with the nucleus of the body towards 17–18 years.

The ring (or annular) apophysis is a secondary ossification nucleus (not a cartilage) with a delayed action, frequently implicated in conditions of abnormal growth.

It is located between the vertebral body and the discs [15]. It partially ensures the growth of the body in height. It is very adherent to the peripheral annulus (Sharpey's fibres), to the peripheral ligaments, the anterior and posterior longitudinal ligaments, and to the nucleus of the vertebral body, whose surface is irregular ("scallop shell"). This explains the possibility of apophyseal detachment in the context of traumatic shear which, instead of causing a disc herniation as in adults,

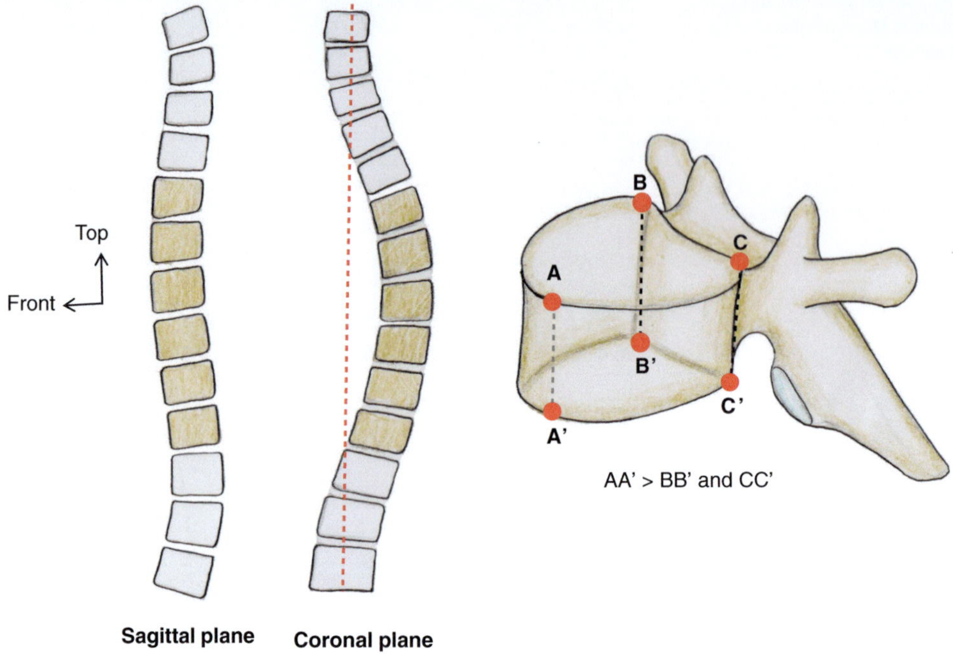

Fig. 21 Deformation in the sagittal plane of the thoracic vertebra according to Dickson et al. [12]; The vertebra at the apex is higher anteriorly than posteriorly and thus participates in the flattening of the thoracic sagittal curvature in kyphosis

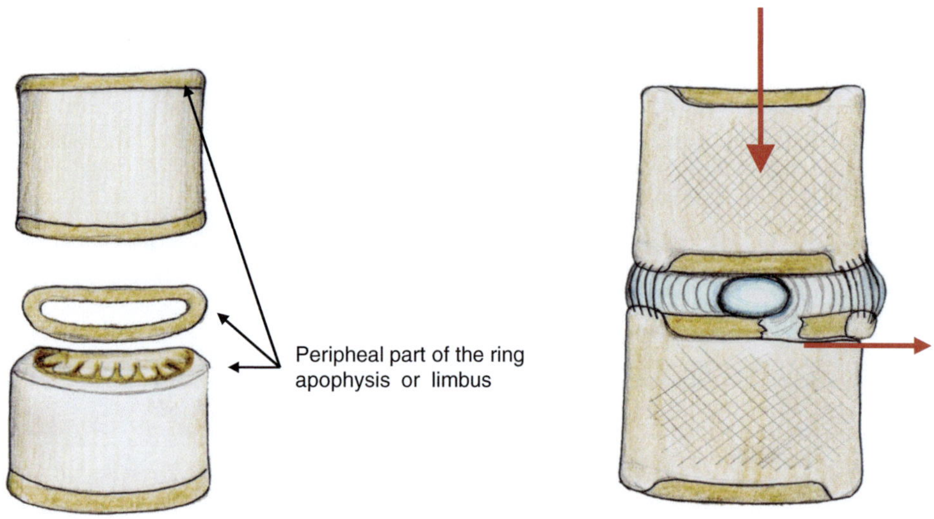

Fig. 22 Anatomy of the ring apophysis: more adherent to the annulus than to the body (**a**); A compression stress causes (**b**) part of the ring apophysis to be pulled away, not a disc herniation

part of the ring is detached causing acute low back pain and sometimes neurological disturbances (Figs. 22 and 23).

Mallet, as early as 1975 [16], has described the different stages of ossification of the vertebral body in his article on spinal dystrophy of growth, classically called Scheuermann's disease with inspiration from Schmorl's work [1] (Fig. 24): at birth, the primary ossific nucleus of the body has a coffee grain shape equal in size to the intervertebral space. The vertebra at the age of 4 years is rectangular with bevelled anterior corners. The intervertebral space decreases in height. At 7 years, the anterior corners of the vertebra each resemble 2 steps of the stairs. Secondary ossification from the ring apophysis begins according to Mallet et al. [16] at 6–8 years in the girl and 7–9 years in the boy; It is under the dependence, according to this author, of the discal apparatus which comprises the nucleus pulposus, annulus fibrosis and cartilaginous plate.

Discs and endplates are of similar embryological origins and are vascularized by the same polar arteries. The clear space corresponding to the ring apophysis will ossify from front to back to constitute a bony line which ends in dotted lines ("comet's tail"), which is continuous at 12 years in the average girl and 15 years in the boy. The final ossification of the vertebral body is the attachment of the vertebral body to the ring. This fusion starts at 14 years and ends very late, at 25 years. The edges of the endplate at the boundary of the

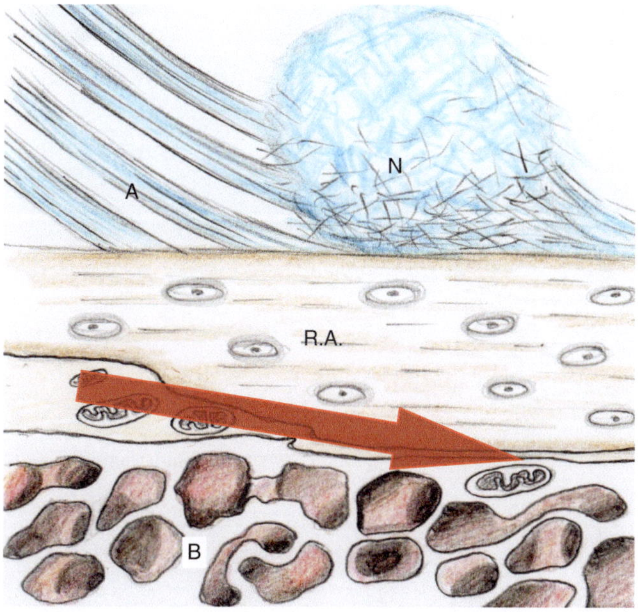

Fig. 23 Microscopic diagram of delamination of the apophysis (according to the red arrow). A: annulus, N: nucleus, L: ring apophysis, O: bone (as per Roberts et al. [15])

primary ossification nucleus of the body resemble a scallop shell, according to Schmorl. When the fusion is complete, the cartilaginous circular border between the body and the ring apophysis disappears. All these evolutionary stages are described both radiologically and histologically by Bick and Copel [17]. Radiological monitoring of ossification of the ring apophysis is more difficult to recognize on X-rays, especially in the thoracic spine, than on Risser's staging.

Mallet et al. [16] describes an early radiological sign of Scheuermann's disease, a bulbous appearance of the anterior corners of the vertebral bodies where the initial ossification of the central aspect of the ring apophysis occurs outside of the horizontal endplate (Dimeglio's "flotation line") (Fig. 25). The anterior ring apophysis should never insert into the anterior marginal area of the vertebral body. An apophysis that has an "overgrown finger nail" appearance invariably portrays, as suggested by Mallet et al. [16], pathology of the ring apophysis or cartilaginous plaque.

Diard et al. [18] in their description of the disco-epiphyseal complex specify that the most peripheral fibres of the annulus of Sharpey anchor at the peripheral cartilaginous margin which later becomes ossified. When the peripheral ossifica-

Fig. 24 The different stages of ossification of the vertebral body as per Mallet et al. [16]; The top ages are from Schmorl and Junghanns [1]

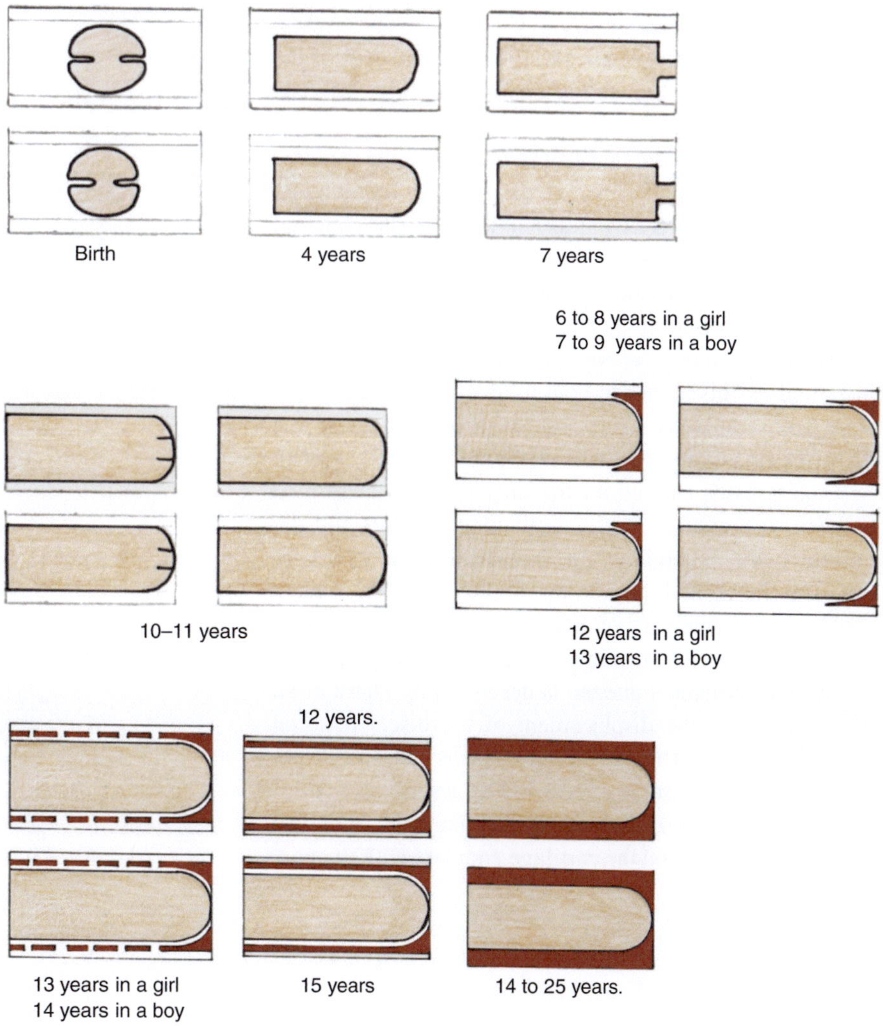

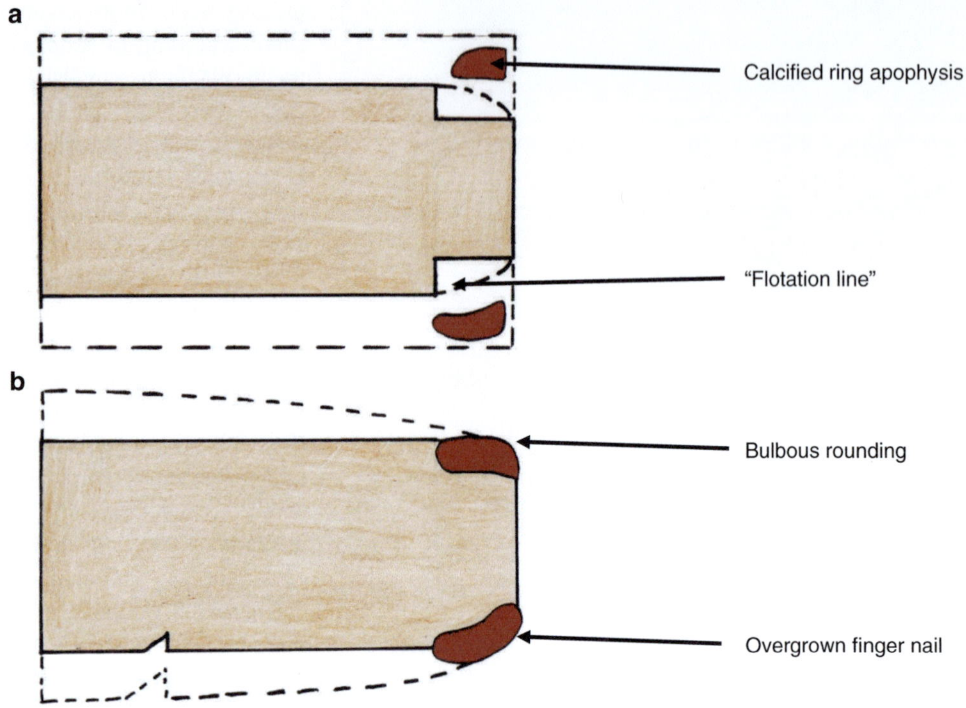

Fig. 25 Early radiological sign of spinal dystrophy of growth (Mallet et al. [16]) (**a**) normal vertebra, (**b**) dystrophic vertebra

tion is complete, Sharpey's fibres insert into the vertebral body and the cartilage occupies only the central part of the vertebral body (cartilage of the endplates) (Fig. 26). The adherence of the important anterior longitudinal ligament is more evident to the vertebral body and less so to the annulus, while on the contrary adherence of the posterior longitudinal ligament is greater to the annulus and lesser to the vertebral body.

Alexander [19] describes the biomechanics of the stresses applied to this disco-epiphyseal complex which explains many of the lesions observed in Scheuermann's disease, understood by this author to be a traumatic secondary dystrophy from repeated micro-trauma (overloading of the body in the case of obesity or excessive mechanical stresses). The axial stresses exerted on the nucleus are transformed into positive pressures on the cartilaginous plates and the vertebral body. In addition to this vertical compression, there is a horizontal tensioning of the annulus, which, through the intermediary of Sharpey's fibres, causes fragmentation of the ring apophysis (Fig. 27). The pathoanatomy of Scheuermann's disease is described by Diard et al. [18] (Fig. 28): if the displacement of the discal material (nucleus or annulus) in the spinal canal is not specific to Scheuermann's disease, it is possible to describe the intra-cancellous herniation (Schmorl's cartilaginous nodules) through the annulus and the cartilage endplate with the possibility of:

- Central displacement (superior or inferior), classical Schmorl intra-cancellous herniation, potentially more

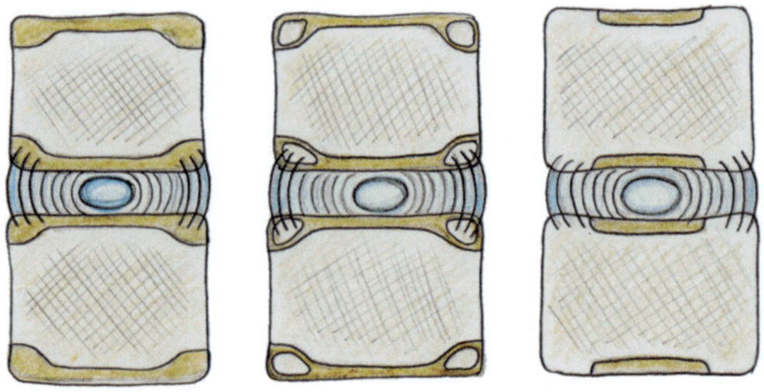

Fig. 26 Growth evolution of the ring apophysis and the ratios of the fibers of the annulus, notably the most peripheral fibers of Sharpey (Diard et al. [18])

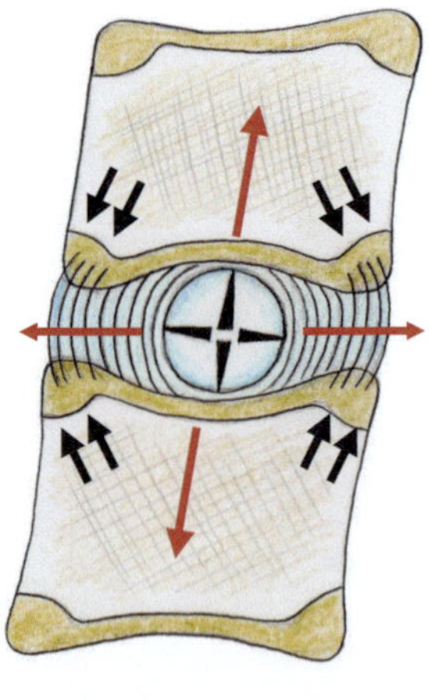

Fig. 27 Compression constraints explaining the endplate discal herniation and traction acting on the ring apophysis (Diard et al. [18])

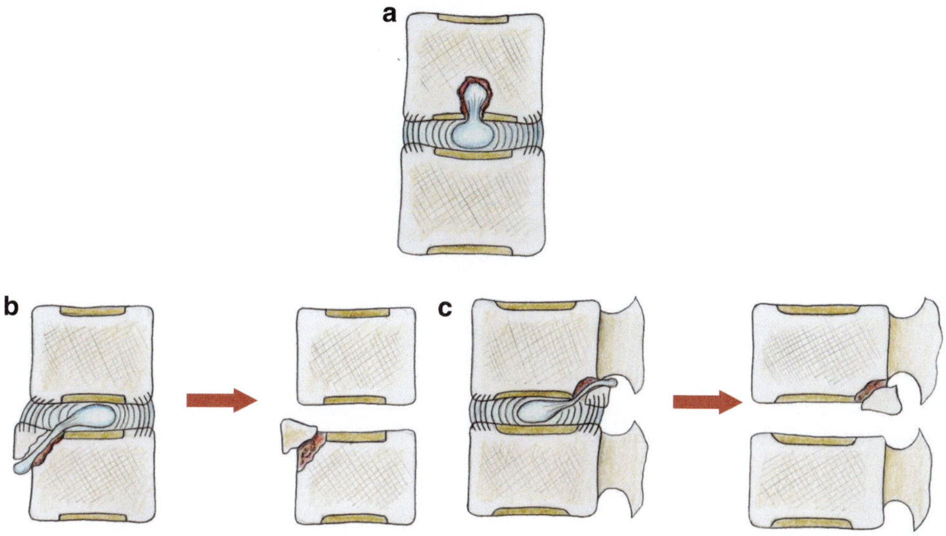

Fig. 28 (**a**) Endplate discal herniation, (**b**) posterior marginal endplate discal herniation, (**c**) pre-marginal intra-cancellous endplate herniation which evolves into a posterior limbic vertebra (Diard et al. [18])

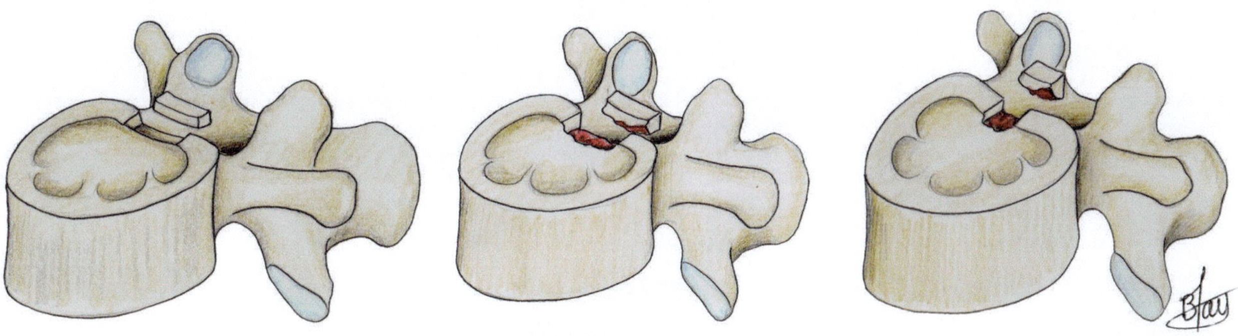

Fig. 29 Classification according the three types of limbus detachment (Takata et al. [20])

likely in an area of physiological weakness: the remnant of the notochord canal, an ossification defect or a vascular channel. An initial severe inflammatory reaction may give a similar impression to an infectious process; a sclerosing osteoblastic reaction will follow.

- Anterior displacement (retro-marginal anterior hernia). The limbus (or peripheral part of the ring apophysis) is torn by the tension of the Sharpey's fibres. The anterior fragment of the limbus, triangular, is ossified and can merge or remain separated from the vertebral body and gives the appearance of a limbic vertebra. After several years, one can observe the fusion of the two adjacent vertebral bodies.
- Posterior displacement hernia (posterior pre-marginal hernia) with the classic detachment of the posterior limbus as described in athletes who have not completed growth and have undergone a lumbar trauma. Takata et al. [20] describes three types of epiphyseal fracture-detachment of the posterior limbus (Figs. 29 and 30):

  – type 1, pure detachment of the cartilaginous ring without bone loss (equivalent to a Salter-Harris 1 stage);
  – type 2, total cartilaginous and bony detachment (equivalent to a Salter-Harris stage 2 or 3);
  – type 3, localized and medial cartilaginous and bone detachment.

All such posterior lesions can lead to the posterior limbic vertebra with a triangular or rounded bone fragment, which may be fused or not to the posterior angle of the vertebral body and which can lead to secondary canal narrowing.

From a histological point of view, Ippolito et al. [21] note from 7 specimens carried out in Scheuermann's disease operations that at the point that the endplate cartilage disappears, the annulus usually inserts directly into the

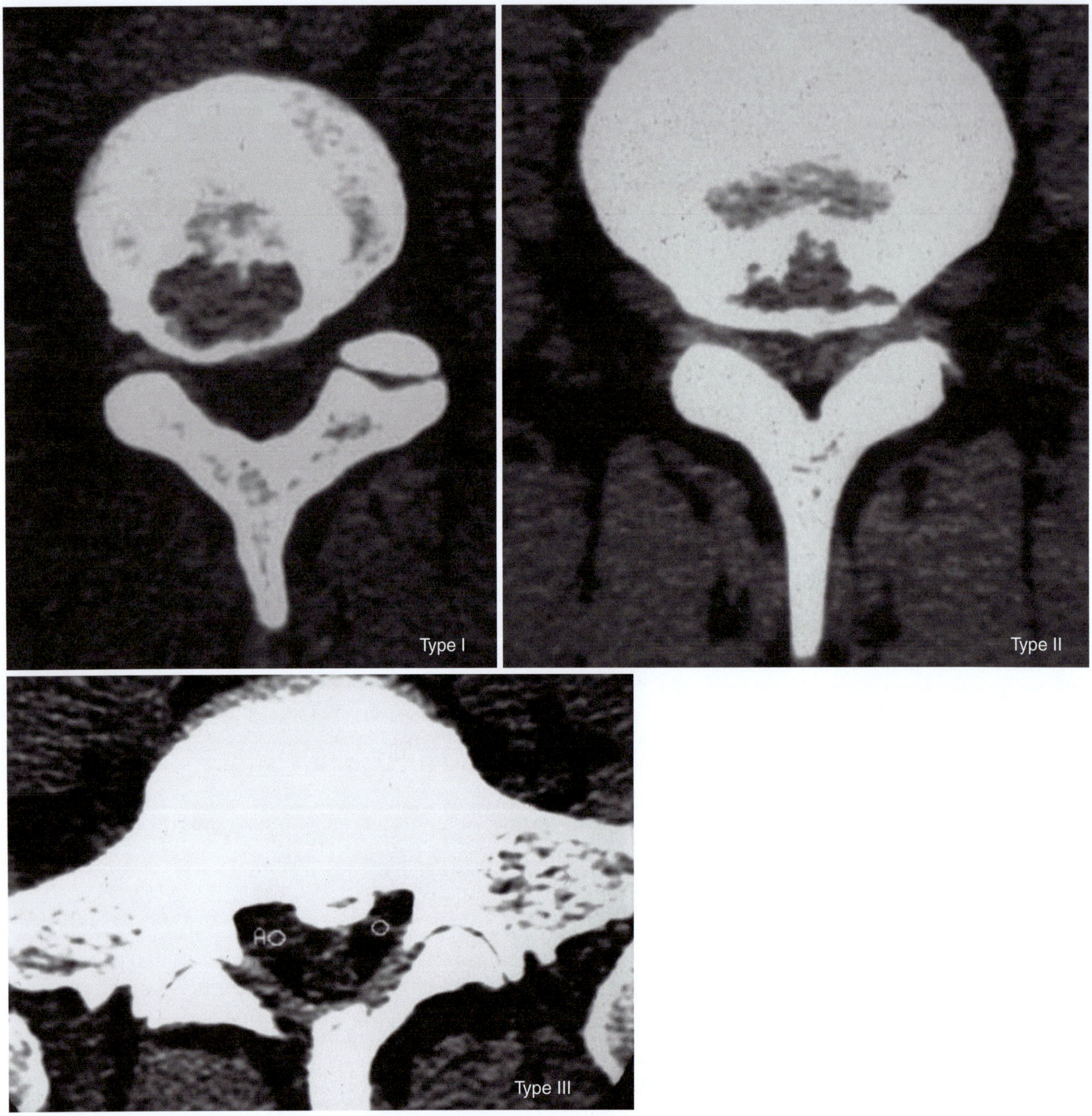

Fig. 30 Radiographs of the three types of limbus detachment Takata et al. [20]

subchondral bone. Studies by electron microscopy show an abnormal cartilage with a matrix rich in proteoglycans and very fine collagen fibrils. Mineralization and ossification of the vertebral plates are irregular.

Ossification of the Pelvic Vertebra

A single radiograph of the pelvis is sufficient to differentiate between the major stages of puberty.

Two cartilages can be studied to monitor the growth of the scoliotic child: the Y cartilage (triradiate), at the junction of the ossification nuclei of the ilium, the ischium and the pubis and the iliac apophysis or what is also termed the ossification nucleus of the iliac wing, evaluated by the Risser test as described in 1958 [22].

We have studied these two pelvic growth cartilages in the same way as the ossification nuclei of the proximal end of the femur in 70 girls and 70 boys of bone age ranging from 9 to 18 years [23]. In this series, the Y cartilage begins to close from inside out at the onset of the growth spurt to close completely as the growth spurt begins; we can describe three suc-

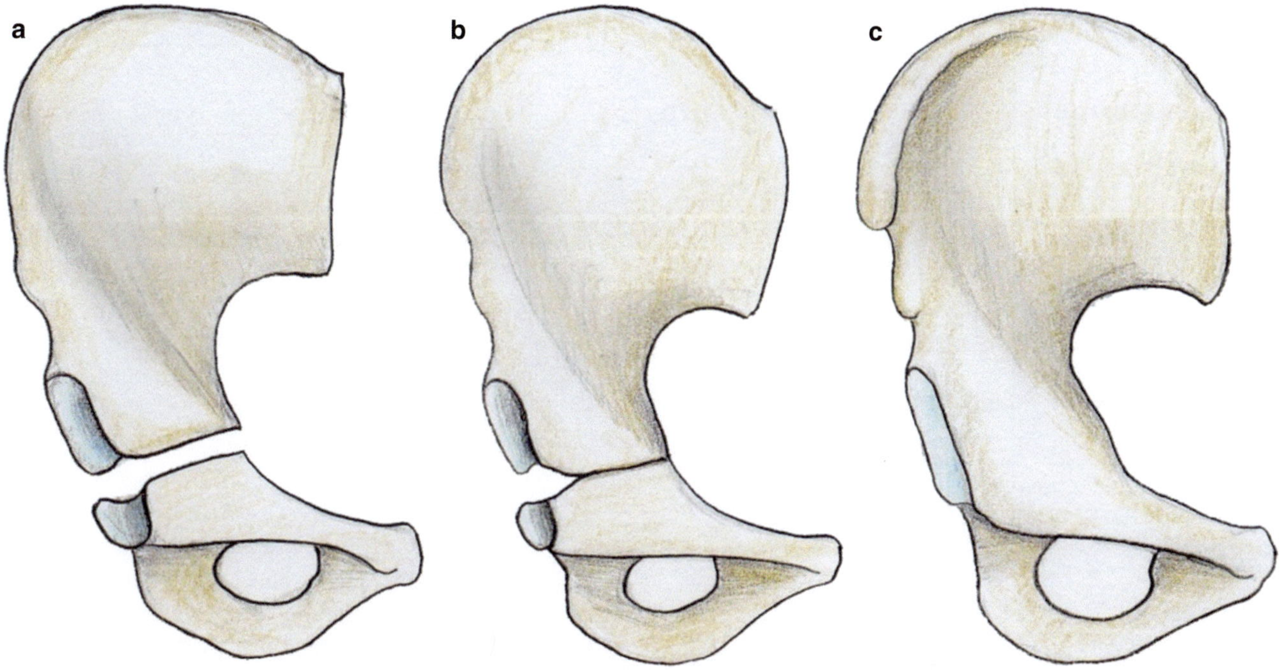

Fig. 31 Evolution of the horizontal portion of the Y cartilage according to three stages: (**a**) open cartilage, (**b**) internal closure, (**c**) complete closure

cessive stages: open cartilage, internal closure at 10 years in the girl and complete closure at 12.5 years in the boy (Fig. 31). Dimeglio et al. [24, 25] states that the Y cartilage is closed 1 year after the onset of puberty. Ryan et al. [26] has described the severity of scoliosis starting with an open Y cartilage. The risk of evolution of scoliotic deformity in the case of an early posterior arthrodesis with open Y cartilage is well known (crankshaft effect of Dubousset). In reality, this crankshaft effect, even if it is less marked, can be expressed after the closing of the Y cartilage. The epiphyseal nucleus of the iliac wing passes from stage 0 to stage 1 long after the closing of the Y cartilage. It was noted in our series that the ossification of the nucleus of the ischium was parallel to that of the epiphyseal nucleus of the iliac wing with better visibility on the anteroposterior radiograph (Fig. 32). Table 2 shows the evolution of the cartilages of the pelvis and the upper extremity of the femur.

In the literature, the principal description by the US-based Risser indicates five stages (Fig. 33):

- Stage 0 where the nucleus does not appear—not ossified,
- Stage 1 where ossification appears laterally, near the anterior superior iliac spine,
- Stage 2 with extension of the ossification towards the median line,
- Stage 3 with the ossification which reaches the top of the iliac crest,
- Stage 4 with the ossification that reaches the sacro-iliac joint,

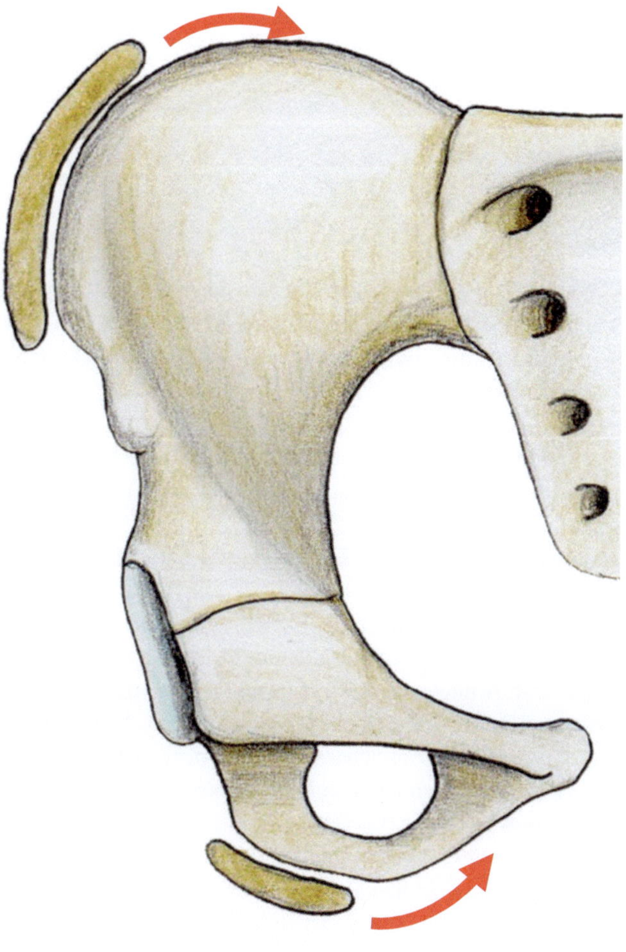

Fig. 32 Parallel evolution of the ossification of the epiphyseal nuclei of the iliac wing and of the ischium

Table 2 Evolution of the ossification nuclei of the pelvic vertebra and the proximal femur

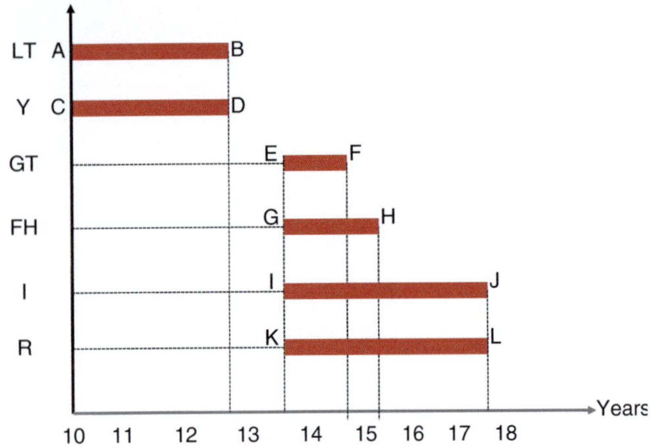

PT: Lesser Trochanter	A visible with cartilage B visible without cartilage (closed)
Y: Y cartilage (horizontal portion)	C internal closure D full closure
GT: Greater Trochanter	E physeal border present F full closure
T: Femoral head	G physeal border present H full closure
I: Ischium	I ossification of outer aspect J closure
R: Risser Test	K Risser 1 L Risser 5

- Finally, stage 5 with complete fusion of the epiphyseal nucleus with the iliac wing and disappearance of the edging from within outwards—without direction of ossification.

Bitan et al. [27] described a French interpretation of the evolution of the Risser test (Fig. 33). The difference is at stages 3 and 4, as the French stage 3 corresponds to the American stage 4 and the French stage 4 corresponds to the beginning of the internal fusion of the epiphyseal nucleus to the iliac wing. Nault et al. [28] differentiates these two descriptions (American and French) of the evaluation of the Risser test. A new group, Risser 0 with closed triradiate cartilage and Risser 1, was the best predictor of the beginning of the curve acceleration phase. From a prognostic point of view, all authors agree that only the Risser 5 test signifies the end of growth.

Kotwicki [29] suggests that lateral radiographs of the pelvis allow a better analysis of the posterior and medial part of the iliac epiphysic nucleus to distinguish the stages of Risser 3 and 4 in the 2 classifications (Fig. 34).

Dimeglio et al. [24, 25] has correlated the Risser test with the evolution of the hand and elbow bones (Figs. 35, 36, and 37).

Dimeglio describes 4 growth zones by evaluating the Y cartilage, the Risser test, and the cartilage of the greater trochanter (Fig. 38):

- Zone 1: Risser 0, Y open,
- Zone 2: Risser 0, Y closed,
- Zone 3: Risser 1–2, Greater Trochanter open,
- Zone 4: Risser 3–4, Greater Trochanter closed.

This is how he summarizes his vision of growth and growth indicators: "Growth is manifested in multiple registers or axes. It is three-dimensional and volumetric. It is made up of phases of acceleration and deceleration".

For example, it is established that by 2 years after menstruation, there is a cessation of spinal growth. Must one wait for a Risser 5 before removing a teenager's corset?

The evaluation of skeletal maturation is a valuable parameter but it is not the only one to consider! It is necessary to correlate all the information gathered:

- The growth rate of the annual sitting height
- The growth of the trunk
- The secondary sexual characteristics.

Cleveland's anatomical pieces showed that in many cases the secondary osseous nucleus of the iliac crest, in other words the Risser test, did not merge with the iliac wing.

Finally, the best criterion is to ensure that the child no longer grows in sitting height using, of course, always the same measurement stick!

The study of the maturation of the skeleton is useful to help with surgical strategy. It is worth considering that only 50% of children have a bone age in line with their chronological age.

Bone Age During Puberty

The ascending slope of the pubertal peak, acceleration phase.

Between 11 and 13 years of bone age in girls, between 13 and 15 years of bone age in boys, the olecranon and Y cartilages are reliable markers to explore Risser 0.

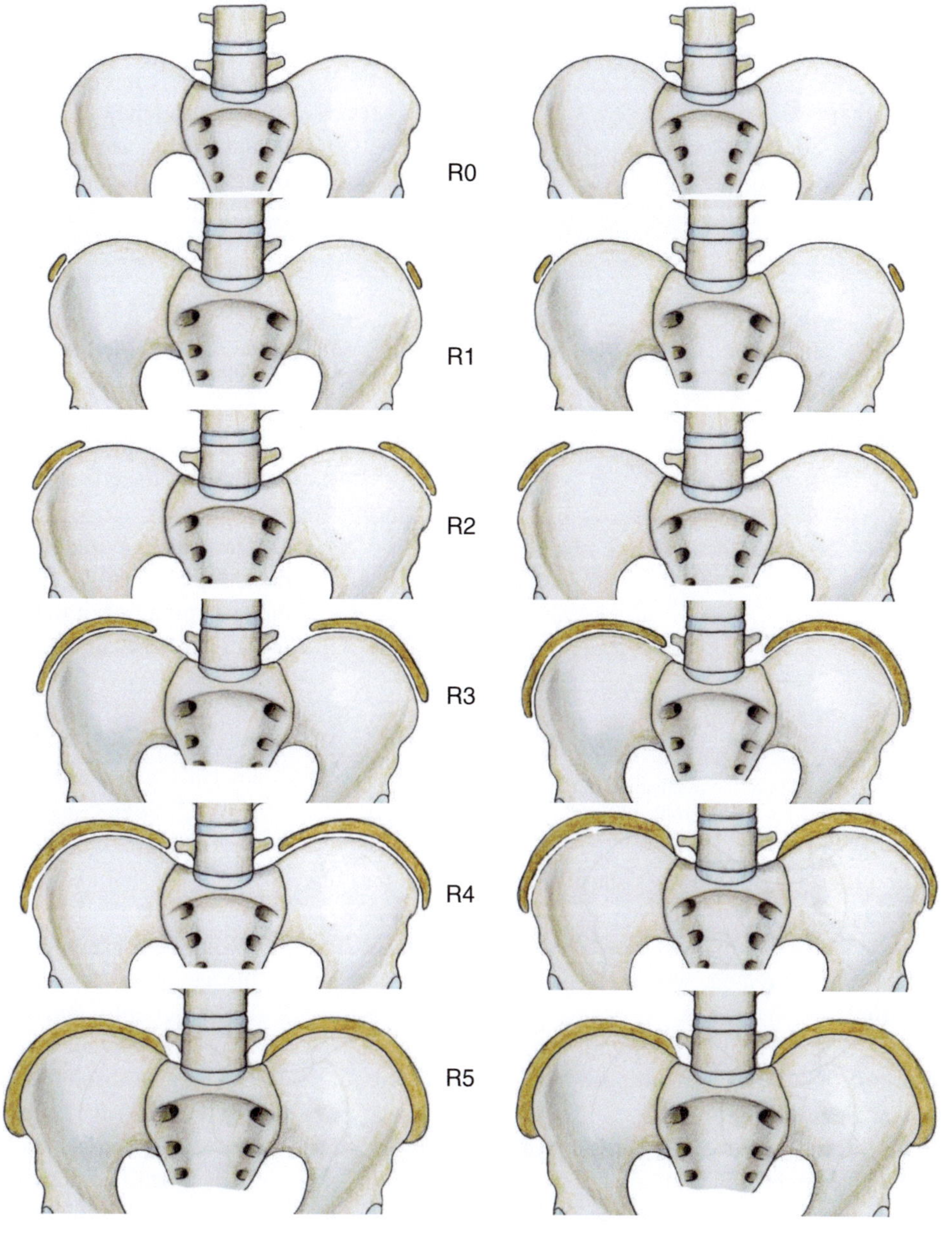

Fig. 33 Risser stages as accepted in the United States on the left and France on the right

On the descending slope of the pubertal peak, deceleration phase.

Bone age at the level of the hand may be correlated with the sign of Risser. The greater trochanter divides the Rissers into two parts. Risser 1/Risser 2: greater trochanter open; Risser 3: the greater trochanter closes; Risser 4/Risser 5: The greater trochanter is closed (Fig. 38).

> One radiograph of the pelvis is enough to differentiate between the main stages of puberty.

The Y cartilage is a radiological marker. But when it closes at 12 years in girls, and at 14 in boys, remaining growth is still 3 years; truncal growth is still 8 cm.

If opting to instrument a scoliosis after closure of the Y cartilage, the risk of crankshaft deformity occurrence is low but certainly not impossible. According to Dubousset, this risk is constant, and omnipresent in a growing spine. The crankshaft effect materializes not only by an angular deterioration but can also be achieved through a morphological distortion of the thorax, caused by spinal imbalance. One must not forget that between Risser 1 and Risser 5 there is a growth of the thorax. The crankshaft effect is present and persistent, as there are a multitude of growth plates in the spine and they are active.

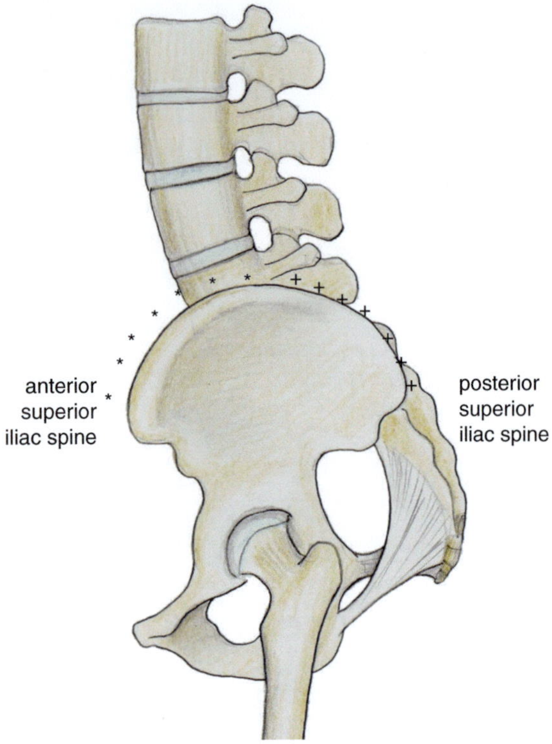

Fig. 34 Evaluation of the ossification of the epiphyseal nucleus of the iliac wing through a lateral profile [29]

In a Risser 0, with open Y cartilage, on the first part of the ascending slope of puberty, the risk for scoliosis of 20° must be multiplied by 3. In other words, a curvature of 20° is likely, if untreated, will worsen to 60° by the end of growth.

In a Risser 0, with closed Y cartilage, the risk of scoliosis curvature of 20° must be multiplied by 2. In other words, the final angle may be 40°.

In a Risser 1 with a 20° curvature, multiply this by 1.5, thus a final angle of 30°.

In contrast when the Risser sign is 3 and the curvature is 20°, the risk of progression is 2%.

Similarly, scoliosis risk must be assessed at Risser 0 during the ascending slope of puberty; when scoliosis increases by 10° per year, one must recognize that this is a malignant scoliosis and may warrant surgical treatment. Thus one must quickly anticipate the inefficiency of bracing and convey realistic expectations to the family. The mistake is to wait as the growth of the spine promotes the scoliosis!

A simple mnemonic is useful for reference:

- Risser 1 to 5 lasts about 2 years.
- At Risser 1, there is a further 4 cm remaining of increase in sitting height,
- Risser 2, there is 3 cm,
- Risser 3 there is 2 cm,
- Risser 4, there is 1 cm.

The Tanner-Whitehouse III method specifically uses the distal radial and ulnar epiphyses and the metacarpal and phalangeal epiphyses of the first, third and fifth digits for determination of skeletal age.

> Any growth produced is absorbed by the scoliosis to the detriment of the sitting height. The scoliosis transforms positive growth into negative growth. Instead of growing, the child loses sitting height.

1. Do not be concerned with the central neuro cartilage after the age of 5 years.
2. Do not confuse annular apophysis and cartilage growth. This is only a secondary growth feature.
3. Do not give absolute legitimacy to the Y cartilage to identify the crankshaft effect.
4. Do not depend on the Risser sign to make the big decisions. Identify other clinical and radiographic parameters.
5. Consider the signs of Tanner.
6. Risser 0 represents 2/3 of puberty.

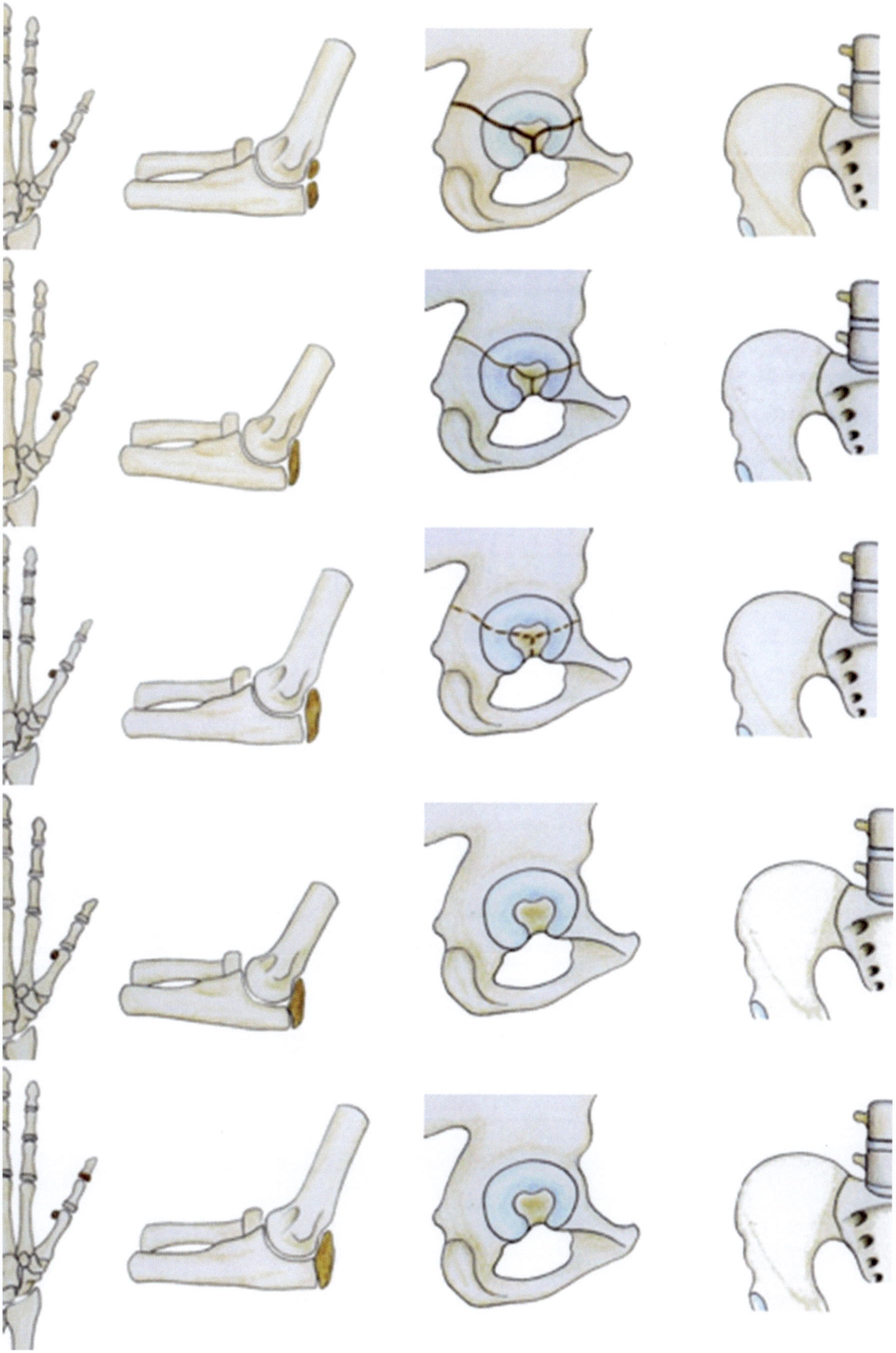

Fig. 35 Relationship between the evolution of the cartilages of the fingers, the elbow, the Y cartilage and the Risser test between 11 and 13 years [24]

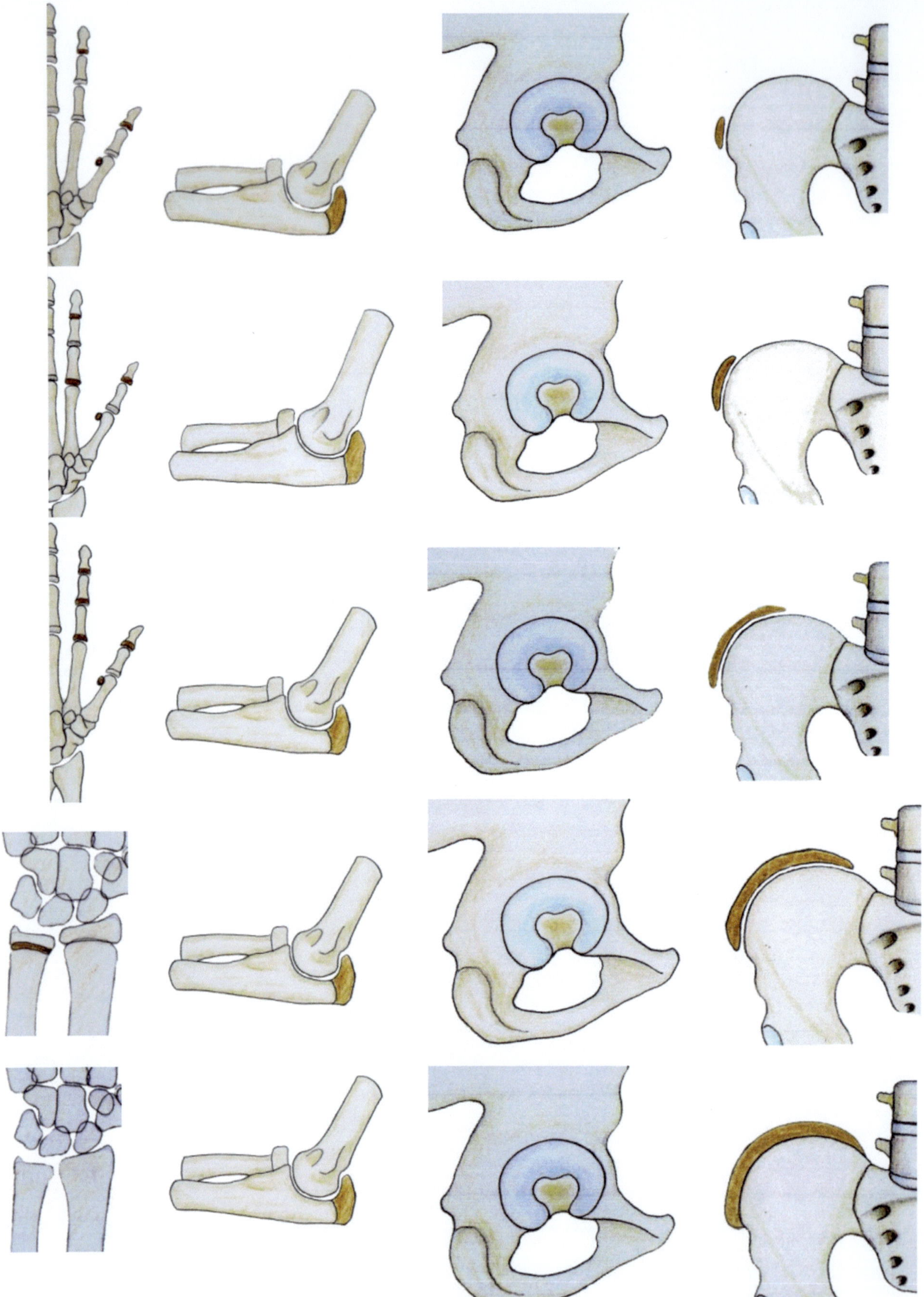

Fig. 36 Relationship between the evolution of the cartilages of the fingers, the elbow, the Y cartilage and the Risser test between 13 and 18 years [24]

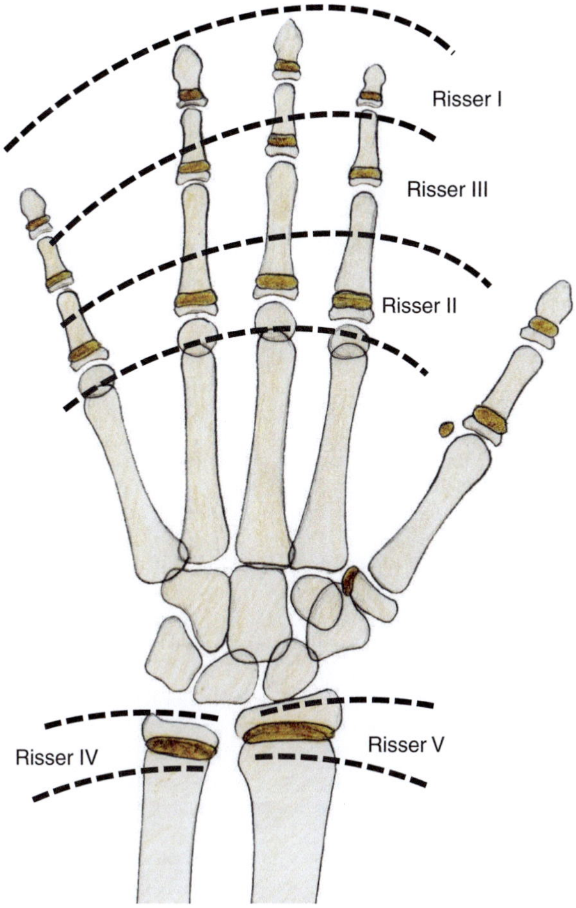

Fig. 37 Correlation between the closure of the phalanges cartilages and the Risser test; The sesamoids dwindle at the beginning of puberty (Dimeglio et al. [24])

Fig. 38 The 4 growth zones (with permission of the author) [24, 25]: Zone 1: Risser 0, Y open; Zone 2: Risser 0, Y closed; Zone 3: Risser 1–2, greater trochanter open; Zone 4: Risser 3–4, greater trochanter closed

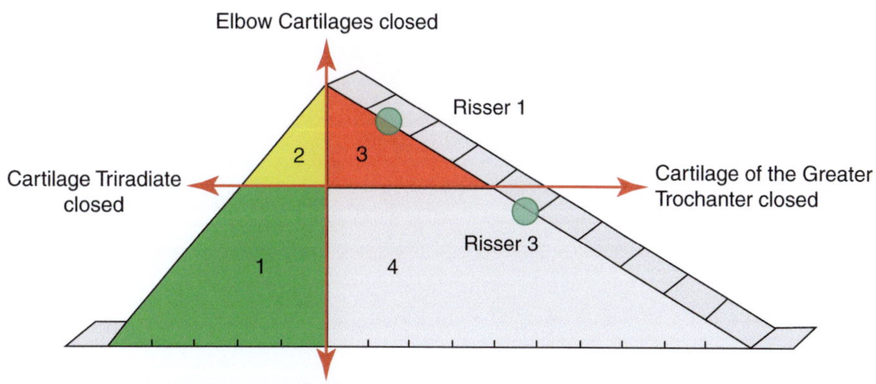

References

1. Schmorl G, Junghanns H. Die gesundeund die kranke Wirbelsaüle. Stuttgart: Thieme Verlag; 1932.
2. Knutsson F. Growth and differentiation of the postnatal vertebra. Acta Radiol. 1961;55:401–8.
3. Nicoladoni C. Anatomie und mechanicus der skoliose. Munich: Urban and Schwrzenberg; 1909.
4. Ottander HG. Experimental progressive scoliosis in a pig. Acta Orthop Scand. 1963;33:91–7.
5. Bouillet R. Pathogénie de la scoliose idiopathique. Acta Orthop Belg. 1967;33:533–46.
6. Mineiro JD. Coluna vertebral humana. Alguns aspectos da sua estrutura e vascularização: Lisboa Sociedade Indudtrial Grafica; 1965.
7. Canadell J. Lesiones del cartilago de crecimiento. Pampelune: Ediciones Universidad de Navarra; 1976.
8. Vital JM, Beguiristain JL, Algara C, Villas C, Lavignolle B, Grenier N, Senegas J. The neurocentral cartilage: anatomy, physiology and physiopathology. Surg Radiol Anat. 1989;11:324–8.
9. Yamazaki A, Mason DE, Caro PA. Age of closure of the neurocentral cartilage in thoracic spine. J Pediatr Orthop. 1998;18:168–72.
10. Beguiristain JL, De Salis J, Oriaifo A, Canadell J. Experimental scoliosis by epiphysiodesis in pig. Int Orthop. 1980;3:317–21.
11. Zhang H, Sucato DJ. Unilateral pedicle screw epiphysiodesis of the neurocentral synchondrosis. production of idiopathic-like scoliosis in an immature animal model. J Bone Joint Surg. 2008;90(A):2460–9.
12. Dickson RA, Lawton JO, Archer IA, Butt WP. The pathogenesis of idiopathic scoliosis biplanar spinal asymmetry. J Bone Joint Surg. 1984;66(B):8–15.
13. Zhang H, Sucato DJ, Nurenberg P, Mcclung A. Morphometric analysis of vertebral growth using magnetic resonance imaging in the normal skeletally immature spine. Spine. 2010.
14. Olgun ZN, Demirkiran G, Ayvaz M, Karadeniz E, Yacizi M. The effect of pedicle screw insertion at a young age on pedicle and canal development. Spine. 2012;37:1778–84.
15. Roberts S, Evans H, Trivedi J, Menage J. Histology and pathology of the human intervertebral disc. J Bone Joint Surg. 2006;88(A):10–4.
16. Mallet J, Rey JC, Raimbeau G, Senly G. Dystrophie rachidienne de croissance. Annales Ortho Ouest. 1975;7:95–116.
17. Bick EM, Copel JW. The ring apophysis of the human vertebra. J Bone Joint Surg. 1951;33(A):783–7.
18. Diard F, Chateil JF, Vital JM, Moinard M. Discopathies et maladie de Scheuermann. Dans "Le rachis lombaire dégénératif". Montpellier: Sauramps Médical; 1998. p. 141–55.
19. Alexander CJ. Scheuermann's disease. A traumatic spondylodystrophy? Skeletal Radiol. 1997;1:209–21.
20. Takata K, Inoue SI, Takahashi K, Ohtzuka Y. Fracture of the posterior margin of a lumbar vertebral body. J Bone Joint Surg. 1998;70(A):589–94.
21. Ippolito E, Belloci M, Montanaro A, Ascani E, Ponseti V. Juvenile kyphosis: an ultrastructural study. J Pediatr Orthop. 1985;5:315–22.
22. Risser JC. The iliac apophysis: an invaluable sign in the management of scoliosis. Clin Orthop Res. 1958;11:111.
23. Vital JM, Martins F, Martins L, Lavignolle B, Chateil JF, Grenier N, Diard F, Senegas J. Etude de l'évolution radiologique des cartilages de croissance du bassin et de l'extrémité supérieure du fémur pendant la croissance. Chir Pédiatr. 1989;30:103–8.
24. Dimeglio A, Bonnel F, Canavese F. The normal growing spine. In: Arkbania BA, editor. The "Growing spine": Springer; 2010.
25. Dimeglio A, Canavese F, Charles YP. Growth and adolescent idiopathic scoliosis; when and how much? J Pediatr Orthop. 2011;31(Suppl 1):28–36.
26. Ryan PM, Puttler EG, Stotler WM, Ferguson RL. Role of the triradiate cartilage in predicting curve progression in adolescent idiopathic scoliosis. J Pediatr Orthop. 2007;27:671–6.
27. Bitan FD, Veliskakis KP, Campbell BC. Differences in the Risser grading system in the United States and France. Clin Orthop Relat Res. 2005;436:190–5.
28. Nault ML, Parent S, Phan P, Roy-Baudry M, Labelle H, Rivard M. A modified Risser grading system predicts the curve acceleration phase of female adolescent idiopathic scoliosis. J Bone Joint Surg. 2010;92:1073–81.
29. Kotwicki T. Improved accuracy in Risser sign with lateral spinal radiography. Eur Spine J. 2008;17:1676–85.

Morphologic and Functional Evolution of the Aging Spine

J. Sénégas, H. Bouloussa, D. Liguoro, G. Yoshida, and Jean Marc Vital

The aging process, often considered to be a specific problem concerning multicellular organisms, is now acknowledged as a general biological phenomenon that does not spare unicellular organisms. Even bacteria age [1].

Aging refers to elapsing time while the occasioned structural and functional alterations are referred to as *senescence*. In fact, in most of the current scientific literature, aging most frequently encompasses the two definitions.

According to the French National Institute of Statistics and Economic Studies (INSEE), the portion of the European population over 65 years old has exponentially increased, from 12.7% in 1910 to 18% in 1970, 20.6% in 2000, and 23.7% in 2012. Forecasts for 2050 average 50% in the majority of modern societies. Longevity increases along with active life years thanks to technological progress. We are now facing a temporal drift in traditional landmarks that structured life steps (education, active life, old age without handicap, and eventually with handicap).

Even though the aging process undoubtedly appears to be deterministic at the scale of the entire body and organs, the alterations it causes and their functional expression arise in a stochastic fashion in various subjects and at different ages. Consequently, some have put forward the "normal aging" concept. In fact, normative criteria are impossible to clearly determinate. At best, it refers to a state of optimal tolerance of biological alterations that gradually and inexorably *weaken* all living systems. This refers eventually to the fundamental concept of *robustness* specific to each system that automation specialists have developed long ago.

In fact, aging should be integrated as a multi-scale biological process, equally genetic/epigenetic and intracellular/matrix molecular or tissue-related, eventually affecting all organs. Level by level and component by component analytic approaches, when considered exclusively, fail to explain the entire process. Aging is actually a complex dynamic process with circular causalities, animated by constant information, energy, and matter flows. All these interactive variables easily account for the fact that wide variations exist between each one of us along the aging process.

Admittedly, the entire musculoskeletal system presents with varying degrees of tissue degeneration signs with aging. Yet their clinical expression is usually clearly more marked at the level of specific joints, hips, or knees for example. In contrast, most spinal degenerative processes are poorly symptomatic and fairly well tolerated because of a better distribution of mechanical stresses on multiple segments of the axial skeleton.

This study features two components:

- Firstly an analytical review of age-related structural alterations, component by component
- Secondly a synthetic study of systemic functional alterations which objective is the description of their interactions.

Age-Related Structural Alterations

The Intervertebral Disc

Structural Modifications

The intervertebral disc is subjected to very important constraints throughout life. Its well-organized fibro-cartilaginous structure is highly exposed to aging as

J. Sénégas (✉) · H. Bouloussa · J. M. Vital
Spinal Unit, University Hospital, Bordeaux, France

D. Liguoro
Neurosurgical Department A, University Hospital of Pellegrin, Bordeaux, France

G. Yoshida
Department of Orthopedic Surgery, Hamamatsu University School of Medicine, Hamamatsu, Japan

J. M. Vital, D. T. Cawley (eds.), *Spinal Anatomy*, https://doi.org/10.1007/978-3-030-20925-4_5

numerous disc alterations occur throughout one's lifetime. According to Roughley [2], the center of embryonic disc is rich in water, proteoglycans, and notochordal cells that gradually disappear and become cartilaginous cells, while the periphery is rich in collagen and fibroblasts. At maturity, the nucleus pulposus cell density averages 4×10^6 cells/cm^3, while the annulus fibrosus cell density reaches 9×10^6 cells/cm^3. The intervertebral disc cell content, however, is the lowest in the entire body. Iatridis et al. [3] showed in a cadaveric biomechanical study on subjects aged 16–88 years that as the shearing forces within the nucleus pulposus increased with age; energy dissipation was less. Disc composition changes with age: in early adulthood and middle age, it is rich in chondroitin-4-sulfate, chondroitin-6-sulfate, and keratan sulfate; in the elderly, dermatan sulfate is predominant.

A Fragile Avascular Tissue

The intervertebral disc is generally considered to be an avascular tissue in adults. However, vessels within the annulus fibrosus without penetration into the nucleus pulposus are found in the fetus and children up to 2 years old. Roberts et al. [4] reported that newborn discs are indeed vascularized initially but that the vascularization typically decreases in adulthood and may be increased with pathology. According to this author, "vascular aging" starts early in the first decade of life with a drastic decrease in vascularity between 6 and 30 months. They describe an alteration of vertebral endplates such as cracks, thinning, and microfractures of subchondral bone; the peripheral annulus densifies secondarily.

Nutrition is therefore precarious by diffusion through the vertebral vascular network at the level of vertebral endplates. The nucleus pulposus is most vulnerable, being the farthest away from vessels. According to Urban et al. [5], a diffusion decrease within the disc by subchondral bone sclerosis or through calcified endplates necessarily translates into a decrease in blood flow and cell nutrition; this typically contributes to nucleus pulposus degeneration, affecting the spinal hydraulic damper.

With final avascular disc architecture being obtained from early childhood, the conditions are consequently met for a rapid aging depending on local and regional biomechanical factors, and also genetic or nutritional properties interfering with the diffusion of micronutrients to the nucleus pulposus.

A Genetic Predisposition?

The role of genetics has been studied by Battie and Videman [6]. They were able to perform MRI studies of identical twins' spines: very similar disc lesions were observed in those twins in spite of varying physical activity levels (profession and sports). Obviously, they suggested that genetic background prevails over mechanical overuse. Two genotypes of metalloproteinase-3 were determined: COL 9 A2 and COL 9 A3.

Sambrook et al. [7] estimated, from a cohort of over 300 twins with cervical assessment and lumbar MRI, that disc degeneration was inherited in 74% of them at the lumbar level and 73% of them at the cervical level, surprisingly concluding that genetics demonstrated a more influential role in aging, as opposed to traditional mechanical theories.

If this genetic factor is truly preponderant, then aging will logically occur in tandem in the cervical and lumbar spine. Following this principle, Matsumoto et al. [8] analyzed 94 asymptomatic subjects aged 48 years on average. 78.7% of them presented with cervical and lumbar tandem degeneration. However, one may notice that only 21.3% of them displayed loss of disc height and 12.8% central canal stenosis, which is consistent with current literature. The last two parameters are relatively infrequent in asymptomatic populations despite a discreet increase with age.

Genesis and Contributions to Aging on Histomorphological Features

Disc degeneration is marked by decreased disc hydration, in parallel with glycosaminoglycan concentration decrease. Cracks form gradually and may constitute nitrogen pockets. Considerable loss of elasticity of the intervertebral disc usually ensues even before loss of disc height. Comparative analysis between *nucleus pulposus* and *annulus fibrosus* along one's lifetime demonstrates important macroscopic and microscopic histological structure variations and a substantial change in the molecular and cellular organization. Vernon-Roberts et al. [9] showed a decrease in disc cellularity with age on L4-L5 discs. This decrease was especially pronounced when cells were in the vicinity of a disc crack or a cartilaginous abnormality of vertebral endplates.

There is a fragile balance within discs between matrix synthesis and destruction; numerous molecular mechanisms upsetting this equilibrium (metalloproteinases, apoptosis pathways, pro-inflammatory interleukins) have been proposed. To this date, none of them has been attributed a cause and effect relationship. Gruber and Hanley [10] reported a significant increase of cell apoptosis incidence within the annulus fibrosus in elderly control discs (73% ± 5.1%) compared to a group requiring discectomy (53.5% ± 5.6%), with an age difference of only 13 years.

It is commonly acknowledged that the key of the aging spine is the intervertebral disc. Its lesions such as radial tears and of concentric fissures begin during the first decade of life (Fig. 1). Indeed, Weiler et al. [11] showed histological alterations of the intervertebral disc starting at the age of 3 compared to intact newborn discs. The nucleus pulposus alterations in the lumbar region are greater in subjects over 60 years old.

It remains difficult, so far, to clearly differentiate aging from pathological disc degeneration. However, it is considered that disc lesions are the *primum movens* of the aging spine impacting zygaphophyseal joints, ligaments, and muscles. Haeffeli et al. [12] sequentially showed macroscopic morphological disc modifications in a cadaveric study of 248 subjects of various ages (7 months to 88 years). Specimens included lumbar vertebrae and discs in sagittal and parasagittal sections. They confirmed that the fibrous transformation of the nucleus pulposus associated with annulus and endplate disorganization anticipate fissures within the nucleus followed by more extensive tears. In subjects aged between 30 and 40, they found fissures of the nucleus and tears of the annulus, cracks that extend with time. According to them, disc lesions are more common in the lumbar spine (Figs. 1, 2, and 3).

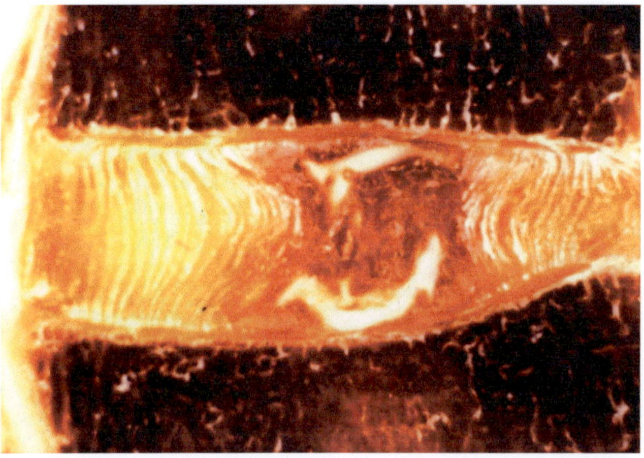

Fig. 1 Lumbar disc, sagittal section; early degeneration, dehydrated and unstructured nucleus pulposus

During aging, both the *nucleus pulposus* and *annulus fibrosus* become more fibrous and rich in collagen so that distinguishing them becomes less obvious in the elderly. Calcifications are formed preferentially at the level of annulus fibrosus but sometimes also affect the nucleus pulposus. Neo-angiogenesis recruiting pro-inflammatory cells was shown by Roberts et al. [4]. It occurs through damaged vertebral endplates and discal tears and consequently accelerates intervertebral disc ossification.

Thus, a cascade of events affects the disc including an early dehydration well-described in the MRI degeneration stages by Pfirmann et al. [13]. In 2001, they proposed a five-stage MRI classification based on T2 sequences according to the following criteria: structure and color (white/black), nucleus/annulus distinction, signal intensity, intervertebral disc height (Fig. 4).

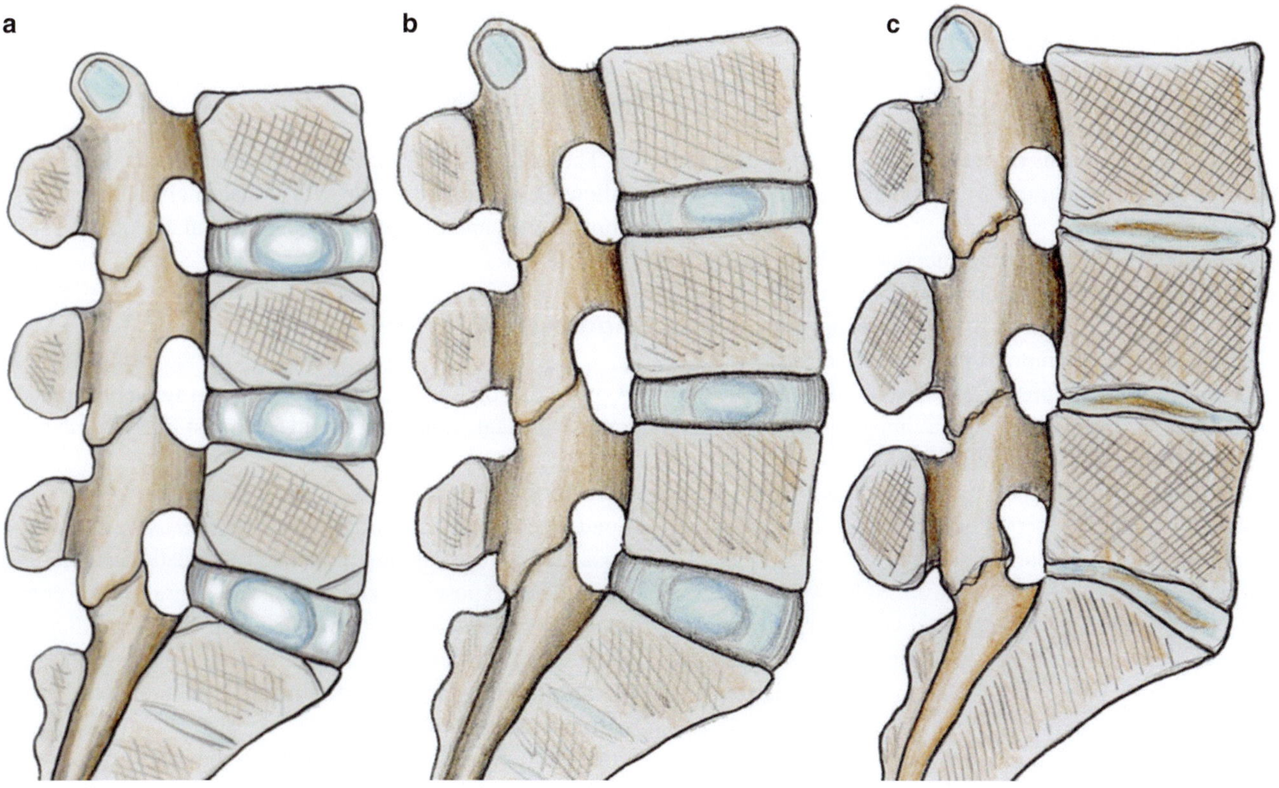

Fig. 2 Sagittal sections of lumbar spines in the newborn (**a**), young adult (**b**), and older adult (**c**)

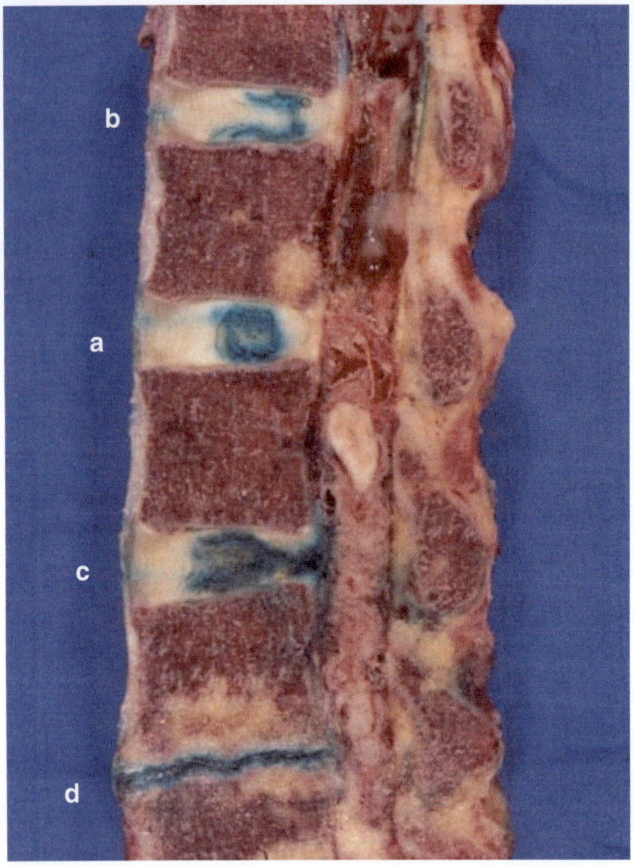

Fig. 3 Sagittal sections displaying various stages of degeneration in the same subject: L2-L3 normal disc (**a**), Medial fissure in L3-L4 disc (**b**), Posterior fissure in L4-L5 disc (**c**), and Loss of disc height in L5-S1 disc (**d**)

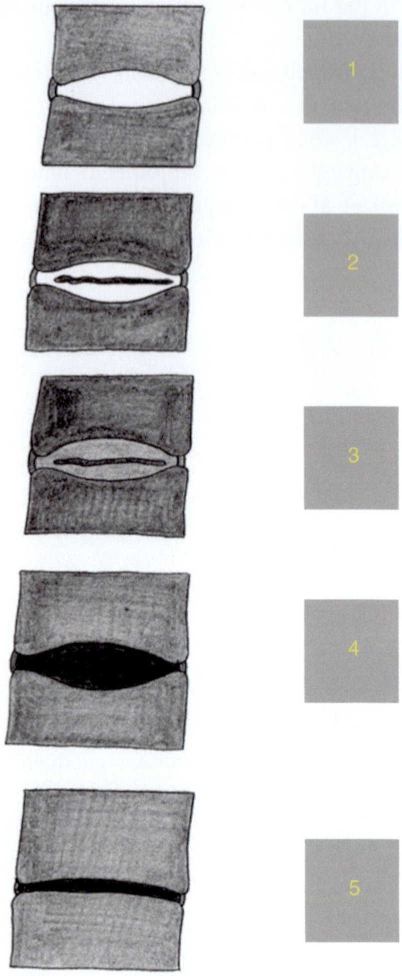

Fig. 4 Pfirmann MRI classification [13]

Cracks in the nucleus and annulus appear, hence causing disc rupture and nucleus ejection responsible for a herniated disc. The latter can therefore be considered as skipping a step in the aging process.

Cartilaginous endplates and subchondral bone display an inflammatory process (Modic 1 sign) with microfissures, probably caused by increasing constraints with reduced intervertebral disc damping: endplate lesions seem to be secondary to disc failure though several authors believe it could be a primary process via impaired disc nutrition through cartilaginous endplates (Fig. 5).

In 1988, Modic et al. [14] proposed a classification based on the inflammatory reaction of vertebral endplates and vertebral bone marrow in particular.

- *Type I* combines a T1 hyposignal with T2 hyperintensity, which demonstrate hypervascularization and edematous inflammatory reactions adjacent to the bone marrow.
- *Type II* comprises both T1 and T2 hyperintensity demonstrating a fatty involution of the bone marrow.
- *Type III*, which is rarer, corresponds to fibrosis with poor vascularization and marked hyperostosis, equivalent to osteocondensation (Figs. 6, 7 and 8).

The last stage of disc degeneration represents disc fusion following hypomobility due to disc space narrowing and disc fibrosis, then anterior, posterior, and lateral osteophytosis.

Aggravating Factors

Aggravating or accelerating factors of such aging phenomena are mechanical, vascular, genetic, and most likely combined.

Mechanical Factors

Load repetition both in intensity and rhythm as well as vibrations leads to cartilaginous endplate calcification. Rotational movements expose to annular tears and aggravate the previously described fissuration phenomenon. According to Stokes and Iatridis [15], underuse may also display detrimental effects by decreasing cellular stimulation and altering nutrient transport. Disc overuse may also lead to degeneration. Examples include sudden shifts between mobile and stiff segments as seen in lumbosacral hinge anomalies (Bertolotti's syndrome) or at surgical fusion extremities (junctional syndromes).

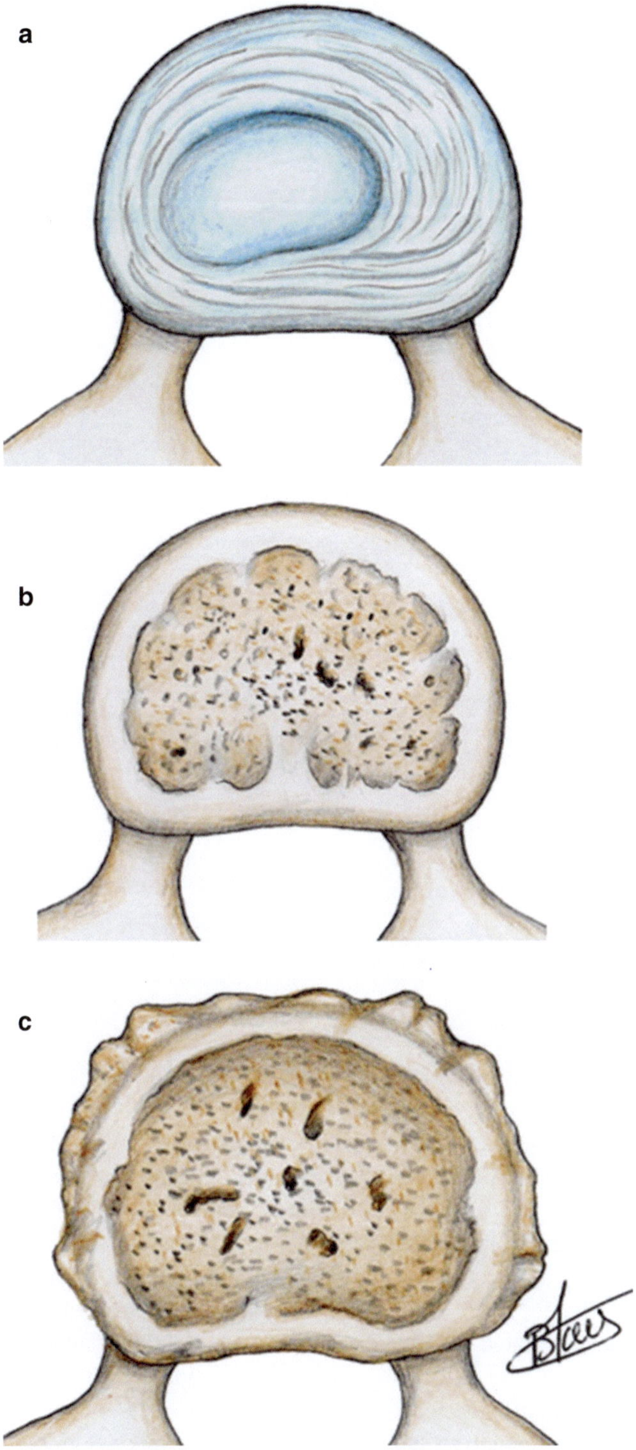

Fig. 5 Disc and vertebral endplate modifications (**a**) Axial section of an intervertebral disk in a symptomatic subject: concentric annulus and laminate, eccentric nucleus pulposus. (**b**) Vertebral endplate showing a porous bone surface with annular ossification. (**c**) Changes due to aging: major circular osteophytes of the vertebral endplate giving a very irregular aspect

Experimental studies have permitted a better understanding of the effect of mechanical stresses on the intervertebral disc and its components.

Hutton et al. [16] showed the production increase of type 1 collagen in nucleus pulposus under the effect of compressive stresses. At the same time, they reported a decrease in type 2 collagen and proteoglycans production.

Handa et al. [17] reported from disc samples a decrease in proteoglycan production under high hydrostatic pressure (10 MPa), while synthesis was increased under low pressure (1 MPa).

Mechanical stresses that are directly applied to cells can modulate matrix protein synthesis [18]. The observed effects are likely to be dependent on the type of stress, its intensity, frequency, and duration.

Inflammatory Factors

The major role of inflammation was well-described by Rannou et al. [18]: certain metalloproteinases, cytokines, and growth factors are involved in disc degeneration with direct correlation between mechanical constraints and metalloproteinase activity. The production origin of these different factors is still debated: disc cells, neovascularization, or inflammatory granuloma.

Vascular Factors

Hypovascularization, especially microvascular disease, is also a factor of accelerated degeneration according to Kauppila et al. [19]. According to Urban et al. [5], smoking and vibrations also interfere by a vascular mechanism.

To date, studies reporting clinical and MRI observations of asymptomatic cohorts concerning the aging of the intervertebral disc mainly use disc-based classifications (derived from the Pfirmann classification [13]) without taking account of the endplate inflammatory reaction. Indeed, Modic types, often attributed to pathological mechanisms, are less studied in the context of asymptomatic subjects with aging spines.

A classic MRI observation is based on the dehydration of lower lumbar discs (L4-L5 and L5-S1) occurring early compared with higher lumbar discs followed by disc space narrowing seen on lateral X-rays. Indeed, the aging of the lumbar spine is "propagated" from the bottom up because of the pivotal position of the L5-S1 segment, or even L4-L5 with respect to the pelvis (Fig. 9). This results in a major loss of lordosis between L4 and S1 where two-thirds of the lumbar lordosis are normally located. The same phenomenon exists at the cervical level: disc space narrowing first occurs on the lower cervical discs (C7-T1, C6-C7, and C5-C6), while disc height is maintained on the discs above. They classically remain hypermobile, especially in extension, to maintain the horizontal gaze (Fig. 10). This phenomenon, which only appears on dynamic X-rays, can create myelopathy, by the underlying degenerated levels in terms of spinal cord compression.

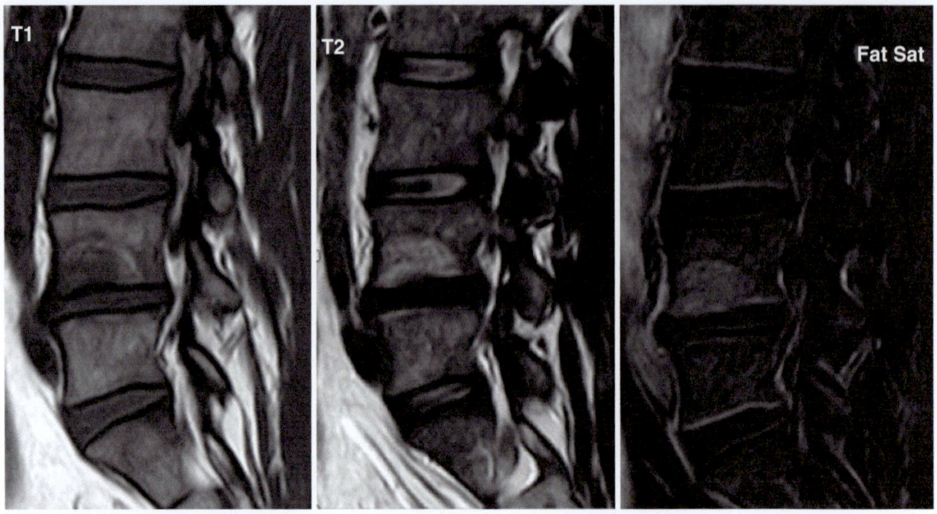

Fig. 6 Modic classification: Modic 1 on MRI [14]

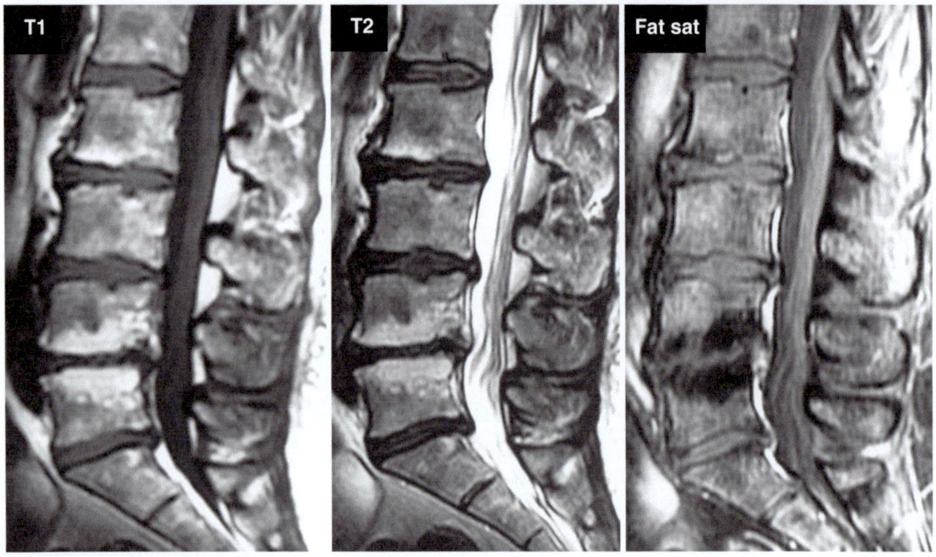

Fig. 7 Modic classification: Modic 2 on MRI [14]

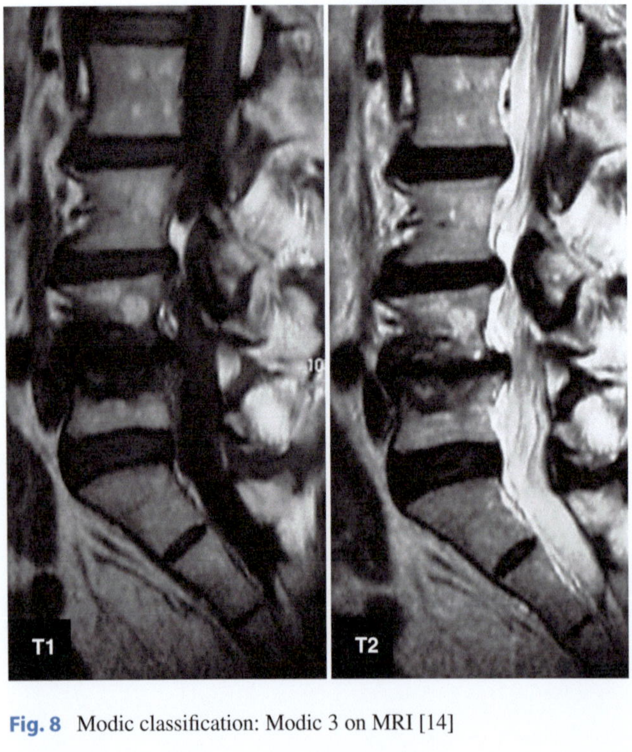

Fig. 8 Modic classification: Modic 3 on MRI [14]

Zhang et al. [20] proposed, in a pilot study, the use of diffusion MRI to detect early disc behavioral abnormalities due to aging on a series of asymptomatic subjects at the molecular scale and in the absence of any morphological abnormality on T2 sequences. They suggested that the diffusion coefficient could decrease in degenerated discs and that it was correlated with the disc water content and the integrity degree of the disc matrix. It could also further specify the direction of the possible disc injury.

A meta-analysis published in 2014 by Brinjikji et al. [21] collected data on 3310 asymptomatic subjects with radiographic data (CT or MRI). Signs of disc degeneration were found as early as 20 years old (37% of asymptomatic subjects of that age group) and in 96% of subjects over 80 years old. A disc signal intensity decrease on T2-weighted images was present in more than half of the subjects over 40 years and 86% of the subjects over 60 years old. The disc height loss was correlated with age but to a lesser extent; however, 1% per year prevalence increase was noted. In contrast, the prevalence of disc protrusions and annular fissures did not seem to increase with age.

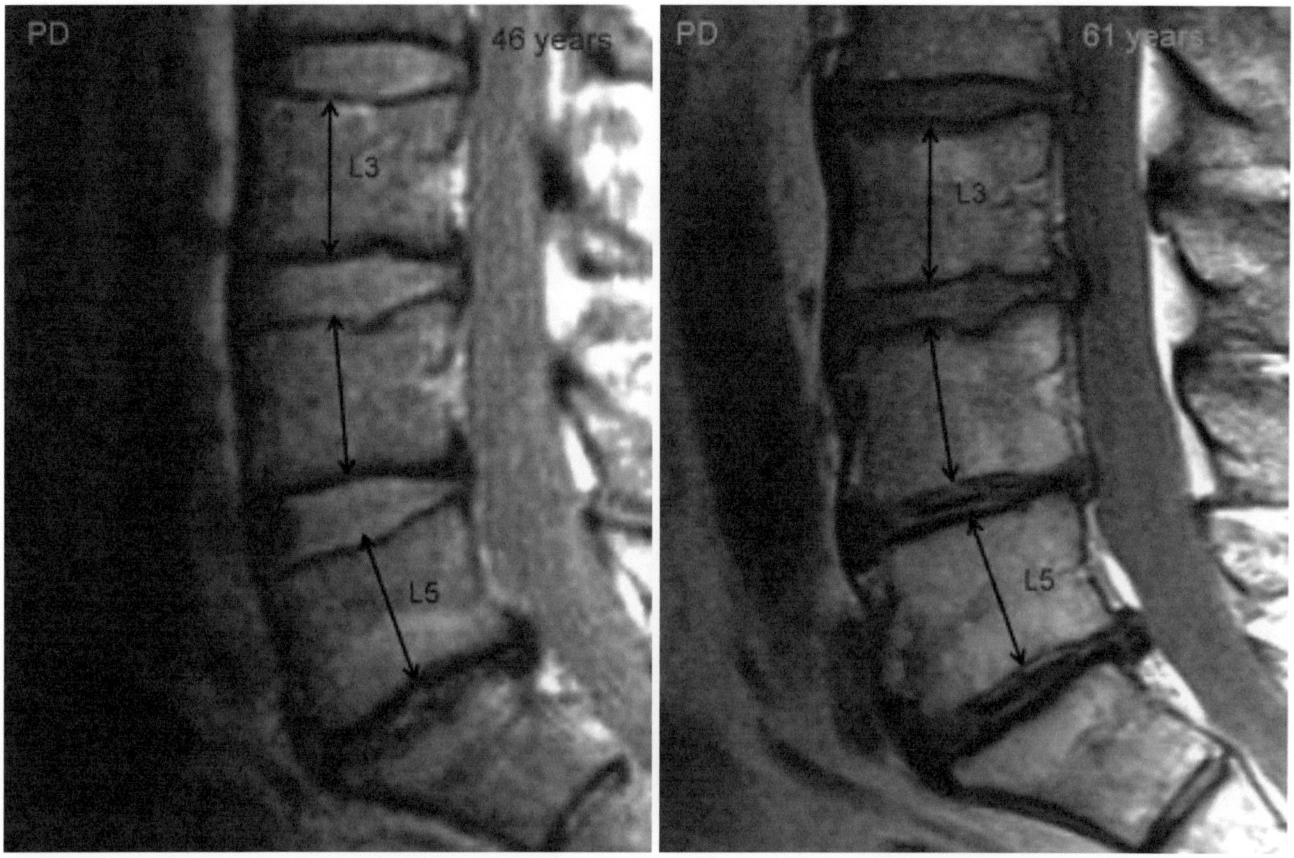

Fig. 9 Natural history of lumbar disc degeneration on MRI: loss of disc height and dehydration of lower discs, L5-S1 disc being affected first

Pollintine et al. [22] highlighted an innovative biomechanical hypothesis regarding the absorption of compressive forces on the spine of elder patients. His cadaveric study on thoracolumbar pieces showed that aging caused a deformity of both vertebral bodies and intervertebral discs under compressive loads. Both structures displayed a substantial "creep." The lower the disc pressures were, the more deformed the vertebrae were when placed under mechanical load.

Videman et al. [23] showed the natural history of lumbar intervertebral disc MRI morphology over 15 years on a large series of asymptomatic Finnish twins. The authors report a decrease in disc height averaging of 3.4% at 5 years and 8–11% at 15 years on MRIs performed during follow-up. An original aspect of that work consisted of showing a compensation by a vertebral height increase on incriminated levels of 3.1% (0.8 mm) in the higher lumbar spine and 4.7% (1.1 mm) in the lower lumbar spine. These preliminary results suggest a height increase of vertebral endplates compensating for multilevel disc height loss and thereby support Pollintine's hypothesis.

Specific Features in the Cervical Spine

Disc degeneration plays a major role in the aging of the cervical spine. Okada et al. [24] showed a significant cervical spine morphological aging on MRI after a 10-year follow-up from a series of 223 asymptomatic subjects aged 39 ± 15 years. 34% of patients that were followed developed clinical symptoms including neck pain, shoulder stiffness, or subjective sensory disorders of their lower limbs; the onset of these symptoms was correlated disc degeneration visualized on MRI.

The same authors [25] analyzed the relationships between sagittal balance and disc degeneration in the cervical spine on a large cohort of asymptomatic subjects at a 10-year follow-up. There was no correlation between clinical symptoms and cervical spine sagittal balance. In their cohort, loss of disc signal intensity, posterior disc protrusions, and disc space narrowing were found in 64.6%, 65.5%, and 28.3%, respectively, of subjects at a 10-year follow-up. Subjects over 40 years old without cervical lordosis were the most likely to develop posterior disc protrusions.

Lumbar and Cervical Tandem Lesions

Okada et al. [25] demonstrated a higher prevalence of disc degeneration in the upper cervical spine in patients who already had lumbar disc herniations compared with asymptomatic controls.

This association between lumbar disc herniations and multilevel cervical disc degeneration suggests a "systemic"

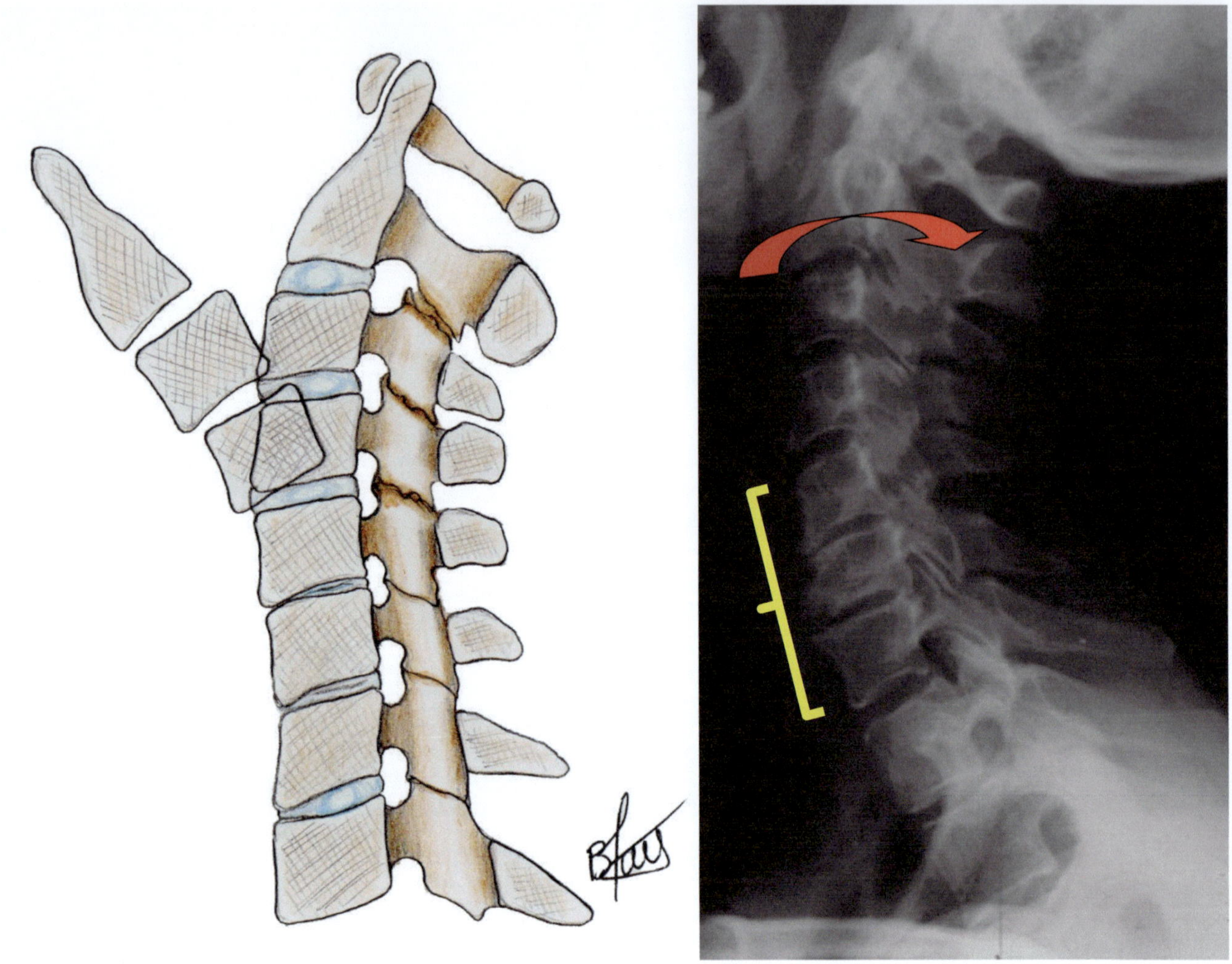

Fig. 10 Natural history of cervical discs on plain X-ray: initial loss of disc height in the lower cervical spine and hypermobility of higher discs

effect of disc aging and a significant participation of genetics (Fig. 11).

Few studies were published regarding the aging of *thoracic intervertebral discs*. Of note, Matsumoto et al. [8] reported on MRI degeneration of thoracic intervertebral discs in 46.8% of subjects from an asymptomatic series of 94 subjects. Of these subjects, patients displayed a decrease in disc signal intensity on T2-weighted images, posterior disc protrusions, and compressions of the dural sac, respectively, 37.2%, 29.8%, and 30.9%. Only 4.3% presented disc space narrowing in the thoracic spine.

The thoracic spine, which has little mobility, therefore does not seem to be spared by these degeneration phenomena, despite greater mechanical constraints than in the cervical and lumbar spines, which are conversely lordosed and mobile.

The Posterior Arch

Facet Joints or Zygapophyseal Joints

The second constituent of the mobile segment of Junghanns, they follow the disc aging process with a natural involution featuring fissures of the articular cartilage (Fig. 12), sometimes erosion, subchondral geodes and, as in any joint affected by osteoarthritis, hypertrophy with osteophytosis and eventually spontaneous fusion with time.

Weishaupt et al. [26] described on CT and MRI four stages of facet joint evolution: *stage 0* normal, *stage 1* with simple narrowing, *stage 2* with small geodes and osteophytes, and finally *stage 3* with significant osteophytes, geodes, and synovial cysts (Fig. 13).

Joint space narrowing is inexorable. Wang and Yang [27] has also shown progressive sagittalization of the lower lumbar facet joints, probably by increased constraints on the anterior and superior thirds of the superior facet of the lower vertebra, potentially leading to a degenerative spondylolisthesis (DSL).

Joint capsules can also be become hypertrophied along with a formation of posterior or anterior synovial cysts which may cause cauda equina with nerve root compression.

Cysts are associated with DSL in 60–89% of cases. A facet joint degeneration classification was proposed by Grogan et al. [28]. They distinguished four MRI stages of cartilaginous degeneration and four MRI stages of subchondral sclerosis.

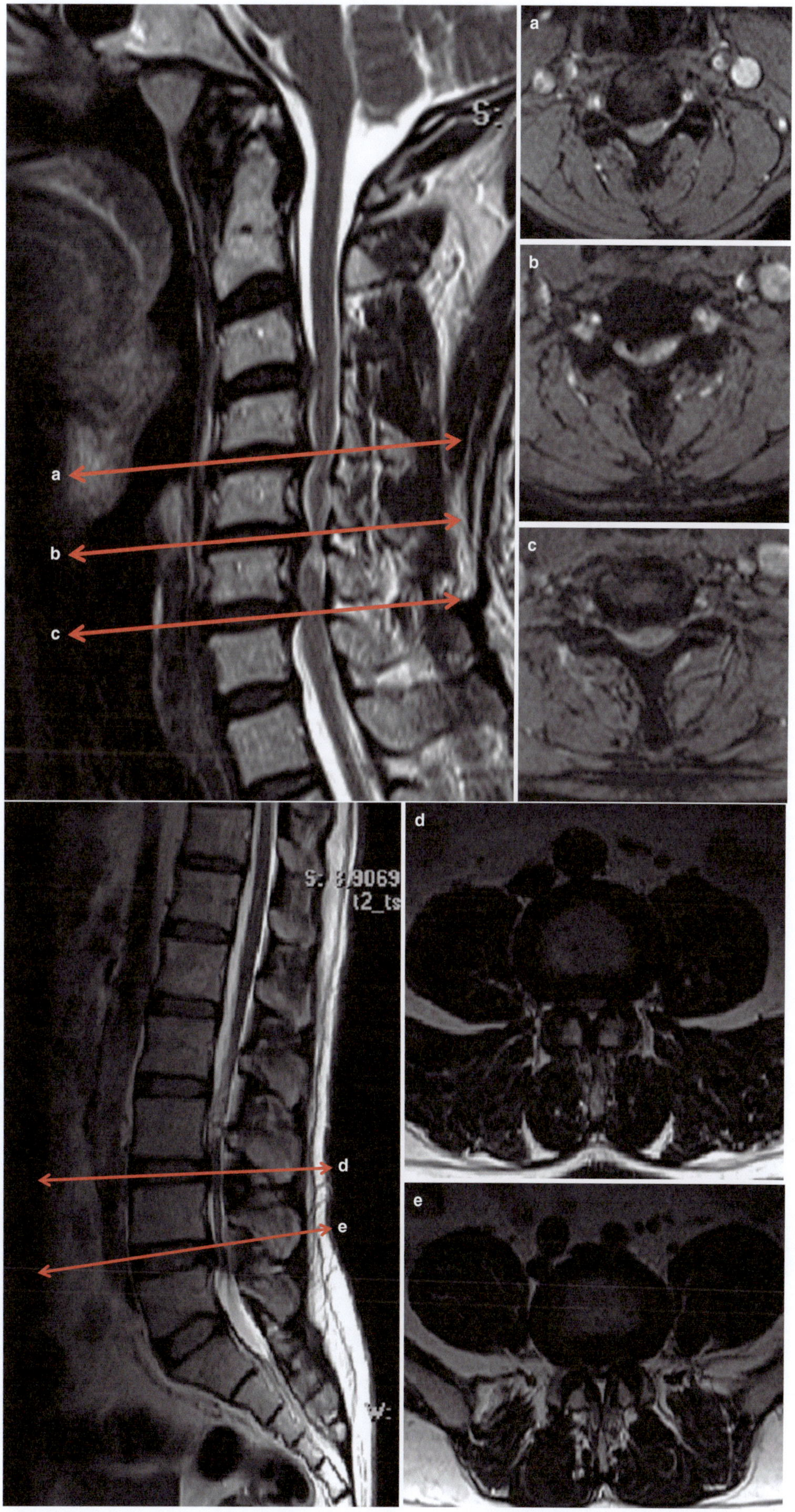

Fig. 11 Tandem lesions with cervical spinal stenosis (**a**, **b**, and **c**) with lumbar spinal stenosis (**d** and **e**)

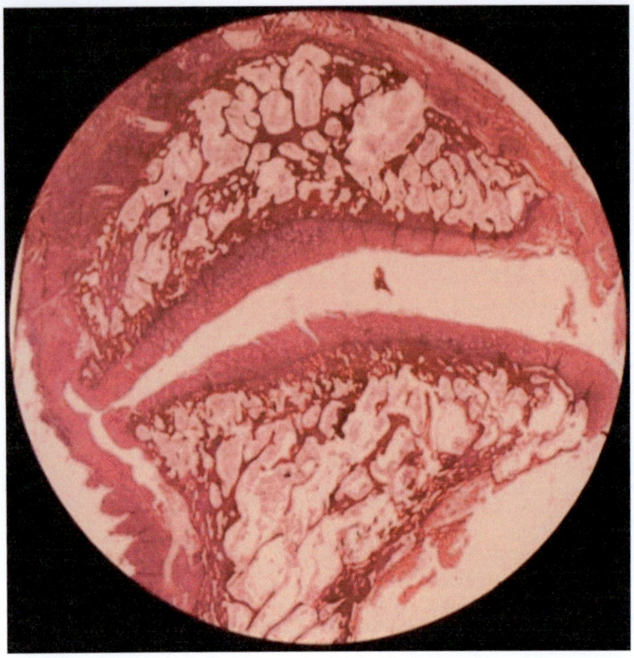

Fig. 12 Fissuring (cracking) of articular cartilage in the cervical spine, first stage of articular aging

Spinous Processes

Aylott et al. [29] demonstrated on a longitudinal CT study that spinous process height increased with decades; this evolution leads to a posterior encumbering phenomenon which reduces extension capacities in the same way as concomitant anterior disc space narrowing (Fig. 14).

Ligaments

The ligament flavum has the highest elastin content in the human body and contains numerous proprioceptive fibers similarly to the multifidus muscle overlying its posterior aspect. As people age, its elastin content, and hence elasticity, decreases. Spinal ligaments can not only become hypertrophied and buckled due to disc height loss and facet joint overlap but they may also present with calcium pyrophosphate or hydroxyapatite deposits which are frequently found in lumbar spinal stenosis. Such deposits are not necessarily always associated with a history of chondrocalcinosis, hyperparathyroidism, or hemochromatosis.

The posterior longitudinal ligament and especially its midline fibers may become calcified, especially in the context of diffuse idiopathic skeletal hyperostosis (DISH).

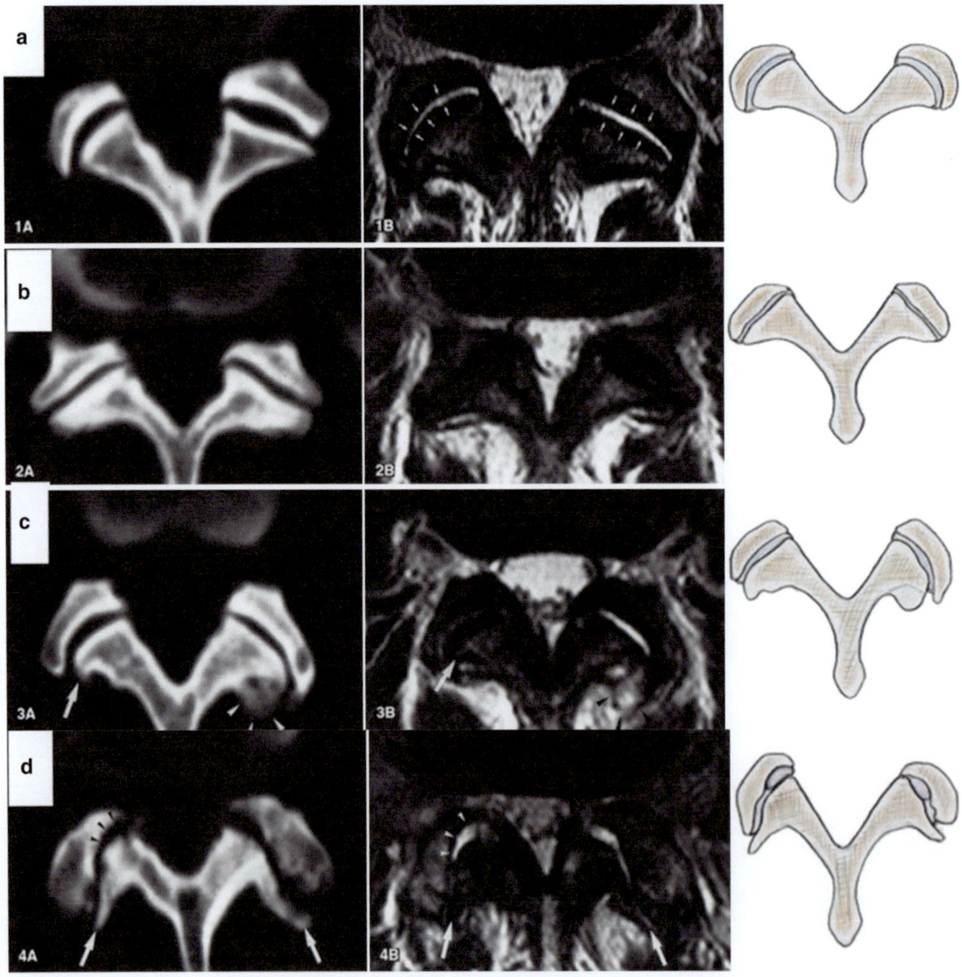

Fig. 13 Degeneration of the posterior articular muscles after Weishaupt et al. [26]: (**a**) normal articular space, (**b**) joint space narrowing, (**c**) geodes and osteophytes, (**d**) irregular cartilage and synovial cysts

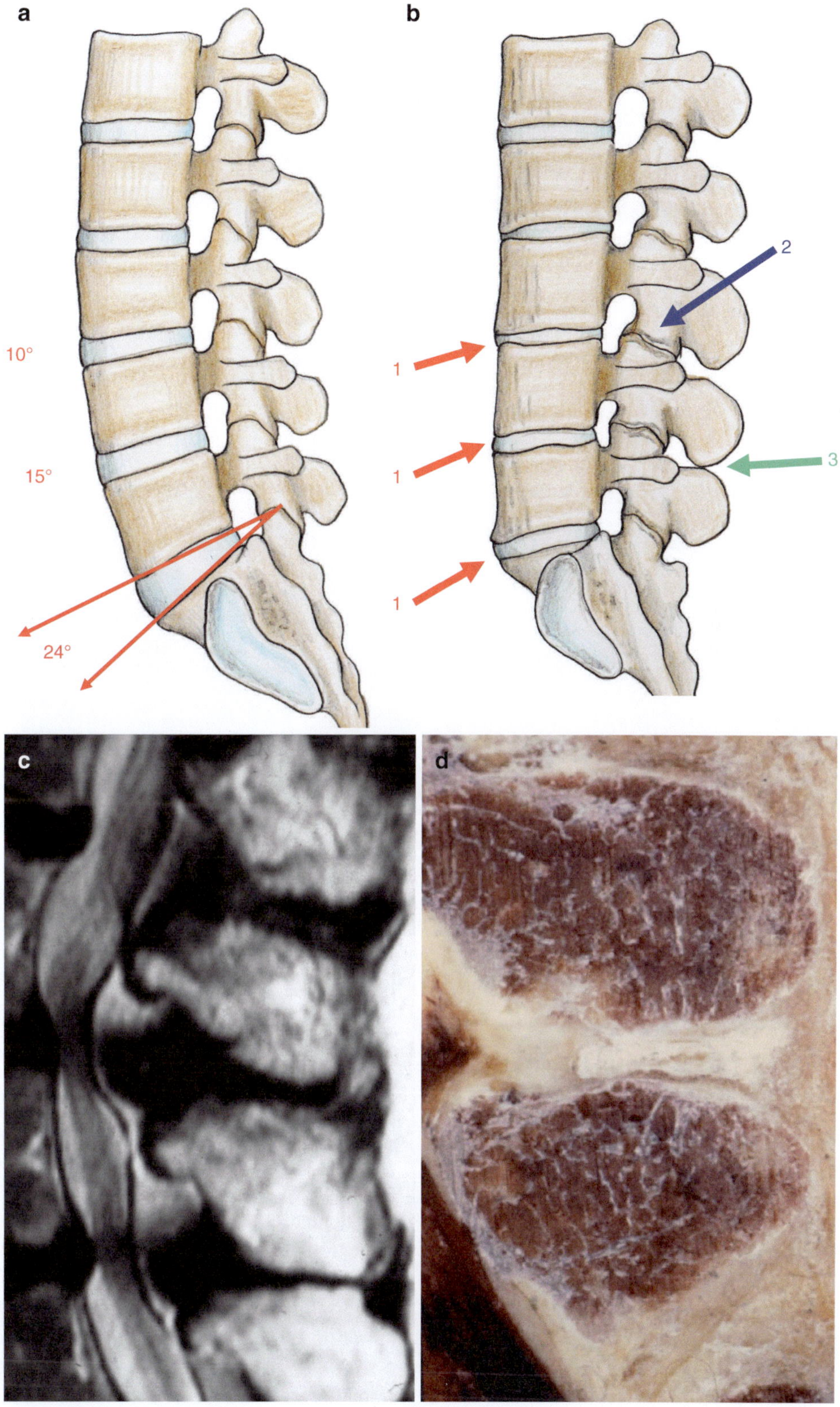

Fig. 14 Evolution toward kyphosis (**b**) with respect to the initial state (**a**) by disc narrowing (1), articular hypertrophy (2), hypertrophy of the spinous processes (**c** and **d**) with interspinous contact (3)

Muscles

Sarcopenia is a geriatric syndrome characterized by loss of muscle mass and therefore decreased physical performance and strength. Spinal muscles are no exception to this. This phenomenon starts in the early thirties and accelerates after 50 years old: muscle mass decreases by 1–2% per year from this age while strength decreases by 1.5% per year. This corresponds to a loss of strength of 30% by decade after 60 years old. Both type I and type II muscle fibers are rarefied. Fiber atrophy is also observed and mostly affects fast type II fibers.

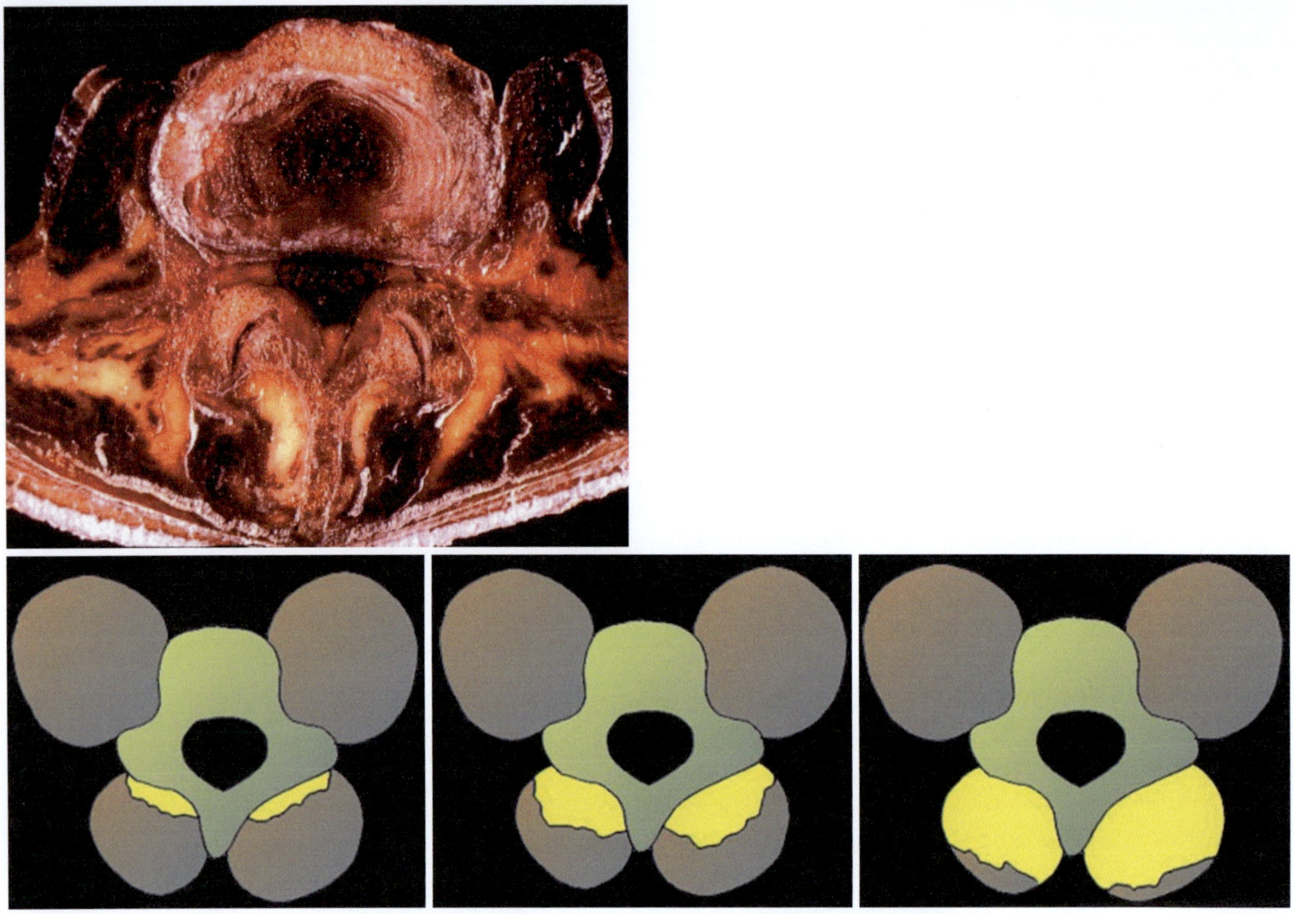

Fig. 15 Fatty muscle degeneration in three stages according to Hadar et al. [30]

Degeneration or fatty infiltration is a recognized phenomenon of natural muscle aging; it was quantified on the lumbosacral muscle mass by Hadar et al. [30] who described three stages of fatty degeneration of paraspinal muscles:

- *Stage 1:* less than half the surface of affected muscles,
- *Stage 2:* 50% fatty infiltration,
- *Stage 3:* more than 50% of fat replacement (Fig. 15).

Interestingly, this fat replacement occurs from deep to superficial, the multifidus muscle being the first affected, and from the bottom up, that is from the lumbosacral junction to the thoracolumbar junction. Cruz et al. [31] demonstrated that there was a direct correlation between aging, loss of lumbar lordosis, and the importance of fatty infiltration of paraspinal muscles.

Fortin et al. [32] performed a 15-year longitudinal MRI study on the multifidus muscle: during this rather short timeframe, multifidus was more markedly atrophied at the L5-S1 level than at the L1-L2 level along with fatty infiltration. These findings were independent of physical activity (work status or sports) but dependent on the body mass index. In degenerative or arthrogenic kyphosis, we found more pronounced signs: near complete disappearance of type II fibers, major fibroadiposis affecting both lumbar and thoracolumbar muscles, the presence of an abnormal number of motheaten fibers, targetoid/core fibers and *ragged red fibers*. All these histological features are found in myopathies [33] (Fig. 16).

Lumbar paraspinal muscle ultrasound allowed Singh et al. [34] to identify a modification in fiber orientation, especially in multifidus, leading to loss of extension power (Fig. 17). This technique also evaluated atrophy and fatty infiltration of the psoas muscles and erector spinae muscles taking into account sagittal balance: in the presence of thoracic hyperkyphosis, erector spinae muscles are atrophied; in the case of pelvic retroversion, the psoas muscles are atrophied and overall the non-contractile tissue content inside multifidus increases [35]. Thanks to the contribution of surface electromyography of paraspinal muscles, authors showed that there was an endurance decrease using the Sorensen test [36] and delayed paraspinal reflex latencies after sudden flexion stimulations of the trunk [37].

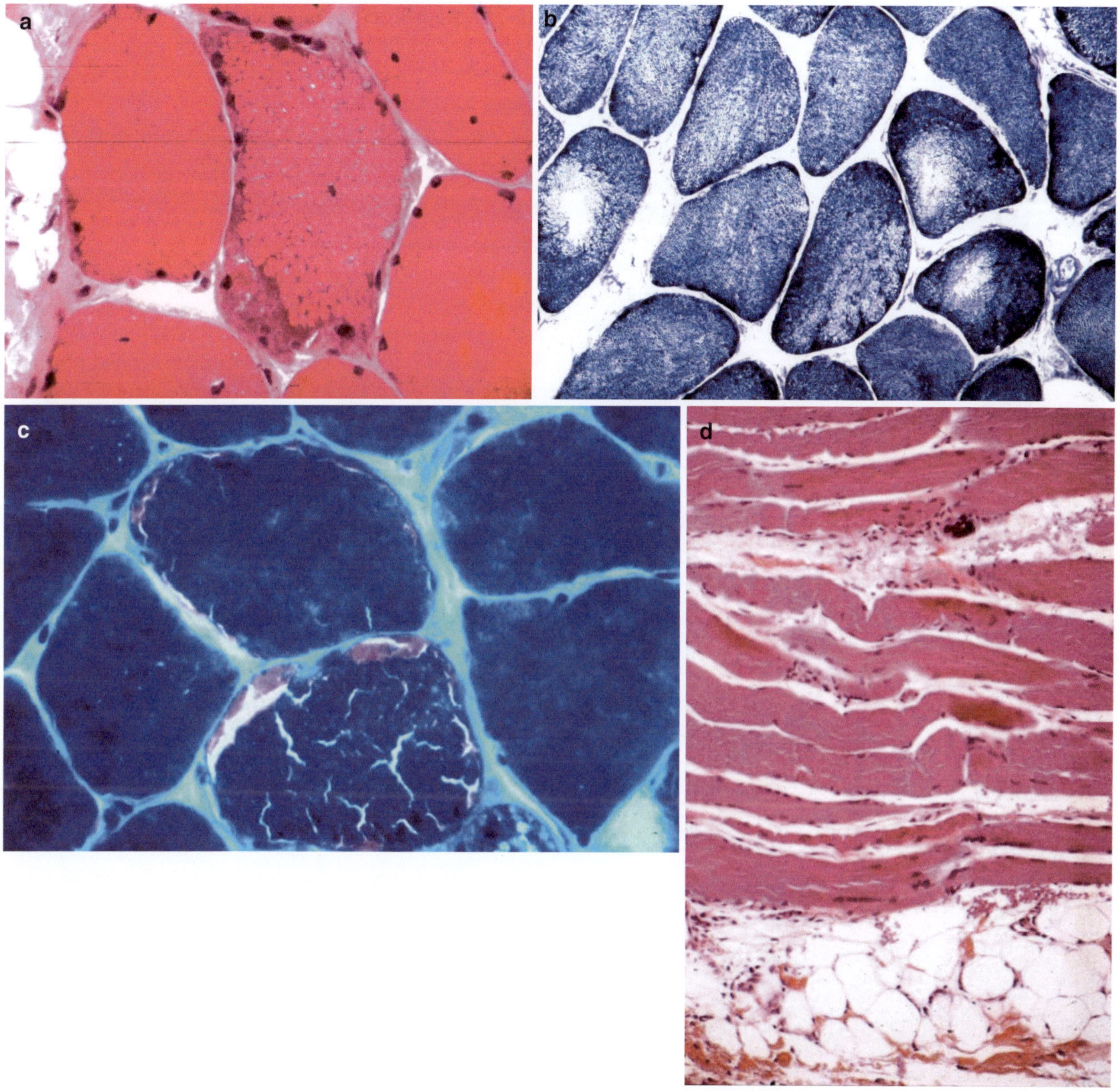

Fig. 16 Histological abnormalities: (**a**) mitochondrial, (**b**) targetoid core, (**c**) ragged red fibers, (**d**) fibro-adipose

In summary, it should be remembered that aging is responsible for a reduction of muscle strength, especially in the lower limbs, of 1.5% per year after the age of 65. This is achieved by muscle fiber atrophy and type II fiber reduction with a power decrease of 3.5% per year. The same phenomena apply to the spine in conjunction with fatty infiltration of extensor muscles. The multifidus muscle, which is the most paramedian and closest to the lumbosacral junction structure, is first affected. Then, fatty replacement propagates laterally and cephalad. The psoas muscles remain unaffected for a long time.

Bone

Bone mineral density decreases with age due to hormonal and mechanical factors: type II or senile osteoporosis is distinct from type I postmenopausal osteoporosis or secondary osteoporosis.

Axial loads are absorbed in the spine by the intervertebral disc with cartilaginous endplates (1–1.5 mm thick) allowing exchanges between discs and vertebral bodies. The latter are composed of cancellous bone surrounded by a thin layer of cortical bone. This cancellous tissue contains vertical, horizontal as well as oblique trabeculations stretched according to force lines that extend:

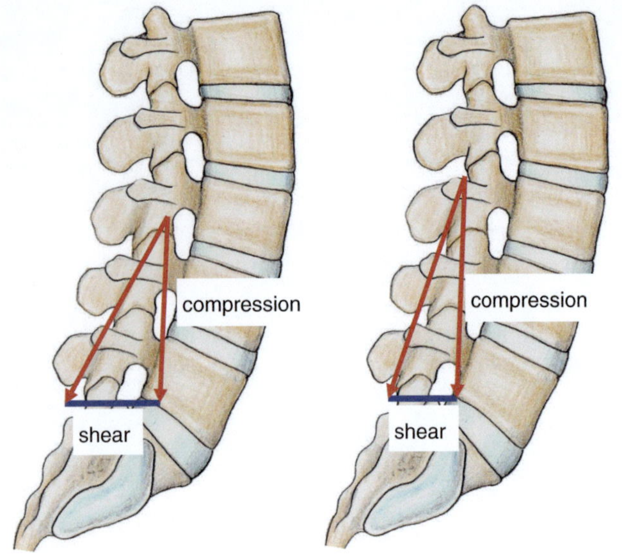

Fig. 17 Modification of muscle fiber orientation on ultrasound with reduction of muscular fiber angle with age from (**a**) to (**b**) [33]

- *in the sagittal plane*, one drawn from the superior endplate toward the lamina and the inferior articular process, the other from the superior articular process to the inferior endplate (Fig. 18),
- *in the horizontal plane* in a circular fashion around the spinal canal.

Bone strength depends on its density which directly depends on its thickness and number of bone trabeculae.

Osteoporosis reduces vertical trabeculae thickness and reduces the number of horizontal trabeculae, which leads to vertical trabeculae lengthening. The strength of a cylindric bone specimen is proportional to its diameter and inversely proportional to the square of its length. Figure 19 displays the resistance decrease by a factor of four if the length is divided by two or if one of two horizontal trabeculae disappears. The compressive strength of vertebral bodies decreases with age, especially after 40 years old. Before the age of 40, the cortex supports 45% of the load, compared to 55% for

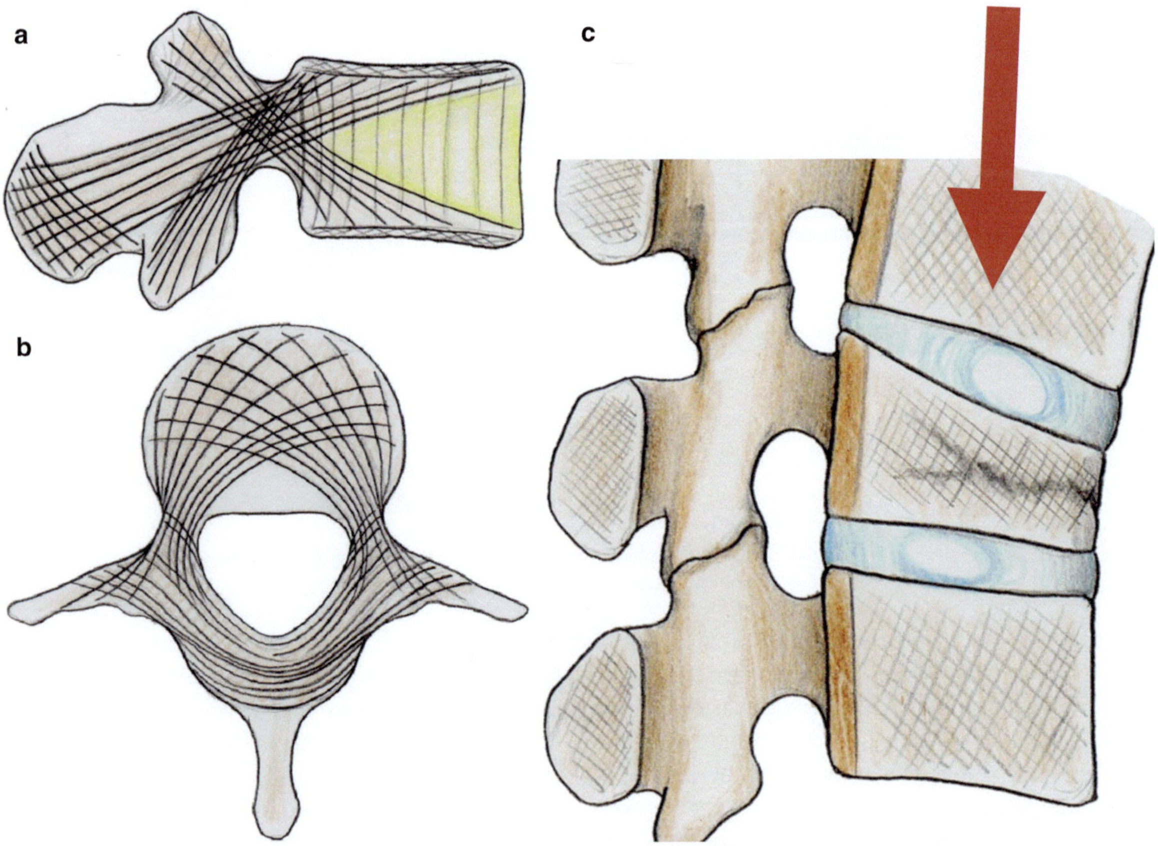

Fig. 18 Bone trabeculae in the sagittal plane (**a**) and in the axial plane (**b**); the weak anterior triangle in bone trabeculae, the very anterior constraints explain the frequency of the anterior wedge-shaped vertebrae (**c**)

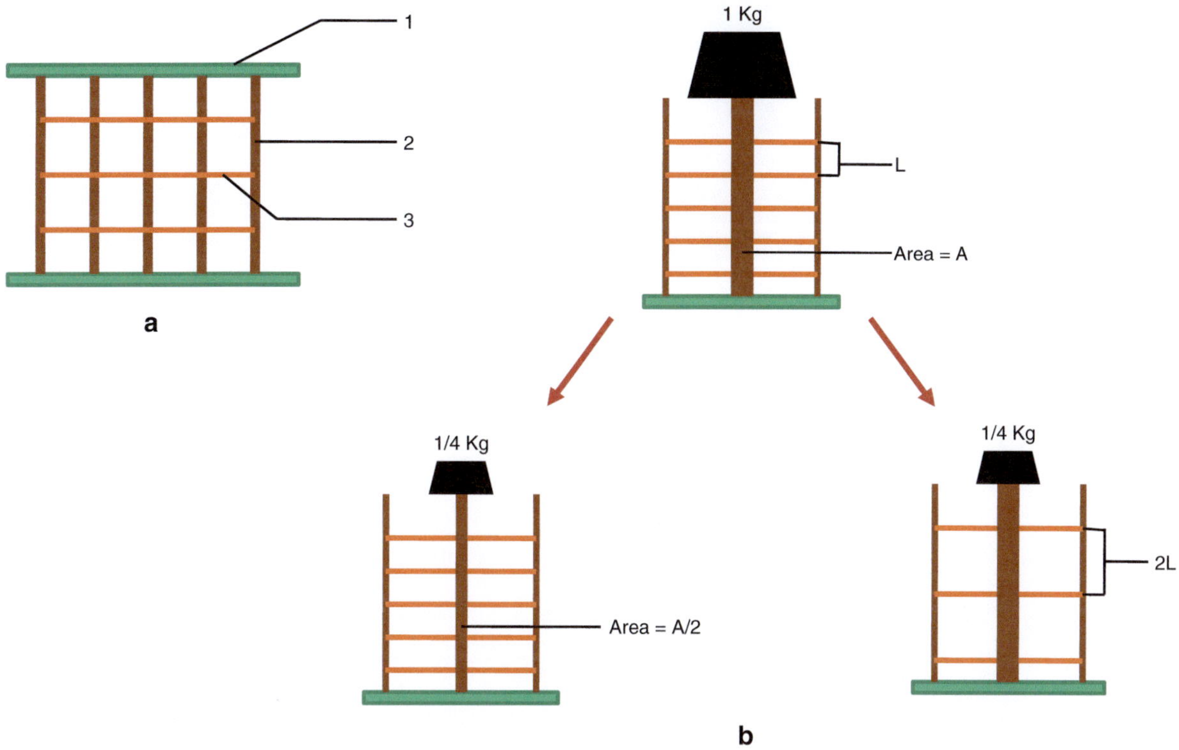

Fig. 19 Evolution of the bony trabeculae: on a normal vertebra (**a**), on an osteoporotic vertebra (**b**); 1 = cartilage endplates, 2 = vertical trabeculae, 3 = horizontal trabeculae

the cancellous bone; after 40 years old, the cortex supports 65% of the load.

Itoi [38] described in 1991 the sagittal profile of 100 elderly osteoporotic subjects (Fig. 20). Lumbar and thoracolumbar osteoporotic fractures were the most severe because they are associated with the most significant loss of lordosis. The domino effect of vertebral compressions, associated with disc space narrowing as described above, leads to a loss in height of up to several centimeters and severe anterior imbalance that can cause falls, therefore new fractures hence constituting a real vicious circle.

Aging and Neurological Control of Posture

With aging, apart from any pathology, deterioration of the neurological mechanisms responsible for postural stability occurs. The frequency and amplitude of postural oscillations increases along with a greater deviation from the gravity line. Visual, proprioceptive, and vestibular functions are altered. In the case of new sensory information, postural adjustments and the integration of sensory feedback loops are less effective. This leads to postural rigidification and alteration of the posture-movement coordination. Postural control is not only linked to spinal reflexes (muscle tone) and sensory information quality but also depends on cortical and subcortical systems involved in motor control and sensory integration. Aging requires a reorganization of cortical and spinal postural control. The aging subject will compensate via neurological and mechanical strategies.

Proprioception

Epicritic sensibility (touch and proprioception) provides important information for postural maintenance and necessary readjustments whether the subject is mobile or immobile.

Numerous factors are involved in proprioceptive aging [39]: decrease of intrafusal muscle fibers, muscle fiber modification, especially at the expense of type II fibers, reduction of receptors within muscles, tendons, joints, and skin, particularly in the foot arches, structural modification of peripheral nerve fibers (myelin reduction), especially for distal sensory fibers, with prolonged nerve conduction times; on examination, deep tendon reflexes are reduced or absent (the ankle jerk or Achilles reflex is absent in more than one-third of subjects over 70).

Plantar sensitivity decreases especially after the 7th decade. Receptors undergo morphological changes and their density decreases. Glabrous skin elasticity and nerve con-

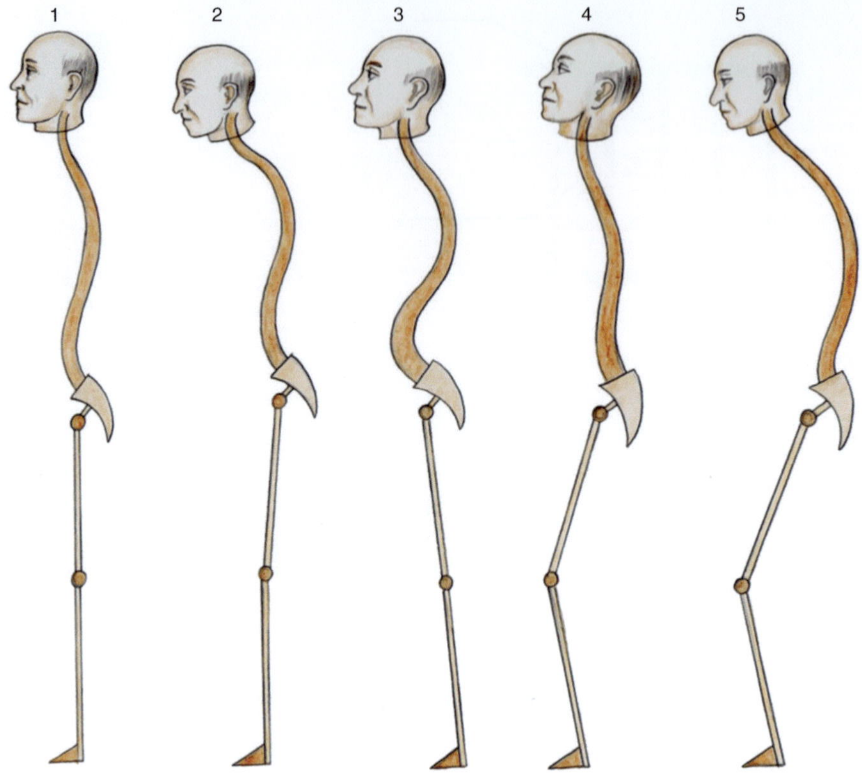

Fig. 20 Profiles of 100 elderly osteoporotic subjects according to Itoi [38]; types 4 and 5 are the most severe with compensation phenomena including pelvic retroversion and knee flexion

duction decrease. The alteration of plantar sensitivity begins at the heel and secondarily affects the forefoot [40]. Visual conditions do not alter the distribution of plantar pressure. An adaptation strategy was proposed by moving plantar pressure to the forefoot [41]. The epicritic afferents from the foot arches constitute an important feedback for postural control for walking and even more so, orthostatism (orthostatic hypotension) [42].

Both plantar sensitivity and ankle dorsiflexors play a role in postural control. Elective vibratory stimulation of certain areas of the foot produces oriented postural responses with a displacement of the body to the opposite side. Plantar afferents could be a source of anticipation of the movements of the line of gravity during the oscillating phase of the step [40, 44].

The cervical spine: the receptor density within cervical muscles, especially in the suboccipital muscles, is largely higher than in most other muscles of the body.

With age, axial stiffness results in underuse of the oculocephalogyric system and loss of the head–trunk dissociation. Joint limitations and pain lead to a lack of proprioceptive information. As a result, abnormal information is sent to the vestibules [45]. A recent study showed that vibration exposure to the neck muscles reduces healthy subjects' performance but improves that of the subjects with cervicalgia on postural control [46].

Despite its involvement in age-related postural disorders, the clinical evaluation of proprioception remains limited in the course of life. Several leads have nevertheless been proposed to improve postural control.

The alteration of type 2 fibers is partially reversible with exercise. Postural work (Tai Chi studies) enhances the proprioceptive capacities of the elderly. "Proprioceptive learning" must be done in conjunction with cognitive work [47]. Shoe adaptation is thought to increase proprioceptive feedback [41].

The maintenance of unipedal stance is a long-known indicator of fall risk. When walking, there is a step height and length decrease. Ankles are less solicited with age as balancing strategies reorganize around the hips.

Vision and Visual Motor Control

After 50 years old, there is a decrease in visual acuity, contrast sensitivity, darkness adaptation, accommodation, depth perception, and distance appreciation [48]. In orthostasis, the body oscillates on the ankles depending on the visual field displacement; the area of the postural oscillations increases by 30% standing with eyes closed [39]. Oscillations increase with age due to a poorer integration and interpretation of visuospatial information.

The Vestibule

The vestibulo-ocular reflex allows visual fixation during movements of the head. The vestibulospinal reflex stabilizes the head and posture in orthostasis by its facilitating action on the extensors of the head, trunk, and limbs.

The medial vestibulospinal tract, which projects bilaterally, facilitates the activity of cervical spine extensors. The lateral vestibulospinal tract, which is ipsilateral and fed by labyrinthine afferents, facilitates limb and trunk extensors activity.

However, in the absence of any pathology, as early as 50 years old, there is a decrease in sensory cells in the otolithic and semicircular systems, and in myelinated fibers from the vestibules. More than a third of individuals over 70 have bilateral vestibular disorders without any reported symptoms of instability [49].

Rotatory movements are integrated with more difficulty, due to an alteration of the lateral vestibulospinal tract which controls the thoracolumbar spine extensors, thus causing repercussions on the morphology of the lumbar spine.

Central Integration

All the structures of the central nervous system are involved in postural control: the tone of extensor muscles by vestibular, reticular, tectal, and olivary afferents; the perception of the vertical line (in the sagittal and coronal planes) by vestibular, thalamic, and cortical afferents; postural stabilization thanks to muscle synergy (basal ganglia) and muscular coordination (cerebellum).

The cortical circuits intervene at several levels in postural control:

- Motor control.
- The interaction between sensory information and its integration in the posterior association cortex. The perception of the vertical line is the result of a multisensory compromise. This is the basis of proposed rehabilitation programs: relationship between visual afferents and cervical proprioception [50]; postural exercises to improve vestibular control, with and without visual control, in individuals over 60 [51]. Sensory-motor reprogramming aims at teaching the elderly to use sensory input that was not used preferentially. The age-related quality deterioration of all sensory messages may lead to a real loss of afferent innervation (deafferenciation) [52].
- Cognitive functions, especially by the prefrontal lobe, such as attentional ability, strategic behaviors, and memory processes.

All proprioceptive afferents are integrated centrally, either in the cerebellum or at the subcortical level, essentially in the minor hemisphere. Functional MRI studies have shown that putamen activation is correlated with proprioceptive capacity and decreases with age [53].

Sensorimotor postural control is hierarchized. Little attention is required, except in the elderly as they experience a decrease in information quality, information integration, and a reduction in automatic movement control. Thus, more attention is needed [54, 55]. Postural corrections are slower with a greater activation of the cortical and subcortical circuits required to maintain good performance [56]. The maintenance of the erect posture in the elderly subject negatively interacts with their ability to perform a second task [57, 58]. The deterioration of holokinetic motricity therefore imposes a greater cortical involvement. For example, subjects stop walking when talking.

Postural disturbances are common in Parkinson's disease at an advanced clinical stage. They are associated with an orientation impairment to space, a trunk flexion tendency, and a decrease in postural correction reflexes [59].

Muscles work synergistically on the trunk and lower limbs and similarly on the neck and upper limbs to maintain posture. Muscle synergy corresponds to muscular activation patterns with reproducible and stable spatiotemporal characteristics, which activation threshold and latency are modified according to somatosensory information, thus allowing postural adjustments. Yet certain muscular synergies are thought to be adaptable and flexible [60].

Muscle synergies and their control could be quantified very early in the setting of the diagnosis of Parkinson's disease even before postural problems translate into clinical symptoms.

Numerous tests have been and are being developed to assess the origin of postural disorders and to guide rehabilitation more specifically [61]. This allows the reorientation of rehabilitation in the case of sensory disorders, to compensate for a specific deficit (vestibulo-ocular or proprioception-vision relationships…). This minimizes the mechanical repercussions associated with postural disorders related to age or specific pathologies (static disorders, falls, lumbar spinal stenosis…).

Functional Alterations Associated with Aging

Postures and Dynamic Balances in Normal Adults

In all vertebrates, a *polyarticular structure*, foldable/unfoldable, made of articulated rigid segments was the solution selected by evolution to support the body and allows it to move in an unknown, irregular environment with multiple obstacles. Evolution favors flexibility at the expense of specialization, thus enabling a considerable number of tasks in the three spatial dimensions.

This solution displays the advantages listed below:

- to provide a very strong and rigid frame thanks to the mechanical qualities of bone tissue and its *adaptive remodeling* capacities under the effect of repeated mechanical stresses,
- to impose kinematic *guidance* to each segment and thus to achieve the same coordinate of the distal segment with a

given approach vector, using several configurations of the proximal segments,

- to *amplify* movements by summing angular motions, which leads to a remarkable acceleration of extremities.

Besides, this was the chosen solution to build humanoid robots.

However, despite the existence of numerous devices permitting automatic mechanical stops and cam effects (*close-packed position*), the precise control of the motions of each of the segments in the three spatial dimensions also requires the intervention of a large number of mono- or multi-articular muscles, mobilizing as well as stabilizing. Their programming and activation/coactivation must be constantly measured by nerve centers whose instructions are continuously running in *perception/decision/action/feedback loops*. Moreover, the main difficulty in anthropoid robotics lies precisely in fine task programming.

The stability of the body is not just an elementary mechanics problem that can be solved with some mathematical formulations. This is a much more complex problem involving a considerable number of regulations extrinsic to the musculoskeletal system. The kinematic study of this entire frame, that is the mechanical *point-by-point* calculation of the organization of each body element relative to each other *at a given instant* in the same inertial reference frame, is itself already terribly complex despite the development of new formulations of mechanical equations, modeling, and digital simulation.

Presently, it is illusory, even when limiting oneself to mechanics, to aim a complete representation of such a complex system as a whole at the risk of inducing inaccuracies and combinatorial explosion, i.e., chaotic results by unmanageable multiplication of data. For medical practice, rehabilitation and the analysis of the sporting gestures, the problem must be simplified, *but at a level acceptable for the envisaged application.*

To date, the only operational solution to facilitate data integration remains indirect. It consists of artificially moving information capture toward the projection of real events on each of the *three anatomical reference planes*: sagittal, frontal, and transverse. These planes do not have a physical existence. They are a theoretical construction intended to establish a simplified model of a mobile structure in an inertial reference frame which escapes our senses. These three planes have been favored because they are convenient for the teaching of anatomy (anatomical cross-sections) and also for the frontal and sagittal plane because they are easily accessible to physical examination and medical imaging. Thus, scoliosis specialists were the first to provide surgeons with geometrical parameters of *normality* formalized in these planes for sagittal and frontal balance. On these projections, the same foldable/unfoldable structures are observed. However each of them carries only partial information, yet different from that of other planes. It is from the study of all these data that one can extrapolate, as closely as possible, what can really happen, in particular thanks to 3D simulation and modeling.

Digital tools such as computed tomography, MRI, full-body weight-bearing EOS® 3D imaging, motion capture devices, and virtual reality are significantly enriching data capture. They will enable us, in the near future, to obtain a more and more precise idea of the exact nature of the structural and functional alterations which affect the vertebral system. Therefore, surgeons will be able to "keep a cool head" and predict side effects (or induced effects) of more and more demanding operative techniques. All the more so as in most cases, operative decisions are not urgent, as for the degenerative spinal deformity of the elderly.

However, the multiplicity of the parameters in question, both bony and non-skeletal, must increasingly encourage surgeons to adopt a holistic approach to patients before proposing therapeutic procedures that are in principle ideal and if possible definitive. We believe that only a systemic approach will advance knowledge in this area (cf. Chapter "Anatomy of the Spinal Meninges").

Bipedal Folding Chains

We will refer to *bipedal folding chains* (BFC) as the projection, on each of the three anatomical reference planes, of the same skeletal device that regulates postural kinematics and movements of the erect man (Fig. 21). This denomination seems to us more direct and concise than "lumbo-pelvi-femoral complex" which seems too restrictive for us to describe all the osteoarticular components that contribute to body balance. Moreover, it neglects the essential role of the cervical spine and the distal segments of the lower limbs (knees, ankles, and feet). For example, characteristics of the human foot alone allow an anthropologist to isolate the Homo genus by implicitly evoking permanent bipedalism (Bennett 2009).

Human BFC include the following:

- the entire spine from the foramen magnum to the sacrum,
- the pelvic girdle,
- and all the skeletal components of the lower limbs.

It does not seem justified to oversimplify by equating the skull, or even the pelvis, with a vertebra for the sole reason that these two elements extend the spine and that their movements can be coupled. Indeed, for anatomists, nothing phylogenetically, embryologically, and morphologically authorizes this assimilation.

Sagittal BFC

The Spine

It is composed of multiple segments called "motors," each with six degrees of freedom. From this organization arise original kinematics comparable to that of a *flexible hose*. This

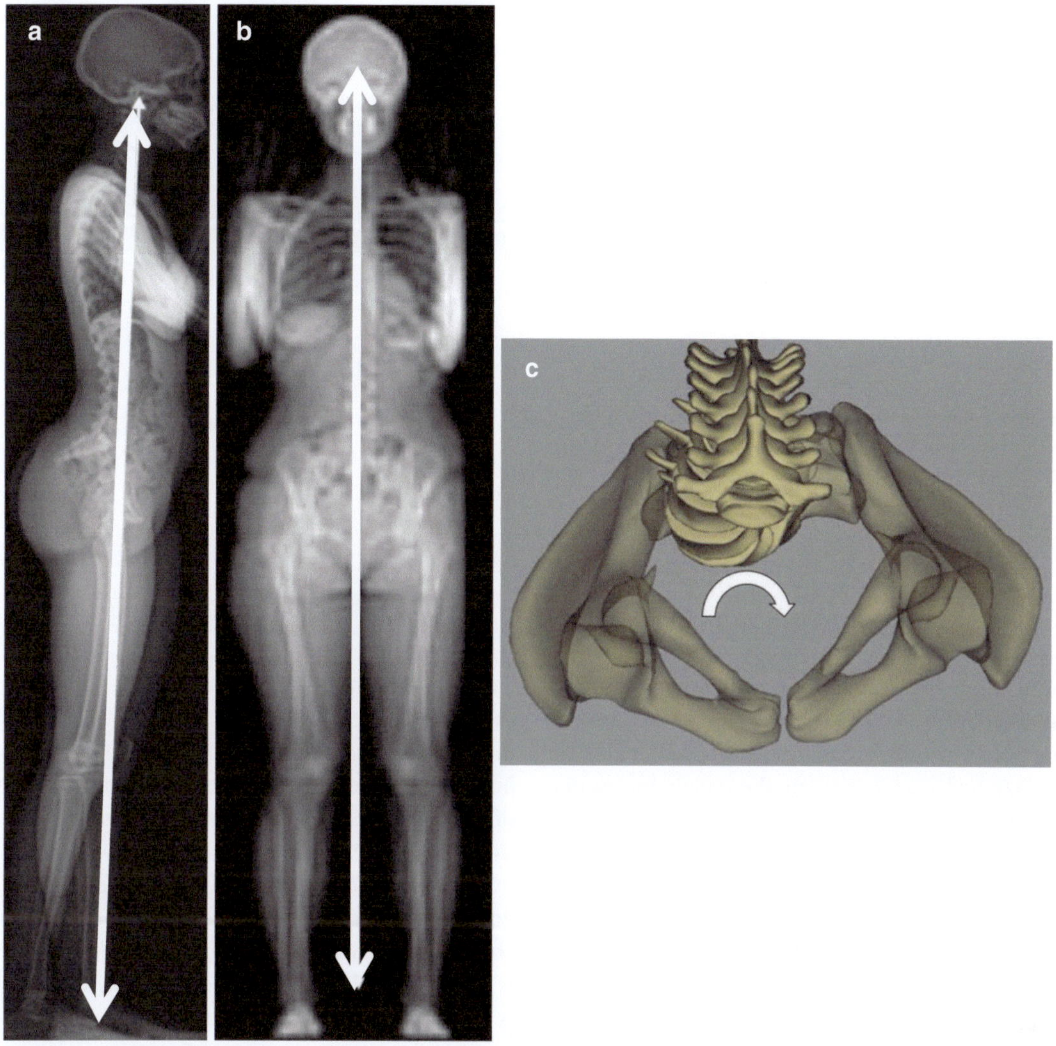

Fig. 21 (**a**) The sagittal bipedal folding chain (BFC). (**b**) The frontal BFC. (**c**) The axial BFC

results in a distribution of mechanical stresses that makes progressive damping possible on several segments. In addition, bone and disc modules turn out to be particularly resistant to compressive mechanical stresses and act as hydraulic dampers. This entire device is made of highly differentiated connective tissues capable of adaptive remodeling in a matter of days.

The *cervical part* and even the first two thoracic segments regulate the head orientation.

In all vertebrates, posture and movement stabilization *favors the horizontal plane* of the exogenous spatial reference frame, that of the environment subjected to gravity and external forces. This plane corresponds to the most explored terrestrial dimension in routine activities. The brain, fed by an information stream from the retina, vestibule, proprioception, and peripheral gravireceptors, controls body balance and maintains it through feedback loops. Wilkie and Wann [62] showed that the sole information from vestibular 3D sensors and proprioceptive receptors in neck muscles is insufficient to develop a precise perception of the body's direction in the environment. Only the access to the retinal streaming signal makes judgment possible [63]. By itself, the retinal streaming signal, which has been enriched in primates by stereoscopic and color vision, constitutes a third reference frame. To prove this point, one only needs to analyze what happens when a subject walks while reading a newspaper or carrying a filled cup in hand. These tests can also be used to evaluate the status of sensory and somatosensory functions in the clinical assessment of the elderly. It follows that, during action, the exogenous and endogenous data subjective perception precision comes from the exploitation of a *qualitative and quantitative information mix*, encoded by all sensory and somatosensory receptors [64].

However, as far as the two major 3D transducers are concerned, evolution resulted in their spatial orientation being not identical. The eye, which developed in Cnidarians during the Precambrian period, moves freely, independently from the skull. The labyrinth, which appeared about 200 M years later in Cyclostomes, is, on the other hand, completely fixed in the temporal bone. The visual field covers on average 45–50° superiorly and 60–80° inferiorly. Therefore, it does not necessarily coincide with the plane of lateral semicircular canals, which is parallel to a fixed cranial reference mark,

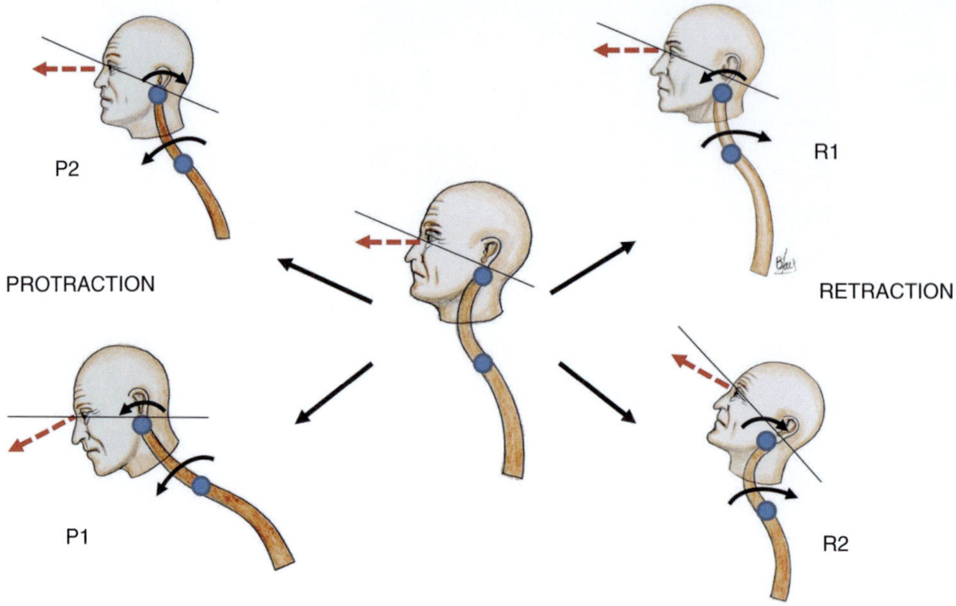

Fig. 22 Movements of Protraction/Retraction of the cervical spine (axis of gaze in red, plane of lateral semicircular canals in black). In protraction, the lower cervical spine is flexed with two variants, one associated with an O-C1 flexion (P1, resting posture), the other associated with an O-C1 extension (P2, sthenic posture). In retraction, the lower cervical spine is in extension with two variants, one associated with flexion O-C1 (sthenic posture (R1)), and the other with extension of O-C1 (R2) which carries look up. P1 and R2 correspond to the classical flexion/extension of the cervical spine

the nasion-opisthion line (nasal root—posterior margin of the foramen magnum) [65]. The specific role of the cervical spine consists of providing a compromise: maintaining the direction of gaze and lateral semicircular canals by oscillations, on demand, *in proximity to the horizontal plane.* This is only made possible by an uncoupling of head movements from those of the rest of the body. Thus head movements refer to a local *inertial reference frame* rather than to the global egocentric spatial reference frame. Ultimately, oculomotricity (vestibulo-ocular reflex) and the head/neck segment inclination adjustment (vestibulocollic and vestibulospinal reflexes) modulate and optimize information capture.

In the sagittal plane (Fig. 22), head orientation is adjusted by two coupled movements, on the one hand flexion/extension of the atlanto-occipital joint, and on the other hand flexion/extension of the lower cervical spine. The coupling of suboccipital joint motions and lower cervical spine motions creates two *natural movement stereotypes* of the head/neck segment in the sagittal plane. Each in turn presents *two variants* according to the mobility direction of CO-C1: *protraction* associates CO-C1 flexion or extension with a flexion of the lower cervical spine, while *retraction* associates CO-C1 flexion or extension with an extension of the lower cervical spine [66].

Anthropological data suggest that, in protraction with suboccipital flexion (P1), the plane of the lateral semicircular canals is established as close as possible to the horizontal plane of the external spatial reference frame, the gaze axis thus being directed downwards by 20–30° [64]. In protraction with suboccipital extension (P2) and also in retraction with suboccipital flexion (R1), the gaze axis in turn becomes parallel to the horizontal line. The plane of the semicircular canals is then inclined upwards by 20–30° (sthenic positions of action or alertness). In fact, when walking and running, the gaze axis constantly changes its orientation between the horizontal plane and 20–30° of downward tilt. The autonomy of the head/neck segment disappears in extreme amplitudes in complete flexion/extension of the whole body. In these extreme situations the perception of the subjective line of gravity becomes problematic because of an intervectorial conflict (*gravity vectorial shift*).

The biomechanics of the orientation settings of the head is known. We were able to demonstrate that the projection locus of the centers of mass of the head (CCG: cranial center of gravity) is closely grouped behind the sella turcica, at the middle of the nasion-inion line (root of the nose to external occipital protuberance). This landmark turned out to show very little variability between subjects [65]. It projects onto the skin, slightly above and in front of the external auditory meatus, at the level of the anterior implantation of the antihelix. In the upright vertical position with a horizontal gaze, the plumb line of the center of mass of the head passes about two centimeters in front of the odontoid (Fig. 23).

The head weight averages 4.5 kg ± 0.7 in both sexes. The head/neck segment weight is 8.3 kg ± 0.8 [67, 68]. This value corresponds respectively to 17, 14, 12, and 6% of the body weight for subjects weighing 50, 60, 70, and 80 kg.

The median theoretical value of the flexion momentums of the head–neck segment is about 40 Nm at 20° flexion, 81 Nm at 30°, 122 Nm at 45°, and 162 Nm at 60°, for an average weight of 8.3 kg of the head/neck segment.

These values are to be compared to the average maximum cervical spine extensor muscle strength. These muscles generate *active muscle* momentums (AMM) in static work, i.e., on average ~200 N in males and ~160 N in females [69–72].

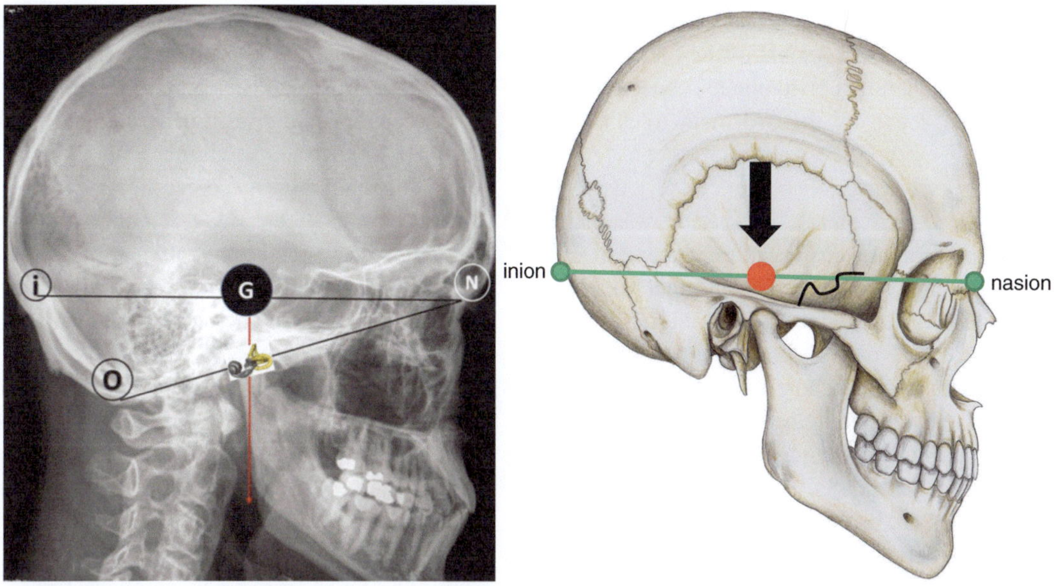

Fig. 23 The center of gravity of the head (G) is located at the middle of the nasion-inion line. When the eye is horizontal, the gravitational line of the head passes in front of the odontoid (in red). The lateral semicircular canals remain constantly parallel to the nasion-opisthion line whatever the position of the head. (N: nasion, I: inion, O: opisthion)

Values are higher, probably by about 80%, for dynamic extension efforts that involve initial acceleration [72].

However, the stretching of head and neck extensor muscles, especially in the nuchal ligament, generates at the same time a *non-muscular passive momentum* (NMPM), which increases *non-linearly* with neck flexion until the movement stops. In maximal flexion (P1), a resting posture adopted for reading or sleeping in a sitting position, non-muscular passive momentums alone ensure the maintenance of the head/neck segment by a *tenodesis effect* as evidenced by the extinction of electromyographic recordings.

Overall, maintaining the head brings into play important active/passive momentums in the maintenance of body balance. It is essential to integrate them into the biomechanical assessment of postural controls.

The *thoracolumbar and sacral* regions of the spine intervene in sagittal balance by varying thoracic and lumbar curve angles and by driving the pelvis. The adaptation of the axial skeleton to bipedalism causes a volume increase in lower vertebrae and restricts the locomotor role of the spine to the lumbar region, as opposed to what is observed in quadrupeds.

By means of a lever arm, the shortening of the lumbar segment in extension pulls the pelvis upwards and projects it forward in anteversion. This provides, *relative to the vertical line* (there is, of course, no real angular gain in the hips), an apparent additional femur extension of about 25° and *vice versa* for lumbar flexion which carries the pelvis in retroversion and creates an equivalent "flexion reserve."

In all quadrupeds, the lumbosacral angle (L.S.A.) is minimal, while it becomes important in primates and especially hominids.

Abitbol [73] studied the variations of this angle: in dogs, it varies from 4 to 14° (mean: 9.3°); in the rhesus monkeys, from 20 to 35° (mean: 26.7°); in chimpanzees from 22 to 44° (mean: 32°); and in humans from 71 to 83° (mean: 77°). Lumbar lordosis is thus clearly related to the acquisition of the permanent erect posture and to the ontogeny of bipedal locomotion.

Anthropometric reference data of the thoracic spine and pelvis, corresponding to the vertical comfort posture, *vary with age* [74]. In subjects younger than 35, the ideal spino-pelvic parameters (correlated with a physical well-being and quality of life score, SF36 PCS), would correspond to:

- Pelvic tilt (PT) angle 10.9°
- Pelvic incidence (PI) angle 52°
- PI-LL gap = −10.5°
- C7 plumb line, SVA (sagittal vertical axis) 4.1 mm. Obviously, these average values should be weighted depending on subjects.

The Pelvic Girdle

It is formed of the two iliac bones, united at the front by the pubic amphiarthrosis, and connected to the sacrum by the sacroiliac joints. It constitutes the *base* onto which the spine rests. It ensures the transfer and distribution of the trunk axial loads on both lower limbs, which creates a sufficient support polygon for an economical center of mass (COM) projection. In addition, the enlargement of the pelvis allows bipeds to support the abdominopelvic organs, especially the gravid uterus. Indeed, these are the two main roles of the pelvic girdle.

The low mobility of the sacroiliac joints under "natural" stresses (0–8° in the sagittal plane) [75] perfectly explains that the pelvis follows the movements of the spine and *vice versa*. However, it is important to understand that these are very particular joints, made to withstand considerable shear stresses. They possess very powerful connections. The most resistant ligament in traction is incontestably the interosseous sacroiliac ligament, unparalleled in the rest of the body. Only forced movements at the extreme may give an exact idea of the range of motion of these joints. The potential for sacroiliac joint motion should not be underestimated. In some subjects, it can exceed 10° according to Smidt [75]. In gymnasts and subjects with joint hyperlaxity, it can even be much higher (*which must make us reconsider the theoretical invariance dogma of pelvic incidence*). This potential can, however, be expressed significantly when flexion/extension stresses increase, for example after a long spinal fusion from T1 down to the sacrum; and explain the non-exceptional instrumentation breakage when the fusion is extended to the pelvis without arthrodesis of the sacroiliac joints [76]. One may fear that it is not only by increasing the diameter of the pedicle screw that these fatigue fractures will be totally eliminated.

The Two Lower Limbs

Their morphology is particularly adapted to walking and fast running, but especially to endurance; which makes the Homo genus champion of the animal world of long distance races (Born to run, Lieberman) [75, 77]. Their length, important compared to the rest of the body, makes it possible to raise the center of mass, which is conducive to accelerations and rapid changes of direction, but, on the other hand, increases motion instability. The long limb segments also increase the *kinetic energy storage-delivery phenomenon* resulting from the passive stretching of the tendons and the elastic molecules of myofibrils, notably titin, during the concentric contraction of antagonistic muscles [78–81]. This phenomenon would make it possible, in fast running, to save about 50% of metabolic energy [79, 82]. Bipedalism thus requires less energy than quadrupedalism, but in return requires more demanding cerebral programming [77].

The lower limbs are the most effective compensators for postural imbalance, especially when they involve significant momentum. Depending on the extent of the support surface, wide or narrow, its hard or soft nature, the carrying of a load or not, and whether it is a static or dynamic balance, a series of three stabilization strategies are possible in the sagittal plane (Fig. 24).

1. The ankle strategy (large, flat and hard support surface, weak acceleration): the balance is stabilized by ankle extension. Hips and knees remain straight. The body, with the exception of the head/neck complex, moves in this case like an inverted pendulum without significant variation in the height of the center of mass.
2. The hip strategy (narrow or compliant support surface, slow movements and low amplitude). The balance is stabilized by hip flexion; knees and ankles are extended. This strategy permits backward movements and to quickly lower the center of mass.
3. The strategy of lower limb flexion (large bearing surface, loaded, static state), the balance is then stabilized by a simultaneous flexion of the three joints. This strategy results in a very effective lowering of the center of mass.

In all three cases, if, despite everything, the imbalance persists, the subject recovers by compensatory stepping.

Coronal BFC

It involves the same skeletal segments as the sagittal chain. The range of motion of the lateral bending of the spine is 60–80° (15–30° in the cervical, 30° in the thoracic, and 45° in the lumbar spine). Regarding hips, the range of motion in the coronal plane reaches 45° in abduction and 30° in adduction. The lateral movements of the knees, with an amplitude of 5–10°, do not appear until after the first degrees of flexion.

In coronal imbalance, the sequence of the three compensation strategies is as follows (Fig. 25):

1. The strategy of the spine: the spine intervenes by bending contralaterally to the pelvic lateral tilt. The balance of the head is restored by ipsilateral bending of the O-C1-C2 joints. It is only suitable for small imbalances.
2. The strategy of the ankle consists of contralateral foot extension, which causes the heel to lift off the ground.
3. The shortening strategy of the ipsilateral lower limb. The hip, knee, and ankle flex. The rotation and the medial bending of the knee are therefore possible.

The foot is placed in inversion. The detachment off the ground of its medial edge augurs imbalance.

If the instability is due to lower limb shortening of less than 2 cm, the subject will still compensate for the pelvic tilt with the sole contralateral spinal lateral bending. Yet beyond and up to about 6 cm, it is the ipsilateral ankle extension that intervenes until the support area on the forefoot becomes too reduced. Beyond this, lateral pelvic tilt is compensated by contralateral limb flexion (Fig. 26).

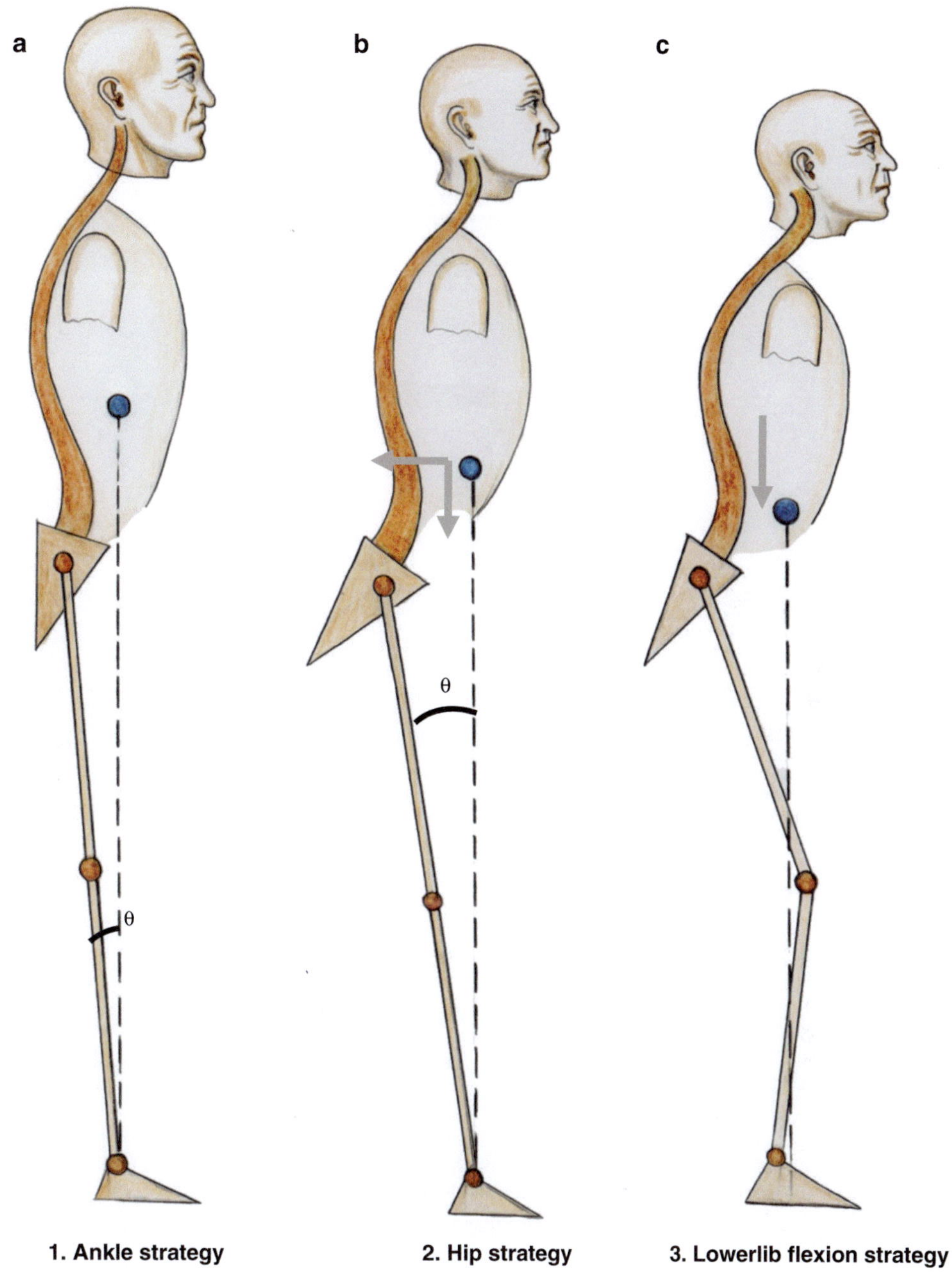

Fig. 24 The three stabilization strategies in the sagittal plane

In the relaxed vertical postures of daily life, there are incessant changes of voluntary support in the coronal plane. These alternating supports from one side to the other use the same stabilization strategies.

Transversal BFC

The transversal BFC controls body rotation. It also involves the entire spine, pelvis, and both lower limbs.

The axial rotation of the trunk reaches 90–95° (averaging 50° in the cervical, 30° in the thoracic, and 10° in the lumbar spine). It is most often coupled to a lateral bending [84]. Coupling occurs in the same direction at the cervical level and in the L5-S1 segment, while it occurs in the opposite direction in the rest of the thoracolumbar spine [78, 82, 84] (Fig. 27).

The stabilization sequence is as follows:

1. The *spinal strategy* by rotation that is inverse of the imbalance.
2. The *hip strategy* of inverse rotation of the pelvis around the ipsilateral lower limb (equivalent to lateral rotation of the hip).
3. The *lower limb strategy* completes the previous two when the imbalance persists. It consists of flexing the ipsilateral

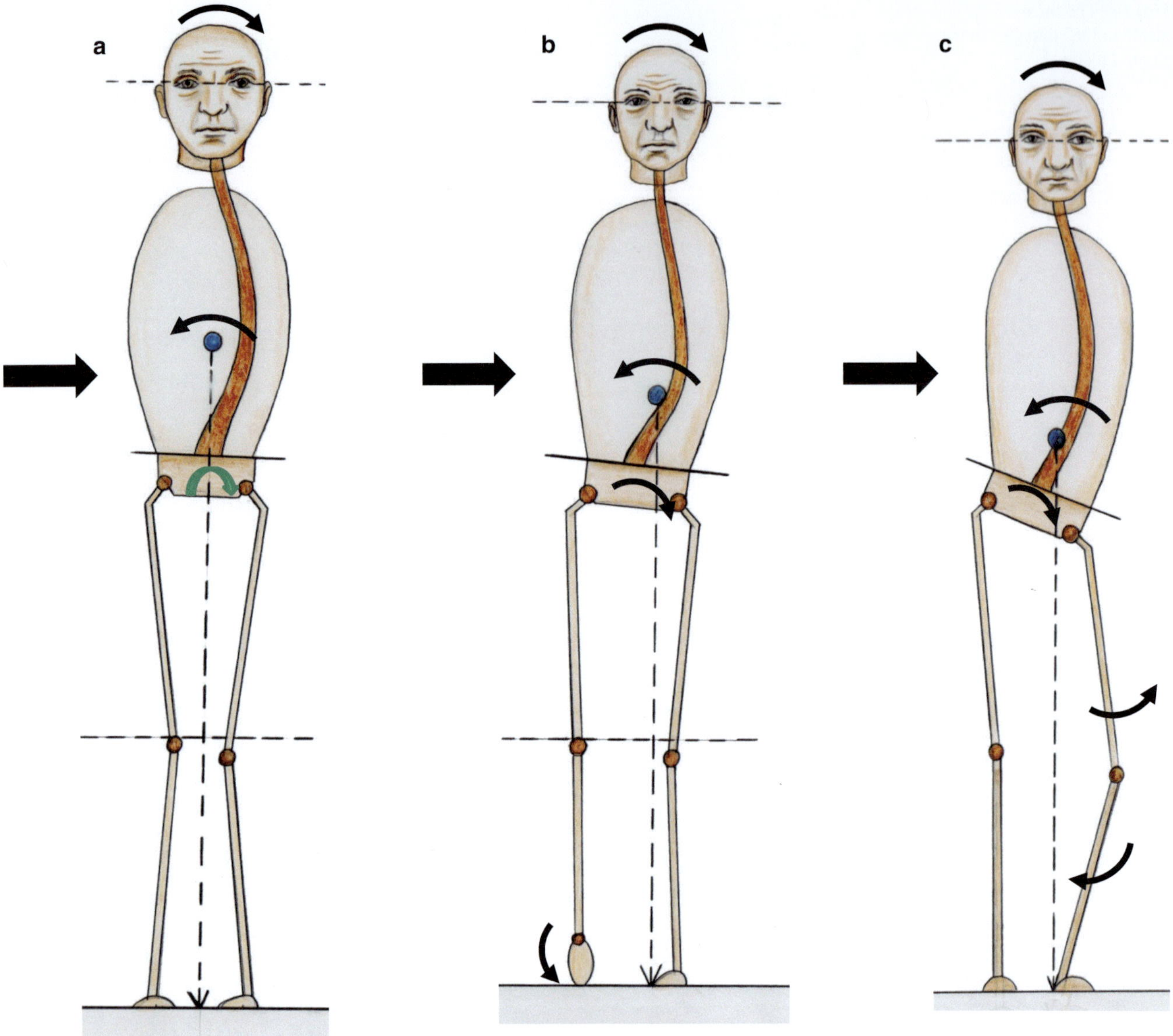

Fig. 25 The three strategies for stabilizing frontal imbalances: (**a**) vertebral strategy, (**b**) contralateral vertebral and ankle strategy (**c**), vertebral strategy, and ipsilateral flexion shortening. If the imbalance is due to the shortening of a limb, the compensations (**b**) and (**c**) are reversed, which prevents too much rocking of the pelvis

limb and extending the contralateral limb. Unlocking the knee, from the first flexion degrees, allows lateral rotation and tilting of the leg. Ankle flexion occurs concomitantly. The foot moves into eversion.

In slow walking, the pelvis and thorax rotate around the supporting leg, in the same direction as the moving leg (*in phase coordination*), whereas, when the speed increases, the thorax moves in reverse direction (*anti-phase coordination*) [78, 82]. In fast walking and running, the angular momentum of the pelvis is therefore counterbalanced by the inverse rotation of the thorax and shoulder girdle. This results in an *axial twisting* of the thoracolumbar spine. According to Gregersen and Lucas [85], the transition between the two inverse rotations would be between the 6th and the 8th thoracic vertebrae. On either side of this neutral point, T1 can reach a rotation of 5°, and L5 of 6° in the *opposite direction.*

According to Gracovesysky et al. [86], the rotation/lateral bending coupling of the trunk is the main motor of bipedal walking.

At this stage, after having artificially decomposed the body kinematics of folding/unfolding in each of the three anatomical planes, it seems important to us to repeat that, under real conditions, most of the postures and motions are the result of more complex kinematics, which constantly use the multi-directional coupling of elementary motions around instantaneous rotation axes of non-linear evolution. Axial rotations are the common denominator of most coupled

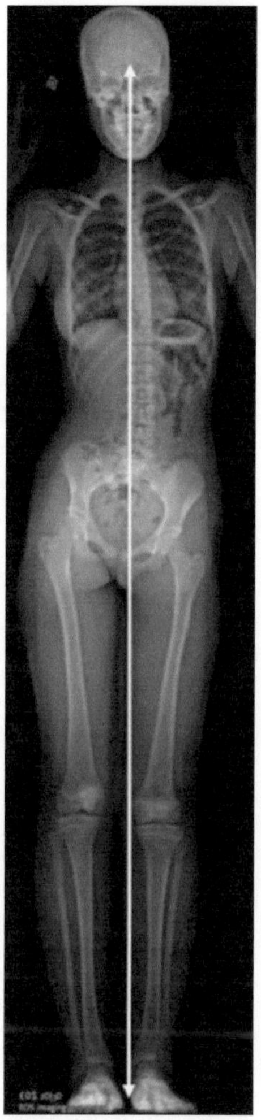

Fig. 26 Compensation of a shortening of the left lower limb of two centimeters purely to a vertebral strategy

motions, a true "groundswell movement" of body kinematics. In instrumented spinal fusions, especially long ones, the neutralization of rotational stresses always poses a complicated problem despite the use of transverse connector's which should be preferably applied at the extremities than at the thoracolumbar junction.

The modern possibilities for movement capture should allow us to renew our knowledge of the moving body balance, starting with normal and pathological walking preoperatively and postoperatively.

Postural Control

For the classical theory of body stability, equilibrium is reached when the projection of the center of mass corresponds to the vertical of the center of pressure (support polygon). This is about *displacement-dependency* or *sway ratio.* It is on this basis that J. Dubousset proposed the existence of a *cone of stability* [87]. In fact, the projection of the center of mass outside the center of pressure does not necessarily cause imbalance at zero or low speed. Inversely, stability is not guaranteed either if the speed of the center of mass exceeds a certain critical value [77]. The position of the center of mass is therefore not the only value which conditions the state of equilibrium. Its displacement, speed, and acceleration are also essential parameters for characterizing each state of equilibrium. This is the concept of *Feasable Stability Region* (FSR) [88, 89]. One may speak of a *useful* pressure surface. Even when the center of mass seems stabilized and the subject motionless, there are always permanent oscillations perfectly visible on a force platform. They are mainly due to changes in neuromuscular instructions, and secondarily to the background noise of functioning viscera and blood circulation. Finally, the standing human is never in stable equilibrium [77].

In a *relaxed standing position*, the gravity axis passes in front of L4 and the center of the acetabulum in 75% of cases [86]. In this situation, in the absence of loading, flexion/extension moments are weak. Spinal extensor muscles generate only 2–5% of their maximal force [85]. Half of the extension moments are passive (NMPM). Balance is adjusted by agonist/antagonist coactivation which increases with higher loads. In the absence of any load, the muscular contractions remain sporadic and brief, essentially recruiting fast fibers (fibers IIa and b).

In a *sthenic standing position* without load, such as standing to attention, the strength of the erector spinae muscles and hip extensors are about 15% of their maximum strength. When this situation persists, there are signs of "relaxation" (creep) at the level of sensorimotor controls rather than muscle fatigue [49].

When lifting loads, subjects flex their thoracolumbar spine, tilt their pelvis in anteversion, and flex their lower limbs. It is important to note that the stabilization of the spinal segments is completely separate from that of the pelvis around the hips. Complete paralysis of the gluteal muscles, as observed in poliomyelitis, condemns patients to quadrupedalism. The thoracolumbar spine is mobilized thanks to the action of the *erector spinae* muscles (*longissimus, iliocostalis, and spinalis* muscles) and also using deep paraspinal muscles (*multifidus* muscles) and superficial muscles which insert away from the spine (*latissimus dorsi, quadratus lumborum, serratus posterior inferior, psoas major* muscles). The essential role of the abdominal muscles is to adjust the symmetry of lifting efforts. The active moments of the erector spinae muscles (about 200 Nm) alone are insufficient to explain the lifting of large loads. NMPM (non-muscular passive moments), including those originating from the thoracolumbar fascia, need to be involved (Fig. 25).

These data are only valid for static balance. In dynamic lifting, trunk acceleration requires a force surplus of about 80% [80]. Pelvic and femoral stabilization is ensured by the extensor muscles of the coxofemoral joints (*glutei and ham-*

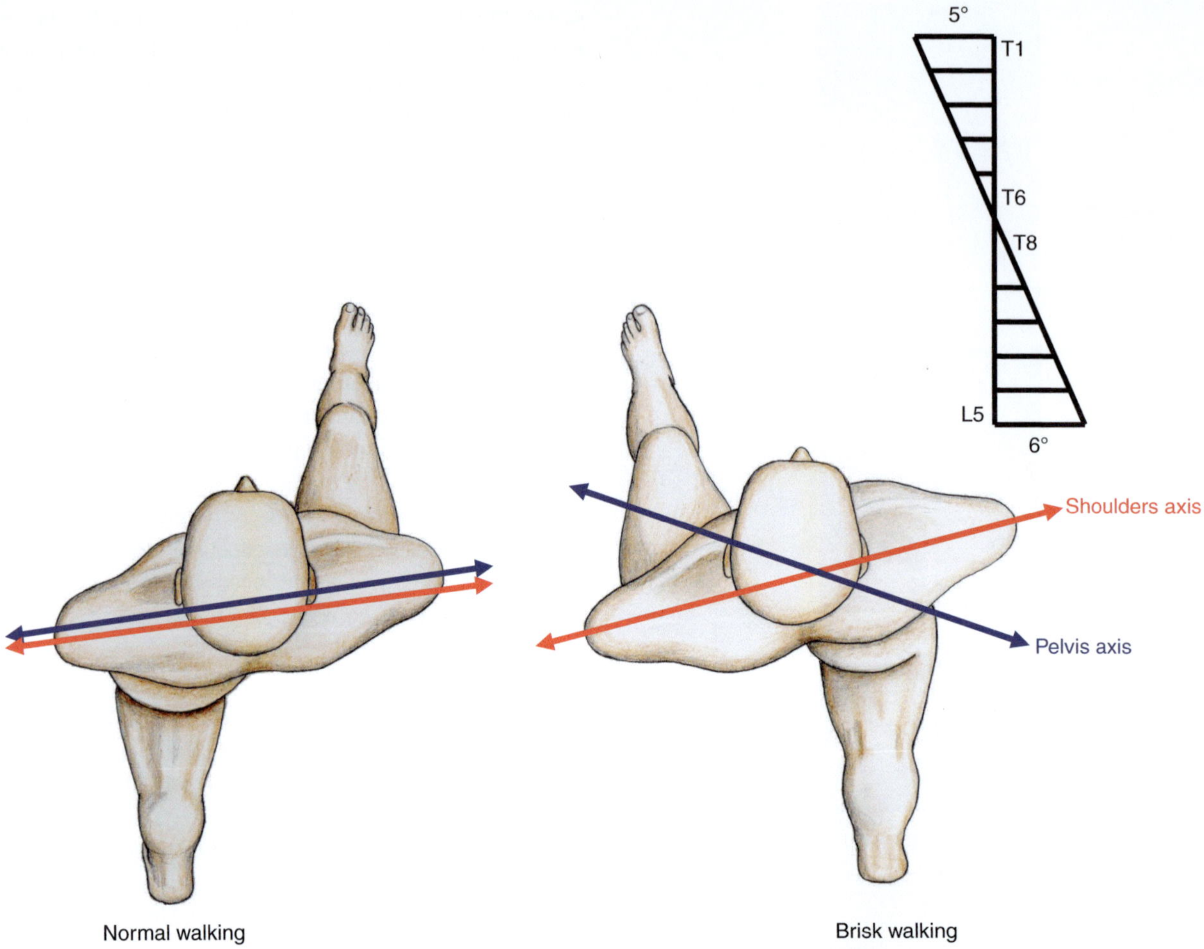

Fig. 27 In normal walking, the chest and pelvis follow the bony limb. In brisk walking the transverse axis of the pelvis and that of the thorax intersect. This results in an axial twisting of the vertebral column

string muscles), the moments of which are considerably increased by pelvic anteversion as well as hip and knee flexion (Fig. 28).

Functional Alterations Related to Aging (Table 1)

Age-related degenerative spinal deformity affects approximately 60% of subjects over 65 years of age [90]. Many are well tolerated, but for some, they become a factor of disability and poor health that can significantly reduce their independence and consequently pose a serious social problem.

In subjects over the age of 60, the volume decrease of the contractile part of muscles (sarcopenia), mostly affecting fast fibers (IIa and IIb), leads to a loss of strength (a decrease in muscular active moments) and endurance when required to make a prolonged physical effort.

On the other hand, perimuscular and intramuscular connective tissue stiffens considerably due to the loss of elastin fibers and the thickening with crosslinking of the collagen fibers. A significant increase in non-muscular passive moments ensues. From a certain amplitude of thoracolumbar flexion and pelvic retroversion, the NMPM alone ensure most of the sagittal balance by a *tenodesis effect.* This mode of postural control has virtually no metabolic cost.

Thus, spontaneously, because of a lower energy cost and also because of an altered representation of the spinal system at the level of the central nervous system, the elderly prefers, between two tasks, keeping the same leaning forward attitude rather than getting up each time as younger subjects would do.

The impact of energy costs on seniors can be appreciated by measuring their VO_2 Max. In the elderly, the decrease in VO_2 Max is one of the most easily observable parameters of the collapse in material/metabolic energy fluxes: at 85, it is on average 18 ml/min/kg for men, and 16 ml/min/kg in women. According to Paterson et al. [91], a value of 14 ml/min/kg corresponds to the minimal physical aptitude necessary to perform the motor activities of daily life. Its measurement should be systematic in the preoperative decision-making process. Indeed, in the postoperative phase, the straightening of an elongated trunk by deformity correction and instrumented fusion theoretically presents much higher energy costs.

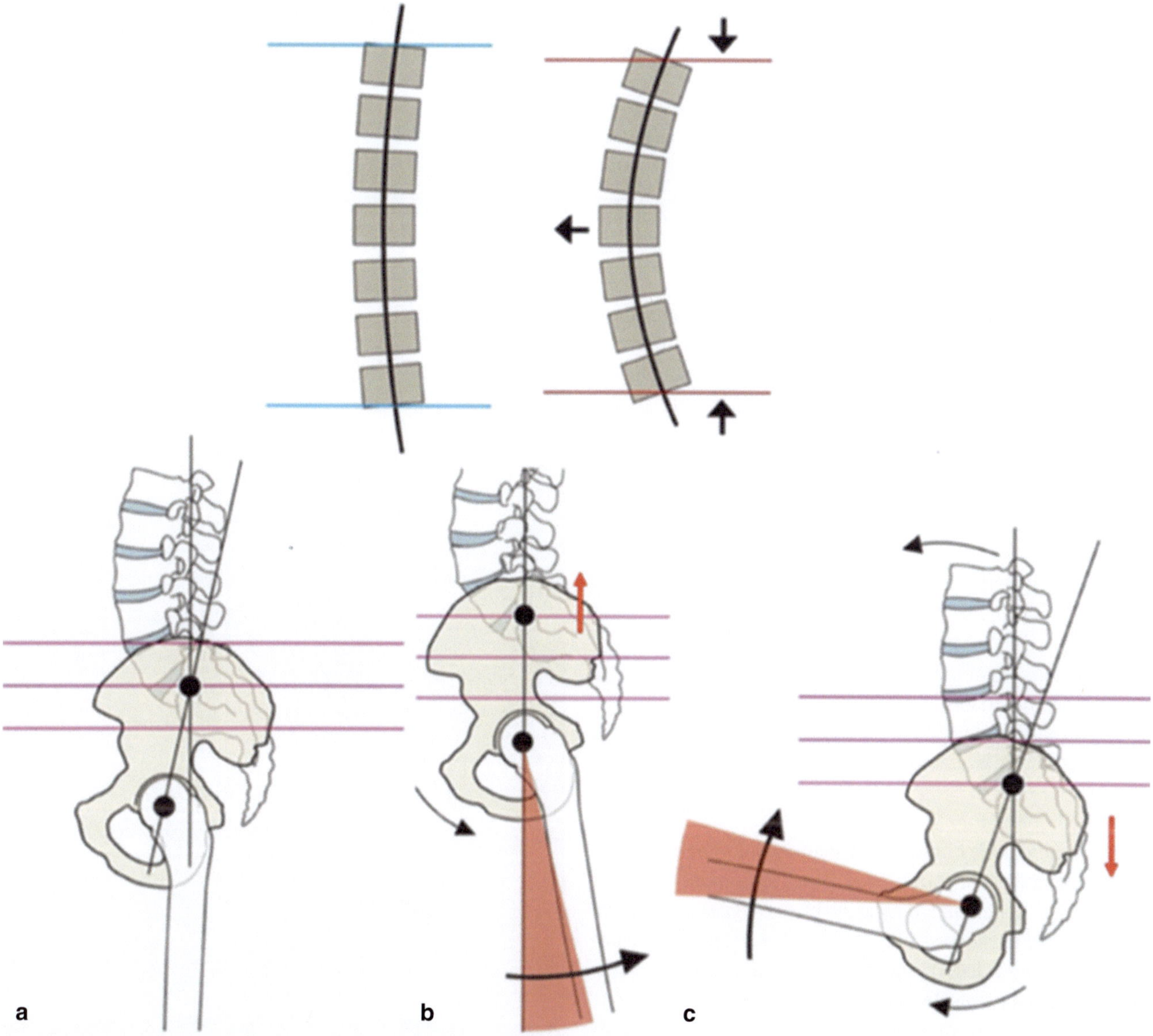

Fig. 28 Kinematics of the lumbar and pelvic couple: The extension of the lumbar spine pulls the pelvis upwards and forwards (anteversion), and thus increases the amplitude of the femur extension compared to the vertical. The flexion of the lumbar segment causes pelvic girdle retroversion and a relative increase in flexion of the femurs

Table 1 Age-related changes in vertebral parameters (with permission of Yoshida et al. [43])

Decades	6th	7th	8th	9th	10th	*p*
Number of subjects	36	176	315	136	8	
Male, number, %	14 (38.9)	73 (41.5)	109 (34.6)	68 (50.0)	3 (37.5)	0.1336
CCG-C7	28.5 ± 13.7	29.2 ± 18.5	29.9 ± 21.7	37.1 ± 22.1	41.1 ± 26.1	0.0006
C7 SVA	29.6 ± 36.4	27.2 ± 31.6	48.9 ± 43.6	80.8 ± 50.7	79.6 ± 42.2	<0.0001
CCG-SVA	58.1 ± 40.2	56.9 ± 37.8	78.8 ± 49.9	117.9 ± 57.9	120.6 ± 56.4	<0.0001
C2-C7 angle	12.3 ± 9.4	12.4 ± 9.1	13.9 ± 9.9	15.1 ± 10.2	18.3 ± 7.8	0.0165
TK (°)	29.5 ± 10.6	33.3 ± 12.4	35.7 ± 13.5	40.0 ± 15.9	39.4 ± 5.5	<0.0001
LL (°)	42.5 ± 10.7	42.5 ± 13.5	40.7 ± 15.6	39.8 ± 17.4	39.3 ± 15.2	0.0002
PI (°)	47.8 ± 8.7	48.3 ± 10.6	49.2 ± 12.5	49.8 ± 10.9	49.2 ± 5.6	0.1471
SS (°)	32.3 ± 7.5	31.9 ± 9.7	30.5 ± 11.6	27.2 ± 10.8	31.3 ± 8.4	<0.0001

Age-related changes in CCG-C7 SVA, CGS SVA, C7 SVA C2-C7 lordosis angle, CT, LL, IP and PS on 671 subjects
CCG cranial center of gravity, *SVA* sagittal vertical axis, *TK* thoracic kyphosis, *LL* lumbar lordosis, *PI* pelvic incidence, *SS* sacral slope

To maintain the balance of the body, each individual spontaneously adopts, according to their own anthropometric data and residual physical performance, *a mechanical and energetic compromise* to ensure that the projection of the center of mass best corresponds to a useful pressure surface. It is important to note that this compromise is dynamic and results from a progressive adaptation that is osteoarticular, neurological, cognitive, and also emotional and social. Adaptation to aging is the adaptation to a loss of margins in the living.

The three BFCs (*bipedal folding chains*) have their respective share of *adaptive compensations*. Standard imaging favors their observation in the sagittal and coronal planes, but 3D reconstructions also display them perfectly in the axial plane, as well as the pathological vertebral translations along the three cardinal axes (Fig. 29).

Compensatory mechanisms for the control of body balance in the sagittal plane include the following:

- Cervical hyperlordosis,
- The displacement of the center of gravity of the head (CCG)
- The extension of the spine,
- Pelvic retroversion,
- Hip extension, knee flexion, ankle flexion/extension, and foot inversion/eversion.

Yet compensatory mechanisms that involve the lower limbs usually elude clinical examination and imaging.

Two compensatory strategies are most commonly adopted by patients, depending on the level and type of thoracic kyphosis, the existence of residual lumbar extension (sometimes at a single level), and especially the residual performance of gluteal muscles and hamstrings.

For example, in some high thoracic kyphoses, with preserved lumbar lordosis (or a single abnormally mobile lower lumbar segment), and a still somewhat effective musculature, the compensatory strategy adopted by the patient consists of straightening the spine as much as possible while keeping hips and knees extended and the ankles flexed. In return, the head/neck segment is carried in R1 retraction, but fatigue can also cause the loss of the horizontal gaze. Only a certain degree of hip and knee flexion can then restore it.

The most usual strategy, however, when there is no possibility of lumbar extension, is to compensate for thoracolumbar kyphosis and pelvic retroversion using maximal femoral extension (while on the imaging, one may believe this is hip flexion). Knees and ankles are stabilized in flexion. This posture lowers the center of mass very efficiently. It is then possible to horizontalize the gaze. However, if patients are asked to extend their knees, they find themselves destabilized forwards.

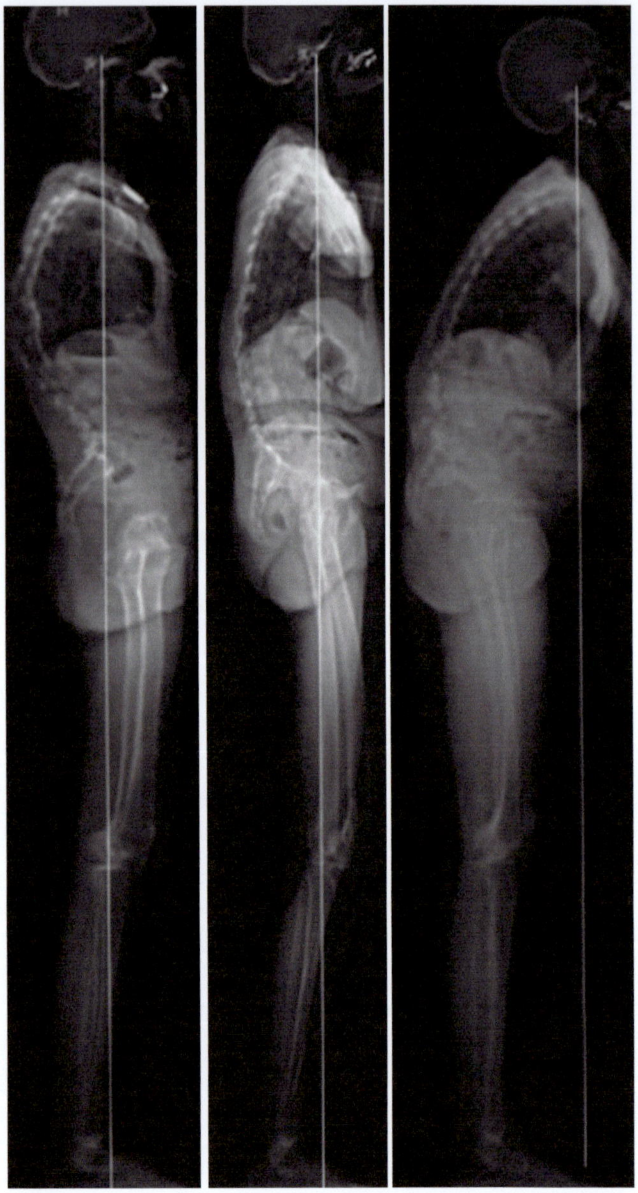

Fig. 29 The two strategies for the compensation of thoracolumbar kyphosis

When spinal curves worsen and cervical as well as thoracolumbar extensor muscles weaken further, gaze horizontalization becomes impossible. There is a cervical collapse in P1 protraction. The gravity line then projects in front of the support polygon. Anterior support becomes indispensable (Fig. 30) [83, 92–95].

- *Balance disorders* described above greatly impede movement and expose elderly subjects to falls. Their walking stiffens and steps shorten. Spinal rotations disappear in walking, and many adopt a lateral sway of the center of mass. Yet the coupling of rotations and other movements persist in the sitting position.

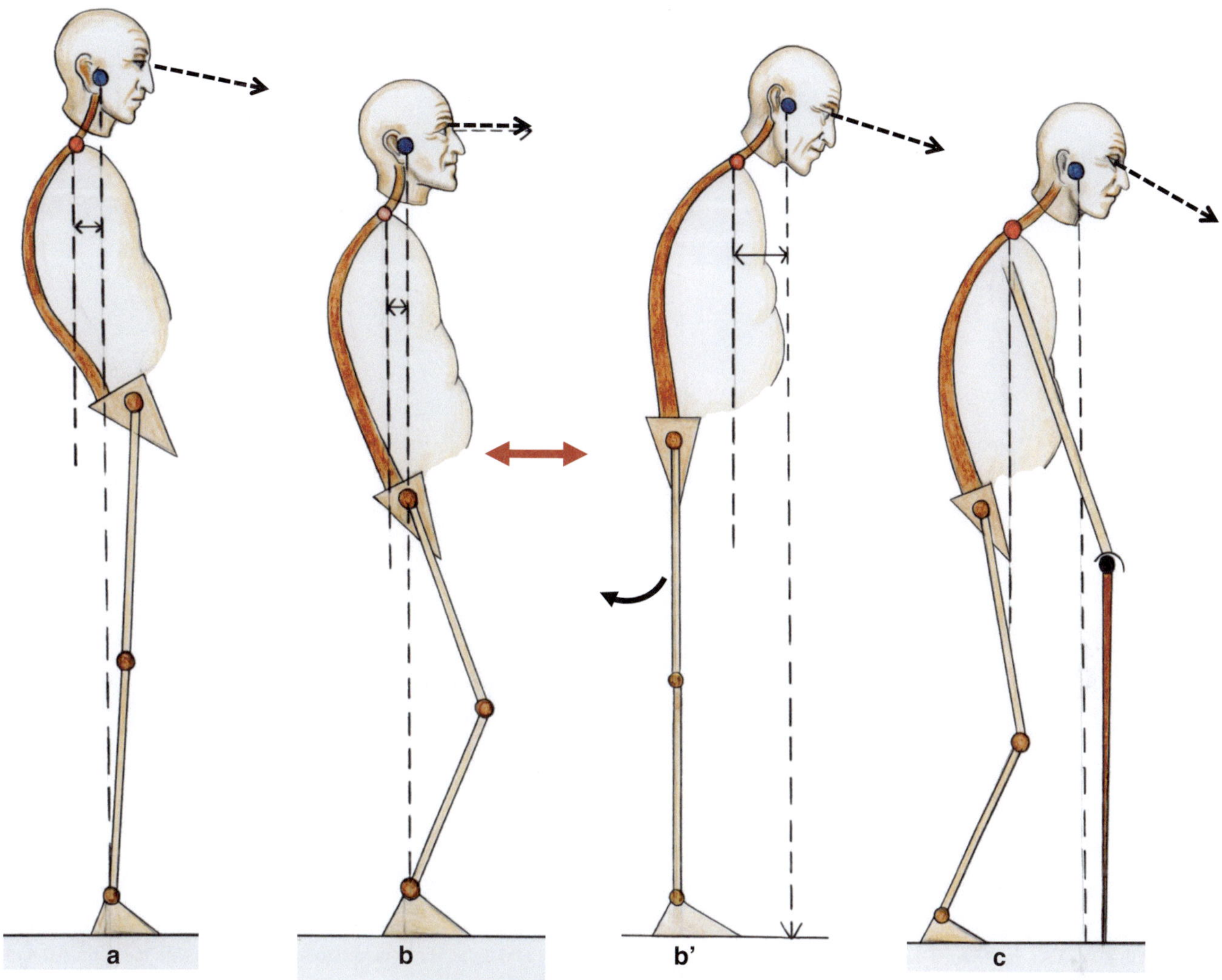

Fig. 30 Evolution of compensations of sagittal imbalance

- *Central or peripheral neurological disorders*, even if discrete, can considerably worsen the situation, especially Parkinson's disease. It should be noted that these disorders can suddenly decompensate postoperatively and compromise the outcome.

Several recent studies have shown that repositioning the center of gravity of the head (CCG) above the femoral heads and maintaining a horizontal gaze are essential aspects of body balance [43, 94, 96, 97]. SVA is useful to estimate the center of body mass projection, but it is only the result of the compensatory mechanisms below C7. Ames et al. [96] have shown that the degree of cervical lordosis to maintain horizontal gaze is clearly correlated with pelvic tilt (PT). This result may seem *a priori* surprising because the maintenance of cervical lordosis is fully active, with no intervention of non-muscular passive momentums (NMPM), contrary to what is observed at the level of the spine and pelvis. However, the analysis of cervical compensatory mechanisms shows that it predominates in O-C1 and therefore solicits muscles which momentum, with respect to this joint, is particularly favorable, such as the occipito-scapular muscles (*trapezius and levator scapularis* muscles) or long muscles, occipitospinous muscles (*splenius capitis* muscle), as well as the *longissimus capitus* muscle. Below a critical value of active moments, the system abruptly collapses to stabilize again, passively, in P1 protraction. From then on, the gaze remains tilted downwards. The only way to turn it upwards is to further flex the knees and ankles (Fig. 31).

Yukawa et al. [90] reported the results of a study on 1230 asymptomatic subjects that showed that cervical lordosis increased in the sixth decade and more so in women.

Finally, it seems that the best compromise for judging sagittal balance is that which combines the parameters of cervical alignment (CCG plumb line) and C7 plumb line (CCG-SVA)

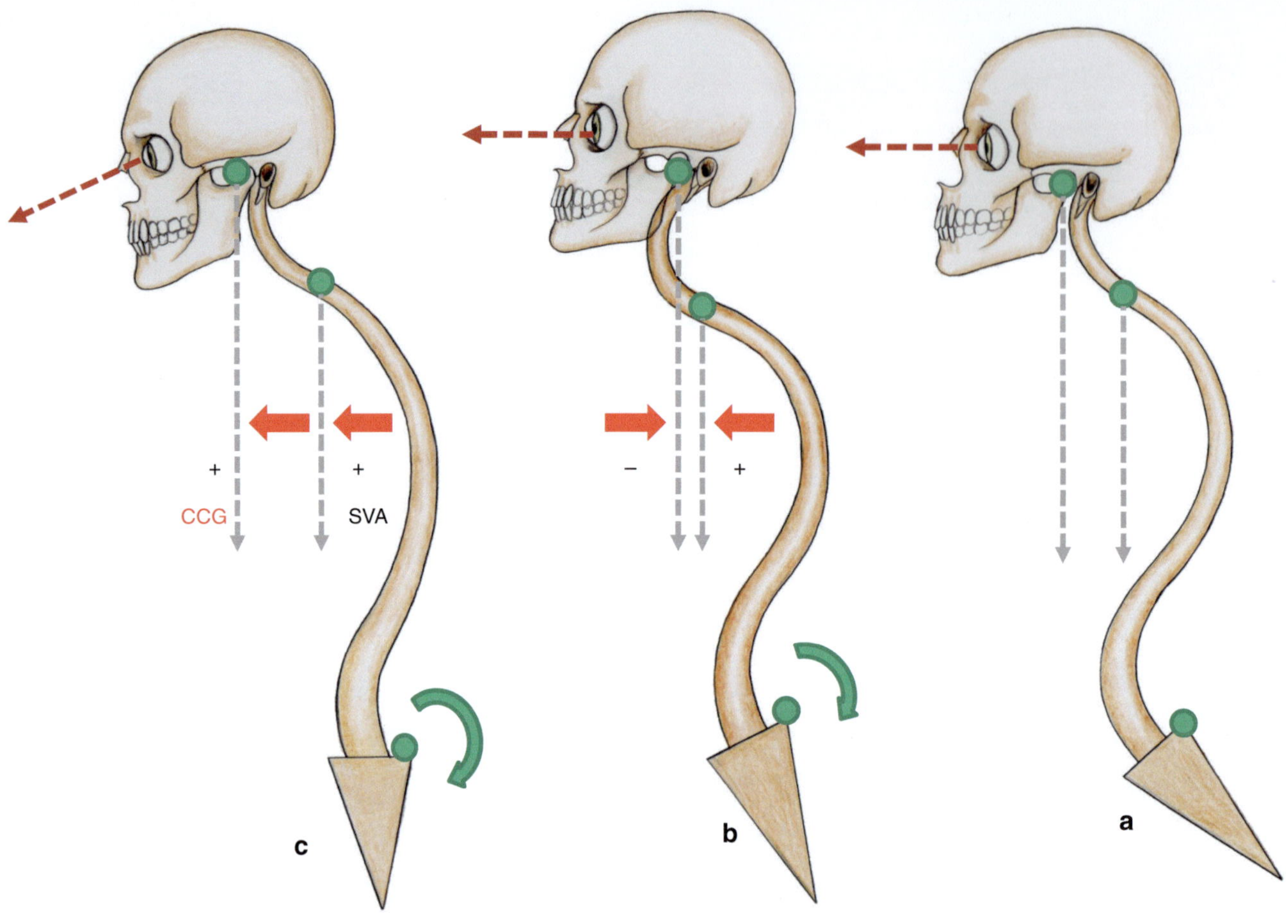

Fig. 31 Projection of the cranial center of gravity (CCG) and the plumb with C7 (SVA). (**a**) Normal equilibrium, without compensation, (**b**) Compensation to bring horizontalize the gaze (retraction R1), it diminishes the two vertical plumb lines. (**c**) The collapse of the cervical spine protraction P1 causes a separation of the two plumb lines. The gaze can no longer be kept horizontal (modified with the permission of Yoshida et al. [43])

[43]. The reduction in the gap between the two plumb lines is indicative of the stabilizing effectiveness of cervical lordosis, first in R1 retraction and then in P2 protraction before the system collapses. Its increase (compared to the gap seen in normal adults) reflects the stabilization in P1 protraction.

Body Balance After Surgical Correction

The correction of thoracolumbar kyphosis by vertebral osteotomy mathematically reduces pelvic retroversion and improves hip extension (Figs. 32 and 33). In contrast, it imposes a long instrumented fusion of T1 down to the sacrum, or even the pelvis, because a shorter arthrodesis would be rapidly exposed to adjacent segment disease (ASD). Deformity correction and its perpetuation by an extensive arthrodesis leads in fact to trunk lengthening and an elevation of the center of mass, which has the effect of significantly increasing the flexion moments of the trunk. On the other hand, the neutralization of the action of the erector spinae muscles imposes an additional effort on hip extensors. On the other hand, when pelvic retroversion correction is sufficient (PT < ~18°), the balancing moments of the gluteal muscles and hamstrings are increased at the same time, which improves stability. When the retroversion correction is insufficient, the moment of these muscles is in no way improved and if they were weak before the intervention, the state of the patient can be even aggravated by the surgery.

At this point in the analysis of postoperative biomechanics, it appears that vertebral osteotomy techniques make it possible to obtain an excellent correction of the spinopelvic parameters in the three anatomical planes. However, they do not have any effect on geometrical or functional anomalies that affect the lower limbs. Yet these are common in the elderly (shortening of a limb, sometimes secondary to a total hip replacement, knee recurvatum or instability, sequelae of foot surgery, and so on). These pathologies, to which patients have often become accustomed, may lead to new adaptation problems after surgical correction of spinopelvic anomalies.

In fact, even if all the bony geometrical parameters are perfectly integrated preoperatively, it appears that the ideal mathematical correction of bony geometry does not always guarantee a satisfactory clinical outcome. This results in a preoccupying uncertainty about the outcome, which we are tempted to attribute to a lack of data on the initial skeletal parameters, and/or to neglected non-skeletal factors, which may compromise the control of postural balance in the elderly.

First of all, should we impose on the elderly an ideal kinematic paragon, calculated on much younger subjects? Lafage et al. [74] studied a cohort of 772 patients aged 35–75 (average age: 53.7 years), 83% of whom were women, and 54% were operated on. She correlated the values of anthropological spinopelvic parameters, those of SF 36 PCS health and quality of life scores, and age. She found that the value of spinopelvic parameters correspond-

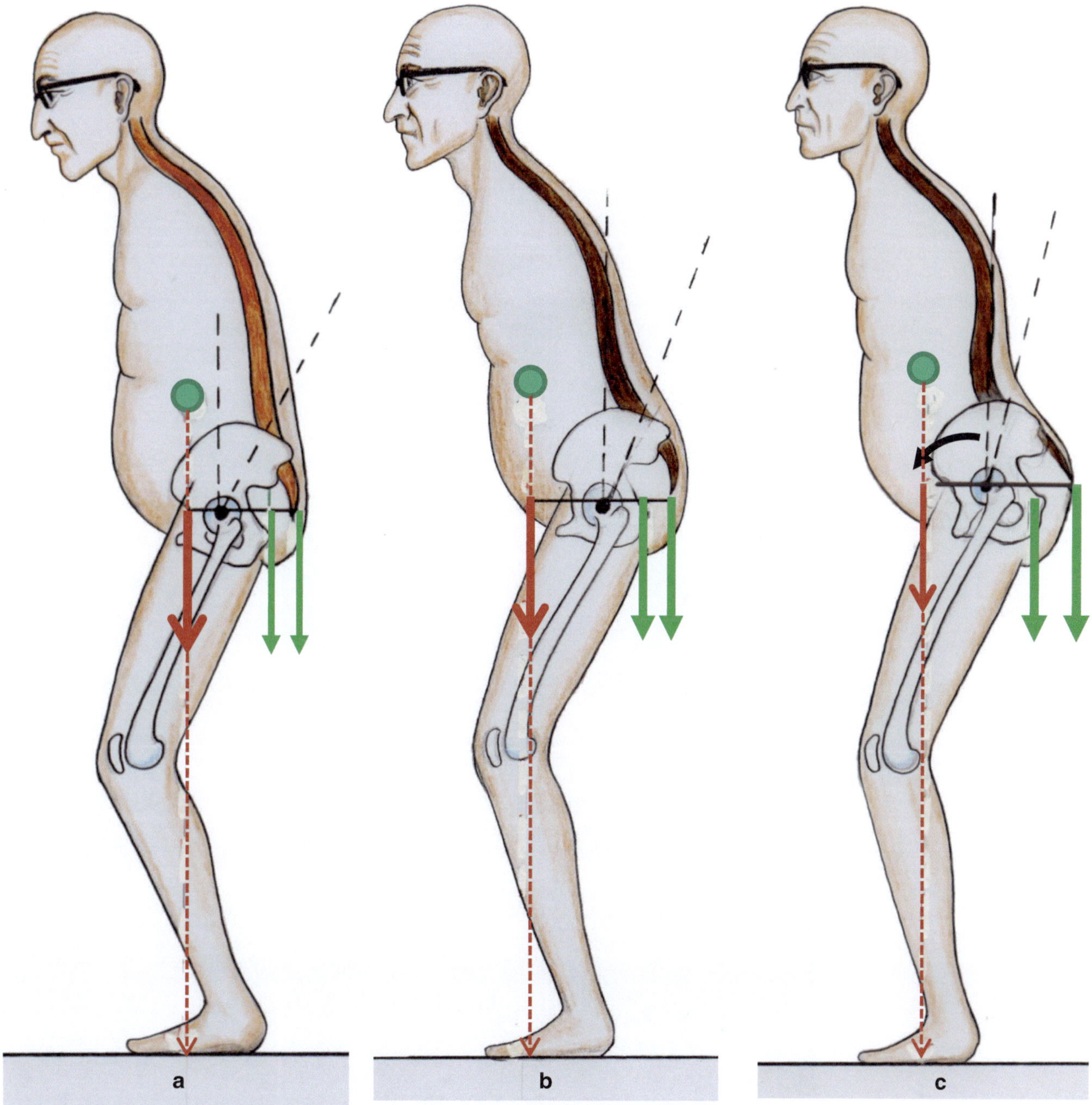

Fig. 32 Theoretical representation of the sagittal balance of the same patient before surgery (**a**), after osteotomy and extensive fusion with an inadequate correction of the reverse version (**b**), and in the case of an ideal correction (**c**)

ing to the best health and physical well-being varied with age, namely:

- *For subjects under 35 years of age*, a pelvic tilt (PT) of 10.9°, pelvic incidence minus lumbar lordosis difference (PI-LL) of −10.5°, and a C7 plumb line (SVA) of 4.5 mm.
- *For subjects over 75 years*, PT = 28.5°, PI-LL = −16.5°, SVA = 78.1 mm.

Older patients operated for degenerative spinal deformity would therefore seem to be accommodating less demanding spinal parameters than younger subjects. For the time being, no satisfactory explanation can shed light on this phenomenon, although it explains why elderly patients prefer the sitting position. In fact, in the elderly, gradually acquired skeletal compensatory mechanisms are probably not the only parameters useful for the adaptive process. The planning of an ideal surgical correction by computer must be contextualized taking into account the numerous non-osteoarticular lesions that also affect the normal functioning of the locomotor system and reduce its robustness.

In conclusion, it is now known that the principles of surgical treatment of idiopathic scoliosis in young subjects, usually equipped with *a robust system* (in the sense of the automation specialists), cannot be simply transposed to the elderly. The problem of these patients is much more complicated. The solution necessarily requires a more complete assessment of the nature and interactions of the multiple defects related to the aging spine.

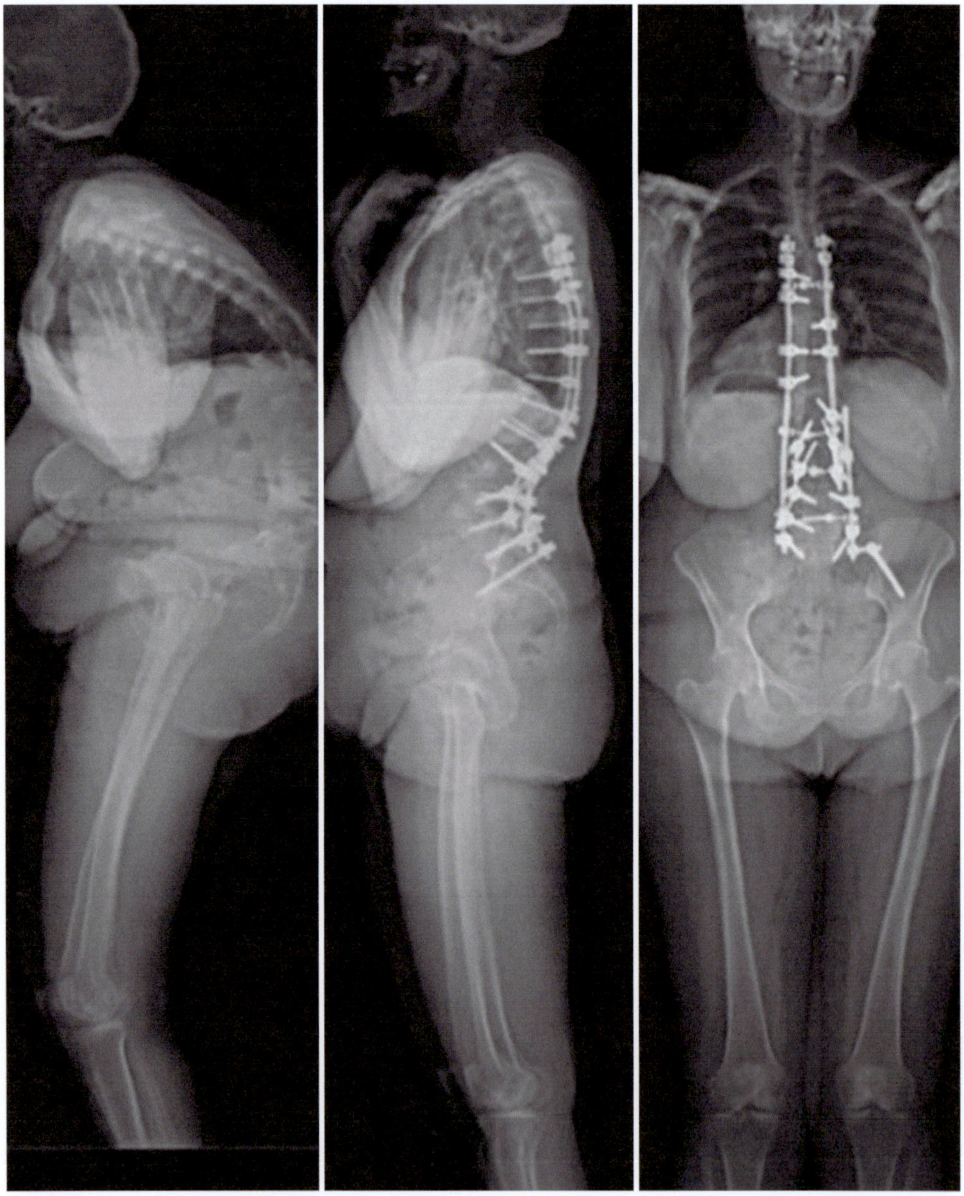

Fig. 33 Correction of deformities in the frontal and sagittal planes (up), and rotations/translations in the transverse plane (down, EOS reconstruction) (from Obeid et al. [83, 95]

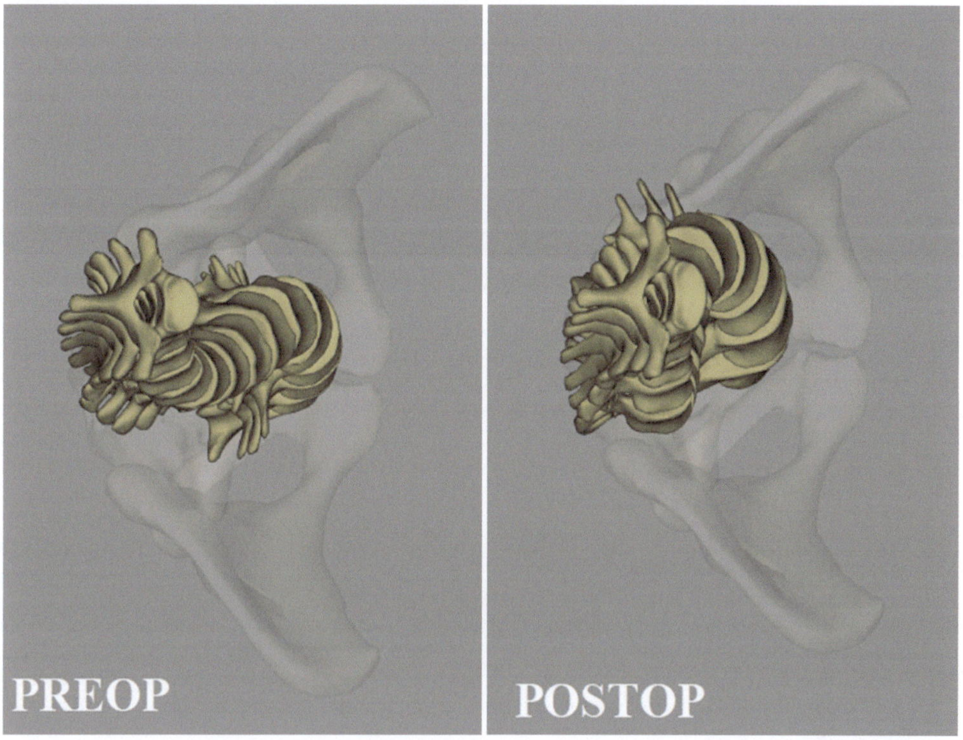

Fig. 33 (continued)

References

1. Stephens C. Senescence: even bacteria get old. Curr Biol. 2005;15(8):R308–1.
2. Roughley PJ. Biology of intervertebral disc aging and degeneration involvement of the extracellular matrix. Spine. 2004;29:2691–9.
3. Iatridis JC, Setton LA, Weidenbaum M, Mow VC. Alterations in the mechanical behavior of the human lumbar nucleus pulposus with degeneration and aging. J Orthop Res. 1997;15(2):318–22.
4. Roberts S, Evans H, Trivedi J, Menage J. Histology and pathology of the human intervertebral disc. J Bone Joint Surg. 2006;88A(Suppl 2):10–4.
5. Urban JPG, Smith S, Fairbank JCT. Nutrition of the intervertebral disc. Spine. 2004;29:2700–9.
6. Battie MC, Videman T. Lumbar disc degeneration: epidemiology and genetics. J Bone Joint Surg. 2006;88A(Suppl 2):3–9.
7. Sambrook PN, Macgregor AJ, Spector TD. Genetic influences on cervical and lumbar disc degeneration: a magnetic resonance imaging study in twins. Arthritis Rheum. 1999;42(2):366–72.
8. Matsumoto M, Okada E, Ichihara D, Watanabe K, Chiba K, Toyama Y, Fujiwara H, Momoshima S, Nishiwaki Y, Hashimoto T, Takahata T, et al. Spine. 2010;35(14):1359–64.
9. Vernon-Roberts B, Moore RJ, Fraser RD. The natural history of age-related disc degeneration: the influence of age and pathology on cell populations in the L4-L5 disc. Spine. 2008;33(25):2767–73.
10. Gruber HE, Hanley EN Jr. Analysis of aging and degeneration of the human intervertebral disc. Comparison of surgical specimens with normal controls. Spine. 1998;23(7):751–7.
11. Weiler C, Schietzsch M, Kirchner T, Nerlich AG, Boos N, Wuertz K. Age-related changes in human cervical, thoracal and lumbar intervertebral disc exhibit a strong intra-individual correlation. Eur Spine J. 2012;21(Suppl 6):810–8.
12. Haeffeli M, Kalberer F, Saegesser D, Nerlich AG, Boos N, Paesold G. The course of macroscopic degeneration in the human lumbar intervertebral. Spine. 2006;14:1522–31.
13. Pfirmann CWA, Metzdorf A, Zanetti M, et al. Magnetic resonance classification of lumbar intervertebral disc degeneration. Spine. 2001;26:1873–8.
14. Modic M, Masaryk TJ, Ross JS, Carter JR. Imaging of the degenerative disc disease. Radiology. 1988;168:177–86.
15. Stokes IAF, Iatridis JC. Mechanical conditions that accelerate intervertebral disc degeneration: over-load versus immobilization. Spine. 2004;29:2224–32.
16. Hutton WC, Elmer WA, Hyon S, Toribatake Y, Tomita K, et al. The effect of hydrostatic pressure on intervertebral disc metabolism. Spine. 1999;24:1507–15.
17. Handa T, Ishihara H, Ohshima H, Osada R, Tsuji H, Obata K. Effects of hydrostatic pressure on matrix synthesis and matrix metalloproteinase production in the human lumbar intervertebral disc. Spine. 1997;22:1085–91.
18. Rannou F, Mayoux-Benhamou MA, Poiraudeau S, Revel M. Disque intervertebral et structures voisins de la colonne lombaire : anatomie, biologie, physiologie et biomécanique. Enc Med Chirg App Locom. 2004;480:A.10.
19. Kauppila LI, Pentilla A, Karnunen PJ, Lalu K, Hannikainen P. Lumbar disc degeneration and atherosclerosis of abdominal aorta. Spine. 1994;8:923–9.
20. Zhang Z, Chan Q, Anthony MP, Samartzis D, Cheung KM, Khong PL, Kim M. Age-related diffusion patterns in human lumbar intervertebral discs: a pilot study in asymptomatic subjects. Magn Reson Imaging. 2012;30(2):181–8.
21. Brinjikji W, Diehn FE, Jarvik JG, Carr CM, Kallmes DF, Murad MH, Luetmer PH. MRI findings of disc degeneration are more prevalent in adults with low back pain than in asymptomatic controls: a systematic review and meta-analysis. AJNR Am J Neuroradiol. 2015;36(12):2394–9.

22. Pollintine P, Van Tunen MS, Luo J, Brown MD, Dolan P, Adams MA. Time-dependent compressive deformation of the ageing spine: relevance to spinal stenosis. Spine. 2010;35(4):386–94.
23. Videman T, Battie MC, Gibbons LE, Gill K. Aging changes in lumbar discs and vertebrae and their interaction: a 15-year follow-up study. Spine J. 2014;14(3):469–78.
24. Okada E, Matsumoto M, Ichihara D, Chiba K, Toyama Y, Fujiwara H, Momoshima S, Nishiwaki Y, Hashimoto T, Ogawa J, Watanabe M, Takahata T. Does the sagittal alignment of the cervical spine have an impact on disc degeneration? Minimum 10-year follow-up of asymptomatic volunteers. Eur Spine J. 2009;18(11):1644–51.
25. Okada E, Matsumoto M, Ichihara D, Chiba K, Toyama Y, Fujiwara H, Momoshima S, Nishiwaki Y, Hashimoto T, Ogawa J, Watanabe M, Takahata T. Aging of the cervical spine in healthy volunteers: a 10-year longitudinal magnetic resonance imaging study. Spine. 2009;34(7):706–12.
26. Weishaupt D, Zanetti M, Boos N, Hodler J. MR imaging and CT in osteoarthritis of the lumbar facet joints. Skeletal Radiol. 1999;28:215–9.
27. Wang J, Yang X. Age-related changes in the orientation of lumbar facet joints. Spine. 2009;34:E596–8.
28. Grogan J, Nowicki BH, Schmidt TA, et al. Lumbar fact joint tropism does not accelerate degeneration of the facet joints. Am J Neuroradiol. 1997;18:1325–9.
29. Aylott CEW, Puna R, Robertson PA, Walker C. Spinous process morphology: the effect of ageing through adulthood on spinous process size and relationship to sagittal balance. Eur Spine J. 2012;21:1007–12.
30. Hadar H, Gadoth N, Heifetz M. Fatty replacement of lower paraspinal muscles: normal and neuromuscular disorders. Am J Neuro Radiol. 1989;141:895–8.
31. Cruz-Jentoft AJ, Baeyens JP, Bauer JM, et al. Sarcopenia: European consensus on definition and diagnosis: report of the European Working Group on Sarcopenia in older people. Age Aging. 2010;39:412–23.
32. Fortin M, Videman T, Gibbons LE, Battie M. Paraspinal muscle morphology and composition: a 15-yr longitudinal magnetic resonance imaging study. Med Sci Sport Exerc. 2014:893–901.
33. Vital JM, Gille O, Coquet M. Déformations rachidiennes: anatomopathologie et histoenzymologie. Rev du Rhumatisme. 2004;71:263–4.
34. Singh DKA, Bailey M, Lee RYW. Ageing modifies the fibre angle and biomechanical function of the lumbar extensor muscles. Clin Biomech. 2011;26:543–7.
35. Mazaki M, Ikezoe T, Fukumoto Y, et al. Association of sagittal spinal alignment with thickness and echo intensity of lumbar back muscles in middle-aged and elderly women. Arch Gerontol Geriatr. 2015;61:197–201.
36. Tsuboi H, Nishimura Y, Sakata T, et al. Age-related sex differences in erector spinae muscle endurance using surface electromyographic power spectral analysis in healthy humans. Spine J. 2013;13:1928–33.
37. Hwang JH, Lee YT, Park DS, Kwon TK. Age affects the latency of the erector spinae response to sudden loading. Clin Biomech. 2008;23:23–9.
38. Itoi E. Roentenographic analysis of posture in spinal osteoporotics. Spine. 1991;16:750–6.
39. Sturnieks DL, St-George R, Lord SR. Balance disorders in the elderly. Neurophysiol Clin. 2008;38:467–78.
40. Perry SD. Evaluation of age-related plantar-surface insensitivity and onset age of advanced insensitivity in older adults using vibratory and touch sensation tests. Neurosci Lett. 2006;392:62–7.
41. Machado AS, Bombach GD, Duysens J, Carpes FP. Differences in foot sensitivity and plantar pressure between young adults and elderly. Arch Gerontol Geriatr. 2016;63:67–71.
42. Zhang S, Li L. The differential effects of foot sole sensory on plantar pressure distribution between balance and gait. Gait Posture. 2013;37(4):532–5.
43. Yoshida G, Yasuda T, Togawa D, et al. Craniopelvic alignment in elderly asymptomatic individuals: analysis of 671 cranial centers of gravity. Spine. 2014;39:1121–7.
44. Kavounoudias A, Roll R, Roll JP. Foot sole and ankle muscle inputs contribute jointly to human erect posture regulation. J Physiol. 2001;532:869–78.
45. Gosselin G, Rassoulian H, Brown I. Effects of neck extensor muscles fatigue on balance. Clin Biomech. 2004;19:473–9.
46. Beinert K, Keller M, Taube W. Neck muscle vibration can improve sensorimotor function in patients with neck pain. Spine J. 2015;15:514–21.
47. Suetterlin KJ, Sayer AA. Proprioception: where are we now? A commentary on clinical assessment, changes across the life course, functional implications and future interventions. Age Ageing. 2014;43(3):313–8.
48. Owsley C. Aging and vision. Vis Res. 2011;51:1610–22.
49. Iwasaki S, Yamasoba T. Dizziness and imbalance in the elderly: age-related decline in the vestibular system. Aging Dis. 2015;6(1):38–47.
50. Bove M, Fenoggio C, Tacchino A, Pelosin E, Schieppati M. Interaction between vision and neck proprioception in the control of stance. Neuroscience. 2009;164:1601–8.
51. Wiszomirska I, Kaczmarczyk K, Blazkiewicz M, Wit A. The impact of a vestibular-stimulating exercise regimen on postural stability in women over 60. J Exerc Sci Fitness. 2015;13:72–8.
52. Manckoudia P, Mourey F, Tavernier-Vidal B, Pfitzenmeyer P. Syndrome de désadaptation psychomotrice. Rev Méd Int. 2007;28:79–85.
53. Goble DJ, Coxon JP, Van Impe A, Geurts M, Doumas M, Wenderoth N, Swinnen SP. Brain activity during ankle proprioceptive stimulation predicts balance performance in young and older adults. J Neurosci. 2011;31(45):16344–52.
54. Papegaaij S, Taube W, Baudry ST, Otten E, Hortobagyi T. Aging causes a reorganization of cortical and spinal control of posture. Front Aging Neurosci. 2014;6(28):1–15.
55. Shumway-Cook A, Woollacott M. Attentional demands and postural control: the effect of sensory context. J Gerontol. 2000;55A(1):M10–6.
56. Boisgontier MP, Olivier I, Chenu O, Nougier V. Presbypropria: the effects of physiological ageing on proprioceptive control. Age. 2012;34:1179–94.
57. Huxhold O, Li SC, Schmiedek F, Lindenberger U. Dual-tasking postural control: aging and the effects of cognitive demand in conjunction with focus of attention. Brain Res Bull. 2006;69:294–305.
58. Redfern MS, Jennings KR, Martin C, Furman JM. Attention influences sensory integration for postural control in older adults. Gait Posture. 2001;14:211–6.
59. Benatru I, Vaugoyeau M, Azulay JP. Postural disorders in Parkinson's disease. Clin Neurophysiol. 2008;38:459–65.
60. Falaki A, Huang X, Lewis MM, Latash ML. Impaired synergic control of posture in Parkinson's patients without postural instability. Gait Posture. 2016;44:209–15.
61. Horak FB, Wrisley DM, Frank J. The balance evaluation systems test (BESTest) to differentiate balance deficits. Phys Ther. 2009;89(5):484–98.
62. Wilkie RM, Wann JP. Judgments of path, not heading, guide locomotion. J Exp Psychol Hum Percept Perform. 2006;32(1):88–96.
63. Le Goic M. Étude du contrôle postural chez l'homme : Analyse des facteurs neurophysiologiques, biomécaniques et cognitifs impliqués dans les 500 premières secondes d'une chute. Thèse Université Paris Descartes; 2013.
64. Berthoz A, Graf W. The head-neck sensory motor system. Oxford: Oxford University Press; 1992.

65. Vital JM, Senegas J. Anatomical basis of the study of the constraints to which the cervical spine is subject in the sagittal a plane. A study of the center of gravity of the head. Surg Radiol Anat. 1986;8(3):169–73.
66. Ordway NR, et al. Cervical flexion, extension, protrusion and retraction: a radiographic segmental analysis. Spine. 1999;24:240–7.
67. De Leva P. Adjustments to Zatsiorsky-Seluyanov's segment inertia parameters. J Biomech. 1996;29:1223–33.
68. Santschi WR, Dubois J. Moments inertia and center of gravity of the living human body. Los Angeles: Northampton America Aviation, Inc. p. 1–62.
69. Ylinen JJ, Malkia EA, Hakkinen AH. Isometric strength of the cervical flexor, extensor, rotator muscles in 220 healthy females aged 20 to 59 years. J Orthop Sports Phys Ther. 2006;36:7.
70. Ylinen JJ, Esko A, Kautianen H, Hakkinen AH. Isometric strength of the cervical flexor, extensor, and rotator muscles in 220 healthy females aged 20 to 59 years. J Orthop Sports Phys Ther. 2006;36:495–502.
71. Portero R. Evaluation des propriétés mécaniques des muscles cervicaux. Analyse du comportement dynamique du segment tête/cou lors de l'application rapide. Thèse de Biomécanique-Université Pierre et Marie Curie, Paris VI; 2010.
72. Vasada A, Siping L, Delp SL. Three-dimensional isometric strength of neck muscles in humans. Spine. 2001;26:1904–9.
73. Abitbol MM. Evolution of the lumbosacral angle. Am J Phys Anthropol. 1987;72:361–72.
74. Lafage V, Renaud MS, Schwab F, et al. Defining spino-pelvic alignment thresholds: should operative goals in adult spinal deformity surgery account for age. Spine. 2016;41:62–8.
75. Smidt G, Wei SH, McQuade B, Sun TG. Sacroiliac motion for extreme hip extension. Spine. 1997;41:2073–82.
76. Ha K-Y, Lee J-S, Kim K-W. Degeneration of sacroiliac joint after instrumented lumbar fusion. Spine. 2008;33:1192–8.
77. Lieberman DE, Vendekasan M, Werbel WA, et al. Foot strike patterns and collision forces in habitually barefoot versus shod runners. Nature. 2010;463:531–6.
78. Pozzo T, Levik Y, Berthoz A. Head and trunk movements in the frontal plane during complex dynamic equilibrium tasks in humans. Exp Brain Res. 1995;106:327–38.
79. Heglund N. Energetics and mechanics of terrestrial locomotion III. Energy changes of the center of mass as a function of speed and body size in birds and mammals. J Exp Biol. 1982;97:41–56.
80. Tsuang YH, Shipplein OD, Trafi JH, Anderson GBJ. Influence of body segment dynamics on loads at the lumbar spine during lifting. Ergonomics. 1992;35:437–44.
81. Asmussen E, Klausen K. Form and function of erect human spine. Clin Orthop. 1962;25:55–63.
82. Jandy B, Schmitt H, Schmitt D, Gregersen G, Lucas D. An in vivo study of the axial rotation of the human thoracolumbar spine. J Bone Joint Surg Am. 1967;49(A):24–8.
83. Obeid I, Boniella A, Boissiere L, Bourghli A, Pointillard V, Gille O, Lafage V, Vital JM. Cervical spine alignment following lumbar pedicle subtraction osteotomy for sagittal imbalance. Eur Spine J. 2015;24:1191–8.
84. Keshner EA, Cromwell R, Peterson B. Head stabilization during vertical seated rotations and gait. In: Woollacott M, Horak F, editors. Posture and gait: control mechanisms. Portland: University of Oregon; 1992. p. 105–8.
85. Gregersen GG, Lucas DB. An in vivo study of the axial rotation of the human thoracolumbar spine. J Bone Joint Surg. 1967;49(A):247–62.
86. Gracovesysky S, Farfan HF, Lamy C. The mechanism of the lumbar spine. Spine. 1981;6:249–62.
87. Dubousset J. Three-dimensional analysis of the scoliotic deformity. In: Weinstein SL, editor. The pediatric spine: principles and practice. New York: Raven Press; 1994. p. 479–96.
88. Hof AL, Gazendam MG, Sinke WE. The condition for dynamic stability. J Biomech. 2005;38(1):1–8.
89. Pai YC, Patton J. Center of mass velocity-position predictions for balance control. J Biomech. 1997;30(4):347–54.
90. Yukawa Y, Kato F, Suda K, et al. Age-related changes in osseous anatomy, alignment, and range of motion of the cervical spine. Part I: radiographic data from over 1,200 asymptomatic subjects. Eur Spine J. 2012;21(8):1492–8.
91. Paterson D, Jones GR, Rice C. Le vieillissement et l'activité physique : données sur lesquelles fonder des recommendations relatives à l'exercice à l'intention des adultes âgés. Appl Physiol Nutr Metab. 2008;34:32(S2F).
92. Roussouly P, Perrin G, et al. Sagittal balance disorders in severe degenerative spine. Can we identify the compensatory mechanisms? Eur Spine J. 2011;20:626–33.
93. Gelb DE, Lenke LG, Bridwell KH, et al. An analysis of sagittal spinal alignment in 100 asymptomatic middle and older aged volunteers. Spine. 1995;20:1351–8.
94. Kobayashi T, Atsuta Y, Matsuno T, et al. A longitudinal study of congruent sagittal spinal alignment in an adult cohort. Spine. 2004;29:671–6.
95. Obeid I, Hauger O, Bourghli A, Pellet N, Vital JM. Global analysis of sagittal spinal alignment in major deformities: correlation between lack of lumbar lordosis and flexion of the knee. Eur Spine J. 2011;20(Suppl 5):S681–5.
96. Ames CP, Blondel B, Scheer JK, et al. Cervical radiographical alignment: comprehensive assessment techniques and potential importance in cervical myelopathy. Spine. 2013;38:S149–60.
97. Stoffegren TA. Flow structure versus retinal location in the optical control of stance. J Exp Psychol. 1985;11:554–65.

Part II

Postural Anatomy

The Standing Position: Its Principles and Spinopelvic Relations

P. Roussouly

Introduction

The standing erect position is specific to humans and the main anatomical differentiation from the animal kingdom. For most terrestrial vertebrates, especially mammals, quadrupedalism is the rule. The four limbs are used to lift and ambulate; bipedalism, when possible, can only be temporary and difficult to maintain. However, bipedalism has found various expressions in vertebrates. Firstly, many dinosaurs were many bipeds, similar to a model that is found in birds today: both lower limbs (or posterior) with short femurs were hinged on a horizontal tank whose mass is distributed over the front and back of the legs. This pendulum effect was increased in some dinosaurs who had a long and heavy tail. This model of bipedalism allows efficient and rapid ambulation. It is unclear whether the release of the forelimbs in these bipedal dinosaurs has diverted their usage for other purposes because they usually became atrophied. In birds, wing development enabled them to fly.

Some demonstrate a postural bipedalism, more akin to a tripod with support from the tail, for example, marsupials whose wandering is by leaps and bounds. Closer to humans, apes convert easily to bipedalism, allowing their forelimbs to perform complex tasks, but biped ambulation remains short, ineffective, and requires forelimb support to compensate for their imbalance. Anatomically, the main differences with humans are a tall, narrow pelvis and a lack of lumbar lordosis.

Man is the only vertebrate capable of maintaining a prolonged upright standing position, and thus becomes more economic. Furthermore, this position can be maintained in ambulation by the lower limbs without support from the upper limbs. Unlike other bipeds, the load distribution is not a balance between the head and the "tail." As shown by Dubousset, the human body while standing oscillates inside a cone whose apex is located at the floor between the 2 ft. This system requires a chain of suitable anatomical elements: feet with a large bearing surface on the ground, vertical lower limbs with knees extended, retroverted pelvis, spinal contours with lumbar lordosis, and the center of the head in the same vertical axis as the pelvis.

In this study, we will analyze the role of the pelvis and its relationship with the lumbar spine. The various forms of the pelvis are identified by geometric parameters as they induce a close interrelationship with the shape and position of the spine.

Form and Position of the Pelvis

Considered by Dubousset as a vertebra, the pelvis bones comprise a rigid ring which connects to the spine by means of the lumbosacral junction and to the legs through the hip joint. If these interfaces are projected on a sagittal plane, we can model the sacral endplate at an inclined line segment limited by its anterior and posterior edges and the bicoxofemoral axis passing through the center of the femoral heads, corresponding to a point. From this model, Duval-Beaupère [1, 2] has defined the pelvic incidence angle and two positional angles, Pelvic Tilt (PT) and Sacral Slope (SS) (Fig. 1).

Pelvic incidence (PI): this is the angle formed by the straight line drawn from the mid-bicoxofemoral axis (center of the line connecting the center of both femoral heads) to the middle of the sacral endplate with the perpendicular bisector of the sacral endplate (mediator). If we consider the pelvis as a rigid structure, this angle is fixed for a given person after the end of growth. The PI is a shape parameter.

Pelvic Tilt (PT): angle formed by a straight line drawn from the mid-bicoxofemoral axis to the middle of the sacral endplate with the vertical. PT characterizes rotation of the pelvis around the heads with femoral diaphyses in a vertical position. PT is a pelvis position parameter.

Sacral slope (SS): angle formed by the direction of the sacral endplate with the horizontal. SS defines the orientation

P. Roussouly (✉)
Spinal Surgery Unit, Croix Rouge Française-CMCR des Massues, Lyon, France
e-mail: chort@cmcr-massues.com

J. M. Vital, D. T. Cawley (eds.), *Spinal Anatomy*, https://doi.org/10.1007/978-3-030-20925-4_6

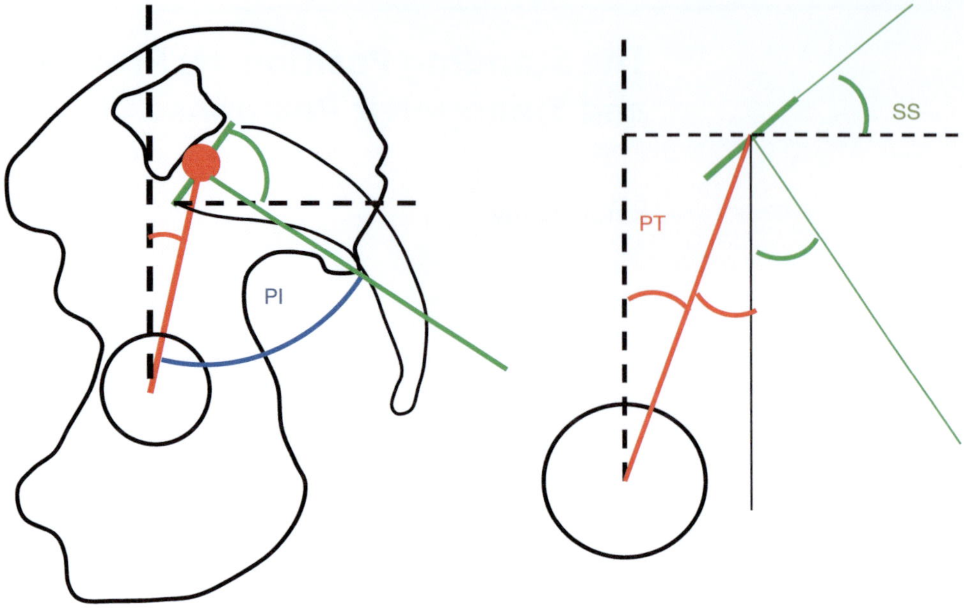

Fig. 1 Pelvic incidence angle, PI (shape angle of the pelvis), is equal to the sum of two positional angles of the pelvic tilt, PT and sacral slope, SSImage: IP = PI VP = PT SS = SS

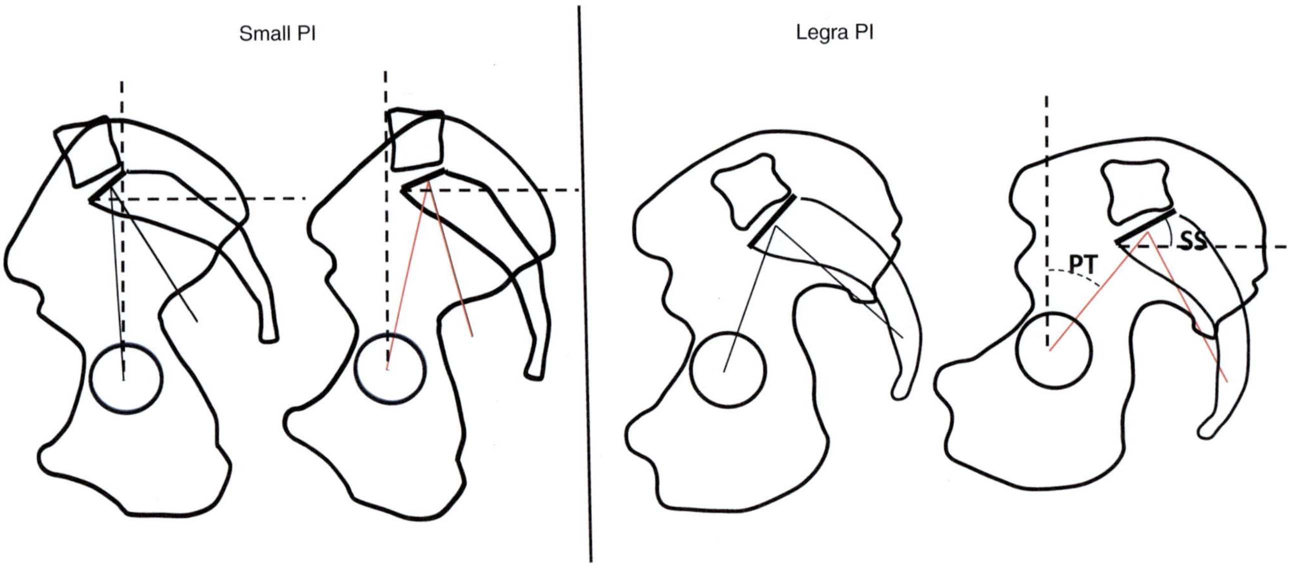

Fig. 2 The pelvis on the left with a low PI allows less retroversion (low PT) than that on the right (high PI). Because of the relationship PI = PT + SS when SS tends to zero, PT tends to PI

of the sacral plate. SS is the second positional parameter of the pelvis.

PI, PT, and SS are related by the geometric relationship: PI = PT + SS. This means that the fixed shape parameter is equal to the sum of the two position parameters. This geometric relationship has two consequences:

- For a given individual, PI is constant. When PT increases, SS decreases and vice versa. In other words, when the pelvis rotates backwards around the femoral heads (retroversion), the sacral endplate horizontalizes. On the contrary, if the pelvis rotates forward (anteversion), the sacral endplate becomes vertical. This is a means of regulating sagittal balance of the human body.
- For two different individuals, one with a large PI and the other with a small PI, the pelvic positioning possibilities are different. Large PI allows higher PT values than smaller PI. By taking 0° as the minimum value of SS, the possibilities to retrovert the pelvis are greater for a high PI. In reality the largest retroversions are limited by the ability to extend the hips (Fig. 2).

Limits for Pelvic Parameters

The values generally accepted in the literature are an average of 52° PI for white Caucasian populations. We have published the largest series (709 individuals) that shows extreme values of 35–85°. There is no gender influence on PI values. In pathology, values can be found within or beyond these limits. The mean values of PT and SS are 12° and 40°, respectively. This does not mean a lot because we have seen that the values of PT and SS are related to PI. Mac-Thiong [3] gives a maximum limit for PT as PI/2. On the other hand, the direct relationship between pelvic positioning and hip amplitudes in extension seems to link the PT and hip limits more closely. Referring to quality of life criteria, Schwab and Lafage [4] propose a PT limit of 20°, irrespective of PI values. Correlations between PT and PI, and SS and PI are $p = 0.65$ and $p = 0.80$, respectively. This shows a stronger relationship between PI and SS. Neither of the two parameters (PT or SS) cannot have a direct linear relationship with PI.

Influence of the Pelvic Incidence on the Shape of the Pelvis [4]

The PI angle is a shape parameter, it affects the shape of the pelvis. The posterior pelvis is formed by the two iliac bones and sacrum, it seems that only the latter is directly impacted by changes in PI. The lower the PI, the longer the sacrum, the higher the sacral endplate projects close to the interiliac (intercrest) line, and the more the sacral endplate is horizontal. On the contrary, the higher the PI, the shorter the sacrum, the lower the projection of the sacral endplate, often well below the interiliac line, and the more the sacred endplate is inclined. This results in a low positioning of L5 with respect to the crests in the high PI and conversely a high L5 in low PI. This is described as an "embedded L5." From the perspective of the overall shape, the low PI pelvis appears more vertical, with a more open pelvic inlet; the high PI pelvis seems more horizontal, with the pelvic inlet opening further up. The pelvis of very low PI approximates the vertical and narrow pelvis of great apes. The functional differences in PI may have obstetric effects: a horizontal pelvic inlet seems best suited to the passage of the fetus by natural means than a vertically oriented canal (Fig. 3).

Another consequence is the position and orientation of the acetabulum. In a low PI pelvis, the femoral heads are positioned just below the sacral endplate. Moreover, there is very little possibility of retroversion of the pelvis.

The orientation of the acetabulum changes minimally in axial rotation. On the contrary, with a high PI pelvis, the acetabuli are generally positioned further forward along the sacral plateau. In addition, the greatest opportunities of

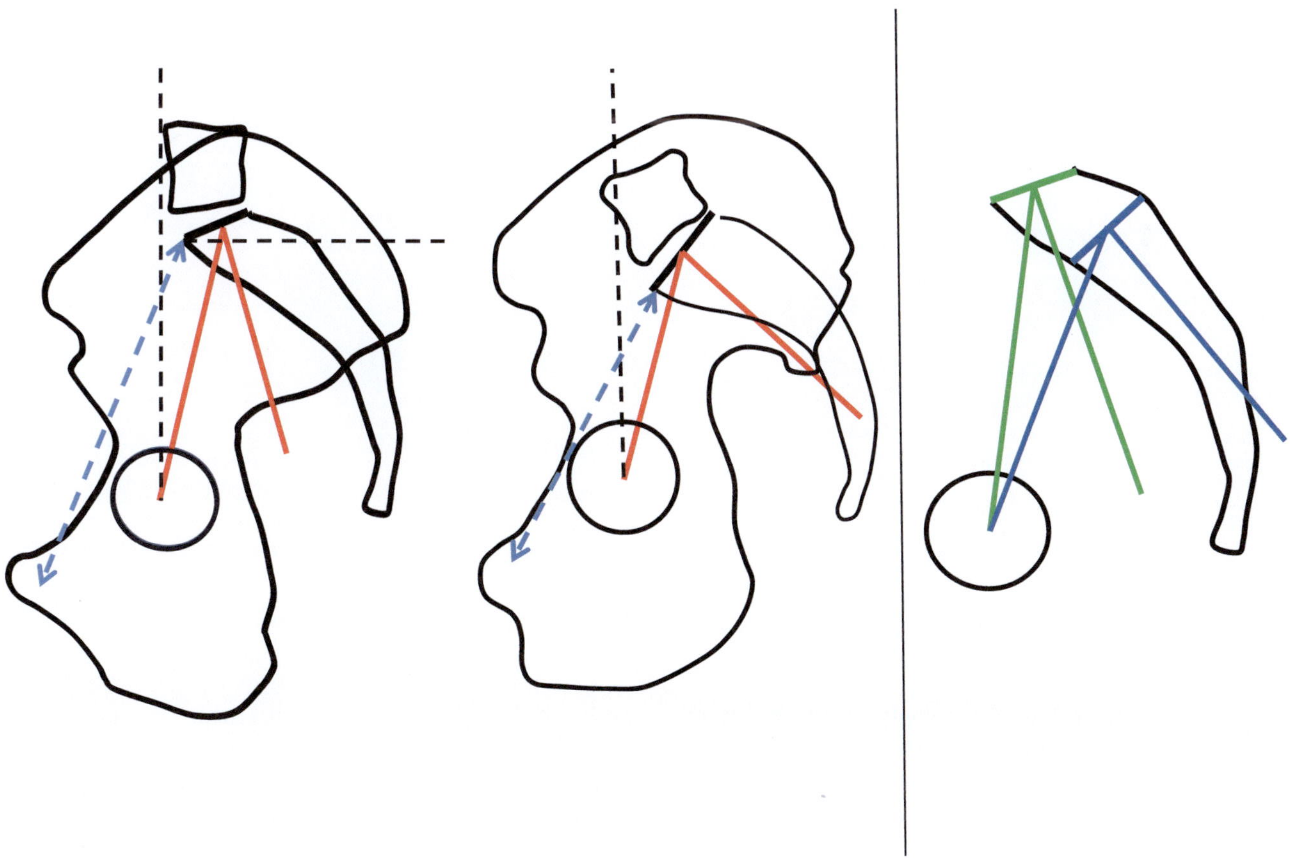

Fig. 3 Left, when PI is low, the sacral endplate is located higher (sacrum elongated) and approaches the horizontal plane passing through the iliac crests. The pelvis appears narrower from front to back; the pelvic inlet is more vertical. Right, when PI is high, the sacral endplate is projected below and behind the plane of the iliac crests. The pelvis appears wider from front to back (horizontal pelvis); the pelvic inlet is inclined further forward

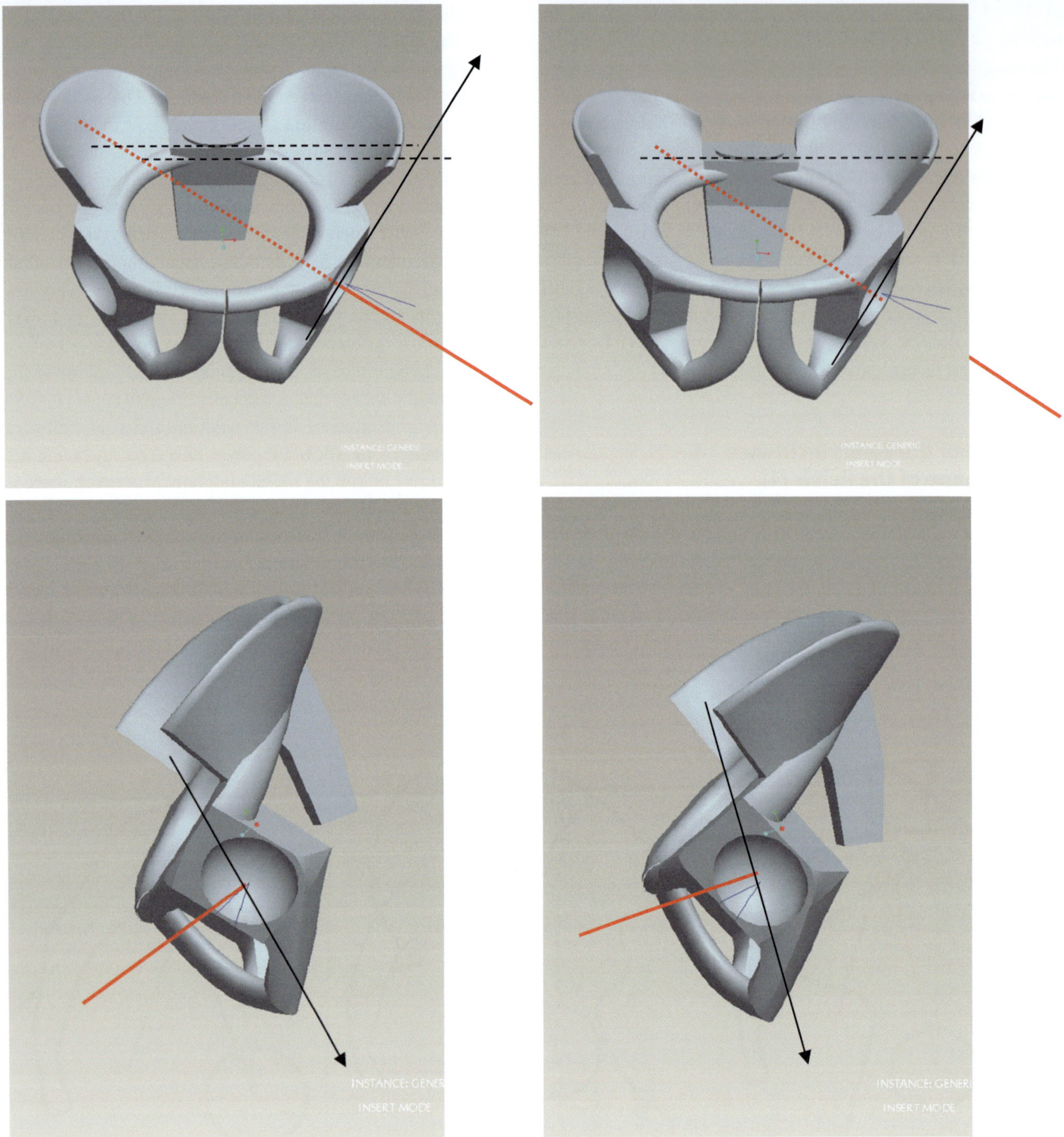

Fig. 4 Variation of the axial positioning of the acetabuli according to pelvic version. Retroversion of the pelvis increases the acetabular anteversion, and vice versa

retroversion of the pelvis will strongly change the orientation of axial rotation of the acetabuli (Fig. 4).

The Lumbar Lordosis

Since Hippocrates, the anatomy of the spine has always been defined as distinct segments characterized by the shape of the vertebrae and the overall direction of the curvature of the vertebrae group concerned. The classic segmentation was cervical lordosis, thoracic kyphosis, lumbar lordosis, and sacral kyphosis. It is thus conceived that lumbar lordosis concerned only the lumbar vertebrae and had to be appreciated as T12L1 to L5S1. However, a pertinent analysis of lumbar lordosis has shown that the anatomical boundaries do not correspond necessarily with the limits of the vertebrae in extension. Short lordoses could be found ending before L1 and long lordoses beyond T12.

Furthermore, Stagnara [5] had shown the influence of the orientation of the sacral endplate on the shape of the spine with a high sacral slope termed "dynamic," and flat sacral slope termed "static."

We propose a functional biomechanical definition of lumbar lordosis [6]. This comprises the vertebral area between the sacral endplate and the inflection point where the curvature in lordosis changes orientation to switch to kyphosis. We propose a model where the geometric curvature of lordosis is divided into two arcs in accordance with a horizontal line passing through the apex of the curve (anterior tangent point of the curve with the vertical). The upper arc is between the point of inflection and the apex. It has been shown that the angular value of the upper arc is relatively constant around 15° for an asymptomatic adult population. The lower arc is between the sacral endplate and the apex. Its angle is equal to the angle of sacral slope (SS). The upper arc is between the apex and the perpendicular to the tangent of the curve at the inflection point. As stated by Stagnara, the orientation of the sacral endplate gives rise to the shape of the lumbar lordosis. Considering the proposed geometric model, the angular variation of SS directly influences the angle of the lower arc and thus its shape. Given the constancy of the upper arc, the sum of the upper and lower arcs can be reduced to SS + 15°. This equation confirms the strong correlation ($R = 0.85$) between the SS and the overall angle of lumbar lordosis (Fig. 5).

From this construction and by segmenting the angular values of SS into three categories (SS <35°, 35° < SS < 45°, SS > 45°), we identified three major types of lumbar lordosis morphologies [7, 8]:

SS < 35°

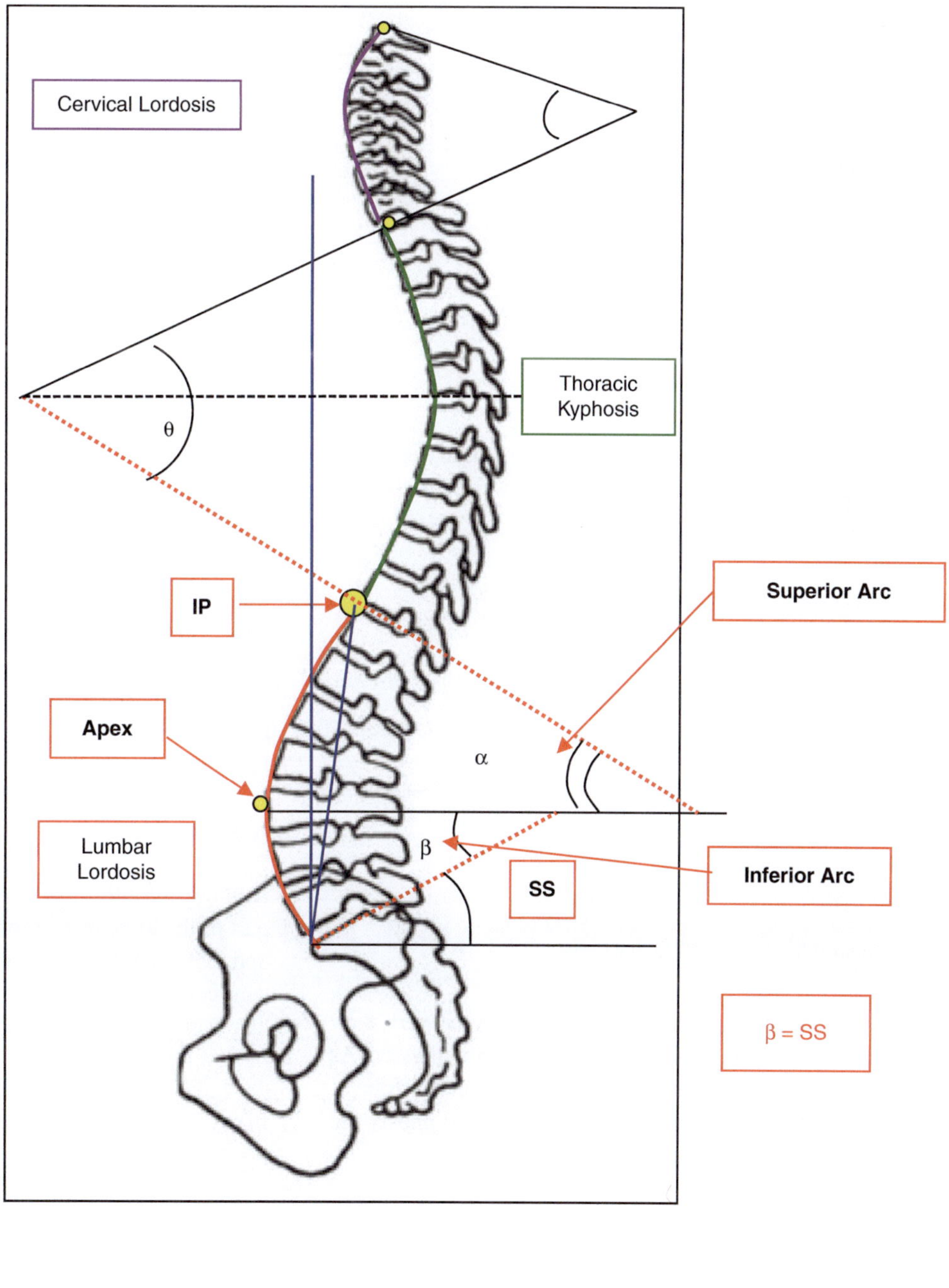

Fig. 5 Vertebral segmentation according to Dimnet, Berthonaud. The inflection point (IP) where the spinal curvatures change direction separates lumbar lordosis (LL) and thoracic kyphosis (TK). Each curve can be divided into two arcs tangential to each apex. The lower arc of LL is equal to the sacral slope

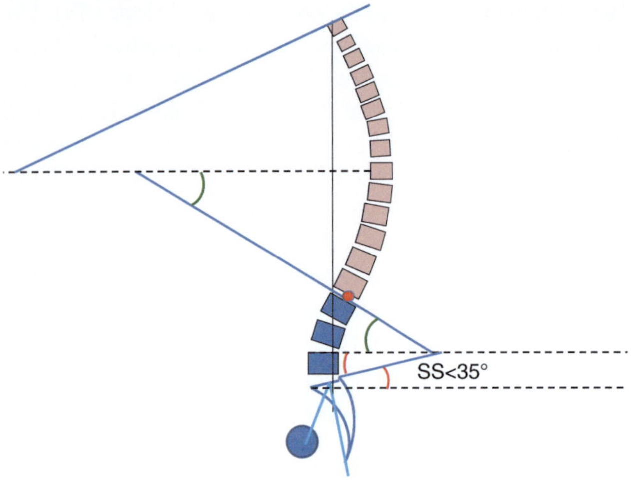

Fig. 6 Type 1: SS is low, <35°; the lower arc of LL is reduced, LL is short with thoracolumbar kyphosis

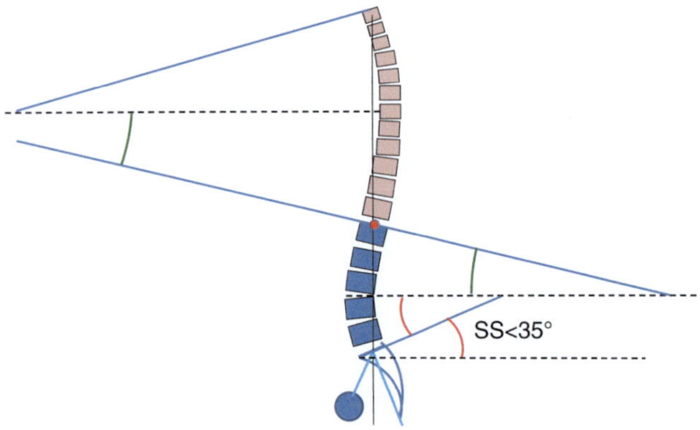

Fig. 7 Type 2: SS is low, <35°; the lordosis angle is small (LL flat)

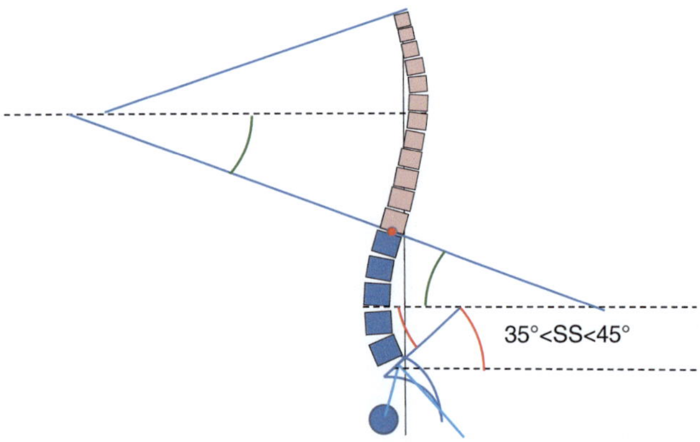

Fig. 8 Type 3: 35° < PS <45°, LL balanced

- Type 1: The lower lumbar arc is a low angle; it is very short or non-existent. Only the upper lumbar arc is expressed. As lordosis is short, kyphosis descends to the lumbar zone to provide a thoracolumbar kyphosis; with more kyphosis, the low lumbar hyperextension increases (Fig. 6).

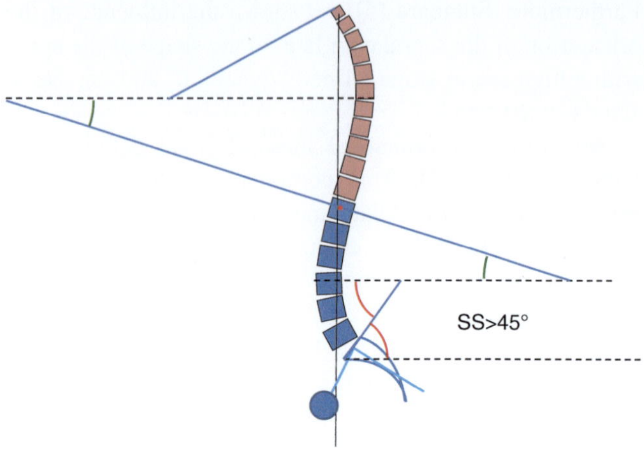

Fig. 9 Type 4: SS > 45°, lordosis has a high angle and is longer because of the proximal extension and angle of increase of the lower arc

- Type 2: The second expression of a low degree arc is to reduce the radius of curvature, the shape of the arc approximates a line segment. Lordosis is longer but very flat. The general form of the thoracic and lumbar spine is generally smooth and minimally curved. The mean angular value of lordosis is <50° (Fig. 7).

35° < SS < 45°

- Type 3: This is the average harmonious type. The lordosis lengthens, the apex is at the level of L4; the average value of lordosis is between 50° and 60° (Fig. 8).

SS > 45°

- Type 4: This is a harmonious hypercurve. The angle of lordosis increases with sacral inclination. As the lower arc lengthens, the number of vertebrae in the lumbar increases. In the highest lordosis, lordosis recruits further vertebrae, by exceeding the L1T12 junction. Moreover, intervertebral hyperextension augments local spinal extensibility. The average lordosis exceeds 60° (Fig. 9).

Remarks

- In more lordotic type 3 and type 4, the most important part of the lordosis rests at the last lumbar segments L4L5 and L5S1 which are necessary to maintain or restore in surgical treatment.
- The flattened shape of the lumbar lordosis in type 2 offers more space for posterior vertebral bone formation, including large volume facet joints and spinous processes. This limits the posterior extensibility and intervertebral flexibility.

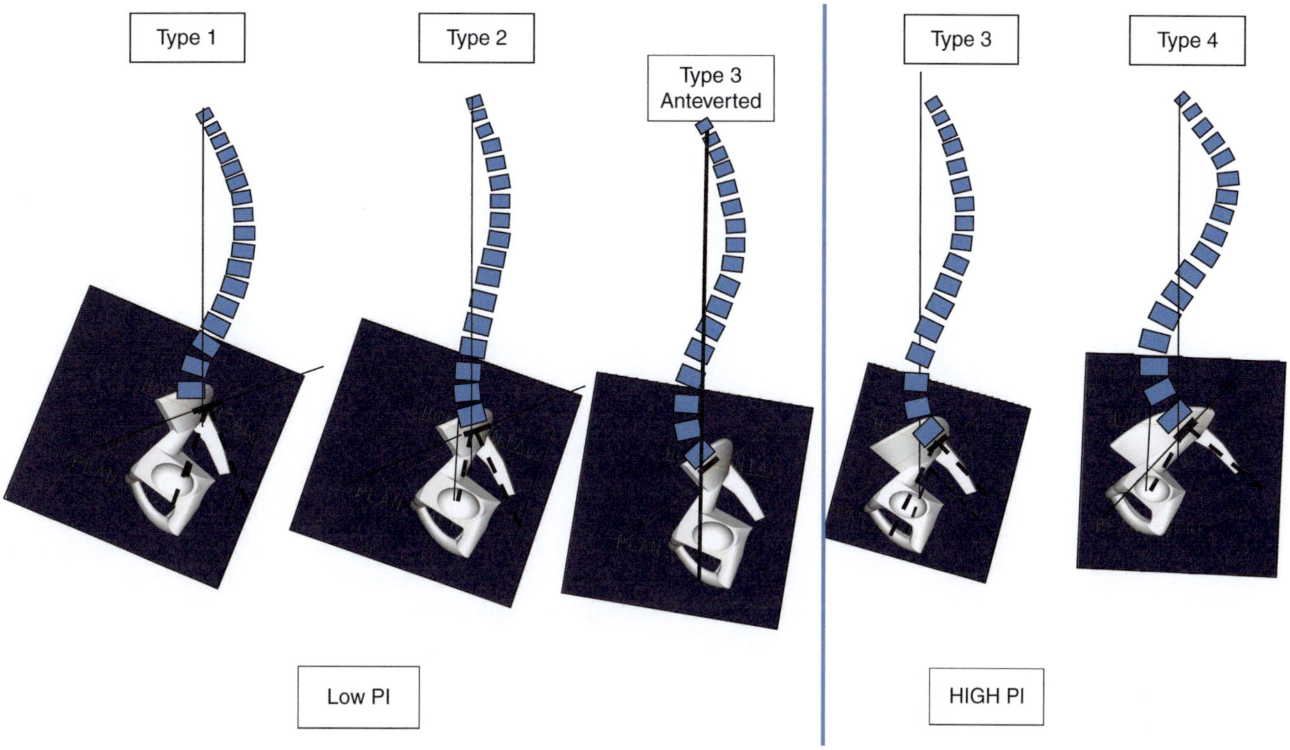

Fig. 10 LL–PI relationship. Types 1 and 2 are always with low PI; types 3 and 4 are with high PI. However, a low PI pelvis with high anteversion can yield a type 3 or 4

- Alternatively, the curvature associated with type 4 has posterior elements with a shorter radius and offers less space for their development. Consequently, joint and spinous process volume are reduced. This anatomy improves extensibility and better spinal flexibility. In return, the small size of articular masses is exposed to risks of intervertebral instability.

Pelvic Incidence Relationship Lumbar Lordosis

All of the literature confirm a strong correlation between PI and SS ($R = 0.80$) and to a lesser degree between PI and LL ($R = 0.65$). The strong PI–SS correlation permits approximation between PI and lumbar morphologies that are indexed from the SS. One can consider that the lowest PI will be found more often in types 1 and 2 lordoses, while with the highest PI one will find types 3 and 4. Here we see the relationship between the shape of the pelvis and lumbar lordosis (Fig. 10).

Global Balance of the Thoracic and Lumbar Spine. Position of C7 (Fig. 11)

The assessment of the overall balance of the human body in a standing position requires analysis of the cranio-cervical position. Until now, the conventional radiographic input on standard 30 × 90 cm formats rarely allowed capture of the skull when evaluating the cervical spine. Since the use of X-ray with EOS scanning, imaging of the body can be grasped in totality. There is no consensus yet to designate a cranial anatomical landmark that identifies the overall balance of the body while standing.

Until now, the consensus has been taken to consider the middle of the C7 vertebral body as the most reliable anatomical landmark in assessing overall balance. On standard radiographs, C7 was the first identifiable vertebra regularly above the shoulders shadow that mostly hid T1. Otherwise, the position at the upper extremity of the thoracic spine reflects the behavior of the entire thoracolumbar spine and pelvis.

The most classical C7 positioning measures [9] were performed from a vertical line through the middle of C7 (Plumb Line). Distance measures on a horizontal projection in relation to an anatomical landmark of the pelvis (sacrum or femoral heads) were proposed. The most widely accepted is the sagittal vertical axis (SVA) as described by Farcy which is the horizontal distance from the C7 plumb line to the posterior edge of the sacral endplate. This radiological distance measurement is questionable because it requires a mandatory calibration of radiographs to ensure the validity of the measures. Finally, a comparison of distance measurements on different sources of X-rays is questionable (Fig. 12). In order to propose a relative rather than absolute measurement

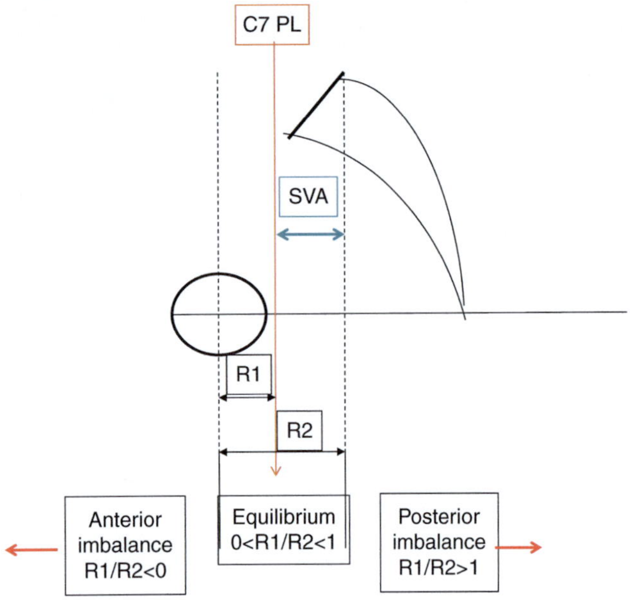

Fig. 11 Evaluation of the overall balance by positioning plumb C7 (C7PL)

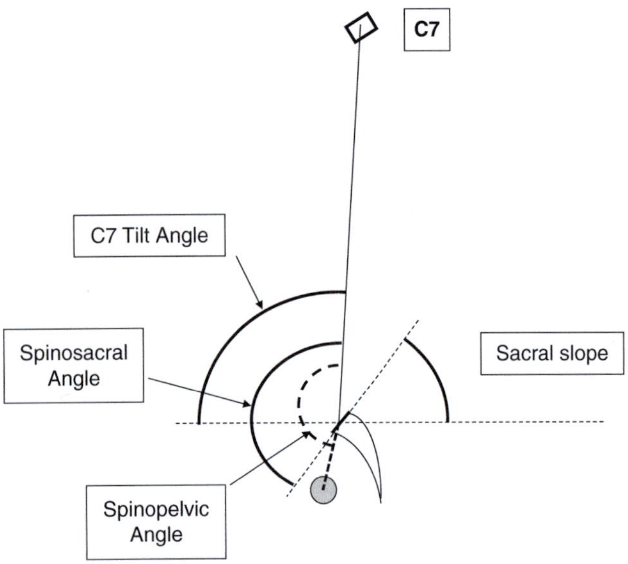

Fig. 12 C7 Positioning angular method

system, Barrey [10] proposed the C7 translation ratio, where the C7 plumb line lies relative to the posterior edge of the sacral endplate and the middle of the bicoxofemoral line. The C7 plumb line to mid-bicoxofemoral point (mid-point between the center of both femoral heads) is then related to the posterior sacral endplate edge to the bicoxofemoral point. Behind the posterior edge of the sacral endplate the Barrey ratio is >1, between the sacrum and femoral heads it is between 0 and 1, anterior to the femoral heads it is negative (Fig. 11).

The angular measure is another C7 positioning measurement mode (Fig. 12). Unlike distance measurements, angle measurements are superimposed on radiographs without calibration.

Three angles are proposed:

- The C7 or spinal tilt angle is formed by the straight line drawn from the middle of the C7 vertebral body to the middle of the sacral endplate, to the horizontal. The C7 tilt angle is a positional angle.
- The sacrospinal angle (SSA) is formed by a line from the mid-C7 point to the mid-sacral endplate and the sacral endplate. SSA is an angle form the sum of two angles position, the C7 and SS. It accounts for the overall kyphosis of the thoracic and lumbar spine. When SSA decreases, the C7 and SS decrease.
- The spinopelvic angle (SPA) is formed by the mid-C7 to sacral endplate line with a line drawn from the middle of the sacral endplate to the femoral heads. It is the sum of the SSA and the PI. Some recent studies attribute a prognostic value to the overall balance.

Values of Overall Balance

It is now generally accepted that the C7 plumb line must fall at the sacral endplate. Specifically, it is just behind the posterior edge of the sacral endplate. This C7 position is stable in an asymptomatic adult population. The average value of the C7-angle is 95° ± 3°. The correlation between SSA and SS is $R = 0.9$. It is almost linear, demonstrating the stability of C7 over the sacrum. Regarding the horizontal projection of C7, Lafage [11] provides a limit of 5 cm for the SVA beyond which the posture is considered unbalanced (or decompensated). Using the Barrey's ratio, one can classify the positioning of C7 as a balance between the posterior sacral endplate and femoral heads or beyond these limits.

Mechanisms for the Compensation of the Spinopelvic Balance

We have seen that the rotation of the pelvis around the femoral heads causes variance of the orientation of the sacral endplate: when the pelvis tilts forward (PT decreases), the sacral endplate increases its inclination (SS increases) and vice versa. In view of its role as liaison between the spine and lower limbs, the imbalance can come from either a subpelvic or a spinal cause. The orientation of the pelvis can be determined by a position change that is coupled to stiffness of the spine, or the lower limbs, hips in particular [10, 12].

We discuss the underlying pelvic causes with relevance to the spine.

Spinopelvic Origin Balance

The classic case is that of flexion of the hip joint. The verticalization of the femur induces, due to the position and stiffness of the hip, a forced anteversion of the pelvis, an increase of SS and increased lordosis. If the possibilities of increasing the lordosis are exceeded, the system becomes anteriorly imbalanced. Forced extension of the spine is painful, which explains the low back pain that can accompany hip pathology. The contracture release from hip arthroplasty is a viable solution, which restores freedom of the pelvis and its repositioning.

Spinal Imbalance

In spinal pathology, equilibrium is always compromised by anterior deflection, even of the whole spine. In the face of this event, the spine-pelvis system puts in place compensations allowing to restore balance to maintain the standing position. Beyond certain limits, the standing position becomes difficult, not very enduring, and at most impossible.

Primary Compensation Mechanisms

In the setting of a local spinal kyphosis (decreased spinosacral angle, SSA), two mechanisms may be involved:

- When adjacent intervertebral mobility around the kyphosis is preserved, affected spinal zones are set in extension. Overall the spinal system seeks to recover the loss of SSA lost in kyphosis by extending the adjacent areas. This forced extension is usually painful and explains many back pains (Fig. 13a).
- When the spine is stiff, SSA decreases, pelvic retroversion (PT increases) occurs. It allows SS decrease to offset the decline in SSA to maintain the C7 balance (SSA = SS + C7 Tilt) (Fig. 13b).

Both mechanisms can be involved, the forced extension leading to the stiffness of the spine.

Influence of the Shape of the Pelvis on Pelvic Version

The shape of the pelvis is characterized by pelvic incidence. It defines the positional parameters by the equation: PI = PT + SS. In absolute terms, the retroversion of the pelvis may be up to the cancellation of SS, or PI = PT + 0. At its maximum PT can match PI. The possibilities of retroversion of the pelvis when compensating are dependent on the value of PI. For large PI, potential version will be greater than for smaller PI. As mentioned, the retroversion mechanism is limited by the extension of the hips. If the femurs remain vertical, increasing PT increases the extension of the hips; when the limit of the latter is reached, the femur must then require bending of the knees. This knee flexion from a spinal cause is often overlooked and can compromise the functioning of a knee replacement.

a b

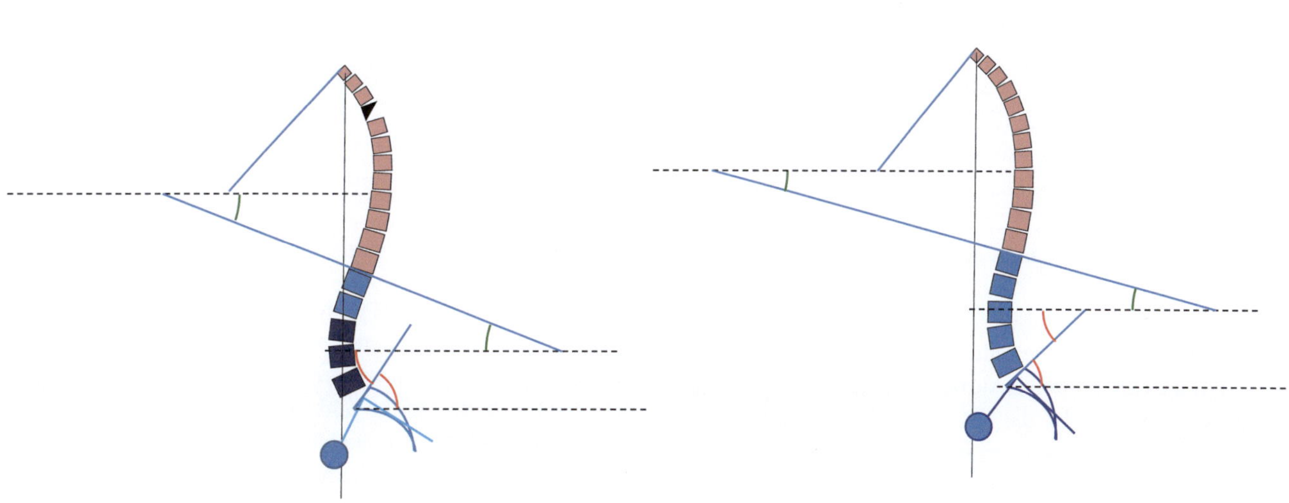

Fig. 13 Balance correction mechanism in the case of increased thoracic kyphosis: (**a**) compensation by lumbar hyperextension, (**b**) compensation by retroversion of the pelvis

Table 1 Algorithm for spinopelvic balance

Pelvic parameters		C7 plumb line	Lumbar lordosis (L3 Apex)
PI	PT	Behind S1	Short LL = TL kyphosis
PI < 55°	Pelvis anteverted	Between S1 and BCFA	Long LL
PI > 55°	normal	In front of BCFA	
	Retroverted		

BFA Bicoxofemoral Axis

- Compensation by increasing distal extension
- Compensation by pelvic retroversion

Although large PI allows better compensation for flexion of the spine, a greater retroversion mechanism is not economical. It is difficult to maintain and often painful. Moreover, it causes great difficulty in walking. The anterior imbalance is then increased during the subsequent step that pushes the pelvis into anteversion and imbalance. That is why large pelvic retroversion patients walk with an anterior carrier such as a caddy or trolley (supermarket syndrome).

Algorithm of Spinopelvic Balance (Table 1)

With the implications of PI, one may define combinations for the level of imbalance, the mildest to the most severe. It is proposed to combine two classes of PI: high (>55°) or low (<55°), then three pelvic positioning levels according to PT (anteverted, normal, retroverted), three positions of C7 (normal, mild imbalance, imbalance), and finally the type of lumbar lordosis (short <3 levels, long >3 levels).

Analysis of Spinal and Discal Constraints: Influence of Spinopelvic Balance

The contact force: the force exerted on each disco-vertebral unit is called contact force (CF). CF is a product of the force of gravity that is usually exerted in front of the spine and its opposing posterior muscular forces. We can compare this force couple to the model of a crane where the two forces counterbalance the weight of each other. If anteriorly imbalanced, the force of gravity moves the spine forward, and opposite moment of muscle forces must increase accordingly. The system can be quickly exceeded, firstly because muscle forces are no longer sufficient, and secondly because the pressure exerted by the CF on the disco-vertebral complex increases and causes it to fail (Fig. 14).

Orientation of the vertebral endplates, force distribution (Figs. 15 and 16): Vertically oriented CF can be divided into two vectors, parallel to the endplate (sliding force) and perpendicular (compression force). With a 40° sloped endplate (average SS) both FC components are practically equal, with a good balance. If the orientation is closer to the horizontal pressure, compression forces increase, otherwise it is the sliding forces that predominate. Furthermore, the contact forces exerted on a highly lordotic spine go through the posterior vertebral elements, the facet joints in particular. By contrast, if CF is exercised on a minimally curved spine or especially in bending, the forces are exerted on the front of the spine (vertebral bodies and discs). The combination of the orientation of the vertebrae and discs and CF impact area shows that in the slightly curved or bending spine, it is the discs and vertebral bodies that are the most stressed. Here we find early disc herniations, degenerative disc disease, or fractures of the vertebral bodies. On the contrary, in the most curved lordosis, discs are spared and CF is on the facet joints, with a predominant sliding component. This is evident in the case of spondylolisthesis (ante or retro), with arthrosis of the facet joints.

If one returns to the classification of the forms of lordosis, one can presume that the effect of the CF is according to the orientation of each of the vertebral shapes (Fig. 17).

Type 1: Low PI, low SS, short lumbar hyperlordosis associated with thoracolumbar kyphosis. The contact forces exerted anteriorly on the intervertebral discs in the kyphotic thoracolumbar area and posteriorly on the facet joints in the lower lumbar region.

Type 2: Low PI, low SS, slightly curved flat lordosis. The intervertebral discs are under compression. This type of back does not support the carrying of heavy loads and thrust forces.

Type 3: Medium to high PI, regular curved lordosis. No negative mechanical features.

Type 4: High PI, high SS, hypercurved lordosis. Stress prevails on posterior elements with large sliding forces. This predisposes to spondylolisthesis, and facet osteoarthritis. As we age, the loss of lumbar disc height may occur with degeneration. This loss of lordosis causes compensation by retroversion of the pelvis. This retroversion is more evident when PI is high.

Conclusion

The organization of the spine and pelvis in the sagittal plane obeys the laws of physics to maintain a biped position that is built to be stable and economical. It is the pelvis that is the fundamental hinge harmonizing the interdependencies between the spine and the limbs below.

The shape of the pelvis characterized by the pelvic incidence angle is probably inherited from our phylogenetic evolution with extreme forms less adapted for a good balance. The impact of the shape of the pelvis on the shape and positioning of the spine allows a better understanding of mechanical phenomena that arise and their repercussion on the spinal and general orthopedic pathologies.

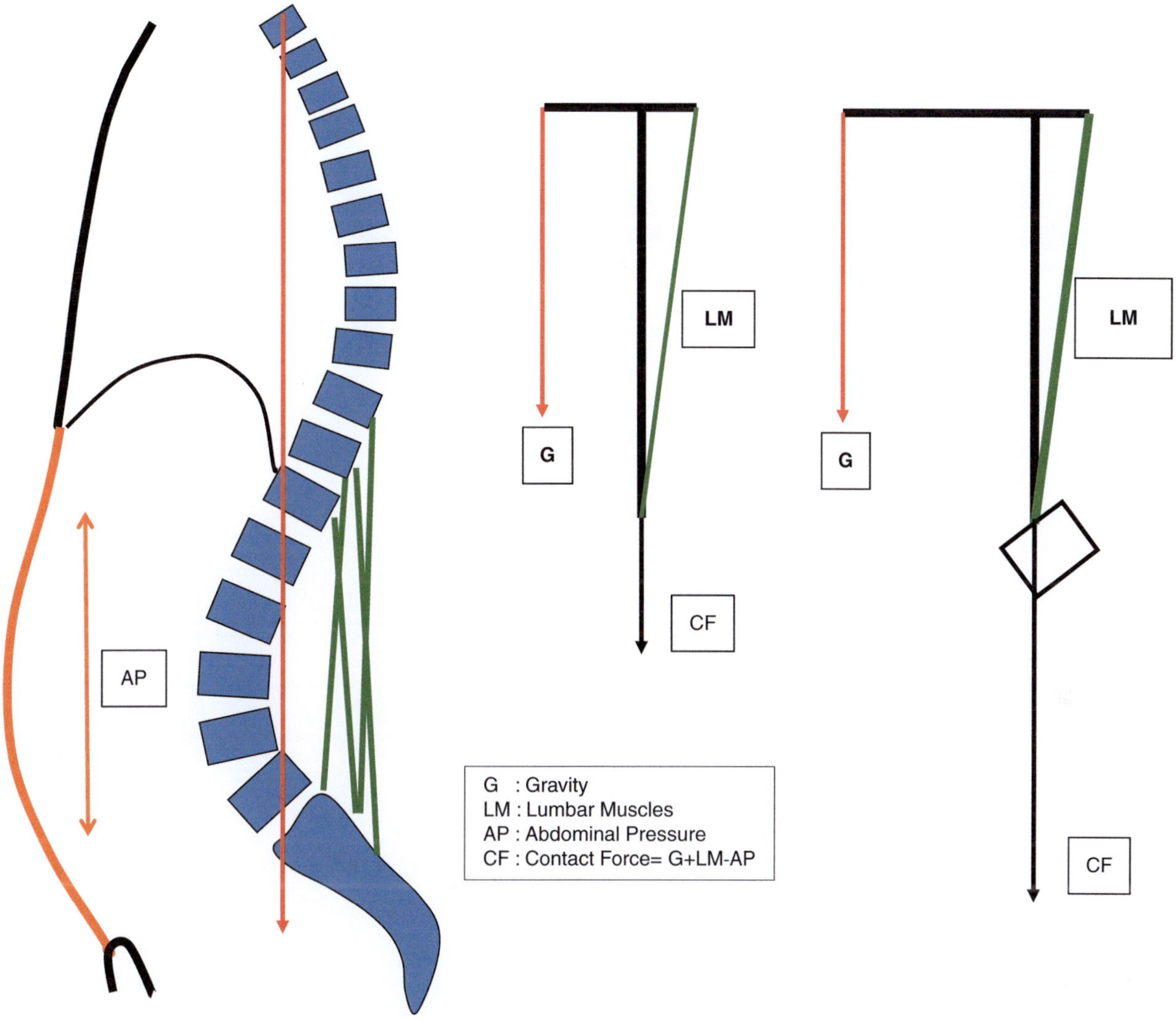

Fig. 14 Modeling the contact force

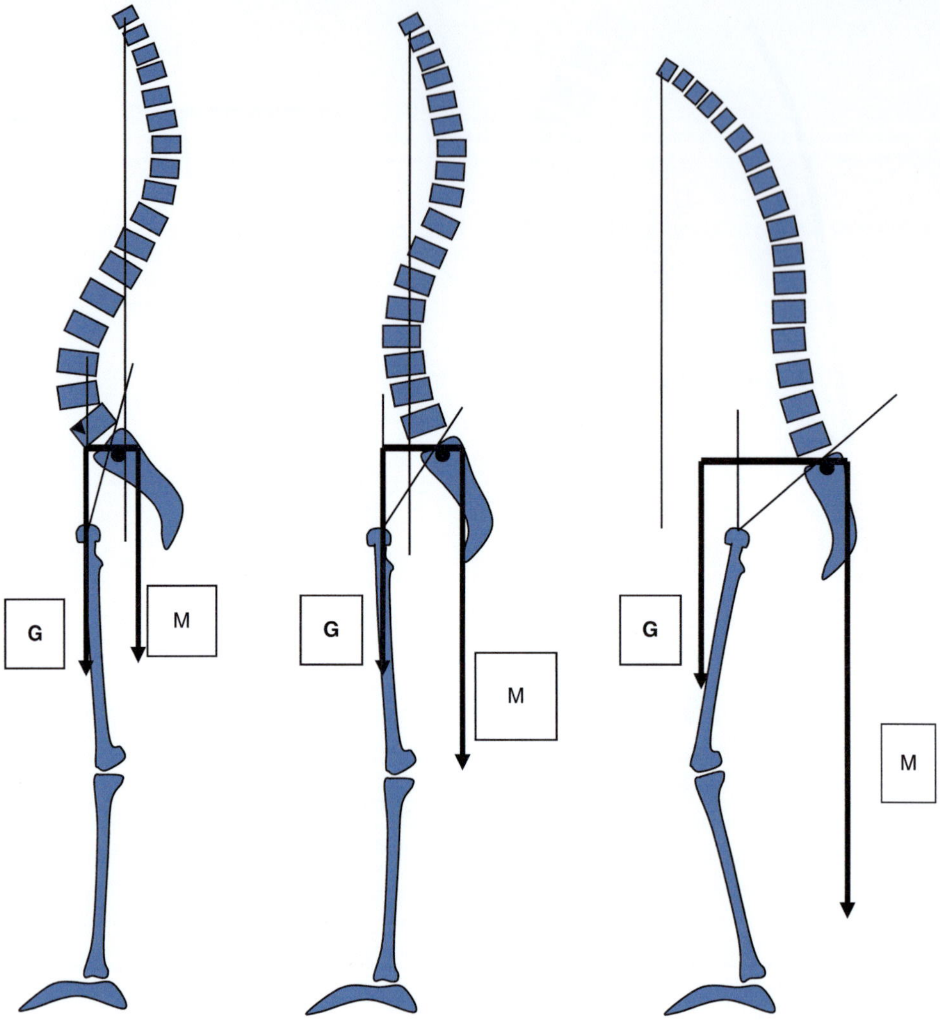

Fig. 15 Evolution of the components of the contact force as a function of spinopelvic balance

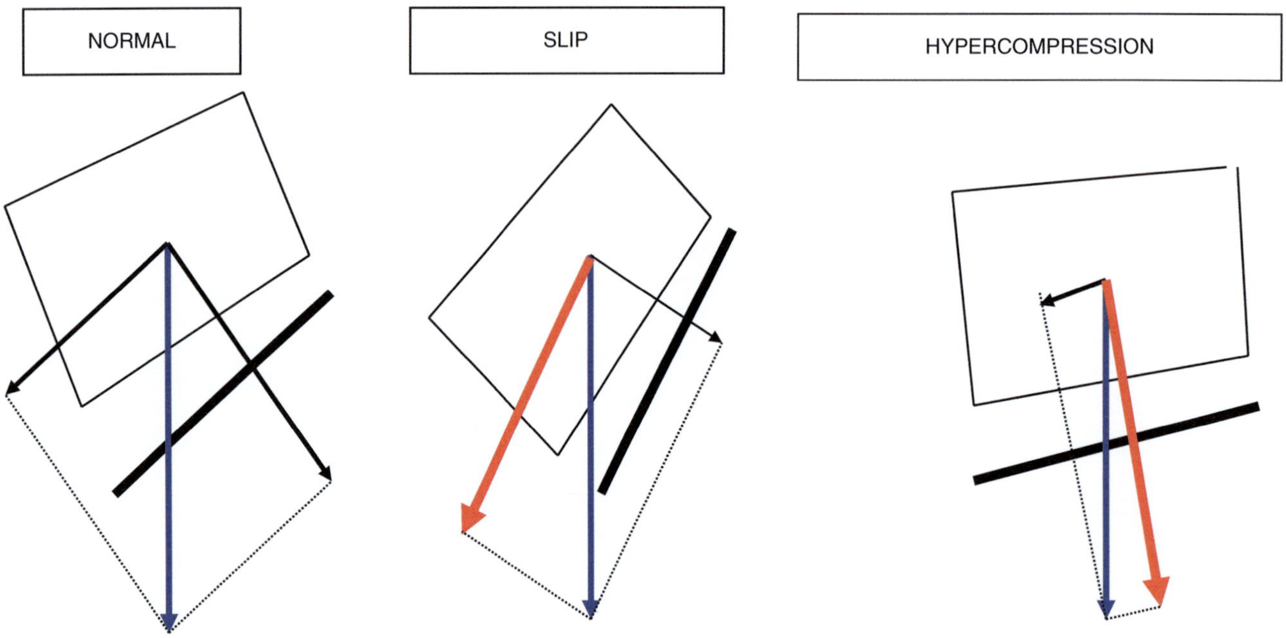

Fig. 16 Distribution of the contact force and effect mechanical depending on the orientation of the vertebral endplates

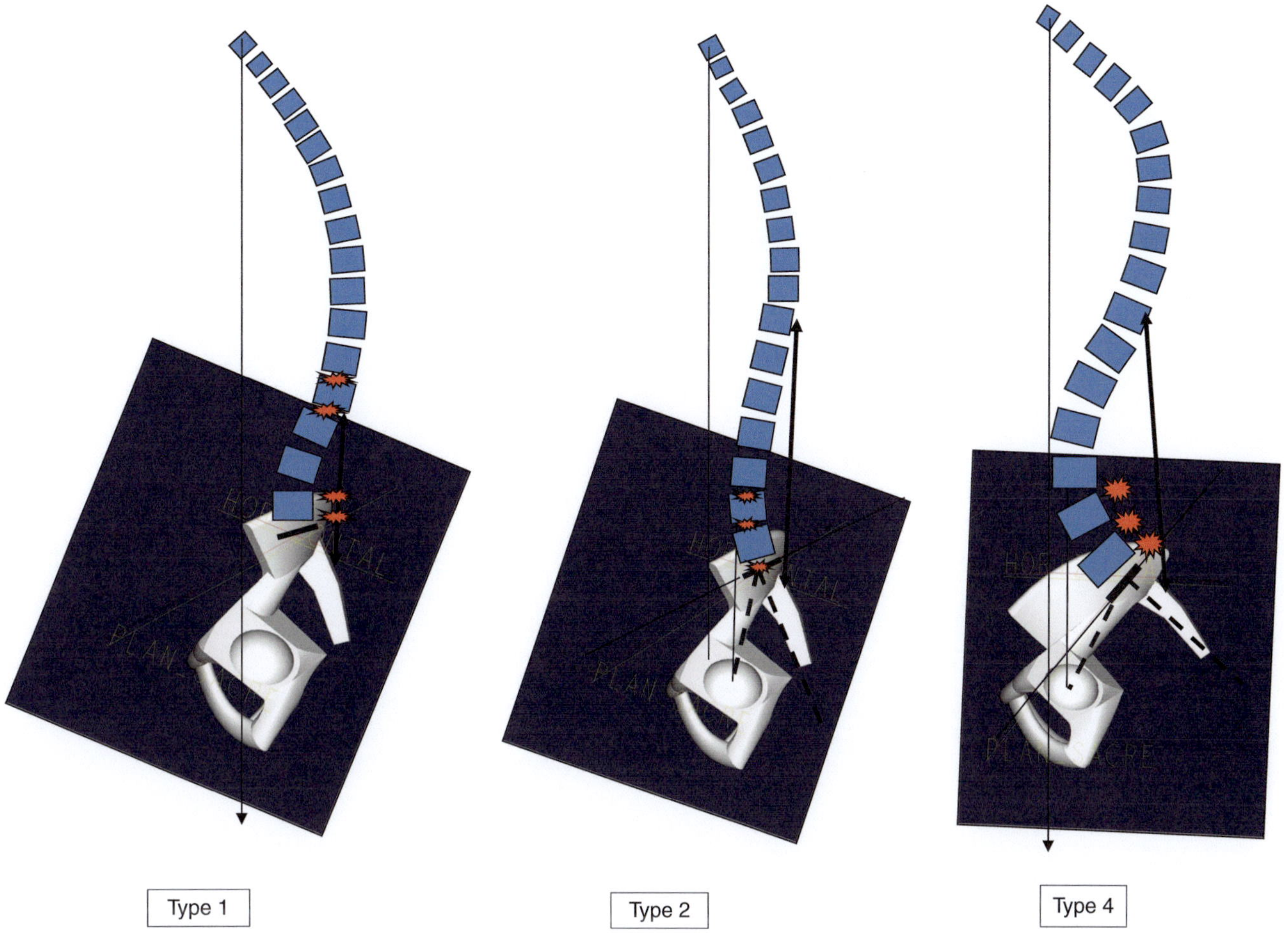

Fig. 17 Location of intervertebral stress depending on the types of spine

References

1. During J, Goudfrooij H, Keessen W, Beeker TW, Crowe A. Towards standards for posture. Postural characteristics of the lower back system in normal and pathologic conditions. Spine (Phila Pa 1976). 1985;10:837.
2. Legaye J, Duval-Beaupère G, Hecquet J, Marty C. Pelvic incidence: a fundamental pelvic parameter for three-dimensional regulation of spinal sagittal curves. Eur Spine J. 1998;7:99103.
3. Mac-Thiong JM, Roussouly P, Berthonnaud E, Guigui P, et al. Spine (Phila Pa 1976). 2010;35(22):E119398.
4. Lafage V, Schwab F, Skalli W, Hawkinson N, Gagey PM, Ondra S, Farcy JP. Standing balance and sagittal plane spinal deformity: analysis of spinopelvic and gravity line parameters. Spine (Phila Pa 1976). 2008;33:15728.
5. Stagnara P, De Mauroy JC, Dran G, Gonon G, Costanzo G, Dimnet J, Pasquet A, et al. Spine (Phila Pa 1976). 1982;7(4):33542.
6. Berthonnaud E, Dimnet J, Roussouly P, Labelle H. Analysis of the sagittal balance of the spine and pelvis using shape and orientation parameters. J Spinal Disord Tech. 2005;18(1):407.
7. Roussouly P, Berthonnaud E, Dimnet J, et al. Rev Chir Orthop Reparatrice Appar Mot. 2003;89(7):6329. (in French).
8. Roussouly P, Pinheiro-Franco JL. Sagittal parameters of the spine: biomechanical approach. Eur Spine J. 2011;20(Suppl. 5):57885.
9. Roussouly P, Gollogly S, Noseda O, Berthonnaud E, Dimnet J, et al. Spine (Phila Pa 1976). 2006;31(11):E32025.
10. Barrey C, Roussouly P, Perrin G, et al. Sagittal balance disorders in severe degenerative spine. Can we identify the compensatory mechanisms? Eur Spine J. 2011;20(Suppl. 5):62633.
11. Blondel B, Schwab F, Ungar B, Smith J, Bridwell K, Glassman S, Shaffrey C, Farcy JP, Lafage V. Impact of magnitude and percentage of global sagittal plane correction on health-related quality of life at 2-years follow-up. Neurosurgery. 2012;71(2):3418; discussion 348. https://doi.org/10.1227/NEU.0b013e31825d20c0.
12. Roussouly P, Pinheiro-Franco JL. Biomechanical analysis of the spinopelvic organization and adaptation in pathology. Eur Spine J. 2011;20(Suppl 5):60918.

The Reserve of Hip Extension and Its Relationship with the Spine

Istvàn Hovorka and Derek Thomas Cawley

With acquisition of the erect posture, limitation of the extension of the hip appears in human development. There are three steps in this process (Fig. 1):

The reserve of hip extension can be defined as the amplitude of maximum extension of the coxo-femoral articulation relative to the vertical neutral position.

This reserve of hip extension is necessary, because if there is a limitation during displacement, the femur would force the pelvis, by ligamentary and muscular tension, to have bending movements, with every step. Thus, it is through repeated hyperlordotic movements that the subject can maintain the fluidity of movements of walking, but when used regularly, it will lead to rapid degeneration of the spine and correlate with low back pain as has been demonstrated by several authors [1–4] (Fig. 2).

This dynamic element must be taken into account in the assessment of clinical and morphological status of patients and in the assessment of abnormalities of sagittal balance.

If there is a sagittal imbalance, it can be represented by two components: anterior spinal imbalance and femoral flexion. To calculate the necessary correction, one must add these two components. However, the subject has a reserve extension which can be called "Actual Extension Reserve ", which should be subtracted from the formula. This formula, in this representation, will allow only a balanced upright position and, as we have seen, a reserve extension is still necessary. This reserve extension, can be called "Theoretical Extension Reserve", should be added to the formula [5] (Fig. 3).

What is the Theoretical Extension Reserve which is necessary for smooth pelvic movement? We do not have a precise figure but based on optoelectronic studies [6–8], we can predict that slow walk requires 10° of extension reserve, for fast walking 15° and to run at least 20°.

This formula which makes it possible to calculate the correction angle necessary in the case of a sagittal imbalance, taking into account the extension reserve, does not give the information if the correction must be made at the level of the spine or pelvis, or even at the femurs. The contribution that can be obtained by stretching was not taken into account either. Thus, in practice, if a correction is necessary, one must assess whether a correction pre- or post-operative stretching could be performed, and this figure is expected to be subtracted from the formula.

How to measure the Extension Reserve? There are two traditional ways: clinical examination and optoelectronics. Clinical examination does not make the difference in a precise way between extension movement at the level of the hip joint or in the lower lumbar spine. Optoelectronics examination is more accurate in lean subjects; however, its application is not feasible in daily clinical practice.

We propose an original method of radiological measurements using specific radiograph images [9]. In Study 1, we compared 37 patients using two methods of measuring the extension reserve. The first method is to achieve an active retroversion movement of the pelvis in an upright position relative to the femur, while the second is to adopt a lunge position where, conversely, it is an active extension of the femur relative to the pelvis that will be applied.

A lateral radiograph with overlapped femoral heads and with a sufficient portion of the femurs as well as the lumbosacral junction allows to calculate the pelvi-femoral angle [10] in the upright neutral position and in two positions tested.

This study shows that the active pelvic retroversion method gives a significantly inferior result compared to the lunge position method. In addition, the implementation of active movement by retroversion of the pelvis presents difficulty for many patients with paradoxical results and measurement failures (Fig. 4).

I. Hovorka (✉)
Institut de la Colonne Vertébrale, CHU Bordeaux, Bordeaux, France

D. T. Cawley
Department of Trauma and Orthopaedic Surgery, Tallaght University Hospital, Dublin, Republic of Ireland

J. M. Vital, D. T. Cawley (eds.), *Spinal Anatomy*, https://doi.org/10.1007/978-3-030-20925-4_7

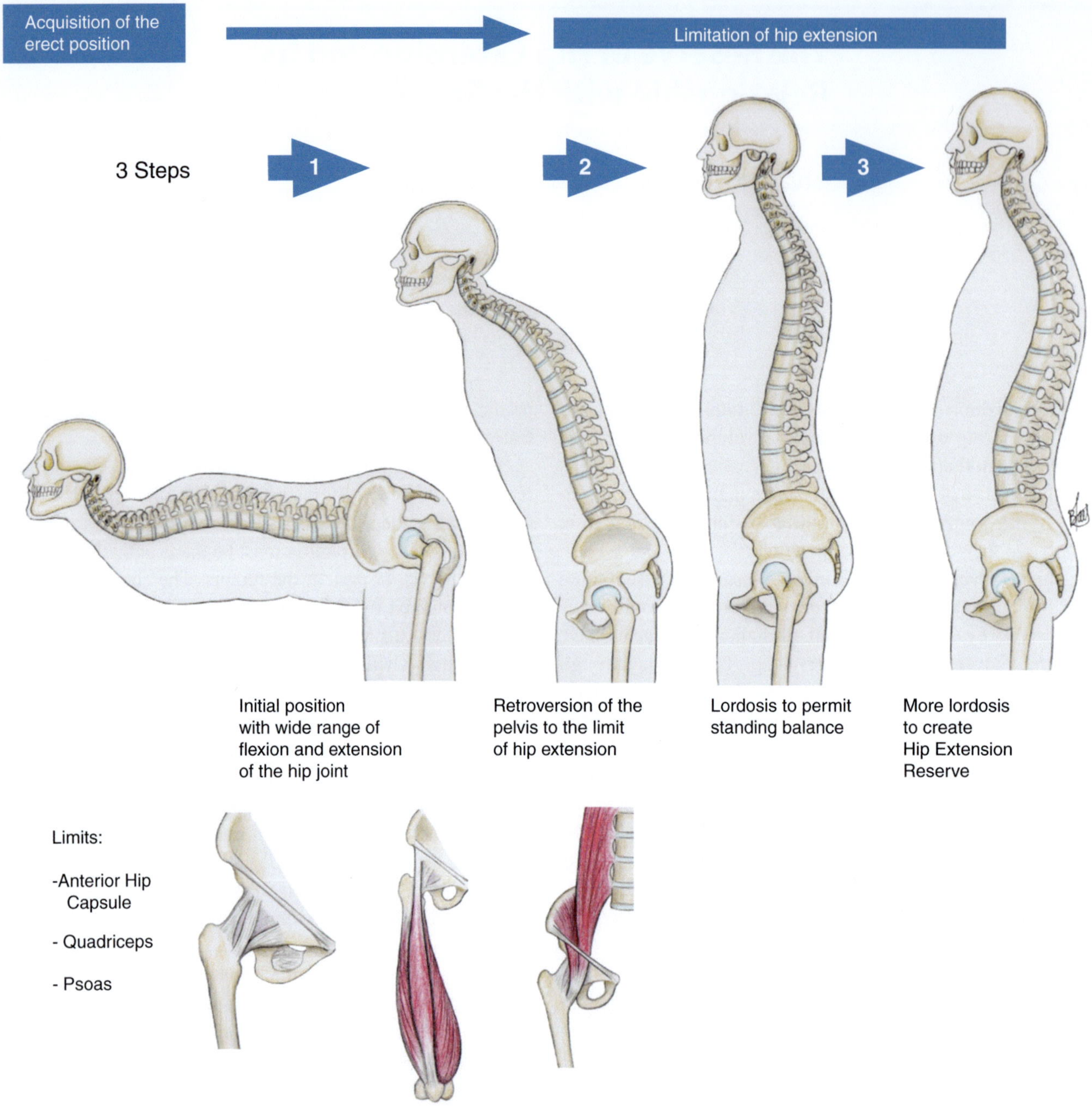

Fig. 1 (1) Active retroversion of the pelvis will help straighten the spine, but it is limited by the extension of the hip. This limit is represented by the tension of the capsule of the hip joint, the quadriceps and psoas muscles anteriorly. (2) The second step is to introduce a lordosis that will permit balance in standing position. However, this will not be enough. (3) A third step is needed with more lordosis that will create the reserve of hip extension

We concluded that only the lunge position radiograph should be used in practice. This is understandable because this is the recommended position for stretching to improve the performance of runners with improving of passive extension of the hip joint.

This is a dynamic radiological assessment that can be criticized for its reliability, repeatability, and the influence of pain. However, this assessment can give information on the reserve of extension so far unknown in clinical applications. Therefore, we have decided to make this assessment systematic for each patient where lumbar surgery could change the sagittal balance. The exploration includes full spine and spinal dynamic radiographs, X-ray in the lunge position for right and left femur as well as in neutral position (Fig. 5).

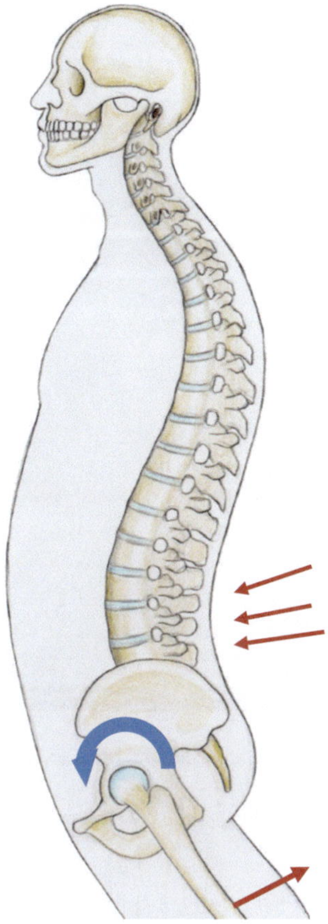

Fig. 2 With repeated end-range extensions of the hip, it forces anteversion of the pelvis and hyperlordotic movements of the lumbar spine, with ensuing degeneration and low back pain

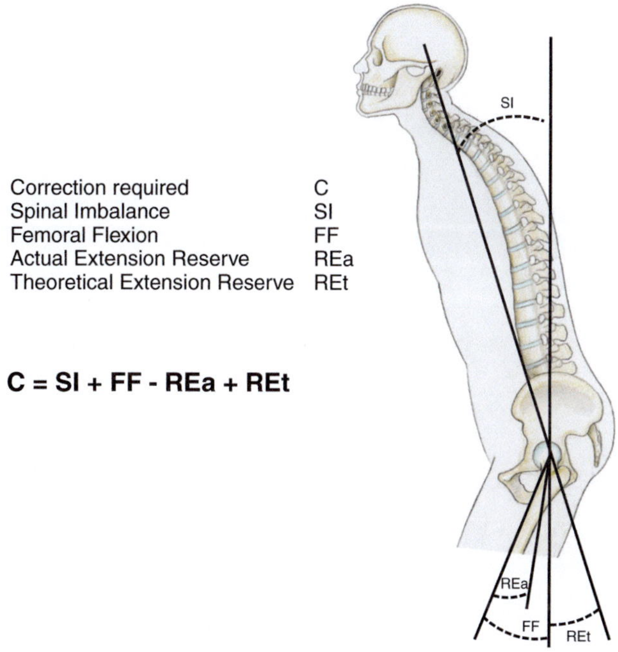

Fig. 3 Calculation of necessary correction of Sagittal Imbalance

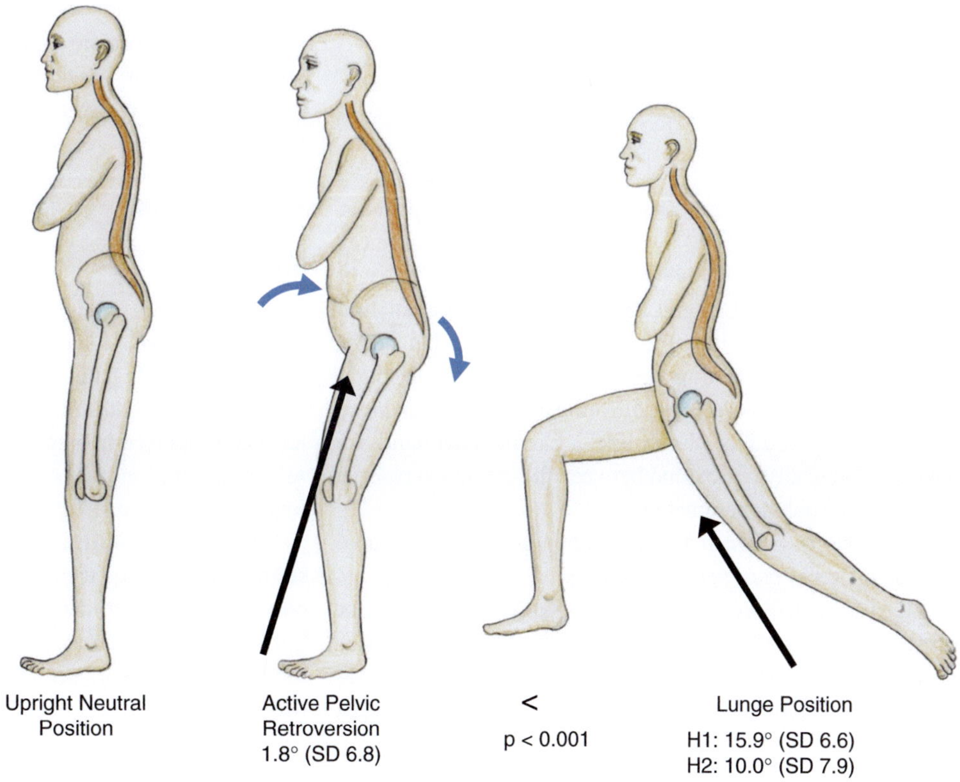

Fig. 4 Profile positions for the neutral pelvis, retroversion and lunge positions. The lunge reliably demonstrates information on reserve of extension

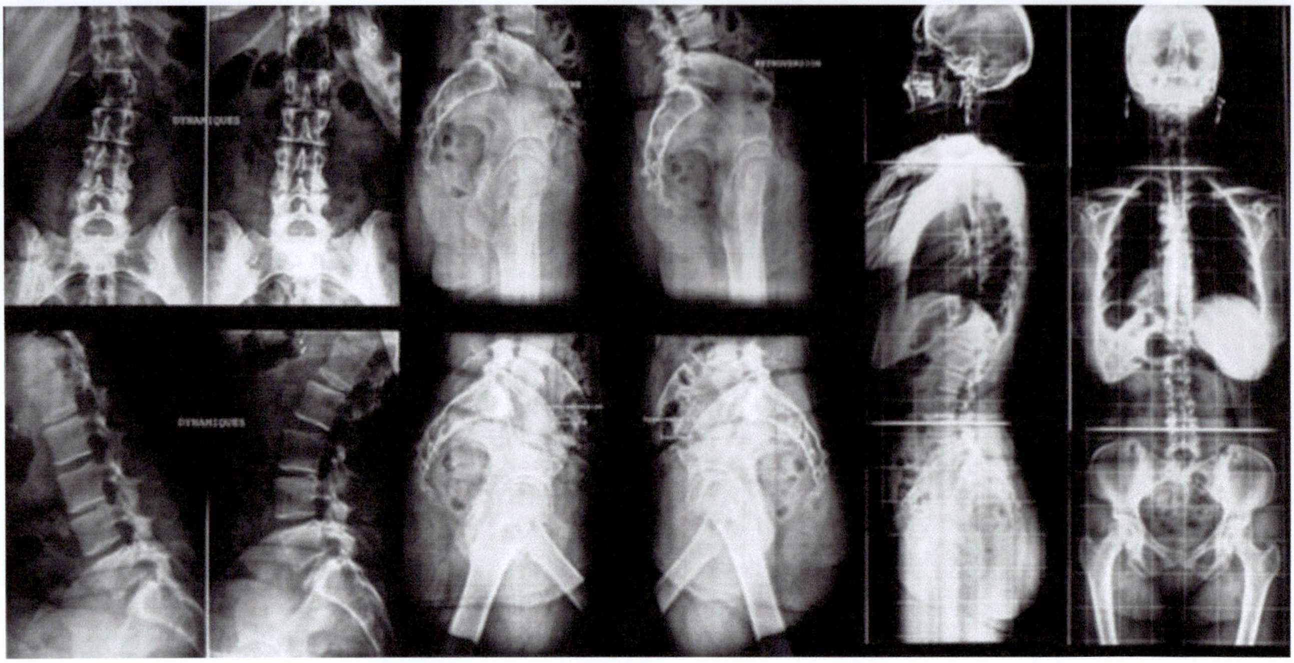

Fig. 5 Series of radiographs, clockwise from top left, postero-anterior views with mild coronal plane abnormality, neutral and retroversion views of the pelvis, full spin radiographs in frontal and sagittal planes, lunge views left and right and lateral views in extension and flexion

Table 1 150 patients with measurements of sagittal balance

Sex	108 women, 42 men	
Age	51.4 years (18/80)	
42 previous operations		
Lumbar lordosis	42.7°	(SD: 16.3)
Sagittal tilt	11.3°	(SD 5.4)
Sacral slope	38.6°	(SD 12.2)
Pelvic tilt	15.7°	(SD 9.2)
Pelvic incidence	51.6°	(SD 13.7)
Extension reserve (right)	11.6°	(SD 8.1)
Extension reserve (left)	12.9°	(SD 8.7)
Calculation of the correction	3.4°	(SD 10.8)

We performed a first analysis on a series of 150 patients. Table 1 shows the results of measurements of sagittal balance.

The measurement of the extension reserve for the right hip in this series is 11.6° and left hip 12.9°. The calculation of the required correction of the defect of sagittal balance is 3.4°. We found a correlation between the angle of correction needed and the age, the angle of lordosis and the imbalance (the angle compared to "plumb-line"). On the other hand, we have not found any correlation between the extension reserve and spinal or pelvic parameters.

Correlations between the correction needed calculated and the different parameters (Table 2).

The extension reserve appears in this study as a single factor that is not closely related to the parameters of sagittal balance.

The study of our patients revealed some specific pathologies. Several patients were found with unequal leg length from a developmental dysplasia in the hip and a limitation of the reserve extension of the dysplastic side, which leads to low back pain. Early orthotic correction of leg length and a stretching programme is hoped to avoid developing back problems in these cases. For some patients, knee conditions with stiffness can also lead to back pain.

Table 2 Correlations between correction and age/lordosis/plumb line

Corr./age	p: 0.008
Corr./lordosis	p: 0.0192
Corr./plumb-line	p: <0.0001

Applications

Stretching

In the literature, it has been reported that stretching programmes provide an improvement in low back pain [11, 12]. However, the angular improvement remains very limited, as has been reported in a series by Kerrigan et al. [13] where a self-rehabilitation protocol over 10 weeks showed only 1.6° improvement on average.

Thus, the rehabilitation with relaxation of sub-pelvic segments appears useful and this programme could be considered in each case where the reserve seems limited, but it appears that one cannot count only on rehabilitation to compensate for extension deficits beyond a certain limit.

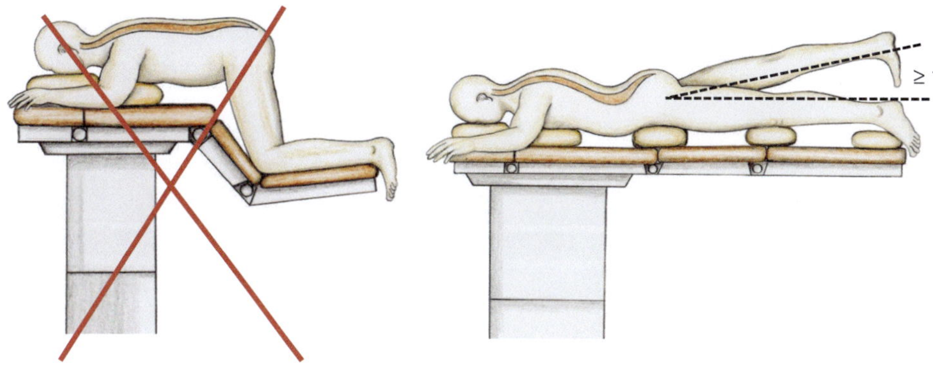

Fig. 6 Kyphoting position on the left, lordoting position on the right

Surgery

1. Prevention is mandatory. To limit the loss of the extension reserve, one must avoid surgical fusions with decreased lumbar lordosis. When positioning the patient for lumbar fusion, femoral flexion should be avoided because in this position a loss of lordosis will occur which not only decreases the patient's extension reserve and disrupts sagittal balance, but in addition limits the possibilities of compensation for the lumbar spine. This may be considered as one of the causes of adjacent segment syndrome and may partly explain why these syndromes appear more frequently after posterior than anterior surgery. In the case where long instrumentation is performed, and specifically with lumbo-pelvic fixation, at the end of the operation, it is imperative that the patient can have at least 10° hip extension compared to the fused spine. This is a prerequisite for post-operative spinal balance and the ability to walk without lumbo-pelvic limitation (Fig. 6).
2. The exploration of Extension Reserve will identify patients who have a hip extension limitation particularly as this does not appear on the full spine radiographs. In this case, an arthrodesis correcting defects of sagittal balance up to the neutral position can cause a failure because it will consolidate a limited extension reserve while removing the ability to compensate with the lumbar spine. Thus, it appears necessary to carry out a more important lordotic correction.

Conclusions and Perspectives

The Extension Reserve appears as an important factor that must be integrated into diagnostic approaches, into surgical correction planning and also into physiotherapy programmes for low back pain patients.

This should also be considered by hip, pelvis and knee surgeons, especially whenever planning a surgical treatment.

In the prevention of low back pain, it is also possible to explore the Extension Reserve to track individuals who represent limitations and avoid back pain that develops later by implementing rehabilitation programmes either through self- or supervised rehabilitation.

The correction formula can help with more precision in the development of the operative strategy for sagittal imbalance.

References

1. Badelon AB, Dumas M, Fabre M. Facteurs constitutionnelles ou acquis favorisant le surmenage du segment mobile vertébral lombaire. Lombalgie et médecine de rééducation. Paris: Masson; 1983. p. 69–78.
2. Ingber RS. Iliopsoas myofascial dysfunction: a treatable cause of "failed" low back syndrome. Arch Phys Med Rehabil. 1989;70:382–6.
3. Kottke FJ, Pauley DL, Ptak RA. The rationale for prolonged stretching for correction of shortening of connective tissue. Arch Phys Med Rehabil. 1966;47:345–52.
4. Offierski CM, Macnab I. Hip-spine syndrome. Spine. 1983;8:316–21.
5. Hovorka I. Extension reserve of the hip in relation with spine. In: Spine concepts. Sauramps: Montpellier; 2007. p. 2007.
6. Dujardin F, Aucouturier T, Bocquet G, et al. Kinematics of the healthy and arthritic hip joint during walking. A study of 136 subjects. Rev Chir Orthop Reparatrice Appar Mot. 1998;84:689–99.
7. Kerrigan DC, Lee LW, Collins JJ, et al. Reduced hip extension during walking: healthy elderly and fallers versus young adults. Arch Phys Med Rehabil. 2001;82:26–30.
8. Lee LW, Kerrigan DC, Della Croce U. Dynamic implications of hip flexion contractures. Am J Phys Med Rehabil. 1997;76:502–8.
9. Hovorka I. Mesure de la réserve d'extension de la hanche en relation avec le rachis. Rev Chir Orthop. 2008;94(8):771–6.
10. Mangione P, Senegas J. Sagittal balance of the spine. Rev Chir Orthop Reparatrice Appar Mot. 1997;83:22–32.
11. Godges JJ, Macrae PG, Engelke KA. Effects of exercise on hip range of motion, trunk muscle performance, and gait economy. Phys Ther. 1993;73:468–77.
12. Winters MV, Blake CG, Trost JS, et al. Passive versus active stretching of hip flexor muscles in subjects with limited hip extension: a randomized clinical trial. Phys Ther. 2004;84:800–7.
13. Kerrigan D, Xenopoulos-Oddsson A, Sullivan MJ, et al. Effect of a hip flexor-stretching program on gait in the elderly. Arch Phys Med Rehabil. 2003;84:1–6.

The EOS System: Overall Assessment of Balance of the Vertebral Column and Its Movements

J. Dubousset

The creation of the EOS system was a confluence of the right people at the right time.

In the first instance where, since 1972, one had noted in the study of the paralytic oblique pelvis [1].

- That radiographs only showed the planar projection of a three-dimensional reality,
- That the whole pelvis could be considered as the "pelvic vertebra" between the lower limbs and the trunk,
- That the whole head, or "heavy cephalic vertebra", the opposite of the support polygon, played a role of inverted pendulum, in posture and the chain of balance, for sitting and standing.

All of this led in 1975 to the three-dimensional notion of the "cone of economy" (Fig. 1) of the muscular work necessary to keep the erect station of the trunk upright or seated.

In this space, joint work had become obligatory between computer engineers and biomechanic engineers, in particular at the LBM (Laboratoire de Biomécanique) of ENSAM (École Nationale Supérieure D'arts Et Métiers) in Paris. This allowed to obtain, from two radiographic planar projections, surface modelling and three-dimensional measurements of scoliotic deformities, until then only confined to 2D planar projections.

Still in the space where the genius of Georges Charpak, rewarded by his Nobel Prize in 1992, allowed, thanks to his invention (multi wires proportionate chamber) with a significant reduction in radiation of each radiograph.

In time, finally, where all these elements were together in the radiography department of Gabriel Kalifa, at Saint Vincent de Paul Hospital, to inspire the team of Georges Charpak to decide to build the prototype of the EOS device, and experimented in 2000 at the same hospital. Jacques Deguise, of LIO Montréal, helped to automate 3D reconstruction [2].

J. Dubousset (✉)
National Academy of Medicine, Paris, France

The device that gives simultaneous anterior-posterior and lateral view radiographs, without distortion or enlargement of the entire standing skeleton, sitting or squatting, gives 2D precise information on the alignment of the different skeletal parts, particularly the lower limbs and trunk. Numerous 3D reconstruction software programmes have since developed based on these raw radiographic data. This allowed at the level of the spine, thorax, pelvis, lower and upper limbs and also the global skeleton to have an exact idea, not only the alignment but also the 3D static morphology and in particular the stacking of skeletal parts in the horizontal planes, with considerably lower radiation compared to the same reconstructions obtained from CT sections whilst maintaining precision.

Despite availability of the first EOS devices for more than 10 years, orthopaedic surgeons, especially spinal, have largely remained using 2D imaging, very centred on the sagittal plane, oblivious to the rotatory aspect, often coupled elsewhere, which happens in the horizontal plane. This suggests a familiarity that has occurred with the various classifications of Lenke for scoliosis or Roussouly for sagittal morphology, which have their merits, but who have neglected this third horizontal dimension that is nevertheless fundamental for function especially the movement despite being "hidden" at first glance.

Information Provided for 2D Alignment of the Body (Fig. 2)

It is understood that with EOS, the X-rays exiting the emitter have the advantage of not being deformed as they are collimated and are always perpendicular to the target. They require a perfect position of the upper limbs, fingers of each hand placed on the corresponding cheekbone of each cheek (so as not to interfere with the posture) and immobility of the patient during the duration of the scan—which may be a possible difficulty in the young child. It takes about 10 s for an adult, less of course for a purely spinal simple sweep, but then we would

J. M. Vital, D. T. Cawley (eds.), *Spinal Anatomy*, https://doi.org/10.1007/978-3-030-20925-4_8

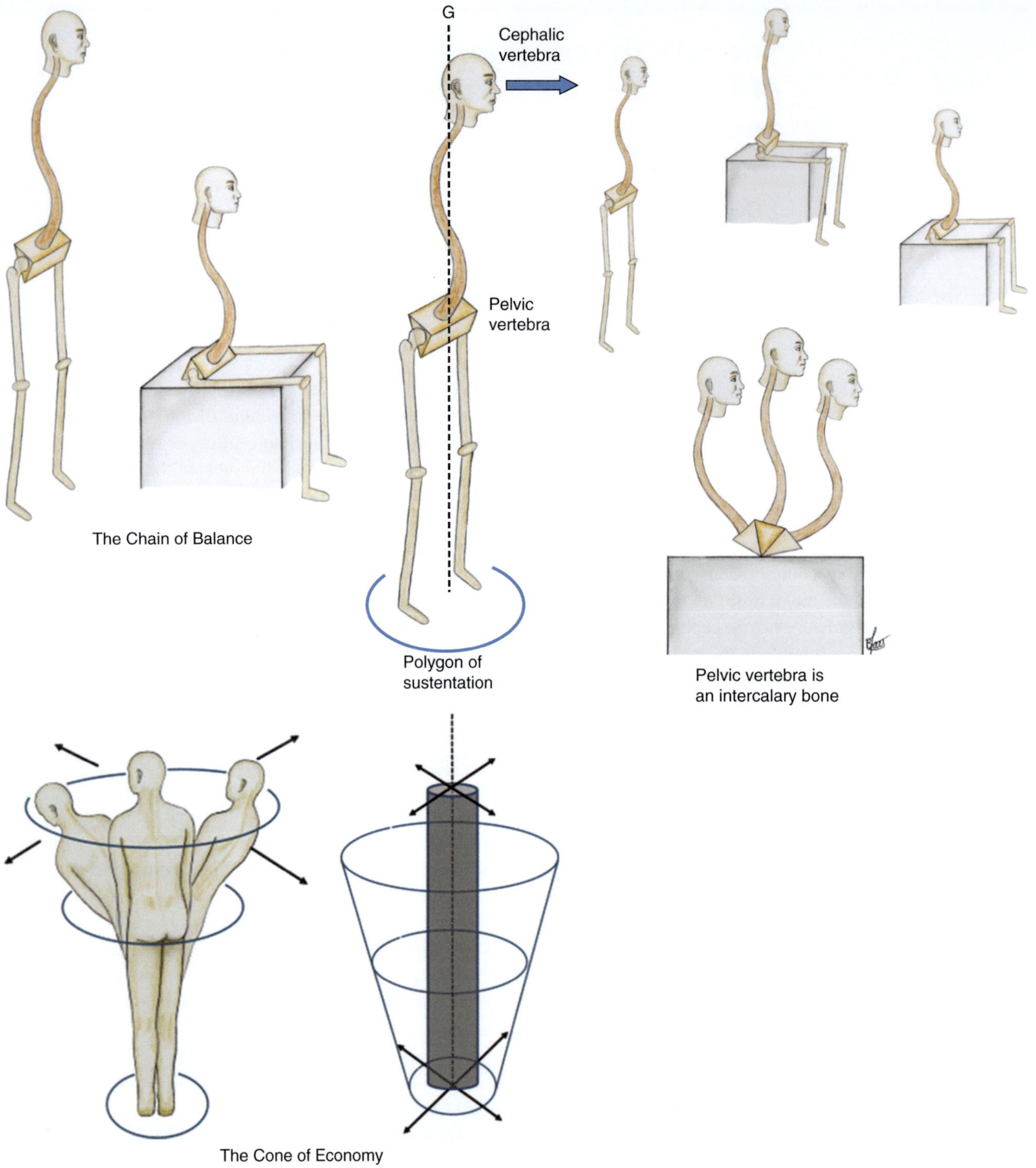

Fig. 1 The Chain of Balance, the cephalic vertebra, the intercalary pelvic vertebra, and the "Cone of Economy"

lose a lot of postural information. These 2D images, obtained with a single shot, thus allow, from a line perpendicular to starting point from the centre of the "Polygon of Support" to give precise measurements on frontal and sagittal body alignment. By measuring the reference points, various bone parts with respect to this axis of reference have been shown to be even more precise and reliable than the no less famous plumb line. They are commonly used for preoperative and post-operative static measurements of orthopaedic surgical procedures involving lower limbs or trunk, and especially the spine.

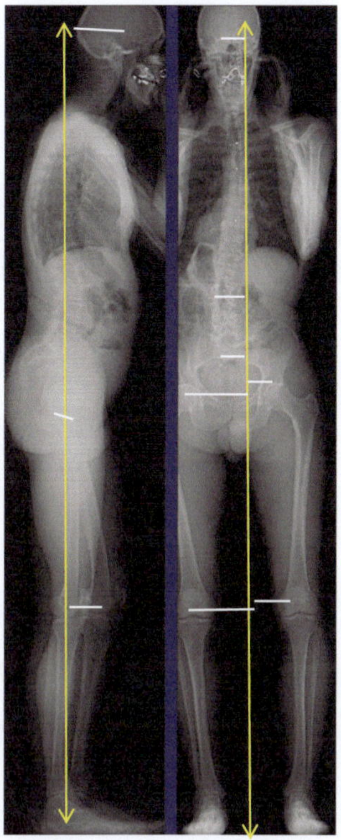

Fig. 2 Two-dimensional (2D) measurements of alignment to the vertical axis drawn from the centre of the Polygon of Support, made from simultaneous images both of the coronal and sagittal profiles of the entire standing skeleton

Information Provided by 3D Volumic Surface Reconstructions Obtained Through Computer Software

They give the same static information as before (Fig. 3), with better reliability because the measurements are generated from well-defined points or reference lines (e.g. mechanical axes of the lower limbs, leg length inequalities and Cobb angle).

Above all, this makes it possible to understand the spatial position of the skeletal elements, especially in the horizontal plane: thus the measurement of the vertebral rotation of each vertebra, and also intervertebral relationships within a scoliotic curvature, with this unique vision of the vertebral column seen from above or below (which demonstrates and visualizes the true basal torsional phenomenon of scoliotic deformity) (Fig. 4).

This approach to the horizontal plane, for the moment, has not been the object of extensive research. It is in stark contrast to the planar radiographic material used for more than a century. The development of 3D CT reconstruction has been used mainly for local morphological purposes and not for a postural and functional approach.

It is therefore easy (Fig. 5) to compare the post-operative and preoperative states in 3D, with reconstruction seen from above, clearly demonstrating the spatial disorder often minimized on simple X-ray images.

However, thanks to dedicated software, EOS makes it possible to perform simulations of scoliosis surgery in 3D (Fig. 6) by varying the implantation levels of the patient.

Similarly, one can simulate levels and values of vertebral osteotomies of large deformities of the child or adult, which minimize or even eliminate malalignment.

EOS allows measurement of anteversion or retroversion of the acetabulum and has direct applications in preoperative simulation and intraoperative navigation of total hip prostheses.

EOS measures the torsional and malalignment phenomena at the level of the lower or upper limbs allowing planning in 3D correction with osteotomies or prosthetic replacement. One has to account for the limitations of intraoperative navigation that this presupposes. The assessment of the anatomical results is then carried out according to real 3D criteria.

EOS allows measurement of thoracic morphology before and after scoliosis surgery, or before and after bracing. EOS can also measure more thoracic data such as thoracic volume (Fig. 7) and/or the spinal penetration index (quantifies the portion of the rib cage occupied by vertebrae) and its outcome after scoliosis surgery, for example [3].

Moreover, EOS perfectly shows the areas at risk of instability or potential rotational dislocation, provided that we analyse the deformed spinal morphology, vertebra by vertebra or disc after disc, favoured by the influence of gravity. The traditional global Cobb angle, with its lumbar and thoracic measurements, which measure only the collapse, are far from the 3D reality [4].

Nothing prevents a surgeon and their computer engineer from developing their own benchmarks and their own software for such a personal study, for the spine or for any other skeletal sector.

For example, Tamas Illès [5] developed the concept of "vertebral vector" (Fig. 8) that quantifies exactly what happens in the horizontal plane at the level of the scoliosis, developed during childhood—regardless of aetiology, or developed in adulthood under the effect of degenerative discs.

We propose that the systematic measurement of this vector during the evolution of childhood or adolescent ("ascending") just as much as for degenerative ("descending") scoliosis will predict its occurrence and if they are only seen once the deformity has been established, the correction strategies are improved.

Finally, EOS is the essential step to understand and measure adequate postural alignment. It should not be confused with the assessment of spinal balance, although it causes confusion everywhere in the spinal world!

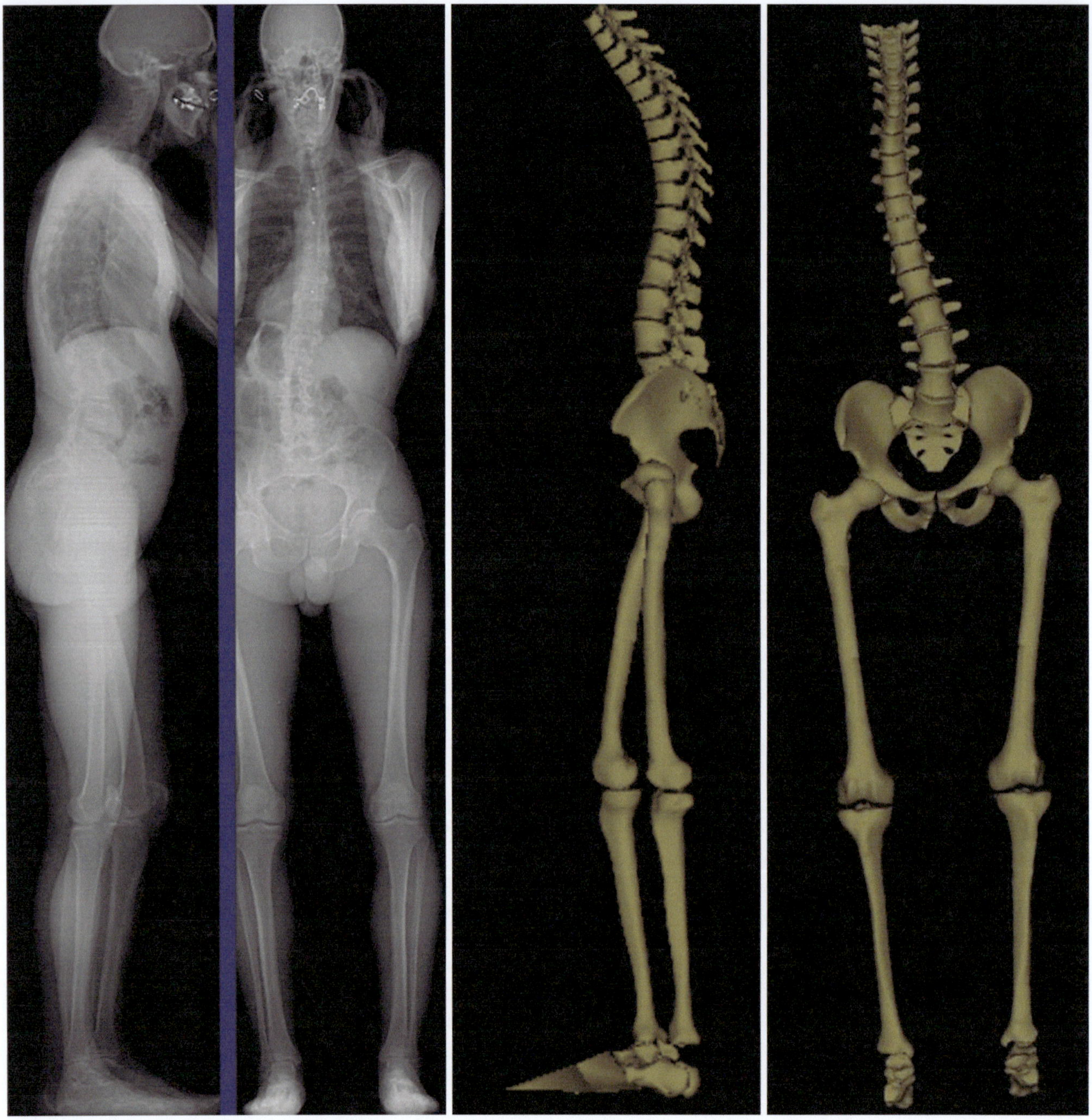

Fig. 3 3D Reconstruction of the entire skeleton while standing

Balance is not a static image as seen on a radiograph. Balance is dynamic, it can be defined as stability in movement. Laboratory measurements require sophisticated multiple systems applied to posture and segmental body mobility, plantar pressures observed on a platform of forces using monopedal or bipedal support, etc. It can only really be learned during dynamic events, causing the movement of the whole body, such as sitting or standing, propulsion or retropulsion, running and up or down the stairs.

The equilibrium of an individual depends in fact on many neurological factors, be they sensory (ocular, vestibular, proprioceptive), motor or automatic reflexes of cerebromedullary origin, where the cognitive implications are relevant. It is therefore understandable that to measure this equilibrium (which when it deteriorates becomes more and more energy consuming), multiple tests are necessary, but do not always require an ambulatory assessment in the laboratory. They can and must be performed in the clinic in the consult-

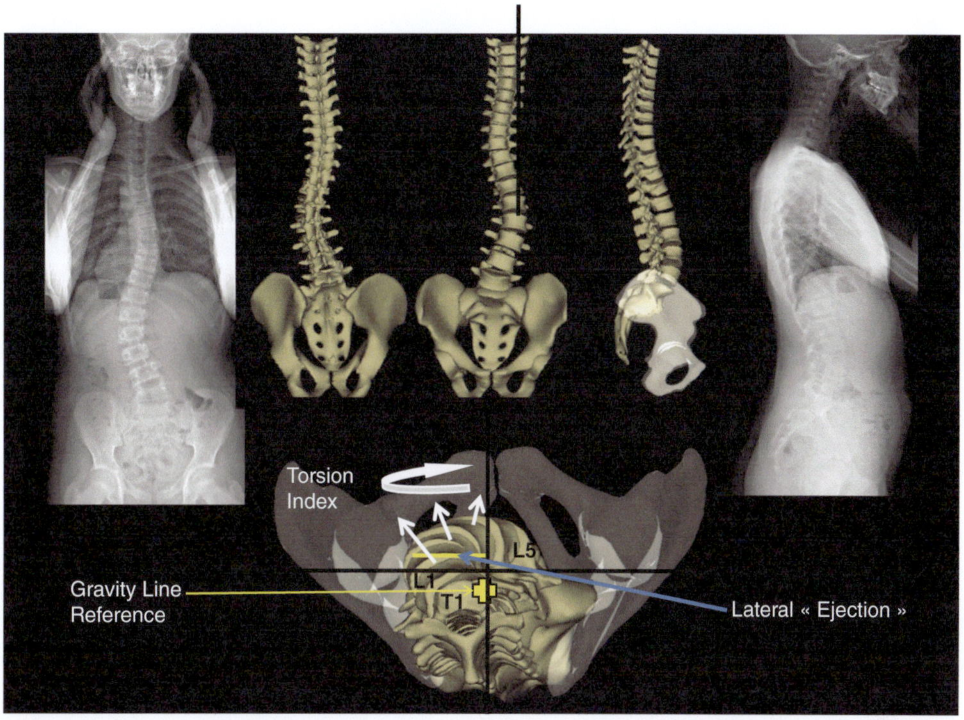

Fig. 4 3D reconstruction of a scoliotic patient's spine, with the axial view from above demonstrating the spinal torsion. This opens a vast field of research

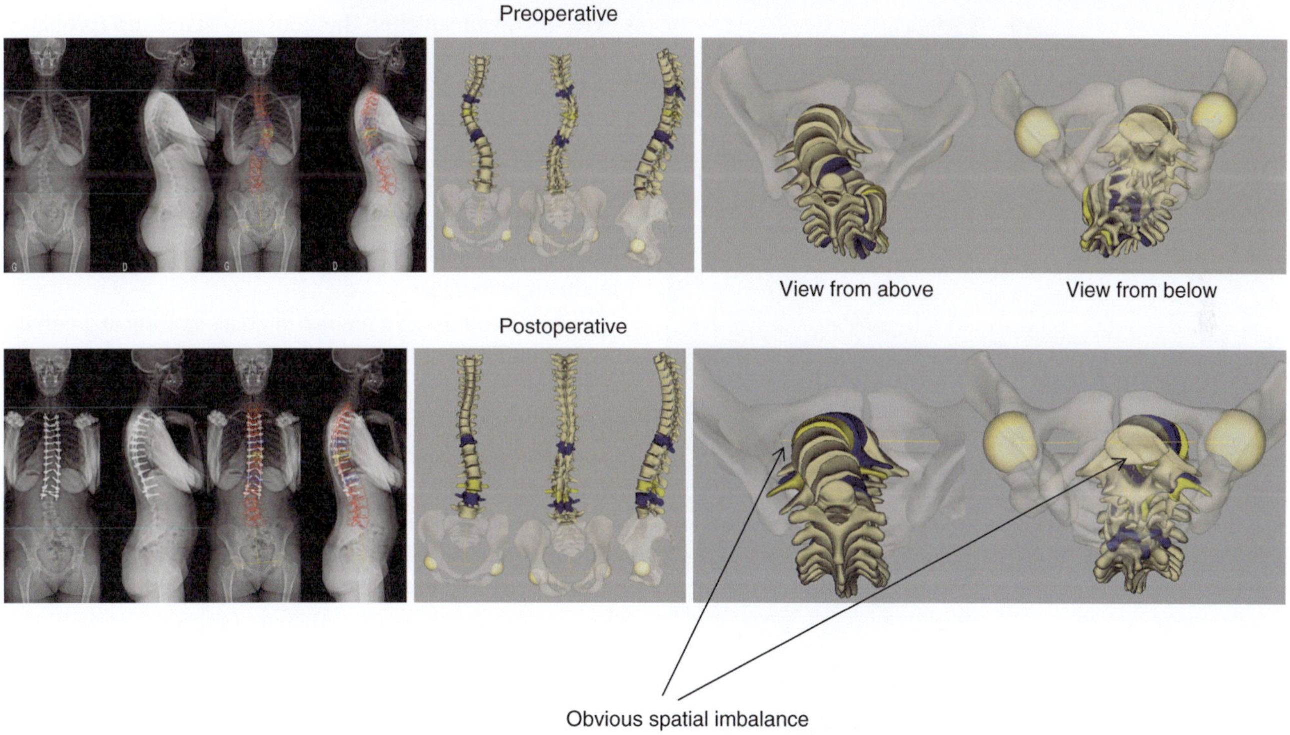

Fig. 5 Preoperative and post-operative comparisons of the 3D correction of scoliosis with the importance of axial reconstruction demonstrating the spatial alignment of the construct

ing room, usually based on a timed speed to perform reference exercises, including when performing a dual task, such as walking by phoning or counting backwards from 100 to 90. Personally, four timed tests seem to be sufficient:

- The patient gets up from the chair and walks 4 m forward and backward and sits back.
- He goes up and down three steps.

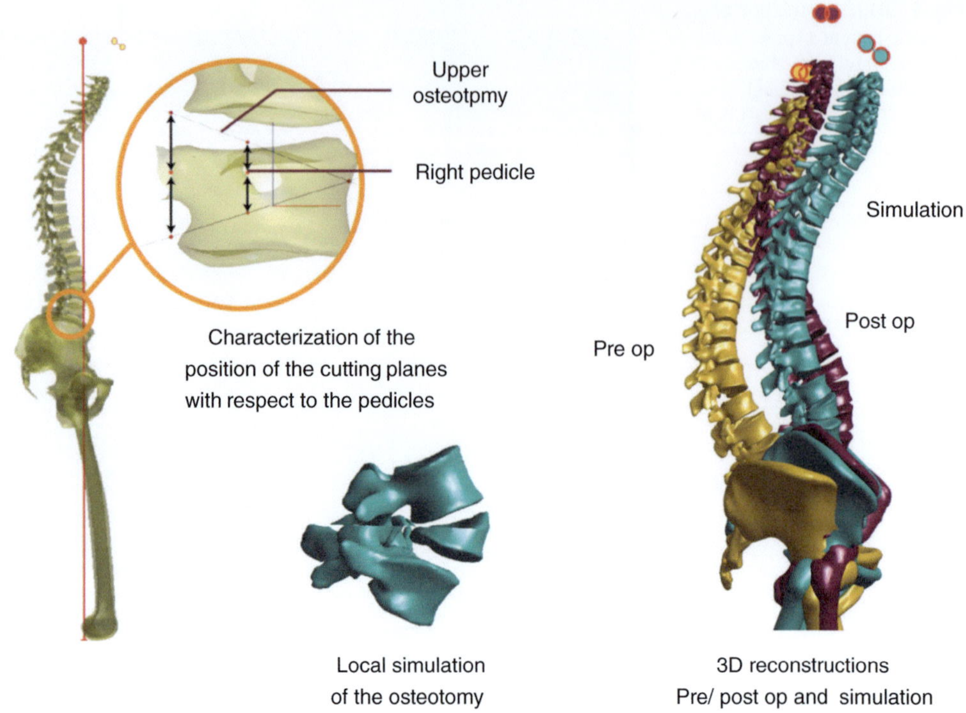

Fig. 6 Planning of the sagittal correction performed by a transpedicular osteotomy on a 3D reconstruction, and comparison in 3D of the result obtained compared to the preoperative simulation

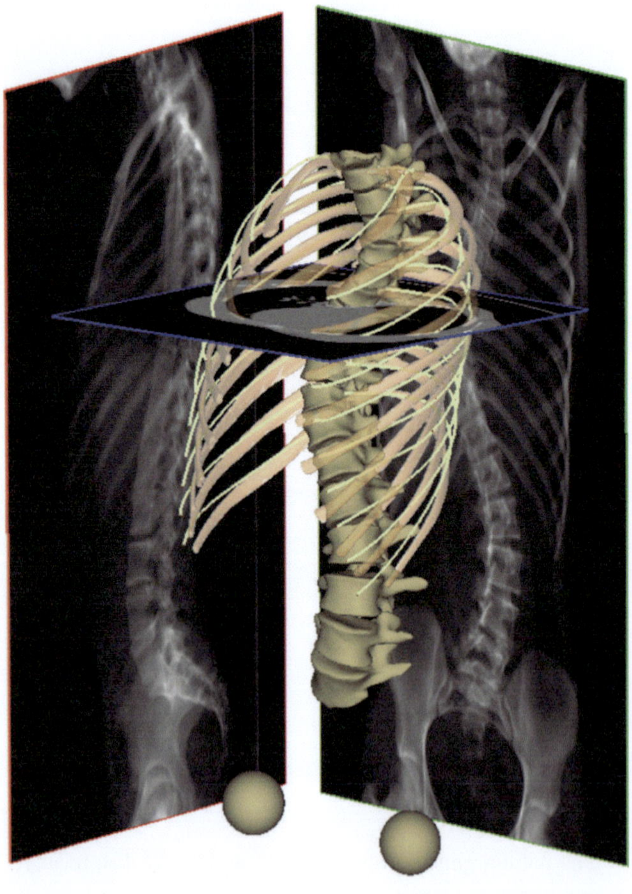

Fig. 7 3D reconstruction of the skeleton of the trunk and in particular, the thoracic cage

- He sits down squat on the floor and stands up (probably the most discriminating test), but this test is refuted by some for very old people because of the risk of falling
- The double-task test.

All this makes it possible to appreciate the relevance of the "cone of economy" at each point of assessment-preoperatively, and on follow-up to appropriately judge the functional outcome.

When performed at a regular interval, starting at a certain age, longitudinally for a given individual with a spinal disorder, a rate of deterioration can be assessed and the appropriate time for a possible realignment surgery can be discussed, encompassing the cardiovascular, nutritional and renal function of the patient.

It is true that the improvement of sagittal alignment is a condition often necessary, even essential to improve balance in kyphotic or kyphoscoliotic collapse of degenerative deformity patients, but it is not sufficient. Ignoring the reality of the multiple mechanisms that comprise the vertical equilibrium can lead to very disappointing functional results despite excellent spinal realignment. Thus (Fig. 9) our current research involving EOS is applied to a mix of static 3D information with data obtained from movement.

I think you have understood that alignment and balance are two elements that are not opposed but complementary.

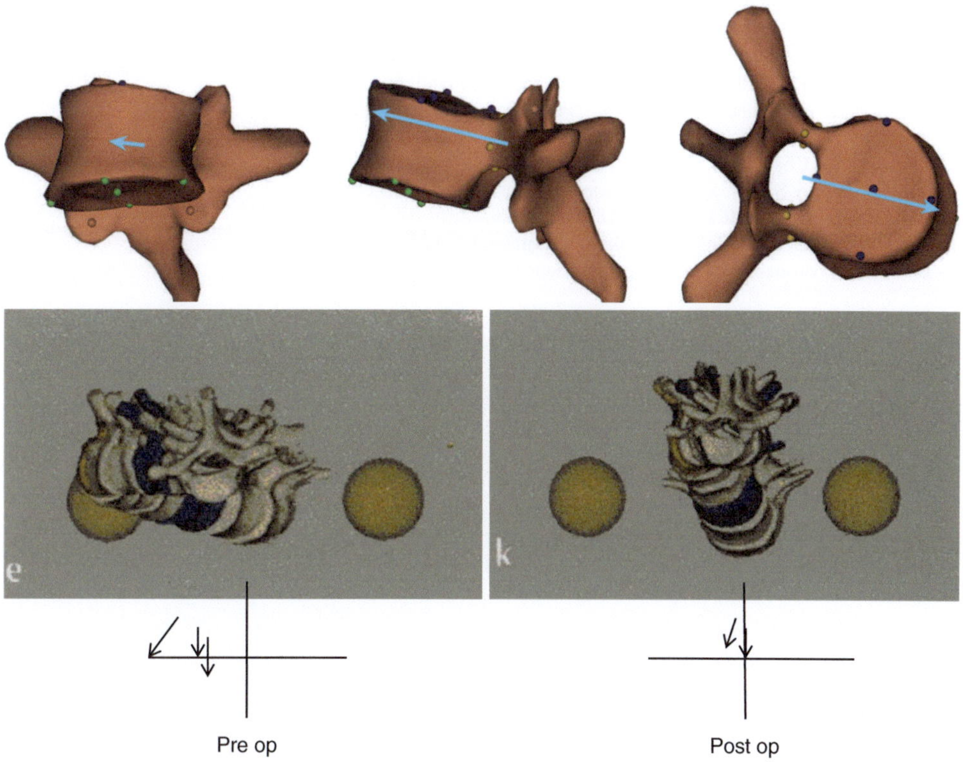

Fig. 8 The "Vertebral Vector" (T. Illes). It is the precise spatial measurement of the 3D orientation of each vertebra, with preoperative and post-operative examples

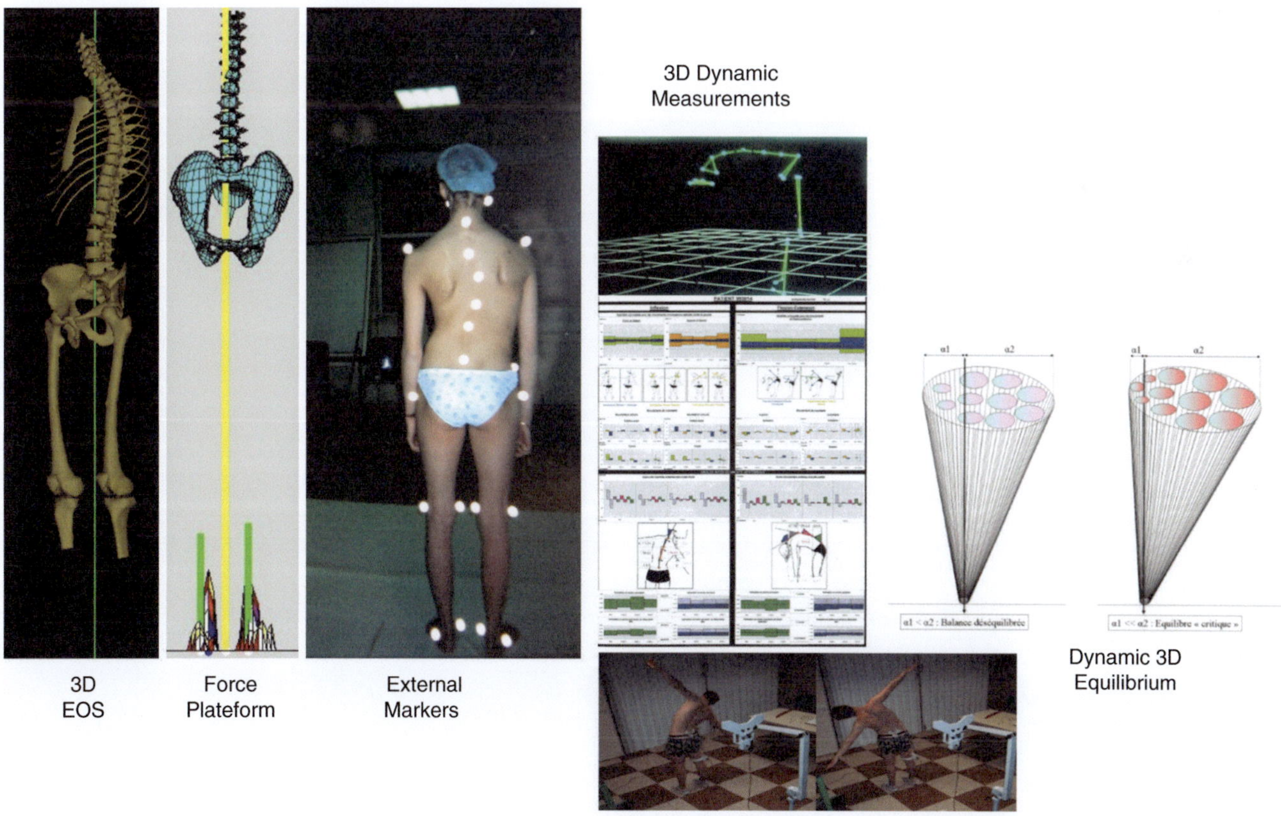

Fig. 9 This is the future: an attempt to mix the static information provided by the EOS system with 3D dynamic movement recordings, to appreciate the dynamic balance of the individual and its evolution over time, either spontaneously or post-operatively

References

1. Dubousset J. Three dimensional analysis of the scoliotic deformity. Chapter 22. In: Weinstein SL, editor. "Pediatric spine" principles and practice. New York: Raven Press; 1994. p. 479–96.
2. Dubousset J, Charpak G, Dorion I, Skalli W, Lavaste F, Deguise J, Kalifa G, Ferey S. A new low dose osteoarticular imaging: the EOS system. Bull Acad Natl Med. 2005;189:287–300.
3. Schwab F, Patel A, Ungar B, Farcy J, Lafage V. Adult spinal deformity-postoperative standing imbalance: how much can you tolerate? An overview of key parameters in assessing alignment and planning corrective surgery. Spine (Phila Pa 1976). 2010;35(25):2224–31.
4. Dubousset J. The aging of the musculoskeletal system with special attention to the aging of the spine. Bull Acad Natl Med. 2009;193:1211–21.
5. Illés T. Comparison of classical 2D measurement of scoliosis and 3D measurement using vertebral vectors; advantages for prognosis and treatment evaluation. Bull Acad Natl Med. 2011;195(3):629–42.

Part III

Descriptive Anatomy

The Cranial Vertebra

Jean Marc Vital and L. Boissière

The skull can be likened to a so-called cranial vertebra, located above the cervical spine with the main function of maintaining in the biped a horizontal gaze. As demonstrated in the chapter of phylogeny, evolution has ensured this important visuo-spatial principle. If one wants to appreciate the sagittal balance of the cervical vertebral column, it is necessary to recognize the radiological references of the cranial vertebra and especially to determine from these reference marks a position, reproducible on lateral radiographs. We will also see in this chapter that it is important to recognize the centre of gravity of the head to locate it above the neck, the trunk, the pelvis and in particular the acetabulum and femoral heads.

Phylogenesis

> We can consider that the nasion-opisthion line is the reference of the horizontal plane.

Many angles have been described by anthropologists to study the evolution of the skull shape according to animal species and in the evolution of hominids, and also to better specify the orientation of the occipital foramen (or foramen magnum) and the orbital cavity. Thus, the occipital angle of Broca (Fig. 1) is delimited by a line joining the nasion (point at the root of the nose) and the opisthion (posterior edge of the occipital foramen) and a line joining the same opisthion at the basion (anterior border of the occipital foramen); this angle decreases when comparing a quadruped skull (45° in a carnivore) to a human skull (10°). This decrease in the occipital angle of Broca corresponds to a horizontalization of the occipital fossa that could be called "intracranial" horizontalization. This horizontalization of the occipital fossa is very clear, moreover, when we compare a primate skeleton with global, cervical, thoracic and lumbar kyphosis and the human skeleton with lumbar lordosis and cervical lordosis. The second angle described by anthropologists is the orbito-occipital angle drawn between the axis of the orbit and the line joining the basion and the opisthion. This angle is

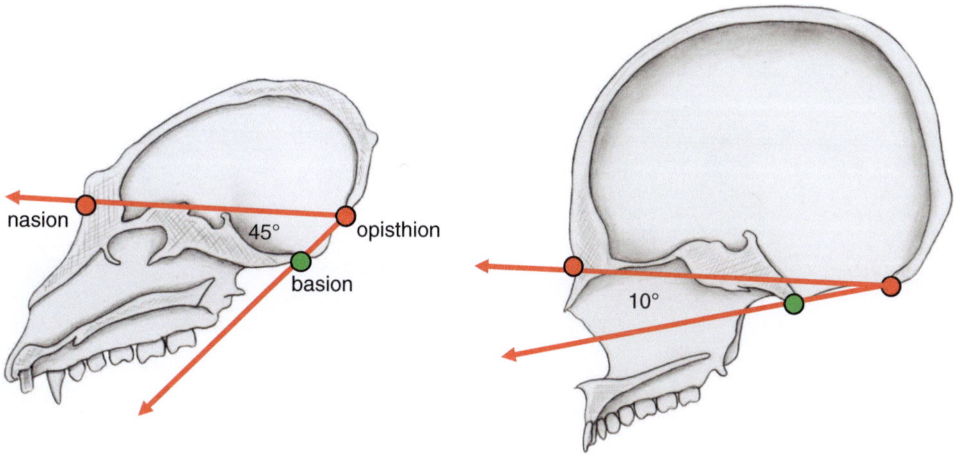

Fig. 1 Occipital angle of Broca; horizontalization of the foramen magnum in the skull

J. M. Vital (✉) · L. Boissière
Spinal Unit, University Hospital, Bordeaux, France

J. M. Vital, D. T. Cawley (eds.), *Spinal Anatomy*, https://doi.org/10.1007/978-3-030-20925-4_9

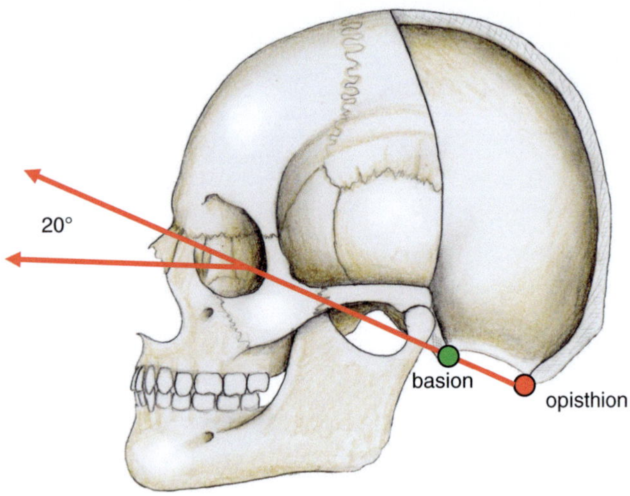

Fig. 2 Orbito-occipital angle in humans: 10°; monkeys: 30–69°, carnivorous: 63–90°

63–90° in carnivores, decreases to a value of 30–69° in monkeys and reaches 20° in humans (Fig. 2). Beauvieux, a Bordelaise anatomist, demonstrated that the nasion-opisthion line is parallel to the lateral semicircular canal of the inner ear. We can therefore consider that the nasion-opisthion line is the reference of the horizontal plane. The axis of the orbit (and therefore that of the gaze) is oriented at 30° downwards and forwards, corresponding to the reference position of the head proposed by many ergonomists (Figs. 3 and 4).

Finally, François Clarac (CNRS, Timone, Marseille) has shown that the foramen magnum has become more and more anterior in the evolution of primates, which tends to increase the leverage of the extensors on the occiput, an essential phenomenon for keeping the head and the eyes horizontal (Fig. 5).

Fig. 3 The lateral (or horizontal) semicircular canal is parallel to the nasion-opisthion plane (Beauvieux)

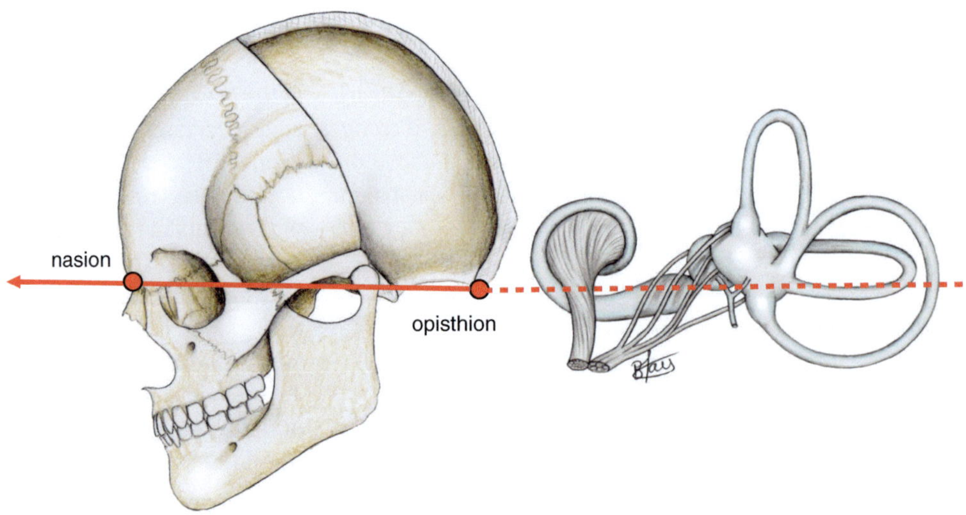

Fig. 4 Reference position; the nasion-opisthion line is horizontal and the axis of the orbit is 30° to this line

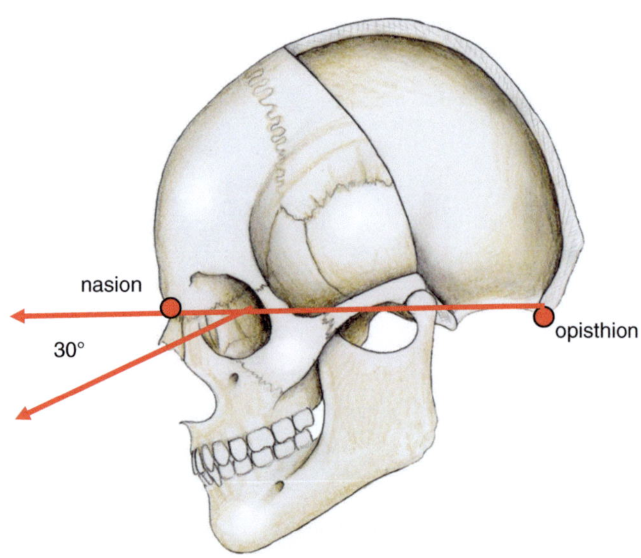

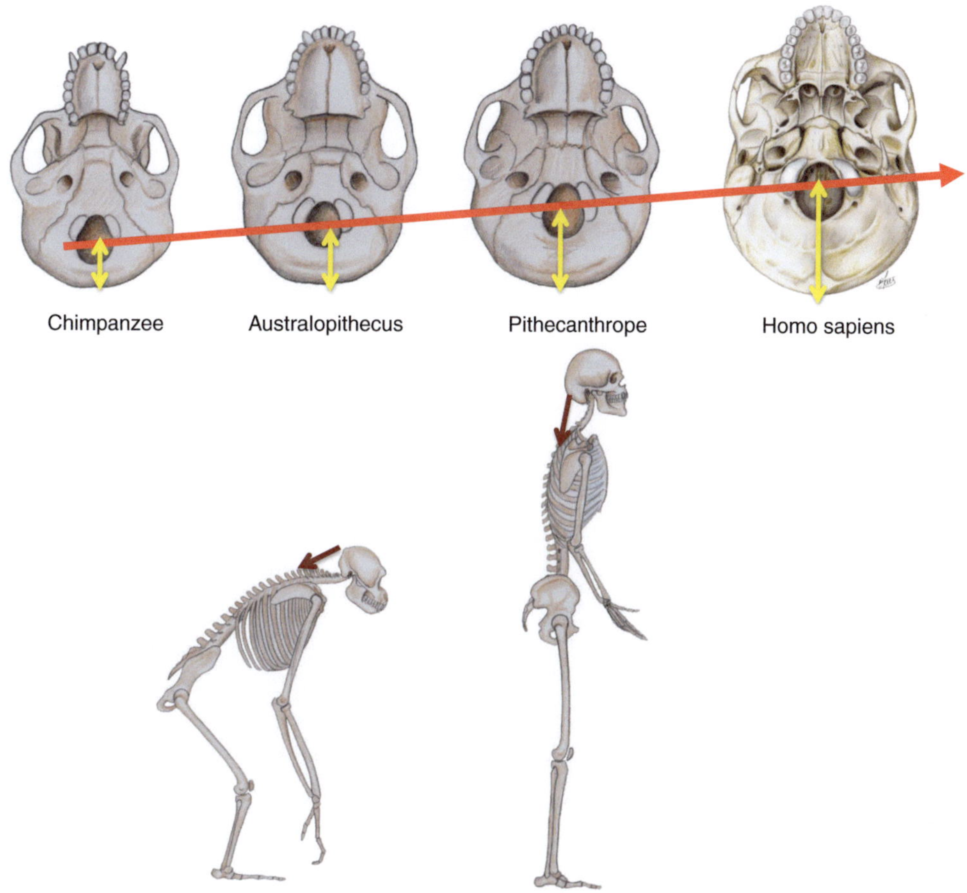

Fig. 5 Evolution of the foramen magnum position in primates (Clarac)

Centre of Gravity of the Head

The centre of gravity of the head is projected directly above the external auditory canals.

This centre of gravity was the subject of an anatomical study published in Surgical Radiology Anatomy in 1986 [1]. The so-called suspension method was applied to six cadaveric skulls from three women and three men weighing between 3.7 kg and 5.2 kg, with cranial indices ranging from 72 (dolichocephalic) to 85 (brachycephalic). The penetration points of Gardner's tongs that allowed the centre of gravity of the head to be recognized were all projected over an area of one square centimetre above the tragus. Radiologically, the centre of gravity projected in the middle of the nasion-inion (external occipital protuberance) line. Slightly behind the sella turcica and directly above the external auditory canal (Table 1 and Figs. 6, 7, and 8). It is interesting to note in Fig. 9 that in the reference position, antagonizing anterior and posterior muscles maintain the head above the cervical spine. The lever arm of the weight of the head applied to the centre of gravity, previously described, is strictly equal to the lever arm of the extensor muscles inserted on the occipital aspect (Fig. 9); on the other hand, when the gaze is horizontal, the leverage of the extensors is greater than that of gravity (Fig. 10).

Table 1 Centre of gravity of the head; characteristics of studied skulls

Specimen number	Sex	Head weight (kgs)	Cranial index	Type
1	F	3.67	85	Brachy
2	F	3.73	76	Dolicho
3	F	4.03	72	Dolicho
4	M	4.33	80	Brachy
5	M	5.21	83	Brachy
6	M	4.82	73	Dolicho

How to Recognize the Exact Position of the Head on Lateral Radiographs?

Since the cranial vertebra is located above a cervical spine that has a certain flexibility and mobility, it has always been difficult to determine a reference position. Thus some prefer to study the sagittal balance of the vertebral column only from

Fig. 6 Description of the suspension method

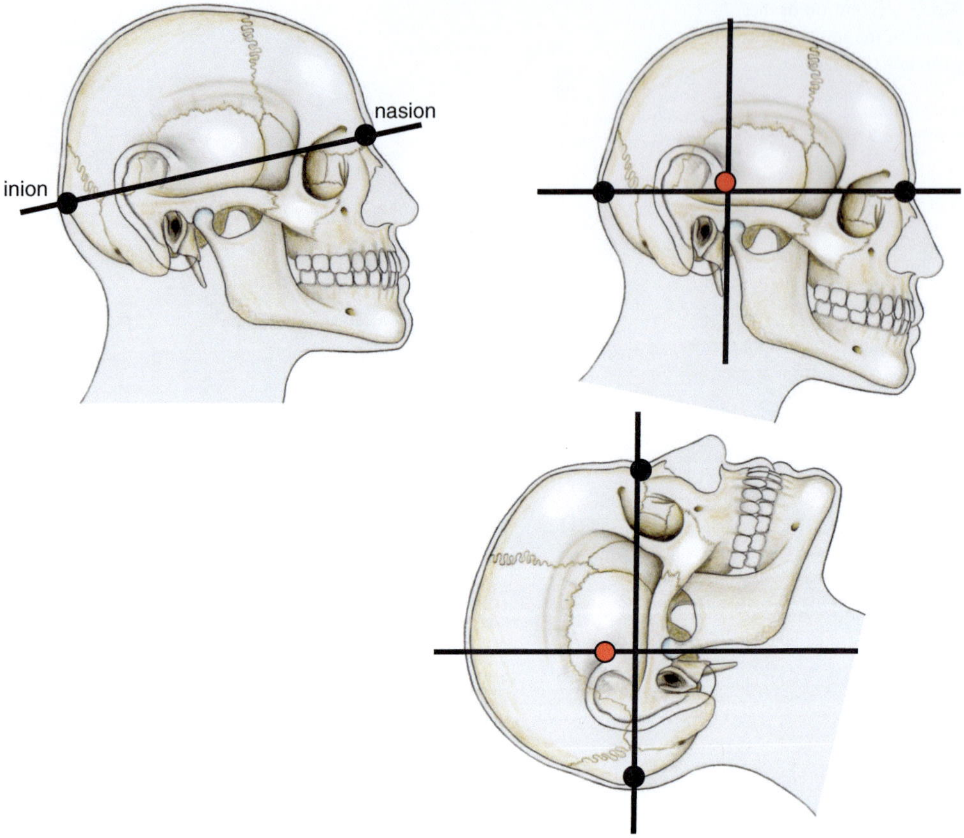

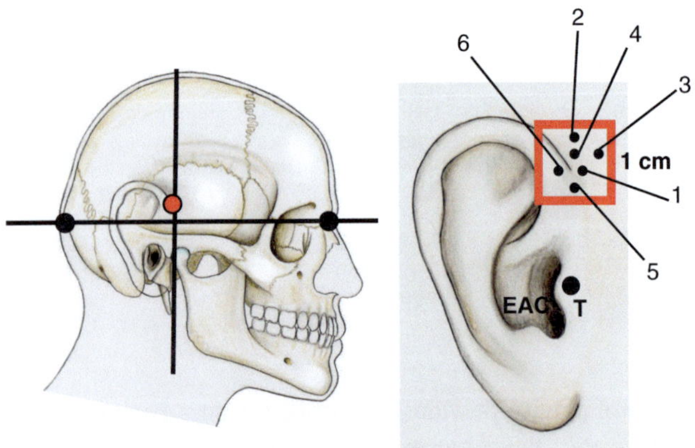

Fig. 7 Demonstration of the centres of gravity of the six specimens. *EAC* External Auditory Canal, *T* Tragus

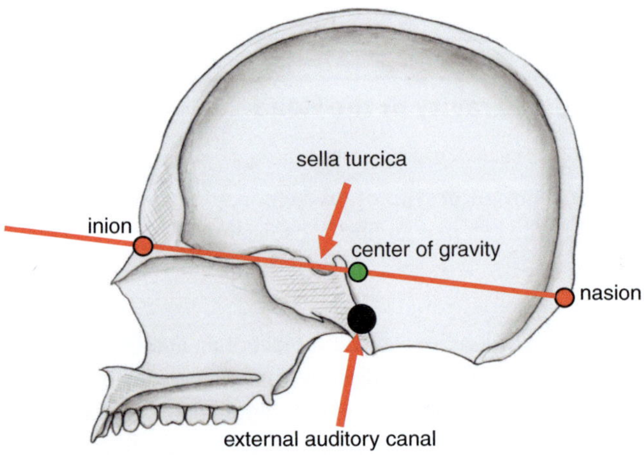

Fig. 8 Projection of a lateral radiograph of the skull with the centre of gravity

the vertebra C7, using in particular the C7 plumbline or vertical line lowered from the middle of the body of C7. Nevertheless Sokolov [2] and Peng [3] have studied the reproducibility of the natural position of the head in the standing position using a mirror placed in front, with which the subject will fix his eyes. They advocate the use of a mirror placed in front, with which the subject will fix his eyes. This mirror can be applied at the EOS system panel in front of the X-rayed subject (Fig. 11). More recently, Sugrue [4] proposes to position the head of the X-rayed subject by aligning the nasion-inion line along the horizontal (Fig. 12). This technique requires repeated snapshots to ensure the correct position of the head. We undoubtedly prefer the use of the mirror. It should be noted that this reference position of the head on the radiograph corresponds to a horizontal gaze, contrary to the ergonomic reference position with a look that is at 30° downwards.

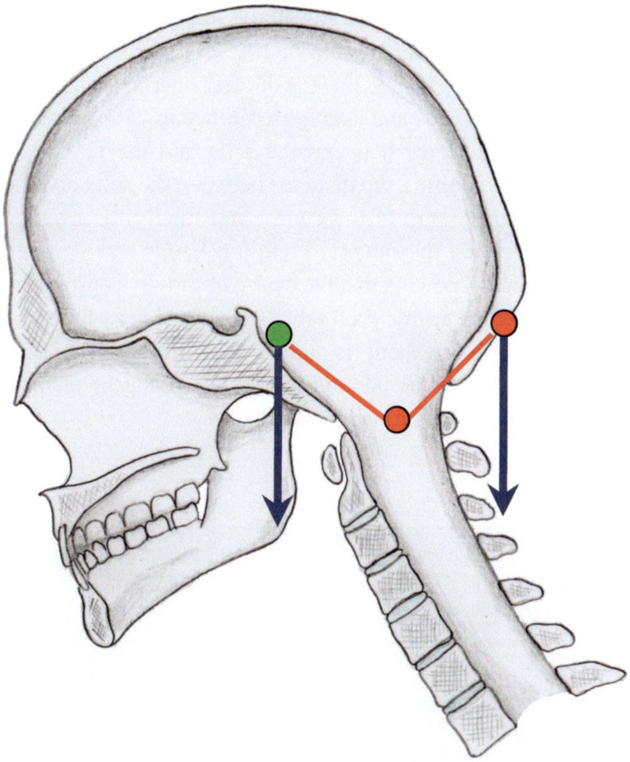

Fig. 9 Inter support lever system in the reference position with equivalent loads

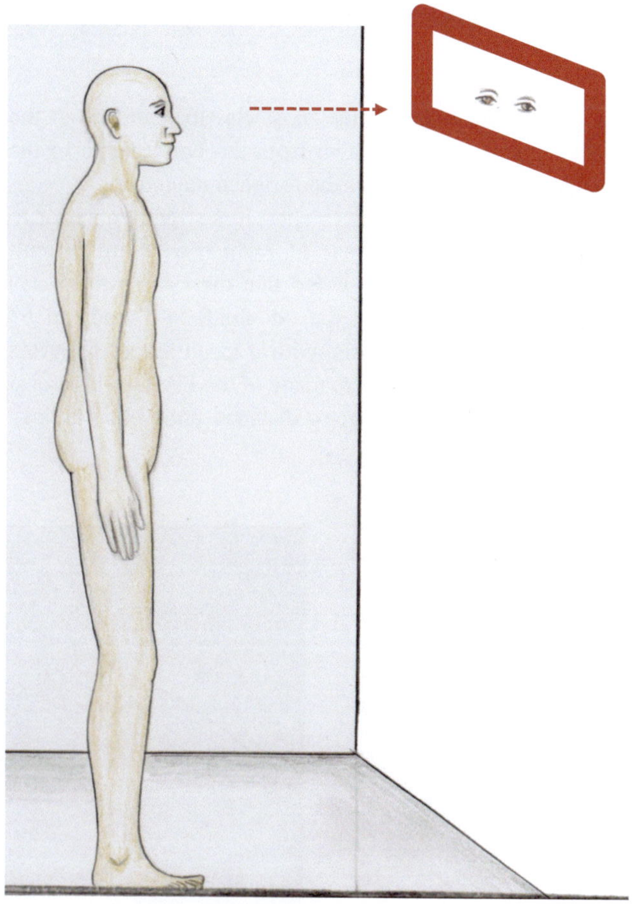

Fig. 11 Control of the position of the head by a mirror

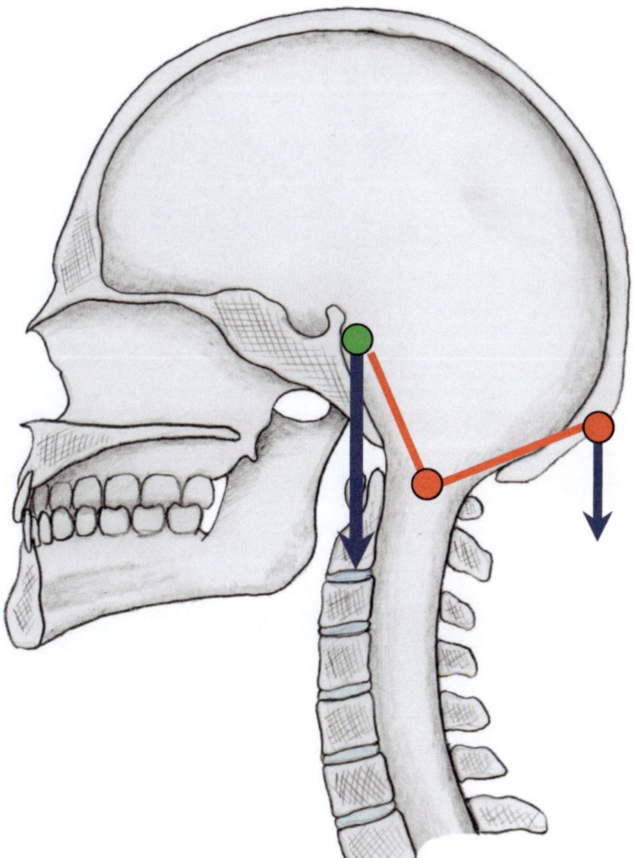

Fig. 10 Inter support lever system with horizontal gaze

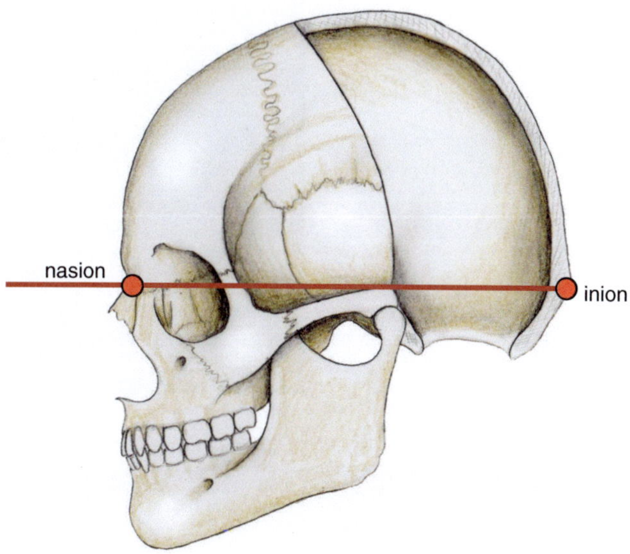

Fig. 12 Horizontal reference nasion-inion line (Sugrue [4])

What Radiological References May We Use? (Fig. 13)

The line of McGregor is the most classic reference at the level of the skull: it is drawn from the bony palate to the opisthion (posterior edge of the foramen magnum).

The sella turcica is easy to spot; it is slightly anterior to the external auditory canals (EAC) which are more difficult to recognize. It should be noted that the EACs are always vertically above the tip of the odontoid. In a study of 53 patients treated for scoliosis, with a mean age of 61 years (27–81), measurements were made of the EAC–sella turcica distance, EAC–odontoid apex distance and sella turcica–odontoid apex distance. In this study, the sella turcica was visible and clearly identifiable in 100% of cases, while the EACs were poorly visible in 41% of cases, perfectly identifiable in 25% of cases and average visibility in 24% of cases. The average distance between the sella and the EAC was 21.8 mm (10–34 mm), the distance between the sella and the odontoid was 19 mm (4.6–34 mm) and finally the average distance between the odontoid and the EACs was 2.7 mm (1.3–8.7 mm). Knowing that the centre of gravity is projected near the EAC, it seems preferable to retain this as the main landmark with, if there is a difficulty of identification, recourse to that of the odontoid apex which is projected, as we have said, vertically below these EACs.

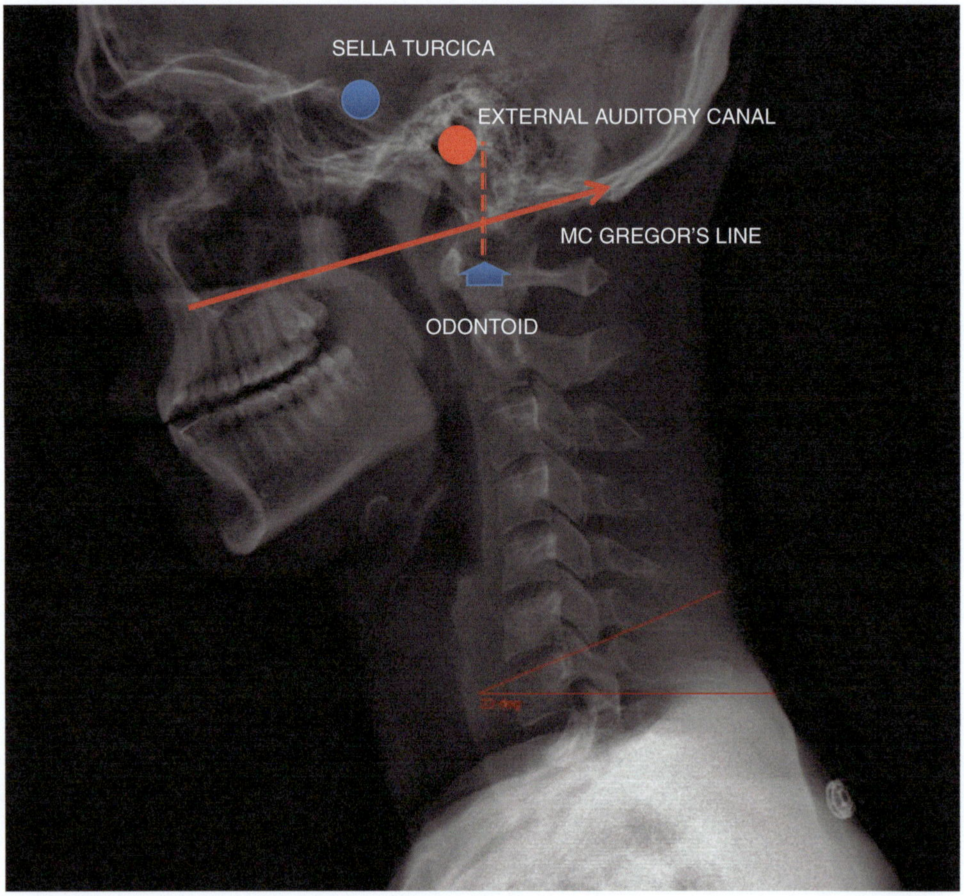

Fig. 13 Main cranial landmarks

How Is the Sagittal Cervical Balance Below the Cranial Vertebra?

> The cervical spine functions as an adjustment rod, upwards to ensure the horizontal gaze and downwards to accommodate the thoracic kyphosis.

The cervical spine adapts its position between the horizontality of the gaze at the top and the orientation of the vertebra C7 (or T1) at the bottom. The so-called slope of C7 (or T1) drawn between the horizontal and the upper endplate of C7 (or T1) is determined by the value of thoracic kyphosis, which is determined by the type of patient's profile, static (with low curvatures and small pelvic incidence) or dynamic (with large curvatures and high pelvic incidence). Vidal and Marnay [5] noted, in 1984, that a small C7 slope is associated with cervical hypolordosis, or even kyphosis, and that, conversely, a large C7 slope is associated with hyperlordosis (Fig. 14). In fact, this cervical lordosis is unequally distributed between a lordosis of the high cervical spine (C1C2),

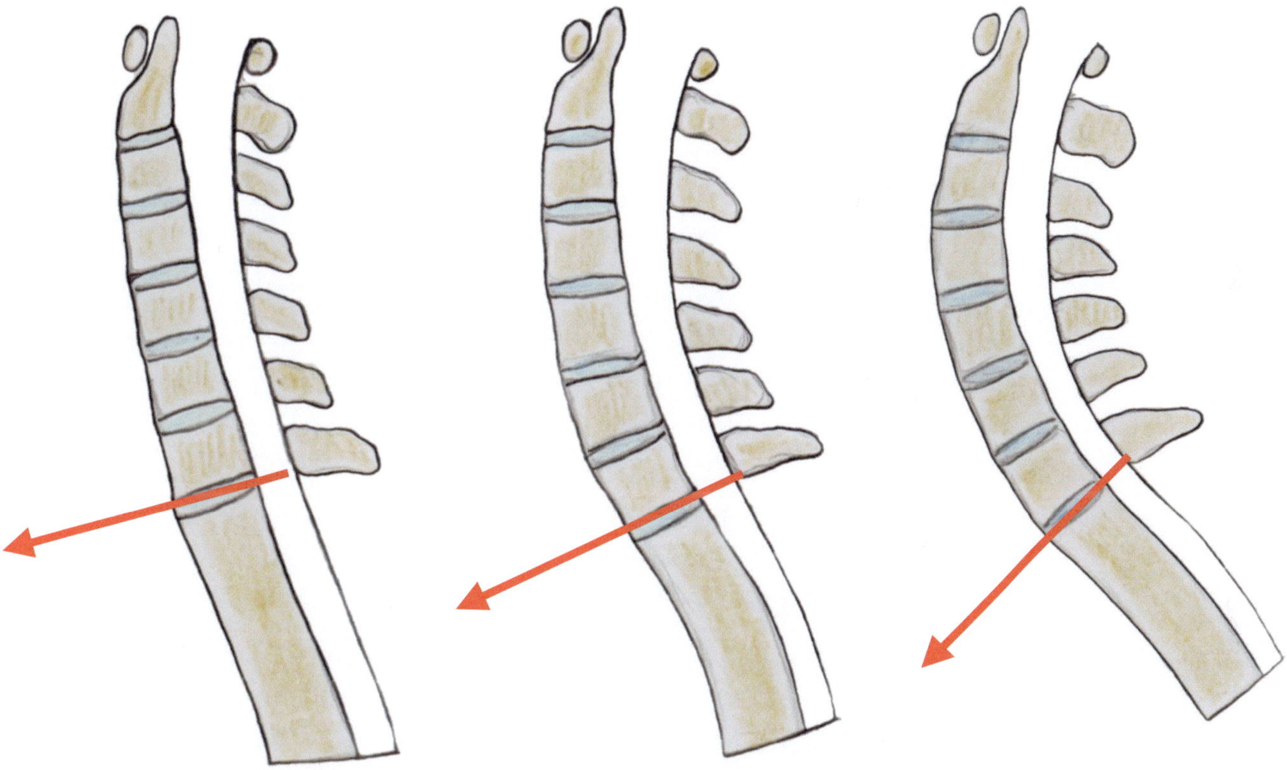

Fig. 14 Relationship between the C7 slope and cervical lordosis (Marnay [5])

Fig. 15 The upper cervical spine functions as an inverted pendulum above the lower cervical spine

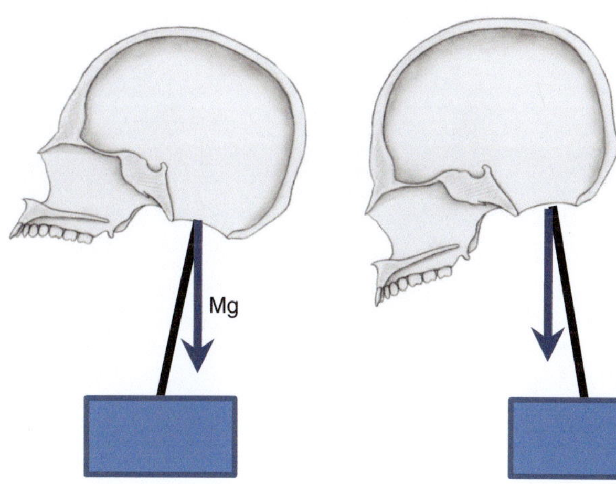

with a mean value of 26–29°, and a lordosis of the low cervical spine (C2C7), much lower since it varies between 5 and 6°. The upper cervical spine functions as an inverted pendulum above the lower cervical spine to ensure the horizontality of the gaze (Figs. 15 and 16). The cervical spine, therefore, as a whole, can be thought of as an upward adjustment rod to keep the gaze horizontal and downward to fit the cervicothoracic junction (Fig. 17), all of which aims to ensure a correct vertical alignment between the cranial vertebra and its centre of gravity, which is the EAC and the pelvic vertebra with its femoral heads, as suggested by Braune and Fischer in 1936 (Fig. 18).

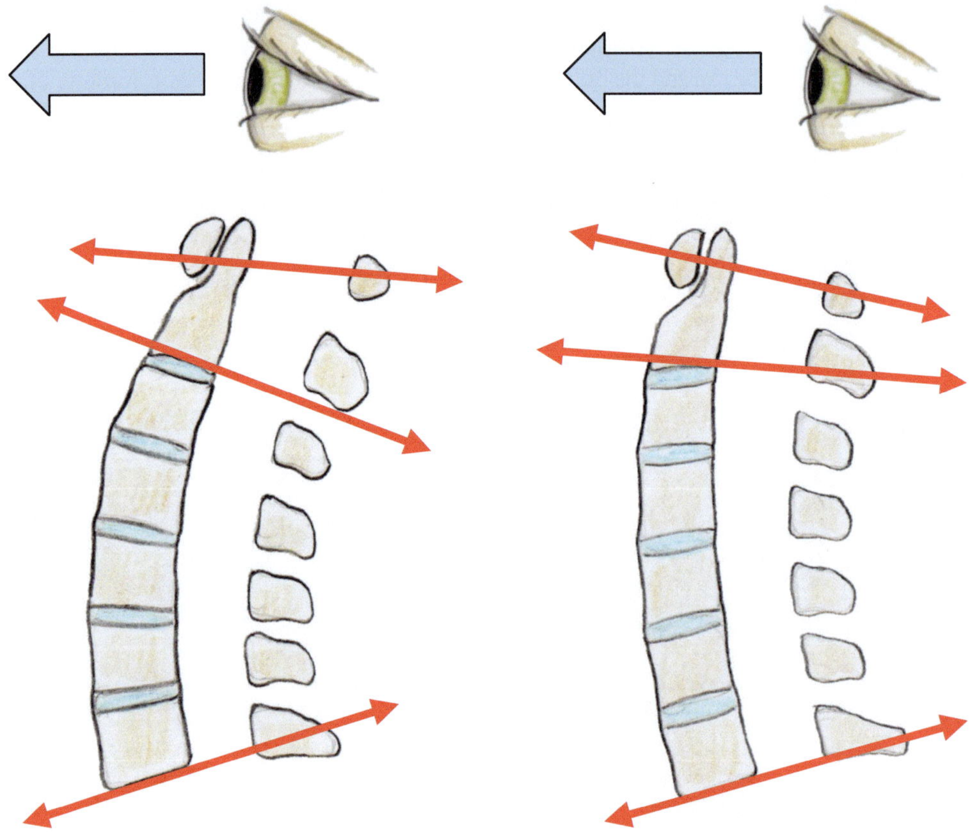

Fig. 16 Compensation of the upper cervical spine above the lower cervical spine to maintain horizontal gaze

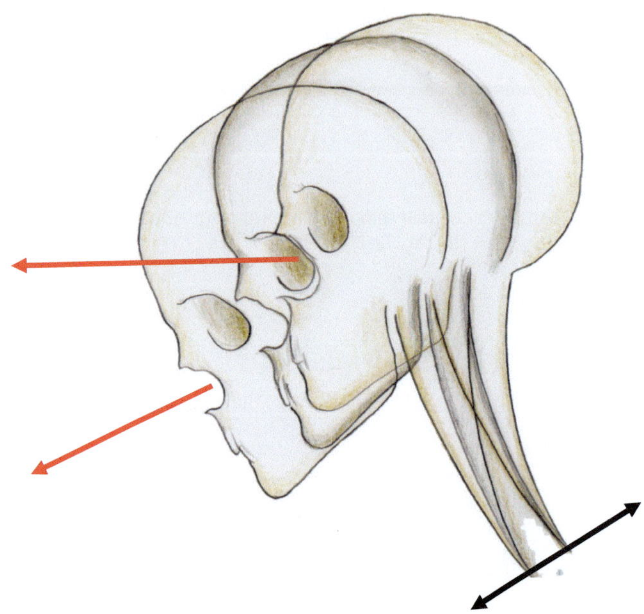

Fig. 17 The cervical spine functions as an upward adjustment rod to ensure horizontal gaze and downward to accommodate thoracic kyphosis

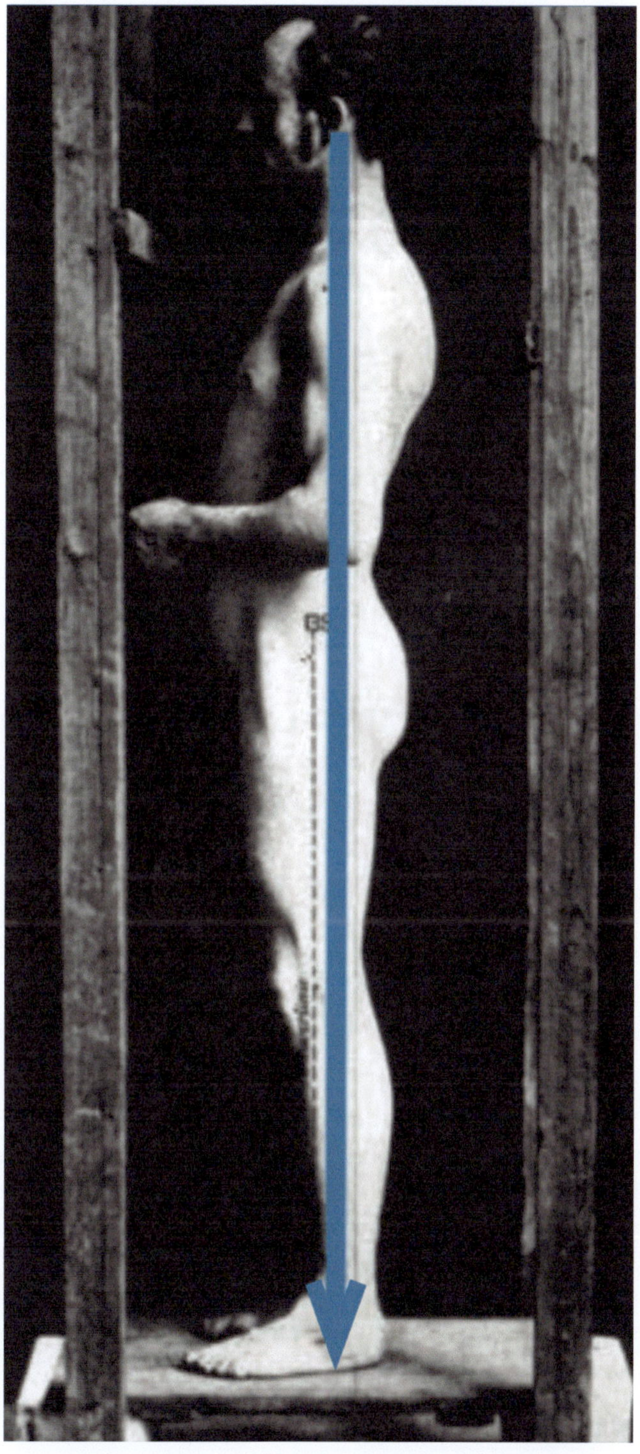

Fig. 18 Relatively constant alignment between the EACs (centres of gravity of the cranial vertebra) and the femoral heads in the centre of the pelvic vertebra (Braune and Fischer)

References

1. Vital JM, Sénégas J. Anatomical bases of the study of the constraints to which the cervical spine is subject in the sagittal plane. A study of the Centre of gravity of the head. Surg Radiol Anat. 1986;8:169–73.
2. Solow B, Tallgren A. Natural head position in standing subjects. Acta Odontol Scand. 1971;29:591–607.
3. Peng L, Cooke MS. Fifteen-year reproducibility of natural head posture: a longitudinal study. Am J Orthod Dentofac Orthop. 1999;116:825.
4. Sugrue PA, McClendon J Jr, Smith TR, Halpin RJ, Nasr FF, Oshaughnessy BA, Koski TR. Redefining global spinal balance: normative values of cranial Centre of mass of a prospective cohort of asymptomatic individuals. Spine. 2013;38:4849.
5. Vidal J, Marnay T. Sagittal deviations of the spine, and trial of classification as a function of the pelvic balance. Rev Chir Orthop. 1984;70(suppl 2):124–6.

Surgical Anatomy of the Vertebral Pedicle

I. Obeid and Jean Marc Vital

The vertebral pedicles are an anatomical structure that connects the posterior arch to the vertebral body. The pedicle has a cylindrical shape with an oval section and flared ends. The exterior is of cortical bone and within is cancellous bone, which may be more or less dense but is sometimes non-existent. The pedicle is an essential element of stability in the vertebra and its involvement, particularly in tumour pathology, is a major sign of instability and increases the risk of fracture, as shown in recent vertebral tumoural classifications.

The pedicle is an essential element in spinal instrumentation as it provides a strong anchorage for osteosynthesis that allows a satisfactory correction of spinal deformities as well as a rigid stabilization of traumatic, degenerative, infectious, iatrogenic or tumoural instability. Direct instrumentation of the pedicle can be performed either through a pedicle screw, which was introduced by Roy-Camille in the early 70s [1, 2], or by a "pedicle" hook which rests on the posterior edge of the pedicle, but which can only be used at the level of the thoracic vertebral column. The pedicle also plays a role of indirect stability in the instrumentation of the vertebral body (anterior and lateral osteosynthesis) or of the posterior arch (hooks, wires or laminar links) while ensuring the transmission of the stresses between the posterior and anterior columns of the vertebra; thus a fixation of the vertebral body or of the posterior arch can be solid only where this structure is intact.

Many recent studies have focused on the morphology and biomechanics of the pedicles. Knowledge of the dimensions and orientation of pedicles is important in order to adapt the spinal instrumentation and reduce iatrogenic risk. The anatomical variations depend on the spinal segment and the presence or not of a deformity, in particular scoliosis.

I. Obeid (✉) · J. M. Vital
Spine Surgery Department, Bordeaux University Hospital, Bordeaux, France

We will, in this article, study the anatomy of the thoracic and lumbar vertebral pedicle on both a normal and deformed spine.

Anatomical Studies, Dimensions and Orientation of Vertebral Pedicles in a Normal Spine

Overview

The tubular-shaped pedicle bridges the anterior vertebral body to the posterior structures at the confluence of the lamina, the transverse process, the superior and inferior articular processes. It is bordered proximally by the overlying intervertebral foramen at the retrodiscal aspect and distally by the next underlying intervertebral foramen in its retrocorporeal part. The outgoing root is in contact with the inferior edge of the pedicle. The medial side of the pedicle forms the lateral wall of the lateral recess; which is therefore in contact with the neurological structures. At the proximal thoracic and lumbar level, the medial wall is in contact with the dural sac, at the middle lumbar level and at the lumbosacral junction, it is in contact with the nerve root at its lateral recess. The lateral wall of the pedicle is in contact with the psoas muscle at the lumbar level and with the costal heads at the thoracic level (Fig. 1).

Lateral or proximal escape of a screw during transpedicular instrumentation results in decreased mechanical strength, while a medial or distal breakage may be more likely to result in or spinal nerve root or cord injury, depending on the region.

The width of the pedicle is defined by the narrowest transverse diameter, and the height by the narrowest sagittal diameter. The transverse angle is defined by the obliquity in the transverse plane between the axis of the pedicle and the anteroposterior axis of the vertebra; this angle often has an anterior apex, thus convergent. The sagittal angle is defined by the obliquity in the sagittal plane between the axis of the

J. M. Vital, D. T. Cawley (eds.), *Spinal Anatomy*, https://doi.org/10.1007/978-3-030-20925-4_10

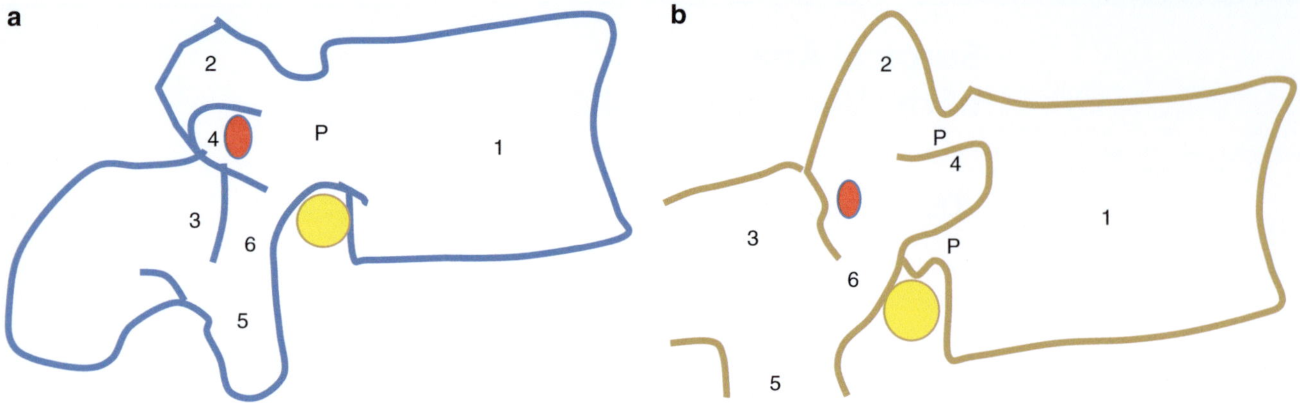

Fig. 1 (**a**) Schematic of a right-side view of a lumbar vertebra showing the position of the pedicle (P) between the vertebral body in front (1) and posterior arch. The posterior point of entry to the pedicle is located at the junction of the upper facet joint (2), the lamina (3) and the transverse process (4); it is separated from the lower facet joint (5) by the isthmus (6). We note the relationship of the pedicle with the exiting root from the intervertebral foraminal position (yellow circle). (**b**) Schematic oblique view of a lumbar vertebra showing the position of the pedicle (P) between the vertebral body anteriorly (1) and the posterior arch

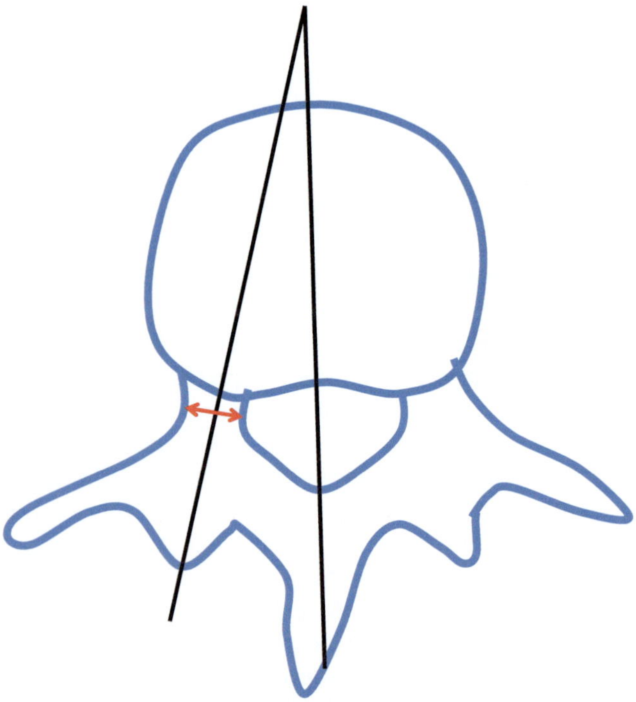

Fig. 2 Diagram of a vertebra, from above showing the transverse angle of the pedicle (between the two lines in black) and the transverse diameter of the pedicle (double red arrow) which is its smallest dimension

pedicle and the superior endplate of the vertebra (Figs. 2 and 3). The transverse interpedicular distance is the distance between the centres of the pedicles of the same vertebra and the vertical interpedicular distance is the distance between the pedicles of two adjacent vertebrae.

The lateral and proximal cortices of the thoracic pedicles extend beyond the limits of the vertebral bodies and endplates, respectively, while at the lumbar level the vertebral bodies and endplates are beyond these same pedicular cortices [3].

Comparative Anatomy by Location

The height but especially the pedicle width are essential elements to know in order to adapt the diameter of the pedicle screw. Several cadaveric and radiological CT anatomical studies have been conducted to identify pedicle dimensions [3–5].

Pedicle width is the essential and determining element. It reaches its minimum at the level of T4 and T5 with an average pedicle diameter of 4.5 mm, sometimes with values <3 mm. This dimension increases by moving away from T4 and T5 to reach 8 mm at T1 and at T11.

At the lumbar level, the pedicle of L2 has the smallest width with an average of 6 mm but can sometimes fall well below this; the lumbar pedicle width increases progressively to reach 15 mm at L5. The pedicle height increases gradually from the T1 up to T12 where it reaches its maximum then decreases until L2 remaining similar through to L5. The height at T1 is on average 8 mm; the height at T12 is 17 mm; at the level of the lumbar region it is around 15 mm. Pedicle height is therefore not a limiting factor in pedicle screw instrumentation.

Orientation [6] (Figs. 2 and 3)

It is essential to know the orientation of the pedicle to optimize the quality of the pedicle screw.

In the sagittal plane, the sagittal pedicle angle is maximal at the thoracic level: it varies between 15 and 20° with a posterior and proximodistal (descending) orientation and then decreases very rapidly between T12 and L1 to reach 5° in L1 and a direction almost parallel with the endplate at L5. For an anatomic trajectory the thoracic pedicle screws are thus oriented more downward than lumbar screws.

In the transverse plane, the convergence is minimal at the level of the 12th thoracic vertebra with a transverse angle which is sometimes negative—a divergent pedicle; the average remains 5° of convergence nevertheless. This convergence increases progressively from T12 to reach 25° on average in T1 and L5. It should be noted that the pedicles between T10 and L1 have a mean convergence of <10°: the orientation when inserting a pedicle at these levels is "straight ahead", without convergence.

Interpedicular Dimensions [3, 6]

The vertical interpedicular distance gradually increases from T1 to S1; this corresponds with the increase in the height of the vertebral body as well as the increase in the height of the intervertebral disc. This distance decreases with age especially at the lumbar level, due to natural disc narrowing.

The interpedicular transverse distance is minimal at the level of the mediothoracic region (T4 to T8) where it measures 20 mm on average. It increases gradually to T1 where it reaches 30 mm, and it also increases towards L5, where it reaches almost 40 mm.

To these quantitative parameters should be added qualitative parameters concerning the abundance of the cancellous bone within the pedicle; indeed in some cases the outer and inner cortices touch each other and there is no presence of cancellous bone between the two, which makes a classical pedicle target impossible (Fig. 4).

Radiological Assessment of Pedicle Dimensions

All the elements just mentioned and analysed vary according to each individual. This anatomical variability depends on the patient's age, size and morphology.

In order to plan a surgical procedure in which a pedicle fixation is required, one should conduct a radiological estimation of these different dimensions and orientations. Standard radiography can be used which is sufficient in the majority of cases, especially when the pedicle width exceeds 5 mm. This corresponds with the anteroposterior radiographs that show well rounded pedicles with dense cortical and clearer cancellous bone, clearly visible inside. For this, radiography of good quality is necessary. EOS radiography meets these objectives. CT imaging allows a more accurate measurement of the pedicle dimensions but with much greater irradiation of the patient. It is useful in cases where standard radiography does not allow visualization of the pedicles. MRI with fine cuts, much more expensive, also allows morphological analysis of the pedicles without the drawbacks of the irradiation of the scanner. Up to date, the reference method remains CT. All these examinations

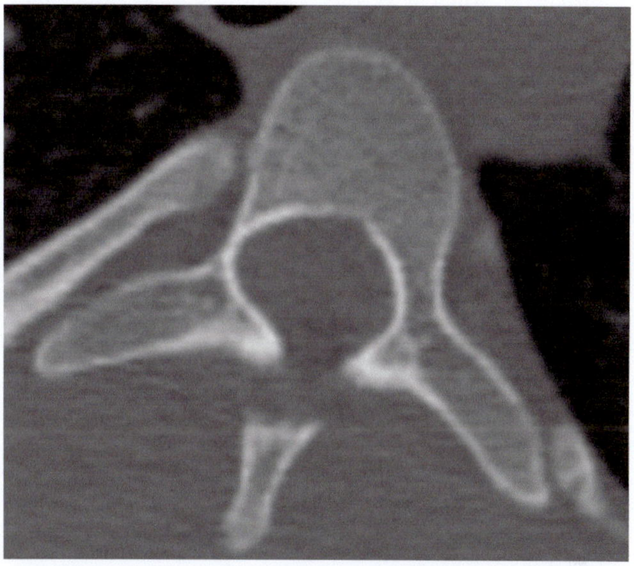

Fig. 4 CT scan of a teenage girl with idiopathic scoliosis. We note the complete disappearance of the cancellous bone and the thin diameter of the right pedicle. This is the anatomical level where the pedicles are the thinnest; to this complexity must be added the effect of the scoliotic concavity. Classic pedicle screw insertion is impossible on the right whereas it is easy to access on the left

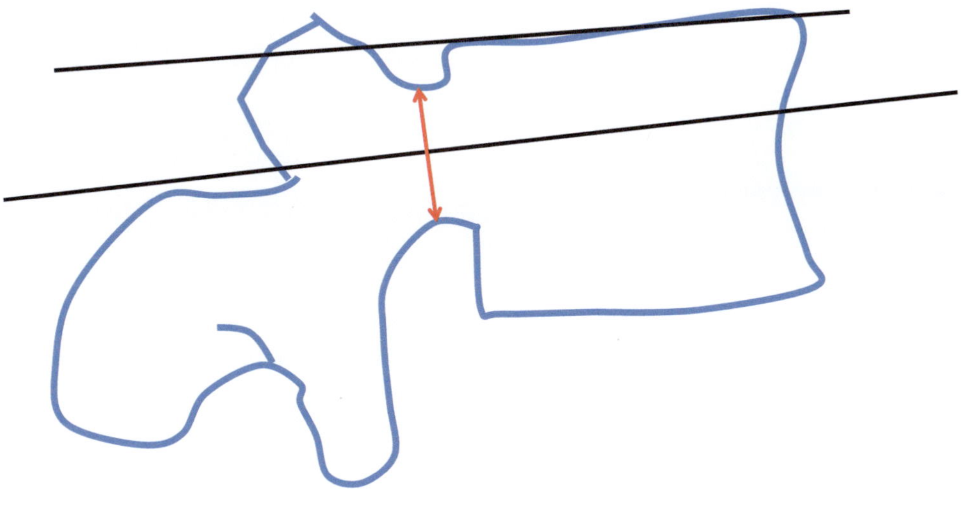

Fig. 3 Diagram of a lateral view of a lumbar vertebra. The sagittal pedicle angle (between the two black lines) is almost nil. The double red arrow indicates the vertical diameter of the pedicle

will allow preoperative planning of the instrumentation and will determine the possibility of free hand screw insertion or with radiological or navigation assistance.

Applications to the Target Pedicle and Contribution of Navigation

The classic transpedicular trajectory is through the spongiosa or cancellous bone present in the pedicle canal. It requires the presence of this cancellous canal through which a perforator can find the path. The drill or probe will follow the path of least resistance and thus allows the cannulation of the pedicle without breaking the walls. When this channel is absent or when it is very thin, the classic direct path becomes impossible, and it may be necessary to replace it either by a hook at the level of the posterior arch or through an extrapedicular that will end in the vertebral body—the "in-out-in" technique. When the anatomical landmarks at the level of the posterior arc are intact and when the pedicle diameter permits, using a free hand technique, without the use of special technology, is very possible and gives satisfactory results with extremely low risk of screw mal-placement. Where this is not possible, the use of fluoroscopic guidance or even better with navigation guidance, it is possible to increase the precision of this technique.

Point of Entry to the Pedicle [7] (Fig. 5)

The posterior entrance of the pedicle lies at the junction of the superior articular facet, the transverse process and the

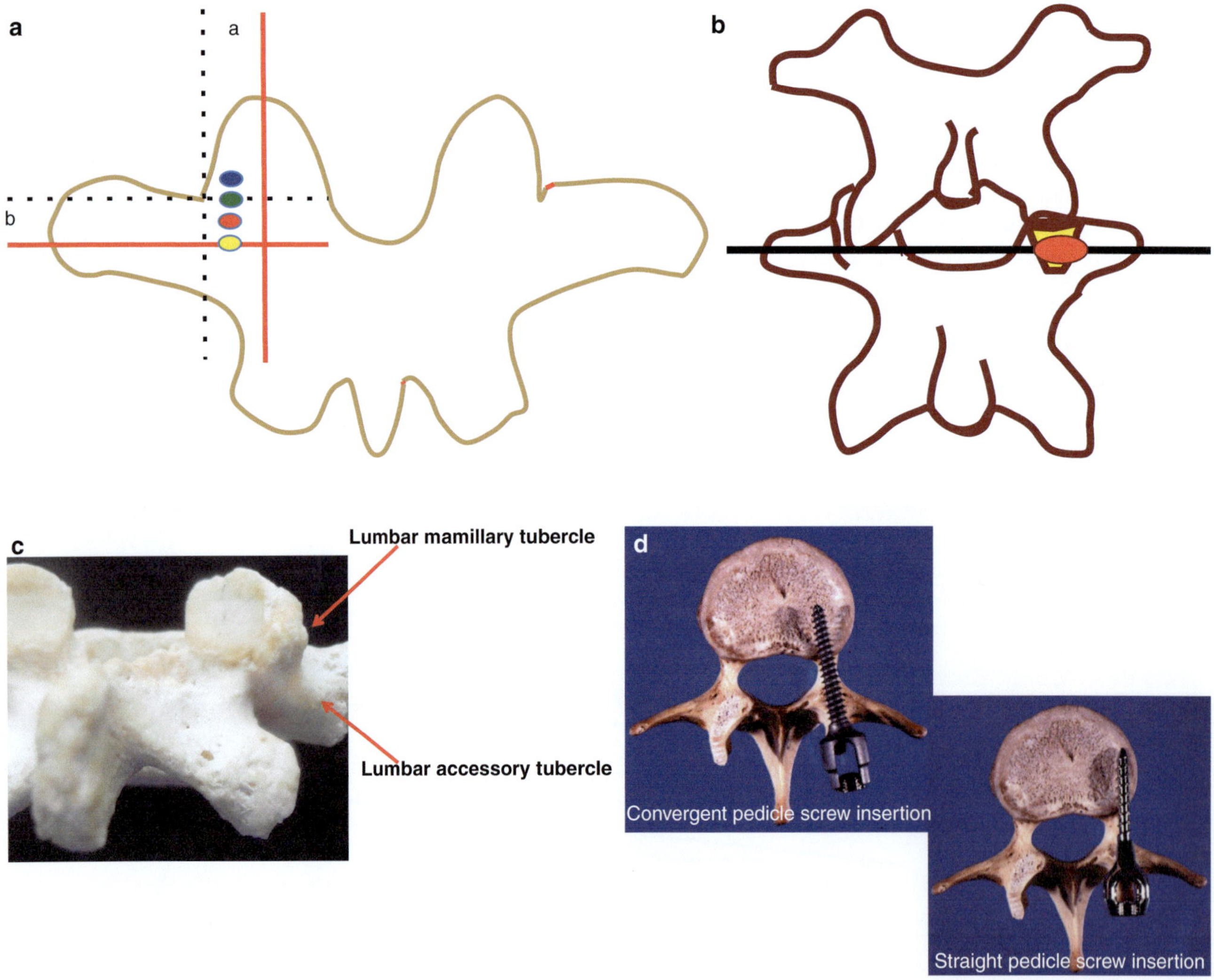

Fig. 5 (**a**) (*a*) Vertical lines passing through the middle (red line) and the lateral edge (black dashed line) of the base of the superior articular facet; the point of entry is always between these two lines. (*b*) Horizontal lines passing through the middle (red) and the upper edge (black dashed line) of the base of the transverse process. The point of entry of the pedicle (coloured dots) is in the superexternal quadrant; the height is variable according to the vertebral level: yellow for T1, T2, T12 and the lumbar vertebrae, red for T3, T4 and T11, green for T5, T6 and T10 and blue for T7, T8 and T9. (**b**) After the resection of the inferior articular facet and exposure of the base of the superior articular facet, a cancellous zone is evident (in yellow); the point of entry is located at the middle of the base of the transverse process (black line) and mediolateral entry depends on the type of trajectory desired, straight anterior or anatomical convergence (red ellipse). (**c**) The point of entry is near the mammillary tubercle and medial to the accessory tubercle. (**d**) The 2 types of pedicle screw insertion, convergent and straight ahead

lamina; its exact position is variable according to the vertebral level. The exact knowledge of the point of entry and the orientation of the pedicle is necessary.

In general, the point of entry is located in the proximal and lateral quadrant of a cross drawn between a transverse line passing through the middle of the base of the transverse process and a vertical line passing through the middle of the base of the superior articular facet. This leaves little choice on positioning in the transverse plane where the point of entry is limited by two vertical lines passing through the middle and the lateral edge of the base of the superior articular facet. On the other hand, several possibilities exist in the vertical direction and depend on the vertebral level.

The height is variable depending on the level: we must first imagine two transverse lines passing through the middle and the upper edge of the base of the transverse process. In the lumbar spine the point of entry is located at the level of the lower line. In the thorax, the pedicles of T12, T1 and T2 are the lowest located at the level of the lower line. The pedicles of T7, T8 and T9 are the highest located just above the top line. The rest of the pedicles have intermediate positions: T3, T4, T11 between the two lines, T5, T6 and T10 at the top line.

This entry point is hidden by a cortex that must be removed in order to access the pedicular cancellous bone.

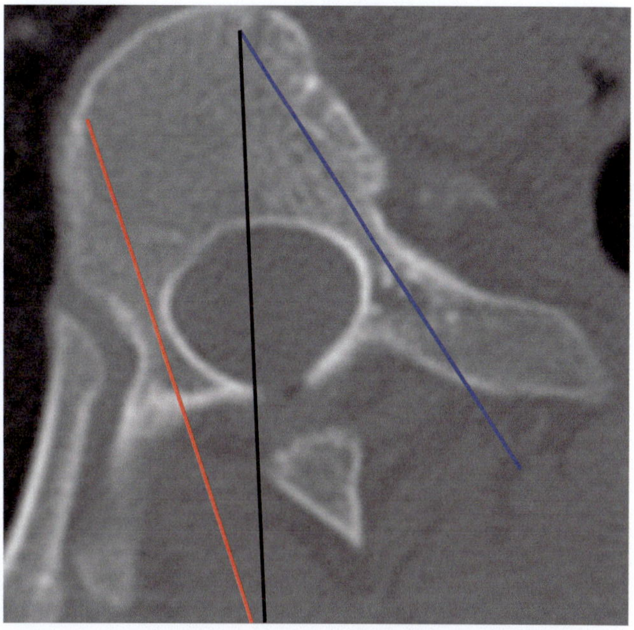

Fig. 6 Pedicles of a T9 vertebra, the apex of a thoracic scoliosis. The black line is the sagittal axis of the patient, the direction of the pedicle screw of the concave side (red) is divergent to 30° while that of the concavity (blue) is convergent to 40°

Special Cases

The Pedicle in Scoliosis (Figs. 6 and 7)

Scoliotic deformation causes a change in the shape, dimensions and orientation of the pedicles.

The pedicle on the concave side becomes thinner, longer and denser with less cancellous bone in its interior. Estimation of its dimensions on standard radiographs is also more difficult because of the rotation of the vertebrae. The dimensions of the pedicles of the concave side are underestimated with respect to their actual dimensions because the rays are oblique with respect to the pedicular axis, whereas on the convex side the rays are parallel to this same axis. It is therefore easier to estimate the width of the pedicle of the side of the convexity. The presence of a rotation should be taken into consideration in the orientation of the pedicle trajectory. This aim is much more convergent on the concave side than on the convex side. In fact, from a concave side it is necessary to add the angle of vertebral rotation to the transverse angle and on the convex side, it is necessary to subtract the angle of rotation. The convex trajectory can therefore sometimes be divergent. Knowing the anatomy and dimensions of the pedicles on the normal spine and knowing that the most important limiting factor is the width of the pedicle, it is understandable that in a right-side thoracic scoliosis, it is at the level of the concavity against the high thoracic curve we will find thinner pedicles and therefore more difficult to instrument, often corresponding to the right-side pedicles of T3, T4 and T5.

In lumbar curvatures, the concave pedicles of L1 and L2 are the narrowest.

Dysplastic Pedicles of Neurofibromatosis [8]

In the vertebral dysplasia of neurofibromatosis, all structures of the vertebrae can be affected—giving rise to thin pedicles, or even their complete disappearance. The vertebral body is often also marked with an anterior and especially posterior scalloping. Dural ectasia fills the void (Fig. 8). Significant destabilization may result in subluxation or even complete spinal dislocation; the appearance of neurological disorder is not uncommon.

A dislocation of the rib head through the intervertebral foramen is regularly observed in dysplastic scoliosis of neurofibromatosis (Fig. 9); particular attention must be observed in order to avoid any neurological event during the surgical procedure and preoperative CT is required to precisely evaluate all these anatomical structures before considering screw insertion.

Dysplastic pedicles may exist in other diseases such as Marfan's disease or Larsen syndrome [9].

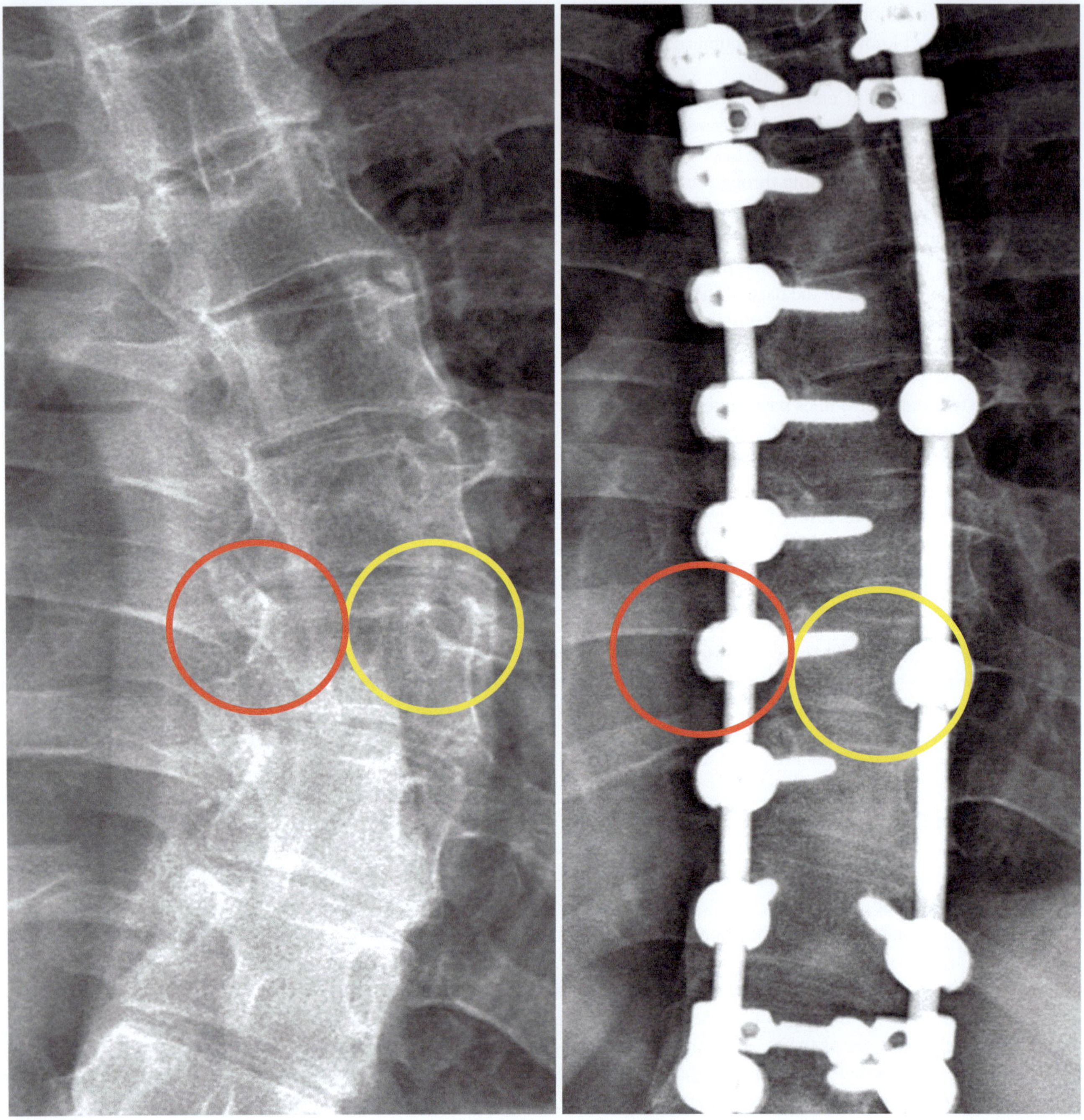

Fig. 7 Left: Posteroanterior radiograph of a thoracic scoliosis with high vertebral rotation: convex and visible pedicles because the rays are parallel to the axis (yellow circle), while the concave pedicle is impossible to see and especially to assess its dimensions (red circle). Right: Screw insertion of these two pedicles was nevertheless possible; we can see the difference in orientation between the convex pedicle screw which is parallel to the radiograph (yellow circle), whereas the concave screw is oblique to the radiograph and more convergent (red circle)

The Pedicle in Vertebral Malformations

In vertebral malformations, pedicles may be normal but may be normal or equally could be small or even absent. The detailed description of pedicle malformations is beyond the scope of this article.

In practice, an assessment of the pedicle morphology using a CT reconstruction parallel with the discs is required each time a surgery is planned; intraoperative navigation can also be useful.

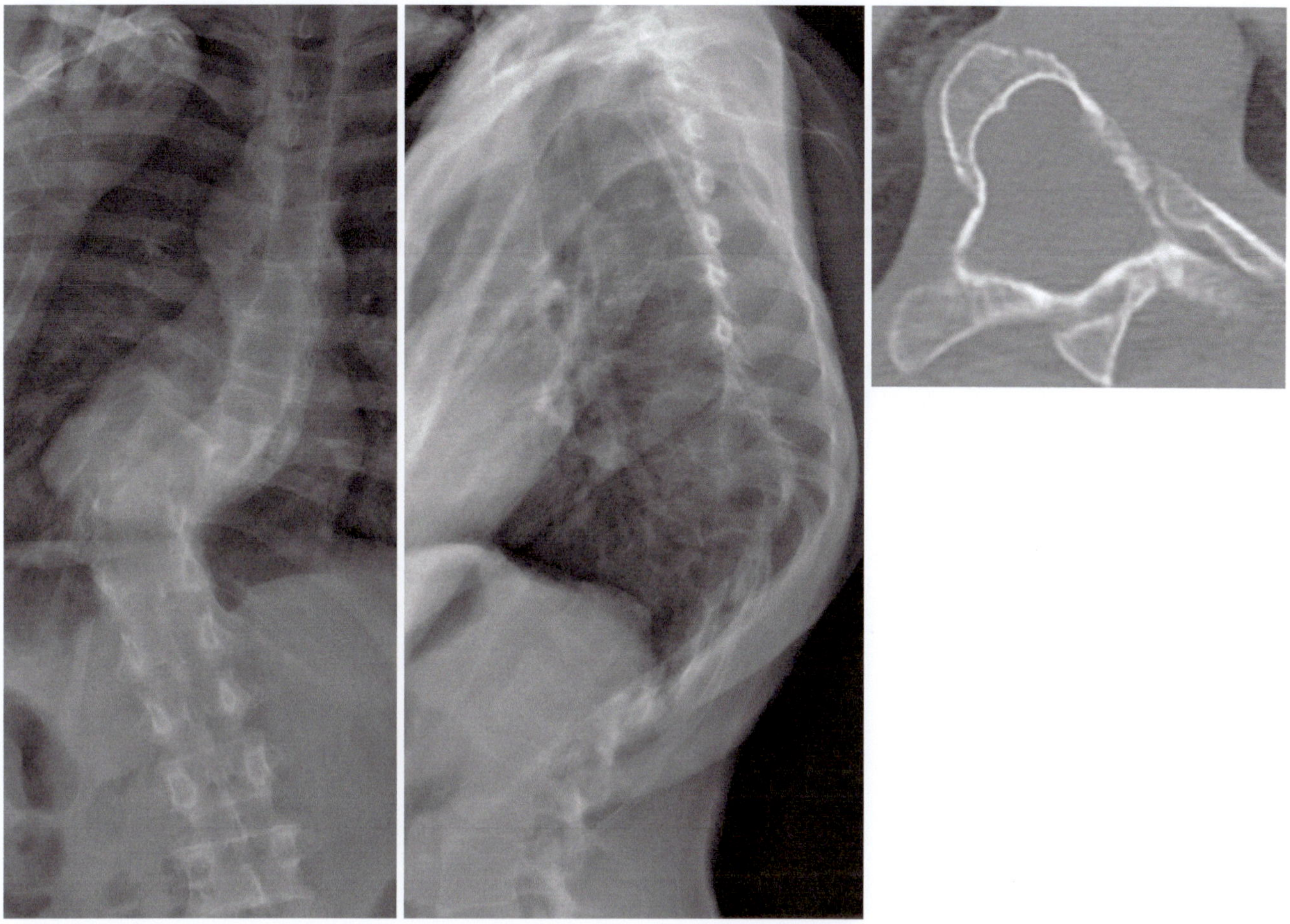

Fig. 8 Example of kyphoscoliosis with spinal subluxation in a 32-year-old patient with type 1 neurofibromatosis. Standard X-ray analysis fails to assess the pedicle anatomy from the seventh to the tenth thoracic vertebrae. CT shows the presence of dural ectasia with disappearance of two-thirds of the vertebral body and dysplastic pedicles reduced to thin strips

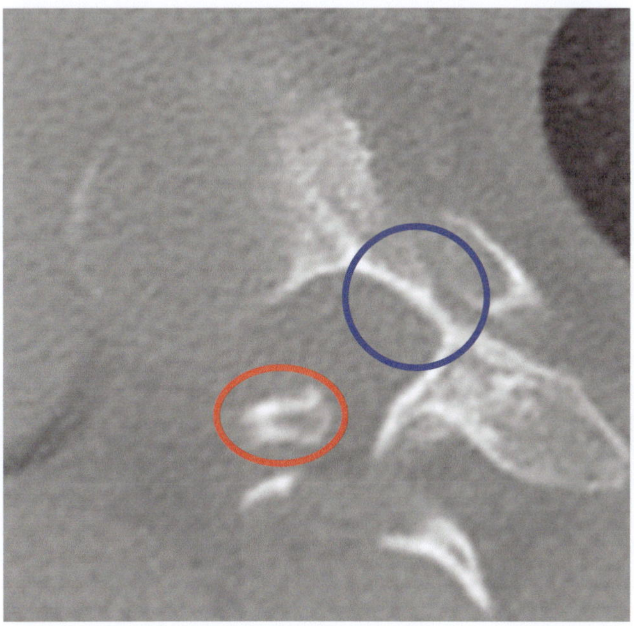

Fig. 9 16-year-old with a scoliosis from neurofibromatosis type 1; we note the dislocation of the rib through the intervertebral foramen on the right (red circle) as well as the dysplasia of the left pedicle (blue circle)

Conclusion

The vertebral pedicle is an essential structure in spinal stability. Its mechanical importance is widely studied in the literature. The pedicle screw is today considered the cornerstone of spinal osteosynthesis. The anatomical and morphological study of the pedicles has thus become an indispensable prerequisite for pedicle screw insertion. A preoperative multimodal image analysis is essential and makes it possible to analyse the difficult cases for which the use of intraoperative fluoroscopy or navigation guidance is desirable.

References

1. Roy-Camille R. Ostéosynthèse du rachis dorsal, lombaire et lombo-sacrée par plaques métalliques vissées dans les pédicules vertébraux et les apophyses articulaires. Presse Med. 1970;78:1447.
2. Roy-Camille R, Saillant G, Berteaux D, Salgodo V. Osteosynthesis of the thoracolumbar spine fractures with metal plates screwed through the vertebral pedicles. Reconstr Surg Traumatol. 1976;15:2–16.
3. Lien SB, Liou NH, Wu SS. Analysis of anatomic morphometry of the pedicles and the area zone for through-pedicle procedures in the thoracic and lumbar spine. Eur Spine J. 2007;16:1215–22.
4. Vaccaro AR, Rizzolo SJ, Allardyce TJ, Ramsey M, Salvo J, Balderston RA, Cotler JM, et al. J Bone Joint Surg. 1995;77(A):1193–9.
5. Cotton C, Wolfram-Gabel R. Pedicles of lumbar vertebrae. Surg Radiol Anat. 1993;15:295–300.
6. Weinstein JN, Rydevikm BL, Auschningm W. Anatomic and technical considerations of pedicle screw fixation. Clin Orthop Relat Res. 1992;284:34–46.
7. Lenke L, Rinella A, Kim Y. Freehand thoracic pedicle screw placement. Seminars in spine surgery. Philadelphia: WB Saunders; 2002. p. 48–57.
8. Cho SK, Stoker GE, Bridwell KH. Spinal reconstruction with pedicle screw-based instrumentation and rhBMP-2 in patients with neurofibromatosis and severe dural ectasia and spinal deformity: report of two cases and a review of the literature. J Bone Joint Surg. 2011;93(A):e86.
9. Sponseller PD, Ahn NU, Ahn UM, Nallamshetty L, Rose PS, Kuszyk BS, Fishman EK. Osseous anatomy of the lumbosacral spine in Marfan syndrome. Spine (Phila Pa 1976). 2000;25:2797–802.

Sacrum Anatomy: New Concepts

O. Gille and T. Chevillotte

Rather than revise concepts of anatomy already known and searchable in the literature, we aimed, in the spirit of this book, to answer some new questions that emerge in the current management of pathologies of the lumbosacral spine.

1. *The importance of the study of posture through the pelvic angle of incidence* as described by Duval-Beaupère is now well recognized. Numerous studies have shown that pelvic incidence, an anatomical parameter, conditions pelvic positional parameters (pelvic tilt and sacral slope) as well as lumbar lordosis. Thus, a new dogma has gradually emerged in spinal surgery: to align the lumbar lordosis angle with the pelvic incidence using regression equations or other simplified formulae. Nevertheless, these studies have always been performed while standing. Also, we were interested in other positions of everyday life, the sitting and supine positions, to analyse the value of the pelvic incidence in these additional two postures.
2. *Screw insertion at S1* is a routine surgical procedure to fix the lumbosacral junction. However, essential data of morphometric anatomy are not known or have never even been studied. We will recall the neurovascular risks during instrumentation of the S1 target. We also measured, on the one hand, the distance of S1 bicortical screws to the anatomical structures that could potentially be injured and, on the other hand, the distance between the S1 screw and the S1 root in the first sacral foramen.
3. *Extension of spinal osteosynthesis to the sacrum*: these fixations are usually done with screws implanted in the first sacral vertebra. But to correct a sagittal deformity of the spine or in the lumbosacral arthrodesis extended to more than five functional units, it is now recommended not to finish the assembly with two sacral screws but to reinforce this grip by extending the instrumentation to the pelvis. Also, we will report on the different surgical possibilities of pelvic fixation.

O. Gille (✉) · T. Chevillotte
Spinal Unit, University Hospital, Bordeaux, France
e-mail: olivier.gille@chu-bordeaux.fr

Study of Radiological Correlation of Pelvic Parameters and Lumbar Lordosis in Standing, Sitting and Lying (Supine) Positions (Fig. 1)

Introduction

Pelvic incidence is an anatomical parameter that, conventionally, does not vary. Correlations between pelvic parameters (PI: pelvic incidence, SS: sacral slope and PT: pelvic tilt) and lumbar lordosis (LL) in an erect position are well known and widely described [1]. In the literature, a fundamental role is given to the PI for the adjustment of the lordosis for lumbar arthrodesis. A large LL must accompany a large PI. This surgical paradigm, which has imposed itself, only takes into account of the static erect position. We can ask whether this PI/LL correlation persists in the other positions of daily sitting or lying down and therefore if relevant to refer to the pelvic incidence in the planning of lumbar or lumbosacral arthrodesis. The adaptation of the lumbopelvic spine during the transition from standing to sitting shows a decrease in lumbar lordosis and sacral slope and a pelvic retroversion [2]. The aim of this study is to analyse the correlations between lumbar lordosis and the different lumbopelvic parameters in the three positions: standing, sitting and supine.

Patients and Methods

We included healthy volunteers aged 18–50 years, non-lumbalgic, with no history of surgery, infection or pelvic or spinal tumoural pathology. This study was approved by a local ethics committee.

J. M. Vital, D. T. Cawley (eds.), *Spinal Anatomy*, https://doi.org/10.1007/978-3-030-20925-4_11

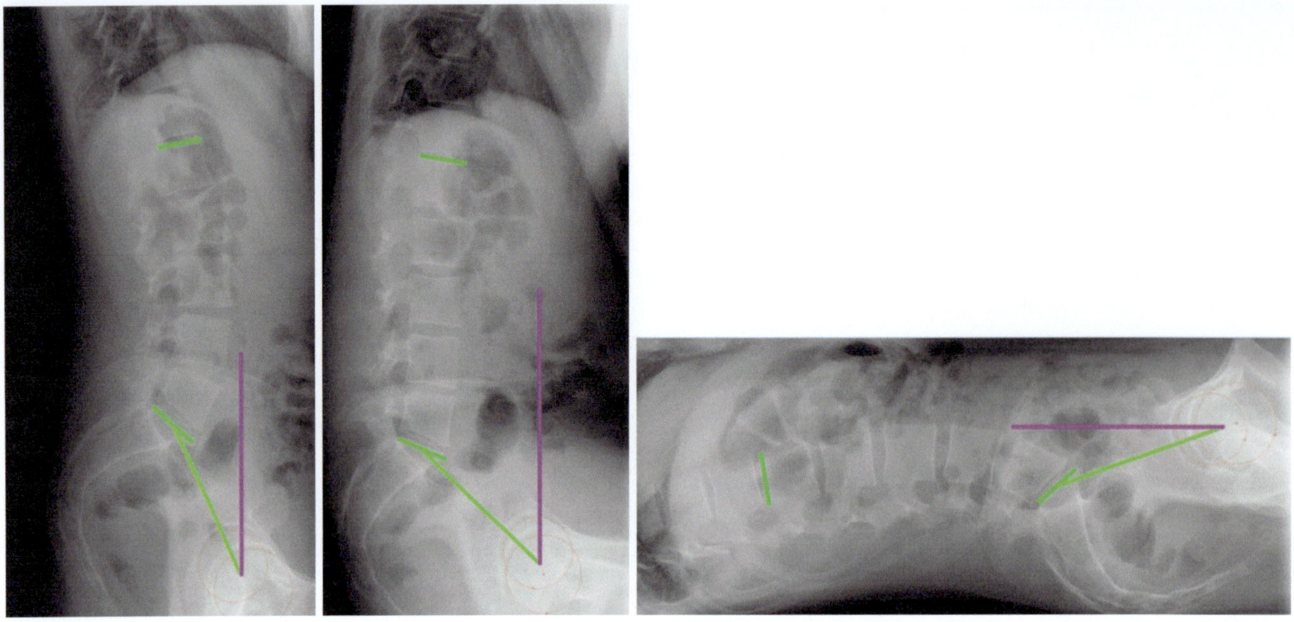

Fig. 1 XRays in standing, sitting and supine position; measurements of pelvic parameters and lumbar lordosis

Radiography

A strict standard radiograph of the twelfth thoracic vertebra (T12) to the femoral heads was performed in the following three positions:

- Standing: erect and relaxed, hands on the clavicles, horizontal gaze.
- Sitting position: patient in a comfortable, natural position, with variable height seat, horizontal thighs, knee flexion at 90°. The upper limbs also relaxed, hands placed and crossed on the thighs to allow visualization of the lumbar spine.
- Supine position: strict supine position on horizontal radiology table. Hands crossed on the chest, in a comfortable and natural position.

Radiological and Statistical Analyses

Pelvic parameters and lumbar lordosis from L1 to S1 were calculated using Surgimap 2.1.1. In the supine position, the sacral slope was calculated with respect to the vertical and the pelvic tilt in relation to the horizontal. Statistical analysis was performed using SPSS software. For each parameter we calculated the means with standard deviation. Normality of distribution of values was verified by the Shapiro–Wilk test. The correlation test used was the Spearman test.

Results

Radiographs of 15 patients, five women and ten men, with an average age of 42.9 years were analysed.

The PI is stable in the standing, sitting and lying positions with respective measurements of 49.3° ± 8, 48.7° ± 8 and 50.4 ± 7°. The LL is 54. 8° ± 10 in the standing position, decreases to 15.9° ± 15 in the seated position and increases to 50.2° ± 10 in the supine position. The PT is 12.1° ± 6, 37.7° ± 10 and 9.5 ± 5.1 in standing, sitting and supine, respectively. The standing SS is 37.1° ± 6.3, decreases to 11.3° ± 11 in sitting and increases to 41° ± 7 in supine (Table 1) (at the end of the text). We checked the normality of distribution of the values. Correlation coefficients between LL and pelvic parameters are shown in Table 2 (at the end of the text).

Discussion

The majority of studies on spinopelvic balance are done in a static erect position. These studies have shown strong correlations between pelvic incidence and sacral slope, pelvic incidence and lumbar lordosis or lumbar lordosis and thoracic kyphosis. In fact, in real life, when standing, the human is most often in motion. He adopts other static postures in daily life, but most often in a sitting or lying position. The time spent during the day while sitting or lying down varies according to the individual, which depend in particular on socio-economic factors and age [3]. Some elderly

Table 1 Mean values of spinopelvic parameters (in degrees)

	Pelvic incidence	Pelvic tilt	Sacral slope	Lumbar lordosis
Standing	49.3	12.1	37.1	54.8
Seated	48.7	37.7	11.3	15.9
Supine	50.4	9.5	41	50.2

Table 2 Correlation coefficients

	LL/PI	LL/SS	PI/SS	PI/PT
Standing	0.57*	0.67**	0.63*	0.54*
Seated	0.68*	0.80**	0.23	0.43
Supine	0.72**	0.9**	0.84**	0.72*

*Significant for $p < 0.05$; **Significant for $p < 0.01$

people spend <10% of a day while standing [3]. In addition, disability may limit a patient to only seated and lying positions. So it seems restrictive to refer exclusively to the erect position for the study of the relationships and correlations between the pelvis and the lumbar spine.

Nevertheless, there has never been a study into the correlation between lumbar lordosis and pelvic incidence in other positions of daily life, particularly sitting or lying. However, it is important to know if this correlation persists in order to confirm the importance of pelvic incidence in posture, whether it is standing, sitting or lying down. It therefore seemed necessary to know if there is a correlation between pelvic parameters and lumbar lordosis in the sitting or lying position. A lack of correlation could suggest that much too much attention has been paid to the PI, for example in the planning of lumbar spinal fusion.

PI, a parameter specific to an individual [4], is nevertheless used in the calculation of theoretical lumbar lordosis when planning lumbar arthrodesis. Its importance is recognized: the suboptimal adjustment of lumbar arthrodesis can accelerate the degeneration of the adjacent level [5] and cause muscle pain. The lack of approximation between postoperative lumbar lordosis and pelvic incidence is correlated with poor clinical outcomes [6, 7].

In a standing position, the values of the pelvic and spinal parameters in our study are comparable to large data from the literature [8]. Similarly, the correlation coefficients PI/LL, LL/SS and PI/SS are superimposable on the coefficients found in the literature. The correlations found in the literature between PI/SS and LL/SS are statistically stronger, i.e. with a coefficient greater than 0.7 than the LL/PI correlation [2, 9–15]. Our population is therefore representative of the general population concerning the lumbopelvic complex.

In the sitting position, the coupled movements of the coxofemoral joints and the lumbar spine have been well described in the literature and specified by Lazennec [16]: hip flexion is accompanied by flexion of the lumbar spine, pelvic retroversion (increased PT) and decreased SS. These changes in pelvic parameters and lumbar lordosis are well documented in our study. These modifications are done harmoniously, with persistence of a strong correlation between PI/LL and SS/LL. The pelvic floor therefore also conditions the posture while seated.

In the supine position, we find a strong correlation PI/LL and very strong LL/SS. It is in a supine position that the PI/LL, LL/SS and LL/PT correlations are the strongest. Presumably, the suppression of gravity excludes the mechanisms of pelvic adaptation to gravity which appear when standing or sitting and must distort the excellent correlation found in the supine position. Nevertheless, surprisingly, we find an increase in the sacral slope and a decrease in PT and LL, which does not correspond to the coupled movements previously described. Perhaps while lying on the X-ray table, there is a discreet extension of the coxofemoral joints that has not been studied in this article. This hyperextension of the hips, which induces an increase of SS by coupled movement, cannot possibly be coupled with hyperextension of the lumbar spine because the back of the patient rests on the table. We had not considered this hypothesis, which should be confirmed by the measurement of the pelvifemoral angle. In our study, this angle could not be measured because the supine radiographs did not include the upper third of the femurs. The other potential explanation for this asymmetric variation of PT and LL in the supine position is secondary to the suppression of gravity constraints on the lumbopelvifemoral complex.

The PI is therefore an essential parameter not only in the erect position but also in sitting or lying. It is therefore essential to regulate lumbar arthrodesis according to the value of PI [1, 17–19], *even in elderly patients with reduced physical activity.*

The limitation of this study concerns especially the absence of analysis of the subpelvic sector, in particular the pelvifemoral angle which could have helped us in the understanding of certain angular variations.

Neurovascular Risks During the Insertion of the S1 Screw: An Anatomical Study

Introduction

The placement of sacral screws in S1 is routinely practiced in spinal surgery. The surgical technique of introducing these screws is known:

– The point of entry of the S1 screw is located at the lateral portion of the lower edge of the upper articular facet of the sacrum [20–26]. The aim is classically convergent from 30° to 40°, targeting the anterosuperior corner of the sacrum. According to a cadaveric study [23], the ideal convergence would be 35° ± 4. Roy-Camille [27] initially described screw insertion parallel to the vertebral endplate of S1 in 1983. De Peretti [28] describes a better bone fixation if the screw is upward of 10°.

Nevertheless, the behaviour of these screws depends on the quality of the bone, as the quality may be poor in osteoporotic patients. In addition, it has been shown that taking the anterior sacral cortex (bicortical screw) significantly enhances this sacral screw strength. But these bicortical screws expose the risk of damage to neurological and vascular structures located in the inner pelvis [29–31]. Also, we wanted to define the safety zone for these sacral screws and measure the distance between an ideally placed screw and the vascular and nerve structures that could potentially be injured by the screw.

In Vivo CT Measurements

In order to evaluate the risk of neurological or vascular injury during S1 screw insertion, we simulated the positioning of an S1 screw on ten pelvic CT scanners. Measurements were performed on CT scans of patients with no traumatic, tumour or infectious condition on the L5, S1 and S2 vertebrae. There were 6 men and 4 women with a mean age of 56 years.

Measurement of the distance of the S1 screw from the first sacral foramen. We simulated the implantation of two S1 right and left screws of 6.5 mm diameter on each scanner, for a total of 20 screws, using the Osirix Viewer® software. The entry point of the screw was classically located at the lateral aspect of the base of the upper articular facet of S1. The angle of convergence of the screw was determined in the axial plane with respect to the axis of the pedicle of S1. Then, in the sagittal reconstruction plane, this angle of convergence was reported to lie exactly in the plane of the pedicle. The path of the screw was then simulated by a 6.5-mm-thick line. We then measured the distance separating the line simulating the screw of the first sacral hole.

Measurement of the distance of the S1 screw with respect to the lumbosacral trunk. On these same scanners we simulated by a line of 6.5-mm-thick with the implantation of two S1 screws on the axial section passing below the upper plate of S1. We then measured the distance separating the end of the line simulating the head of the lumbosacral trunk screw.

Measuring the distance of the screw S1 from the iliac vessels. On these same scanners we simulated a line of 6.5-mm-thick for the implantation of two screws S1 on the axial section passing below the upper plate of S1. We then measured the distance between the end of the line and the common iliac artery screw on the right and the common iliac vein on the left.

The measurement for the medial sacral artery was hardly feasible since it is too small a vessel to be viewed on a standard scanner.

Results

On average, the S1 screw goes to 5.2 mm from the first sacral foramen (±0.75 mm). It can be considered that screw insertion of S1 is a low risk procedure for the S1 root if it is inserted appropriately. In our experiment, we recommend performing S1 screw under fluoroscopy magnification in order to target the anterosuperior corner of the vertebral body of S1.

The distance between a bicortical S1 screw and the iliac vessels is on average 22 mm ± 2 mm. The average distance between a bicortical S1 screw and the lumbosacral trunk is on average 8.5 mm ± 0.8 mm.

Discussion

Mirkovic et al. performed an anatomical study to define the anatomical lesions that can be damaged when inserting a screw to S1 [30]. They defined two safety zones for S1: a median zone and a lateral zone (Fig. 2). The median zone is situated between the medial sacral artery on the one hand and the lumbosacral trunk and the primary iliac vessels on the other. The lateral zone is located outside the internal iliac vessels. The median area should be preferred because of the better bone quality for holding the screw. At this point, the

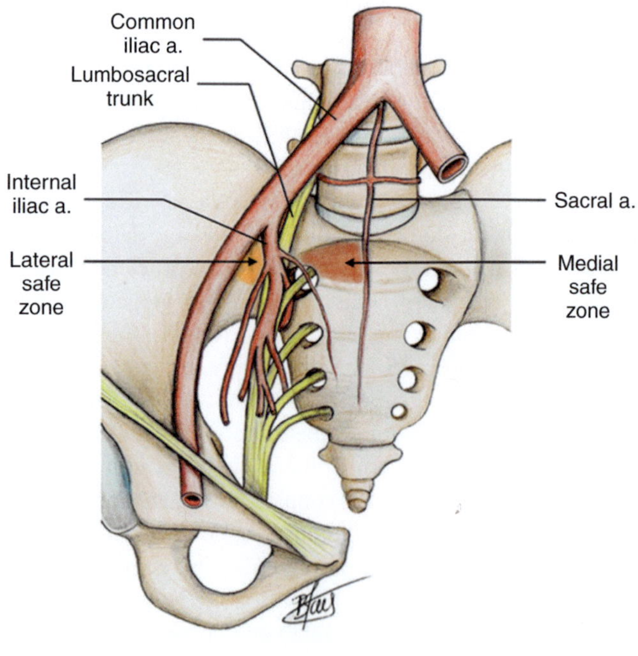

Fig. 2 Safe zone for S1 and S2 screws

S1 screw can cross the anterior cortex of the sacrum to obtain a greater resistance to pull out.

The common iliac vessels can be reached if the screw in S1 is insufficiently convergent. On the right, the common iliac artery is in contact with the bone surface. The vein is located just in front of the artery. On the left, it is the common iliac vein which is located against the bone and which could therefore be reached. In another cadaveric study of 30 cadavers, screwing S1 with the entry point at the foot of the articular facet of S1 and a median convergence of about 10° did not produce injury of the iliac vessels. In this study, the medial sacral artery was reached in 4 out of 30 cases.

In our study, we were able to measure the distance between an ideally located S1 screw and the iliac vessels and the lumbosacral trunk. In case of a bicortical screw, the risk of vascular injury is very low, the distance between a converging screw of about 30° and the iliac vessels being >20 mm. On the other hand, the distance between the tip of the screw and the lumbosacral trunk is much smaller, 8.5 mm. It is therefore sufficient that the aim is not sufficiently convergent for a S1 screw to cause conflict with the lumbosacral trunk. The lumbosacral trunk is bulky, 8 mm wide, applied to the anterior surface of the sacral ala (wing). In addition to its volume, its vulnerability is increased by the fact that it is adherent to the bone to which it is attached by fibrous tissue [26].

Finally, the distance between the S1 screw and the S1 foramen had never been measured. Presumably, the breach of the sacral foramen by the S1 screw is rare; the S1 foramen can be visualized on the posterior aspect of the sacrum during the placement of the screw. Nevertheless, the distance between the ideally positioned S1 screw and the S1 foramen is small, of the order of 5 mm.

One must therefore be particularly careful when inserting a screw at S1 not to have a point of insertion that is too low and/or a downward trajectory that would risk compression of the S1 root.

Pelvic Fixation: Surgical Techniques

The Biomechanical Zones at the Level of the Sacrum (Fig. 3)

Achieving fusion of the lumbosacral junction is a complex problem in spine surgery, a source of mechanical (mobility segment, screw or rod fracture, screw pull-out), neurological or even vascular complications (lesion of a nerve structure or a vessel by an extra-heavy or malplaced screw) [32]. In addition, the sacrum does not have a uniform fixation quality for instrumentation. At the level of S1, De Peretti [33] recalls the postero-anterior screw insertion techniques including the "straight ahead" trajectory as described by Roy-Camille and the oblique anteromedial pediculo-corporeal convergent screw trajectory. In an in vitro biomechanical study, De Peretti showed that the latter is the most resistant to pull out. The density of the S1 and S2 vertebrae was measured by CT and expressed in Hounsfield units (UH) in 20 healthy subjects of mean age of 32 years. At the level of S1, the best bone density is found in the pedicles (335 HU), followed by the body (281 HU), and then the sacral ala (60 HU). At S2, the bone density is lower: pedicles (108 HU), body (108 HU), then the sacral ala (42 HU) [33].

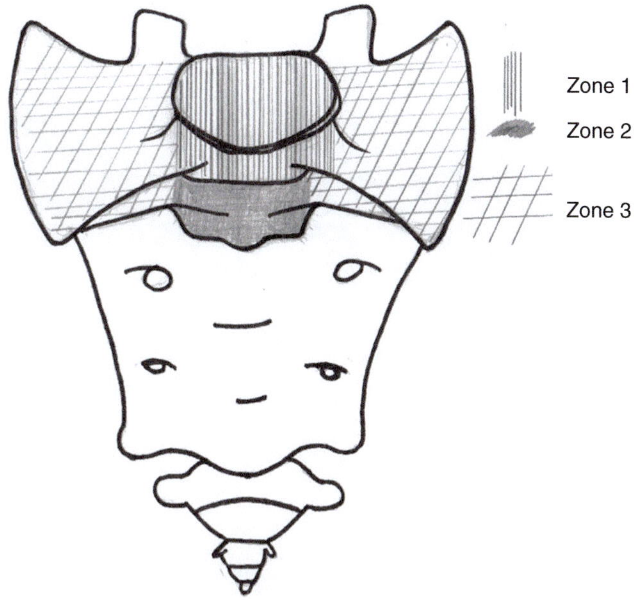

Fig. 3 Bone density in the sacrum

According to Dubousset [34], the sacral screw insertion directed forward and outward at 45° would allow a solid anchoring and with easy access provided that the bone is not too porous. The cadaver study of De Peretti clearly shows that the divergent aim in the sacral ala does not have a good anchorage in the elderly person.

Moshirfar et al. described the lumbosacral pivot point [32]. This point belongs to the middle column between the L5 and S1 vertebrae. Implants that attach anterior to this point provide greater rigidity [32, 35]. Note that a triangular assembly improves the pull-out resistance [8]. Finally, a second point of attachment to the pelvis is more effective than S1 fixation alone [35].

We define three biomechanical zones at the level of the sacrum. The mechanical resistance decreases from zone 1 to zone 3. Zone 1 corresponds to the vertebral body of S1, zone 2 corresponds to the vertebral body of S2. Zone 3 corresponds to the ala of the sacrum.

We propose the following scheme (Fig. 3):

Screw Insertion at S1 and S2 (Fig. 4)

The addition of an S2 screw increases the rigidity of the assembly with respect to S1 alone but minimally increases the

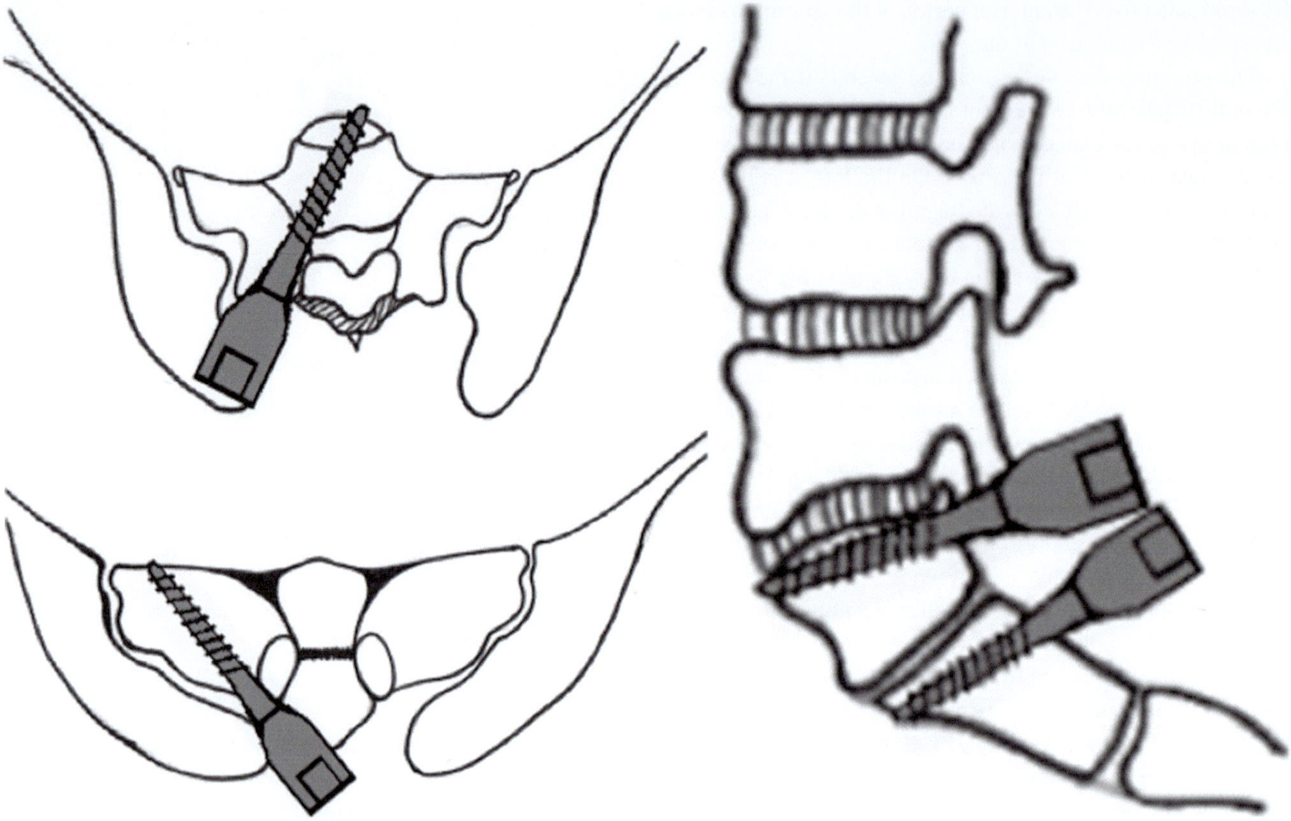

Fig. 4 Position of S1 and S2 screws

flexural strength with respect to S1 alone [36]. This assembly is mechanically weaker than an iliac screw [37]. This arrangement allows good control of the sagittal plane but less so in the frontal (coronal) plane because of the more medial position of the screws compared to an iliac anchor [38].

Anatomically, the S1 and S2 screws are in the same axis, but the passage of the rods though the S1 and S2 screw heads can be difficult [36]. There are several types of sacral plates to position these two screws with a single anchorage for the rod.

Jackson's Intrasacral Rod (Fig. 5)

It is an intrasacral rod introduced through S2 [39]. This rod is attached to an S1 pedicle screw. It rests on the anterior cortex of the sacrum [39]. This rod has a supportive effect that is effective in osteoporotic patients [38]. In fact, the posterior cortex of the sacrum and the two cortices of the posterior part of the iliac wing will resist flexural forces. It provides a stiffness in bending, rotation [40] and a long lever arm. It therefore spares sacroiliac fixation [41]. As for S1 and S2 screws, the medial position of this fixture would make it less effective on frontal correction [38]. Like the Galveston rod, it can have a "windscreen wiper" effect [42]. It poses a risk of fracturing the sacrum [41].

The Galveston Stem (Fig. 6)

This technique consists of attaching to the iliac wing with a point of entry in the posterior superior iliac spine [40] via a curved rod. This rod is fixed in front of the pivot point [37]. It affords a good resistance in torsion [37] and flexion movements [42]. It allows the incorporation of the pelvic bone into the assembly [32] while maintaining a small footprint [40]. On the other hand, the fixation being ensured by a smooth stem, it can create a wiper effect in the iliac bone. The triple contouring of this rod can present a technical difficulty.

Iliac Screw Insertion (Fig. 7)

This is an evolution of the Galveston technique. The point of entry is at the posterior iliac spine [43]. The path of the screw is oblique downward, outward and forward, at a variable angle with the sagittal plane depending on the orientation of the iliac wing. This orientation can be calculated on preoperative imaging. Downward, the orientation is at an angle of 30° to the horizontal, towards the greater trochanter which is a good external marker. This iliac screw is perpendicular to the screw of S1, allowing a triangulation assembly resistant to pull-out forces [32]. As for other

Fig. 5 The Jackson's Rod

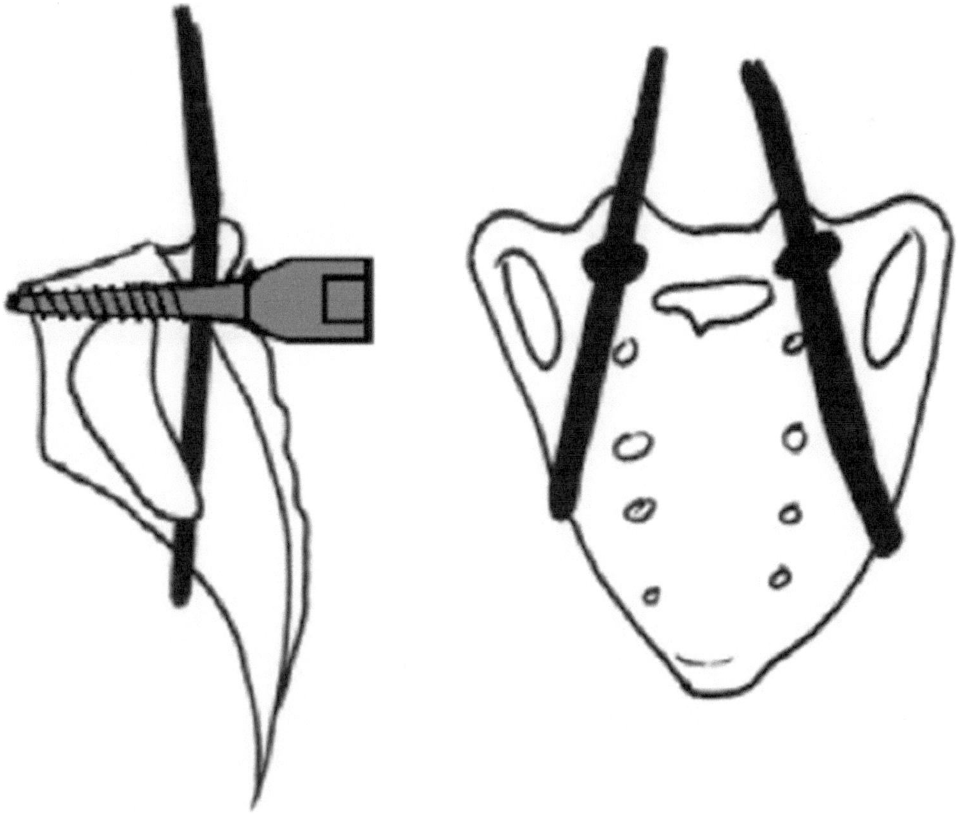

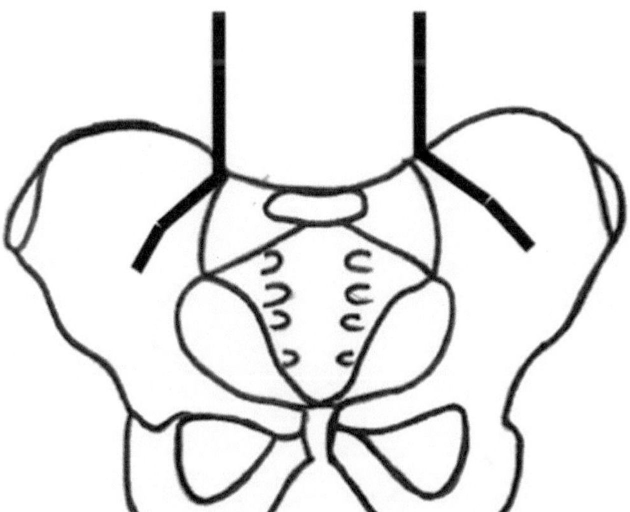

Fig. 6 The Galveston Stem

means of fixing to the pelvis, the iliac screw makes it possible to reduce the stresses on the sacral screws [44], reduce the risk of lumbosacral pseudarthrosis [32] and provide loosening resistance three times greater than the Galveston rod. Iliac screw fixation shows better efficacy in correcting pelvic obliquity compared to Galveston rods [37]. Similarly, the use of sacral S1 screws decrease the forces exerted on the iliac screws [38].

Side connectors are required [43]. The placement of this iliac screw connector proximally or distal to the S1 screw does not alter the biomechanics [37]. Adding a transverse connector can reduce pull-out of the iliac screws [42, 44].

Iliosacral Screw Insertion (Fig. 8)

There are ancillaries for the easy placement of this screw: the point of entry is above and in front of the posterior superior iliac spine, 2 cm from the posterior edge of the iliac crest [38]. This entry point is addressed by a counter skin incision. The screw is positioned towards the centre of the S1 body, with a reference angle of 30° to the horizontal. A connector is inserted in a bone box created at the level of the sacral ala. This iliosacral fixation allows a very solid anchoring. It is a tricortical fixation. The lateralised position of the iliosacral screw allows an Eiffel tower assembly, resulting in a large lever to correct the frontal plane, in particular any pelvic obliquity [45]. This technique has a small footprint. The screw does not cross the sacroiliac joint but remains posterosuperior. Harrington had described a similar technique using Steinmann pins.

S2 Iliac Screw Insertion (Fig. 9)

The entry point is between the first two sacral holes 1 mm below and outside the first sacral foramen [43]. The S2 iliac

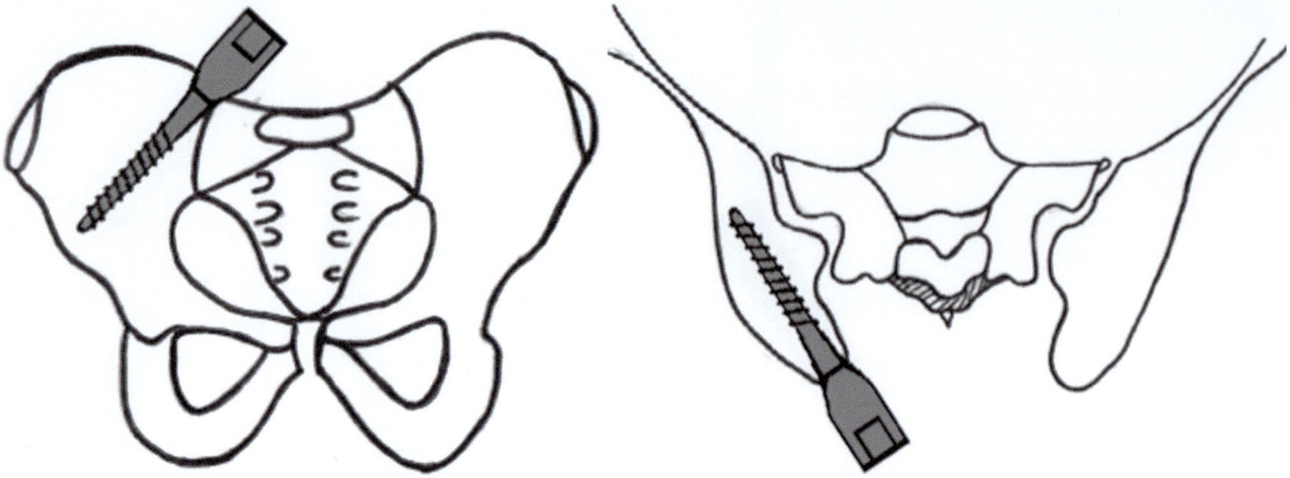

Fig. 7 The iliac screw

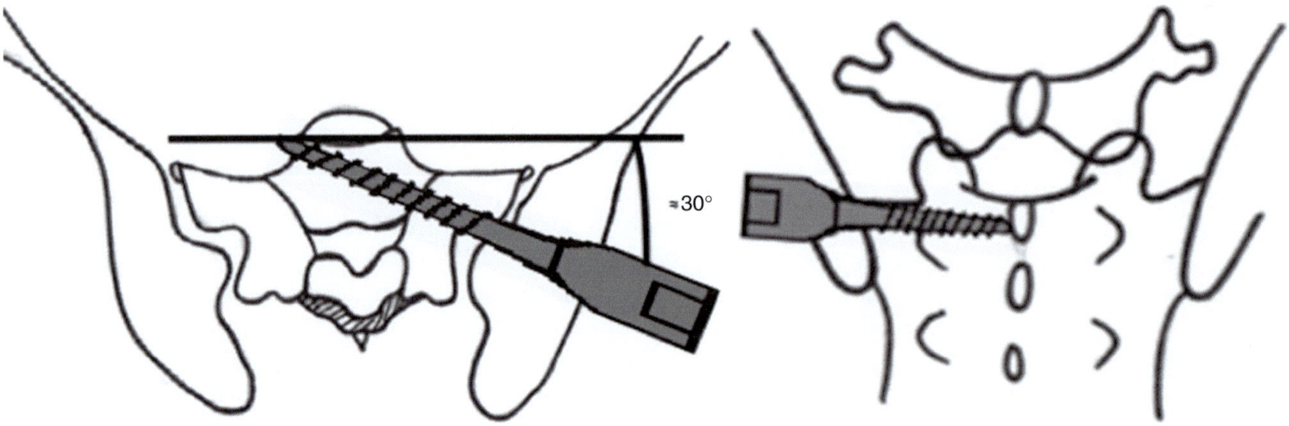

Fig. 8 The iliosacral screw

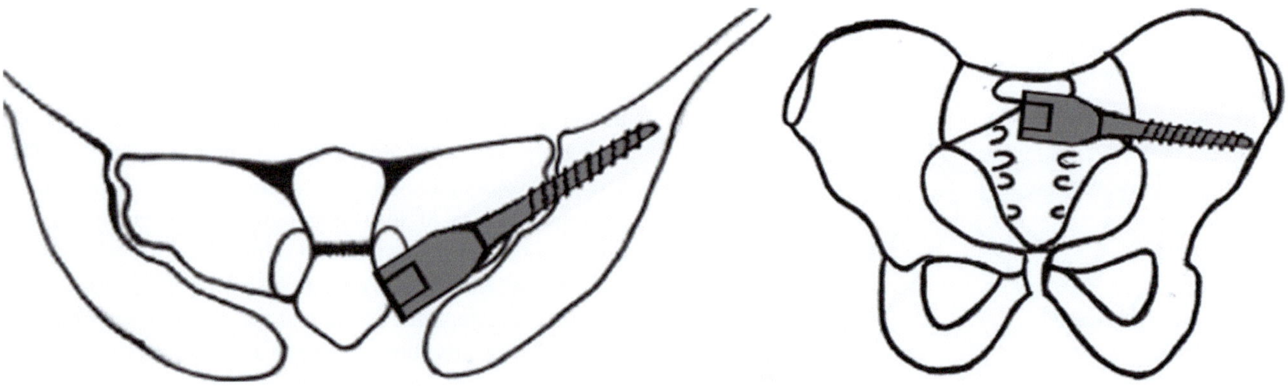

Fig. 9 The sacroiliac screw

screw is tricortical and passes through the sacroiliac joint in 60% of cases [46]. The quadricortical character does not increase the biomechanical strength of the assembly [41]. This screw has excellent pull-out resistance [47]. The length of the screw is shorter than that of an iliac screw. A 65-mm S2 iliac screw is biomechanically equivalent to a 90-mm iliac screw [46].

The S2 iliac screw does not require a lateral connector [37], it is aligned with the screw heads of L5 and S1 [41] facilitating the introduction of the rod. This technique is

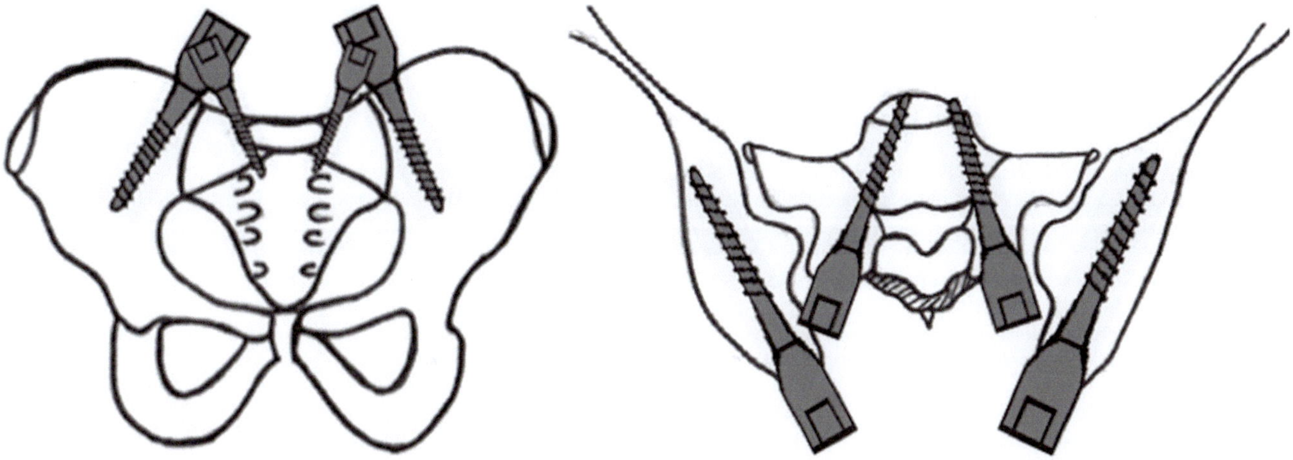

Fig. 10 T-Construct

more difficult when the patient is in hyperlordosis [42]. This screw is less prominent than the iliac screw, does not require dissection of the pelvic bone and has little effect on the possibility of iliac cresting for autograft [41]. But according to Guler [45], in cases of insufficient correction of a sagittal imbalance, the S2 iliac screw has an increased risk of short-term material fracture compared with iliac screwing.

"T-Construct" by Vialle (Fig. 10)

This assembly is based on two standard iliac screws and two standard S1 sacral screws [48]. A horizontal rod connects the four screws. This horizontal rod is connected by 90° connectors to the upper construct [49]. At the time of correction, the correction forces apply to the four implants simultaneously. The forces are transmitted to the two iliac wings with a large lever arm. This fixation concerns the three pelvic bones with fixation in the different planes [50].

References

1. Boulay C, Tardieu C, Hecquet J, Benaim C, Mouilleseaux B, Marty C, et al. Sagittal alignment of spine and pelvis regulated by pelvic incidence: standard values and prediction of lordosis. Eur Spine J. 2006;15(4):415–22.
2. Vaz G, Roussouly P, Berthonnaud E, Dimnet J. Sagittal morphology and equilibrium of pelvis and spine. Eur Spine J. 2002;11(1):7.
3. De Cocker K, Duncan MJ, Short C, Van Uffelen JG, Vandelanotte C. Understanding occupational sitting: prevalence, correlates and moderating effects in Australian employees. Prev Med. 2014;67:288–94.
4. Legaye J, Duval-Beaupere G, Hecquet J, Marty C. Pelvic incidence: a fundamental pelvic parameter for three-dimensional regulation of spinal sagittal curves. Eur Spine J. 1998;7(2):99–103.
5. Umehara S, Zindrick MR, Patwardhan AG, Havey RM, Vrbos LA, Knight GW, et al. The biomechanical effect of postoperative hypolordosis in instrumented lumbar fusion on instrumented and adjacent spinal segments. Spine. 2000;25(13):1617–24.
6. Schwab FJ, Smith VA, Biserni M, Gamez L, Farcy JP, Pagala M. Adult scoliosis: a quantitative radiographic and clinical analysis. Spine. 2002;27(4):387–92.
7. Kumar MN, Baklanov A, Chopin D. Correlation between sagittal plane changes and adjacent segment degeneration following lumbar spine fusion. Eur Spine J. 2001;10(4):314–9.
8. Cord MC. Biomechanical analysis of lumbosacral fixation. Spine. 1992;17:S235–43.
9. Marty C, Boisaubert B, Descamps H, Montigny JP, Hecquet J, Legaye J, et al. The sagittal anatomy of the sacrum among young adults, infants, and spondylolisthesis patients. Eur Spine J. 2002;11(2):119–25.
10. Lee ES, Ko CW, Suh SW, Kumar S, Kang IK, Yang JH. The effect of age on sagittal plane profile of the lumbar spine according to standing, supine, and various sitting positions. J Orthop Surg Res. 2014;9(1):11.
11. Cho IY, Park SY, Park JH, Kim TK, Jung TW, Lee HM. The effect of standing and different sitting positions on lumbar lordosis: radiographic study of 30 healthy volunteers. Asian Spine J. 2015;9(5):762–9.
12. Mac-Thiong JM, Roussouly P, Berthonnaud E, Guigui P. Age and sex-related variations in sagittal sacropelvic morphology and balance in asymptomatic adults. Eur Spine J. 2011;20(Suppl 5):572–7.
13. Berthonnaud E, Dimnet J, Roussouly P, Labelle H. Analysis of the sagittal balance of the spine and pelvis using shape and orientation parameters. J Spinal Disord Tech. 2005;18(1):40–7.
14. Vialle R, Levassor N, Rillardon L, Templier A, Skalli W, Guigui P. Radiographic analysis of the sagittal alignment and balance of the spine in asymptomatic subjects. J Bone Joint Surg. 2005;87(A):260–7.
15. Jackson RP, McManus AC. Radiographic analysis of sagittal plane alignment and balance in standing volunteers and patients with low back pain matched for age, sex, and size. A prospective controlled clinical study. Spine. 1994;19(14):1611–8.
16. Lazennec JY, Brusson A, Rousseau MA. Lumbar pelvic femoral balance on sitting and standing lateral radiographs. Orthop Traumatol Surg Res. 2013;99(1 Suppl):S87–103.
17. Yamato Y, Hasegawa T, Kobayashi S, Yasuda T, Togawa D, Arima H, et al. Calculation of the target lumbar lordosis angle for restoring an optimal pelvic tilt in elderly patients with adult spinal deformity. Spine. 2016;41(4):E211–7.
18. Legaye J, Duval-Beaupere G. Sagittal plane alignment of the spine and gravity: a radiological and clinical evaluation. Acta Orthop Belg. 2005;71:213–20.

19. Schwab F, Lafage V, Patel A, Farcy JP. Sagittal plane considerations and the pelvis in the adult patient. Spine. 2009;34(17):1828–33.
20. Basaloglu H, Turgut M, Taser FA, Ceylan T, Baloglu HK, Ceylan AA. Morphometry of the sacrum for clinical use. Surg Radiol Anat. 2005;27(6):467–71.
21. Candan Arman A, Sait Naderi B, Amaç Kiray A. The human sacrum and safe approaches for screw placement. J Clin Neurosci. 2009;16:1046–9.
22. Ebraheim NA, Lu J, Yang H, Heck BE, Yeasting RA. Anatomic consideration of the second sacral vertebra and dorsal screw placement. Surg Radiol Anat. 1997;19(6):353–7.
23. Esses SI, Botsford DJ, Huler RJ, Rauschning W. Surgical anatomy of the sacrum. A guide for rational screw fixation. Spine. 1991;16(6 Suppl):S283–8.
24. Kubaszewski L, Nowakowski A, Kaczmarczyk J. Evidence-based support for S1 transpedicular screw entry point modification. J Orthop Surg Res. 2014;9:224.
25. Robertson PA, Plank LD. Pedicle screw placement at the sacrum: anatomical characterization and limitation at S1. J Spinal Disord. 1999;12(3):227–33.
26. Matejcik V. Anatomical variation of lumbosacral plexus. Surg Radiol Anat. 2010;32(4):409–14.
27. Roy-Camille R. Journée d'Orthopédie de la Pitié; Spondylolisthésis L4L5 et L5S1. Paris: Masson Ed; 1983. p. 91–148.
28. De Peretti F, Argenson C, Bourgeon A, Omar F, Eude P, Aboulker C. Anatomic and experimental basis for the insertion of a screw at the first sacral vertebra. Surg Radiol Anat. 1991;13(2):133–7.
29. Ergur I, Akcali O, Kiray A, Kosay C, Tayefi H. Neurovascular risks of sacral screw with bicortical purchase: an anatomical study. Eur Spine J. 2007;16(9):1519–23.
30. Mirkovic S, Abitbol JJ, Steinman J, Edwards CC, Schaffler M, Massie J, Garfin SR. Anatomic consideration for sacral screw placement. Spine. 1991;16(6 Suppl):S289–94.
31. Pierchon F, Fontaine C, Mestdagh H. Injury to pelvic vessels and nerves during ostheosynthesis of the sacrum. Rachis. 1994;6:3–8.
32. Moshirfar A, Rand FF, Sponseller PD, Parazin SJ, Khanna AJ, Kebaish KM, et al. Pelvic fixation in spine surgery. J Bone Joint Surg. 2005;87:89–106.
33. De Peretti F. Bases anatomiques et expérimentales de la mise en place d'une vis dans le sacrum. In: Conférence d'enseignement de la SOFCOT. 1995.
34. Dubousset J. Correction et fusion jusqu'au sacrum des bassins obliques avec une instrumentation C.D. chez l'enfant et l'adulte. In: SOFCOT Réunion annuelle. 1986.
35. Lebwohl N, Cunningham B, Dmitriev A, Shimamoto N, Gooch L, Devlin V, et al. Biomechanical comparison of lumbosacral fixation techniques in a calf spine model. Spine. 2002;27(21):2312–20.
36. Tis JE, Helgeson M, Lehman RA, Dmitriev AE. A biomechanical comparison of different types of lumbopelvic fixation. Spine. 2009;34(24):E866–72.
37. Early S, Mahar A, Oka R, Newton P. Biomechanical comparison of lumbosacral fixation using Luque-Galveston and Colorado II sacropelvic fixation: advantage of using locked proximal fixation. Spine. 2005;30(12):1396–401.
38. Saigal R, Lau D, Wadhwa R, Le H, Khashan M, Berven S, et al. Unilateral versus bilateral iliac screws for spinopelvic fixation: are two screws better than one? Neurosurg Focus. 2014;36(5):E10.
39. Guler UO, Cetin E, Yaman O, Pellise F, Casademut AV, et al. Sacropelvic fixation in adult spinal deformity (ASD); a very high rate of mechanical failure. European Spine Study group. Eur Spine J. 2015;24(5):1085–91.
40. Dubousset M. Iliosacral screw fixation for pelvic obliquity in neuromuscular scoliosis. Spine. 1997;22(15):1722–9.
41. O'brien JR, Yu W, Kaufman BE, Bucklen B, Salloum K, Khalil S, et al. Biomechanical evaluation of S2 alar iliac screws: the effect of length and quadcortical purchase as compared to iliac fixation. Spine. 2013;38(20):E1250–5.
42. Dayer R, Ouellet JA, Saran N. Pelvic fixation for neuromuscular scoliosis deformity correction. Curr Rev Musculoskelet Med. 2012;5(2):91–101.
43. Bachy M, Kabbaj R, Bouyer B, Mary P, Vialle R, et al. EMC Tech Chir Orthop Traumatol. 2014;9(1):1–16.
44. Desrochers-Perrault F, Aubin C-E, Wang X, Schwend RM. Biomechanical analysis of iliac screw fixation in spinal deformity instrumentation. Clin Biomech. 2014;29(6):614–21.
45. Jain A, Hassanzadeh H, Strike SA, Menga EN, Sponseller PD, Kebaish KM. Pelvic fixation in adult and pediatric spine surgery:historical perspective, indications, and techniques: AAOS exhibit selection. J Bone Joint Surg. 2015;97(18):1521–8.
46. Chang TL, Sponseller PD, Kebaish KM, Fishman EK. Low profile pelvic fixation: anatomic parameters for sacral alar iliac fixation versus traditional iliac fixation. Spine. 2009;34(5):436–40.
47. Jost GF, Walti J, Mariani L, Cattin P. A novel approach to navigated implantation of S2 alar iliac screws using inertial measurement units. J Neurosurg Spine. 2015;24(3):447–53.
48. Bouyer B, Bachy M, Zahi R, Thévenin-Lemoine C, Mary P, Vialle R. Correction of pelvic obliquity in neuromuscular spinal deformities using the "T construct": results and complications in a prospective series of 60 patients. Eur Spine J. 2014;23(1):163–71.
49. Dubory A, Bachy M, Bouloussa H, Courvoisier A, Morel B, Vialle R. Screw augmentation for spinopelvic fixation in neuromuscular spine deformities: technical note. Eur Spine J. 2015;24(11):2580–7.
50. Zahi R, Thévenin-Lemoine C, Rogier A, Constantinou B, Mary P, Vialle R. The "T-construct" for spinopelvic fixation in neuromuscular spinal deformities. Preliminary results of a prospective series of 15 patients. Childs Nerv Syst. 2011;27(11):1931–5.

The Pelvic Vertebra, the Cephalic Vertebra and the Concept of the Chain of Balance

J. Dubousset

Introduction: Foundation for the Concept

In 1972, my teacher Pierre Queneau asked me to study the " Paralytic pelvic obliquity" for the meeting of the 1973 GES scoliosis study group. It then appeared obvious to me the concept of "Pelvic vertebra" [1].

Indeed, there was a surprising contrast between what we saw on the radiograph of the spine with the obliquity of the pelvis in relation to the horizontal and what was seen when looking at the patient. It was found that the pelvis was displaced in three planes of space and that the radiograph showed us only the "Chinese shadow" of reality. It was then easy to consider the pelvis, as a whole, as the last piece of the truncal skeleton (Fig. 1) and that it was displaced in space as were the different skeletal parts of the spine. The reality of the three dimensions was at the same time obvious (Fig. 2).

The anatomical reality of the concept quickly appeared to me when both White and Panjabi [2] showed that the mobility of the sacroiliac joint was minimal (approximately 1.5° and up to 3.5° in peripartum women to facilitate natural delivery). In addition, the book by RJ and P. Ducroquet [3] on "la Marche et les Boiteries" (literally "the Walk and Limps") demonstrated to me "the pelvic step" where the whole pelvis during walking is moved not only up and down but also rotated in the horizontal plane from right to left, as walking progresses. Finally, to comfort me in this concept, I frequently visited the Anatomical Museum, located in the slightly abandoned basement of the Parisian Baudelocque Maternity Hospital, in front of the Saint Vincent de Paul hospital where I worked. There I found a collection of pelvic and spinal skeletons where it could be noticed that many of them had considerable deformities of pelvic morphology

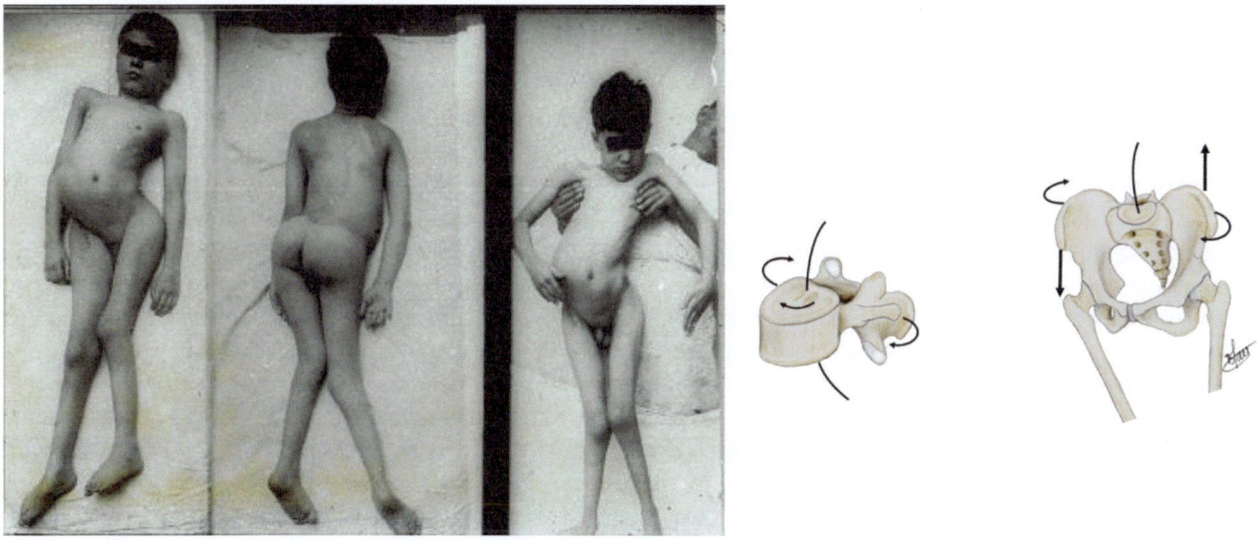

Fig. 1 Oblique pelvis of poliomyelitis. The pelvis is displaced in the three dimensions of space: frontal, sagittal, horizontal

J. Dubousset (✉)
National Academy of Medicine, Paris, France

J. M. Vital, D. T. Cawley (eds.), *Spinal Anatomy*, https://doi.org/10.1007/978-3-030-20925-4_12

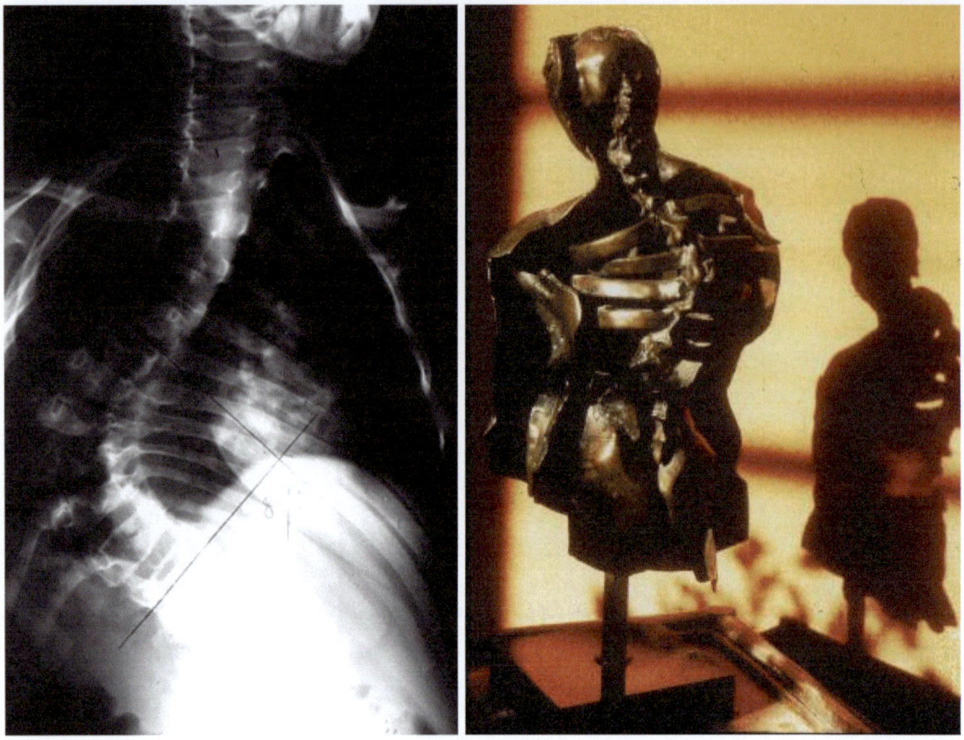

Fig. 2 The radiograph depicts the 3D reality as a "Chinese shadow"

which explained why they were there in this museum, for example, because of labour dystocia (obstructed labour) in parturients (females about to give birth) which often did not survive at that time.

So, it seemed appropriate to me to consider the pelvis as the last vertebra of the spinal skeleton and therefore to explain why, when one looked at a complete skeleton of the human body, how much this element played a role (interposed between trunk and lower limbs) in the erect posture of the human being. And it is with this same vision that appeared to me, around the same time, an identical but perhaps even more subtle role in the erect skeleton, of the "cephalic vertebra" (the whole head considered as a vertebra) where only the weight of the head at the other end of the articular chain played the role of the weight of a pendulum, provided that standing is regarded as the function of an "inverted pendulum"(Fig. 3).

Once I understood that, the remainder of my intentions would only serve to support and refine this concept according to multiple practical applications.

Anatomical Basis for the Pelvic Vertebra

Morphologically

The best studies come, as appropriate, from obstetric services, where very precise and complete descriptions relate to the different pelvic anatomy in women compared to men in the form of the outer pelvic ring (which is wider in females) at the opening of the iliac wings, antero-posteriorly and transversely. We know that pelvimetry is part of the armamentarium of the obstetrician. Moreover, recent work by Christophe Boulay [4] has shown a frequent prevalence of right–left asymmetry—if one refers to the respective size of the two iliac bones. Above all, the works of Duval-Beaupère et al. [5] have shown the individual variation of the angle of pelvic incidence (according to the name she gave to this angle), measured in sagittal projection between the perpendicular of the middle of the sacral endplate and the line uniting the centre of this endplate with the centre of the femoral head(s) (Fig. 4).

This angle is variable from one individual to another, it is generally lower for a newborn and increases steadily during the first 5 or 6 years to reach a plateau, but actually stabilizes only at the end of growth with an average around 50°.

It represents the spatial relationship of the two components of the sacroiliac joint. If we look at the evolution of species, we see that in quadrupeds, the angle of incidence is very low, is increased in some primates, then in the first hominids (for example Lucy, the 3.2-million-year-old skeleton) and finally in the human, as the erect standing position becomes dominant (Fig. 5).

This is well understood when we examine pelvises of various kinds, dysplastic or not, where the anteroposterior distance, variable between the sacrum and the pubic symphysis, will be a determining factor in this angle. Similarly, the anteroposterior or lateral variation in the position of the centre of the acetabulum makes it possible to understand the individual variations of the angle of incidence.

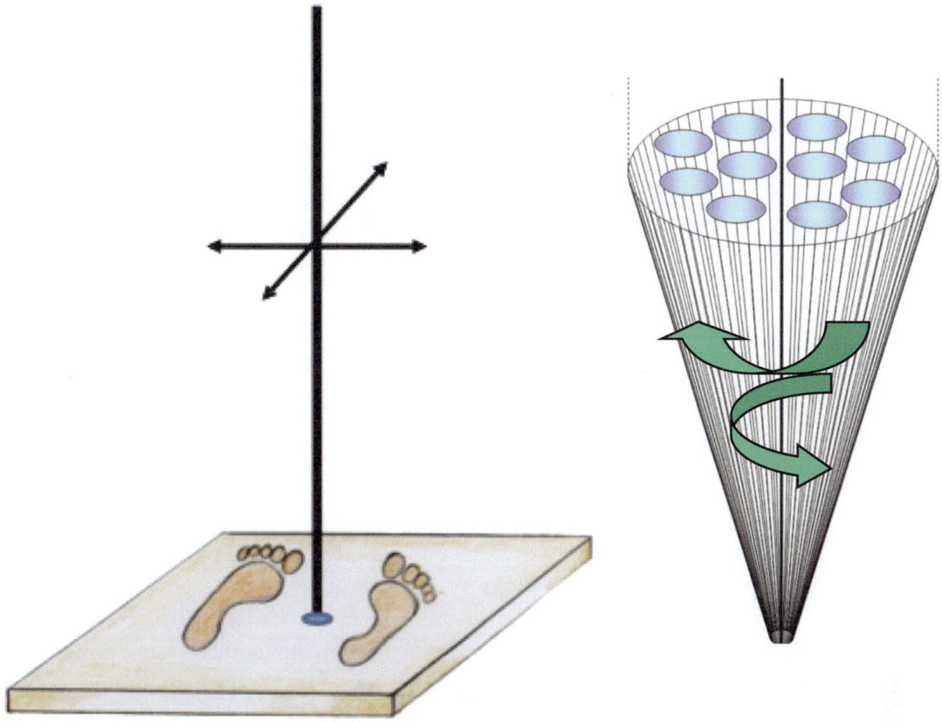

Fig. 3 The erect human functions as an inverted pendulum from a Polygon of Support

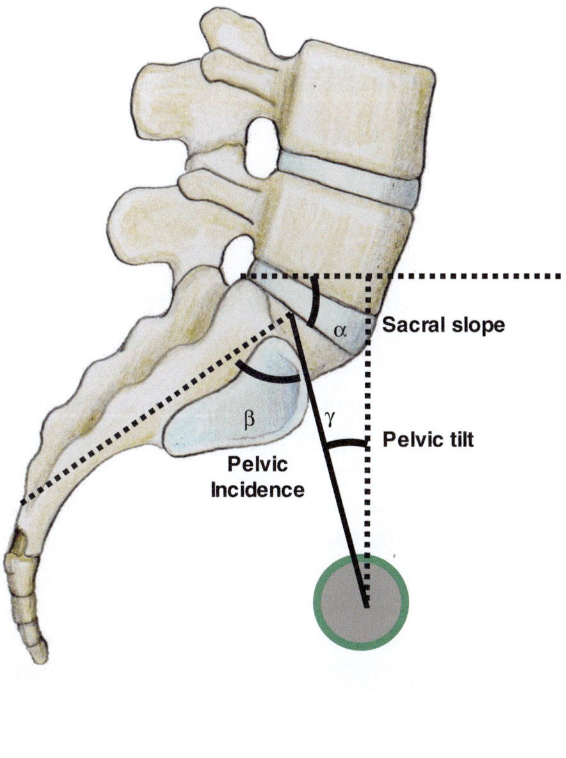

Fig. 4 From barycentrometric studies, Duval-Beaupère defined the (anatomical) angle of pelvic incidence (β) with its postural corollaries, sacral slope (α) and pelvic version (Y)

On the other hand, when a lumbosacral fusion (L5S1 or L4L5S1) is performed, the starting point of this angle is prolongated upwards since the fused vertebrae form a block with the pelvis, and this automatically reduces this angle of incidence by creating a new pelvic vertebra (Fig. 6).

Intrapelvic Degrees of Freedom

The work of White and Panjabi [2] has perfectly demonstrated that the movements of the sacroiliac joint were minimal but real, of the order of 1.5° up to 3.5°. Due to the hollow rail shape of the lateral sacrum and its articulation with the solid rail shape of the medial ilium and the inverted L- or C-shaped articular surfaces of this joint, these so-called nutation or counter-change movements are relatively weak, locking together the unit at this point. The pelvic entity is created by the juxtaposition of the two right and left iliac bones to the sacrum posteriorly and which meet each other anteriorly at the pubic symphysis. The transverse axis of these movements of nutation (anterior tilting of the promontory, posterior tilt of the coccyx) and of counter-nutation (posterior tilt of the promontory and anterior of the coccyx) is located behind the articular surfaces (hollow rail/solid rail) at the level of insertion of the interosseous ligament or axillary ligament.

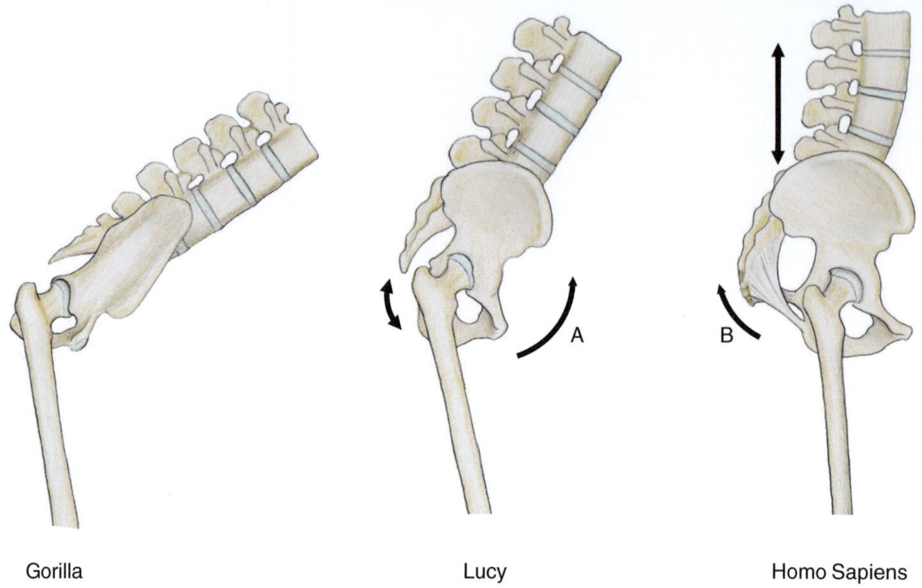

Fig. 5 Pelvic incidence has changed with the evolution of the species, with concomitant changes in pelvic tilt

This explains why this movement combines sliding at the level of the hollow rail/solid rail with anteroposterior rotation around this transverse axis: it is the nutation against the wobble!

The pubic symphysis, in reality a diarthro-amphiarthrosis joint, has a particularly resistant structure with a vertical elliptical central zone. This looks like an intervertebral disc with an oval cleft in the centre (often virtual), but circumferentially surrounded by strong ligaments, which explains why its mobility is negligible in the normal state, and only during pregnancy can one observe some minimal mobility.

On the Other Hand, the Degrees of Freedom Around the Pelvic Vertebra Are Quite Considerable

At the level of the lumbosacral joint, there are six degrees of freedom in three planes of space (flexion/extension, right/left Inclination and right/left axial rotation), not to mention a minimal up/down axial mobility, according to the vertical axis coming from the compressive elasticity of the L5S1 disk.

Moreover, at the level of each hip joint, there are also six degrees of freedom. So, we understand how the pelvic vertebra, by these mobilities at the level of the upper and lower points of support of the elements which surround it, will be able to adapt to almost all spatial situations which it will meet during the various functions of human life, within the limits allowed by these degrees of freedom [6].

Plasticity of the Pelvic Vertebra

It must also be remembered that according to various pathologies, either congenital malformations or acquired paralytic or infectious origins, affecting each of the components of the pelvis (especially during a period of growth), we will be able to observe considerable morphological changes which will, of course, affect the function it represents in the equilibrium of the skeleton as well as in its function of transmission of supra- and sub-jacent forces and moments working on the joints.

The visit to the old obstetrical museum located in the basement of the Baudelocque Maternity Hospital was enlightening for me and made me discover not only the entity of the pelvic vertebra but also the formidable capacities of adaptation and compensation of the human machinery.

The Texture and the Bone Architecture of the Pelvis

By studying this point, it is quite easy to identify the best possible anchor points for inserting implants of instrumentation material [7, 8].

As for the sacral skeleton, it is certain that the solid zones are represented by the central body of the sacrum, whereas the wings (ala) are much more cancellous (spongy) and have low anchoring capacity (Fig. 7). Of course, the screws bearing on the two anterior and posterior cortices will have the best screw hold. Finally, the extreme solidity of the sacroiliac periarticular ligaments must be noted, including that of the iliolumbar ligament to understand that concomitant use of the two iliac wings with sacroiliac screw fixation considerably increases the lever arms and thus the rigidity of a lumbosacral assembly. Screws along this trajectory, between the inner and outer bony iliac cortices spanning as far as overlying the roofs of the acetabulii and aligned along the lines of force from the acetabulum to the sacroiliacs, create a very robust anchor.

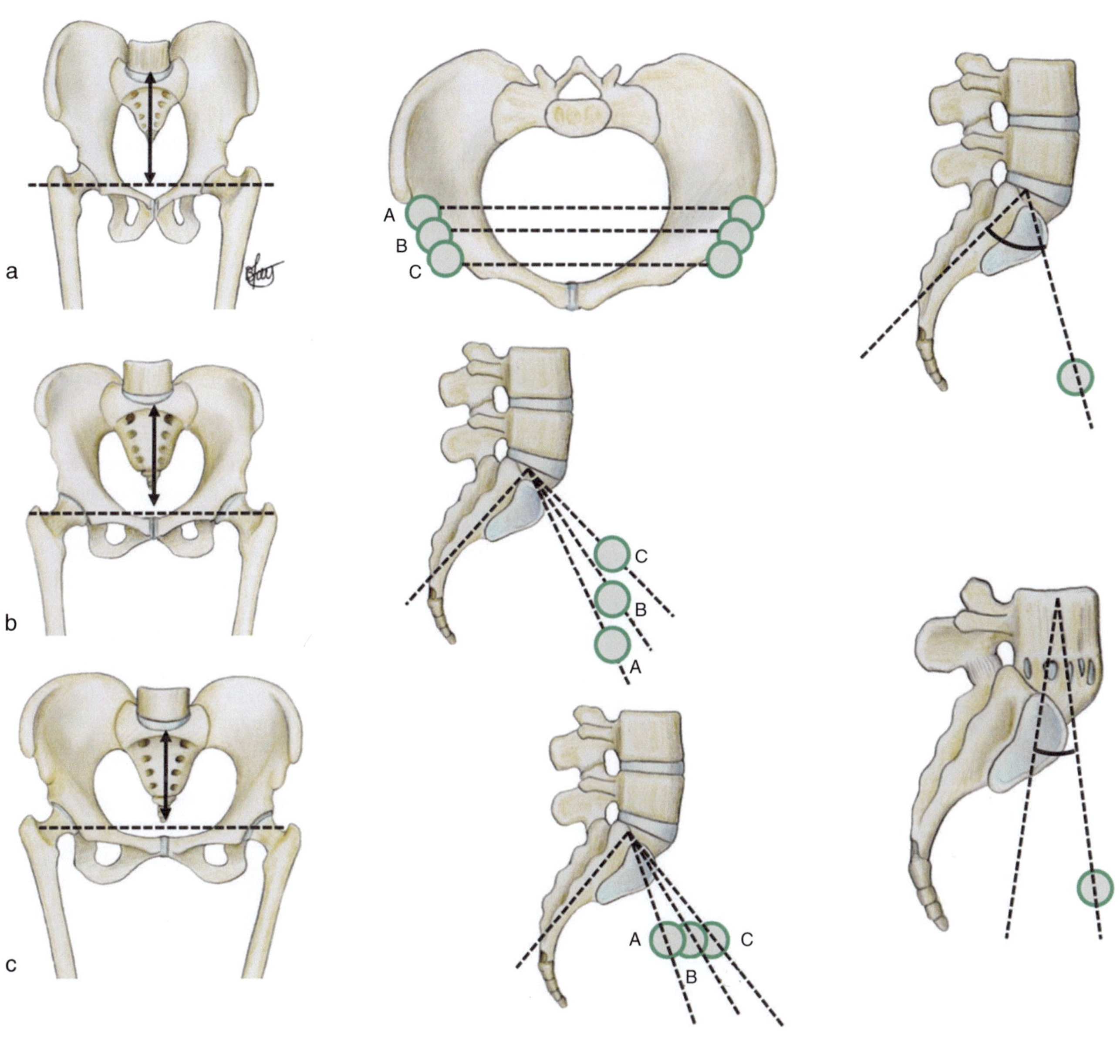

Fig. 6 Pelvic morphology changes the pelvic incidence. Lumbosacral fusion automatically decreases the angle of incidence

Physiological, Pathophysiological and Mechanical Implications of the Pelvic Vertebrae

The Pelvic Vertebra as an "Intercalary Bone"

The pelvis will play this role between the skeleton of the trunk (essentially spine) and the skeleton of the lower limbs.

1. Here again is *the study of the paralytic pelvic obliquity* which has been decisive in the understanding of this role—the "3 planes of space" as mentioned, and also that in can be "deformed in its morphology".

It was originally caused by sub-pelvic causes (below the pelvis contractures or paralysis of the hips, knee, etc.), intrapelvic causes (congenital or infectious deformities, such as childhood sacroiliitis associated with paralysis, which if occurring early in infancy, would result in a torsional deformity of the pelvis +/− femoral head growth deformity and asymmetry of the peri-pelvic muscular elements) and finally, supra-pelvic causes, i.e. all spinal deformities, scoliosis and kyphosis (Fig. 8).

Thus it was clear that a contracture of the hip in flexion-abduction forced the pelvis to move in the frontal plane with an inclination on the side of the hip anomaly, whereas if the hip was retracted in adduction or inversion,

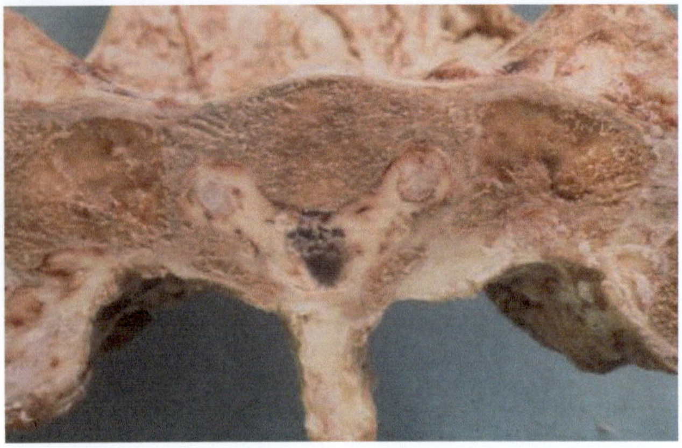

Fig. 7 On this cross section of the sacrum (S1), note the lack of resistance of a possible osteosynthesis at the level of the sacral ala

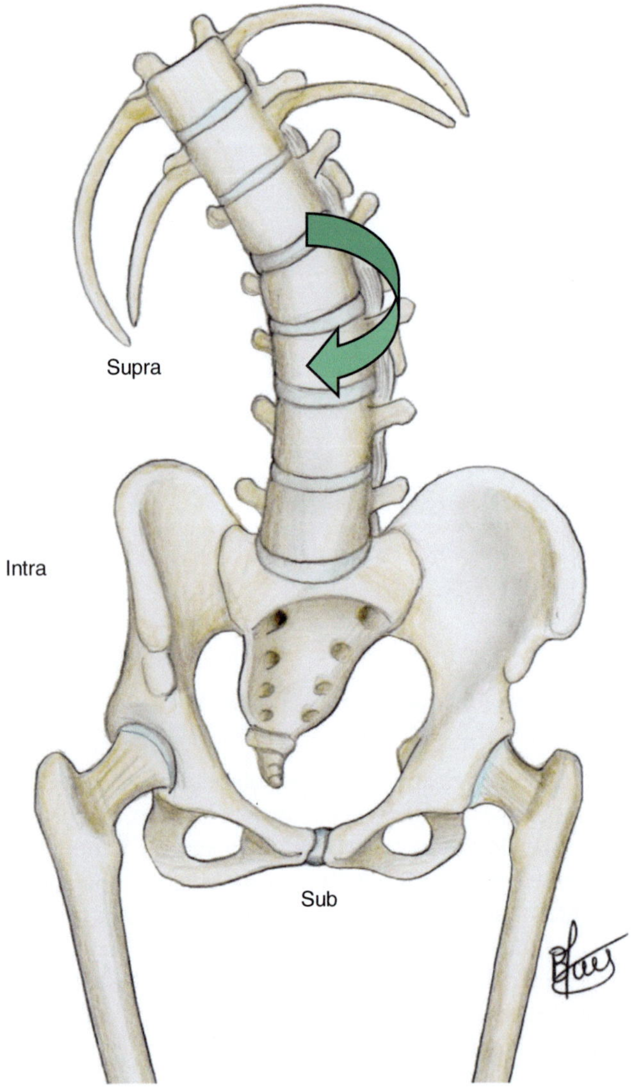

Fig. 8 Supra, intra and sub-pelvic causes of paralytic oblique pelvis are found with their own components adapted from the causal pathology

the pelvis was moving in the opposite direction and migrated superiorly in the frontal plane on the side of the hip anomaly.

Similarly, in the sagittal plane, any "flexion contracture" of the hip (vicious attitude in flexion) caused a rocking of the pelvis forward or anteversion, while a deficit of flexion (by contracture of the gluteus for example) produces an automatic retroversion during tested sitting. Similarly, in this sitting or standing position, the anteversion of the pelvis was automatically associated with a greater lumbar lordosis as the pelvis tipped over while inversely its retroversion was always associated with a lumbar kyphosis; the causes of these disorders are secondary to peri-pelvic contractures or paralysis.

In the horizontal plane, displacements in axial rotation were observed in the clockwise or counterclockwise direction as a function of the distribution of retractions or paralysis (Fig. 9).

2. So there were two phenomena that came together:
   (a) that of musculotendinous contractures or paralysis which forced the pelvis to move in space;
   (b) the effect of gravity which, according to the situations created by the first phenomenon, amplified the deformity in one direction or another.

Each of these elements could be found in the deformities and the three-dimensional pelvic expression, both physiological and whatever the pathology involved: the pelvis was indeed an "intercalary bone" (Fig. 10).

3. Studies in the sagittal plane by many authors have reinforced this point of view
   (a) The work of Duval-Beaupère demonstrated that in standing there was a close relationship on a lateral spine radiograph, between the angle of pelvic incidence and the amount of lumbar lordosis required to have a normal erect posture (small angle of incidence = small lordosis, wide angle of incidence = large lordosis) (Fig. 11). This has provided a practical measure that is essential to the orthopaedic world by confirming this notion of "intercalary bone" and "pelvic vertebra" [4, 5].
   (b) The work of Roussouly on the normal population has come to demonstrate the reality of this notion again creating a practical classification of the sagittal balance of individuals, in four major categories that have now become standard [9].
   (c) The influence of sub-pelvic causes, in non-paralytic cases but for example in the so-called "normal" aging population, has been demonstrated by the works of

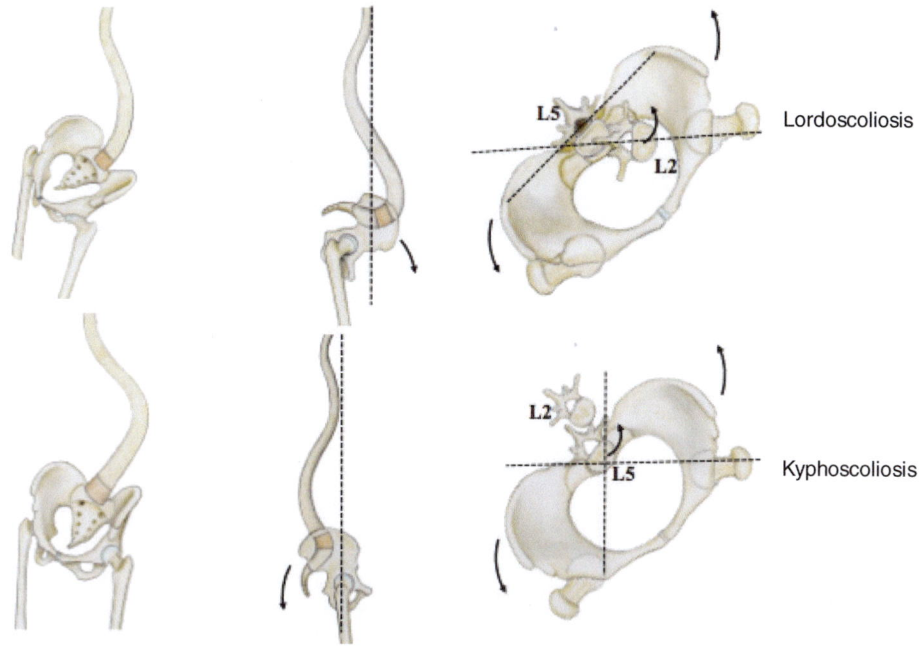

Fig. 9 The study of the paralytic oblique pelvis demonstrates that the pelvic vertebra had to be studied in the three dimensions

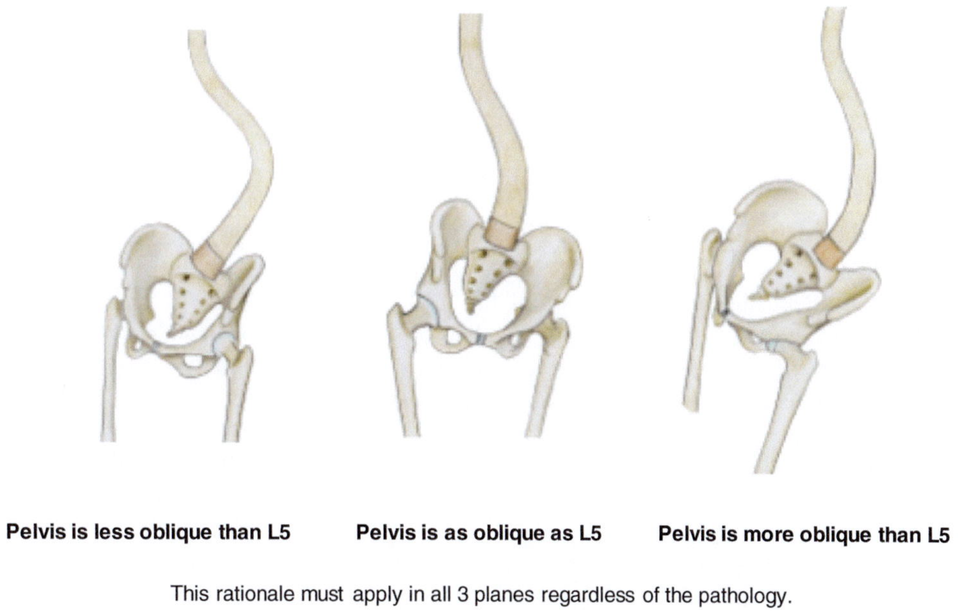

Fig. 10 The relationships of the pelvic vertebra with the lumbar spine are fundamental to establish a strategy of correction in the three planes of the space (example here in the frontal plane)

Hovorka who describes the loss of the reserve of extension of the hip (Fig. 12), an initiating factor of lumbar kyphosis in the elderly [10].

Finally, from a practical point of view, another proof: it is well known that when one has hip osteoarthritis associated with low back pain, the correction of the severe hip attitude by total hip arthroplasty often leads to the disappearance of low back pain.

4. *In the horizontal plane, we must also remember the original work of the Ducroquets*, who had perfectly defined the oscillating movements of the pelvis during walking, not only from top to bottom but also from front to back alternated with a reverse movement of the shoulders, called "the Pelvic Step"; the Ducroquets had perfectly observed it in space by walking the patients in a large room covered with mirrors, on the floor, on the ceiling and on the four walls [3].

It is also interesting to note that if one carefully examines an idiopathic scoliosis, especially when it involves a lumbar curvature, it is not uncommon to note that the curvature extends to the pelvis, which itself is asymmetric. Large 30 × 90 radiographs have already shown it in the form of an asymmetry of the pelvic projection (width asymmetry of the iliac wings, and the asymmetric appearance of the sciatic notch).

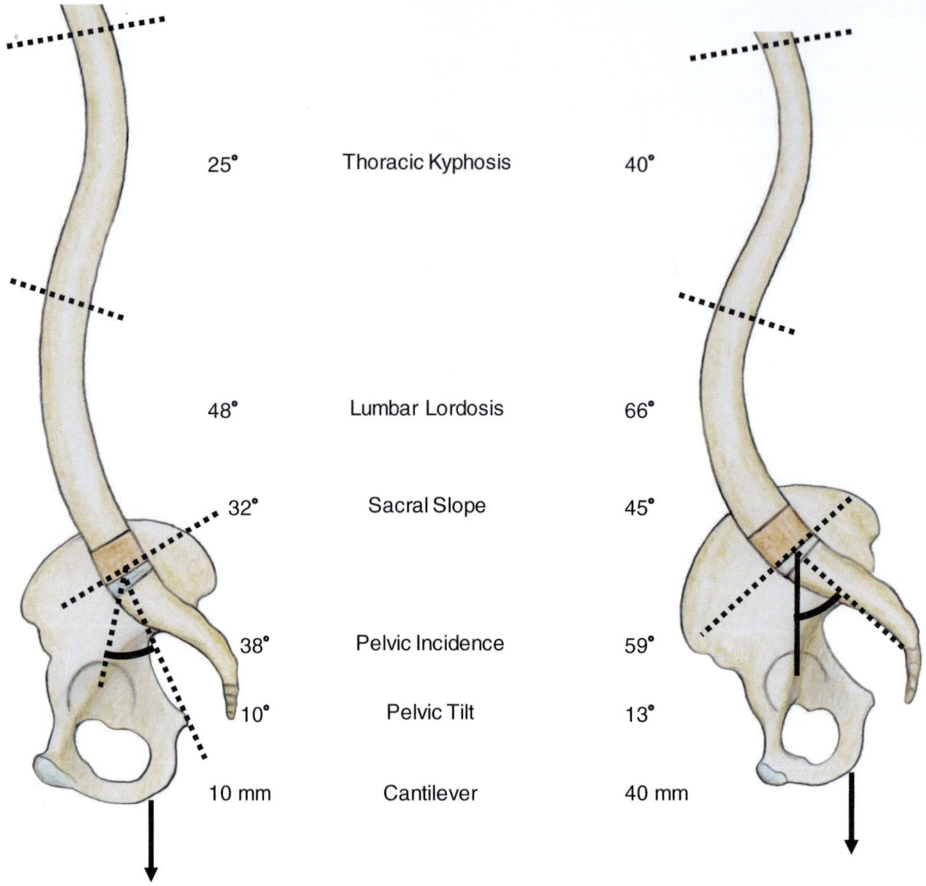

Fig. 11 Pelvic incidence determines the importance of the lumbar lordosis

Practical Consequences of These Findings

This is the establishment of the notion of the " Chain of "Balance " of the erect posture, whether standing or sitting (Fig. 13). The pelvic vertebra plays a central role in both orientation and compensation, given its privileged status as an "intercalary bone".

This global vision of the individual, standing or sitting, led us inevitably to go to the other end of the chain, i.e. to the head, considering it (because of its weight and its spatial context) as a true "Cephalic Vertebra", the upper end of the inverted pendulum characteristic of erect species.

The purpose of this characteristic being, on the one hand, to ensure the horizontal gaze, and on the other hand, to process visual, vestibular, auditory, and proprioceptive inputs. It is the place of automatic analysis and quasi-instantaneous efferences, thanks to the cerebral computer which houses and governs this Chain of Balance.

The *Polygon of Support* represents the following:

- Standing up by the support of the soles of both feet (spaced or close together), thus realizing a large surface whose geometric centre will represent the reference point of departure of the vertical gravity line.
- Sitting, which will be the same surface corresponding to the support of the two ischial tuberosities, buttocks and often from the posterior aspect of the thighs from which one will determine a geometric centre of reference. Recording of this pressure surface will probably be the best reliable measurement of the correction of a pelvic obliquity.

Standing or sitting, these elements will be best determined by a platform of forces to measure the support exercised at each point and also to determine this gravity reference centre.

If the plumb line remains a practical way to represent a vertical line of gravity, the reasoning is made from "top to bottom", whereas it seems to us preferable to reason from "bottom to top" starting from the centre of the polygon of sustentation using the force platform [10, 11].

It is common to note, in practice, that due to the minimal but almost permanent movements of the human being while standing or sitting, the projection of the centre of gravity of the human body varies according to a cloud of points around this geometric centre of the polygon of support. Above this polygon, there will be the succession of an " chain of joints" of about 30 levels of mobility passing through the bones of the skeleton of the lower limbs, with major importance of the large joints, ankle, knee, hip, then the pelvic vertebra, and the lumbar, thoracic and cervical vertebral parts, according to an harmonious state alternating in sagittal plane, kyphotic

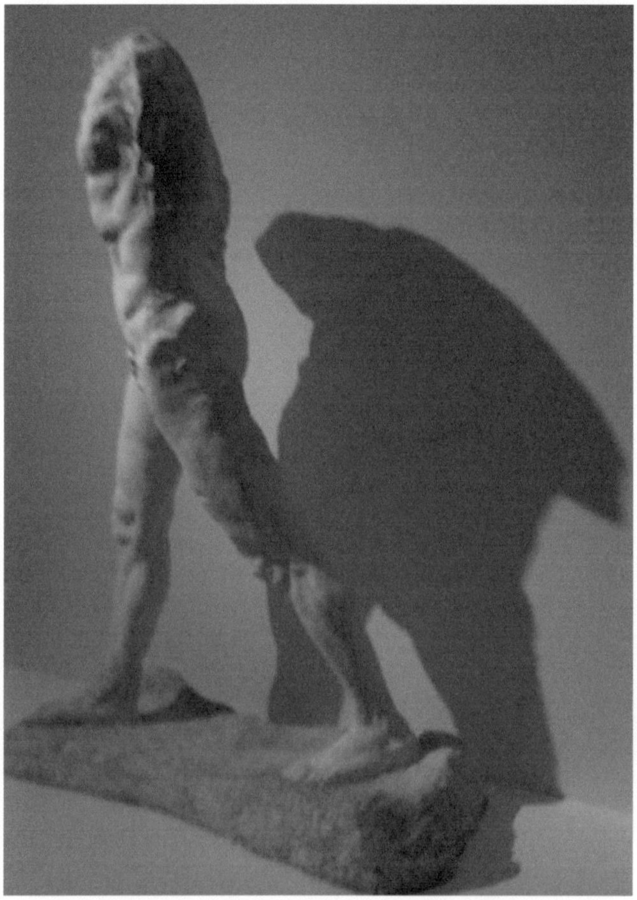

Fig. 12 "The Walking Man" by Auguste Rodin (1840–1917); note the clear extension of the left thigh of the model (as noted hip extension reserve by Hovorka)

and lordotic curves, ending with the cephalic vertebra with its weight of 4.5–5.5 kg, adjusting the equilibrium of this chain to obtain the physiological harmony of erect human balance.

Multiple static measurements of the various elements of this chain have been made and give average values for the human species which have only a relative value for an individual's skeletal anatomy, but muscular and metabolic processes also play a part.

It seems more important to take into account the dynamic values of this balance and the capacities of movement in the three planes of space around this axis of gravity starting from the polygon of support to establish a true muscular "*Cone of Economy*" (Fig. 14) allowing a harmonious and useful erect posture.

In this "Cone of Economy", we can consider that if we are inside a small cone, that is where there is little or no spinal or peri-vertebral muscular effort to stand up, the balance will be considered economical. On the contrary, if one is outside, it will require much more muscular work and fatigue factor to bring the various parts of the chain of the joints to a harmonious and stable posture. This is where the pathology of postural fatigue may even result in fatigue of possible spinal or other orthopaedic implants that will eventually give way to permanent stresses against them.

I cannot fail to mention the experience I had with Pol Le Coeur and the skeleton (mounted by the small assemblies of bones with wire) that he had in his cabinet: having detached it from the gallows where it was in suspension, he meticulously attached two non-extensible strings between the posterior aspect of the femoral condyles and the calcaneus, then he fixed a strip of leather between the anterior surface of the acetabulum above the roof and the anterior surface of the femurs just below the femoral neck. He puts his skeleton thus equipped on the 2 ft on the ground; he adjusts head, spine, knee and hip, so that strings and strips are taut and allow the skeleton to stand for a moment (half a second) without any other support!

It was at this moment that I imagined what I later called the "Cone of Economy".

All these considerations, pelvic vertebra, intercalated bones, cephalic vertebra and balance chain, were important reasons for me to participate in the design and implementation of the EOS imaging system [12]. Thanks to Georges Charpak's invention of the multiwire chamber, which considerably reduces the radiation dose needed to obtain a radiograph, thanks to the joint work of the ENSAM Paris Biomechanics and the Montreal LIO laboratories and to the work of the radiology department of the Saint Vincent de Paul Hospital in Paris, this machine was created for imaging the whole body in a standing or sitting position. It allows a pair of digital radiographs—simultaneous front and side profiles of the entire skeleton in the upright or sitting functional position with a dose reduction of the order of ten times for 2D radiography in comparison with conventional radiographs.

In addition, thanks to the computer program developed in the biomechanical labs, a 3D surface reconstruction of the entire skeleton can be obtained in a relatively short time with a precision equivalent to that obtained with the contiguous sections of sequenced radiographs.

Thus, we can perfectly understand this joint balance and measure the deformities in three planes at all levels simultaneously and appreciate exactly the compensation phenomena that occur at different joint levels. This quantification is essential to really judge the results of orthopaedic interventions, in particular at the level of the spine but also at the level of the lower limbs.

Therapeutic Consequences

The Paralytic Pelvic Obliquity Correction Strategy

This derives from the concept of the pelvic vertebra as applied to all surgical spinal pathology. Indeed, the compensation or aggravation capacities given by the position of the pelvic vertebra will directly reflect the outcome.

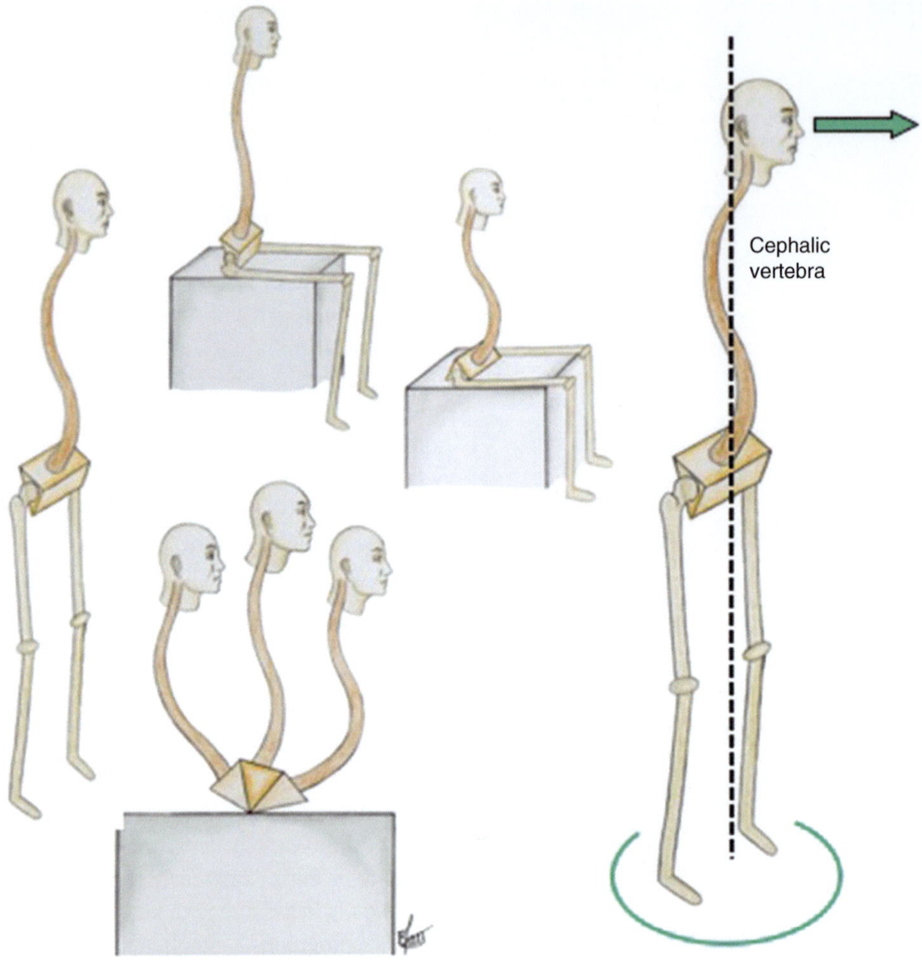

Fig. 13 The "*Joints Chain of Balance*" (note the constant horizontal gaze)

For example, we have shown that in the paralytic spine, there were two situations in which the need to include the pelvis in the spinal fusion was mandatory under penalty of recurrence of the pelvic imbalance for the sitting position (Fig. 10):

- The pelvis is *more* inclined than the lumbar curvature in the same direction as it had an irreducible lumbosacral junction;
- The pelvis is *less* inclined than the lumbar curvature but displays a fixed iliolumbar angle on the side of the convexity of the lumbar curvature.

On the other hand, when one has a lumbar curvature but with a neutral L5L1 coronal-plane orientation, one can avoid including the sacrum in the fusion provided that the peri-pelvic elements (above and below) are symmetrical in spatial equilibrium (contractures or amplitudes of mobility) and in balance of muscular strength to achieve anteroposterior (abdominal, gluteus maximus, and hip flexors, rectus abdominis) and horizontal (common sacrolumbar mass (iliocostalis, longissimus and multifidus), gluteus medius, quadratus lumborum, tensor fascia lata) balance.

If we apply these principles to the adult degenerative spine, for example, by studying both passive and active mobility, to judge of the supra- and sub-pelvic balance, we arrive at the same conclusions.

Another application of this concept of the pelvic vertebra is provided by the notion of inclusion or exclusion of the pelvis that accompanies the thoracic and lumbar idiopathic curvature and that we have fully explained with Salanova [13].

In a frontal view, the pelvis is considered "included" in the lumbar curvature when the iliac wing is elevated on the side of the concavity and in this case the lumbar curvature must be included in the fusion, generally down to L4. The pelvis is considered "excluded" when the pelvic bone is elevated on the side of the convexity of the lumbar curvature (there is in this case as a short lumbosacral countercurve at L4-Sacrum). In this case, one can simply merge only the

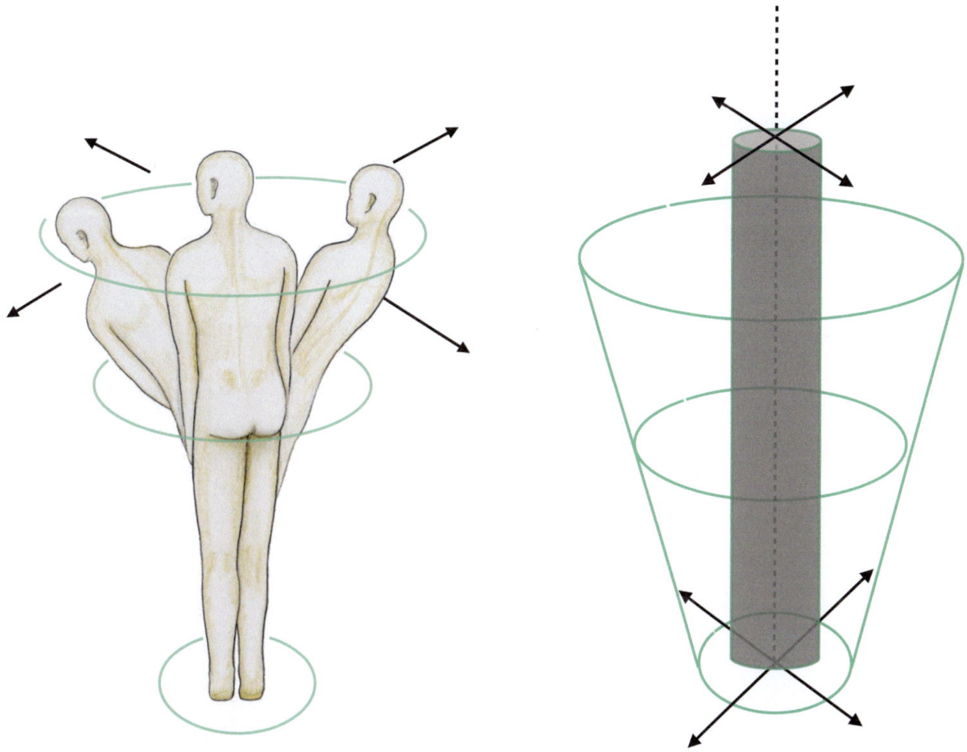

Fig. 14 The concept of the muscular "cone of economy"

thoracic curvature, and the lumbar curvature tends to reduce itself then spontaneously.

This implies in addition to our static angular analyses and passive mobility or reducibility (lordosis, kyphosis, pelvic angle of incidence, hip mobility, etc.) to have a quantitative assessment of active muscle factors.

This is the reason why we must strive to have active lateral flexion R&L radiographs preoperatively to establish a Cartesian planning.

Therefore, the decision to include the pelvis or not in an extensive spinal fusion whatever the etiology will depend on the analysis of these three factors:

- *Relative anatomy in the three planes,*
- *Passive reducibility and at what level*
- *Active peri-pelvic muscular environment, in three planes*

The Three-Dimensional Equilibrium of High Grade Spondylolisthesis

It is still obvious that this concept of pelvic vertebra exists, since in these cases, which can go as far as spondyloptosis (anterior displacement of L5 past the body of S1), it is not so much the importance of the sliding as measured by Meyerding that determines the pathology and prognosis, but the existence or not of a lumbosacral (lumbopelvic) kyphosis which, resulting in a considerable retroversion of the pelvis, explains not only the typical posture of these patients with an anterior abdominal fold, hip flexion relative to the pelvis and compensatory knee flexion, in order to protect the tension of the nerves of the cauda equina (Fig. 15).

It is therefore understandable that it is the angular displacement in lumbosacral kyphosis of the pelvic vertebra which will be the main factor of not only the improvement of the posture but also the relaxation of the neural structures.

This explains why some authors, including myself, use a technique of progressive reduction of kyphosis of the pelvic vertebra by external means (as shown by Scaglietti). This involves longitudinal traction in slight hip flexion but pelvic suspension, followed by hip progressive extension. The reduction of the spondylolisthesis is maintained by a plaster cast followed by a purely posterolateral fusion alone without opening the canal, when the obtained correction brought the balance of the pelvic vertebra in the "Cone of Economy" (lumbosacral angle ≥110°). An additional anterior lumbosacral graft (L5/S2) is only done in the case where this lumbosacral angle was ≤100°.

In the first case, the posterior fusion mass would only be aligned according to the stress lines and the anterior degenerate disk, discharged from its stabilizing role, while in the second case, the posterior fusion mass would not be sufficiently aligned, the disc would undergo destabilizing stresses and must be processed and fused.

The results of over 20 years ago, with the maintenance of the restoration of a harmonious and normal lumbopelvic morphology, are there to prove the value of these reasonings.

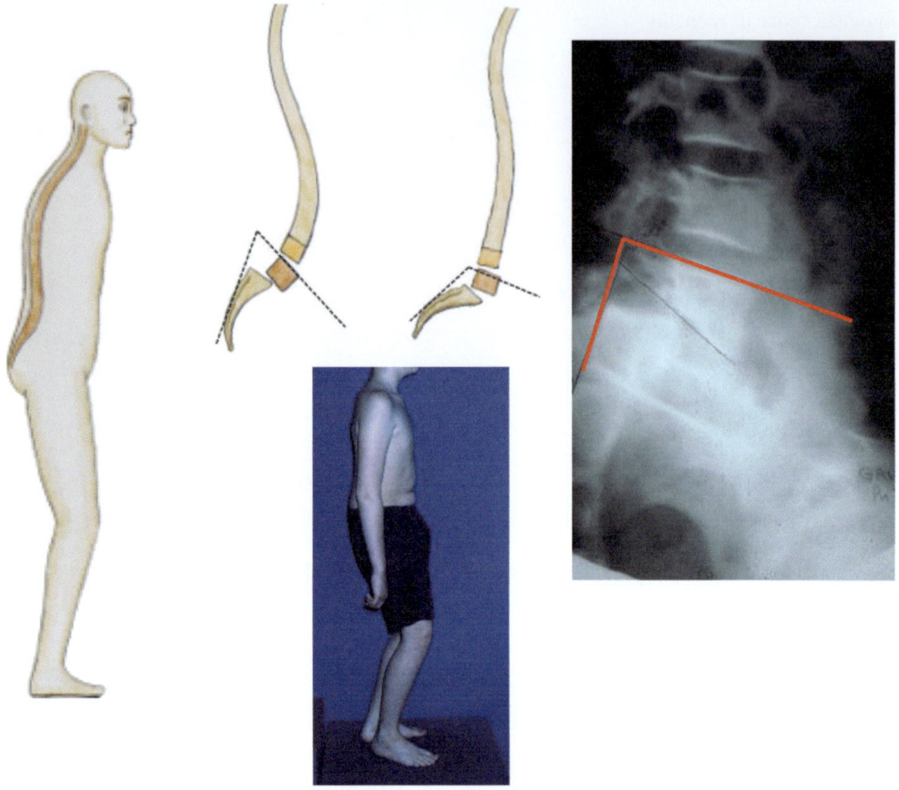

Fig. 15 Vertical sacrum with spondylolisthesis is a kyphosis of the pelvic vertebra (with its typical nerve root protection posture)

Compensation Phenomena Occurring at the Level of the Pelvic Vertebra

This occurs not only with posture but with mobility after spinal fusion for scoliosis, another proof of this concept [14, 15].

In a series of 30 idiopathic scoliosis fused in the thoracic region only (fusion & instrumentation stopped above L3) compared to 30 adolescents of the same age without any spine pathology as controls, the studies of posture, mobility and 3D reconstruction of the skeleton were performed at 3 months, 1 year and 3 years post-operatively, and they showed very interesting results.

FOR POSTURE: no difference between preoperative pelvic posture for the scoliosis group and controls. But there is a clear difference for the posture of the shoulders with a constant antepulsion in the scoliotic group, of the shoulders on the side of the convexity of the thoracic curvature.

On the other hand, after surgery, a frequent modification of the pelvic posture was observed compared to preoperatively: anteversion increased in 35% of the cases, decreased in 35% of cases and a change of orientation in 30% of the cases, demonstrating perfectly the compensation of pelvic origin of the spatial equilibrium in each individual.

FOR MOBILITY: in the postoperative group, a clear decrease in all trunk mobility was observed (which is logical after extensive arthrodesis of the spine), but this decrease was found to be strictly parallel to the decrease in pelvic mobility. For example, for the pelvic participation in the overall flexion of the trunk, it was increased in 18 patients, unchanged in nine of them and decreased in only one patient: again, evidence of compensation of pelvic origin.

Finally, even more surprisingly, a change in the angle of incidence of more than 5° was observed between pre- and postoperative in 50% of cases (10/21): four have increased (between 5 and 18°), six have decreased (between 7 and 14°) and 11 remained unchanged.

This again testifies to the mobilization of the pelvic vertebra which, after having exhausted its possibilities of purely postural compensation, will modify the very structure of the pelvis at the level of its sacroiliac joint (particularly as the procedures were carried out before the completion of spinal maturation).

The Possibilities of Anatomical Changes in the Pelvic Vertebra with Bilateral Pelvic Osteotomies of Sagittal Reorientation of the Trunk

In fact, when spinal surgery fusion & instrumentation including the pelvis is not in equilibrium with anterior tilt of the trunk, the correction of the imbalance can be obtained by a vertebral osteotomy, for example transpedicular extension of the upper segment. But this can also be achieved by performing a bilateral anterior opening supra-acetabular iliac osteotomy giving extension in the upper part of the pelvis with the overlying spine fused to it (Fig. 16).

It is thus possible to obtain up to 30° correction whilst remaining careful not to over-distract the femoral nerve as I

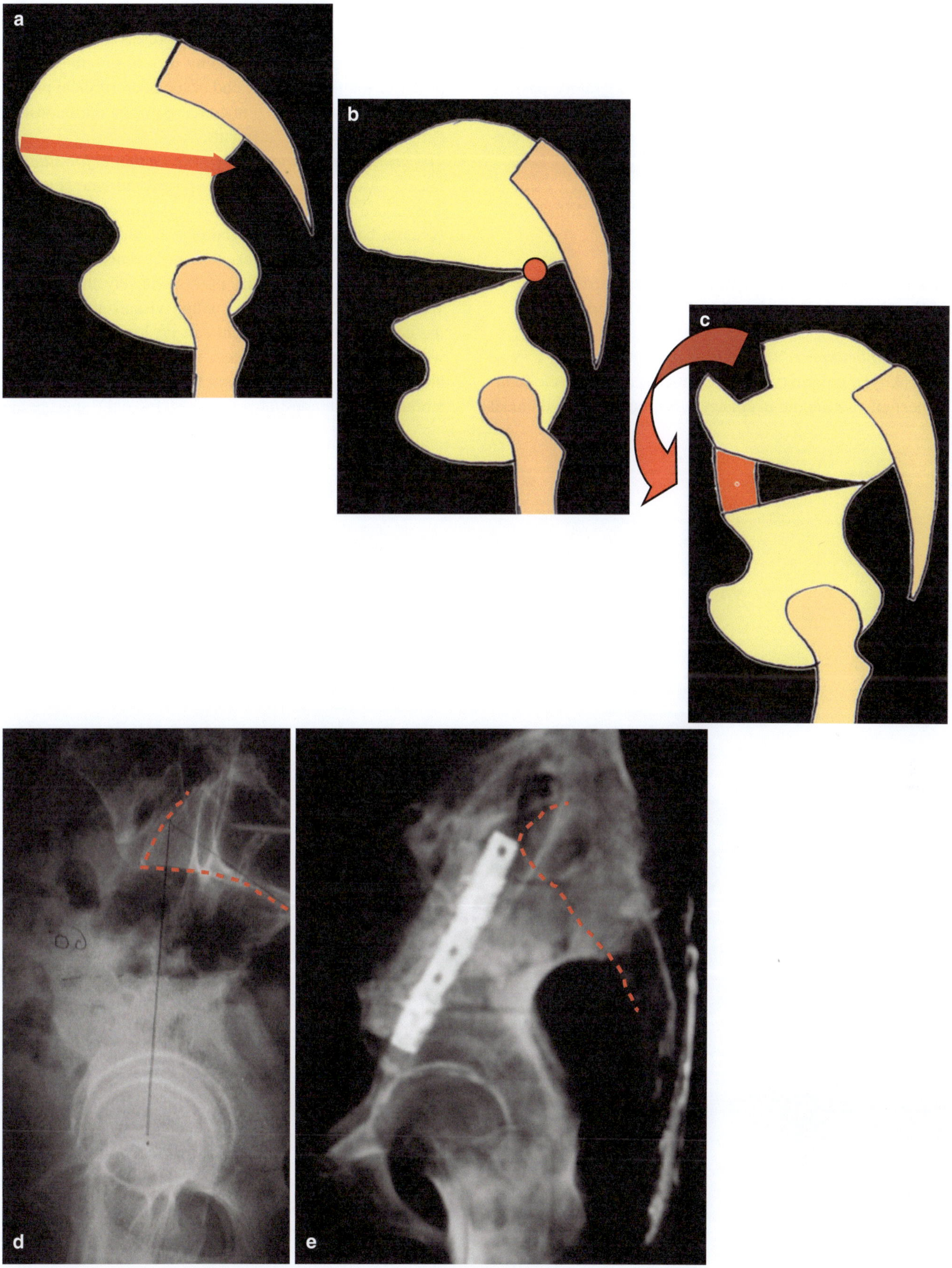

Fig. 16 Supra-cotyloid or pelvic addition osteotomy: (**a**) osteotomy tracing, (**b**) opening of the osteotomy, (**c**) graft in the opening, (**d**) preoperative radiograph and (**e**) postoperative radiograph (pelvic incidence decreases)

observed in my first case, resulting in bilateral quadriceps paralysis which fortunately recovered in 3 months.

But the goal had been reached, allowing the patient when in a standing position to have the line of gravity passing behind the femoral heads and to be in an economic position, whereas before the osteotomy, it passed anteriorly and created a sagittal imbalance.

One can also imagine a series of unilateral pelvic osteotomies, for example as shown by Hall to correct a difference in length of the lower limbs.

The Therapeutic Consequences of the Notion of the Cephalic Vertebra Are Just as Important

- *The explanation of the creation and prevention of* a swan neck-type deformity (Fig. 17) after cervicothoracic laminectomy for tumour in infancy is obvious for the individual to maintain a horizontal vision. Its prevention has now become well established by laminar preservation with laminoplasty instead of laminectomy or repositioning of the posterior joint cover at the end of the neurosurgical procedure and its maintenance in correct position until consolidation of the posterior elements.
- *The arthrodesis to address kyphotic lumbar deformities* in muscle diseases such as Rigid Spine Syndrome (Fig. 18) can reduce the lumbar kyphosis and project the cephalic vertebra backwards. The syndrome includes contractures of the muscles of the neck, thus it prevents any anterior flexion of the head so that post-operatively the cephalic vertebra tilts backwards permitting visualization only of the ceiling. Thus, the patient can no longer see his feet when standing and sometimes requires the wearing of a high posterior corset to support the neck and cephalic vertebrae. This demonstrates the need for only appropriate

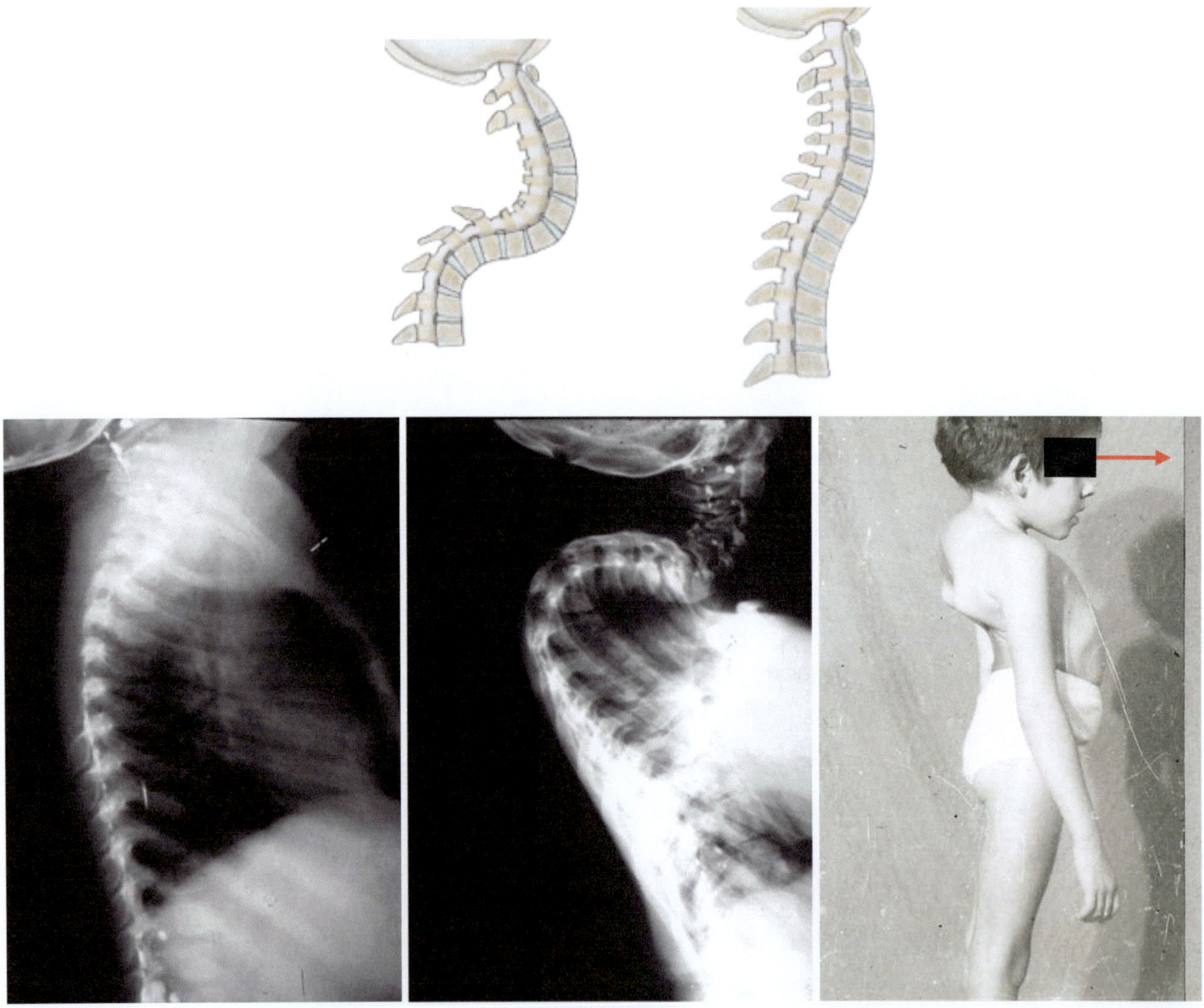

Fig. 17 The Swan neck deformity post-laminectomy of the cervicothoracic region in juveniles is a reflection of the role of the cephalic vertebra in the maintenance of balance and horizontal vision

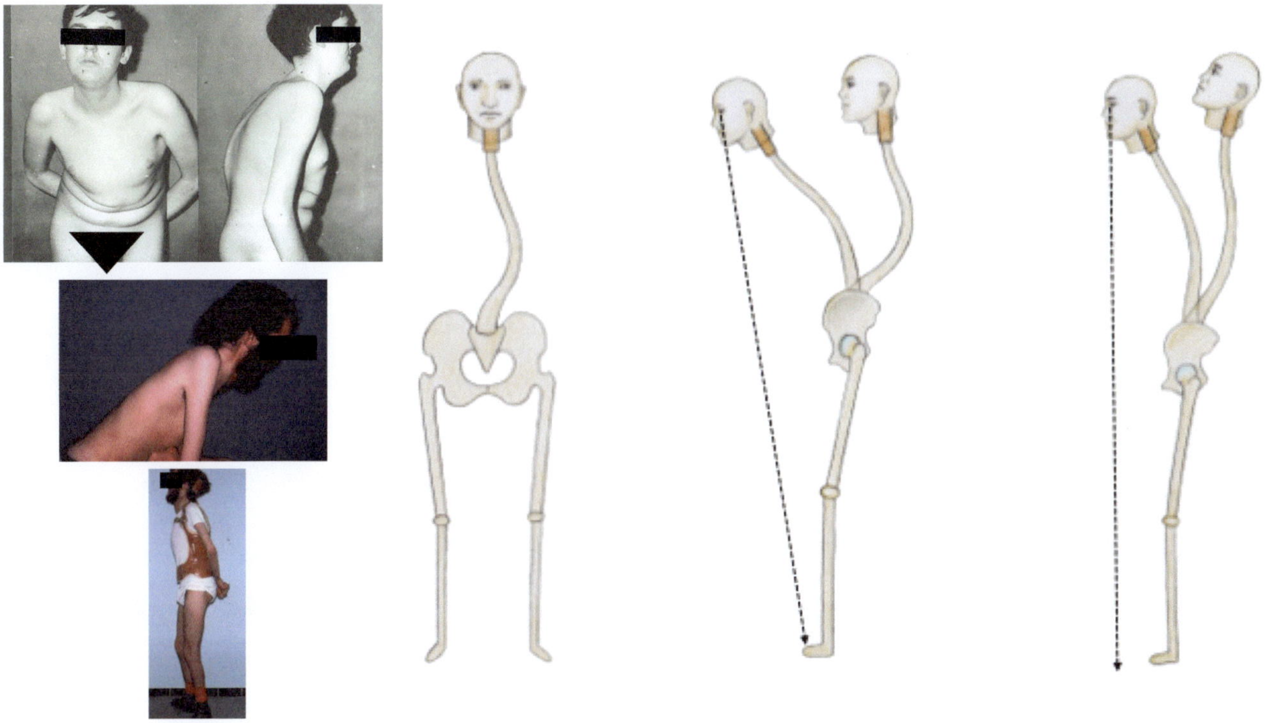

Fig. 18 "Rigid Spine Syndrome" (a slowly progressive childhood-onset congenital muscular dystrophy): the lumbar kyphosis compensates for the absence of anterior flexion of the cephalic vertebra, its suppression propels the head back and the patient cannot see his feet when standing

partial correction of the lumbar kyphosis or requires a cervical flexion vertebral osteotomy, which carries high risk of neurological injury.

- The proximal junctional kyphosis accompanying long extended vertebral fusions (Fig. 19);
- This is a frequent problem, observed more and more with the extensive use of rigid and powerful instrumentation, resulting in a significant modification of sagittal balance. It is observed particularly in neurological etiologies such as Parkinson's disease or cerebral motor conditions or muscular diseases, and also in a certain number of idiopathic cases in a normal neuromuscular context. This may be attributed to insufficient consideration of the spatial equilibrium of the cephalic vertebra:
  - The first reason is the lack of awareness of a small, high structural curvature at the level of an apparently pure thoracic scoliosis. The assembly stops at a junctional vertebra undergoing flexion and torsion as the fulcrum is carried by the most unstable vertebra which in fact was part of a "hidden" double thoracic curvature.
  - The second reason is the failure to maintain a harmoniously kyphotic curvature of the thoracic region; the loss of this kyphosis will propel the upper part of the spine and the cephalic vertebra backwards. To regain its balance above the polygon of sustentation, the mass of the cephalic vertebra is projected forward, resulting in major kyphotic constraints on the end of the posterior instrumentation and thus the junctional kyphosis.
  - The third reason, especially for long osteosynthesis extended to the sacrum, is the exaggeration of the lumbar lordosis, often with acute correction (especially in case of transpedicular osteotomies) and the posterior projection of the upper end of the assembly. Here again, the loss of the progressive physiological harmony of the sagittal plane, given by the alternation of cervical lordosis, thoracic kyphosis, lumbar lordosis and pelvic anteversion, associated with the extent of the instrumentation, leads to overwork of the only possible compensation zone, i.e. the upper junction zone just above the upper instrumented vertebra).

This brings us, when faced with this risk, to consider three main prevention factors:

1. Never stop the upper aspect of a construct at the junctional vertebra of a structural curvature (preferably stopping at one level below), taking care not to over-correct the underlying thoracic curvature, staying within the limits allowed by the flexibility of the upper curvature.
2. Study preoperatively the active mobile segments, for example in flexion/extension of the cephalic and cervical segments at the same time, and also those of the upper thorax, including the shoulders, based on the displacement of the humeral heads in sagittal projection when the upper limbs are placed parallel to the body.

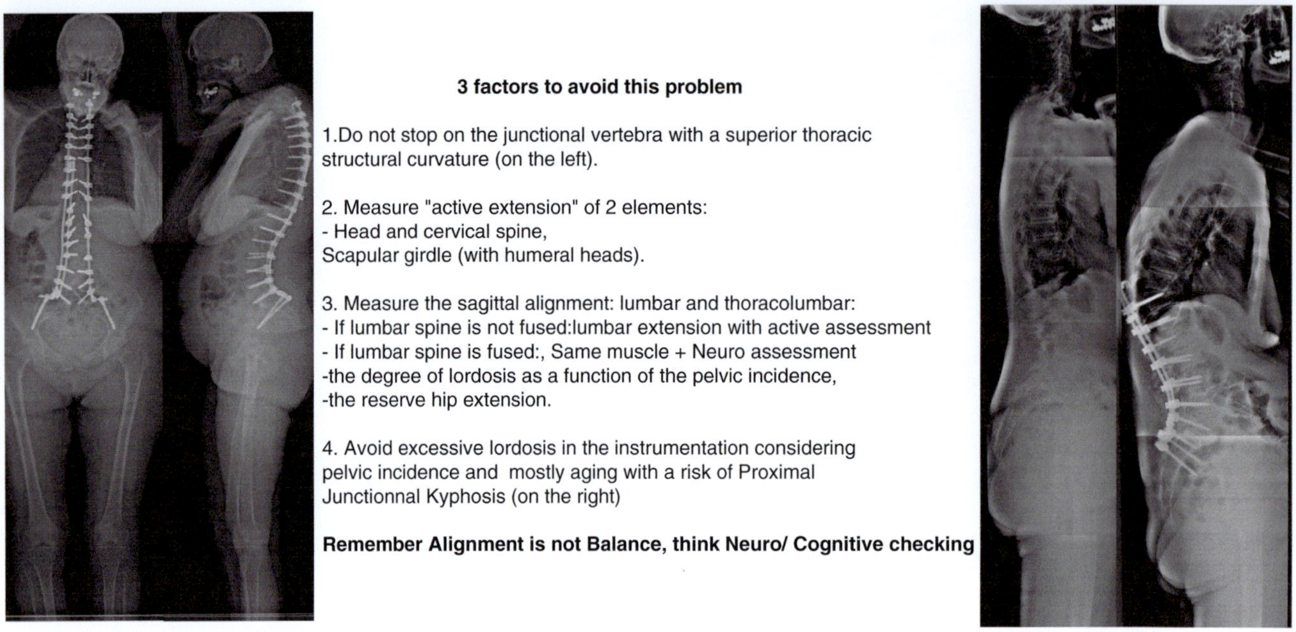

Fig. 19 Proximal junctional kyphosis: three factors to avoid this problem

3. Study the thoraco-lumbo-pelvic sagittal alignment with an active muscle assessment.
   (a) If the lumbar spine is not fused, look at the active lumbar mobilities in flexion/extension.
   (b) If it is fused and *a fortiori* if the fusion extends to the sacrum, one must know the following:
   The amount of lordosis required according to the pelvic angle of incidence,
   The amount of extension reserve at the hip joint level.

All this is to affirm even more clearly that in the case of spinal fusion, extended or not, what matters most for the quality of the result is not about the fused area but the areas left free below or above the fusion.

Conclusion

The notion of the “Chain of Balance”, in which the “Pelvic and Cephalic Vertebrae” play for us a primordial role, is a concept that any spinal orthopaedic surgeon, as any practitioner dealing with the musculoskeletal system, must permanently have in mind.

It signifies a static and dynamic system of permanent adaptation of all the bones and joints of the human being within a polygon of support from the cephalic vertebra passing through all the spinal pieces, the pelvic vertebra to the skeleton of the lower limbs,, harmoniously distributed (particularly in the sagittal plane), realizing a succession of curves separated by progressive junction zones, the assembly allowing mobility and stability that can be adjusted at any moment.

With pathological alteration of an element of this particular chain, the ability of adaptation and compensation given by the other elements of this chain is considerable; to keep them to the maximum and to know how to use them according to the pathologies are one of the bases of the therapy of the affections of the spinal axis.

References

1. Dubousset J. Le bassin oblique paralytique. In: Proceedings GES Paris. 1973.
2. White A, Panjabi MM. Clinical biomechanics of the spine, vol. 1. New York: Lippincott; 1978.
3. Ducroquet RJ, Ducroquet P. La marche et les Boiteries, vol. 1. Paris: Masson; 1965.
4. Boulay C, Tardieu C, Hecquet J. Sagittal alignment of spine and pelvis regulated by pelvic incidence: standard values and prediction of lordosis. Eur Spine J. 2006;15:415–22.
5. Legaye J, Duval-Beaupère G, Hecquet J. Pelvic incidence: a fundamental pelvic parameter for three-dimensional regulation of spinal sagittal curves. Eur Spine J. 1998;7:99–103.
6. Dubousset J. The pelvic vertebra 3D concept for physiopathology, classification, and management of pelvic obliquity. In: Zielke farewell symposium meeting, Bad Wildungen. 1989.
7. Dubousset J. CD instrumentation for paralytic & neuromuscular spinal deformities with particular emphasis on pelvic obliquity. In: Bridwell KH, Dewald RL, editors. Textbook of spinal surgery. New York: Lippincott; 1991. p. 347–64.
8. Dubousset J. Three-dimensional analysis of the scoliotic deformity. In: Weinstein SL, editor. The pediatric spine: principles and practice. New York: Raven Press; 1994. p. 479–96.

9. Roussouly P, Gollogly S, Berthonnaud E. Classification of the normal variation in the sagittal alignment of the human lumbar spine and pelvis in the standing position. Spine. 2005;30:346–53.
10. Hovorka I. Current concepts in spine surgery. In: Nice spine course 2007, vol. 1. Montpellier: Sauramps; 2007.
11. Lafage V, et al. Standing balance and sagittal plane spinal deformity. Analysis of spinopelvic parameters and gravity line parameters. Spine. 2008;33(14):1572–8.
12. Dubousset J, Charpak G, Skalli W, Lavaste F, Deguise J, Kalifa G, et al. Bull Acad Natl Med. 2005;189(2):287–300.
13. Salanova C, Dubousset J-F, Moreno P, Boulot J. Instrumentation segmentaire dans la scoliose idiopathique. Rôle du cliché de face debout dans la détermination de la zone à fusionner. Rev Chir Orthop. 2000;86:441–51.
14. Skalli W, et al. Importance of pelvic compensation in posture and motion after posterior spinal fusion using CD instrumentation for idiopathic scoliosis. Spine. 2006;31(12):E359–66.
15. Schwab F, et al. Gravity line analysis in adult volunteers: age related correlation with spinal parameters, pelvic parameters and foot position. Spine. 2006;31:E959–67.

The Cranial and Pelvic "Vertebrae" Are They Real Vertebrae?

Jean Marc Vital, M. Laurentjoye, A. Dimeglio, and T. Chevillotte

Introduction

Jean Dubousset knew, through his vast clinical experience, to integrate the skull and the pelvic ring into the vertebral column proffering thus the cranial and pelvic vertebrae. This concept, accepted by all, makes it possible to better understand the complex spinal pathological entities such as deformity or sagittal or coronal imbalances.

We would therefore like in this chapter to focus rather on the formation and growth of craniocervical and lumbopelvic joints, remembering that only the occipital condyles and the sacrum are actually part of the spine.

Formation and Growth of the Skull

The cephalic extremity bone is likened to a "cranial vertebra" resting on the cervical spine. In reality, this vertebra is composed of different bones whose assembly constitutes the calvaria (the upper part of the neurocranium and covers the cranial cavity containing the brain), separated from the facial skeleton by the base of the skull. In adulthood these bones are fused together except for the mandible, the only mobile craniofacial bone.

During its formation, the skull develops from the mesenchyme surrounding the brain. Bone derivatives are from endochondral ossification, typically forming long bones, and/or membranous, directly from the mesenchyme. We distinguish the neurocranium, enveloping the brain from the viscerocranium, the origin of the facial skeleton. The neurocranium is composed of a cartilaginous base (chondrocranium) and a membranous calvarial portion (desmocranium). Thus, the bones of the base of the skull derive from the chondrocranium by endochondral ossification. During organogenesis and until the end of growth, the bones of the skull base are separated not synchondrosed. These will be at the origin of growth and in particular, the morphology of the skull base.

We could therefore consider the base of the skull as a stack of welded cephalic vertebrae. The analogy between the vertebrae and skull base is remarkable as to the somites origin, mode of ossification, the presence of a mirrored intervertebral growth area but also the similarities in their protective roles of the central nervous system. Having no place in locomotion, the basicranial bone structures are immobile but provide a stiffness between the bones of the base of the skull for the protection of encephalic structures. Some consider nevertheless some "cranial mobility" essential in the architectural balance of the cranial puzzle! [1–3].

Somites

Towards a vertebral and basicranial common origin: the pro-atlas.

Derived from the differentiation of somatomeres, somites are set up along the notochord from the occipital region to the embryonic tail. They differentiate into sclerotomes, myotomes, and dermatomes. Sclerotomes from the first four pairs of somites or occipital sclerotomes contribute to the establishment of the basicranial skeleton, while those that follow are involved in the formation of the spinal skeleton.

The proatlas is considered as a vertebra between the atlas and the occipital bone [4]. From a phylogenetic point of view, it is often found in vertebrates below the apex of the odontoid process or in the region of the foramen magnum. Described in other species, it is not usually found in humans. From a morphogenetic point of view, the proatlas,

J. M. Vital (✉) · T. Chevillotte
Spinal Unit, University Hospital, Bordeaux, France

M. Laurentjoye
Anatomy Laboratory, University Hospital Bordeaux, Bordeaux, France

A. Dimeglio
Department of Pediatric Orthopedic Surgery, Polyclinique Saint Roch, Montpellier, France

J. M. Vital, D. T. Cawley (eds.), *Spinal Anatomy*, https://doi.org/10.1007/978-3-030-20925-4_13

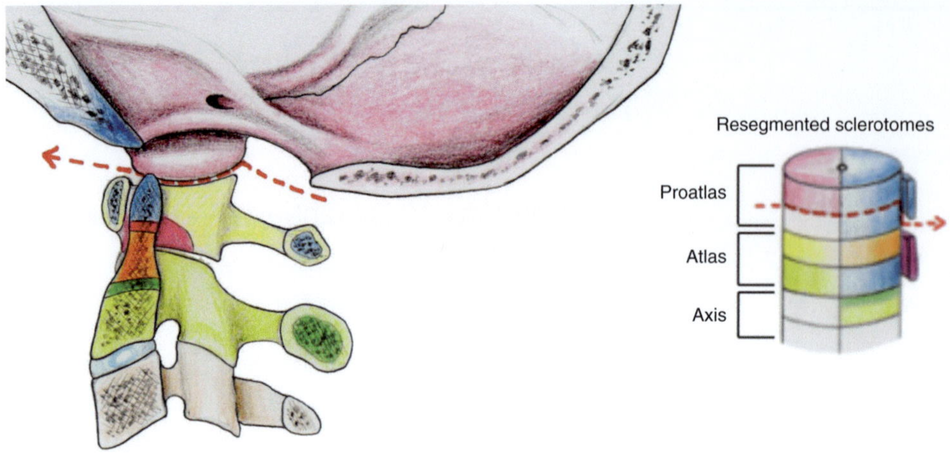

Fig. 1 Re-segmentation of the craniocervical region. Embryological origin of the base of the skull and the cranial part of the cervical spine. Note the contribution of the proatlas in the formation of the occipital bone (pink and blue) (Bernard [6])

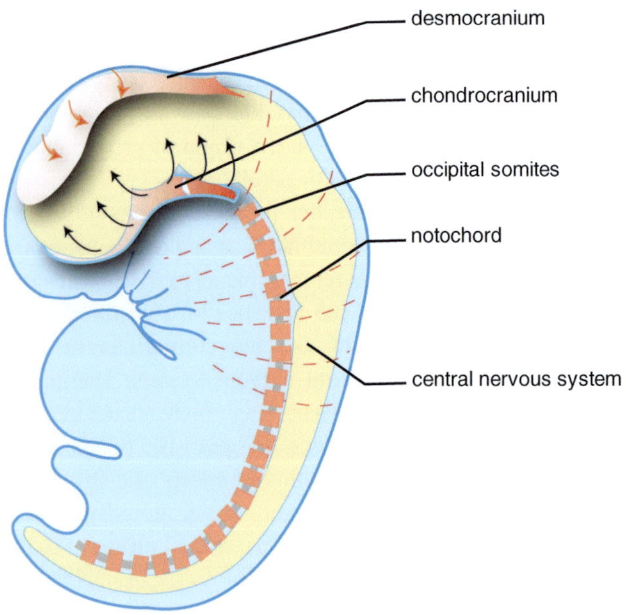

Fig. 2 Segmentation of the chondromesoblast at 4 weeks, occipital somites and notochord

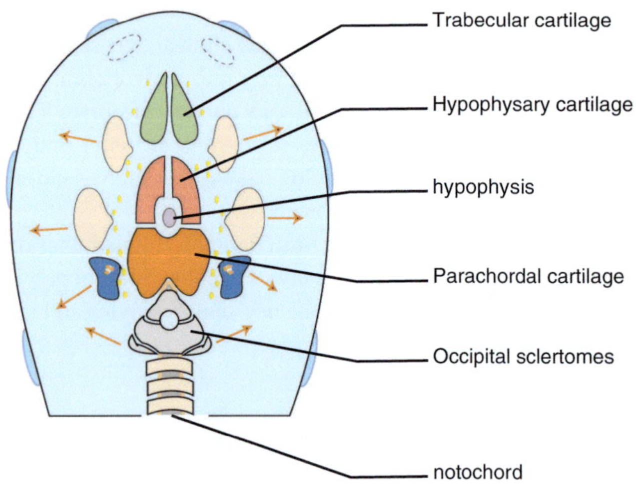

Fig. 3 Formation of the chondrocranium at 6 weeks

which derives from the first four occipital sclerotomes and the cranial part of the first cervical sclerotome, participates in the formation of the basioccipital and at the craniovertebral joint [5] (Fig. 1).

Basicranial Chondrogenesis (Figs. 2, 3, 4, and 5)

The basic basicranial skeleton appears in the form of cartilage islands in the basicranial mesenchyme. This mesenchymal tissue has two origins: the cells of the neural ridges and the paraxial somitic mesoderm [8].

The notochord, surrounded by parachordal cartilages, terminates at the level of the pituitary gland at the level of the future sella turcica, a true center of the base of the skull where we find pituitary cartilages. Rostrally prechordal cartilages (trabecular cartilage) and their lateral expansions (otic capsule and chondroethmoid) derive from the neural ridges. Thus the chondrocranium is formed from three pairs of cartilaginous foci that will fuse to form the basement of the brain: the prechordal cartilages, the pituitary cartilages, and the parachordal cartilages.

Dorsally, around the seventh week, the perinotochordal mesenchyme becomes the parachordal cartilages that become the postsphenoidal part of the base of the skull. The parachordal cartilages represent the outline of proatloid vertebrae: basipostsphenoid and basioccipital, separated by future synchondroses, characteristically modified intervertebral discs.

The skull protects the brain from the outside via calvarial and facial membranous bones. The base is the border traversed by the peripheral cranial nerves and the spinal cord. Thus, between the cartilaginous drafts circulate neurovascular structures. The expansion of the cartilaginous parts until their fusion will organize the foramina of the skull base to the input or output of these elements of the cranial cavity.

Finally, the cephalic skeleton of the fetus is in place at 3 months and includes a cartilaginous chondrocranial chassis whose anterior and posterior parts have a different origin [8, 9]. The base of the postsphenoid skull has a common somitic origin with the spine. The presphenoidal part depends on the neural ridges such as lateral expansions or capsules in relation to the sense organs.

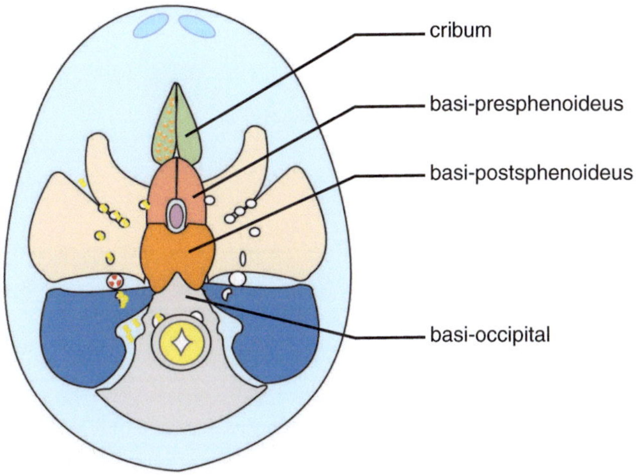

Fig. 4 Fusion of chondrocranium cartilage at 12–13 weeks

Craniofacial Ossification (Figs. 6 and 7)

Some bones have a double origin such as the occipital bone: endochondral for its basilar part around the foramen magnum and membranous for its flat part.

The ossification of craniofacial bones has two origins: endochondral, from cartilaginous and membranous tissues, from the ectomesenchymal cells of the cephalic neural crest.

The calvarium and many bones of the facial skeleton are from membranous ossification. Ossification points appear within the ectomesenchyme constituting the embryonic skull. Ossification is centrifugal to create conjunctive boundaries between bone parts.

These junctions are synfibroses or cranial sutures which allow the passive and functional secondary [11] growth of the bones controlled by the neighboring structures (brain, eyeball, muscular tension, nasal ventilatory flow…).

The base of the skull develops as an enchondral ossification, starting from the cartilaginous base. Its growth is inde-

Fig. 5 Chondrocranium and its expansions (according to Mugnier [7])

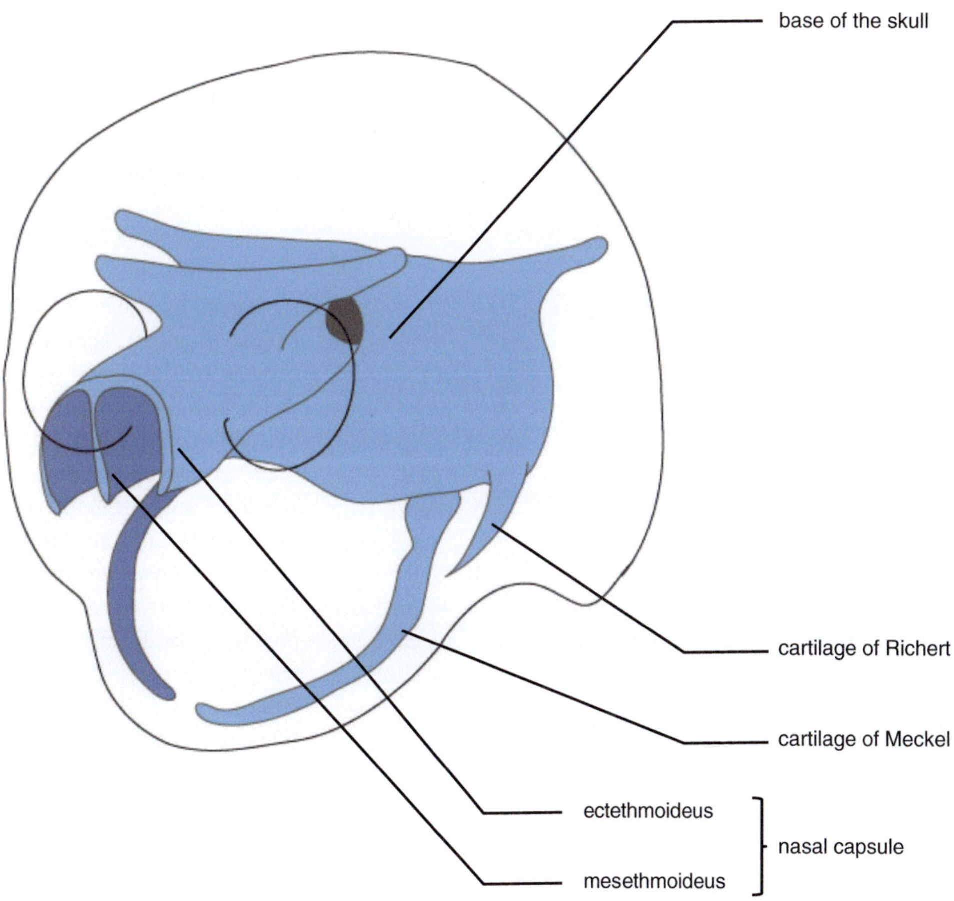

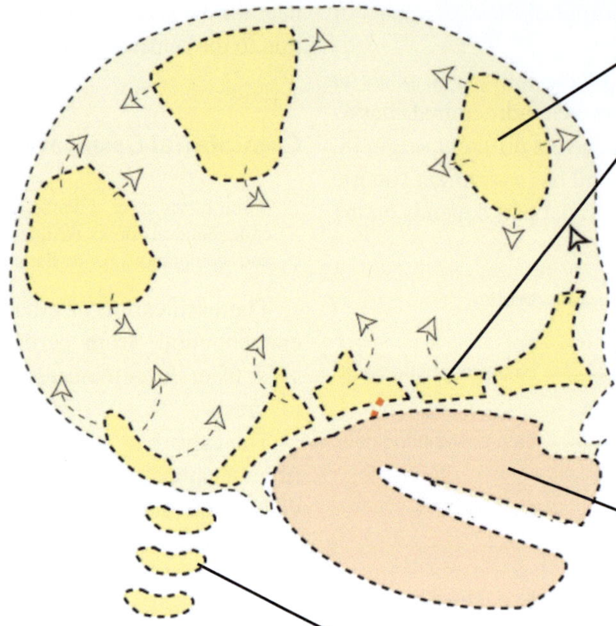

Fig. 6 Different modes of ossification

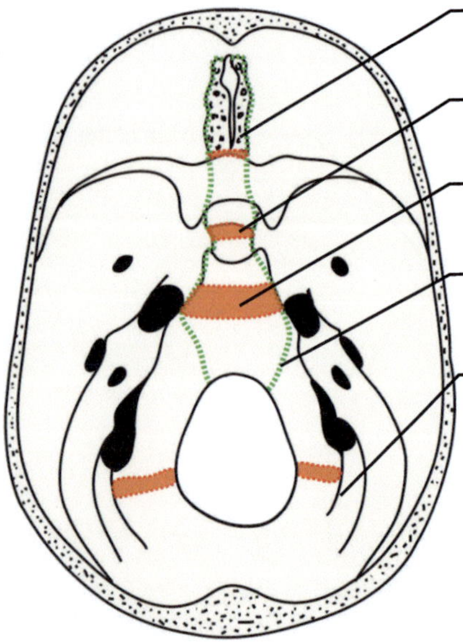

Fig. 7 Synchondrosis of the base of the skull (Couly [9], Stricker [10])

pendent, or primary, determined genetically and under hormonal control [9, 11]. The borders between the bony parts of the base of the skull are synchondroses which are areas of growth by endochondral ossification whose structure is comparable to that of the epiphyses of the long bones. They have a bilateral growth area or mirrored "dual action epiphysis" according to Scott [12].

The occipital bone has a double origin: endochondral for its basilar part surrounding the foramen magnum and membranous for its squamous (flat) part [6].

Craniofacial Growth

Synchondroses determine the growth of the base of the skull in three planes of space. They remain active for some until the end of growth [3]. The sphenoethmoidal, intrasphenoidal, and intraoccipital synchondroses mainly involved in sagittal growth come from the base of the skull. The spheno-occipital synchondrosis contributes to the sagittal and vertical growth of the base. The latter disappears at the age of 20 and constitutes, with exosuboccipital and exobasioccipital synchondroses, evidence of the multi-vertebral origins of the basipostsphenoid and occipital bones [9].

During human evolution, the brain grows and bipedalism, subject to gravity, appears. The head is balanced on top of the column of the biped. The column pulls the occiput backwards bringing the foramen magnum horizontally. The cranial volume increases, and the basicranial angle closes. The face, very dependent on the skull base to which it is attached, involutes proportionally to the increase in brain capacity and in parallel with changing dietary constraints.

During morphogenesis, one can observe the flexion of the skull base between the basi- and presphenoid. This curvature begins at the level of spheno-occipital synchondrosis [13] and will depend on phenomena of periosteal apposition-resorption. Finally, from a phylogenetic and morphogenetic point of view, a counterclockwise rotation of the occipital bone and a clockwise rotation of the sphenoid bone are observed.

The superficial skeleton (upper skull) exhibits membranous ossification and adaptive growth under the influence of

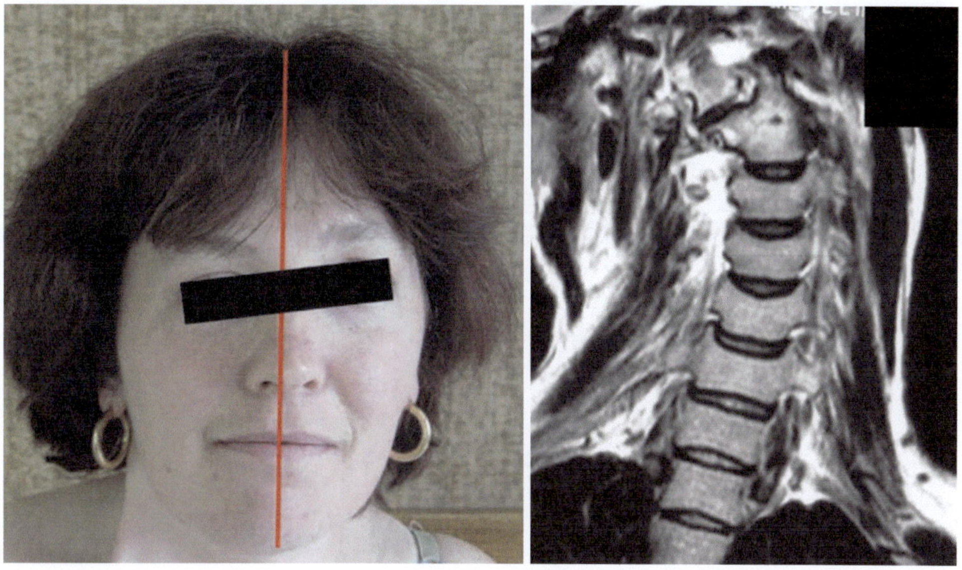

Fig. 8 Facial asymmetry following a congenital torticollis

extrinsic forces such as encephalic expansion on the calvarium resting on the basicranial base. Facial growth depends on the growth of the base of the skull in its middle and anterior part. The flexion phenomena of the base of the skull affect the sagittal maxillomandibular balance [14].

The chondroethmoid emits extensions that support facial intra-membranous ossification. The mesethmoid (future nasal septum) and ectoethmoid (future lateral masses) [9] are at the origin of the vertical sutural growth and by the nasofrontopremaxillary and palatal facial sagittal thrust [10, 15]. Laterally, the otic capsules emit ventral extensions: the cartilages of Meckel and Richert. Meckel's cartilage will serve as a guardian of mandibular morphogenesis (Fig. 5).

Facial growth is equally dependent on the manducatory and ventilatory functions. Normal mandibular growth is dependent on that of the middle level of the face via the dental occlusion (the relationship between the maxillary (upper) and mandibular (lower) teeth when they approach each other). The nasal breathing flow also has a considerable influence on the growth of the middle floor of the face and maxillomandibular harmony.

Thus vertebral and facial growths are linked within the base of the skull as the vertebral column is postsphenoidal and as the face is presphenoidal. Moreover, in clinical practice, there are many facial asymmetries related to basicranial and/or vertebral asymmetry (Fig. 8).

Conclusion

If the center of gravity of the head is just behind the turcica sella area [16], we can consider that it separates the vertebral column at the back from the face in front. Indeed, the postsphenoidal portion of the base of the skull and the craniocervical vertebral junction is of somitic origin. The ossification is of endochondral type through synchondroses, essentially basicranial intervertebral discs. The ventral part of the skull base contributes significantly to the morphology of the face. Morphological growth abnormalities are associated with each other: facial scoliosis, asymmetries of the skull base, cervical postural disorder, vertebral or pelvic abnormalities.

Formation, Growth, and Aging of the Pelvic Ring

The pelvic ring includes the sacrum (constituted by the fusion of the five sacral and the four coccygeal portions) and the two coxal bones (articulating with the sacrum at the level of the sacroiliac joints, considered as quite immobile and coming from the fusion of the three bones: ilium, ischium, and pubis). At this articulation with the inferior limb, the pelvic girdle is not detached from the spine, as opposed to the scapula at the origin of the superior limb due to the disappearance of the basilar bone (Fig. 9).

Phylogenesis

> With man's evolution to bipedalism, there is an increase of the angle of pelvic incidence, which expresses the size of the pelvis and the sacrococcygeal angle, which measures the curvature of the sacrum.

Fig. 9 Comparison of pelvic and thoracic (superior and inferior) limb girdles

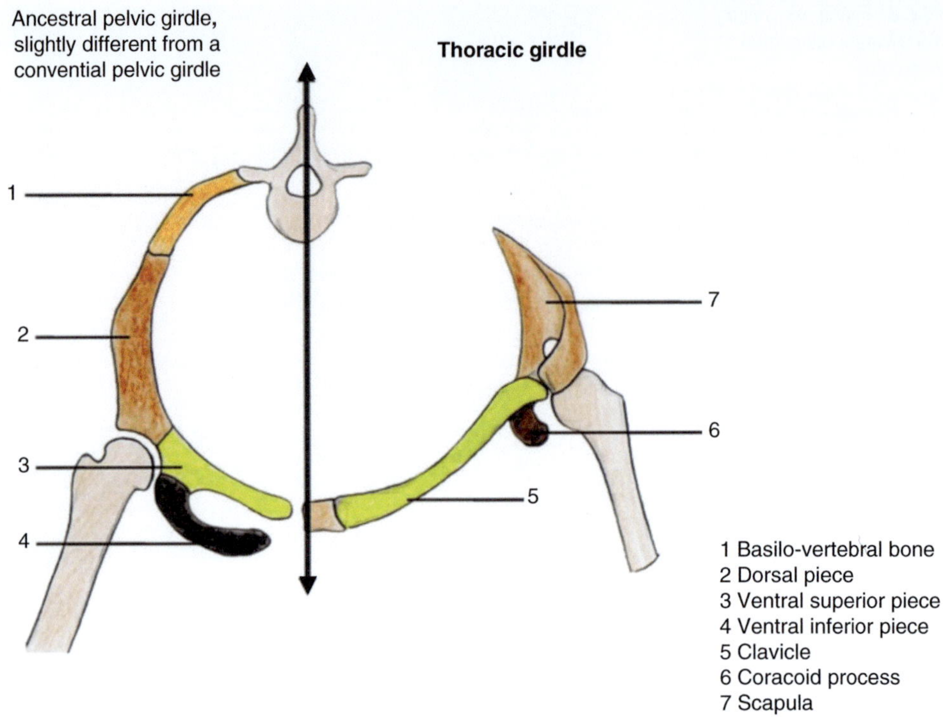

Tardieu [17] made a 3D study of the pelvic ring of hominoid fossils, 19 newborns and 50 adults. She was interested in the evolution of the shape of the hip bone and the sacrum during the acquisition of walking and, as we will see later, during growth. This analysis focussed on the angle of pelvic incidence [18] and also an original angle, entitled the " bow angle" or iliopubic angle, formed by a mid-sacral endplate to a midacetabular line and a line from the mid-acetabulum to the anterior aspect of the pubis (Fig. 10). This angle, which measures the anteroposterior width of the pelvis, increases during primate evolution to bipedalism as well as pelvic incidence that evaluates the width of the pelvis at its middle part.

According to Tardieu [17], as for Morvan [19], the iliac wings widen and become sagittalized (Fig. 11) in the evolution of bipedalism. The pelvis thus widens in the anteroposterior direction (from where the pelvic incidence increases) (Fig. 12), towards the front (where the iliopubic angle increases) and finally opens superiorly to facilitate the viscera and the trunk.

The sacrum evolves by curving forward. Abitbol [20] uses the angle between the sacral curvature along the anterior wall of the body of the S1 and the anterior wall of L5. The sacrococcygeal angle (Marty [21]) is traced between a line perpendicular to the upper endplate of S1 and a second perpendicular to the endplate of S5; this angle increases with the acquisition of bipedalism (Fig. 13), according to Tardieu [17]. The widening and sagittalization of the iliac wing, and the curvature of the sacrum in the acquisition of bipedalism parallel with the increase of lumbar lordosis are explained by the action of the extensor muscles (lumbosa-

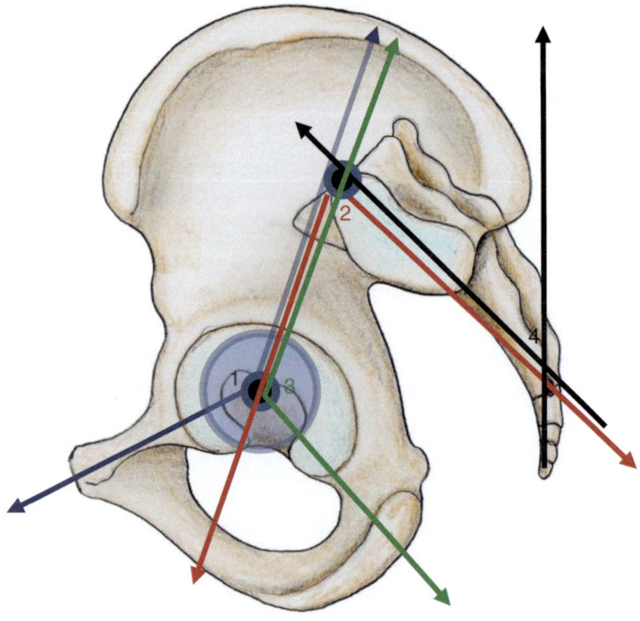

Fig. 10 Iliopubic angle (1), pelvic incidence (2), ilioischial angle (3), sacrococcygeal angle (4)

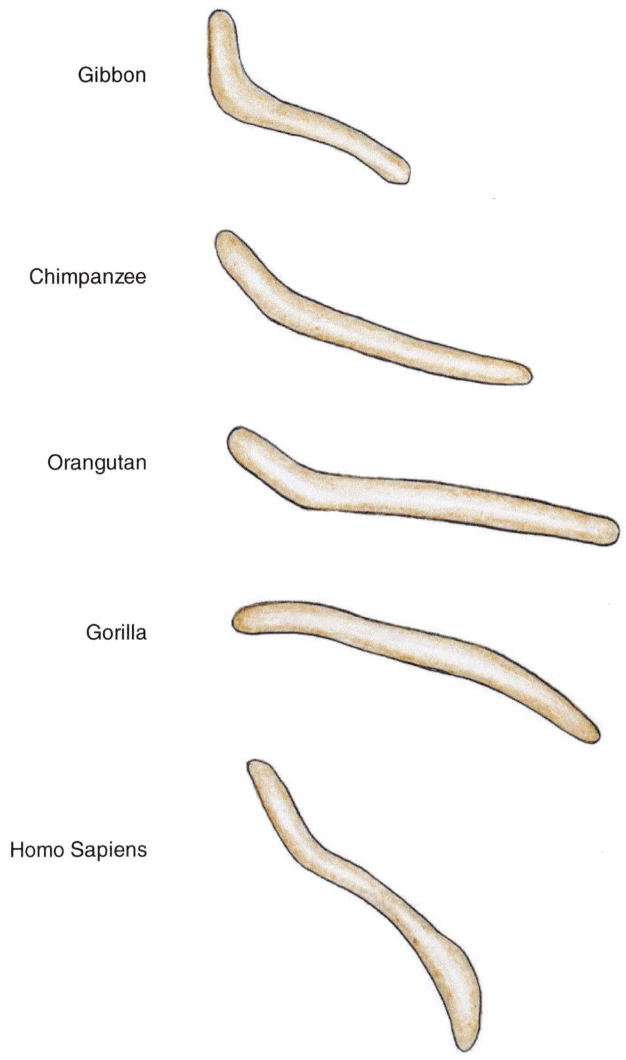

Fig. 11 Sagittalization of left iliac wings from gibbon to homo sapiens on superior view

cral mass, glutes, and hamstrings) but also, especially for the sacrum, by the tension of strong ligaments such as sacrospinal ligaments (Figs. 14, 15, and 16). Finally, to complete this work (Tardieu [17]), we are reminded of the study performed on the pelvic ring of Lucy, the Australopithecus africanus, three million years old: where the pelvis is tilted backwards, with a small pelvic incidence and shape and orientation of the intermediate iliac wings between chimpanzee and Homo sapiens (Fig. 17).

The recent works of Schlosser and Castelain [22] show a new ilioischial angle (Fig. 10), drawn between a line that connects the middle of the sacral endplate to the center of the acetabulum and a line passing through the middle of the ischium: this angle increases with the acquisition of bipedalism and also with growth; the thickness of the pelvis in its posterior part in addition to the iliopubic or " bow angle" of Tardieu [17] which evaluates the thickness of the pelvis in its anterior part and the pelvic incidence angle which evaluates the thickness of the pelvis in its middle part. The increase of the ilioischial angle is in the direction of an increase of the lever arm of the hamstrings, essential to maintain the extension of the standing femurs (Fig. 18).

Formation and Growth of the Sacrum

> In severe dysplastic spondylolisthesis of L5 there is a distortion between a strong pelvic angle of incidence (wide pelvis) and a weak sacrococcygeal angle (flat sacrum).

The sacrum comes from somites 31–44 starting from S2. It will evolve like superjacent vertebrae from a mesenchymal and then cartilaginous model and finally bone with primary ossification nuclei of the body anteriorly, laterally (costally) to give rise to the sacral ala and posteriorly, to the arch [23] (Fig. 19).

According to Dimeglio [24], 35–40 centers of ossification participate in the formation of the sacrum. The sacrum is in fact the fusion of five independent primitive vertebrae.

Each sacral vertebra, like the other vertebrae of the spine, has three centers of ossification: an anterior median and two lateral centers for the posterior arch. The ossification center in the vertebral body appears around the fourth month of the fetal life. The centers of ossification for the lateral arches appear towards the sixth month, which is much later than for the thoracolumbar vertebrae.

The first three sacral vertebrae are very characteristic. They cover the posterior part of the transverse processes, two centers of ossification that match rudimentary sacral ribs (hence "costal").

These five centers of ossification, called primary ossification centers, are supplemented by centers of secondary ossification.

One appears in the upper part of the vertebral body, another in the lower part, and a third in the spinous process.

The first two centers of secondary ossification appear at puberty, the third not until the age of 18!

The fusion of the different ossification processes is the same as for the other vertebrae. Two lateral centers merge posteriorly on the midline. Then, the costal centers unite with the lateral mass and finally merge with the vertebral body.

The merging of the various sacral elements does not occur at the same time:

- The posterior fusion is more precocious. It begins around the age of 3 for the first and second sacral vertebrae and at the age of 4 for the third vertebra.

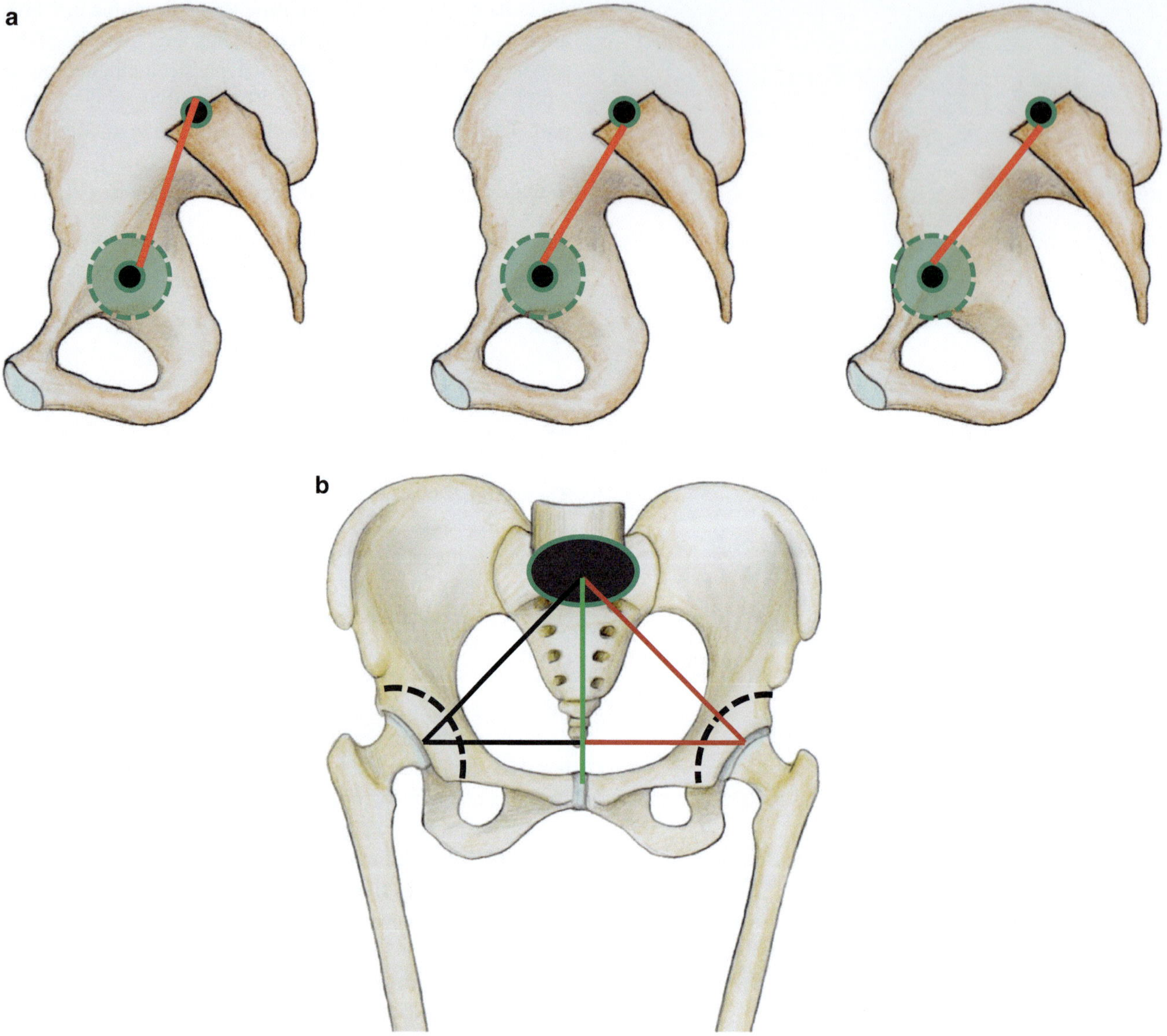

Fig. 12 Pelvic incidence increases with sacrocotyloid distance in lateral (**a**) and frontal (**b**) views (Tardieu [17] and Morvan [19])

- At the age of 7, the closing of the sacral arch is theoretically complete. However, there are dehiscences of these posterior arches that one need not necessarily consider as abnormal.
- At birth, the posterior arch is largely open, not ossified. The posterior wall of the sacrum is represented by a thin fibrous membrane.
- In contrast, fusion is progressive and ascending. It begins towards the fifth sacral vertebra and continues upward to the first sacral vertebra. The discs disappear from the bottom up and no longer exist in the third decade (Fig. 20).

Finally, the multiplicity of sacral cartilages explains that a serious pelvic trauma at a child's sacroiliac joints may be responsible for an epiphysiodesis that may lead to an asymmetric pelvis.

Thus, the fusion process is different anteriorly and posteriorly.

Very late, at the end of growth, secondary ossification centers appear. They complete lateral ossification of the sacrum of each sacral "rib."

The coccyx is made of four or five completely atrophied vertebrae. It has persistent disc structures between these remnants of vertebrae which remain mobile.

Marty [21] describes the evolution of the sacrococcygeal angle which increases with pelvic incidence (Fig. 21). During the phylogenetic evolution and postnatal growth, which we describe here, the coxal bone widens and in parallel, the sacrum is probably curved under the effect of

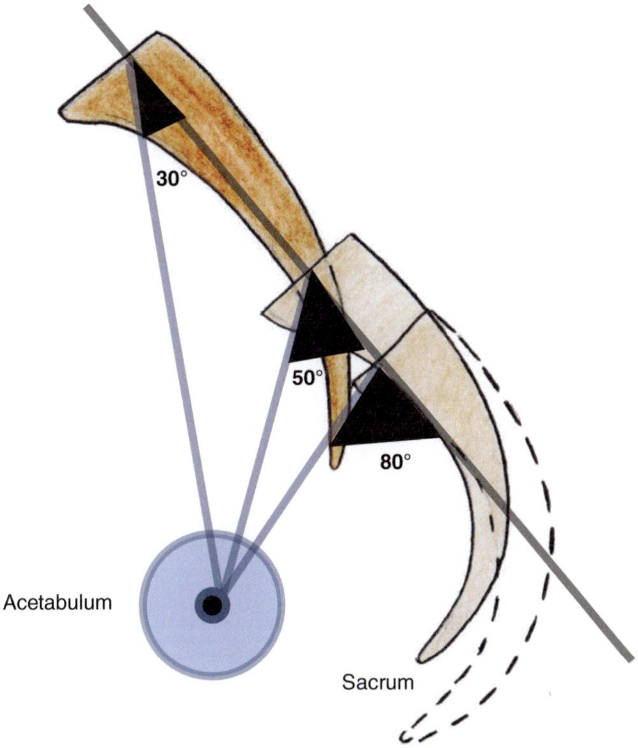

Fig. 13 Parallel evolution of the sacrococcygeal angle and the pelvic incidence (Tardieu [17])

harmonious constraints on this sacral model. On a series of 15 severe dysplastic spondylolisthesis (SPLD) we have noted a very elevated pelvic incidence (78° vs. 51.4°) and a weak sacrococcygeal angle (58° vs. 89°) for the high pelvic incidence (Table 1). It is as if there is an anomaly in the growth of the pelvis with a coxal bone too wide for a sacrum which is too flat with a small sacrococcygeal angle. This leads to a shift of the femoral heads anterior to L5 and therefore a forward trunk rocker with a risk of collapse and a decrease in the posterior lever of the extensors of the spine so that the hip which goes in the same direction of anterior imbalance (Fig. 22).

Formation and Growth of the Coxal Bone [24–26]

According to Dimeglio [24], the acetabulum, a three-dimensional structure, is at the center of gravity of the coxal bone.

This coxal bone is a field of energy modeled or punctuated by the growth cartilages of the sacrum, the acetabulum, the cartilages of the ischium, ischia, and pubic bone; the pressure of the two femoral heads in their reciprocal acetabulii contributes to the formation of the pelvis. Furthermore, the acetabulum is actually at the "junction"

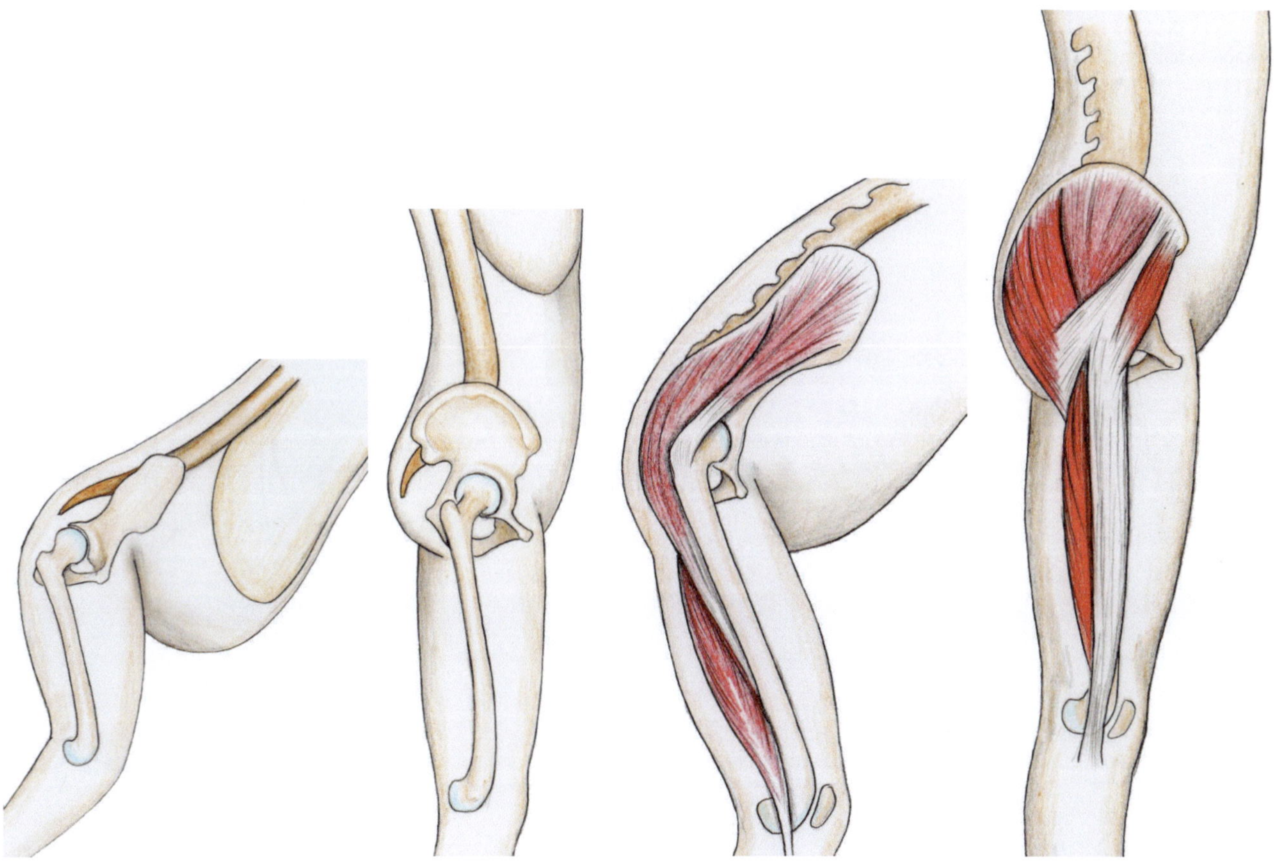

Fig. 14 Widening of the iliac wings in parallel with thickening of the gluteus maximus when comparing the chimpanzee to the human

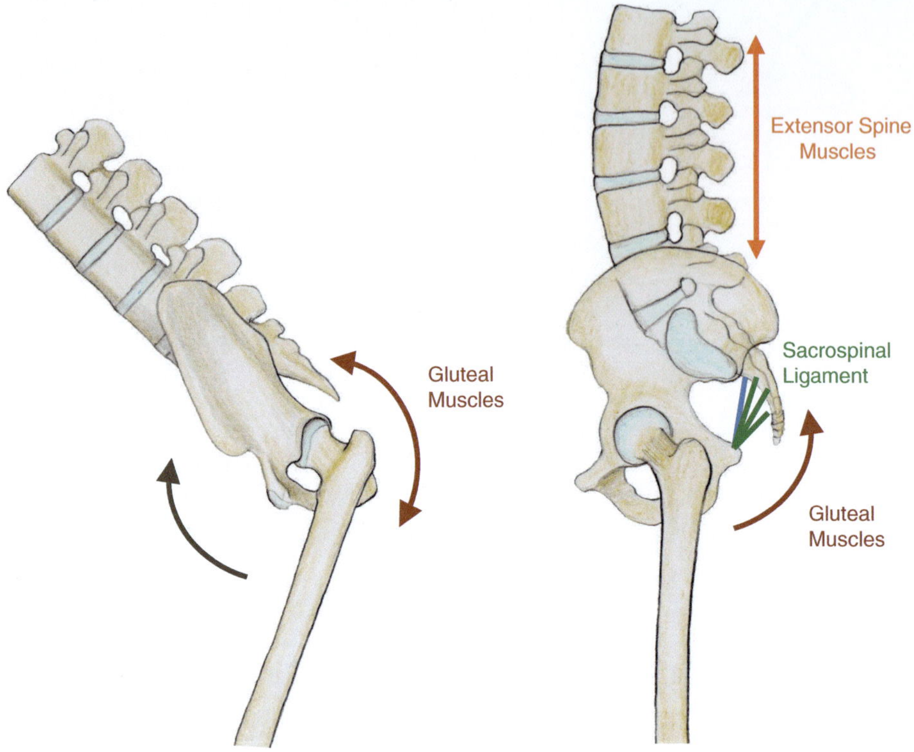

Fig. 15 Acquisition of lumbar lordosis, enlargement of the iliac wing and curvature of the sacrum

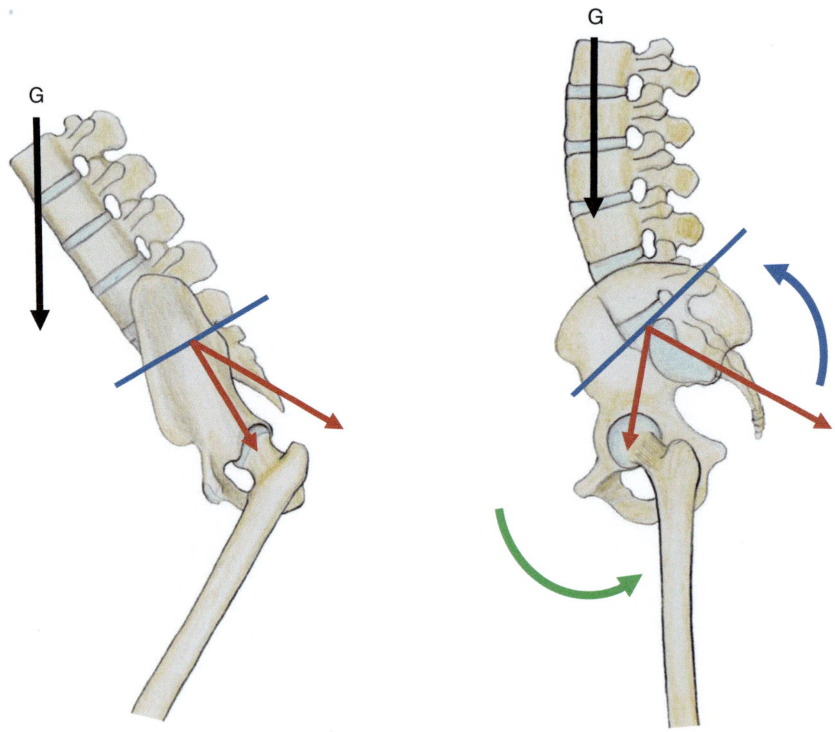

Fig. 16 Increased lumbar lordosis and femur extension parallel to the morphological changes of the hip bone and the sacrum as described in Fig. 14

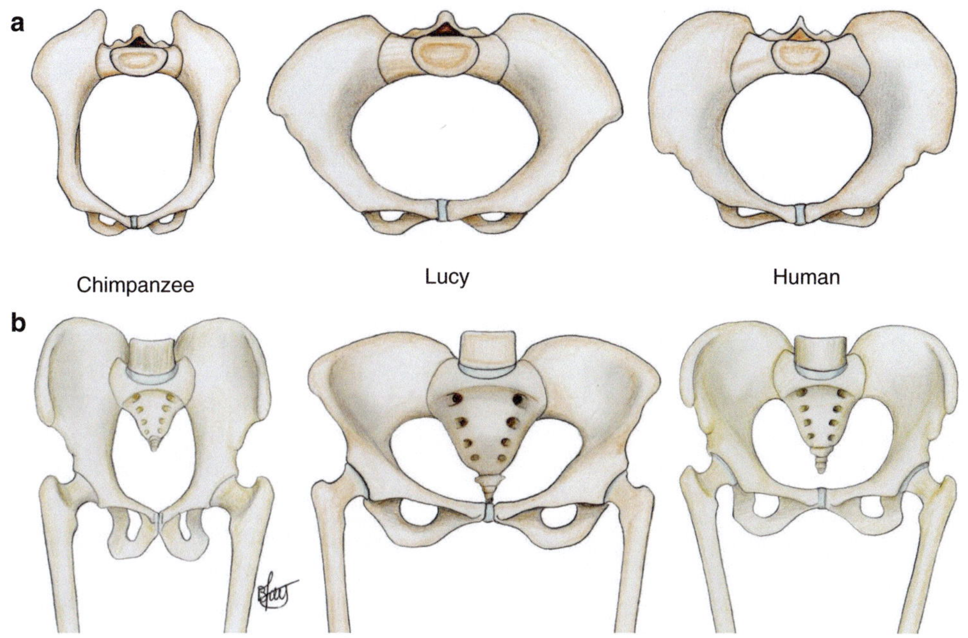

Fig. 17 Lucy's pelvic ring seen from above (**a**) and from the front (**b**) compared to those of the chimpanzee and the human

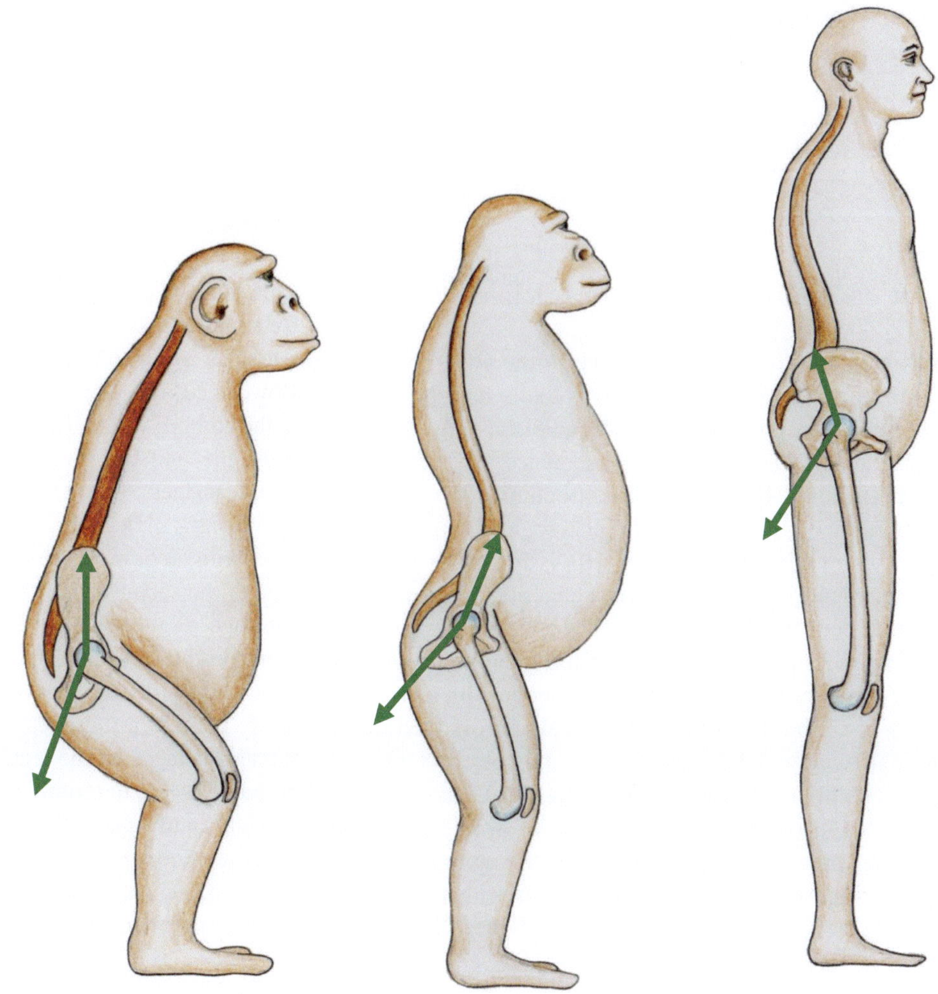

Fig. 18 Evolution of the ilioischial angle (Schlosser [22])

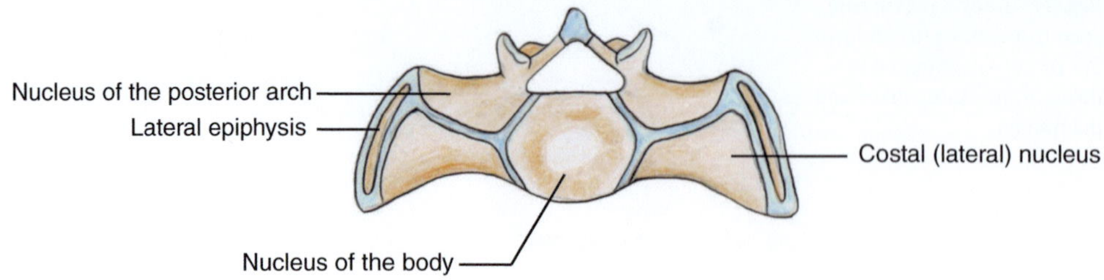

Fig. 19 Primary ossification nuclei of the sacrum on a superior view

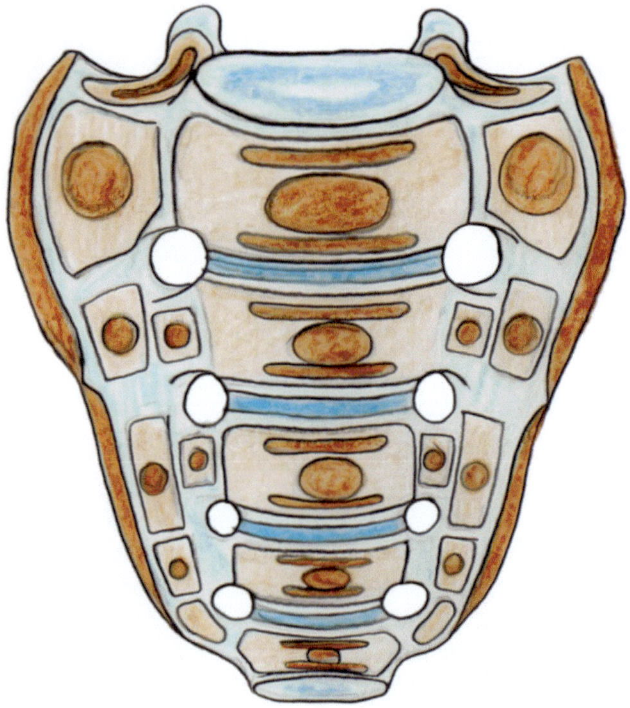

Fig. 20 Ossification of the sacrum (Dimeglio [24])

of three pieces of bone that belong to the pubis, ischium, and ilium; each bone piece behaves like a long bone with two epiphyses, one proximal and one distal (Fig. 23). The Y-cartilage is the point of convergence of these three pieces of bone. The histological structure is the same for all three pieces of bone but the histological configuration of the germ cells and column cells is higher in the iliac bone element; therefore, there is a quantitative growth differential between the three pieces of bone.

Delaere [26], on a prenatal histological study, recalls the enchondral ossification of the hip bone with a hip joint which is visible from the eighth week, an ossification of the iliac wing which begins at the ninth week and the acetabulum which is formed at 28 weeks. For Dimeglio [24], the cartilage replaces the mesenchyme from the second month of life in utero and this will extend up to the end of growth. Figure 24 shows the evolution of primary and secondary ossification nuclei of the coxal bone. The closure of the Y (triradiate) cartilage, the synchondrosis presenting histologically as bipolar cartilage is 1 year after the beginning of puberty. This closure is better detailed in the chapter on growth cartilages of the spine and pelvic vertebra.

The volumetric, three-dimensional growth of this coxal bone is considerable; the pelvic morphology changes from birth to the end of growth as it flares outwards, according to Dimeglio [24].

Mangione [27] studied the pelvic incidence in 30 fetuses, 30 neonates, and 30 adults: it shows that the pelvic incidence value increased up to the age of 10 (Fig. 25). Mac Thiong [28] noted this increase in the pelvic incidence from 4 to 18 years.

It should be noted, moreover, that Legaye [29] has demonstrated that the pelvic incidence could vary by increasing even after the end of growth and particularly after 60 years in healthy and painful backs, a phenomenon related to a laxity of the sacroiliac joint (Fig. 26).

Formation and Growth of the Sacroiliac Joint (SIJ)

This joint, synchondrosis or motionless cartilaginous joint for some, synovial-type diarthrosis for others, is rather classified as an amphiarthrosis, with weakly mobile joints. Bowen [30] notes on dissections of 40 SIJ of ages different to the embryo where the joint is flat, that the anterior capsule is fragile and the iliac surface is more serrated than the sacral surface. The SIJ deepens at around 17 years and shows signs of degeneration from 40 years. Kampen [31] on 25 SIJ dissections of ages 1–93 years shows that the cartilage of the sacral surface is more hyaline and thick than the cartilage of the iliac surface. The fibrous degeneration is more on the iliac side that best protects the sacral surface from shear stresses. Vleeming [32] notes that at 8 weeks in utero, there is a mesenchymal zone between the iliac and sacral cartilages; at the tenth week, a central cavity appears, probably due to micromovements. A ridge separates the cranial and caudal parts. Even before birth, Vleeming [32] also notes a smooth sacral surface, covered with hyaline cartilage and 2–3 times thicker than the irregular iliac surface and covered with fibrocartilage.

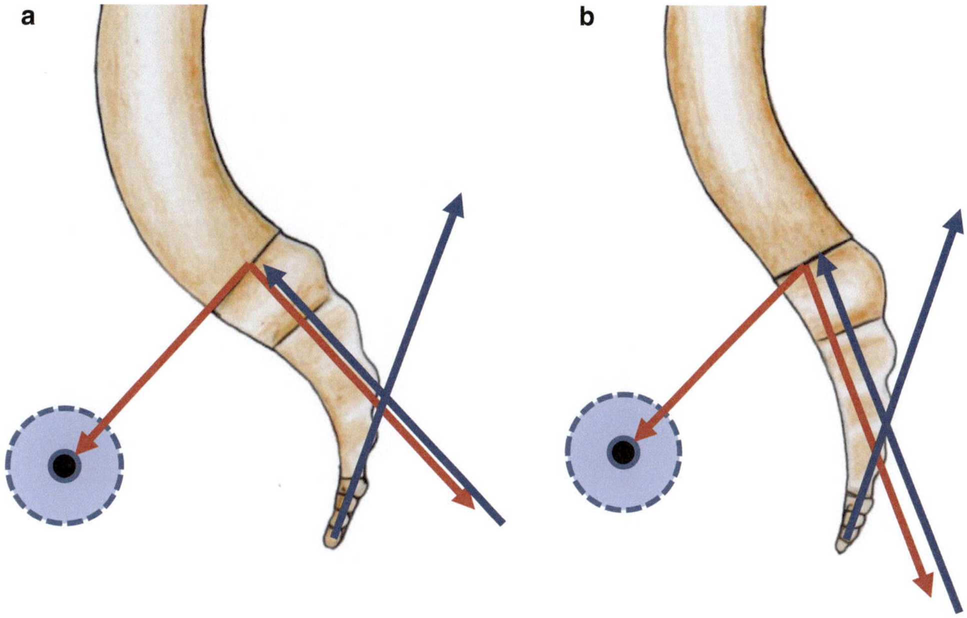

Fig. 21 Pelvic incidence (red) and sacrococcygeal (blue) angles in a subject with high pelvic incidence in (**a**) and low pelvic incidence in (**b**)

Table 1 Values of the abnormal sacrococcygeal angle with respect to the pelvic incidence in dysplastic spondylolisthesis

	Average	Minimum	Maximum	Dysplastic SPL (15 cases)
Pelvic incidence	**51.4°**	33.4°	77.7°	**78°**
Sacrococcygeal angle	**74.3°**	47.7°	88.9°	**58°**

Bold values are the more interesting values

How Is the Acetabulum Oriented According to the Pelvic Position?

Lazennec [33] described an angle called "anatomical anteversion" defining the orientation of the acetabulum in the axial plane and formed by the line joining the anterior and posterior edges of the acetabulum and the anteroposterior line drawn from the posterior edge of the acetabulum (Fig. 27). This angle increases when anteversion of the acetabulum increases and decreases as anteversion decreases. Thanks to the comparison of seated radiographs (retroversion of the pelvis) and standing (anteversion of the pelvis) and to a 3D study, Lazennec [33] reported the version of the acetabulum with the version of the pelvis (pelvic tilt): in pelvic retroversion, the acetabulum is more anterior (anteverted), whereas in anteversion, the acetabulum is more posterior (retroverted) (Fig. 27). Orthopedic surgeons inserting hip implants must therefore appreciate the preferential orientation of the pelvis in ante- or retroversion.

In conclusion, this chapter, which is based on phylogenetic and ontogenetic data, makes it possible to recall that only the occipital condyles and the sacrum are actually part of the spine. The terms cranial and pelvic vertebrae have become a clinical connotation as developed by Jean Dubousset.

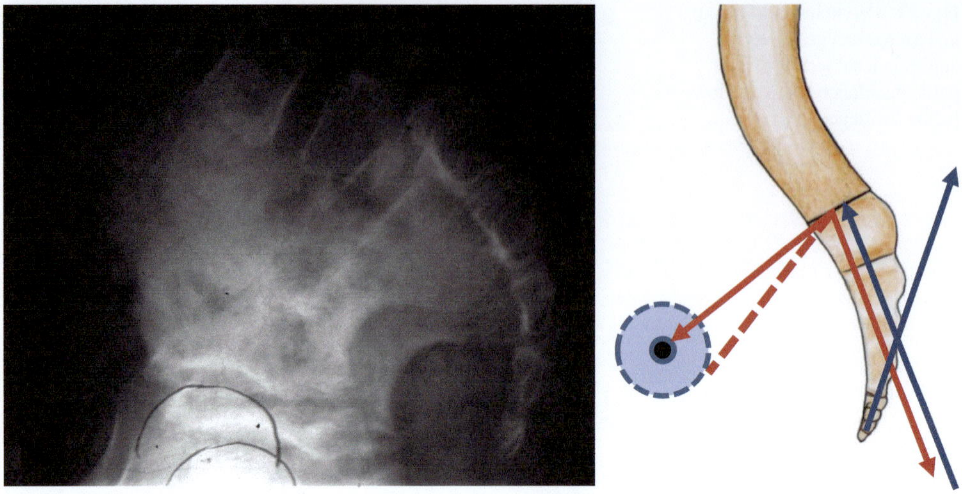

Fig. 22 Low sacrococcygeal angle (blue) for high pelvic incidence (red) on a severe dysplastic SPL

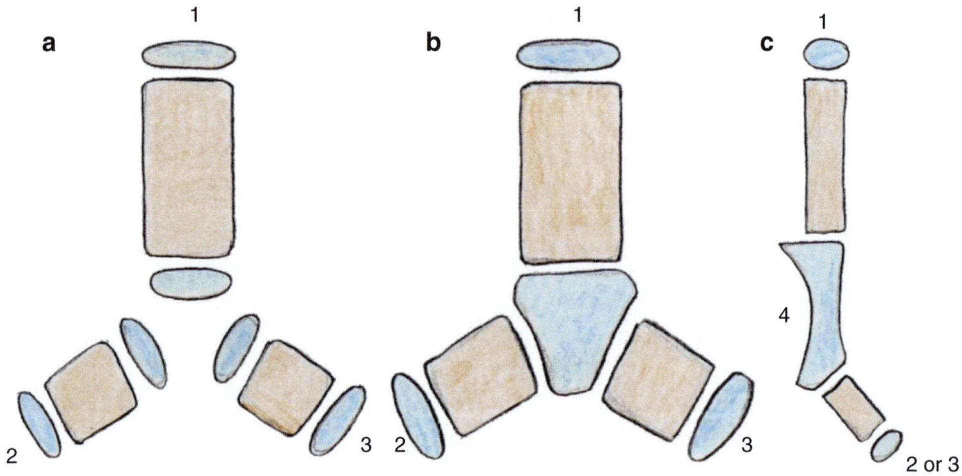

Fig. 23 Ilium (1), ischium (2), and pubis (3) are like long bones with diaphyses and epiphyses which join at 4 (Y cartilage); (**a**) initial frontal view, (**b**) frontal view at a more advanced stage, (**c**) coronal section (Dimeglio [24])

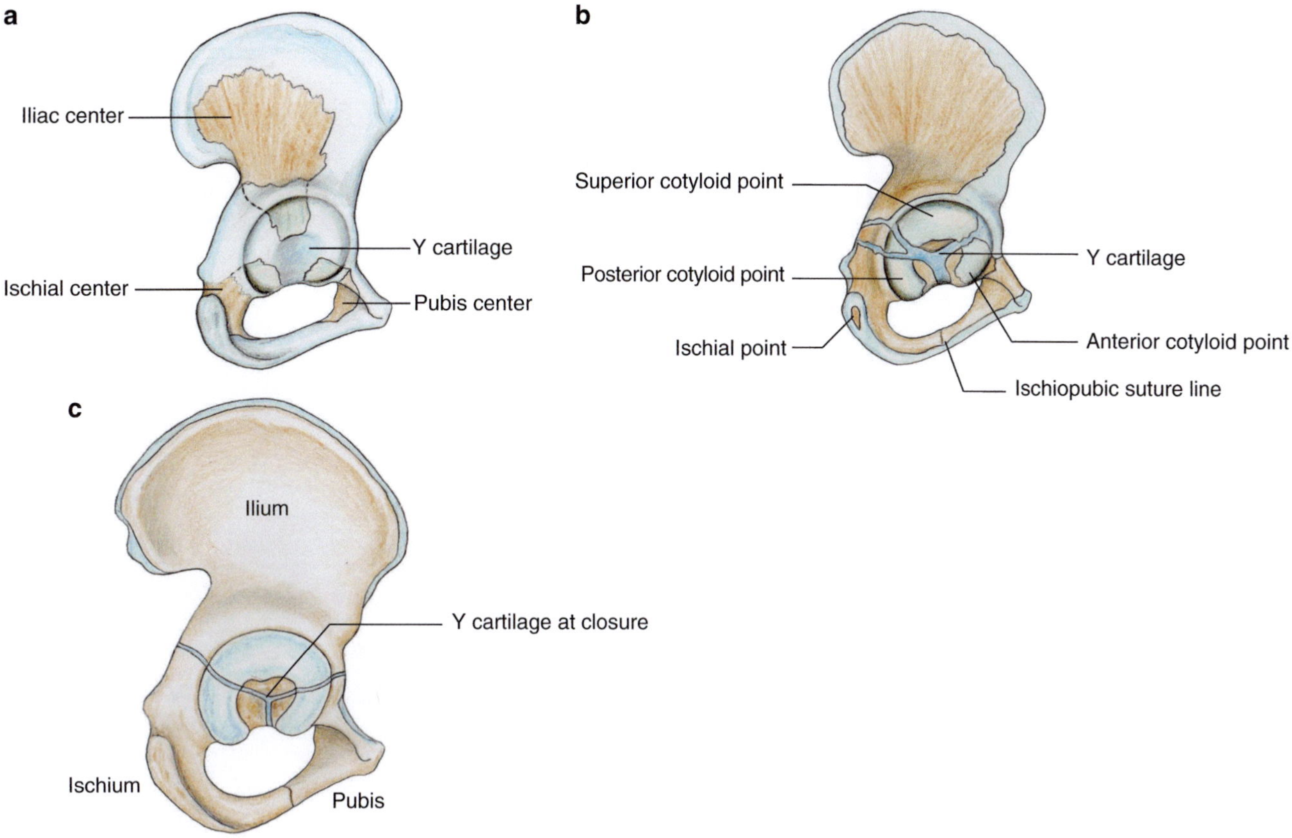

Fig. 24 Ossification of the coxal bone (Dimeglio [24]). (**a**) at birth. (**b**) 10 years. (**c**) at 12 years

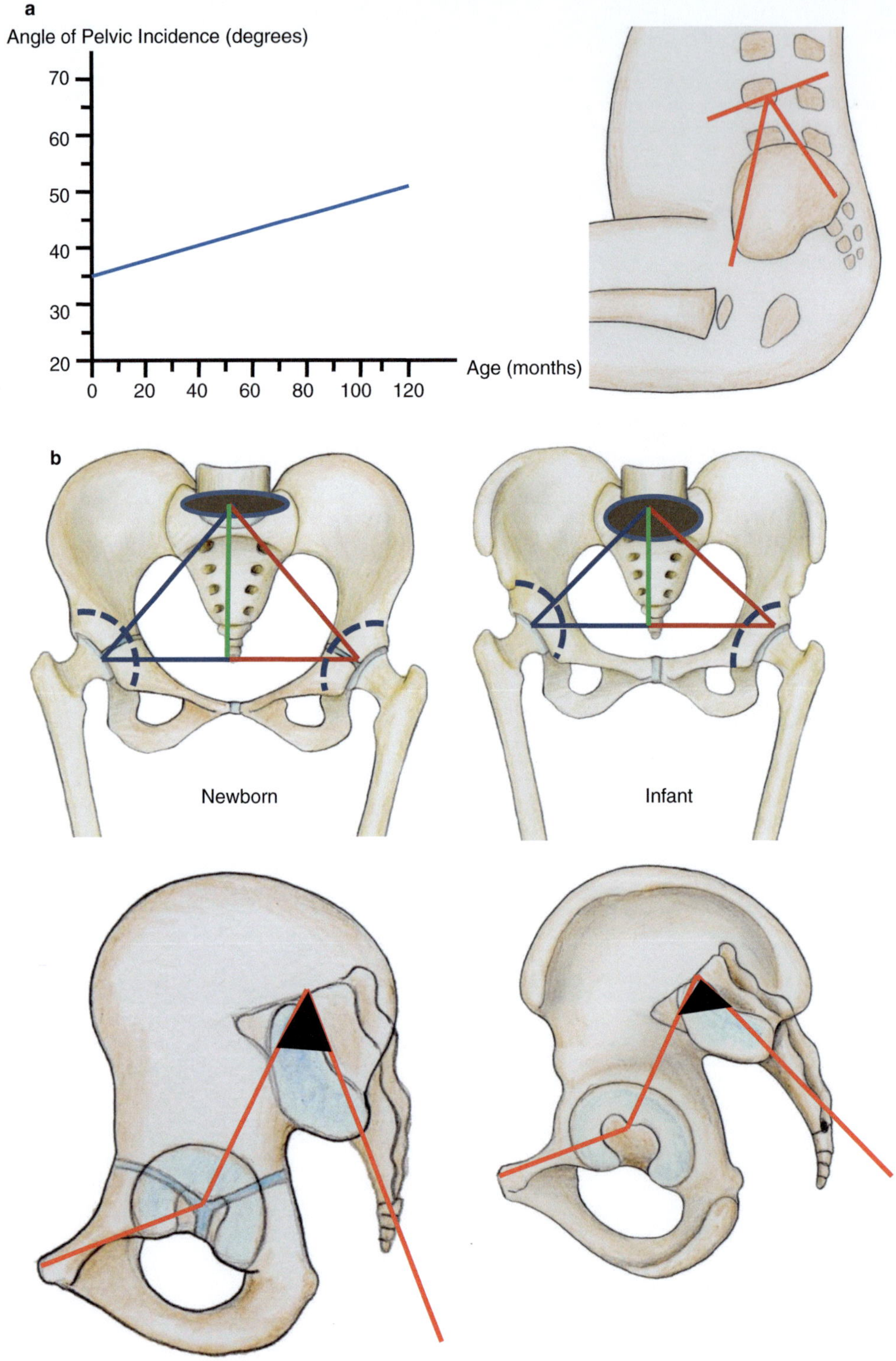

Fig. 25 (**a**) Evolution of pelvic incidence as a function of age (Mangione [26]). (**b**) Evolution of the pelvis in frontal view and in profile in a newborn and in an infant (Tardieu [17])

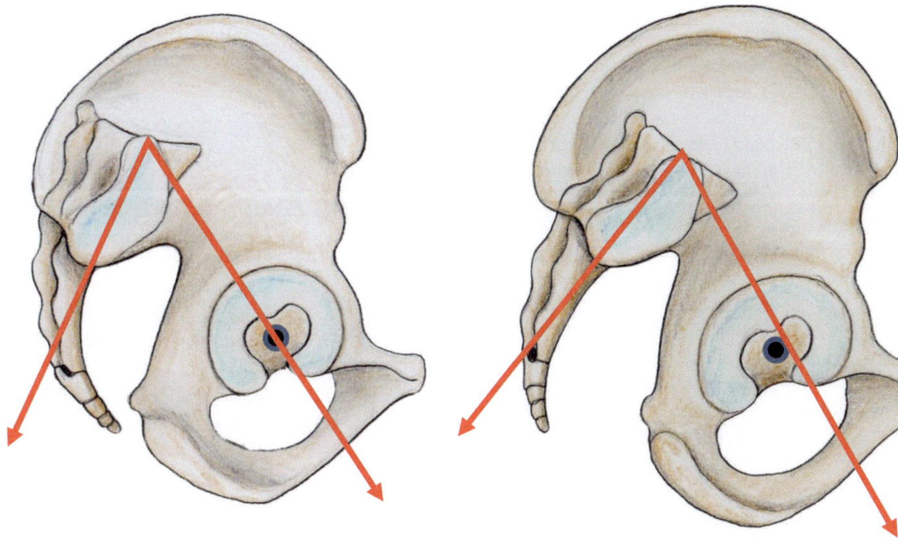

Fig. 26 Increased pelvic incidence by mobility of the sacroiliac joint (Legaye [28])

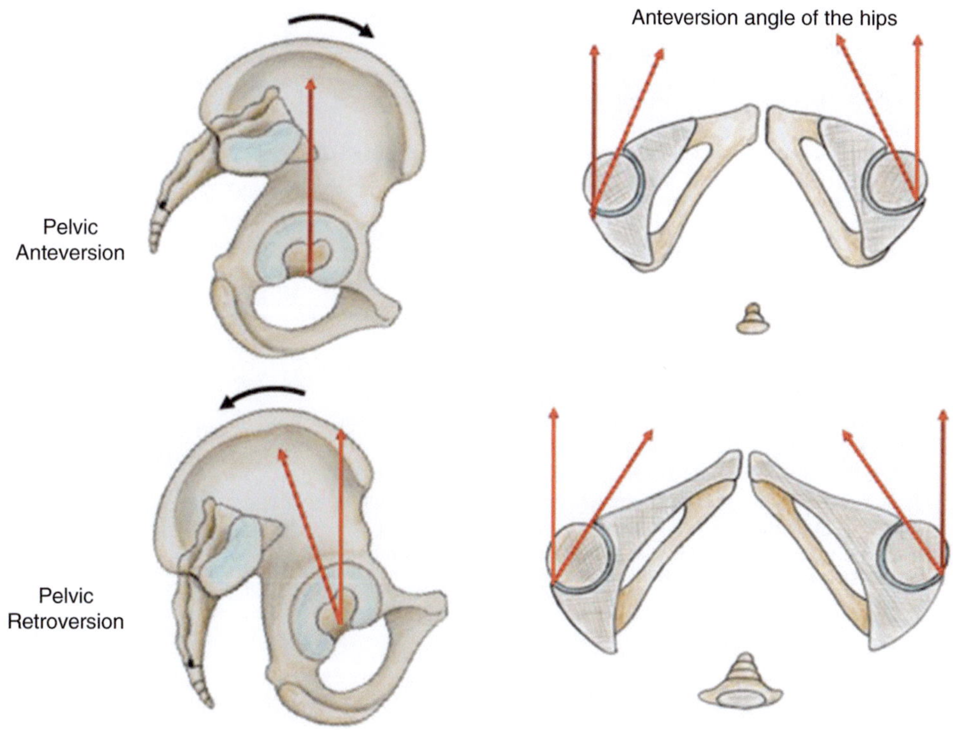

Fig. 27 In retroversion, there is an increase in the inclination and anteversion of the acetabulum and vice versa (Lazennec [33])

References

1. Sutherland WG. The craniofacial bowl. Mankato: Free Press; 1939.
2. Deshayes MJ. Croissance craniofaciale et orthodontie. Paris: Masson; 1996.
3. Aknin JJ. La croissance craniofaciale. Paris: Édition SID; 2007.
4. Wolling DG. The Os odontoideum, Separate odontoid process. J Bone Joint Surg Am. 1963;45(A):1459–71.
5. Muhleman M, Charran O, Matusz P, Shoja MM, Tubbs RS, Loukas M. The proatlas: a comprehensive review with clinical implications. Childs Nerv Syst. 2012;28:349–56.
6. Bernard S, Loukas M, Rizk E, Oskouian RJ, De-Lashaw J, Tubbs RS. The human occipital bone: review and update on its embryology and molecular development. Childs Nerv Syst. 2015;31:2217–23.
7. Mugnier A. Embryologie et développement bucco-facial (introduction à la stomatologie infantile). Paris: Masson; 1964.
8. Couly G, Coltey P, Le Douarin N. The triple origin of skull in higher vertebrates: a study in quail-chick chimeras. Development. 1993;117:409–29.
9. Couly G. Développement céphalique: embryologie, croissance, pathologie. Paris: CDP Édition; 1991.
10. Stricker M, Raphael B. Croissance cranio-faciale normale et pathologique. Reims: Éditions Morphos-France; 1993.
11. Petrovic A. Analyse biologique des processus de croissance postnatale de la mandibule et du maxillaire. In: Château M, editor. Orthopédie detto-faciale. Bases fondamentales. Paris: CDP Édition; 1993. p. 43–84.
12. Scott JH. Dentofacial development and growth. Oxford: Pergamon Press; 1967.
13. Melsen B. Time and mode of closure of the spheno-occipital synchrondosis determined of human autopsy material. Acta Anat. 1972;83:112–8.
14. Boileau MJ. Orthodontie du jeune enfant et du jeune adulte. Principes et moyens thérapeuthiques. Paris: Éditions Elsevier Masson; 2011.
15. Delaire J. Comment le septum influence-t-il la croissance prémaxillaire et maxillaire ? Rev Stomatol. 1977;78:214–54.
16. Vital JM, Sénégas J. Anatomical bases of the study of the constraints to which the cervical spine is subject in the sagittal plane. A study of the center of gravity of the head. Surg Radiol Anat. 1986;8:169–73.
17. Tardieu C, Bonneau N, Hecquet J, Boulay C, Marty C, Legaye J, Duval-Beaupere G. How is sagittal balanced acquired during bipedal gait acquisition? Comparison of neonatal and adult pelvises in three dimensions. Evolutionary implications. J Hum Evol. 2013;65:209–22.
18. Legaye J, Duval-Beaupere G, Hecquet J, et al. Pelvic incidence: a fundamental pelvic parameter of three-dimensional regulation of spinal sagittal curves. Eur Spine J. 1998;7:99–103.
19. Morvan G, Wybier M, Mathieu P, Vuillemin GH. Clichés simples du rachis: statique et relations entre rachis et bassin. J Radiol. 2008;89:654–66.
20. Abitbol MM. Evolution of the lumbosacral angle. Am J Phys Anthropol. 1987;72:361–72.
21. Marty C, Boisaubert B, Descamps H, Jp M-G, Hecquet J, Legaye J, Duval-Beaupere G. The sagittal anatomy of the sacrum among young adults, infants and spondylolisthesis patients. Eur Spine J. 2002;11:119–25.
22. Schlosser TPC, Janssen MMA, Vrtovec T, Per-Nus F, Oner FC, Viergever MA, Vincken KL, Caste-Lein RM. Evolution of the ischio-iliac lordosis during natural growth and its relation with the pelvic incidence. Eur Spine J. 2014;23:1433–41.
23. Cheng JS, Song JK. Anatomy of the sacrum. Neurosurg Focus. 2003;15(2):1–3.
24. Dimeglio A, Kaelin A, Bonnel F, De Rosa V, Cou-Ture A. The growing hip: specifications and requirements. J Pediatr Orthop. 1992;3:135–47.
25. Ponsetti IV. Growth and development of the acetabulum in the normal child. J Bone Joint Surg. 1978;60(5):575–85.
26. Delaere O, Dhem A. Prenatal development of the human pelvis and acetabulum. Acta Orthop Belg. 1999;65:255–9.
27. Mangione P, Gomez D, Senegas J. Study of the course of the incidence angle during growth. Eur Spine J. 1997;6:163–7.
28. Mac-Thiong JM, Berthonnaud E, Dimar JR, Betz RR, Labelle H. Sagittal alignment of the spine and pelvis during growth. Spine. 2004;29:1642–7.
29. Legaye J. Influence of age and sagittal balance of the spine on the value of the pelvic incidence. Eur Spine J. 2014;23:1394–9.
30. Bowen V, Cassidy JD. Macroscopic and microscopic anatomy of the sacroiliac joint from embryonic life until the eighth decade. Spine. 1981;6:620–8.
31. Kampen WU, Tillmann B. Age-related changes in the articular cartilage of human sacroiliac joint. Anat Embryol (Berl). 1998;198:505–13.
32. Vleeming A, Schuenke MD, Masi AT, Carreiro JE, Danneels L, Willard FH. The sacroiliac-joint: an overview of its anatomy, function and potential clinical implications. J Anat. 2012;221:537–67.
33. Lazennec JY, Charlot N, Gorin M, Roger B, Arafati N, Bissery A, Saillant G. Hip-spine relationship: a radio-anatomical study for optimization in acetabular cup positioning. Surg Radiol Anat. 2004;26:136–44.

The Intervertebral Disc

B. Lavignolle

General Characters

Biomechanical Specifications

In fish and marine mammals, intervertebral joints have a shape close to the ellipsoid with a concave portion and a convex portion and movements in all three planes to provide propulsion.

In humans, primates, and most mammals, there is a strong but deformable layer of soft tissue between the vertebral bodies in the form of an intervertebral fibrocartilaginous disc. Mechanically, the disc must be strong enough to support the load, deformable to accommodate the movements of the vertebra without compromising its strength and rigid enough not to be injured during movement and effort.

Anatomical Structure [1–3]

The intervertebral disc (IVD) has a biconvex shape separated from the vertebral bodies by the hyaline cartilage of the vertebral end-plates and the fibrocartilage disc. Classically, the disc has a central gelatinous core or nucleus pulposus and a peripheral fibrous ring, made of dense collagen or annulus fibrosus. The vertebral end-plate separates the disc from the adjacent vertebral bodies and is considered a component of the intervertebral disc (Figs. 1, 2).

The *nucleus pulposus* (NP) of young adults is a semiliquid mass of mucoid material with the consistency of toothpaste. NP is a remnant of the notochord and cartilage cells with a few irregular collagen fibres disseminated in a semiliquid medium. The fluidic nature of NP allows it to deform under pressure but its volume cannot be compressed, similar to a

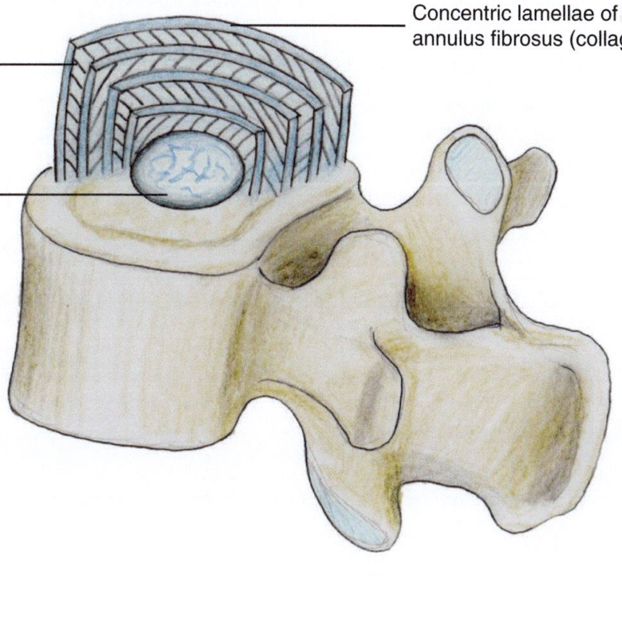

Fig. 1 Concentric lamellae of collagen surrounding the nucleus with fibres running at 65° to the horizontal

B. Lavignolle (✉)
Anatomy Laboratory, Bordeaux University Hospital,
Bordeaux, France

J. M. Vital, D. T. Cawley (eds.), *Spinal Anatomy*, https://doi.org/10.1007/978-3-030-20925-4_14

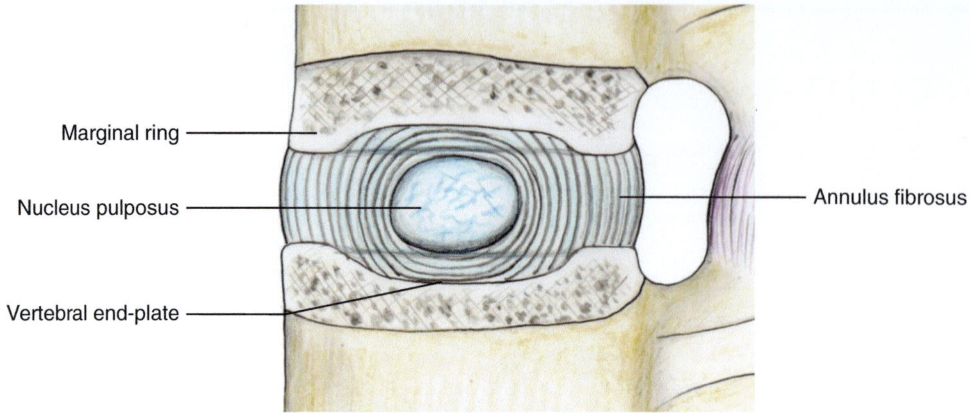

Fig. 2 Structure of the disc and the vertebral end-plate

balloon filled with water. Subject to multidirectional pressures, the NP deforms and stretches the collagen walls of the IVD. In fact, histological studies show that the nucleus is almost indistinguishable from the annulus in a young IVD (Fig. 3). Subsequently, after bone maturation in the spine, the articular cleft is an acquired fissure.

AF is composed of collagen fibres arranged in 10–20 lamellae (Latin lamella: small leaf) [2], organized in concentric rings surrounding the NP. The lamellae are thicker on the ventral and lateral slopes of the annulus and thinner on the dorsal side. The orientation of the fibres is constant—at 65° to the vertical with an alternating direction for each lamella [3–6].

The end-plates (EP) are formed of a layer of cartilage 0.6–1 mm thick. The two EPs of each disc cover each vertebra, except at the periphery of the disc at the level of the marginal or peripheral bone ridge in the adult. Hyaline cartilage is present in newborns and children. In adults, the EPs are fibrocartilaginous and formed by the insertion of AF collagen fibres into bone.

The collagen fibres of the lamellae penetrate the EP and turn parallel to the EP. The NP is thus surrounded by a spherical "capsule" of collagen; EPs are attached to the disc via the AF [4]. EPs are poorly attached to the vertebral bodies [5, 6] and can become detached in certain traumas in the growing child (scallop type detachment and rupture of the EP limbus) and in growth dystrophies at the marginal non-ossified apophyseal ring (see chapter "The Cranial and Pelvic "Vertebrae" Are They Real Vertebrae?").

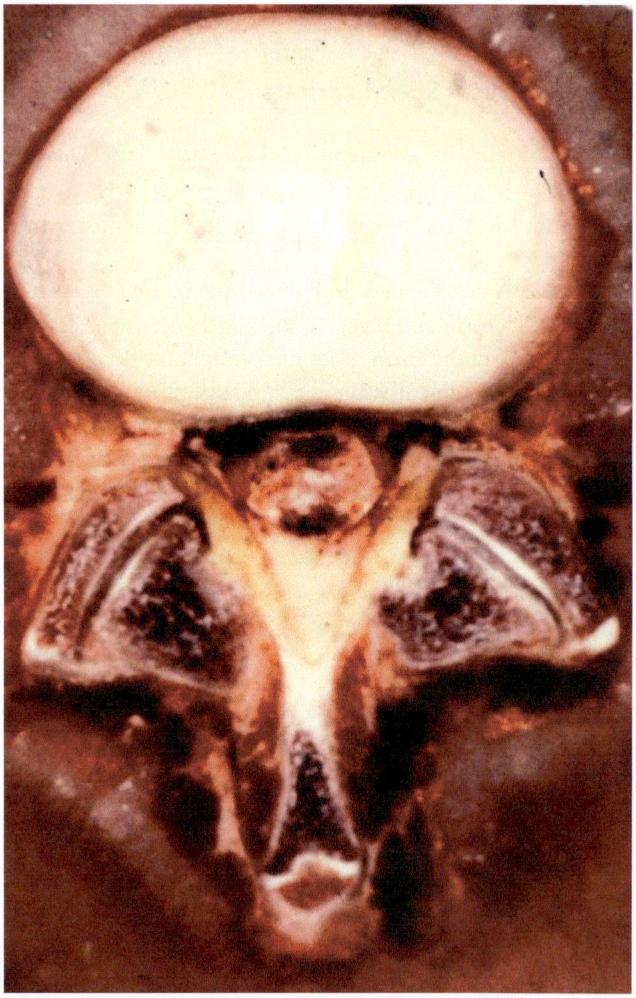

Fig. 3 Microtome section of a lumbar disc of a young subject; it is difficult to macroscopically distinguish nucleus and annulus

IVD Ultrastructure (Fig. 4)

The IVD is composed of glycosaminoglycans, collagen, and water.

Glycosaminoglycans (GAG) [7–13]

They are present in the skin, bone, cartilage, tendons, synovial fluid, the aqueous humour of the eye, and especially at the level of NP in the IVD. They form chains of polysaccharides composed of 20 repeating units (disaccharides hexoses) of sugar–amine–sugar.

In the disc, the dominant GAG are chondroitin sulphate (CS), keratan sulphate (KS), and hyaluronic acid.

Proteoglycans (PG) are 20–100 chains composed of GAG bound to hyaluronic acid by binding proteins. The hydrophilic

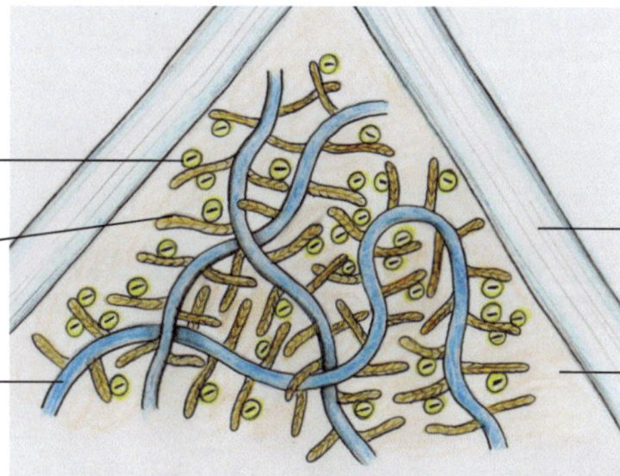

Fig. 4 Schematic view of the structure of the interstitial space of the disc

capacity of PGs depends on the size and spiral shape to form 3D molecules akin to the entanglement of cotton with similar absorbent properties as a cotton ball. The hydrophilic strength of the PGs, however, depends on the sulphate and carboxylate radicals. CS has both sulphate and carboxylate radicals while KS has only sulphate. These GAG have fixed negative charges [9] that attract positive sodium and calcium ions. The sodium concentration in the disc is higher than in the plasma and adjacent tissues, the excess of ions is responsible for the significant osmotic pressure in the IVD matrix and its ability to withstand high loads. The hydrophilic capacity of a PG is proportional to the structural density of the ionic radicals.

The swelling pressure of the disc is equal to the osmotic pressure of the PGs minus the tensile force in the collagen fibres which is, in general, very low.

Collagen [14–16]

The basic unit of collagen is the tropocollagen molecule (15 Angstroms) consisting of three polypeptide chains helically wound and linked by hydrogen bridges. The joining of several chains of tropocollagen results in a large fibril (0.04 μ). The collagen fibre (0.1–0.5 μ) is formed by the association of several large tropocollagen fibrils. There are 11 types of collagen determined by the chemical nature of the polypeptide chains:

- Type 1 of elastic nature is found in tissues subject to tension and compression (skin, bone, tendon, meniscus) and type 2 more elastic is found in tissues exposed to pressure (articular cartilage). These two types are present in the IVD. Type 1 is the predominant form in AF and Type 2 is dominant in NP.
- Type 3 (dermal vessels, synovium) is in the NP and in trace elements in the AF.
- Type 9 (cartilage) is found with type 2 (2% collagen type 2 concentration) in NP.
- Type 6 (vessels, viscera, muscles) and type 10 (growth cartilage) are present in the IVD in very small amounts.

The chemical structure of the vertebral end-plate corresponds to that of the disc with PGs and collagen fibres with cartilage cells aligned along the collagen fibres.

Water and Chemical Composition of Human Discs [8]

The water and the chemical composition of the human disc represent 70–90% of the NP. PG represents 65% of the dry weight of the NP with only 25% of the PGs linked to the hyaluronic acid. The PGs of the NP are smaller than those of articular cartilage with 8–18 units of PG on a small chain of hyaluronic acid.

Water forms a gel with PGs. The concentration of PG is four times greater in the central part of the disc than in its periphery with twice the amount of hydration.

Collagen represents 15–20% of the NP, disseminates in the PG medium, and serves as a support for the PGs. Water represents 60–70% of the AF and collagen 50–60% of the dry weight of AF, a quantity twice as large at the peripheral level (Table 1) (at the end of the text). Between the collagen fibres, the spaces are filled by PGs forming a fine network between which very fine pores of 30–100 angstroms persist. The disc loses fluid under pressure only very slowly.

The chondrocytes are located in the NP near the vertebral end-plates and provide PG synthesis and collagen type 2 for the NP.

Proteolytic Enzymes [17]

Proteolytic enzymes are the matrix metalloproteinases (MMP) with collagenase (MMP 1), gelatinase (MMP 2), and stromelysin (MMP 3).

Collagenase can cleave collagen type 2, and stromelysin is the most destructive for collagen type 2 and PG.

Under normal conditions, enzymes allow the addition of new components.

Table 1 Chemical composition of the various components of the intervertebral disc (Maroudas [8])

Parameter	External annulus	Internal annulus	Nucleus
Hydration (mg H_2O) mg of dry weight	1–2	2–3	3–4
Concentration of GAG (CS & KS) mg of dry weight	5–7	10–15	22–30
Collagen (% of dry weight)	50	25–30	15–25
Ratio KS/CS	0.2–0.3	1.0	1–2

By removing the worn components of the disc matrix, the chondrocytes synthesize collagen and PGs forming the matrix and retain water. Enzymes are controlled by activators such as plasmin and inhibitors such as tissue inhibitors of MMPs. The state of the matrix is based on a delicate balance between synthesis and destruction activities.

The swelling pressure of the disc decreases with the level of PG. Water content decreases with age and degeneration. The hydration of the aged discs decreases as the discs are subjected to physiological pressures of 6–10 atmospheres in an active subject. Discs lose water when exposed to higher loads. The liquid flow is made more rapidly when the pores are larger and as the swelling pressure is lower. An aged or degenerate disc dehydrates faster during a day of work than that a young disc.

The cells in the centre of the disc are remote from blood vessels, thus do not receive significant glucose or other nutrients. The lactic acid concentration is ten times higher than plasma. The pH, decreasing to 6, can promote the action of proteolytic enzymes with progressive degradation of the disc matrix and in particular the PGs responsible for the hydrophilic power.

The equilibrium hydration under a load of 78 atmospheres (0.7–0.8 NM/m^2) is 1.5–2.2 g of water/g of dry weight for an aged or degenerate disc as opposed to 3 g of water/g of dry weight for a young disc (Maroudas [8], Urban [9, 10]). A less hydrated and thinned disc is less able to perform its mechanical functions. The functional deterioration of IVD leads to an overload of other structures such as the facet joints whose degeneration follows that of IVD.

Vascularization and Innervation of the Disc

Classically, the IVD is non-vascularized and non-innervated. In fact, the periphery of the disc is a real “living area”.

During growth, the epiphyseal vessels at the marginal apophysis provide some peripheral vascularization of the disc.

In degenerate discs, neoangiogenesis allows penetration of the disc with an inflammatory membrane and disc cavitation clearly visible on endoscopy. According to Bogduk [5], the sinuvertebral nerve resulting from an anastomosis of a branch of the anterior branch of the spinal nerve and grey communicating branch of the paravertebral sympathetic lymph node chain gives a direct branch or Roofe nerve which is distributed to the dura mater, dorsal longitudinal ligament, and commonly at the annulus.

The outer 1/3 of the periphery of the disc thus has a radicular and sympathetic segmental innervation. Disc cracking is the trigger for neovascularization and neoinnervation of the disc. It is the characteristic of intradiscal rupture, which is an acquired traumatic condition rather than linked to degeneration.

The nerves seem to accompany the vessels that grow in the cracks.

These discs are symptomatic and painful enough on discography–manometry which gave rise to coblation with thermomodulation radiofrequency of the fissure zone.

Role of the Disc

The IVD is hydrophilic and a hydraulic damper.

Under pressure during the day, the water leaves the disc for the vertebra through the vertebral end-plate and the subject can lose up to 2 cm in height during the day (the height of the discs represents a quarter of the spine height).

With age, the hydrophilicity decreases; after 65 years, the disc contains only 65% of water versus 90% in children. The size of the subject is reduced by up to 5 cm.

Osteoporosis bone compression is associated with disc compression.

The NP and AF are involved in the load with transmission of load from one vertebra to another.

The mechanism of load transfers in the disc is as follows:

- The compression increases the pressure in the NP which is exerted radially on the AF and increases the tension of the AF. The disc is a model of tensegrity (tensile integrity) where there is a balance of compressive and tensile stresses (Fig. 5).
- The tension in the AF is applied to the NP, preventing it from widening radially, hence the importance of the AF tension forces. The NP pressure is then exerted on the vertebral end-plate.

This prestressed system represents a structure that deforms and returns to the initial state once the external constraint has been removed.

The load is supported by AF and NP. The radial pressure in the NP puts the AF under tension and the pressure in the EP transmits the load from one vertebra to the other.

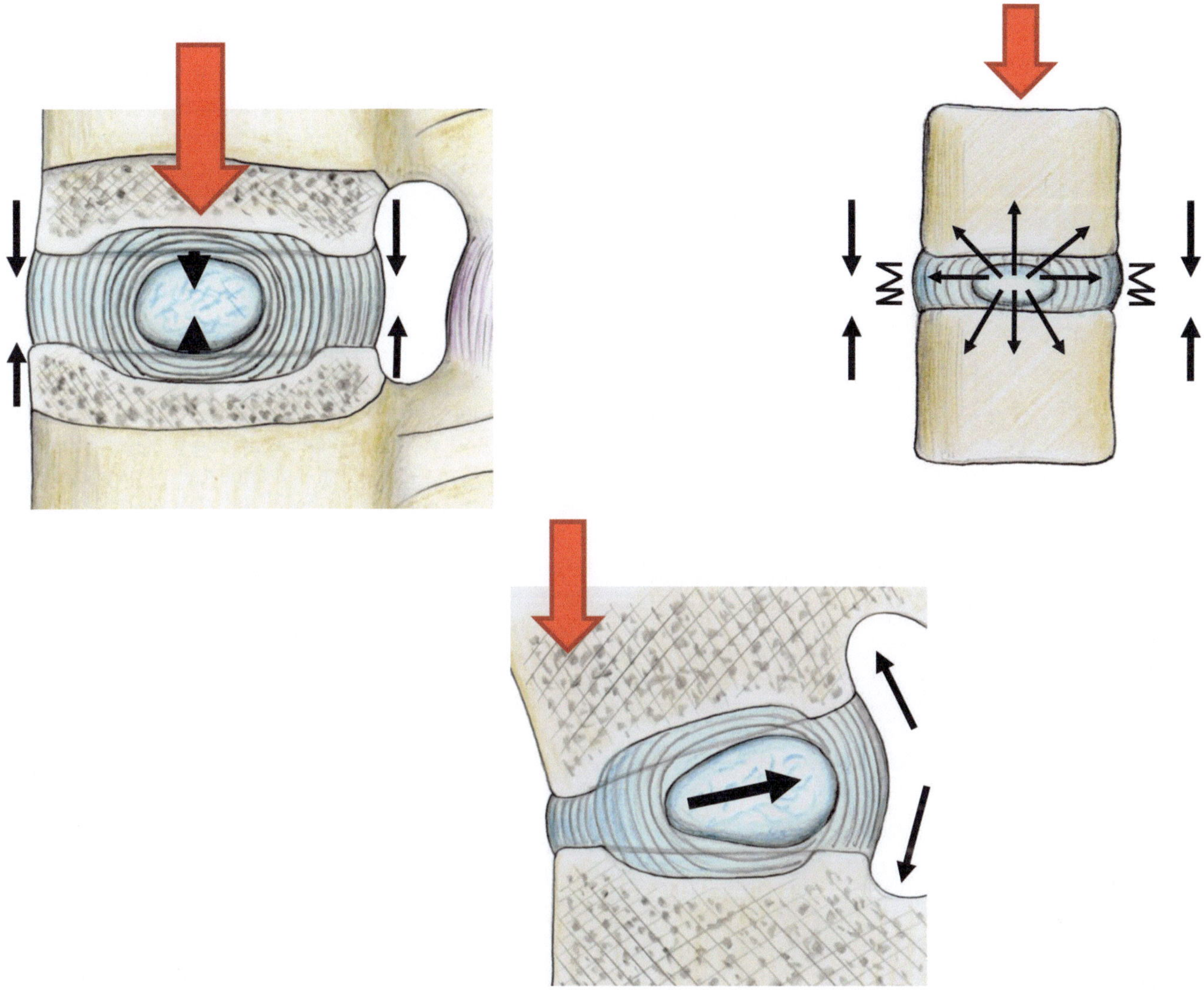

Fig. 5 Compression constraints on the nucleus pulposus and tension on the annulus fibrosus

The balance is achieved with minimum radial expansion of the NP of a healthy disc with intact collagen lamellae. The application of a load of 40 kg on the IVD creates a compression of 1 mm and a radial expansion of 0.5 mm. The very strong AF resists the protrusive tendency of the IVD (Fig. 5).

A disc without NP maintains the same large capacities under axial loading for short durations, but the disadvantage is that it flattens under prolonged loading with deformation of the AF with expulsion of water. The joint action of NP and AF allows the disc to support load. Any change in the PG and water content inevitably changes the disc properties.

Nachemson's in vivo research on disc pressure measurement [18] shows the disc stresses in the different bodily positions and associated efforts (Fig. 6).

Disc pressure is normally uniform but increased (2 MPa) in the posterior part of the disc. With annular cracking, the pressure is reduced and irregular with pressure drop in discomanometry [19] (Fig. 7).

Movements and Constraints

The IVD allows movements of the vertebral bodies around an amphiarthrosis joint (continuous, slightly movable joint), guided by the synovial posterior facet joints. The whole disco articular tripod is the intervertebral mobile segment of Junghans. Disc deformity allows adaptation to all movements in the three planes (flexion-extension, inclination, and rotation) (Fig. 8).

The instantaneous centre of rotation (ICR) is located for flexion-extension at the level of the posterior part of the disc. In distraction, the separation of the vertebral bodies increases the height of the IVD, and all the collagen fibres of the AF are elongated in tension whatever the orientation of the fibres. Distraction has been studied less, and the studies are contradictory because the disc of the biped is in compression whereas the brachiators (primates who use their arms to move from tree branch to tree branch) use their discs in distraction.

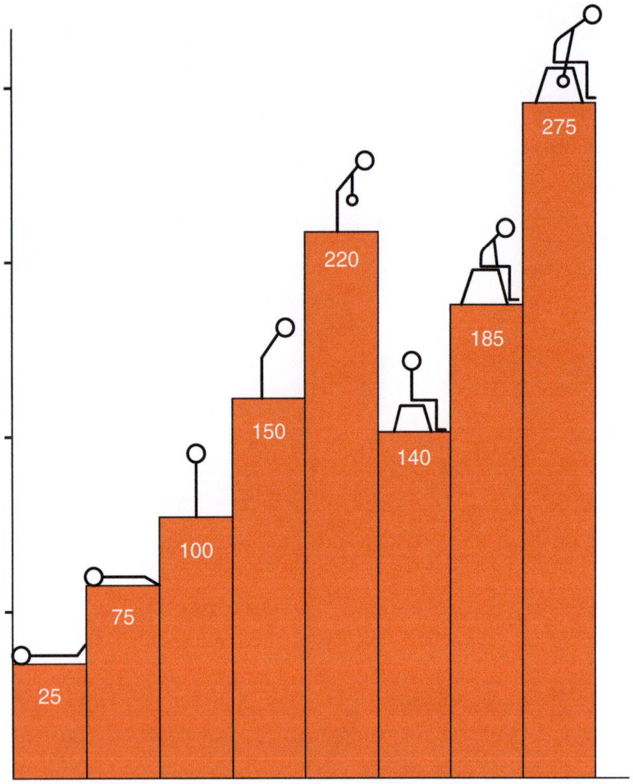

Fig. 6 Discal constraints (kg) in different positions [18]

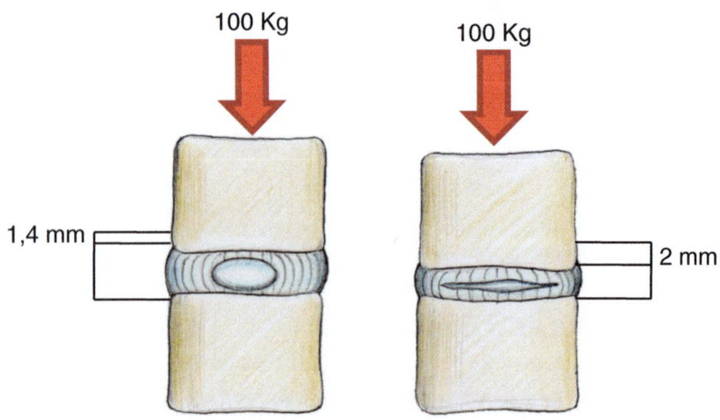

Fig. 7 Effect of a load of 100 kg on a healthy disc and a degenerate disc

The stiffness of the spine falls between 10 and 80 MPa with rupture of the articulations at 600 N. The anterior disc region is more fragile than the posterior distraction. Lumbar traction of 9 kg causes an elongation of 7.5 mm on average and 9 mm, with prolonged traction. Elongation is faster in young people. 40% of the lengthening of the spine is related to the decrease of the curvatures and 80% to the intervertebral joint separation of the order of 0.1 mm, per articular level.

- In sliding or translation, the collagen fibres of the AF oriented in the direction of movement are stretched.
- In the pendulum motion in flexion-extension or left-right lateral inclination, there is a compression of the AF in the direction of the movement and displacement of the NP in the opposite direction with tension of the fibres of the AF in the opposite direction to the movement. The posterior concave discs have a larger portion of the AF posteriorly with better resistance to stretching and therefore less protrusion.
- In extension, there is reduction of disc protrusion with the use of lordosis or extension rehabilitation with protrusive herniation (Cyriax, Mc Kenzie, Troisier).
- In the twisting or rotating movement, the tension of the fibres causes a pinching of the disc with tension of the collagen fibres located in the direction of movement. The annular tear occurs in torsion.

For rotation, there is no match for the ICR of the disc and that of the posterior facet joints as there is a shear disc on the side opposite to the rotation and a facet joint distraction on the side of rotation.

The movements are guided by the posterior articular facets and limited by the intervertebral ligaments. The AF also behaves like a ligament that limits mobility and stabilizes the joint. The directional alternation of the fibres of the lamellae of the AF is an integral part of the torsional disc resistance.

In axial compression stresses, there is a transmission of the load by the NP and the AF. Under a load of 100 KPa, the NP loses 8% of its water and the AF 11% of its water. The loss of water causes an increase in electrolytes and this concentration serves to rehydrate the disc after releasing stress.

The compressive load is supported uniformly by the inner part of the AF and the NP with maximum stress inside the posterior part of the disc (Adams).

With pathology by compression, the AF can support a pressure of 3.2×10^7 Nm^2 and the cancellous bone yields under a pressure of 3.4×10^6 Nm^2. So end-plates give way sooner than the AF.

The vertebral body yields between 3 and 12 KN depending on the bone density of the cancellous bone whereas osteoporotic compression fracture occurs at a compression of <1 KN.

The disc exhibits creep with water loss of 10% of disc fluid with 2% loss of size after 16 h of daily activity. The standing disc pressure is 70 KPa and with 5 kg load, the pressure increases to 700 KPa.

The articular facets support 40% of the load in normal circumstances with isolation of the articular facets on the lower laminae by the inferior articular facets.

Variations According to Spinal Levels

- The height of the discs varies according to the vertebral levels. Disc height is half in the thoracic spine (1/6) than in the cervical or lumbar (1/3). The co-efficient of mobility is therefore twice as low in the thoracic area.

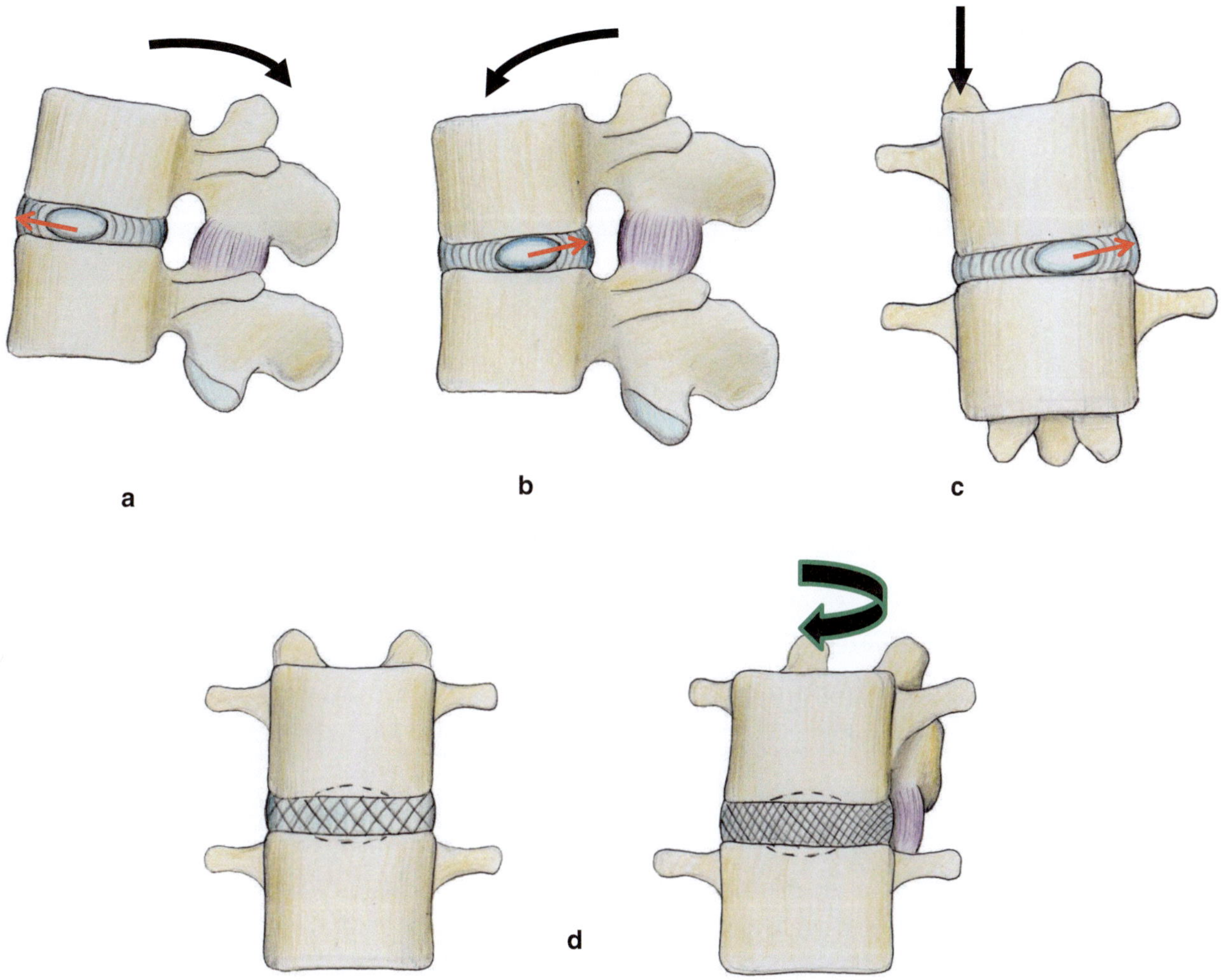

Fig. 8 Motion of the nucleus and annulus in extension (**a**), flexion (**b**), lateral inclination (**c**), and rotation (**d**) movements

- The NP is located slightly behind the centre of the disc but it is more posterior in the lumbar level.
- At the cervical level, there is often in the young adult a phenomenon of lateral cracking arising from the middle part of the disc and moving between the uncus; Hirsch has studied this phenomenon and describes after fissuring, a metaplasia with appearance of chondrocytes without a synovial membrane.
- At the lumbar level, the discs are higher anteriorly than posteriorly, starting from the T12L1 disc: this opening towards the front is all the more marked as one goes down towards the lumbosacral junction.

This orientation is involved largely in lumbar lordosis. In the frontal plane, the discs project to the upper part of the interlaminar space and become lower relative to this space when closer to the lumbosacral junction.

Disc Fissuring and Herniation (Figs. 9 and 10)

Due to ageing and under excessive compressive or shear stresses, the disc can tear in the form of cracks that are often radial and most often project posteriorly into the vertebral or intervertebral foramen; disc material which is usually central (herniated nucleus of pulposus) can pass through these cracks and compress the roots of the lumbar region, most often to cause radicular pain (thigh pain for L3 or L4 roots, and sciatica for L5 and S1 roots).

Lumbar disc herniations are of different patho-anatomical types depending on whether they are:

- Protrusion: focal protrusion of disc material beyond margins of adjacent vertebral body, over <90 degrees of circumference, with a base that is wider than dome

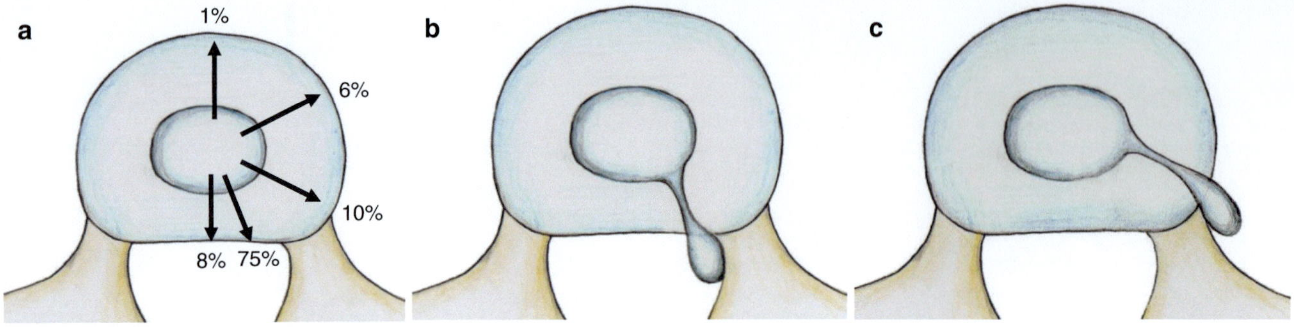

Fig. 9 Topography of cracks and herniated discs (**a**), anterior (1%), lateral (6%), foraminal (6%) and extraforaminal (4%), posterolateral (75%), median (8%). Posterolateral hernia (**b**). Extraforaminal hernia (**c**)

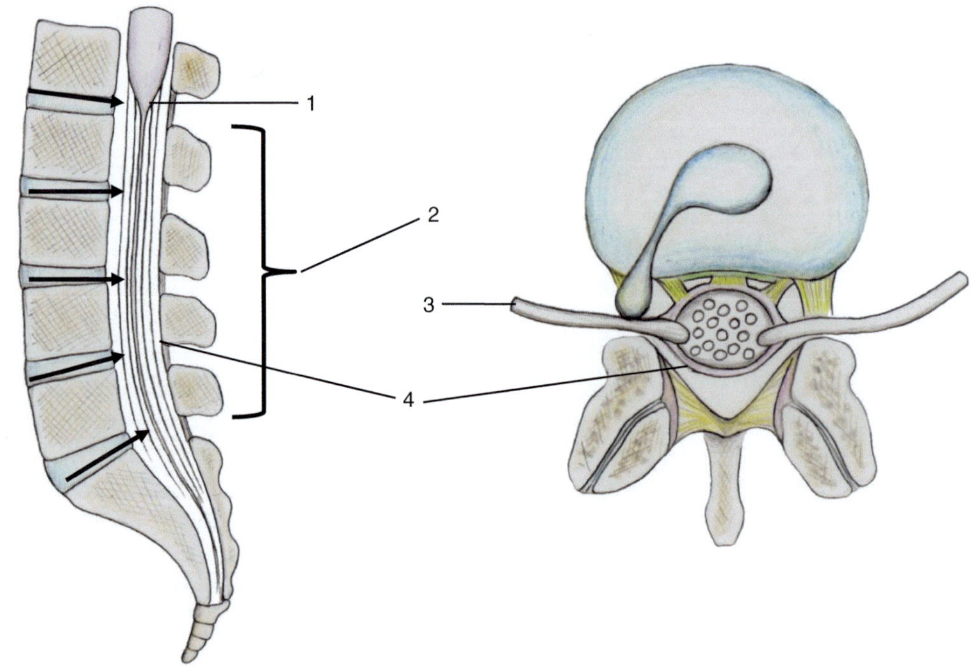

Fig. 10 Possibilities of compression by herniated disc: conus medullaris (1), cauda equina (2), root (3), dura mater (4)

- Extrusion: focal herniation of disc nuclear material through an annular defect, remaining in continuity with the disc, with a base narrower than the dome of the extrusion
- Sequestration: distal migration of extruded disc material away from the disc, with no direct continuation with the adjacent disc (Fig. 11).

At the cervical level, herniations, to be symptomatic (radiculomedullary compression), are most often migrated, transligamentous and sequestered.

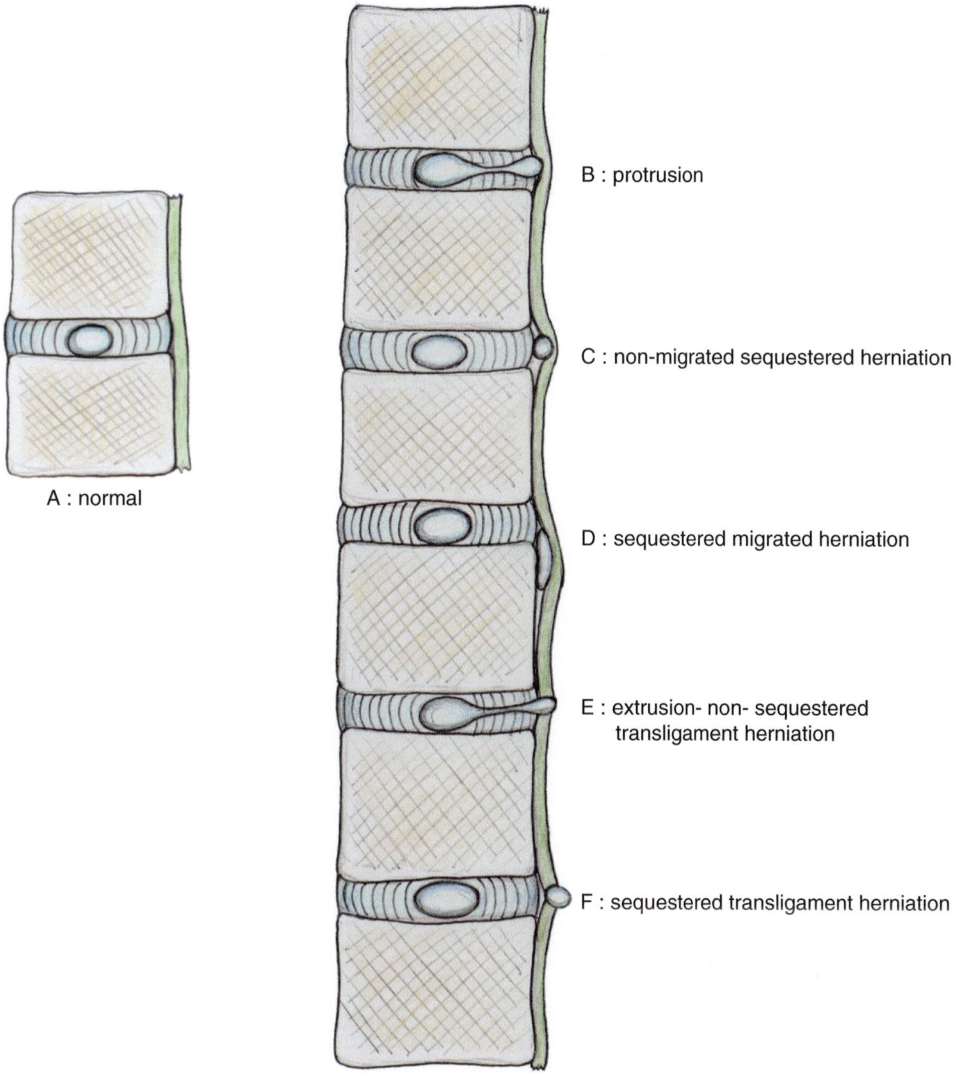

Fig. 11 Different types of herniated discs

References

1. Taylor JR. The development and adult structure of lumbar intervertebral discs. J Man Med. 1980;5:43–7.
2. Macnab I. Anatomy in backache. Baltimore: Williams & Wilkis; 1977. p. 47.
3. Coventry MB. Anatomy of the intervertebral disc. Clin Orthop. 1969;67:9–15.
4. Marchand F. Investigation of the laminate structure of lumbar disc annulus fibrosus. Spine. 1990;15:402–10.
5. Bogduk N. Clinical and radiological anatomy of the lumbar spine. 5th ed. London: Elsevier; 2005.
6. Hickey DS, Hukins DWL. Relation between the structure of the annulus fibrosus and the function and failure of the intervertebral disc. Spine. 1980;5:106–16.
7. Eyring EJ. The biochemistry and physiology of the intervertebral disc. Clin Orthop. 1969;67:16–28.
8. Maroudas A, Nachemson A, Stockwell R, et al. Some factors involved in the nutrition of the intervertebral disc. J Anat. 1975;120:113–30.
9. Urban J, Maroudas A. The chemistry of the disc in relation to its physiological function. Clin Rheum Dis. 1980;6:51–76.
10. Urban J. Fluid and solute transport in the intervertebral disc [Thesis PhD]. University London; 1977.
11. Holm S, Maroudas A, Urban J. Nutrition of the intervertebral disc: solute transport and metabolism. Connect Tissues Res. 1981;8(2):101–19.
12. Maroudas A, Urban J. Propriétés biochimiques du disque lombaire normal et pathologique. In: Simon L, editor. lombalgies et Med Ré-éducation. Paris: Masson; 1980.
13. Johnstone B, Bayliss MT. The large proteoglycans of the human intervertebral disc. Spine. 1995;20:674–84.
14. Roberts S, Menage J, Urban PG. Biochemical and structural properties of cartilage endplate and its relation to intervertebral disc. Spine. 1989;14:166–74.
15. Inoue H. Three-dimensional architecture of lumbar intervertebral discs. Spine. 1981;6:138–46.
16. Eyre D, Muir H. Quantitative analysis of type I and II collagen in human intervertebral discs at various ages. Biochim Biophys Acta. 1977;49:29–42.

17. Kanemoto M, Hukuda S, Komiya Y. Immunohistochemical study of matrix metalloproteinase 3 and tissue inhibitor of metalloproteinase1 in human intervertebral discs. Spine. 1996;21:18.
18. Nachemson A. The influence of spinal movements of the lumbar intra-discal pressure and on the tensile stresses in the annulus fibrosus. Acta Orthop Scand. 1963;33:183–207.
19. Bayliss MT, Johnstone B, Brien O'. Proteoglycan synthesis in the human intervertebral disc variation with age, region and pathology. Spine. 1988;13:972–81.

Anatomy of the Thoraco-Lumbar Facet Joint

Christian Louis and René Louis

Formation of the Posterior Thoraco -Lumbar Joints [1]

The appearance of the vertebral column in the animal series is so important that it alone determines the branching of vertebrates, of which man is the most advanced species. At first simply limited to the notochord, the axial skeleton joins the vertebrae which add to the solidity and the flexibility of its primitive form. In addition, vertebrates are characterized by the constitution of a neural tube developed on the posterior aspect of the notochord and enveloped by the vertebrae. The complete development of the spine includes both prenatal and postnatal periods.

Without going into the details remember that the period of prenatal development is broken down first by the formation of the primitive line (end of the second week), the formation of the notochord (from the 15th day), the formation of the neuraxis and of the sclerotome that will be the original tissue of the vertebral model (from the third week). First precartilaginous or membranous vertebrae (fourth week), it becomes cartilaginous (sixth week) and is composed of three pairs of centers of chondrification, one for the vertebral body or centrum, one for the posterior arch, and the last for the costal or transversal process. From the third month appear the three primitive points of ossification heralding the vertebral bone (Fig. 1). One of the primitive points, median, is destined to the centrum and the other two, lateral, to the posterior arch. The primitive lateral points of the posterior arch are located in the future zone of attachment of articular and transverse processes. Between the primitive points of the arches and the centrum lies the intermediate cartilage of Schmorl. After birth, the formation of the spine continues with the disappearance of the intermediate cartilage of Schmorl and the fusion of the median and lateral primitive points between 4 and 8 years and the fusion of the primitive lateral points between them towards 7 years of age. Other points of secondary ossification occur at the extremities of the upper and lower articular processes and the lumbar tubercles from about 11–18 years of age, and their fusion ends as late as between 21 and 25 years of age!

At all stages of vertebral development there may be an abnormality in the posterior joints but often associated with other vertebral abnormalities or neuropathy. Disorders of segmentation of sclerotomes occasionally concern only the posterior joints (numerical and transitional anomalies), more regularly disorders of the ossification by aplasia (Fig. 2), and especially dysplasia or a malposition that disrupts the orientation of the facet joints, their symmetry, and their ability to cope with their dynamic functions.

Morphology of Posterior Thoraco-Lumbar Joints (TLJ)

Morphology of the Posterior Thoracic Joints

Between the articular processes or zygapophyses are the joints whose articular facet planes are covered with strongly oblique cartilage (65° on average compared to the plane of the discs). The thoracic facets appear to be aligned along a sphere whose center is located in the disc (Fig. 8) [1].

Masharawi performed a morphometric study on 240 normal dry vertebral columns [2, 3] (Figs. 4, 5, and 6). There is no difference in the size of the facet joints according to age, and men have slightly larger dimensions than women. The craniocaudal length and the anteroposterior width of the facets have a parabolic distribution with a progressive decrease in size of T1 (from 10.75 mm and 12.75 mm, respectively) to T8 (10.34 and 9.05 mm) and a gradual increase from T12 (11.45 and 9.83 mm). It is therefore towards the vertex of the thoracic kyphosis that the surface of the facet joints is the weakest. Facet asymmetry is almost constant at the level of the thoracic spine concerning both dimensions and

C. Louis (✉)
HP Casamance, Aubagne, France

R. Louis
4 bis impasse du roc fleuri, Marseille, France

J. M. Vital, D. T. Cawley (eds.), *Spinal Anatomy*, https://doi.org/10.1007/978-3-030-20925-4_15

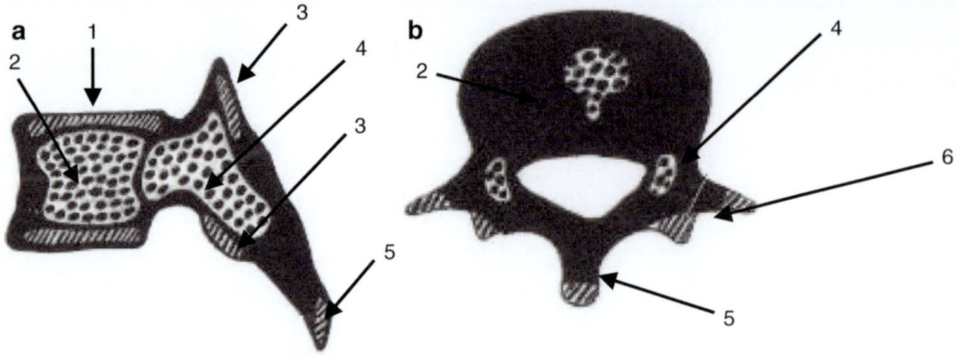

Fig. 1 Embryology: Primary and secondary ossification points of the thoracic (**a**) and lumbar vertebrae (**b**). (1) marginal listel or epiphyseal disc, (2) medial primitive point, (3) articular secondary point, (4) lateral primitive point, (5) secondary spinal point, (6) mamillary secondary point [1]

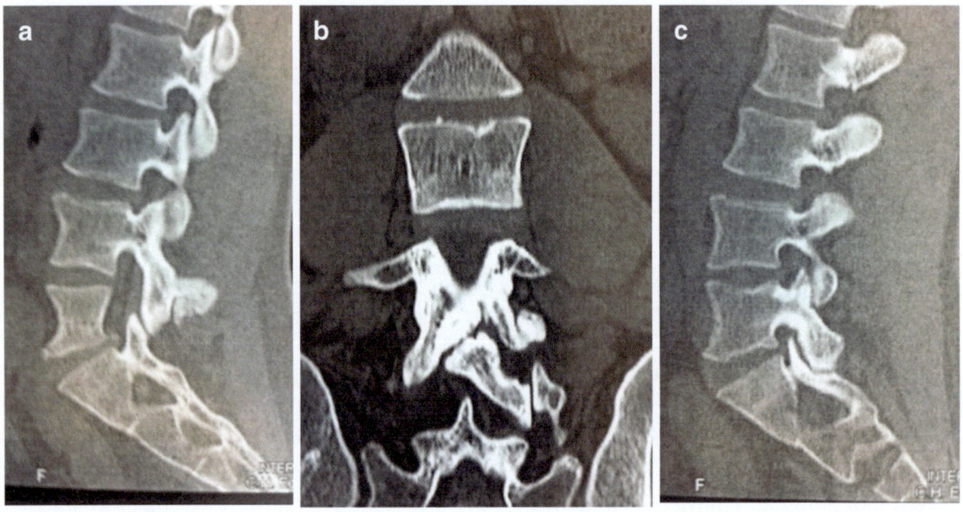

Fig. 2 Posterior articular agenesis. (**a**) right parasagittal CT scan showing the absence of the L4 L5 and L5S1 posterior articulations but only one joint L4S1, (**b**) frontal image, (**c**) left parasagittal CT image with a normal aspect of the posterior joints

orientations. The *craniocaudal length* of the upper left facets is greater than that of the upper right facets from T1 to T11 and that of the lower left facets is greater than that of the lower right facets in T2, and T6–T10 and the reverse in T12. The *anteroposterior width* of the upper right facets is greater than that of the upper left facets of T1–T6 and that of the lower left facets is greater than that of the lower right facets of T6–T8. In posterior view, comparing for each vertebra the distribution of interfacet distances in the horizontal plane and the vertical plane the posterior arches of T1 and T2 have an inverted trapezoidal aspect which becomes a rectangle from T3 to T12. There is also a right /left asymmetry of the facet transverse angle with a greater right-hand transverse angle than that of the left-hand side with respect to the lower and upper facets as well as for the longitudinal angle of the upper facets. The right thoracic facets are therefore a little more vertical and frontal than the left ones. Outside the TL junction, however, the angular values between the lower and upper facets are symmetrical.

The orientation of the facets and therefore of the articular line at the TL junction between T11 and L2 has many varieties according to which side or the other adopts the thoracic (spherical segment) or lumbar (pulley segment with sagittal slopes) (Fig. 9). Singer et al. [4] described these variations (Fig. 12). A sharp transition from frontal orientation to sagittal orientation was noted in 46% of cases in T12 and 33% in T11. Asymmetry >20° between the two joints of the same level is more marked at T11–T12 (21%) than at T12–L1 (9%).

The union of the facets is done by a fibrous capsule reinforced anteriorly by the ligamentum flavum and posteriorly by a posterior longitudinal ligament. A synovial lining on the inner aspect of the capsule with folds that are mistakenly taken on anatomical sections for a small intra-articular meniscus [5].

Morphology of the Posterior Lumbar Joints

The zygapophyseal joints are of the trochoid type (a joint in which one element rotates on its own axis), as the facets are hollow grooves for the upper facets and embossed for the lower facets (Figure 9). The facets covered with cartilage are, after interlocking, anteroexternal for the superior and posterointernal for the inferior. The joint line is vertical in the craniocaudal direction but curved with its center situated at the base of the spinous processes, in the horizontal plane. The orientation of the lumbar articular facets varies in the craniocaudal direction and between the two sides at the same

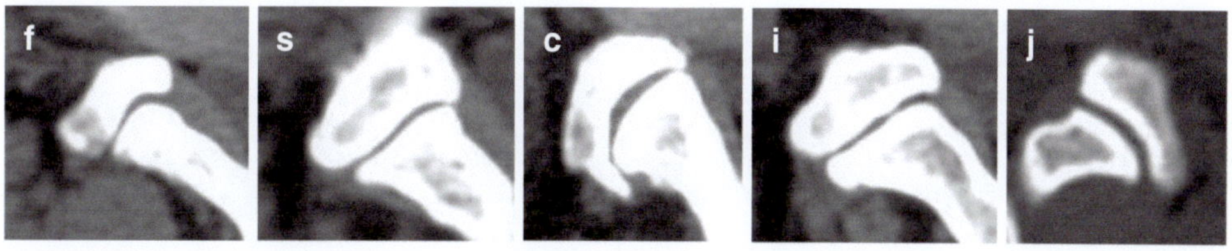

Fig. 3 Morphological variations of the posterior joint space. F: line spacing “F”, S: line spacing “S”, C: line spacing “C”, I: line spacing “I”, and J: line spacing “J”

level. The joint spacing shown on CT sections has large variations in appearance. A personal study of 800 posterior lumbar joints in CT slices showed five different morphotypes from L1L2 to L5S1 (Fig. 3). The facets are oriented more sagittally towards L1 and more frontally towards S1 with at this level a preponderance of “I” morphotype. The asymmetry (or tropism) of the lumbosacral articular facets is very frequent or even constant [1, 3, 6, 7]. Kenesi and Lesur [7] measured at the L4L5 level a mean angle, in a plane horizontal to the median axis of the vertebrae, straight facets of 45.7° and left facets of 51.4° with extreme variations to the right from 28 to 69° and to the left from 30 to 74°. At the L5S1 level, the average angle of the right facets is 47.2° (range 30–71°) and left facets 51.5° (range 30–78°). There is therefore a more important sagittalization on the right of 4.3° on average [1].

In the Masharawi study [2, 3] (Figs. 4, 5, and 6), the craniocaudal length and anteroposterior width of the lumbar facets increased progressively to maximum L5 dimensions (with mean values of 12.5 and 10.6 mm at L1 and 15 and 14.3 mm at L5, respectively). A certain degree of asymmetry also exists in the facet joints of the lumbar spine. Except at L5, the craniocaudal length of the upper right facets is greater than that of the upper left facets and in L1 and L3 that of the lower right facets is greater than that of the lower left facets. The R/L facets on the anteroposterior width are symmetrical except for L1 and L4–L5 where the left facets are wider than the straight lines. There is therefore a kind of asymmetry compensation with respect to the asymmetry observed at the thoracic level. In posterior view, comparing the interfacet distances at each vertebra in the horizontal and vertical plane the posterior arches of L1–L5 have a trapezoidal aspect with a large lower base, unlike T1–T2, which favors the imbrication of facets into each other especially during lumbar extension. Except for L1, there is no right-left asymmetry at the level of the lumbar spine in this study concerning the angular values of the transverse and longitudinal facet angles. Note however that the study stopped in L5 and that the asymmetries are classically found at L5S1. As the longitudinal angle of the upper facets increases progressively, that of the lower facets decreases from L1 to L5, the lower facets thus become more oblique than the upper facets of L1 to L5. This fact is explained by the presence of lumbar lordosis.

The maintenance of joint integrity is the doubled synovial capsule, the ligamentum flavum anterior to the joint, a posterior ligament strengthening the capsule posteriorly, and remote ligaments. As in the thoracic stage, there is no intra-articular meniscus [1].

Participation of the Posterior Articulations in the Overall Stability of the Spine [1]

The factors of stability are different according to whether the spine is considered vertically along its long axis or perpendicular to it in the horizontal plane. The vertebral stability results in fact from the synergy of the factors of axial stability and horizontal stability. The posterior joints participate fully in vertebral stability.

Vertical Stability

In the vertical direction, stability finds its support in the elementary and global architecture of the spine.

The elementary architecture of each TL vertebra is composed of three vertical mini columns: that of the vertebral body in front and those of the articular processes behind. The three columns are joined by horizontal bars: the two pedicles and the laminae behind. The global architecture of the TL spine is composed of three vertical columns. The anterior column, the largest, takes on a quadrangular pyramid appearance formed by the alternation of vertebral bodies and discs to the sacral plateau. The two posterior columns arranged in a frontal plane are constituted by the succession of articular processes. This system of columns is reinforced by horizontal bars (pedicles and laminae), which at each vertebral level, solidify the columns together. This three-column structure is found in the development of the spine from the three primary points of ossification: the centrum for the large anterior column and the two points of ossification of the posterior arch for the two posterior columns. The increasing caliber, in the craniocaudal direction, of the three columns testifies to their bearing function. For the same reasons, the articular surfaces of each of the mobile vertebral segments increase in the craniocaudal direction. If we consider only the articular surfaces of the posterior columns, Masharawi [3] reports a decrease of these surfaces between T4 and T10 which can be explained by the presence at this level of the dorsal kyphosis submitting more vertical stress to the anterior column and to the posterior columns. Thus the posterior columns with their facets should not be considered as simple articulations orienting the

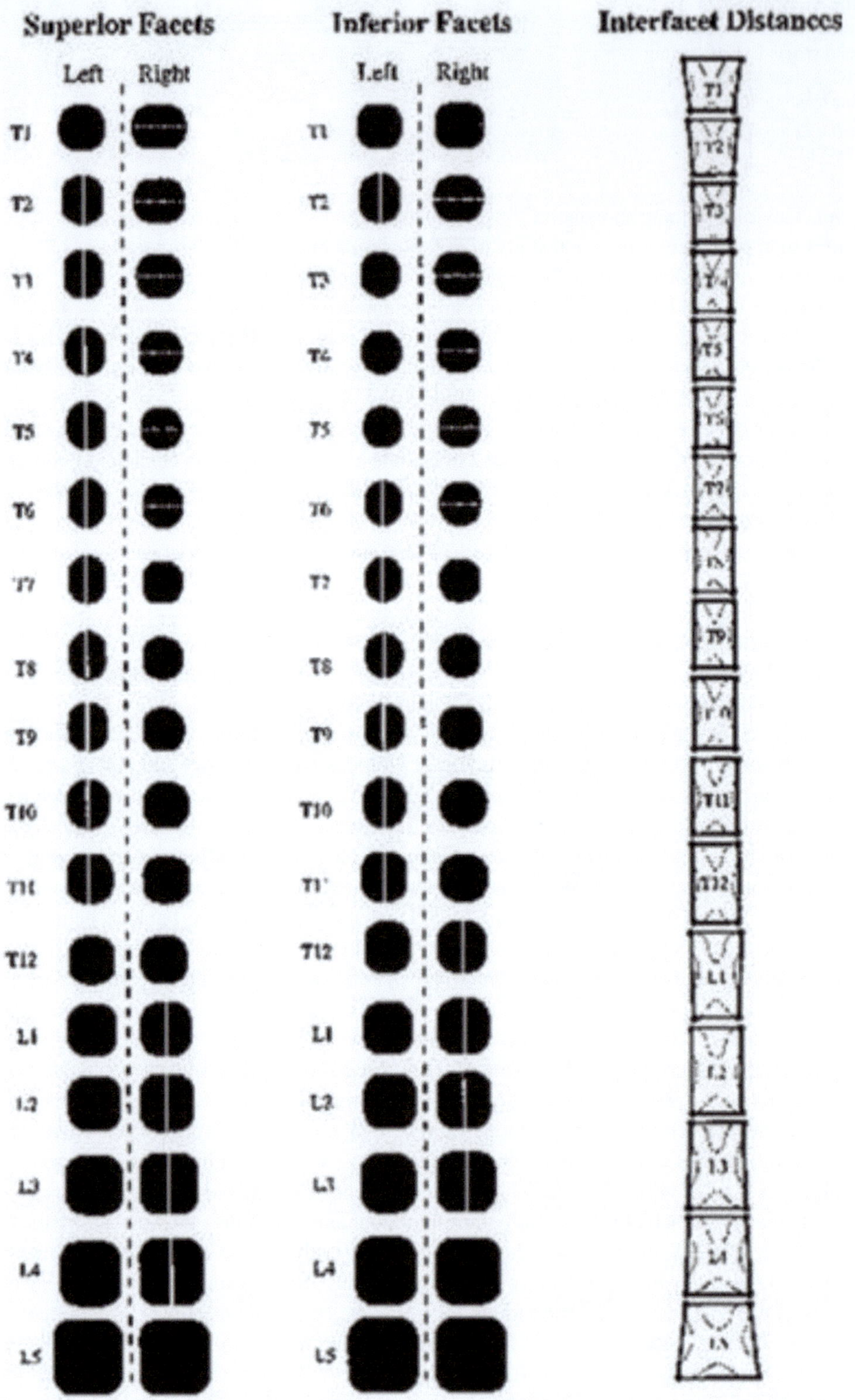

Fig. 4 Representation of facet asymmetries at the TL spine and distribution of interfacet distances. The vertical white line (craniocaudal facet length) and horizontal line (anteroposterior facet width) indicate the longest or widest facet on both sides (which corresponds to facet asymmetry)

Fig. 5 Distribution of facet angulations in the transverse plane at the TL spine. *ITFA* lower facet transverse angle (alpha1), *STFA* superior facet transverse angle (alpha)

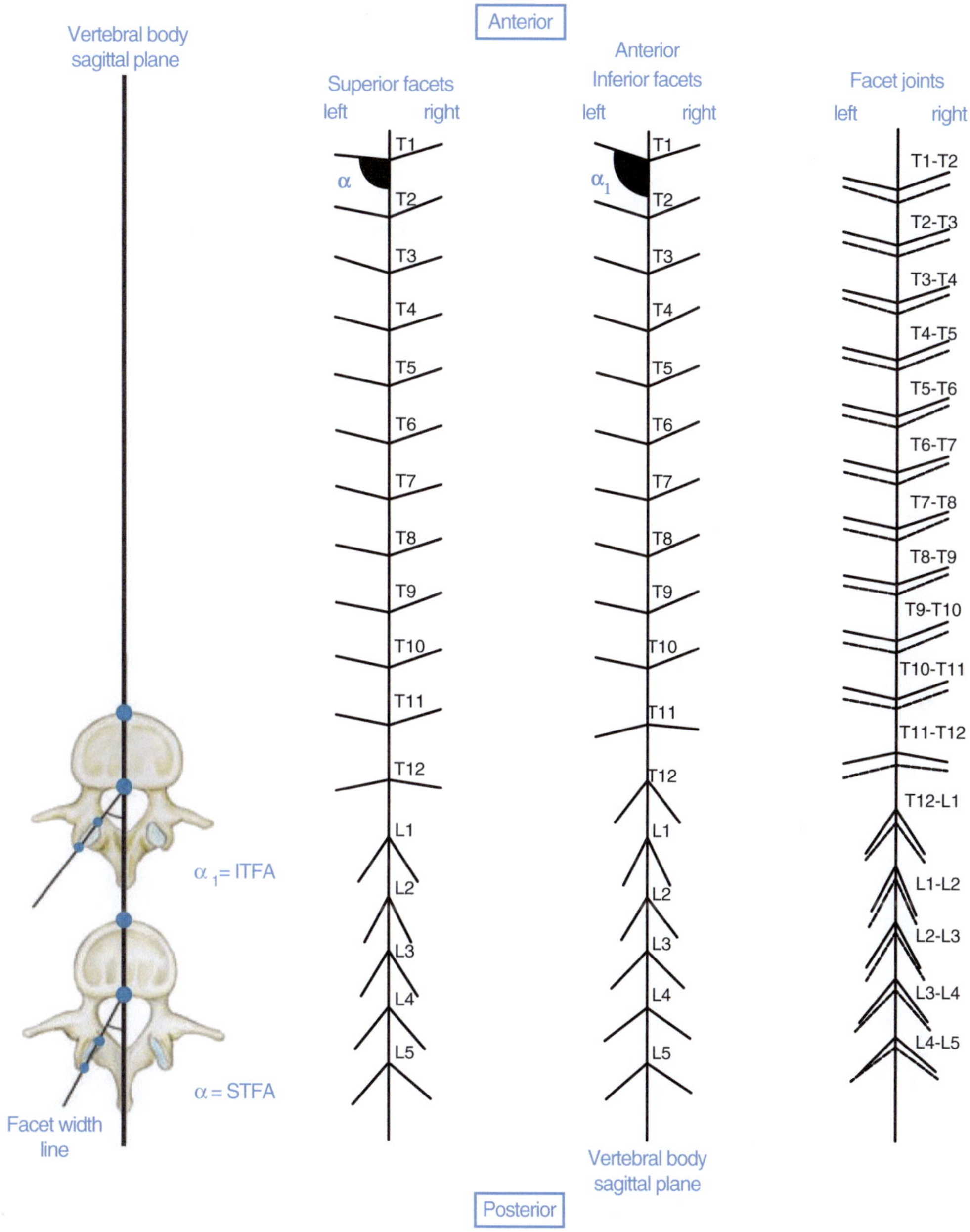

segmental movements of the spine but as true load bearing formations of the spine following the positions of the spine.

Horizontal Stability

When the spine is subjected to forces perpendicular to its major axis, the weak points are situated at the level of the mobile and articular zones. Stability is ensured by the osteo-ligamentary pair of joint stops and ligament brakes (Fig. 7).

In flexion, the articular processes whose facet direction opposes horizontal sliding play the role of bending abutments. The articular capsule, the ligamentum flavum, and all ligaments located behind the nucleus pulposus slow extreme vertebral flexion. The oblique articular facets planes allow a sliding which results in an angulation between two vertebrae but it is the limit of elasticity of the ligament brakes which prohibits the dislocation of the facet joints.

In forced extension, it is the ligaments situated in front of the nucleus pulposus which limit the movement, the capsulo-ligamentary elements of the articular facets do not play a primordial role. The most posterior part of the articular processes, and the spinous processes between them, come in contact and block extension.

Rotation and tilt movements are almost always combined. The inclination of the articular facets between 45° and 80° with respect to the plane of the intervertebral space imposes a simultaneous rocking and rotation movement. When a lower right articular facet rises and advances on the underlying facet, the left facet descends and recedes. Virtually all

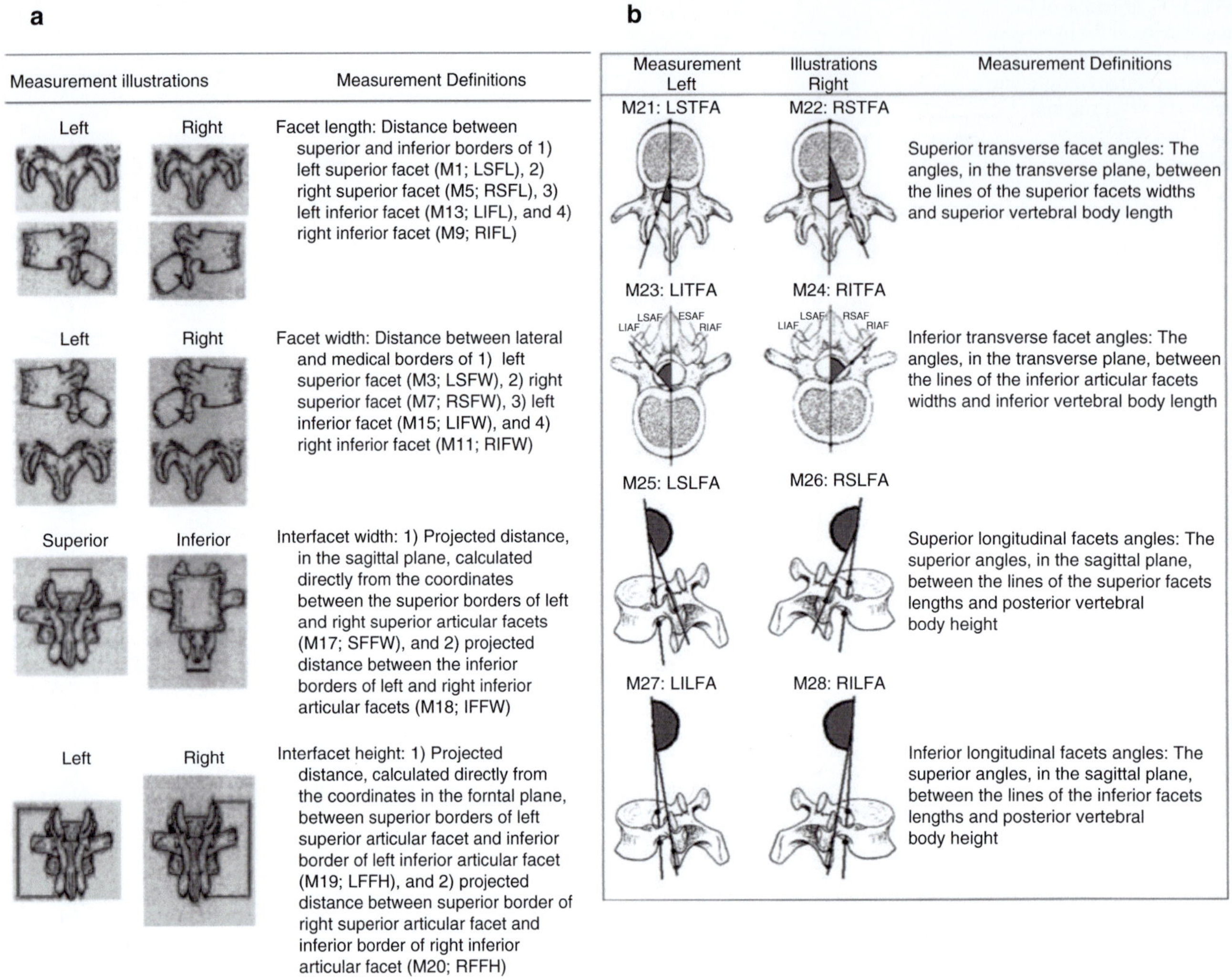

Fig. 6 Definition of the measurements made by Masharawi [2, 3]

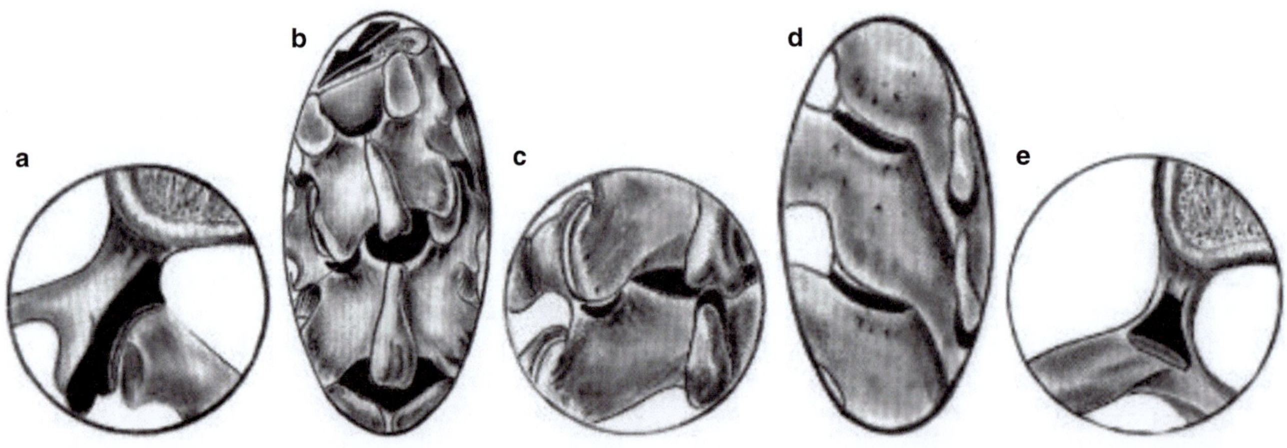

Fig. 7 Bone abutments and ligament brakes. (**a**) lumbar articular abutment, (**b**) lumbar abutments in lateral inclination, (**c**) lumbar abutments in extension, (**d**) thoracic abutments in extension, (**e**) thoracic articular abutment [1]

structures within the intervertebral union participate in the role of rotation and inclination braking. The stops that also limit these movements are always the joints, especially at the level of the lumbar region. In the thorax, the costovertebral joints considerably limit the lateral inclination and the rotation, although the orientation of the articular facets inscribed on a circular arc is favorable to rotation.

Participation of Posterior Articulations in Vertebral Dynamics [1]

Flexion-Extension and Tilt-Rotation (Fig. 8)

Joint mechanics depend on the coexistence of three joints in each mobile segment: the intervertebral disc and the two zygapophyseal joints. Two types of associated movements must be described: flexion-extension and tilt-rotation with regional thoracic and lumbar features. If an isolated disc allows a very wide range of motion between two vertebrae, the existence of the posterior apophyseal joints limits these movements to a sector of space specific to each vertebral region.

Regarding thoracic and lumbar flexion-extension, it is a circular motion around a transverse axis that is not at the nucleus but lower on the superior plateau. The articular cartilages determine an articular spacing fitting well on a circular arc of the same center. The overlying vertebra thus follows a circular arc with arciform sliding of the articular facets and pendulous movement of the disc around the same center. In fact, this center is not unique, but varies during the movement describing an area of instantaneous center of rotation (ICR) [8]. At the lumbar level, the flexion-extension amplitude is variable according to the stages with a minimum of 11° in L1–L2 and a maximum of 24° in L4–L5 for a total flexion of 53°, a total extension of 30°. At the thoracic level, there is no significant difference in amplitude according to the stages and the total flexion amplitude is 30° and total extension of 20°.

With regard to the inclination-rotation, it is the strongly oblique disposition of the posterior articular facets which imposes on every inclination movement a simultaneous movement of rotation and vice versa.

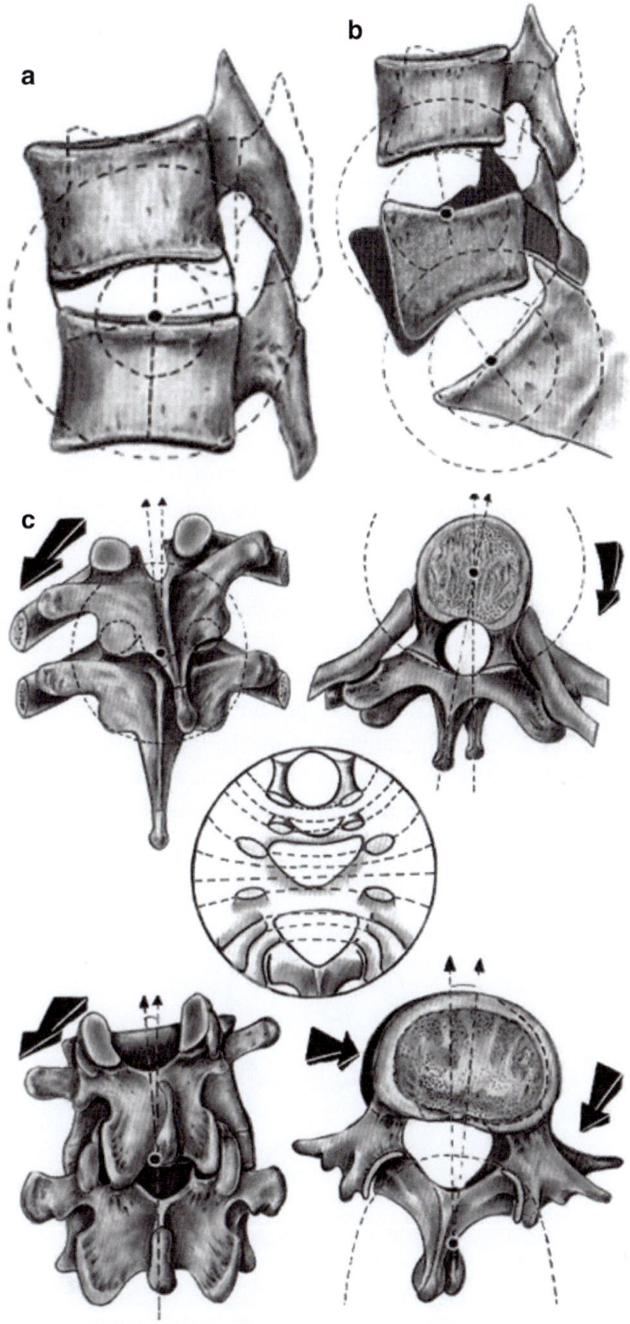

Fig. 8 Rotation centers. (**a**) center of rotation in flexion-extension in D8–D9, (**b**) center of rotation in flexion-extension in L4-L5-S1, (**c**) center of rotation of the lumbar and thoracic vertebrae in lateral inclination and rotation and the range of orientation of the vertebral articular facets [1]

- At the thoracic level, two mechanisms combine to create this dynamic synergy. On the one hand, the inclination of the articular facets (75–85° relative to the horizontal plane) initiates a rotation during inclination, by which the articular facet which rises becomes more anterior and that which lowers becomes more posterior. On the other hand, the existence of vertical and oblique costotransverse and intertransverse ligaments creates by the asymmetrical set of tensions a phenomenon of simultaneous rotation and inclination. Lateral inclination also causes an extension component. It is this mechanism which, associated with the progressive cuneiformity of the growing vertebrae, causes scoliosis, lateral inclination, rotation, and extension. The axis of rotation in the horizontal plane at the thoracic level is part of an arc whose circle is in the middle of the lower vertebral plateau. The inclination-rotation amplitude is <8° per moving segment with small variations depending on the level.

- At the lumbar level, lateral inclination movements are possible but reduced by tilting between the vertical rails of the upper facets. The rotation movements are not favored either by the arrangement of the facets because they are inscribed, in a horizontal plane, on a parabolic curve opened posteriorly. The axis of rotation is on the spinous processes so that the disc must undergo oscillatory movement with lateral shear. The amplitude of inclination-rotation is <5° per moving segment with small variations depending on the level.

Although their center of rotation is different, at the lumbar level, the flexion-extension and inclination-rotation movements are often associated in the gestures of everyday life. To allow for these two very different types of motion, the facet joints are cut at the expense of the slopes of the groove of a pulley (Fig. 9). This is the worst orientation for rotational movements. However, the lumbosacral facets are part of a curvature that is more open and therefore less unfavorable than that of the upper lumbar vertebrae.

At the level of the moving segments, there is therefore a common center of rotation for flexion-extension and inclination-rotation movements. The articular facets thus fit on a spherical circumference (Fig. 9).

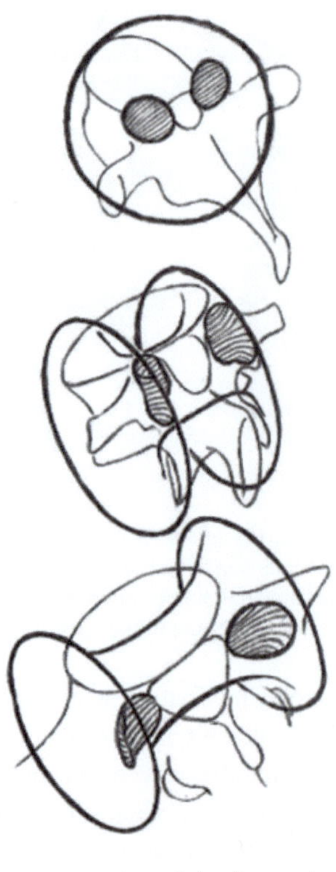

Fig. 9 Volumetric representation of the facets: the articular facets of the various mobile segments are comparable to a segment of geometric volume, variable according to the level [1]

Facet Asymmetry

Ideally the articular facets of the same mobile segment should be symmetrical in shape, size, and orientation, which would promote harmonious movements.

As mentioned by many authors [6, 7], recent works by Masharawi [2, 3] have confirmed that facet, right-left and upper-lower asymmetry is a constant over the entire length of the spine. Despite the adaptability of the intervertebral disc and ligament means, these joint asymmetries can predispose to degenerative processes earlier than for strictly symmetrical joints.

Innervation of the Posterior Articulations

The innervation of the posterior joints is rich and multiradicular. These joints receive innervation via the mediodorsal branch of the spinal nerves, nerve fibers on their lateral side but also from anterior and deep (Fig. 10). Total surgical denervation is therefore difficult to conceive without destruction of the joint or dissection of the ventral root branch. A mini-invasive partial denervation under fluoroscopy by thermocoagulation or cryodenervation [9–11] is however feasible.

Most Common Pathologies of Posterior Lumbar Joints

The pathology of the posterior vertebral joints concerns mostly the lumbar spine.

The orientation of the lumbar articular facets in the sagittal plane will protect the disc from torsional and shear stresses [12].

On an intact mobile segment, it is primarily the outermost fibers of the fibrous ring that will oppose the abnormal movements [13]. They are organized into concentric lamellae consisting mainly of type I collagen fibers, whereas the nucleus pulposus consists of a loose lattice of elastin fibers and type II collagens bathed in a proteoglycan gel [13]. This infrastructure gives the disc the coupled mechanical properties of a ligament (tensile and torsional strength) and articular cartilage (compressive and shear strength). Haefeli et al. [14] have described the chronology of macroscopic changes occurring during physiological disc degeneration. His observations suggest that disc degeneration begins in the nucleus and continues with changes and disorganization of annulus fibers making a series of cracks and nuclear cysts. Butler et al. [15] confirmed the hypothesis previously made by Vernon-Roberts [16] and Bywaters [17] that disc degeneration occurs before facet osteoarthritis. There are, however,

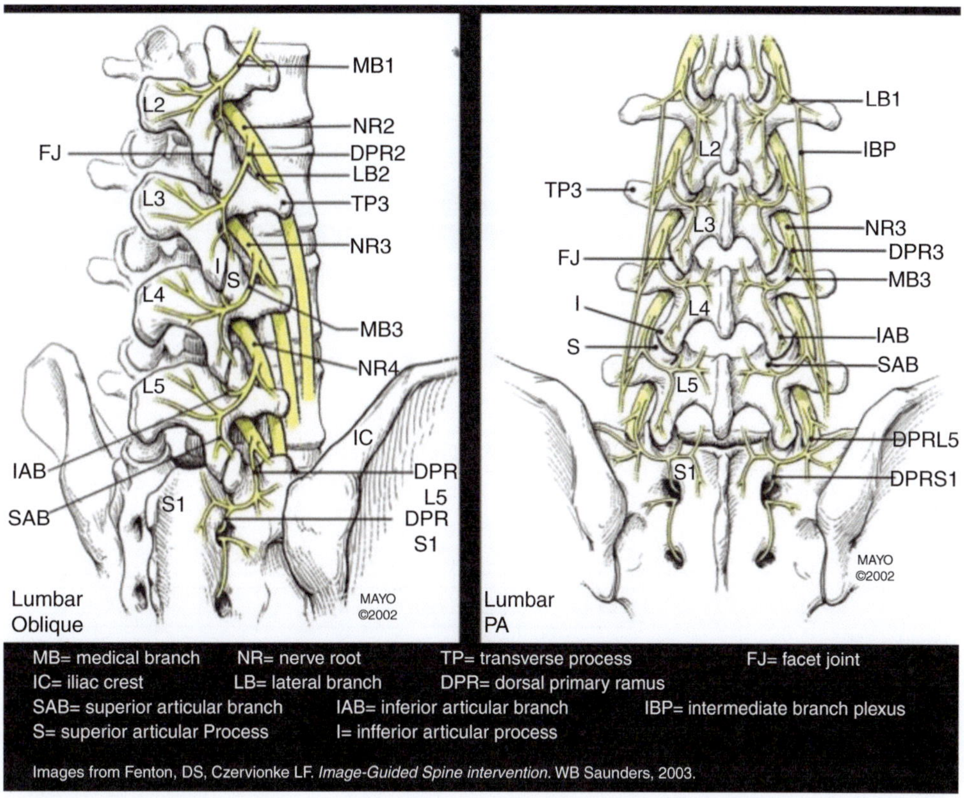

Fig. 10 Innervation of the posterior lumbar joints

facet arthrosis without disc degeneration opposing this theory where other etiologies can be advanced, such as specific arthropathies, activities with high rotational components (e.g., golf). and some lumbar morphotypes favoring hyperstressing posterior columns, as for lumbar hyperlordoses (high-impact spine) of type IV lordosis of Roussouly [18].

Disc degeneration is accompanied by a loss of the mechanical properties of the disc, a reduction of the disc height inducing a mechanical overload at the level of the posterior articulations [1, 19, 20] responsible for a thickening of the articular capsule [21], joint narrowing, and osteophyte formation. A classification of stages of posterior joint degeneration has been proposed by Grogan [22]. He distinguishes magnetic resonance imaging (MRI) four stages of cartilaginous degeneration and four stages of subchondral sclerosis. Capsular thickening and osteophytosis is a process stabilizing the degeneration of the mobile segment [21, 23]. Indeed, the articular cartilaginous degeneration induces an increase in the multidirectional segmental mobility [23] responsible for the formation of osteophytes [24] resulting in the restabilization of the facets [23, 25]. However, the appearance of facet osteophytes may also in some circumstances indicate segmental instability, as is the case in degenerative spondylolisthesis (SPLD). Initially described by Macnab in 1950 [26], the SPLD corresponds to an anterolisthesis of the cranial vertebra on the caudal vertebra without isthmic lysis more particularly concerning menopausal females at the L4L5 level. The controlled slip of a segmental instability is induced by the remodeling of osteoarthritic facet joints. Before the appearance of a slip, an SPLD can be suspected on an MRI in view of the widening of the joint space (>1.5 mm) [27]. The etiology of this remodeling is certainly multifactorial. Osteopenia induced by osteoporosis (postmenopause) can explain the premature wear of the facets in a context of excessive mechanical stresses at the level of the posterior columns, which is the case for lumbar lordosis in type I and IV Roussouly classification [18]. Excess sagittalization of the lumbar facets is commonly accepted as a promoting factor [28–30]. According to Kim [30] patients with facets whose angulation is >78° are 2.5 times more likely to develop a SPLD than patients with lower values. This excess sagittalization of the facets is manifested by articular lines that are abnormally visible on the anteroposterior radiographs [30–32] (Fig. 11).

The facet asymmetry or "facet tropism" was defined in 1928 by Brailsford [33] as an asymmetry of angulation between the two facets of the same mobile segment with a more sagittal facet than the other (Figs. 11 and 12). Although quasi-physiological [1–3, 6, 7] the facet tropism is the bed of disc degeneration [34] and promotes the occurrence of symptomatic disc herniation [28]. According to Hirokazu [6] the presence of a facet tropism advances the age of occurrence of a herniated disc. Farfan and Sullivan [35, 36] found a greater frequency of herniated discs on the sagittal side of the joint line. Sagittal orientation of the facet joints, which is consistently more pronounced on the right side, seems to promote

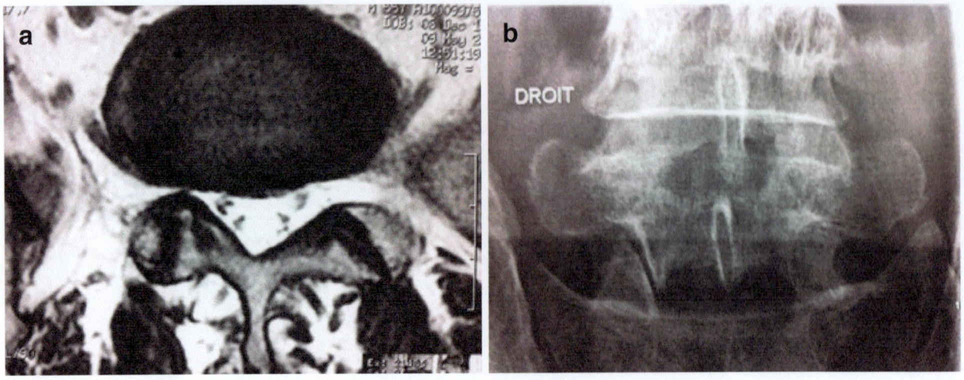

Fig. 11 An example of facet tropism. (**a**) horizontal MRI section in L5S1 with right sagittal and left oblique line spacing. (**b**) frontal X-ray showing a clearly visible line on the right indicating a very sagittal articulation

Fig. 12 Angular variations of joint line at the thoracolumbar junction [4]

Level	Left articular angle	Right articular angle
T10-T11	101.5° (101.1–102.9)	103,1° (101.7–104.6)
T11-T12	69, 0° (64.9°-73.1°)	71,2° (67.1–75.3)
T12-L1	31,3° (29.1–33.6)	33,0° (30.9–35.2)
L1-L2	24,6 (23.1 –25.9)	26,5° (25.2–27.8)

the occurrence of disc prolapse at the lumbosacral level [7]. According to Loback et al. [37] this tropism favors the occurrence of herniated discs rather posterolateral to the opposite of medial hernias occurring on more symmetrical facet morphotypes. On the other hand, for Hagg [38], facetism does not increase the risk of a disc pathology. For Boden [28], facet asymmetry does not seem to play a role in the occurrence of a SPLD.

The degeneration of the posterior joints also induces the formation of posterior or posterior synovial cysts, a source of low back pain, radicular pain, radicular claudication, and even cauda equina syndrome. Cysts are associated with an SPLD in 60–89% of cases [39]. They more frequently concern the L4L5 level (L5S1 > L3L4 > L2L3) and more often in females [40].

The degeneration of the posterior joints may be at the TL junction [41] at the origin of a syndrome well known to rheumatologists and unknown to surgeons, the syndrome of the TLJ (or Maigne's syndrome). This syndrome is manifested either by low back pain, or pain of the outer aspect of the hip or thigh, or pseudo visceral abdominal pain or even pubic pain. The painful manifestations coincide with the distribution of the corresponding spinal nerves (T12 and L1) by their anterior branch (pseudo-visceral and pubic pain), posterior (low back and buttock pain), and cutaneous lateral perforating branch (pseudo-trochanteric pain).

References

1. Louis R. Chirurgie du spine: anatomie chirurgicale et voies d'abord. Germany: Springer-Verlag; 1982, 1993.
2. Youssef M, Rothschild B, Dar G, Peleg S, Robinson D, Been E, Hershkovitz I. Facet orientation in the thoracolumbar spine. Three-dimensional anatomic and biomechanical analysis. Spine. 2004;29(16):1755–63.
3. Youssef M, Rothschild B, Salame K, Dar G, Peleg S, Hershkovitz I. Facet tropism and interfacet shape in the thoracolumbar vertebrae characterization and biomechanical interpretation. Spine. 2005;30(11):E281–92.
4. Singer RP, Breidahl PD, Day RE. Variations in zygapophyseal joint orientation and levels of transition at the thoracolumbar junction. Preliminary survey using computed tomography. Anat Clin. 1988;10(4):291–6.
5. Louis R. Spinal stability as defined by the three-column spine concept. Anat Clin. 1985;7:33–42.
6. Hirokazu I, Matsui H, Osada R, Ohshima H, Tsuji H. Facet joint asymmetry as a radiologic feature of lumbar intervertebral disc herniation in children and adolescents. Spine. 1997;22(17):2001–4.
7. Kenesi C, Lesur E. Possible role in pathology of the intervertebral disc. Anat Clin. 1985;7:143–8.
8. Gonon GP. Etude biomécanique de la colonne dorsolombaire de D10 à S1 [Thèse médecine]. Lyon; 1975.
9. Manchikanti L, et al. Prevalence of lumbar facet joint pain in chronic low back pain. Pain Physician. 1999;2(3):59–64.
10. Manchikanti L, Singh V. Review of chronic low back pain of facet joint origin. Pain Physician. 2002;5(1):83–101.
11. Manchikanti L, et al. Contribution of facet joints to chronic low back pain in postlumbar laminectomy syndrome: a controlled comparative prevalence evaluation. Pain Physician. 2001;4(2):175–80.
12. White AA, Panjabi MM. Clinical biomechanics of the spine. 2nd ed. Philadelphia: Lippincott; 1990.
13. Wong DA, Transfeldt E. Macnab's Backache. 4th ed. Lippincott Williams & Wilkins: Philapelphia; 2007.
14. Haefeli M. The course of macroscopic degeneration in the human lumbar intervertebral disc. Spine. 2006;31(14):1522–31.
15. Butler D, Trafimow JH, Anderson GBJ, Mc Neill TW, Huckman MS. Discs degenerate before facets. Spine. 1990;15:111–3.
16. Vernon-Roberts B, Pirie CJ. Degenerative changes in the intervertebral discs of the lumbar spine and their sequelae. Rheumatol Rehabil. 1977;16:13–21.
17. Bywaters EGC. The pathological anatomy of idiopathic low back pain. In: White AA, Gordon S, editors. Idiopathic low back pain. St. Louis: Mosby; 1982. p. 144–75.
18. Roussouly P. Influence de l'organisation morphologique sagittale de l'ensemble spine-pelvis sur l'évolution des pathologies

dégénératives rachidiennes: Alternatives à l'arthrodèse lombaire et lombosacrée. In: Cahiers d'enseignement de la SOFCOT. Paris: Elsevier Masson SAS; 2007. p. 27–35.
19. Nachemson A. Lumbar intradiscal pressure. Acta Orthop Scand. 1960;43(suppl):1–104.
20. Yang KH, King AI. Mechanism of facet load transmission as a hypothesis for low back pain. Spine. 1984;9:557–65.
21. Tanno I, et al. Morphometry of the lumbar zygapophyseal facet capsule and cartilage with spécial reference to dégénérative osteoarthritic changes: an anatomical study using fresh cadavers of elderly Japanese and Korean subjects. J Orthop Sci. 2004;9: 468–77.
22. Grogan J, Nowicki BH, Schmidt TA, et al. Lumbar facet joint tropism does not accelerate degeneration of facet joints. Am J Neuroradiol. 1997;18:1325–9.
23. Fujiwara A, Lim TH, An HS, et al. The effect of disc degeneration and facet joint osteoarthritis on the segmental flexibility of the lumbar spine. Spine. 2000;25(23):3036–44.
24. Tischer T, et al. Detailed pathological changes of human lumbar facet joints L1-L5 in elderly individuals. Eur Spine J. 2006;15:308–15.
25. Twomey LT, et al. Age changes in the lumbar articular triad. Aust J Physiother. 1985;31:106–12.
26. Macnab I. Spondylolisthesis with an intact neural arch. The so-called pseudospondilolisthesis. J Bone Joint Surg Br. 1950;32:325–33.
27. Chaput C, Padon D, et al. The significance of increased fluid signal on magnetic resonance imaging in lumbar facets in relationship to degenerative spondylolisthesis. Spine. 2007;32(17):1883–7.
28. Boden SD, Riew DK, et al. Orientation of the lumbar facet joints: association with degenerative disc disease. J Bone Joint Surg Am. 1996;78-A:403–11.
29. Grobler LJ, Robertson PA, Novotny JE, Pope MH. Etiology of spondilolisthesis. Assessment of the rôle played by lumbar facet joint morphology. Spine. 1993;18(1):80–91.
30. Kim NH, Lee JW. The relationship between isthmic and degenerative spondilolisthesis and the configuration of the lamina and facet joint. Eur Spine J. 1995;4(3):139–44.
31. Nagaosa Y, Kikuchi S, Hasue M, Sato S. Pathoanatomic mechanisms of degenerative spondylolisthesis. A radiographic study. Spine. 1998;23(13):1447–51.
32. Sato K, Wakamatsu E, Yoshizumi A, Watanabe N, Irei O. The configuration of the laminae and facet joints in degenerative spondylolisthesis. A clinicoradiologic study. Spine. 1989;14(11):1265–71.
33. Brailsford JF. Deformities of the lumbosacral region of the spine. Br J Surg. 1928;16:562–627.
34. Noren R, Trafimow J, Andersson GBJ, Huckman MS. The role of facet joint tropism and facet angle in disc degeneration. Spine. 1991;16:530–2.
35. Farfan HF, Sullivan JD. The relation of facet orientation to intervertebral disc failure. Can J Surg. 1967;10:179.
36. Farfan HF, Huberdeau RM, Dubow HI. Lumbar intervertebral disc degeneration: the influence of geometric features on the pattern of disc degeneration: a post mortem study. J Bone Joint Surg Am. 1972;54:492–510.
37. Loback D, Young-Hing K, Cassidy JD, Tchang S. The relationship between facet orientation and lumbar disc herniation: the role of torsion in intervertebral disc failure. Orthop Trans. 1985;9:560.
38. Hagg O, Wallner A. Facet joint asymmetry and protrusion of the intervertebral disc. Spine. 1990;15:356–9.
39. Vital JM. Processus de dégénérescence lombaire: alternatives à l'arthrodèse lombaire et lombosacrée. In: Duparc J, editor. Cahiers d'enseignement de la SOFCOT N°96. Paris: Elsevier Masson; 2007. p. 1–7.
40. Epstein NE. Lumbar cysts: a review of diagnosis, surgical management, and outcome assessment. J spinal Disord Tech. 2004;17(4):321–5.
41. Maigne R. Le syndrome de la charnière dorsolombaire. Une source d'erreur de diagnostic. Maitrise Orthopédique. Janv 1998;70. maitrise.orthopedique.com.

The Spinal Ligaments

Jean Marc Vital

The ligaments act mainly to limit the movements of the spine. It can be considered that the intervertebral disc constitutes the strongest intervertebral ligament, by the annulus and especially by its posterior peripheral part considered as a full ligament portion; the middle column as described in traumatology by Denis, includes the posterior vertebral wall and the posterior third of the disc [1] (Fig. 1).

Certain ligaments have a protective function of the spinal canal and thus of the neurological elements within (posterior longitudinal ligament (PLL), yellow ligament (ligamentum flavum)).

Figure 2 shows the schematic arrangement of the spinal ligaments. Some are longitudinal and extend from the skull to the sacrum: the ventral (anterior) and dorsal (posterior) longitudinal ligaments (ALL and PLL) and the supra-spinous ligament. Others have a segmental arrangement and interconnect adjacent posterior arches: they have the particularity of being in continuity in the horizontal plane. They are from back to the front, the inter-spinous ligament and the yellow ligament, situated between the laminae, extending laterally to the articular capsules. We will see that there are variations according to the spinal level (especially at the level of the cranio-cervical junction) and that there are specific ligaments (stabilizing the roots or peripheral nerves, especially in the lumbar region).

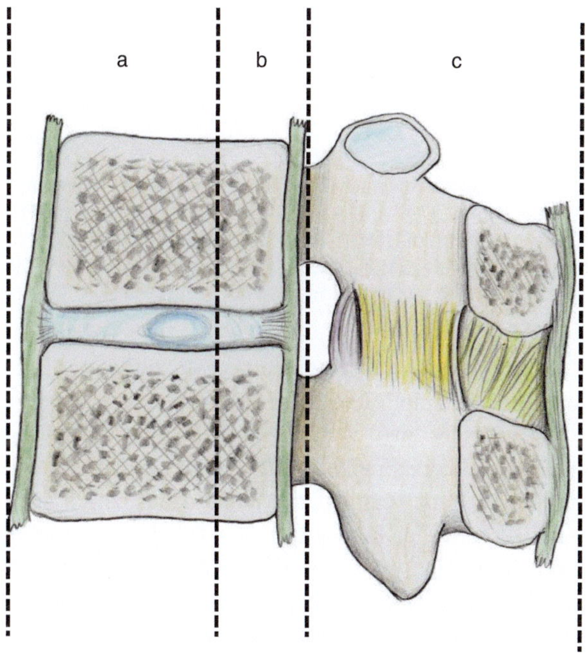

Fig. 1 The 3 spinal columns in traumatology according to Denis [1]: (*a*) Anterior column, (*b*) Medium column (with posterior annulus), (*c*) Posterior column

Ligaments in the Suboccipital Area

A complex ligamentous system around the transverse ligament, which constitues part of the cruciform ligament, with the apical and alar ligaments, stabilizes the odontoid process (peg) behind the anterior arch of C1.

On a strictly sagittal section (Fig. 3), the *PLL and ALL ligaments* are present: the first inserts on the exocranial aspect of the basilar process of the occiput, the second on the endocranial surface. These two ligaments extend to the sacrum and the first coccygeal vertebra. The PLL has an arrangement which varies according to the spinal levels, as discussed later.

The *supra-spinous ligament* does not exist at this level and is replaced by *the posterior cervical ligament or nuchal septum* [2] (Fig. 4). This very resistant sagittal septum inserts superiorly on the inion (or external occipital protuberance) and on the external occipital line, and inferiorly on the spinous process of C7. It separates the posterior muscular masses and consists of rather vertical occipital fibers and

J. M. Vital (✉)
Spinal Unit, University Hospital, Bordeaux, France

J. M. Vital, D. T. Cawley (eds.), *Spinal Anatomy*, https://doi.org/10.1007/978-3-030-20925-4_16

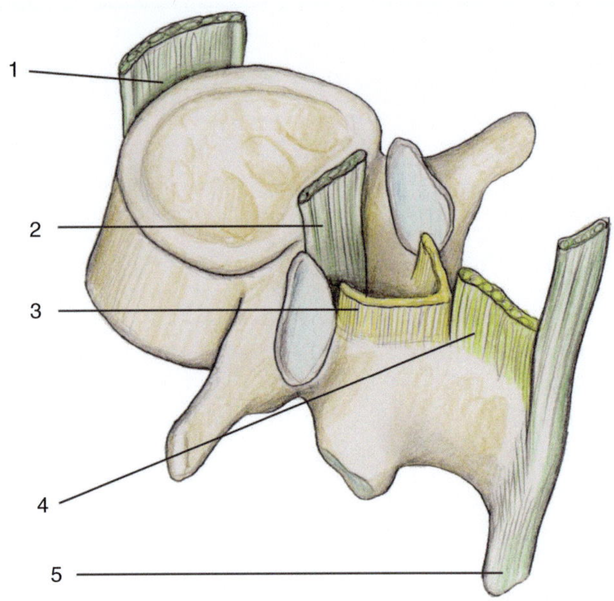

Fig. 2 Schematic presentation of the spinal ligaments: (1) Anterior longitudinal ligament (ALL); (2) Posterior longitudinal ligament (PLL); (3) Yellow ligament; (4) Inter-spinous ligament; (5) Supra-spinous ligament; (3), (4), and (5) are in continuity in the horizontal plane but they are not in continuity in the vertical plane as (1), (2), and (5)

fibers coming from the spinous processes, oblique in a posteroinferior direction. In a more recent description, Mercer [3] distinguishes two components from this nuchal ligament: a dense dorsal raphe formed by fibers from the upper trapezium, splenius capitis and rhomboideus, and a medial sagittal septum. For this author, it is the dorsal raphe that extends from inion to the spinous process of C7. The medial septum extends from the deep side of the raphe to the inter-spinous ligaments and the atlanto-axial and occipito-axial membranes anteriorly (Fig. 5).

The joint capsule and the yellow ligament only exist at C2–C3. Superiorly, there is a *dorsal occipito-atloid* membrane or *ligament* between CO and C1 (as described by Tubbs [4]) and a *dorsal atlanto-axial* membrane or *ligament* between C1 and C2, traversed by the nerve of Arnold (a.k.a. the dorsal branch of the second cervical nerve).

Around the odontoid process of C2 and the anterior arch of C1 there are a multitude of small ligaments.

The strictly median formations are from front to back (Fig. 3):

- The *ventral occipito-atloid ligament* (also called the anterior atloido- (or atlanto) occipital membrane) between the basilar process and the anterior arch of C1.
- The *ventral atloido-axial ligament* between the anterior arch of C1 and the anterior surface of the body of C2.
- The *medial occipito-odontoid ligament* or ligament of the apex of the odontoid process.

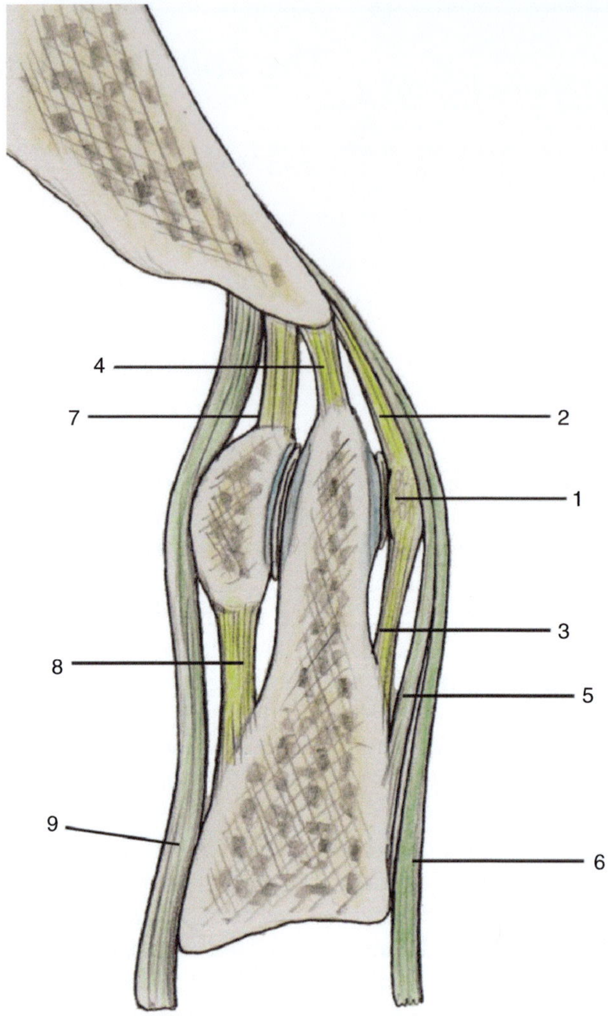

Fig. 3 Sagittal view of the suboccipital region: (1) Transverse ligament, (2) Occipito-transverse ligament; (3) Transverse-axial ligament; (4) Median O–C1 ligament (apex ligament); (5) O–C2 ligament; (6) PLL; (7) Ventral ligament O–C1; (8) C1–C2 ventral ligament; (9) ALL, (1), (2), and (3) = cruciate ligament of C1

- The *occipito-transverse ligament* between the basilar process and the transverse ligament which passes behind the odontoid process, which we shall describe in greater detail.
- The *transverse-axial ligament* which is inserted on the lower edge of the transverse ligament and joins the posterior surface of the base of the odontoid process.

These last two ligaments constitute the *longitudinal bundle* which, together with the *transverse ligament*, forms a true ligamental cross behind the odontoid process (*cruciform ligament of the atlas*).

- Finally, the *median occipito-axial ligament* lies between the longitudinal bundle and the PLL.
- The *membrana tectoria* (tectorial membrane) is the most posterior structure, located directly in front of the dura

mater [4]. Composed of three layers (superficial, medium, and deep), it has an average height of 6 mm between the clivus and the body of C2, a width of 3 mm and a thickness of 1 mm. This membrana tectoria extends to the lower cervical level to constitute the posterior layer of the PLL (as discussed later).

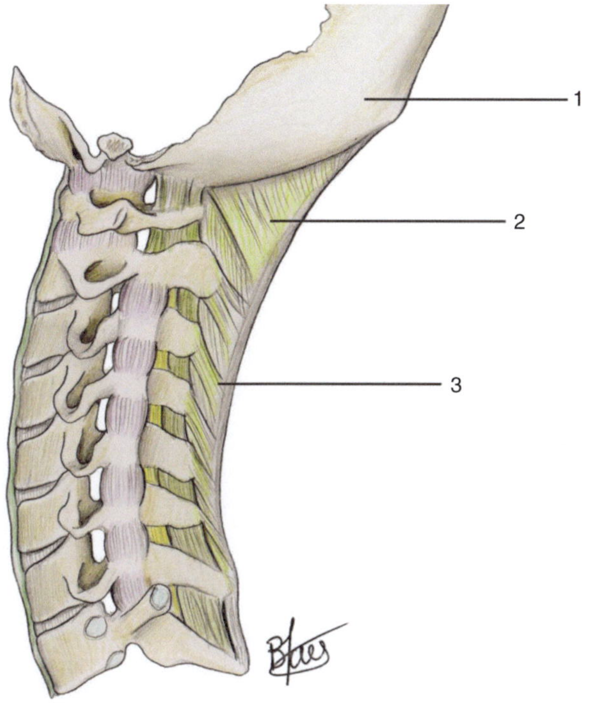

Fig. 4 Nuchal septum: (1) External occipital protuberance (inion); (2) Occipital fibrous fibers: (3) Spinous fibrous fibers

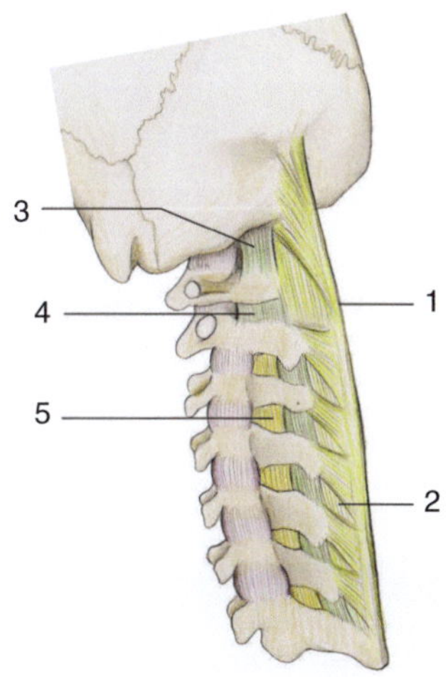

Fig. 5 (**a**) Nuchal septum (left postero-lateral view) (according to Mercer [3]): (1) Dorsal raphe; (2) Segmental portion of the nuchal ligament; (3) Posterior O–C1 membrane; (4) C1–C2 posterior membrane; (5) Yellow ligament. (**b**) Nuchal septum dissection: lateral view (*A*), posterior view (*B*) (Anatomy Conservatory of Montpellier, Pr F. Bonnel)

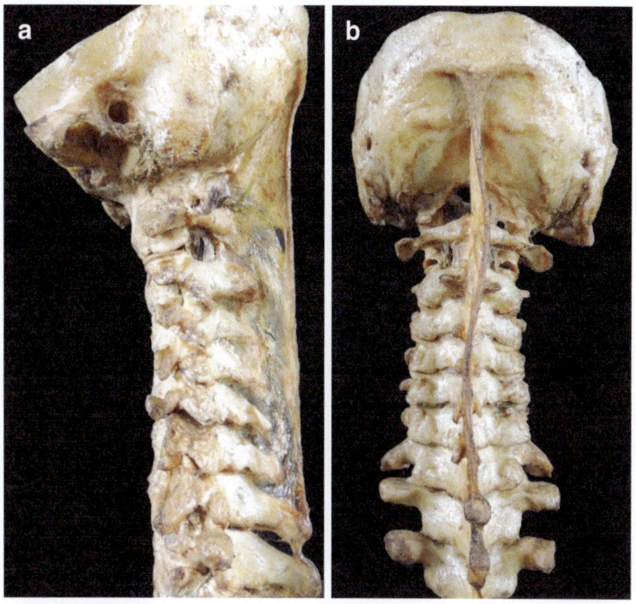

Fig. 5 (continued)

Figure 6 shows that there are paravertebral structures that are not visible on the strictly sagittal section. Those are:

- The *lateral occipito-atloid ligaments* which reinforce the lateral parts of the O-C1 capsules. Tubbs [5] described 20 anatomic specimens, with consistent findings; for this author, these left and right ligaments reduce lateral flexion and rotation of the O-C1 joint and have an essential role in stabilizing the cranio-cervical junction.
- The *lateral occipito-odontoid ligaments*, which insert on the lateral masses of the occiput, and terminate at the apex of the odontoid process, or somewhat below it, according to Osmotherly [6]: These alar ligaments terminate outside the apex ligament (Fig. 7) [7].
- The *transverse ligament* inserts on the medial side of the articular masses of the atlas; it leaves an imprint on the dorsal surface of the odontoid process and receives the fibers of the longitudinal bundle (occipito-transverse ligament at the top and transverse-axoid at the bottom) to form the cruciform ligament. Its rupture, most often traumatic, in a movement of hyperflexion, can sometimes lead to compression of the spinal cord (Fig. 7). Recently, Tubbs [4] described the *transverse occipital ligament* which he finds seven times out of ten between the occipital condyles and above the transverse ligament (Fig. 8).

The *Barkow ligament* is situated horizontally between the occipital condyles, which passes behind the alar ligaments and the apex of the odontoid process: this ligament reinforces the stabilizing effect of the transverse ligament at the level of the median atloido-axial joint.

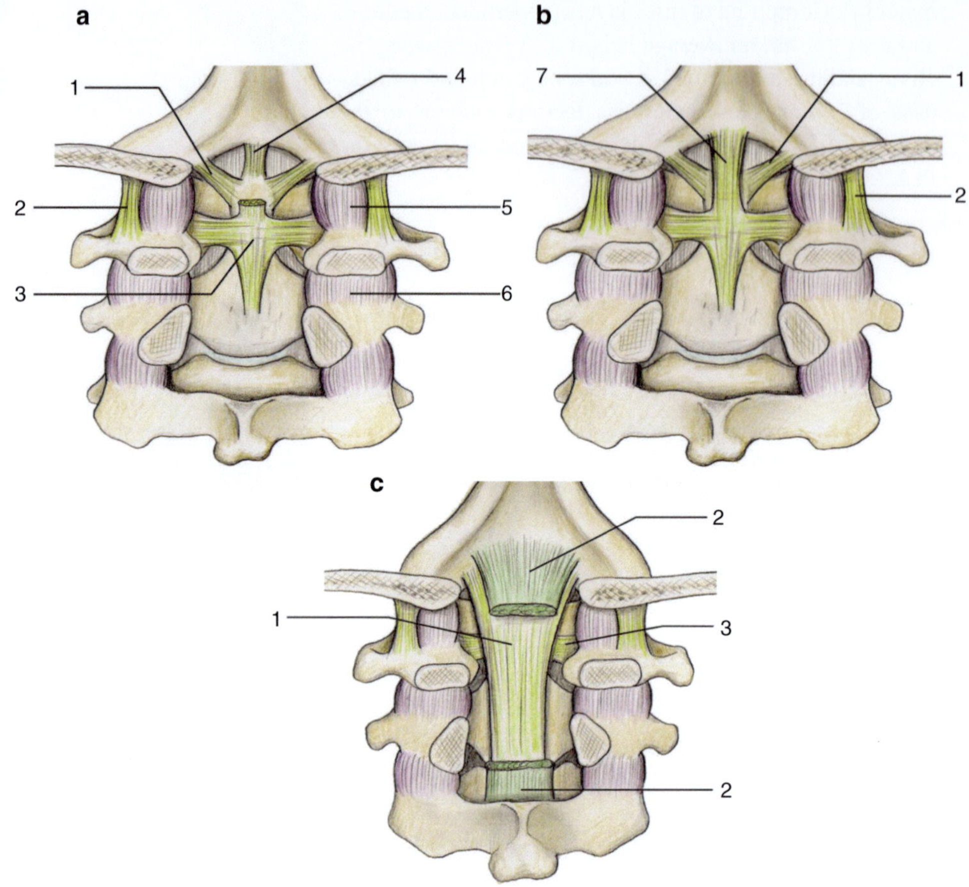

Fig. 6 Suboccipital ligaments (posterior view). After removal of the posterior arches of C1, C2, and C3, sections a to c from front to back. (**a**, **b**) (1) Lateral ligament O–C2; (2) Lateral ligament O–C1; (3) Transverse ligament; (4) Ligament of the apex, (5) Capsule C1–C2; (6) Capsule C2–C3; (7) Occipito-transverse ligament. (**c**) (1) O–C2 ligament; (2) PLL; (3) Lateral O–C2 ligament

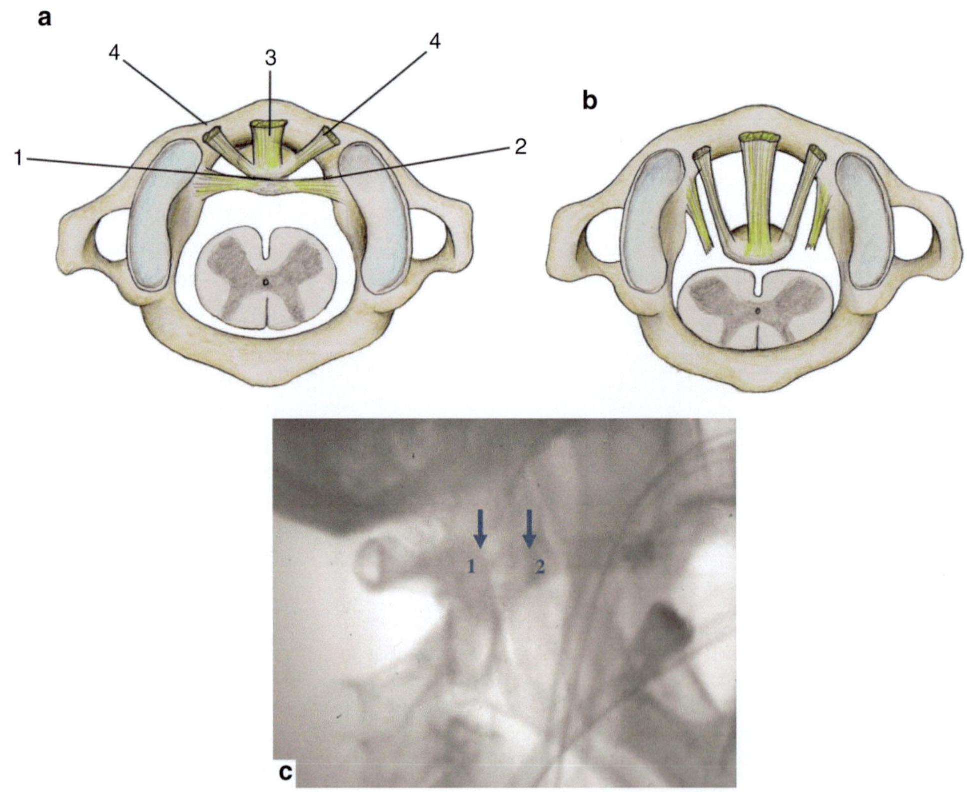

Fig. 7 Traumatic lesion of the transverse ligament with possible medullary compression in the case of stretching of the alar ligaments and of the apex ligament: (**a**) Normal top view: (1) Odontoid; (2) Transverse ligament; (3) Ligament of the apex; (4) Alar ligament. (**b**) Upper view after trauma (direct dislocation C1–C2). (**c**) Lateral X-Ray: (1) Odontoid; (2) Anterior arch of the atlas

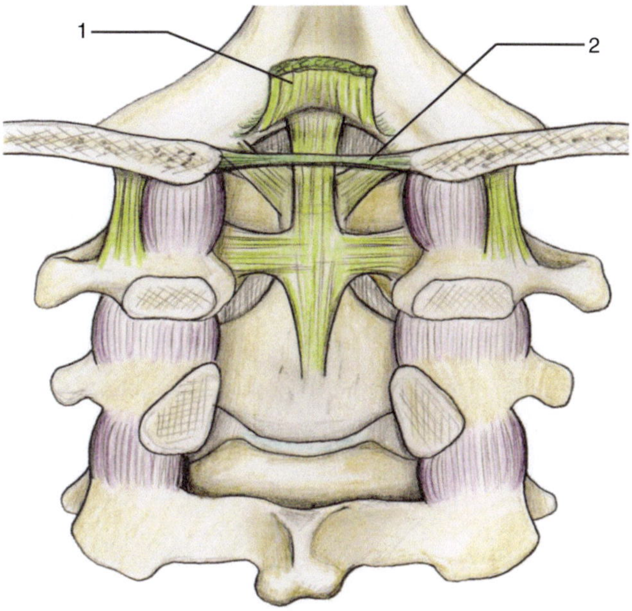

Fig. 8 Suboccipital ligaments (posterior view) according to Tubbs [4]: (1) Membrana tectoria; (2) Occipital transverse ligament

- The *lateral occipito-axial ligaments* (Fig. 6c) frame the median occipito-odontoid ligament, already described on the sagittal section.

Ligaments of the Lower Cervical Area

In a severe cervical sprain, all ligaments excluding ALL are ruptured, including the posterior annulus.

Figure 9 includes a lateral view, a sagittal section, and a cranial view. We find from front to back:

- The *ALL* which adheres to the discs and the vertebral bodies.
- The *intertransverse ligament* with close vertebral artery links.
- The *PLL*: Fig. 10 shows that it is made of two bundles: deep, which is thick and fused to the posterior surface of each vertebra, and superficial, which is thin and a prolongation of the tectorial membrane. Between these two bundles circulate the anterior venous plexus. The deep bundle loses its width from C3 to C7 (Fig. 11).
- The articular capsules extend posteriorly and medially as the *yellow ligament* (ligamentum flavum) between the laminae.
- The *inter-spinous ligament* has slightly oblique fibers in an inferior and posterior direction.
- The *supra-spinous ligament* inserts on the tips of the spinous processes; there is still at this level the thick fibrous *nuchal septum*, separating the posterior right and left muscular masses. Johnson [8], using the plastination technique on eight cadavers, shows that this nuchal septum is formed by aponeurosis of the trapezius, splenius capitis, rhomboideus, and posterior and superior serratus muscles.

The transverse line in Fig. 9c separates the ligamentous system from the discocorporeal complex (with PLL and ALL and intertransverse ligaments) and the ligamentous system of the posterior arch comprising all other ligaments. In a hyperflexion mechanism, the rupture of all the described ligamentous elements (posterior annulus included but excluding ALL) characterizes a *severe cervical sprain* to which we shall return (Fig. 12).

There are *extra-spinal ligaments* in the lower cervical as well as the lumbar level, which tie the spinal nerves to neighboring structures, in particular the transverse processes in the transverse foramina: they have been well described by Kraan [9] with variations depending on root levels.

The Ligaments of the Thoracic Area

There is a group of specific ligaments that firmly anchor the ribs to the vertebral bodies.

This thoracic region is made stable by the presence of the rib cage and therefore of the ribs. Some ligaments are similar to the cervical segment: the PLL, ALL, articular capsule, yellow ligament, inter-spinous, and supra-spinous ligaments which are also evident here (Fig. 13).

Johnson [10] shows by plastination technique on two adult cadavers that the supra-spinous ligament in the upper thoracic region is constituted by the fibers of the trapezius, the rhomboideus, and the splenius cervicis, while in the lower thoracic level it is constituted by the fibers of the thoracolumbar fascia.

What is different at this level comes from the ligaments between the ribs and the vertebrae (Fig. 14). The head of the rib articulates with two facets framing the disc on its posterolateral part: at this level lies the *radiate ligament* with a cranial bundle for the overlying vertebral body, a horizontal middle bundle that reinforces the annulus and a caudal bundle for the underlying vertebral body.

The *upper costo-vertebral ligament* extends between the lower edge of the transverse process and the medial side of the neck of the underlying rib.

The *intertransverse ligament* is situated behind the preceding one and joins, after a vertical path, the two adjacent transverse processes.

The *lateral costo-transversal ligament* is stretched between the top of the transverse process and the tubercle of

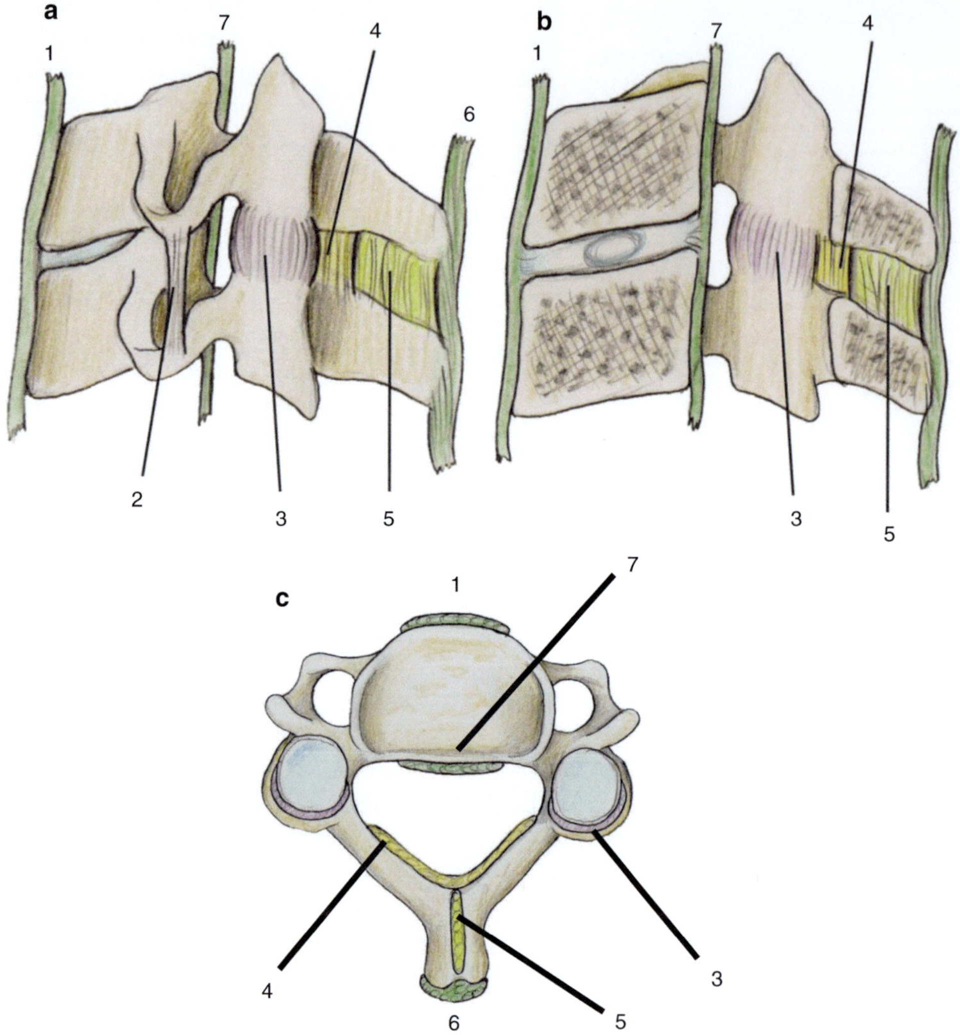

Fig. 9 Ligaments of the lower cervical spine: (**a**) Lateral view, (**b**) Sagittal section, (**c**) Cranial view. (1) ALL; (2) Inter-transversal ligament; (3) Joint capsule; (4) Yellow ligament; (5) Inter-spinous ligament; (6) Supra-spinous ligament; (7) PLL

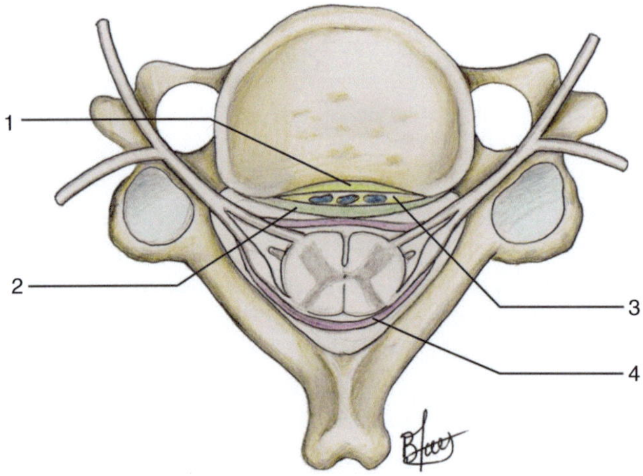

Fig. 10 PLL in the cervical region: (1) Deep layer; (2) Superficial layer (membrana tectoria); (3) Venous plexus; (4) Dura mater

the rib. Ibrahim [11], in a relevant study, describes superior and posterior costo-transverse bundles.

Ligaments of the Lumbar Area

Figures 15 and 16 show that the same ligaments are found here as in the cervical and thoracic areas. Figure 13 shows the oblique inferior and anterior direction of the fibers of the inter-spinous ligament which constitutes a limit on flexion.

Lumbar supra- and inter-spinous ligaments are reinforced, according to Johnson [10], by thoraco-lumbar fascia, longissimus, and multifidus. The PLL merits a specific description because it maintains special relationships with the annulus fibrosus and the anterior epidural venous plexus. Figure 15 shows that this ligament is narrow in relation to the vertebral bodies and that it widens in relation to the discs, which gives it

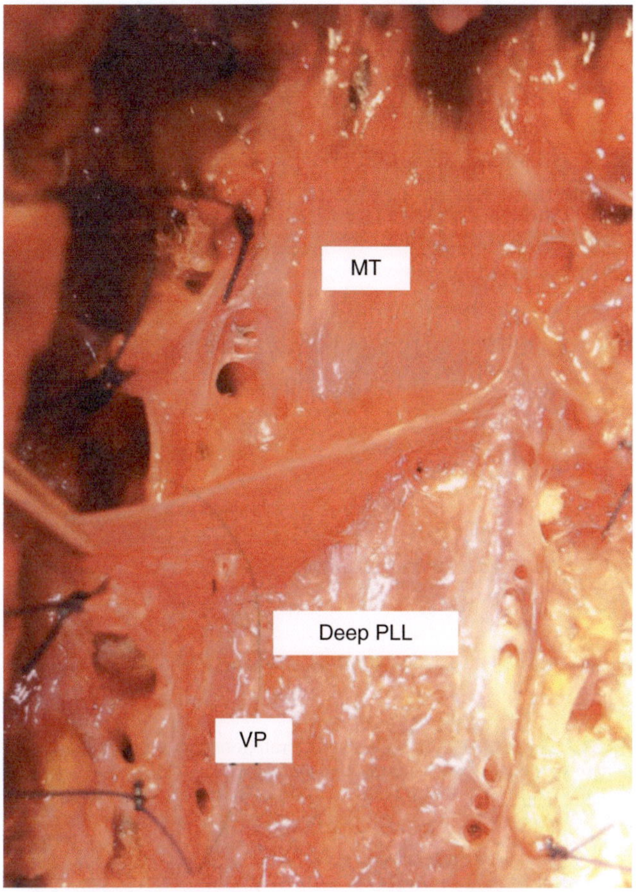

Fig. 11 Posterior view of the PLL in the cervical area with its deep and superficial layers. MT = Membrana tectoria; VP = Venous plexus

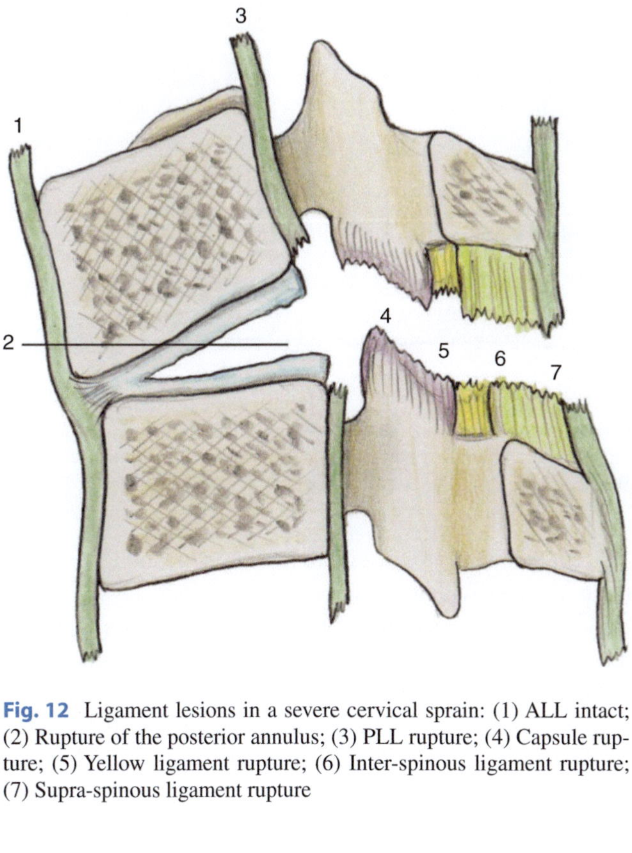

Fig. 12 Ligament lesions in a severe cervical sprain: (1) ALL intact; (2) Rupture of the posterior annulus; (3) PLL rupture; (4) Capsule rupture; (5) Yellow ligament rupture; (6) Inter-spinous ligament rupture; (7) Supra-spinous ligament rupture

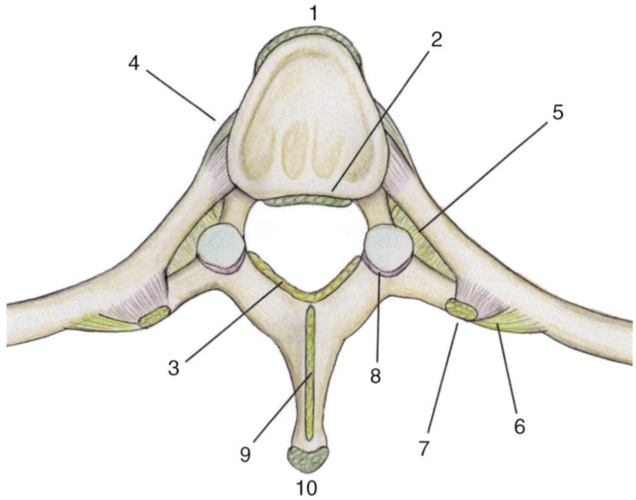

Fig. 13 Ligaments in the thoracic area (cranial view): (1) ALL; (2) PLL; (3) Yellow ligament; (4) Costovertebral radiate ligament; (5) Costovertebral upper ligament; (6) Costo-vertebral lateral ligament; (7) Intertransverse ligament; (8) Capsule; (9) Inter-spinous ligament; (10) Supra-spinous ligament

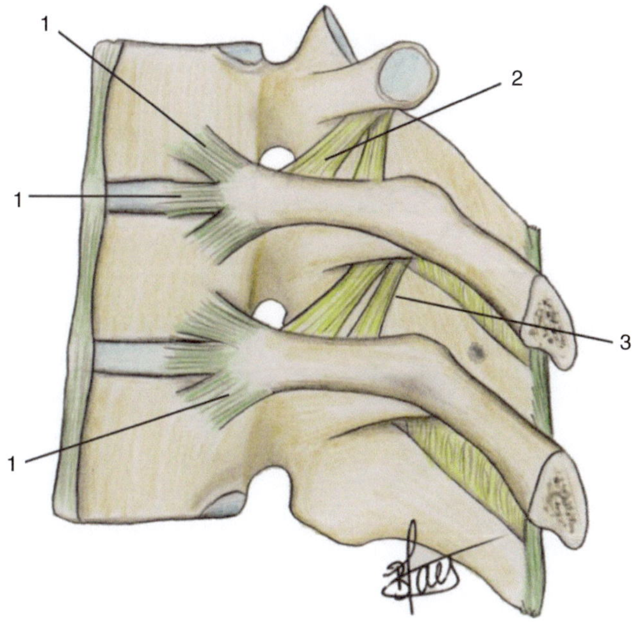

Fig. 14 Costo-vertebral ligaments (left lateral view): (1) Radiate ligament; (2) Upper costo-vertebral ligament; (3) Inter-transversal ligament

a typical scalloped appearance. It is very adherent to the intervertebral disc, less to the vertebral bodies due to the presence of corporeal venous plexuses. Oshima [12] notes a difference in adhesion of PLL to the disc in upper and lower lumbar level: less adhesion in the upper lumbar level, which explains the higher frequency of the median hernias and more adhesion in the lower lumbar level where postero-lateral hernias dominate.

The sagittal section (Fig. 17) shows that this ligament is adherent to the periphery of the disk and thus constitutes a natural barrier to herniation at the mid-line; It is, on the other hand, not very adherent to the vertebral bod-

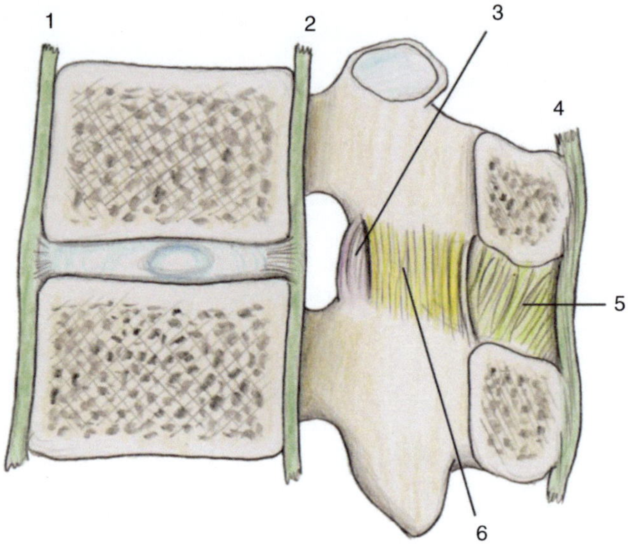

Fig. 15 Ligaments in the lumbar region (sagittal section): (1) ALL; (2) PLL; (3) Capsule; (4) Supra-spinous ligament; (5) Inter-spinous ligament; (6) Yellow ligament

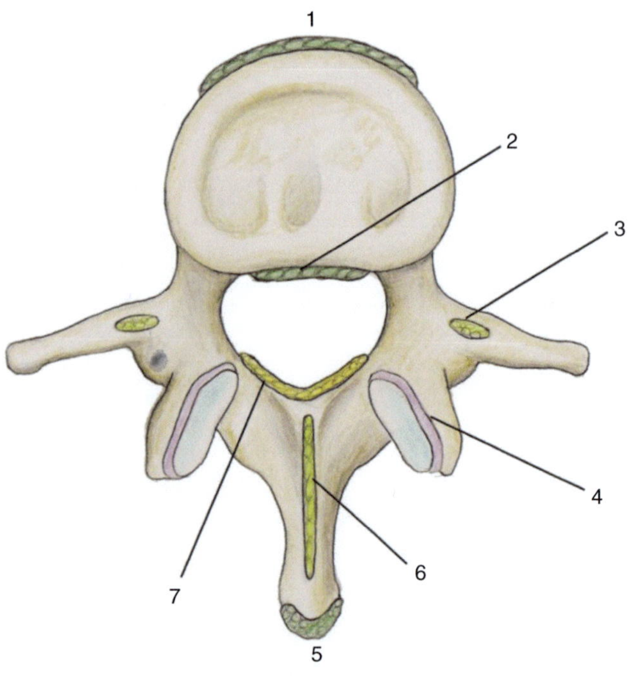

Fig. 16 Lumbar ligaments (upper view): (1) ALL; (2) PLL; (3) Inter-transversal ligament; (4) Capsule; (5) Supra-spinous ligament; (6) Inter-spinous ligament; (7) Yellow ligament

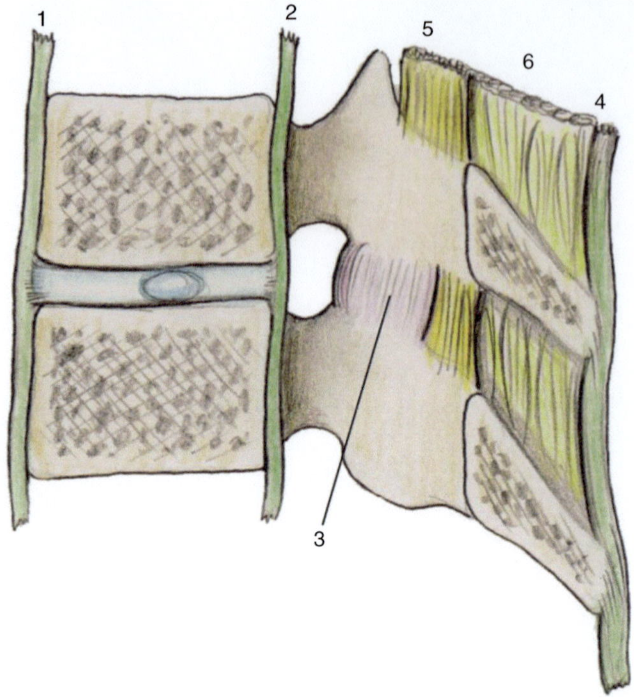

Fig. 17 Sagittal section showing the relationships between ALL: (1) and PLL; (2) and vertebral bodies and discs; (3) Capsule; (4) Supra-spinous ligament; (5) Yellow ligament; (6) Inter-spinous ligament

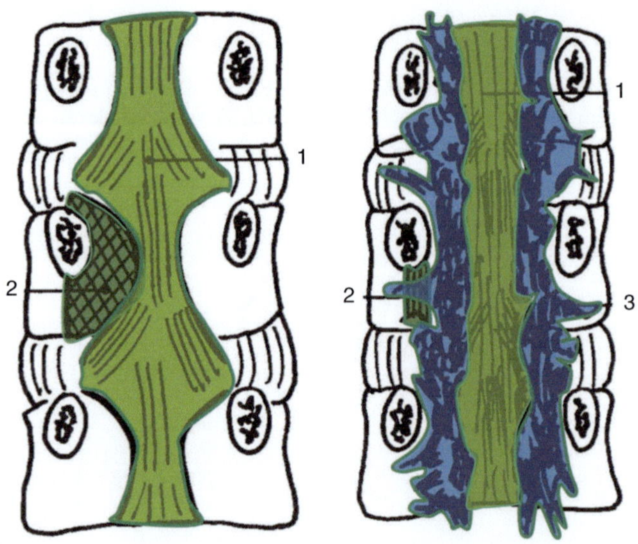

Fig. 18 The 2 layers of PLL in lumbar area (Posterior view after removal of the posterior arch): (1) Superficial layer; (2) Deep layer (epidural membrane); (3) Antero-lateral venous plexus (according to Wiltse [13])

ies, and the anterior venous plexus circulates between the posterior surface of the body and the ligament. Wiltse [13] gave a more detailed description of this ligament and described two bundles: one superficial, median, corresponding to the classic PLL and the other deep (or epidural membrane) which seems to correspond to the periosteum.

The venous plexus is situated between these two bundles (Fig. 18).

Loughenbury [14], in a more recent publication, describes three fascicles with an additional membranous layer.

More recently, Ansari [15] performed a meta-analysis on the anatomy of the *epi- or peridural membrane* assimilated to the peritoneum or pleura.

The ALL, unlike the PLL, adheres to the vertebral bodies and less to the discs, especially near the vertebral endplates.

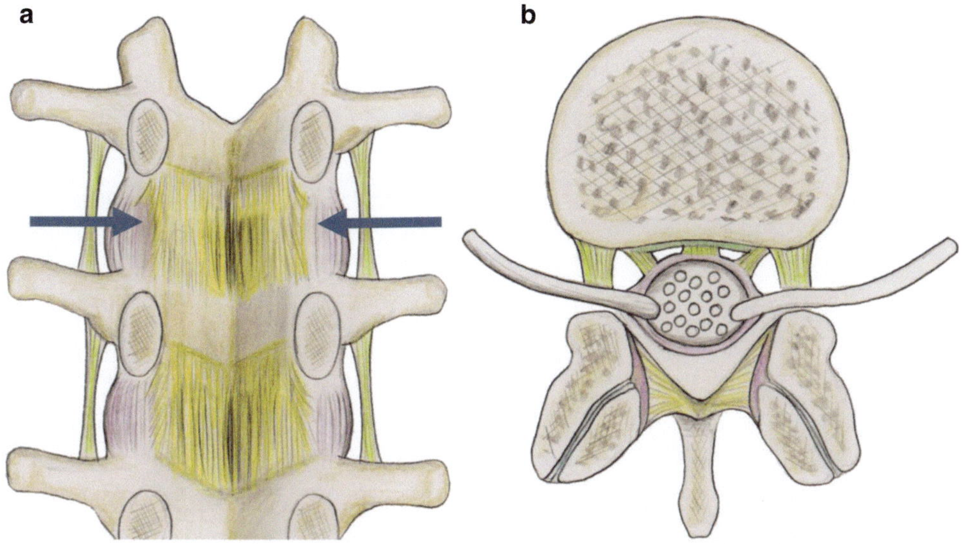

Fig. 19 Yellow ligament in the lumbar area: (**a**) Anterior view: the arrows show the lateral extension of the ligament. (**b**) Horizontal section: continuity between yellow ligament and capsule

The yellow ligament (or ligamentum flavum or interlamillary ligament), which closes the spinal canal behind the laminae, inserts below the cranial border of the lower lamina, above the middle of the ventral surface of the upper lamina (Fig. 19a), and laterally, it merges with the articular capsule (Figs. 19b and Fig. 20).

This ligament has the highest elastin/collagen ratio in the spine; its mean thickness is 3 mm (from 1.5 mm at the cervical level to 6 mm at the low lumbar level).

Olszewski [16], in a study of six fresh lumbar columns, confirms the presence of two layers, the superficial being thicker than the deep.

Some ligaments are specific to the lumbar region or at least have been better described because they may be involved in lumbar degenerative pathology.

The *fibrous formations described by Hofmann* [17] (Fig. 21) fix the middle part of the dura mater at its median part at PLL (medial ligament of Hofmann). The root itself, via the dura mater, is fixed by its anterior surface to the vertebral body (lateral ligament of Hofmann) and laterally, in the foramen, to the underlying pedicle (lateral radicular ligament). Wadhwani [18], on 18 dissected cadavers, has never found these Hofmann formations in the cervical spine but describes them between C7 and L4 in terms of dimensions and orientation. Yaszemski [19] describes these periradicular structures as "discectomy membrane" or "nerve root fibrovascular membrane" on five fresh cadavers; they are always found, as fine structures and limit the movements of the roots. Solaroglu [20] describes a ligament found ten times on 14 dissections (71%) which lies between the deep side of the yellow ligament and the L5 roots (ATA ligament); its presence increases the risk of dura mater tear in discal or arthritic decompression surgery.

Foraminal ligaments (Fig. 22), which exist in both the thoracic and lumbar areas, are in fact partitions creating compartments within the intervertebral foramen around the spinal nerve and the spinal ganglion in the upper part, and around the vessels, in particular the veins in the lower part [23]. These ligaments reduce the space around nerve structures but also protect them during movements [24]. The most classic and oldest description is that of Golub and Silverman: on ten cadavers they describe superior corporeal-transverse ligaments extending from front to back, from the postero-inferior angle of the upper vertebral body to the lower edge of the transverse process, inferior corporeal-transverse ligaments extending from back to front from the postero-inferior angle of the underlying vertebra and the neighboring disc, and finally, purely transforaminal ligaments, practically horizontal at the upper, middle, and lower part of the foramen. It should be noted that these ligaments are more frequently encountered in L1–L2, L3–L4, and L5–S1. They are three times less frequent in L4–L5 than in

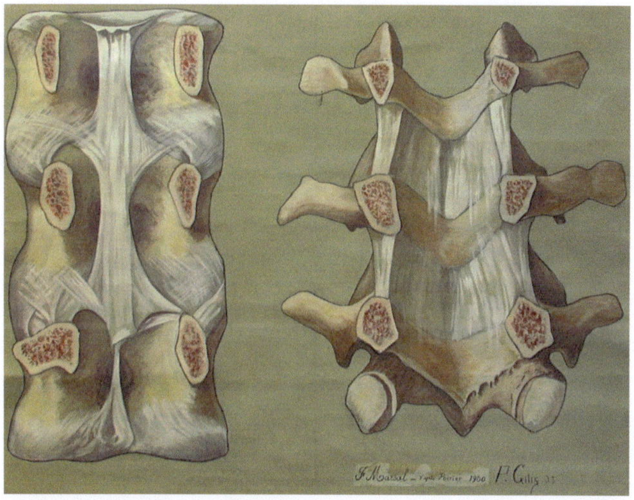

Fig. 20 Lumbar PLL on the left on a posterior view and yellow ligament on an anterior view on the right (Anatomy Conservatory of Montpellier)

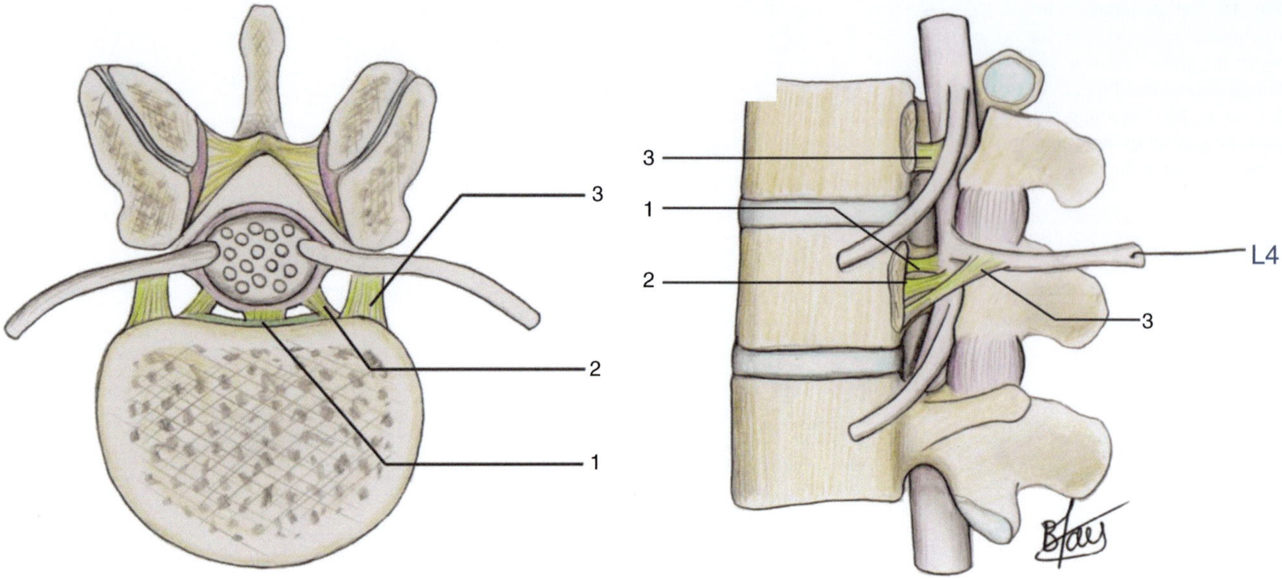

Fig. 21 Ligaments stabilizing roots (root L4 is posteriorly retracted): (1) Median ligament of Hofmann; (2) Lateral ligament of Hofmann; (3) Lateral radicular ligament

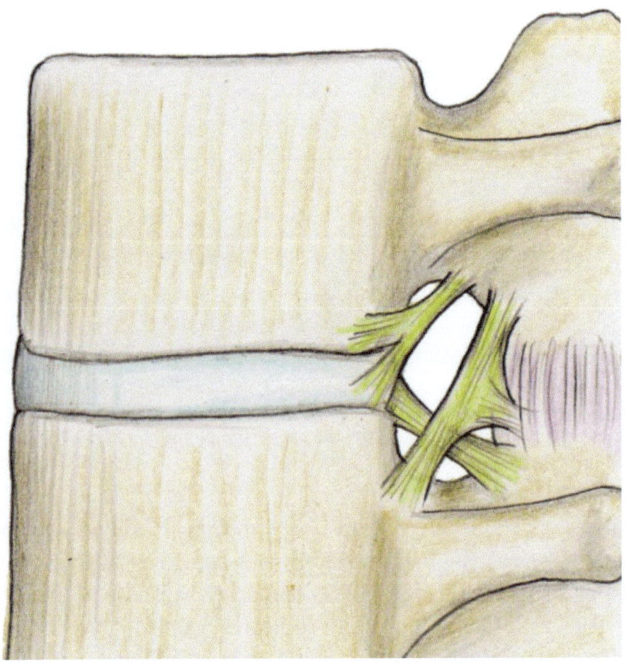

Fig. 22 Ligaments of the intervertebral foramen according to Amonoo Kuofi [21, 22]

L1–L2. More recently, Amonoo-Kuofi [21, 22] described ligamentous bands of the same arrangement but more dense at the top of the foramen. Finally, there is a true fibrovascular tethering around the spinal ganglion which makes it unmovable. Grimes [25] confirms on 12 cadavers the presence of superior, middle, and inferior trans-foraminal ligaments, which are increasingly thick from the upper lumbar to the lower lumbar region and which again limits the movements of the nerve structures.

The following ligaments are *extra-spinal*:

- *The intertransverse ligament* presents as a thin membrane or a thicker strip or a more complex structure with one leaflet joining the vertebral body and the other the articular process [26].
- *The mamillo-accessory ligament*, as described by Bogduk [27] situated between the upper tubercle and the accessory tubercle below, which together with the osseous structures constitutes a vertebral osteo-ligamentary canal for the medial branch of the medial dorsal nerve (Fig. 23); it is calcified in 10% of cases.
- *The transverse-corporeal or corporeal-transverse ligament* of Mac Nab [28] is situated between the L5 transverse process and the vertebral body; it can reduce the space within the L5–S1 foramen in its upper part and can create, for this author, an extra-foraminal compression of the L5 root (Fig. 24).
- Finally, the *iliolumbar ligaments* present three fascicles [29, 30] (Fig. 25):
  - the *upper fascicle* situated between the tip of the L4 transverse process and the iliac crest; this fascicle is oblique downwards and outwards in the frontal plane and is situated in a coronal plane.
  - The *lower iliac fascicle* lies between the lateral part of the transverse process of L5 and the iliac crest.
  - The *lower sacral fascicle* or lumbosacral ligament inserts, more medially, on the transverse process and ends at the anterior surface of the sacroiliac joint. These last two fascicles have the same oblique downward and outward direction in the coronal plane; in the sagittal plane, they are directed forward and downward. They

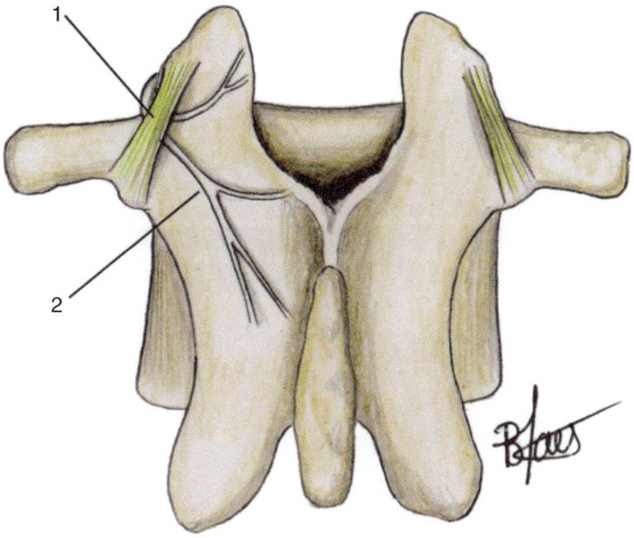

Fig. 23 (1) Accessory mammillary ligament (2) Medial branch of the dorsal ramus of the spinal nerve

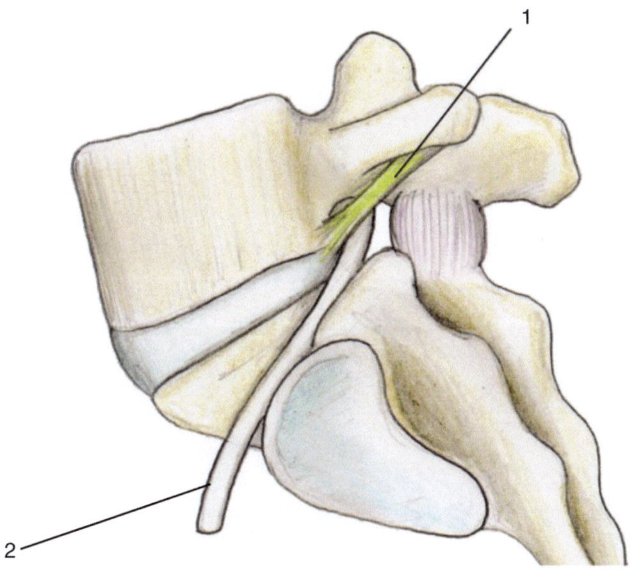

Fig. 24 Transverse-corporeal ligament on right side view: (1) Transverse-corporeal ligament; (2) Root L5

firmly anchor the fifth lumbar vertebra to the pelvic ring and protect the mobile segment (and therefore the disk) between the fifth lumbar vertebra and the sacrum (segment L5-S1), better than the upper fascicle which less protects the L4-L5 segment, thus more exposed to lumbar degeneration. Pool-Goudzwaard [31] describes in detail the two lower fascicles of the iliolumbar ligament. Amonoo-Kuofi [22] and Transfeldt [32] have described the lumbosacral ligament.

In the coronal plane, the fascicles of the iliolumbar ligament limit the contralateral inclination, in the sagittal plane, the upper fascicle limits the flexion, the two lower fascicles limit extension.

The Ligaments of the Sacral Area

The *ligaments of the sacroiliac joint* :

They are described in the specific chapter concerning this articulation.

The *saccrococcygian ligaments*:

They stabilize the sacrococcygeal joint, which is an amphiarthrosis (half-joints). There are anterior, posterior, and lateral ligaments (Fig. 26).

Ligaments in Spinal Pathology

Traumatology

In traumatology, the concept of severe ligamentous lesion from a tear is associated with that of a so-called persistent instability since the ligaments (including the intervertebral disc) have the particularity of poorly consolidating or healing with time.

This notion of instability, which has become persistent due to a severe ligamentous lesion, is the basis of classifications, notably of Magerl, which, in contrast to type A lesions of pure compression, where there is no ligamentous lesion, lesions of compression-posterior distraction (type B) with a possibility of a ligamentous lesion at the level of the ligamentous elements located between the posterior arches; the latter, because of this lasting instability, are much more appropriately treated surgically than type A lesions. Vaccaro [33], more recently, has developed a classification for thoracolumbar fractures where, using CT and MRI, it integrates these recognized ligamentous lesions.

We can retain two characteristic pure ligamentous lesions and thus surgical:

- Isolated lesions of the transverse ligament which is in fact a more complex lesion of both the transverse ligament, the alar ligaments, and probably the ancillary structures described by Tubb [5]; they are treated most often by a C1–C2 posterior arthrodesis.
- Severe cervical sprain (Fig. 27), in relation to a bending mechanism, with a back to front rupture of all the intervertebral ligaments: nuchal ligament, inter-spinous ligament, capsules, yellow ligament, PLL, and the posterior part of the annulus.

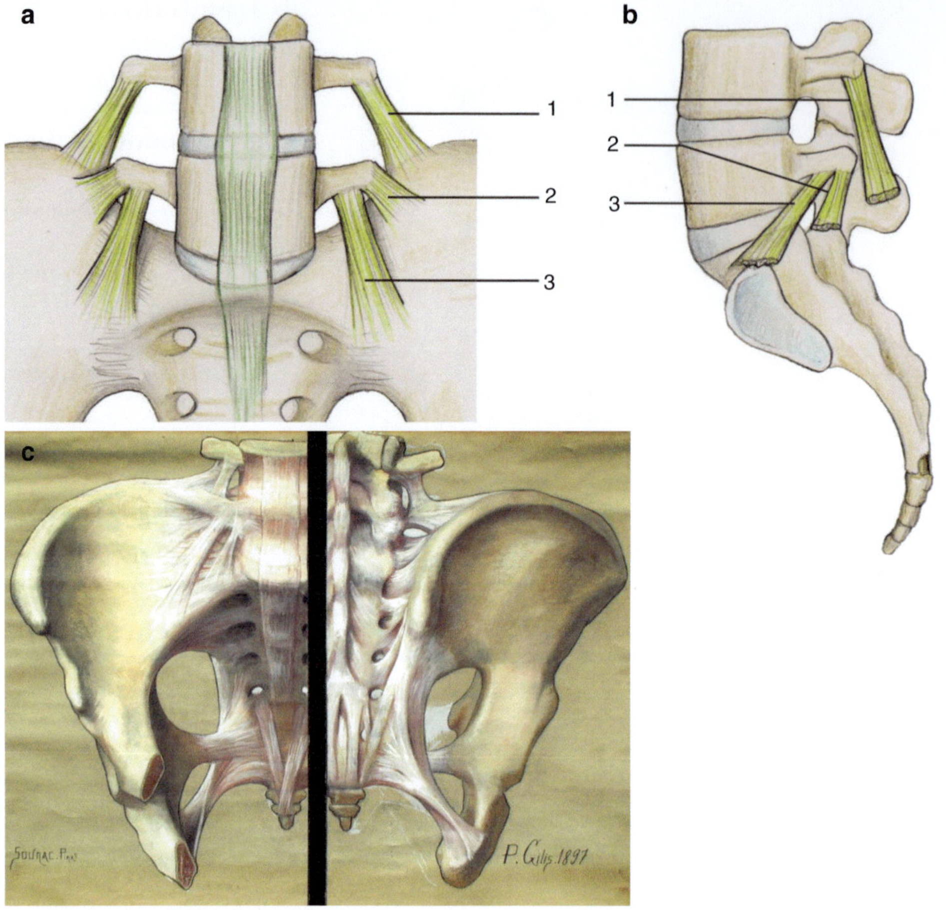

Fig. 25 Iliolumbar ligaments: (a) Anterior view, (b) Left side view, (c) Anterior (on the left) and posterior (on the right) (Anatomy Conservatory of Montpellier—Pr Bonnel): (1) Upper fascicle; (2) Lower iliac fascicle; (3) Lower sacral fascicle

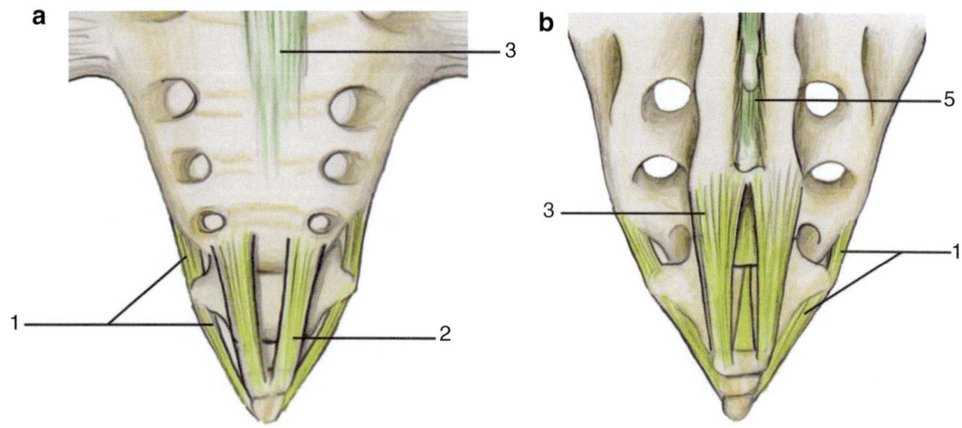

Fig. 26 Sacrococcygeal ligaments: (a) Anterior view, (b) Posterior view. (1) Lateral sacrococcygeal ligament; (2) Ventral sacrococcygeal ligament; (3) Dorsal sacrococcygeal ligament; (4) Termination of ALL; (5) Supra-spinous ligament

These lesions, which are more regularly recognized on dynamic bending images than on MRI, are surgical; the surgery performed anteriorly will detect the rupture of the disc and will be followed by an arthrodesis with graft and plate.

Degenerative Pathology

Cervical Level

- Soft disc herniation is a special entity, which in eight times out of ten demonstrates a postero-lateral fragment that will pass behind the PLL and therefore its posterior layer which is in the prolongation of the membrana tectoria. It is behind these deep and lateral layers that the hernia must be found.
- The PLL, and mainly its median, thick and anterior part, can be ossified in the case of ossifications of PLL. This entity is much more often found in Asian than in Caucasian subjects. There may be predominant factors such as diabetes, obesity, and hyperparathyroidism. These so-called OPLL lesions (ossification of the posterior longitudinal ligament) can cause myelopathy and are invariably associated with an adhesion to the dura mater.

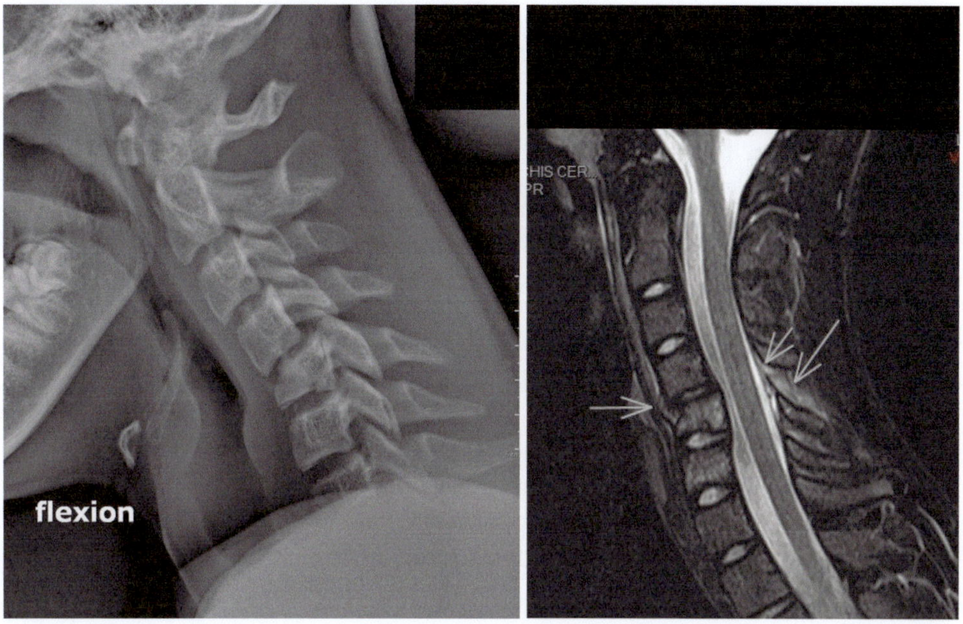

Fig. 27 Dynamic X-rays and MRI images of a severe C7–T1 sprain; all the posterior ligaments and the disc are ruptured

Thoracic Level

Soft disc herniation, or particularly, with calcification, can be approached anteriorly. It is known that the disc level is exactly at the level of the rib head, thus is necessary to disarticulate with dissection of all the described ligaments, in particular the radiate ligament.

Lumbar Level

- The PLL by its anatomy explains the frequency of postero-lateral (para-median) herniations apart from its discal indentations and the possibility also of sequestered pre-ligamentous medial hernias that lead to stenosis of the canal (so-called stenotic herniation). This ligament can become calcified or ossify at the cervical level in the context of an OPLL or Forestier disease (diffuse idiopathic skeletal hyperostosis).
- The yellow ligament is a ligament most often excised during the interlaminar approach, especially for herniated disc surgery. It is also a ligament which can become compressive due to its thickening and infolding in connection with intervertebral telescoping; it can sometimes be loaded with hydroxyapatite. In the context of a complete excision during a decompression, it must be remembered that it inserts on the upper edge of the lower lamina and that it raises high on the anterior surface of the upper lamina where it is best to approach it.
- The ligaments of Hofmann, as well as the ligaments described in the transverse aspect of the cervical area or in the lumbar area (notably at L5–S1), are ligaments which limit root movement and which sometimes explain in case of adhesions, tears of the dura mater.

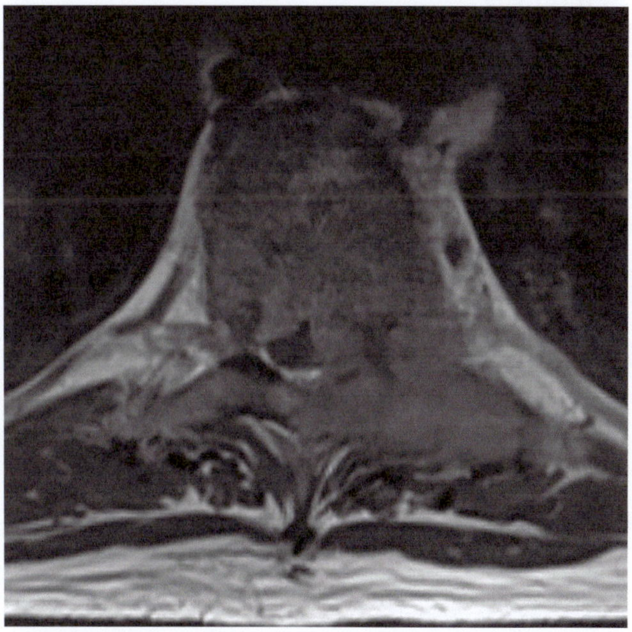

Fig. 28 "Curtain Sign" in a vertebral metastasis enveloping the epidural membrane but is resisted by the firmly attached medial ligament of Hofmann which shield the tumor from herniating in the midline

The ligaments of the intervertebral foramen are numerous and explain the small movements of the spinal ganglion and its easy compression.

Tumor Pathology

It should be noted especially in spinal metastasis that the venous plexus (elements essential in metastatic dissemination) are related to the PLL, and, in particular, its deep and superficial fascicles. The presence of the median Hofmann ligament very often explains the so-called curtain sign in tumoral spread, the superficial structure of the dorsal longitudinal ligament serving as the last shield between the dura mater and the invaded vertebral body (Fig. 28).

Spinal Deformities

In Scheuermann's kyphosis, associated with lesions of the vertebral end plates, there has been described a thickening and retraction of the anterior longitudinal ligament which, for some, made it obligatory in the surgical treatment of these deformities, to cut this ligament. This attitude is currently abandoned in favor of the isolated posterior pathway with the practice of Ponte osteotomies.

References

1. Denis F. The column spine and significance in the classification of acute thoracolumbar injuries. Spine. 1983;8:817–31.
2. Paturet G. Traité d'anatomie Humaine. Tome 1, Ostéologie – Arthrologie – Myologie. Paris: Masson; 1951.
3. Mercer SR, Bogduk N. Clinical anatomy of ligamentum nuchae. Clin Anat. 2003;16:484–93.
4. Tubbs RS, Hallock JD, Radcliff V, Naftel RP, Mortazavi M, Shoja MM, Loukas M, Cohen-Gadol AA. Ligaments of the craniocervical junction. J Neurosurg Spine. 2011;14:697–709.
5. Tubbs RS, Stetler W, Shoja MM, Loukas M, Han-Sasuta A, Liechty P, Acakpo-Satchivi L, Wellons JC, Blount JP, Salter EG, Oakes WJ. The lateral atlan-to-ocipital ligament. Surg Radio Anat. 2007;29:219–3.
6. Osmotherly PG, Rivett DA, Mercer SR. Revisiting the clinical anatomy of the alar ligaments. Eur Spine J. 2013;22:60–4.
7. White A, Panjabi M. Clinical biomechanics of spine. Philadelphie: Lippincott; 1978.
8. Johnson GM, Zhang M, Jones DG. The fine connective tissue architecture of the human ligamentum nuchae. Spine. 2000;25:5–9.
9. Kraan GA, Smitth TH, Hoogland PV. Extraforaminal ligaments of the cervical spinal nerves in humans. Spine J. 2011;11:1128–34.
10. Johnson GM, Zhang M. Regional differences within the human supraspinous and interspinous. ligaments: a sheet plastination study. Eur Spine J. 2002;11:382–8.
11. Ibrahim AF, Darwish HH. The costotransverse ligaments in human. Clin Anat. 2005;18:340–5.
12. Ohshima H, Hirano N, Osada R, Matsui H, Tsuji H. Morphologic variation of lumbar posterior longitudinal ligament and the modality of disc herniation. Spine. 1993;18:2408–11.
13. Wiltse LL, Fonseca AS, Amster J, Dimartino P, Ravessoud FA. Relationship of the dura, Hofmann's ligament, Batson's plexus and fibrovascular membrane lyring on the deep of the posterior longitudinal ligament. Spine. 1993;18:1030–43.
14. Loughenbury P, Wadhwani S, Soames R. The posterior longitudinal ligament and peridural (epidural) membrane. Clin Anat. 2006;19:487–92.
15. Ansari S, Heavner JE, Mcconnel JE, Azari H, Bosscher HA. The peridural membrane of the spinal canal. A critical review. Pain Pract. 2012;12:315–25.
16. Olszewski AD, Yaszemski MJ, White AA. The anatomy of the human lumbar ligamentum flavum. New observations and their surgical important. Spine. 1996;21:2307–12.
17. Hofmann M. Die befestigung der duramater in wirbelkanal. Arch F Anat Physio. 1898:403.
18. Wadhwani S, Loughenbury P, Soames R. The anterior dural (Hoffman) ligaments. Spine. 2004;29:623–7.
19. Yaszemski MJ, White AA. The dissectomy membrane (nerve root fibrovascular membrane): its anatomic description and its surgical importance. J Spinal Disord. 1994;7:230–5.
20. Solaroglu I, Okutan O, Beskonakli E. The ATA and its surgical importance. Spine. 2011;36:1268–972.
21. Amonoo-Kuofi MS, El Badawi MG, Fatani JA. Ligaments associted with lumbar intervertebral foramina 1 L1 to L4. J Anat. 1988;156:177–83.
22. Amonoo-Kuofi MS, El Badawi MG, Fatani JA, Butt MM. Ligaments associted with lumbar inter-vertebral foramina 2 the fifth lumbar level. J Anat. 1988;159:1–10.
23. Akdemir G. Thoracic and lumbar intraforaminal ligaments. J Neurosurg Spine. 2010;13:351–5.
24. Nowicki BH, Haughton VM. Ligaments of the lumbar neural foramina: a sectionnal antomy study. Clin Anat. 1992;5:126–35.
25. Grimes PF, Massie JB, Garfin SR. Anatomic and biomechamical analysis of the lower lumbar forminal ligaments. Spine. 2000;25:2009–14.
26. Behrsin JF, Brigg CA. Ligaments of the lumbar spine: a review. Surg Radio Anat. 1988;10:211–9.
27. Bogduk N. The lumbar mamillo accessory ligament: its anatomical and neurosurgical significance. Spine. 1982;6:162–7.
28. Mac Nab I, Mac Culloch J. Bach ache (2e édition). Baltimore: William and Wilkins; 1990.
29. Kapandji IA. Physiologie articulaire. 3. Tronc et rachis. Paris: Maloine; 1994.
30. Martinez C. Le Rachis, Cahier d'Anatomie Vivante. Paris: Masson; 1982.
31. Pool-Goudzwaard AL, Kleinrensink GJ, Snijders CJ, Entius C. The sacroiliac part of the iliolumbar ligaments. J Anat. 2001;199:457–63.
32. Transfeldt EE, Roberston D, Bradford DS. Ligaments of the lumbosacral spine and their role in possible extra-foraminal spinal nerve entrapment and tethering. J Spinal Disord. 1993;6:507–12.
33. Patel AA, Vaccaro AR. Thoracolumbar spine trauma classification. J Am Acad Orthop Surg. 2010;18:63–71.

Sacroiliac Joints

B. Lavignolle

Descriptive and Functional Anatomy of the Pelvic Girdle

The transition region between the lumbar spine and the lower limbs, the pelvic girdle retains its original character, designed for stability and stress transmission of body weight. Unlike the shoulder girdle, it has very strong connections with the caudal spine and its ventral parts, where it forms a hammock for the abdominal viscera.

This girdle forms a ring comprised of three parts: posteriorly the sacrum, and the two iliac bones or coxa laterally and anteriorly. The coxa consists of three welded parts: the ilium, pubis, and the ischium, joined at the acetabulum after ossification of Y cartilage around the age of 12. These three bones are joined together by three articulations: both sacroiliac joints posteriorly and the pubic symphysis anteriorly (Fig. 1).

The Pubic Symphysis

The pubic symphysis joins both pubic bones and constitutes a fibrocartilaginous articulation of the amphiarthrosis type. The articular surfaces are ovoid, of 32 mm by 12 mm on average, with the long oblique axis aligned anterosuperiorly at an inclination of 40°. An intervertebral, wedge-shaped fibrocartilage disc fills the larger joint space anteroinferiorly.

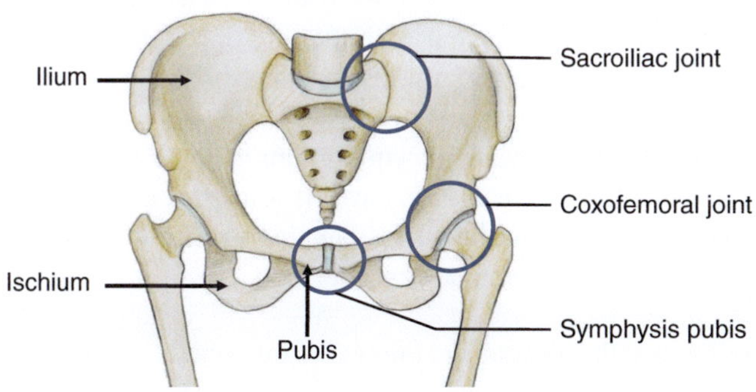

Fig. 1 General arrangement of the pelvic girdle

The ligaments are located on the four sides—anterior, posterior, superior, and inferior (or arched).

Mobility (Walheim [1]) is very low with a craniocaudal displacement of 1 mm for males and 1.6 mm for females; anterior translation of 0.5 mm (males) and 0.9 mm (females); sagittal translation <1 mm and frontal and sagittal rotations <1.5°.

There are small movements during childbirth and sport (football) which can cause pain (pubalgia) and arthropathic deterioration.

In severe trauma of the pelvis, there may be a disruption of the symphysis, sometimes associated with a fracture or a dislocation with sacroiliac instability by rupture of the pelvic ring (Sénégas [2]).

Sacroiliac Joints

The sacroiliac joints are the association of a synovial joint in the anterior part, and a posterior syndesmosis by the interosseous and posterior ligaments. The posterior volume of the interosseous ligament is almost the same size as the anterior articular surface without significant difference in both sexes (Klein [3]) (Fig. 2).

The sacral cartilage is three times thicker than the coxal cartilage, 2.5 mm versus 1 mm on average (Bogduk [4]).

The convex parts refer to the coxal bone and the concave parts to the sacrum (Farabeuf [5], Weils [6]). The aspect is reversed at the bottom third.

The articular surfaces are constituted of the coxa and sacrum in a crescent shape at the posterior concavity whose center of curvature corresponds to the iliac tuberosity and the perforated fossa of the sacrum.

The articular surfaces have an elongated L shape with a long, almost horizontal, upright arm of 5.4 cm ± 0.5 cm, and

B. Lavignolle (✉)
Anatomy Laboratory, Bordeaux University Hospital, Bordeaux, France

J. M. Vital, D. T. Cawley (eds.), *Spinal Anatomy*, https://doi.org/10.1007/978-3-030-20925-4_17

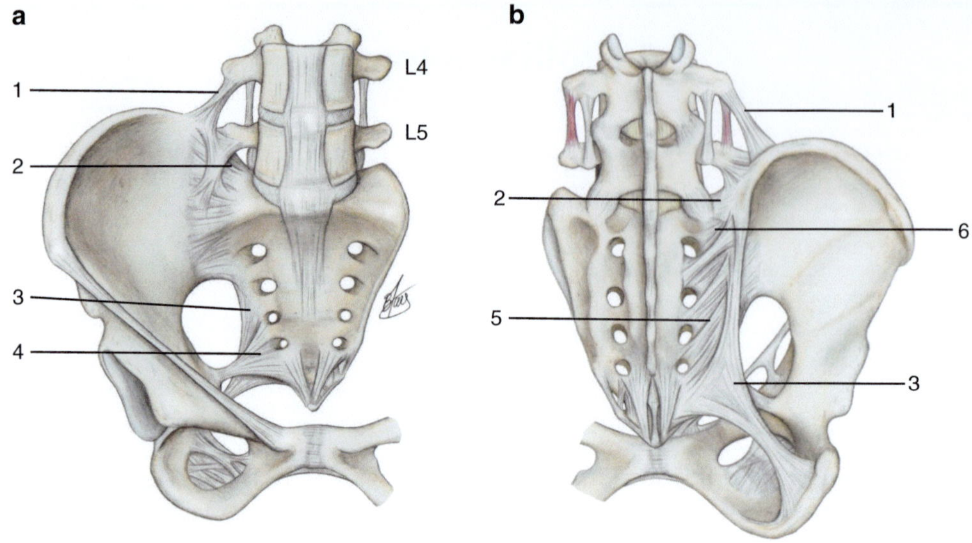

Fig. 2 Ligaments of the sacroiliac joint on a ventral (**a**) and dorsal (**b**) view: (1) iliolumbar ligament; (2) Sacroiliac ligament superior; (3) Sacrotubal ligament; (4) Sacrospinous ligament; (5) Superficial posterior sacrio-iliac ligament; (6) Deep sacroiliac ligament

an almost vertical short arm of 2.9 cm ± 0.6 cm; (Klein [3]), with an open angle backwards of 110° ± 11° (Fig. 3).

The joint space is oblique anterolaterally from 12° to 20° with respect to the sagittal plane (angle of declination) and oblique at the bottom and within 75–85° with respect to the transverse plane (angle of inclination). The line has a double obliquity which favors the isolation of the sacral corner and the stability of non-coaxial sacroiliac joints. This also allows the asymmetrical movements of the two coxal bones with helical oblique axes. The sacroiliac joint extends over three sacral bone segments (S1–S3).

Classically, the innervation is posterior from the posterior branches of L4–S3 and anterior from the anterior branches of L2–S2 (Klein [3]). However, contradictory studies describe an exclusively posterior innervation from the dorsal branches S1 and S2 (Bogduk [4]).

With age, the articular surfaces show erosion and fibrillation of cartilage with a loss of thickness. The capsule and synovium become thicker and more fibrous especially after 50 years (Bogduk [4]). The sacral cartilage decreases by 1 mm and ilium decreases by 0.5 mm, i.e. 50% of the thickness with restriction of mobility. Ankylosis is one of the first signs of pelvispondylitis.

The Sacrococcygeal Joint

The sacrococcygeal joint is an amphiarthrosis with ventral and dorsal interosseous and sacrococcygeal ligaments, remnant of the tail in humanoid primates. The mobility is 15° in flexion while seated and during the contraction of the pelvic floor muscles (Maigne [7]).

This joint has no role in the pelvic girdle but is the origin of coccygodynia from its hypermobility (traumatic or postpartum).

Biomechanical

Static: The Pelvic Girdle Is Hyperstable

Stability in the Frontal Plane

The pelvis forms an arch whose apex is the sacrum acting as a wedge between the two hip bones. The body weight is transmitted to the lower limbs by means of the sacroiliac joints and coxal bones to the hip joint and joints of the ground reaction force towards the symphysis pubis. The interosseous ligament is very powerful as well as the force of the abductor muscles (Klein [3]).

Stability in the Transverse Plane

The pelvis is held between the two coxal bones like a nut between the arms of a nut-cracker. Posterior sacroiliac ligaments ensure the power of the damping system according to a second or third class lever with the pressure of the femoral heads (Figs. 4 and 5). The equilibrium is likened to a torsion bar with the role of the lateral rotator pelvitrochanteric muscles, especially the piriformis muscle.

In the sagittal plane, the equilibrium is unstable (Fig. 6). The lumbopelvic wedge (Klein [3]) joins the lumbosacral junction, pelvis, and hip. This damping system is linked to the evolution of Homo erectus with:

- Levers: the sacrum and the two coxal bones.
- The articular links: sacroiliac joints, symphysis, and coxofemoral with a closed kinetic chain. A movement in one articulation necessarily causes movement in the other articulation. The sacrum cannot move freely.
- The passive brakes of sacral nutation (oscillatory movements within the axis of rotation) are the powerful

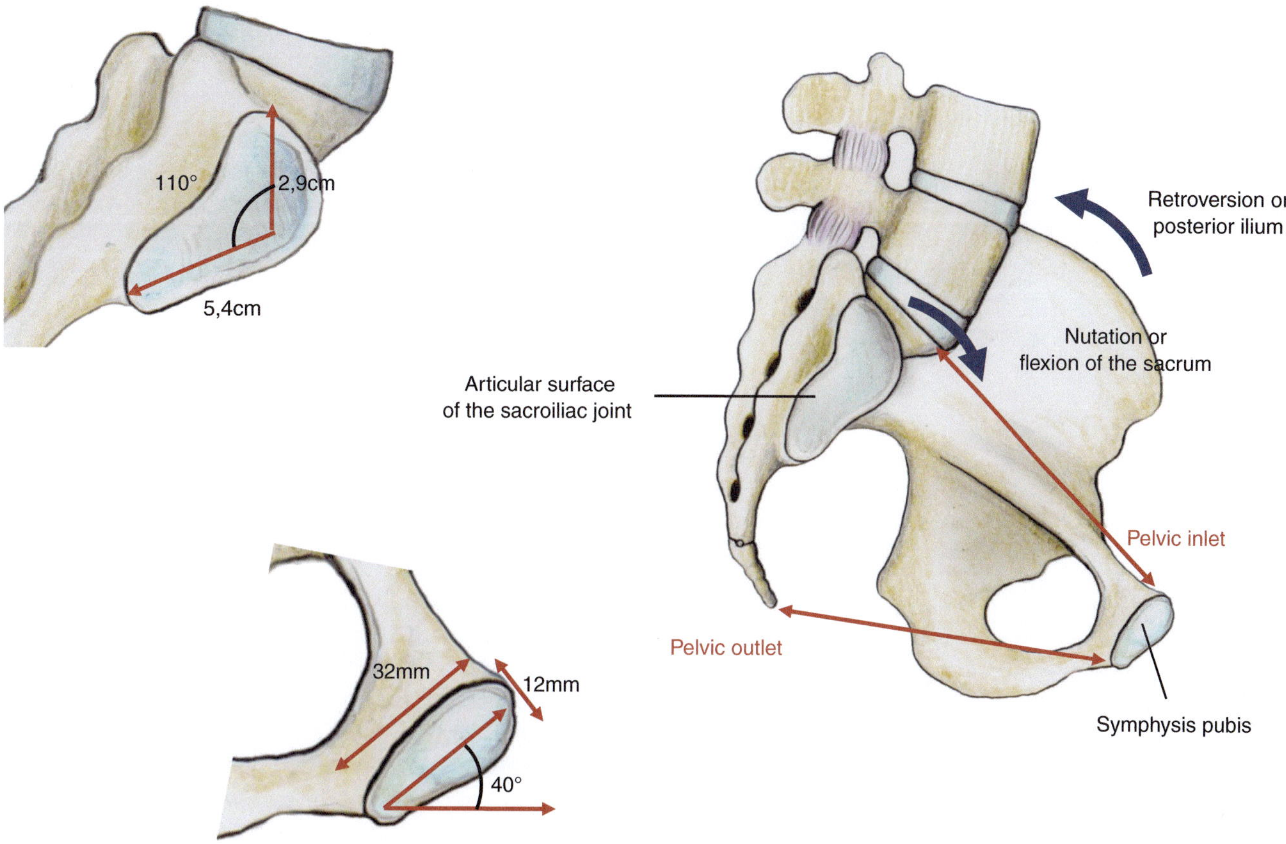

Fig. 3 The joints of the pelvic girdle

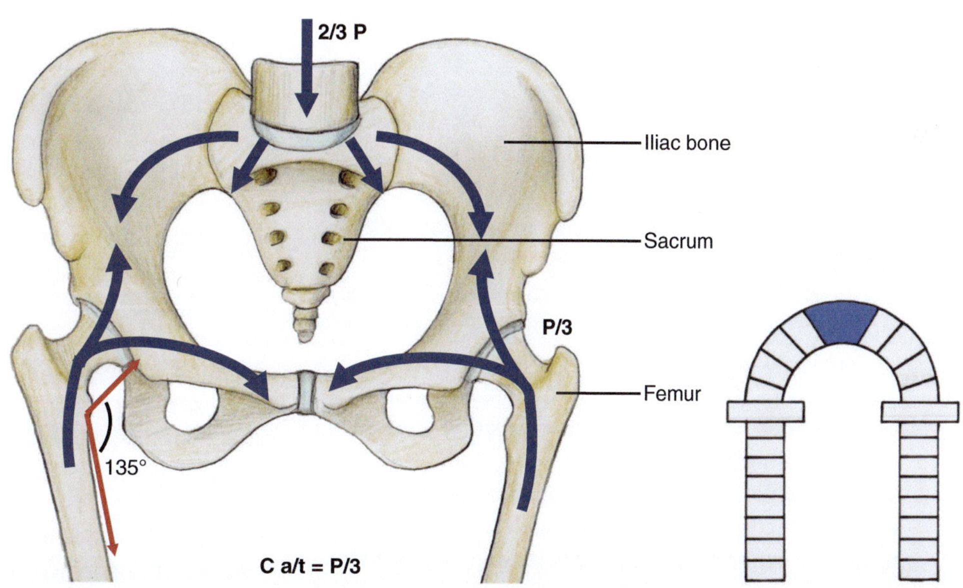

Fig. 4 Static in the frontal or coronal plane, *C a/t* = constraints of the acetabulum on the femoral heads

sacrospinous and sacrotuberal ligaments and the active brakes are the iliac muscles, hip flexors (right femoral, fascia lata tensor, sartorius), piriform muscles, and pelvic floor.

- The psoas muscle induces a moment of flexion on the lumbar spine and lumbosacral junction in the sense of nutation (Sturesson [8]).

Kinematics of the Sacroiliac Joint

Classical Studies

No movement has been described until that of Vesalius:

- Zaglas [9] describes the rotational movements of the sacrum with respect to the coxal bone with changes in the

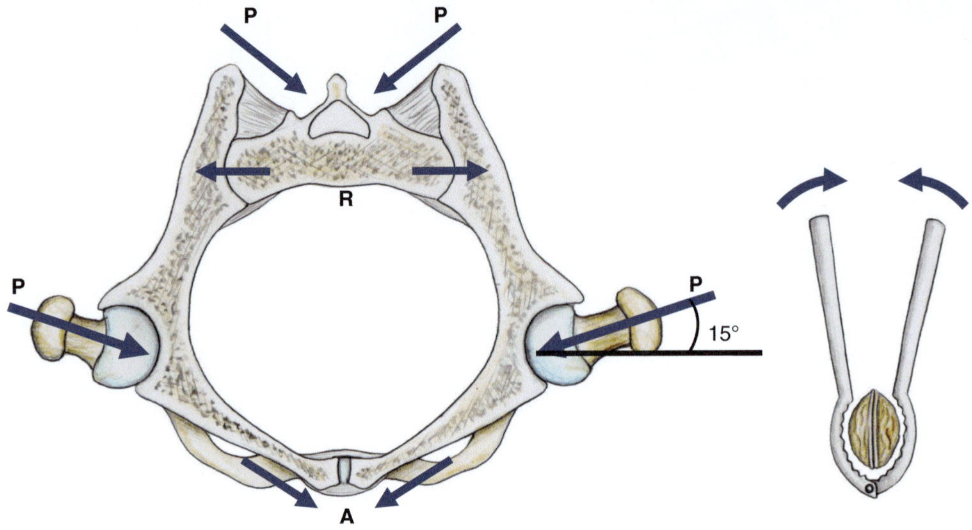

Fig. 5 Static in the horizontal or transverse plane: A = support, R = sacral resistance, P = ligament tension and femoral head pressure

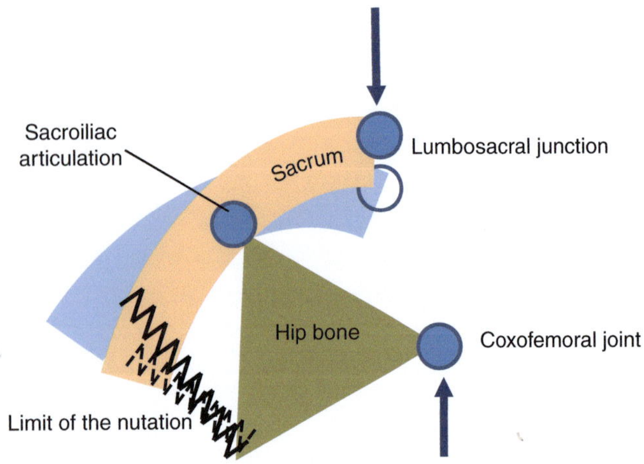

Fig. 6 Lumbopelvic scissors (Klein, Sommerfeld [3])

upper and lower pelvic brims with a transverse axis passing through S2 (Fig. 7).

It is especially during supine childbirth as some mobility is observed with the nutation of the sacrum, a decrease in the diameter of the greater pelvis with a medial tilt of the iliac wings and an increase of the pelvic outlet <1–2.5 cm with a separation of the ischia favoring the release of the fetal head.

This movement is obtained by the position of the thighs in flexion and abduction associated with lumbar flexion or kyphosis and iliac retroversion or posterior ilium (position of Devraigne-Descomps).

The mobility of the sacroiliac joints also exists in walking and running which may be asymmetric while oscillating in young patients.

- Duncan [10], Farabeuf [5], and Gray [11] determine an axis of rotation at the level of the interosseous ligament on the morphological analysis of articular surfaces.
- Bonnaire [12] describes an axis of rotation around an axis located at the point of intersection of the two arms of the articular surfaces at the tubercle of Bonnaire.
- Weisl [6] describes a two-dimensional analysis, an axis of rotation located in front of the sacroiliac joint in the inner pelvis and behind the pubic symphysis. A second study identified a translation of the sacrum along the horizontal arm (Fig. 8).

Recent Studies

- Colachis [13] measured the range of motion in the posterior superior iliac spine using Kirschner wires in 12 volunteers. The maximum amplitude of the posterior superior iliac spine is 5 mm on average.
- Egund [14] used radiostereophotogrammetry, as described by Selvik [15], with tantalum spheres of 0.8 mm diameter implanted in the two coxal bones and the sacrum under local anesthesia in six patients including four low back pain patients. The seven-position analysis shows a maximal amplitude of the sacrum in the sagittal plane of 1–2° according to the position in supine or unipodal support. There is also a sliding movement between the articular surfaces of the order of 2 mm, on average in nutation and counter-nutation.
- Lavignolle [16, 17] performed a preliminary study (1978) on fresh cadavers of both sexes, of age over 40 years, to determine the coefficients of the matrix flexibility and location of the instantaneous centers of rotation (ICR). The pelvises were solicited by forces and torques simulating muscle actions in anteversion and retroversion. The corresponding displacements, rotations, and translations were measured by comparators and a laser optical system. (Figs. 9 and 10). Frigerio [18] confirmed mobility on an identical anatomical study.

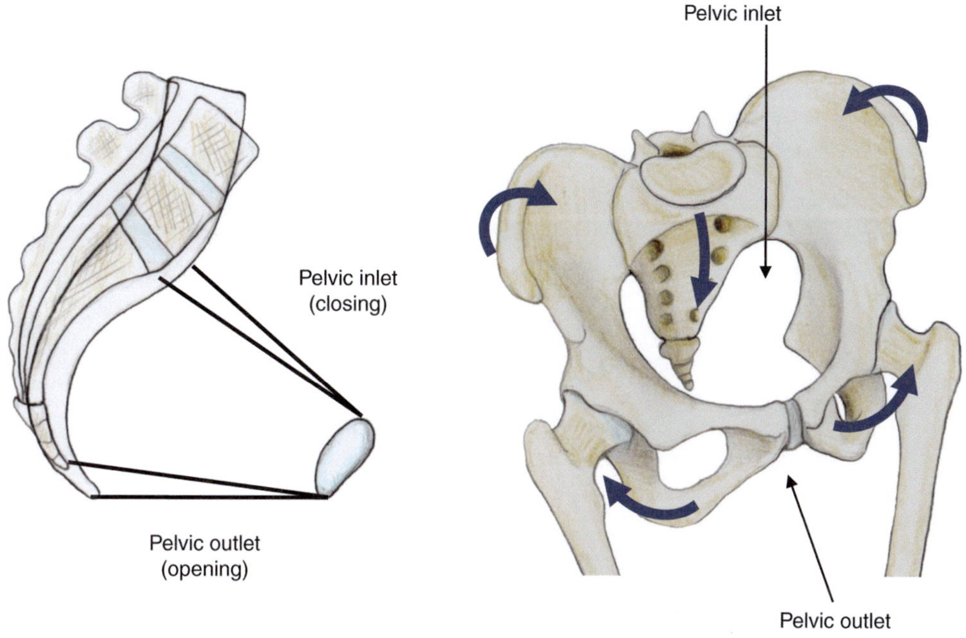

Fig. 7 Rotation of the coxal bones during nutation of the sacrum. Rocks medial iliac wings (closing) side rocker ischial (opening)

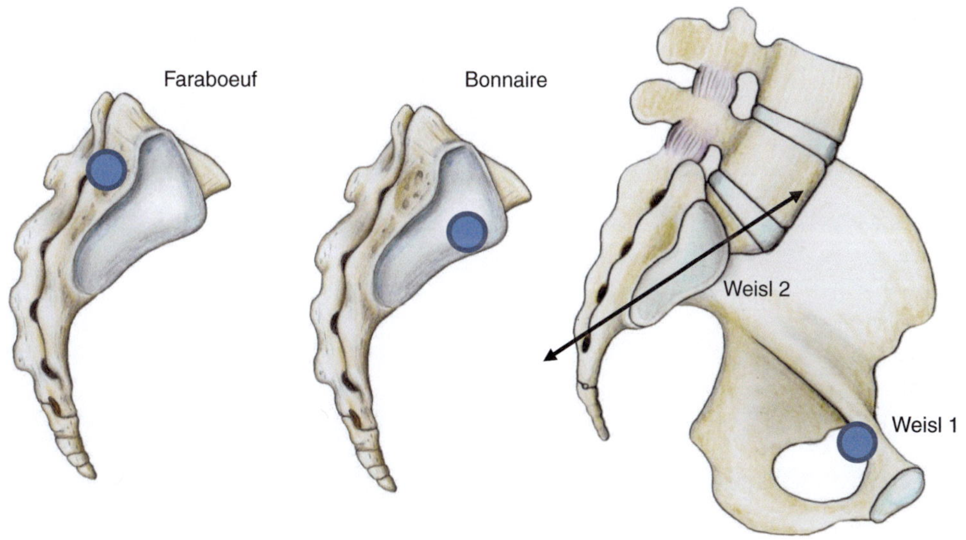

Fig. 8 Centers of rotation in classical studies

Each iliac bone has six degrees of freedom with three rotations and three translations. The position of the ICRs in the sagittal plane is located on a craniocaudal line in front of the sacroiliac joints confirming Weisl's analysis.

The 3D kinematics study, performed in 25 volunteer athletes aged 16–25 years, the relative movements of the iliac bones with respect to the sacrum in asymmetrical movements of the pelvis, simulating walking with 60° of right hip flexion and 15° left hip extension with a wide variation (Figs. 11 and 12).

Data processing was accomplished with a computer program designed to study the relative displacements and to define the position and direction of the screw axes of the sacroiliac joints and the direction and amplitude of the rotation around and the translation along these axes. Given the low amplitudes, a statistical study was needed to acquire the coordinates of the projection of these points on orthogonal radiographs with a significance level estimated at 0.1 and an error of ±0.1 mm. Ten targets were necessary for each point for a satisfactory confidence level.

The objectives included:

- Study the movements of each bone relative to an absolute reference and relative displacements of each pelvic bone relative to the other and to the sacrum which is considered fixed.
- Define the position and the direction of the axes of screw insertion with respect to the sacroiliac joints, the direction and the amplitude of the rotations and translations on these axes.

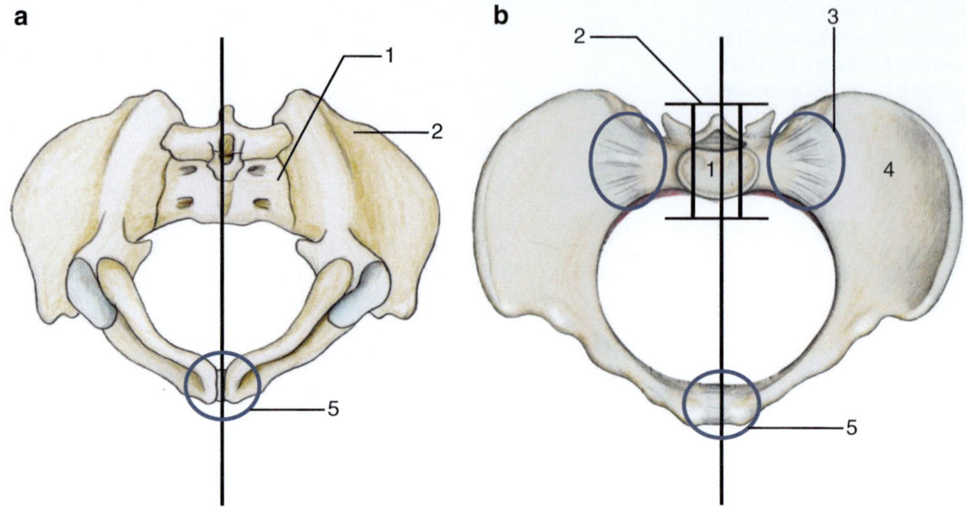

Fig. 9 Study on pelvis of fresh cadavers; (**a**) bottom view, (**b**) top view: (1) sacrum; (2) fixation of the sacrum; (3) sacroiliac joint; (4) iliac bone; (5) pubic symphysis

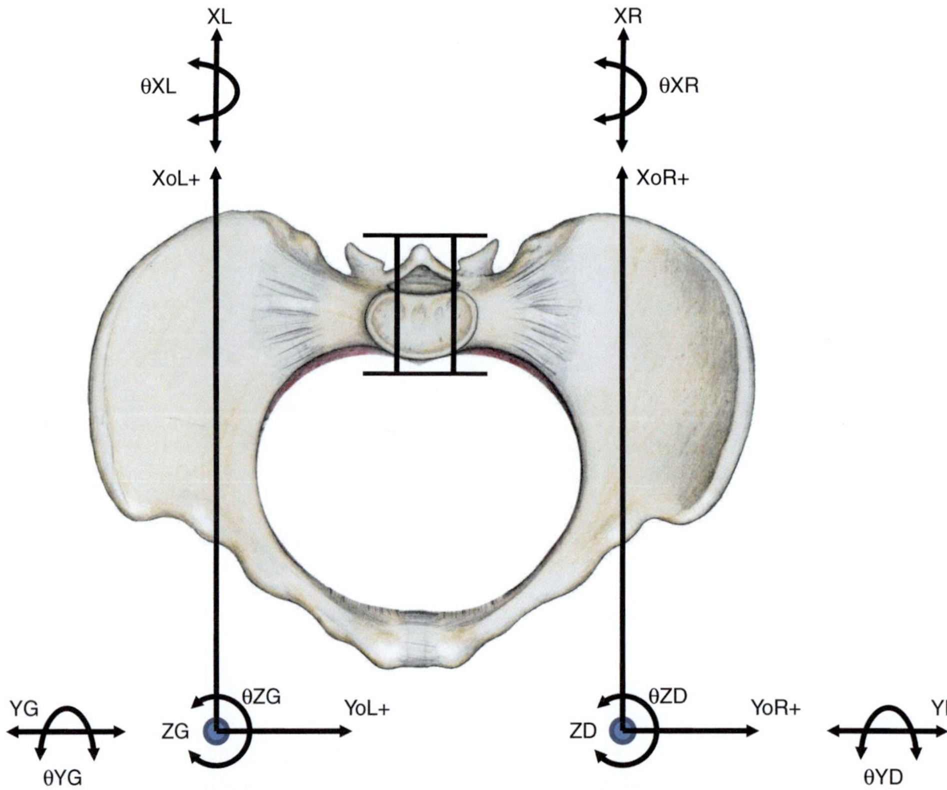

Fig. 10 Modeling of the pelvis and degrees of freedom

The first stage corresponded to the spatial reconstruction of the coordinates of the points in the absolute coordinate system with the need for a registration to ensure the condition of indeformability according to the Lagrange multiplier method.

This condition being assured, a repository consisting of two secant lines and identified by their data Plükériennes was allocated to solid bones. The last stage concerns the modeling of the displacements and the characteristics of the screw insertion according to the work notably of Dimnet [19].

The conclusions of our study are as follows:

- The axes of rotation are oblique, and the position of the axes is variable according to the subjects, but the position is constant in front of and below the sacroiliac articulations and behind the symphysis pubis.
- The amplitude is variable according to the individual, more marked in the hyperlax juveniles, on average around 8° (6–10°) of rotation of the coxal bone compared to the other coxal bone, is half by articulation and 4° (±2) nutation of the sacrum. The translation of the coxal bone relative to the other is 4 mm (±1.8 mm along the axis).

These amplitudes are similar to studies by Decupere [20] and Smidt [21] on the rotation of iliac bones with a large deviation.

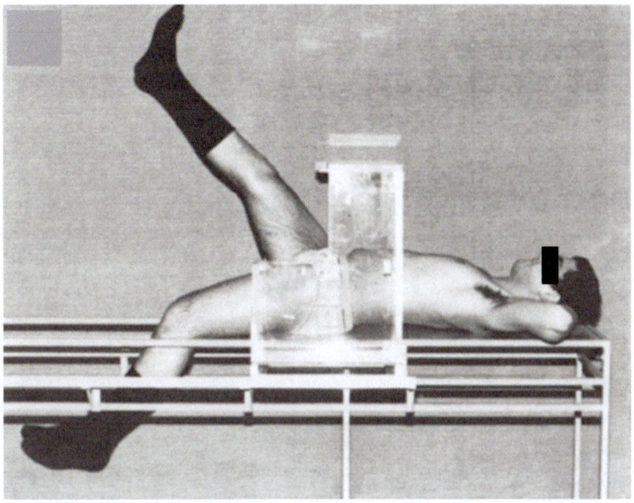

Fig. 11 Dissymmetric movements of the pelvis: right bending and left extension in radiostereophotogrammetry

The acquisition of data on radiographic bone markers undoubtedly contributes to an overestimation of the mobility, but the localization of the helical oblique axes is reliable. Jacob [22], with implanted metal pins, reports a mobility of 8.4° around a transverse and later helical axis.

These values are more reduced in the elderly population. Sturesson [8] reports lower values including 2.5° of rotation and 0.7 mm of translation on a population over 45 years in symmetrical movements of flexion-extension of the trunk. These movements were analyzed from tantalum beads implanted in vivo very close to the joint sites regardless of bone volume and leverage of the pelvic girdle. In the extreme, Tulberg [23], in a stereometric study found no mobility.

Conclusion

The cinematic model cannot be definitively reported, given the low number of subjects studied in vivo, the significant time required to capture data and with the further yield from 3D computerized analysis. The mobility of the sacroiliac

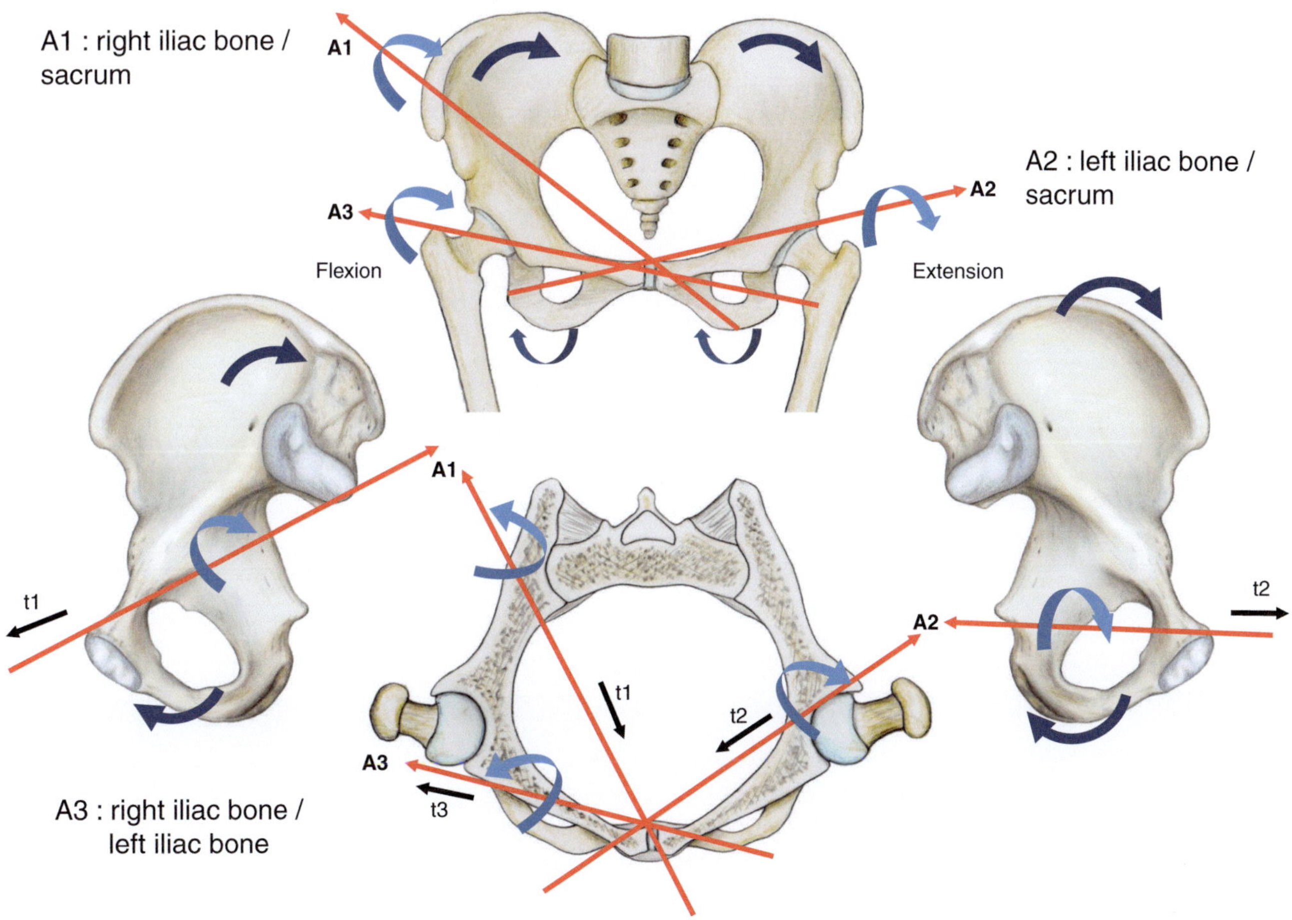

Fig. 12 Instantaneous axes of rotation during asymmetric movements

joint is very low between 2° and 4°, especially outside childbirth.

The sacroiliac joint has above all a role of transmission of the constraints in load during the walk and the run. It locks and unlocks its significant load-carrying ability in unipodal support.

References

1. Walheim GG. Mobility of the pubic symphysis. Acta Orthop Scand. 1984;55(2):203–8.
2. Senegas J, Viale B. Les fractures de la ceinture pelvienne. J Trauma. 1980;1:27–39.
3. Klein P, Sommerfeld P. Biomécanique des membres inférieurs, vol. 437. Paris: Elsevier Édit; 2008.
4. Bogduk N. Anatomie clinique du rachis lombal et sacré, vol. 340. Paris: Elsevier Édit; 2005.
5. Farabeuf LH. Sur l'anatomie et la physiologie des articulations sacro-iliaques avant et après symphysiotomie. Ann Gynecol Obstet. 1894;4:407–20.
6. Weisl H. The movement of the sacro-iliac. Acta Anat. 1955;23(1):80–91.
7. Maigne JY, Molinie V, Fautrel B. Anatomie des disques sacro et intercoccygiens. Rev Med Orthop. 1992;28:34–5.
8. Sturesson B, Selvik G. Uden: movements of the sacro-iliac joints. A roentgen stereophotogrammetric analysis. Spine. 1989;14(2):162–5.
9. Gairdner W, Barlow J. Mechanism of the pelvis articulations. Month J Med Sci. 1851;21:289.
10. Duncan JM. The behaviour of the pelvic articulations in the mechanism of parturition. J Med Sci. 1864;18:60–9.
11. Gray H. Sacro-iliac joint pain. Mobility and axes of rotation. Int Clin. 1938;2:54.
12. Bonnaire E, Bue V. De la mobilité des articulations pelviennes. Ann Gynecol Obstet. 1899;52:296.
13. Colachis SC, Warden RE, Bechtol GO, et al. Movement of the sacro-iliac joint in the adult male; a preliminary report. Arch Phys Med Rehabil. 1963;44:490–8.
14. Egund N, Olsson TH, Selvik GA. Movements of the sacroiliac joints demonstrated with Roentgen stereophotogrammetry. Acta Radiol Diagn. 1978;19(5):833–46.
15. Selvik GA. A roentgen stereophotogrammetric method for the study of kinematics of the skeletal system (Thesis PhD). AV Centralen Lund; 1974.
16. Lavignolle B, Vital JM, Toson B, et al. An approach to the functional anatomy of the sacroiliac joints in vivo. Anat Clin. 1983;5:169–76.
17. Lavignolle B, Toson B, Morlier P. Biomécanique des articulations sacro-iliaques et, Pathologie du sortif. In: Simon L, et al., editors. Rachis et sport. Paris: Masson; 1995. p. 380.
18. Frigerio NA, Stowe RR, Howe JW. Movement of the sacro-iliac joint. Clin Orthop. 1974;100:370–7.
19. Dimnet J. Contribution à l'étude biomécanique des articulations par utilisation des procédés radiographiques [Thèse doctorates Sciences]. n° 7823, Université de Lyon, France; 1978.
20. Decupere Y. Evaluation de la mobilité des articulations sacro-iliaques à l'aide d'un digitaliseur tridimensionnel Metrecom. In: Klein P, editor. Mémoire Réadaptation. Bruxelles: Université libre de Bruxelles; 2000.
21. Smidt GL, Cade MC. Sacro iliac kinematic. Spine. 1995;20(9):1047–54.
22. Jacob H, Kissling R. The mobility of the sacroiliac joints in healthy volunteers between 20 and 50 years of age. Clin Biomech. 1995;10:352–61.
23. Tulberg T. Manipulation does not alter the position of the sacro-iliac joint. Spine. 1998;23:1124–9.

The Normal and Pathological Spinal Muscle

Jean Marc Vital

Introduction

We describe in this chapter a "practical" anatomy with simple description of the various spinal muscles, their actions and their lesions in pathological conditions.

Generaly, we can estimate that the muscles have a function of stabilization (or of tensioning) and of mobilization. They can be classified into 3 topographic groups: anterior, lateral and posterior. We can also, as per Martinez [1], differentiate them into intrinsic and extrinsic muscles. The first originate and end on the spine: they are the deepest. The latter have their origin, and sometimes also their insertion, at a distance from the spinal column; they are therefore long, powerful and more superficial muscles that will have a rather mobilizing action, contrary to the intrinsic muscles, which act primarily as stabilizers.

Normal Descriptive Anatomy

We will somewhat artificially divide the description of the muscles of the vertebral column into cervical muscles and thoracolumbar muscles, and we shall conclude this chapter of descriptive anatomy by describing the thoracic diaphragm, the pelvic diaphragm, the sub-pelvic muscles which participate in the stabilization of the vertebral column, and finally, the muscular aponeurosis.

The Cervical Muscles

They can be distinguished schematically in four groups (Fig. 1) [1].

1. The deep muscles, akin to short cable-stays for bridge suspension, are located near the spine (longus colli, intertransversarius, transversus spinalis).
2. Two long powerful muscles, the sternocleidomastoid and the trapezius, and two long stays, the supra- and infrahyoid muscles.
3. Intermediate muscles in the upper cervical spine with small anterior and posterior muscles located at the craniocervical junction.
4. Intermediate muscles at the lower cervical spine, with muscles projecting towards the scapular girdle or the first pair of ribs.

Deep Muscles

The deep muscles are pure intrinsic muscles.

Longus Colli
Longus colli is an anterior intrinsic muscle of the lower cervical spine.

It is immediately prevertebral and presents three fascicles (Fig. 2).

1. Para-median longitudinal deep fascicle extending from the body of C2 to that of T3,
2. Ascending upper oblique fascicle extending from the transverse processes of C3–C6 to the anterior tubercle of the atlas,
3. Descending lower oblique fascicle which extends from the transverse processes of C4–C7 to the bodies of T2 and T3.

These three fascicles create a diamond construct in which the bodies and discs of the lower cervical spine are inscribed. Longus colli is a flexor which flattens the cervical lordosis. It also has a stabilizing function to which we shall return.

J. M. Vital (✉)
Spinal Unit, University Hospital, Bordeaux, France

J. M. Vital, D. T. Cawley (eds.), *Spinal Anatomy*, https://doi.org/10.1007/978-3-030-20925-4_18

The Intertransversarius

The intertransversarius is a muscle that extends throughout the spine and is considered as an intrinsic lateral muscle.

The Transversarius Spinalis

The transversarius spinalis extends along the entire length of the column; it is a posterior intrinsic muscle divided into three layers: semi-spinous fascicles, long fascicles (multifidus), and short fascicles (rotatores).

The Peripheral Muscles

These are totally extrinsic muscles.

The supra- and infrahyoid muscles are anterior extrinsics.

The mylohyoideus (mylohyoid) is the only suprahyoid muscle; there are, on the other hand, four infrahyoid muscles, thyrohyoid, sternohyoid, sternothyroid, and omohyoid. All these muscles act mainly in phonation but have an action of cervical flexion against resistance. Poisson [2], recently demonstrated by an isometric and electromyographic force study on rugby players, that the protection of the teeth with a buccal protection system had an effect of increase of force of the cervical flexors and thus, a priori, a protective effect of the cervical spine (Fig. 3).

The Sternocleidomastoid (SCM)

The SCM includes a fascicle that originates on the clavicle and a second on the sternal manubrium. It ends on the cranial side at the level of the mastoid but also on the upper occipital line. This muscle constitutes a large muscular band obliquely extending downward and forward and contains three fascicles: a deep cleidomastoideus and two superficial (cleido-occipital posteriorly, covering the deep and sterno-mastoideus anteriorly, ending in a true tendinous attachment to the sternal manubrium (Fig. 4). This muscle, innervated by the accessory nerve (XIth cranial nerve), has an action in the sagittal plane which varies according to whether or not the cervical column is locked in flexion, by the longus colli in particular; the contraction of the two SCM induces in the

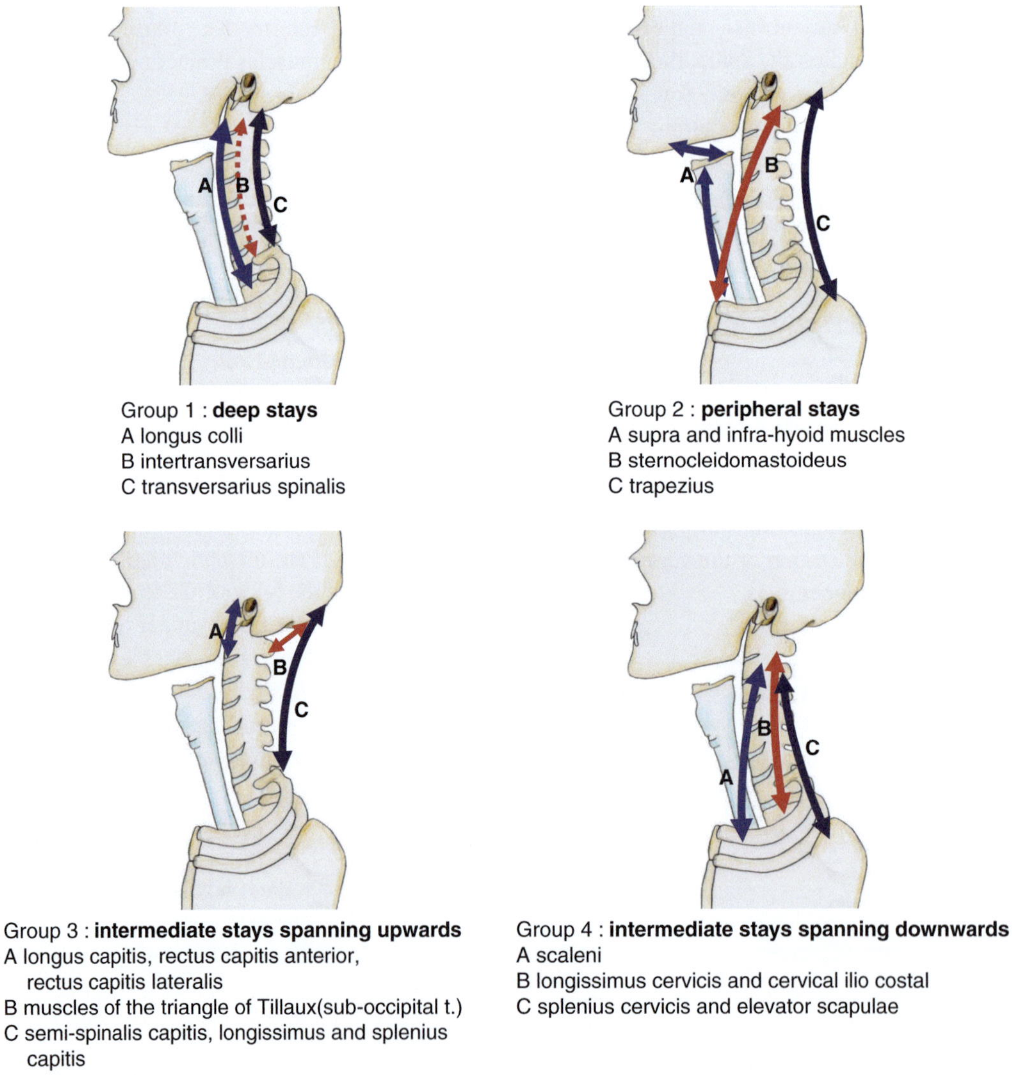

Fig. 1 The four cervical muscle groups [1]

Fig. 2 Longus colli and supra- and infrahyoid muscles: (**a**) left lateral view, (**b**) anterior view

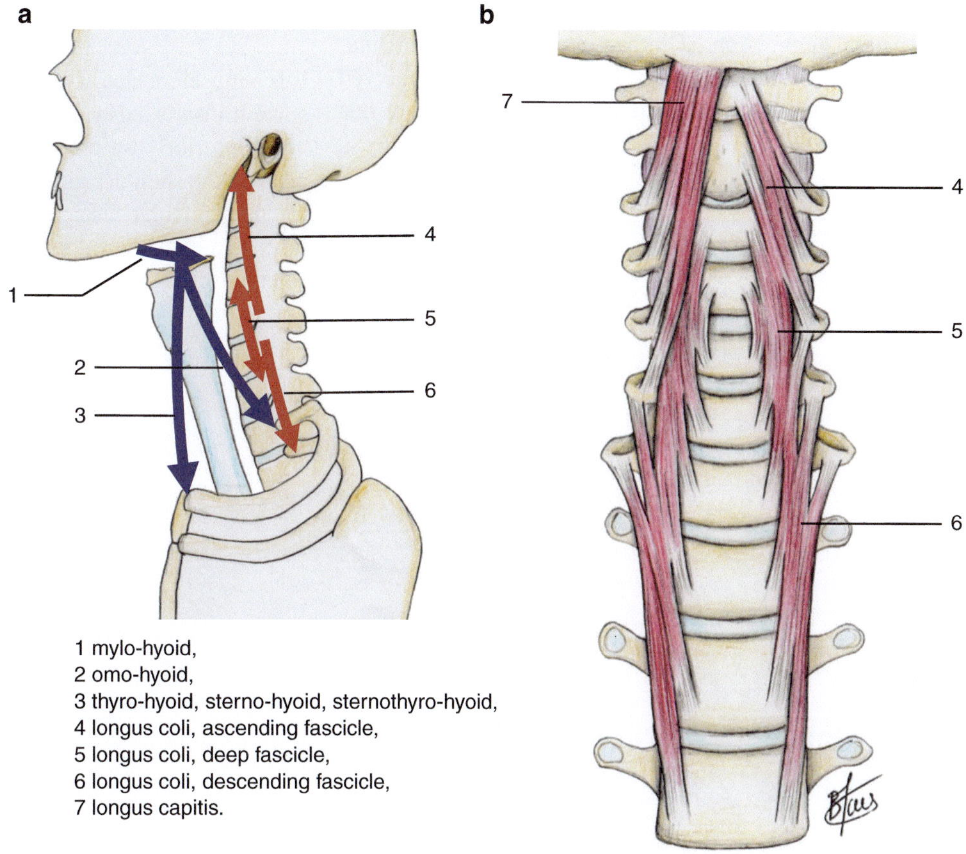

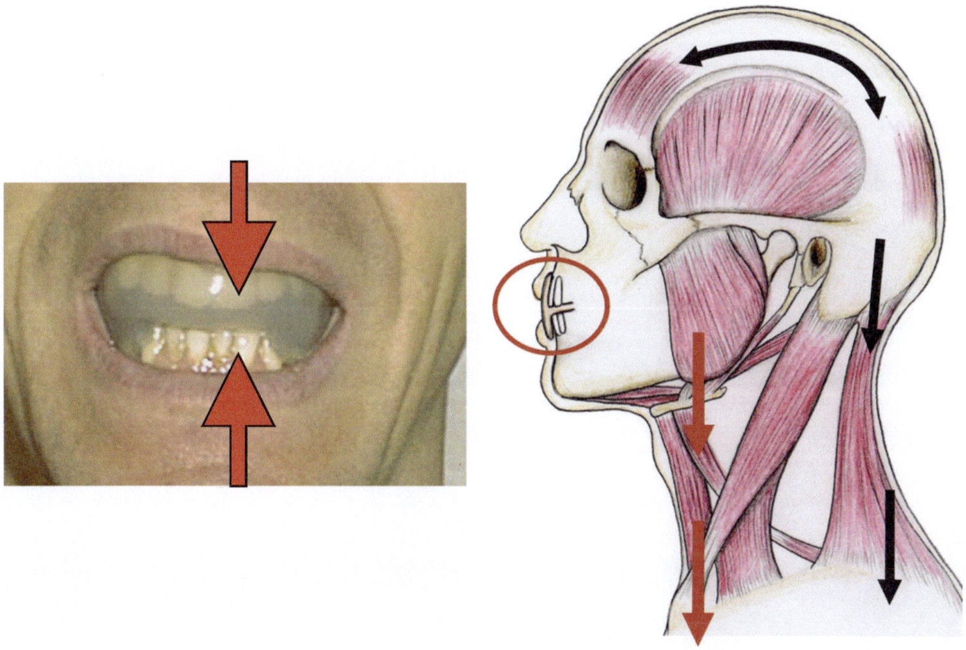

Fig. 3 Activation of the supra- and infrahyoid muscles by clamping on a dental protective gutter [2]

first case a flexion and in the second a hyper-extension [1]. In an unilateral contraction, SCM causes a homolateral inclination and a contralateral rotation: this is the attitude observed in the congenital torticollis where there is retraction of this muscle (Fig. 5).

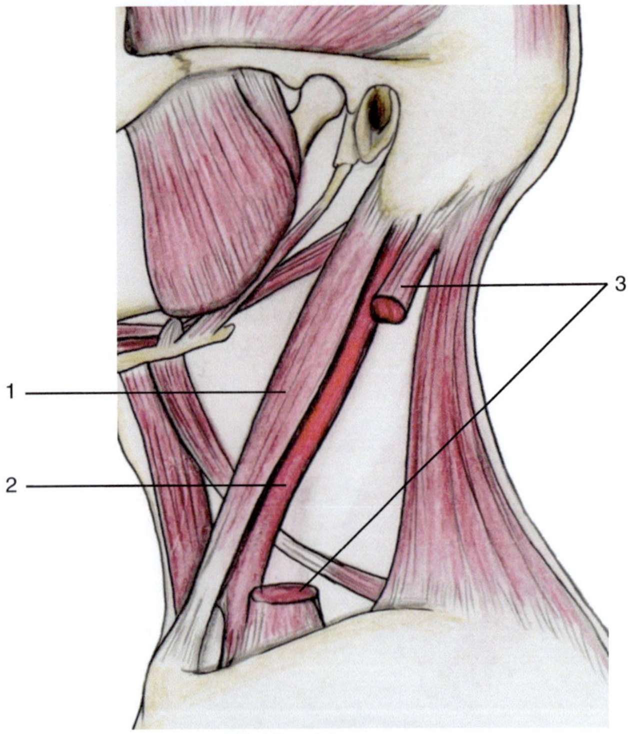

1 superficial sternomastoidal fascicle,
2 deep cleidomastoidal fascicle,
3 superficial cleidooccipital fascicle.

Fig. 4 Anatomy of the sternocleidomastoid muscle (left lateral view)

The Trapezius

It is a muscle which is at the same time cervical and thoracic since it inserts superiorly on the external occipital protuberance, inferiorly on the spinous processes down to T11 and ends on the shoulder girdle on the lateral third of the clavicle for its clavicular fascicle, on the acromion for its acromial fascicle and on the spine of the scapula for its spinal fascicle. This muscle is innervated by the accessory nerve (XIth cranial nerve) and by the cervical plexus (C2 and C3). It is an

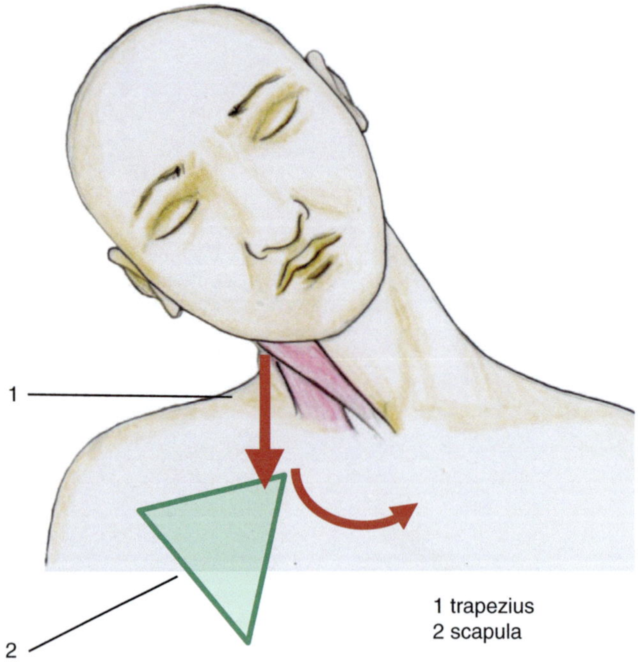

1 trapezius
2 scapula

Fig. 6 Trapezius muscle action in tilt-rotation

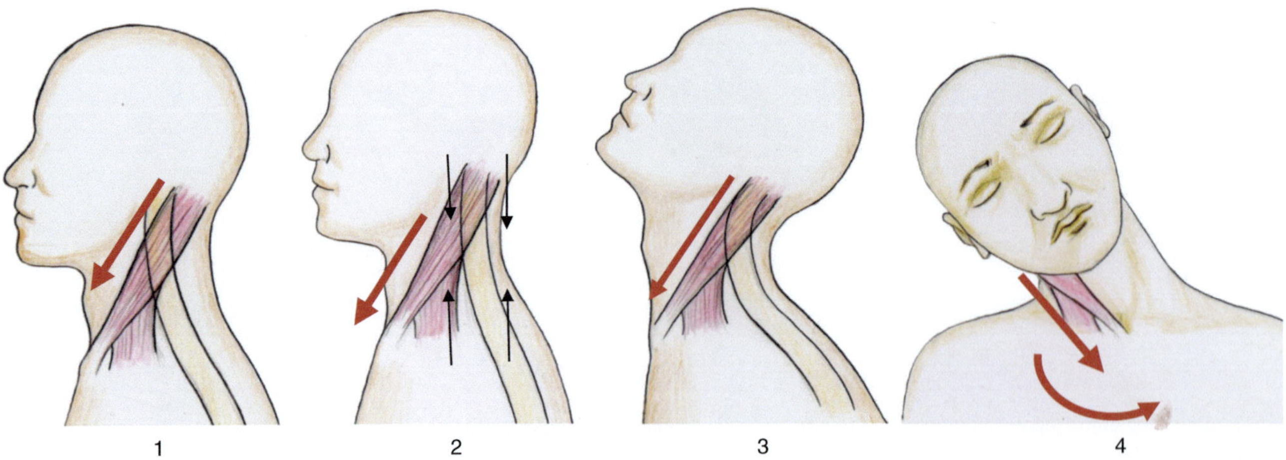

1 overall direction of the muscle,
2 flexion on a locked cervical spine,
3 extension on a non-locked cervical spine,
4 homolateral inclination and controlateral rotation.

Fig. 5 Actions of the sternocleidomastoid muscle

essential stabilizer of the head in the sagittal plane and an extender when the two muscles contract. Like the SCM, its unilateral contraction causes a homolateral inclination and a contralateral rotation (Fig. 6).

The Intermediate Muscles Extending Upwards

These are intrinsic muscles with proximal insertion on the base of the skull and distal insertion on the upper cervical spine.

Three anterior sub-occipital muscles (Fig. 7) [3]:

- The longus capitis which is positioned between the basilar process of the occiput and the anterior tuberculum of C3–C6.
- The rectus capitis anterior located between the anterior limit of the occipital foramen and the lateral mass of the atlas.
- The rectus capitis lateralis, parallel to the preceding one.
- These three muscles are flexors and homolateral rotators.

Four posterior sub-occipital muscles (Fig. 8):

- The rectus capitis posterior major positioned between the inferior nuchal line of the occiput and the axis spinous process; it extends and inclines the head but has no real rotatory action.
- The rectus capitis posterior minor, more medial, situated between the inferior nuchal line and the posterior ring of the atlas; it is an extensor.
- The obliquus capitis inferior positioned between the transverse process of the atlas and the spinous process of the axis and which operates on the atlas, according to Kapandji [3] with the opposite obliquus capitis inferior acting as a pair of reins (Fig. 9). It controls homolateral rotation of the atlas.

The three following muscles are positioned between the skull and the spine and lie between the plane of the posterior sub-occipital muscles which have just been described and the trapezius; those are:

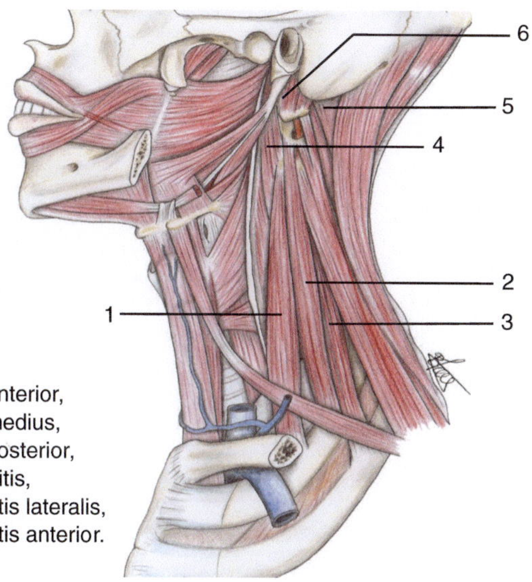

Fig. 7 Anterior sub-occipital muscles and scaleni

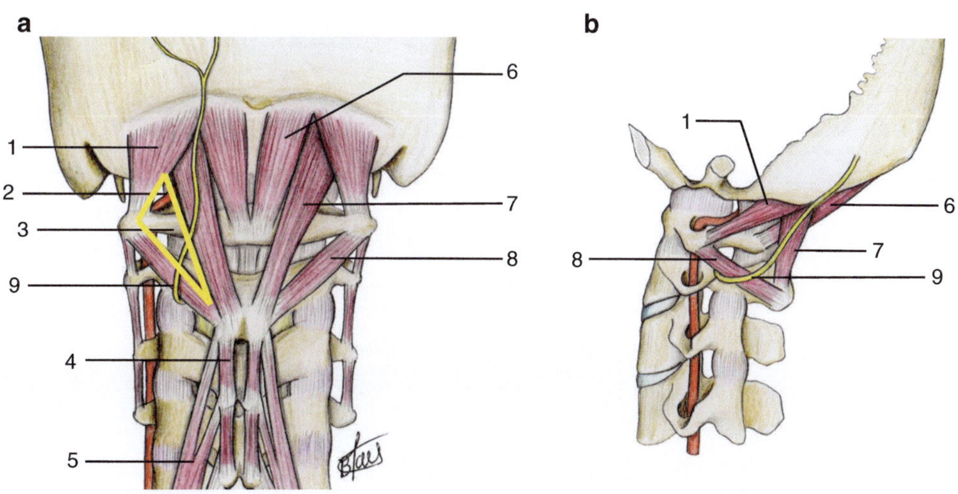

Fig. 8 Sub-occipital posterior muscles: (**a**) posterior view, (**b**) left lateral view

- The semispinalis capitis extending from the superior nuchal line to the transverse processes from C3 to T5 (Fig. 10).
- The longissimus capitis which extends from the mastoid process to the transverse processes from C3 to T1.

These two muscles are pure extensors with a tilt component for the longissimus capitis.

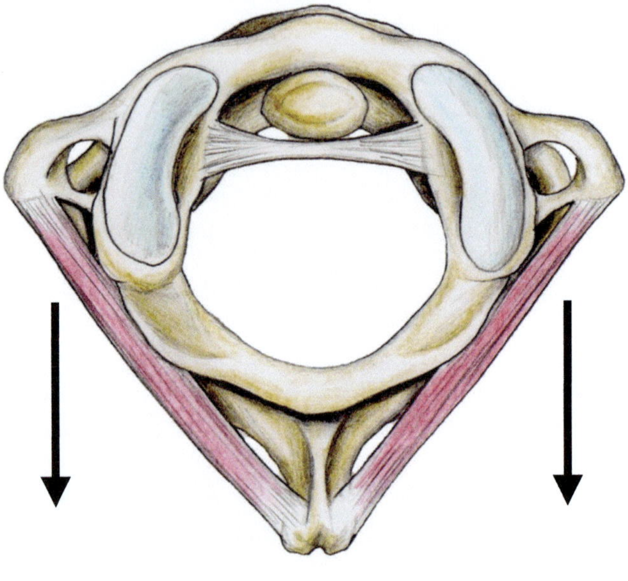

Fig. 9 Stabilizing action on C1–C2 of the obliquus capitis inferior

- The splenius capitis is inserted on the mastoid and the superior nuchal line and ends on the cervical spinous process. It is a powerful extensor and a homolateral rotator; it has in this movement a synergistic action with the controlateral SCM.

The Intermediate Muscles Extending Downwards

These are rather extrinsic muscles with a proximal insertion on the cervical spine but distal insertion at a distance on the thoracic spine, the ribs, or the scapula.

Scaleni

There are three (Fig. 7)

- The scalenus anterior which extends from the anterior tubercle of the transverse processes from C3 to C6 to the upper surface of the first rib.
- The scalenus medius which extends from the edge of the transverse process gutters of C2–C7 and ends on the same first rib behind the subclavian artery.
- The scalenus posterior that extends from the posterior transverse tubercle of C4–C6 and ends on the second rib.

Fig. 10 Posterior muscles from the neck to the head

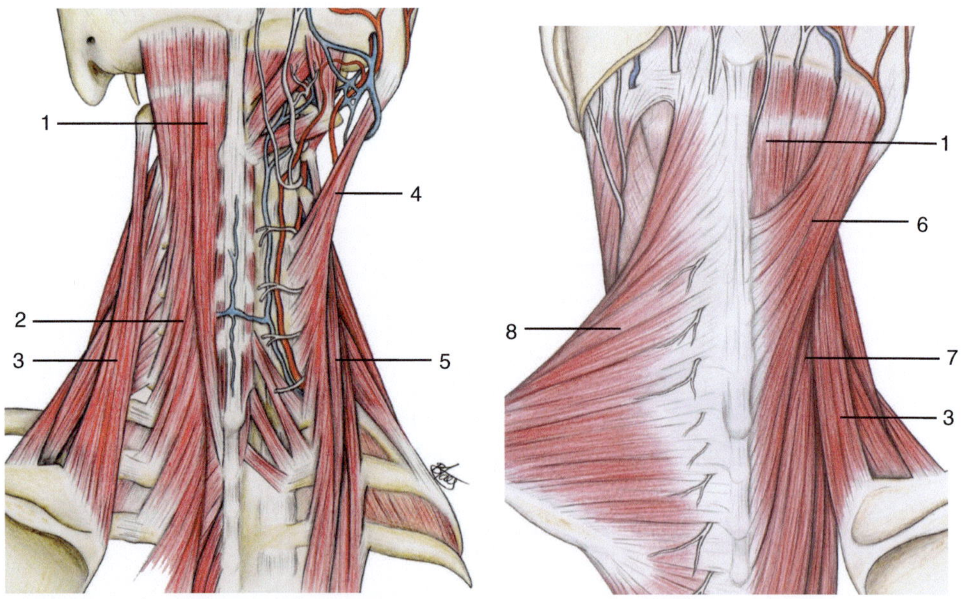

1 semi-spinosus (large complex),
2 longissimus capitis (small complex),
3 elevator scapulae,
4 splenius capitis,
5 ilio-costalis,
6 splenius capitis,
7 transversarius spinosus,
8 trapezius

Besides their respiratory role, these muscles are flexors and lead to a homolateral inclination with contralateral rotation.

The Longissimus Cervicis
It extends from the transverse processes of the last four cervical vertebrae to those of the first five thoracic vertebrae; it is a powerful extensor.

The Ilio-Costalis (Fig. 10)
It has nearly the same origin as the preceding muscle; more lateral, it ends on the posterior arch of the first pair of ribs.

The Epi-Spinalis
It extends between the spinous processes of C2 to C7 and participates in the constitution of the star-like formation of muscles around the spinous process of C2; we have shown only the cranial insertions in Fig. 8.

The Splenius Cervicis
It extends from the transverse processes of C1 to C3 to the spinous processes of the first five thoracic vertebrae; it is a direct extensor.

The Levator Scapulae
It is inserted on the tip of the transverse processes of the first four cervical vertebrae and after a tortuous path joins the superior medial angle of the scapula; if the scapula is fixed, it causes a homolateral extension-inclination.

Thoraco-Lumbar Muscles

The thoraco-lumbar muscles can be simplified by division into three groups (Fig. 11)

1. The posterior or dorsal group which will extends inferiorly towards the lumbo-sacral junction.
2. The lateral group with the psoas and the quadratus lumborum.
3. Finally, the anterior or ventral group with the muscles of the abdominal wall.

The set of posterior and lateral groups envelops the spinal column as the muscles of the thigh envelop the femur to realize a composite beam which has a protective function, we will return to this in the chapter on functional anatomy (Chap. 30) (Fig. 12).

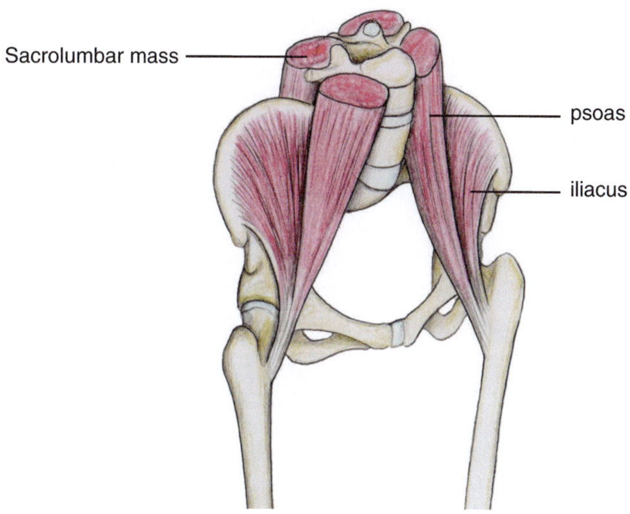

Fig. 12 Composite spinal beam

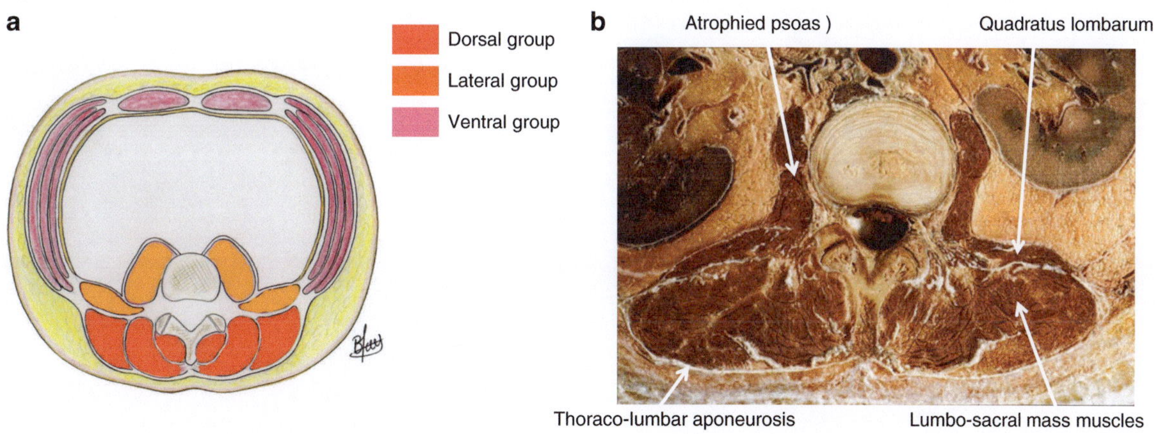

Fig. 11 (**a**) The three groups of thoraco-lumbar muscles. Dorsal group, lateral group, ventral group. (**b**) Horizontal cut at the lumbar level of the posterior thoraco-lumbar muscles; note the difference in surface between the psoas and the paravertebral muscles. (Conservatory of Anatomy, Montpellier—Pr F. Bonnel)

Posterior Muscle Group

The Deep Plane

The deep plane (Fig. 13) consists of the inter-spinous muscles and the inter-transversal muscles, the segmental muscles situated between the spinous processes and between the transverse processes, respectively.

The transversus spinosus that exists at the cervical level is situated, according to Trolard, between the tip of the transverse process and the spinous processes or the laminae of the four overlying vertebrae. They are therefore muscular rafters (like the supports of a roof) which is commonly called the multifidus. More laterally and more superficially, we find the epi-spinalis of the thorax and the semi-spinous. The latter is purely thoracic and is situated between the transverse processes of the thoracic vertebrae and the spinous processes of the lower cervical vertebrae.

The spinalis thoracis also exists in the neck. It is more superficial and extends from the lateral surfaces of spinous processes from the thoracic region to the upper lumbar region where it is very close to the multifidus.

The longissimus thoracis, which extends from the longissimus capitis and the longissimus cervicis, unites downwards with the ilio-costalis to constitute the lumbo-sacral common mass. It inserts into the accessory processes of the lumbar vertebrae, the transverse processes of the thoracic vertebrae, and the posterior arch of the ribs.

The ilio-costal inserts on the posterior arch of the ribs and on the iliac crest.

About these deep posterior muscles, we can make three observations:

- According to Kapandji [3], the third lumbar vertebra at the apex of the lumbar lordosis, horizontal in the sagittal plane, is a true muscular relay (Fig. 14) since it receives from superiorly the longissimus and epi-spinalis thoracis and from inferiorly, the multifidus. This muscular disposition is reminiscent of that of the muscles around the posterior arch of C2.
- Functionally, these posterior deep muscles are extensors and have rather a stabilizing function as shown by their composition in type 1 fibers (slow) and type 2 fibers (fast). Jorgensen [4] and Bagnall [5] demonstrated that these muscles were more rich in slow fibers than the superficial posterior muscles. It is interesting to note that in degeneration (or natural aging) these deep posterior muscles degenerate first and are replaced by fat and this normally occurs, from caudad to cephalad, from the lumbo-sacral junction to the upper lumbar spine.
- Finally, at the base, the ilio-costalis, longissimus, and multifidus, although constituting the lumbo-sacral common mass, are separated by cleavage planes containing fat tissue. The multifidus—longissimus space can easily be dissociated with a finger and thus we can easily reach the articular processes or the transverse processes (classic Wiltse approach [6]) (Fig. 15).

The Intermediate Plane

It consists of the serratus posterior—superior and inferior (Fig. 16). The serratus posterior superior is situated between the spinous processes of the last two cervical vertebrae and those of the first two thoracic vertebrae and the first ribs.

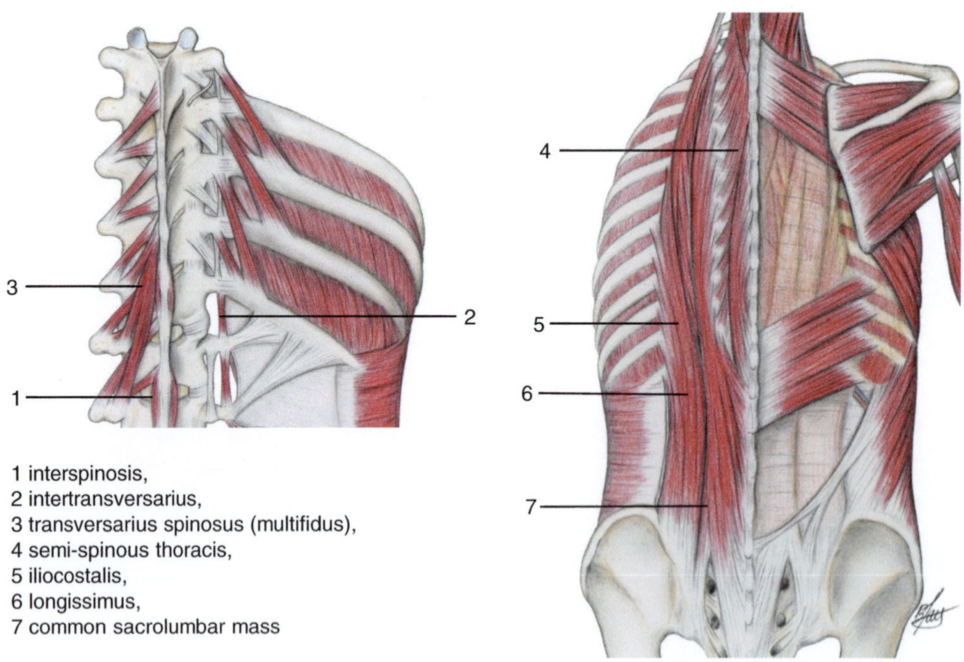

Fig. 13 Deep posterior muscles

1 interspinosis,
2 intertransversarius,
3 transversarius spinosus (multifidus),
4 semi-spinous thoracis,
5 iliocostalis,
6 longissimus,
7 common sacrolumbar mass

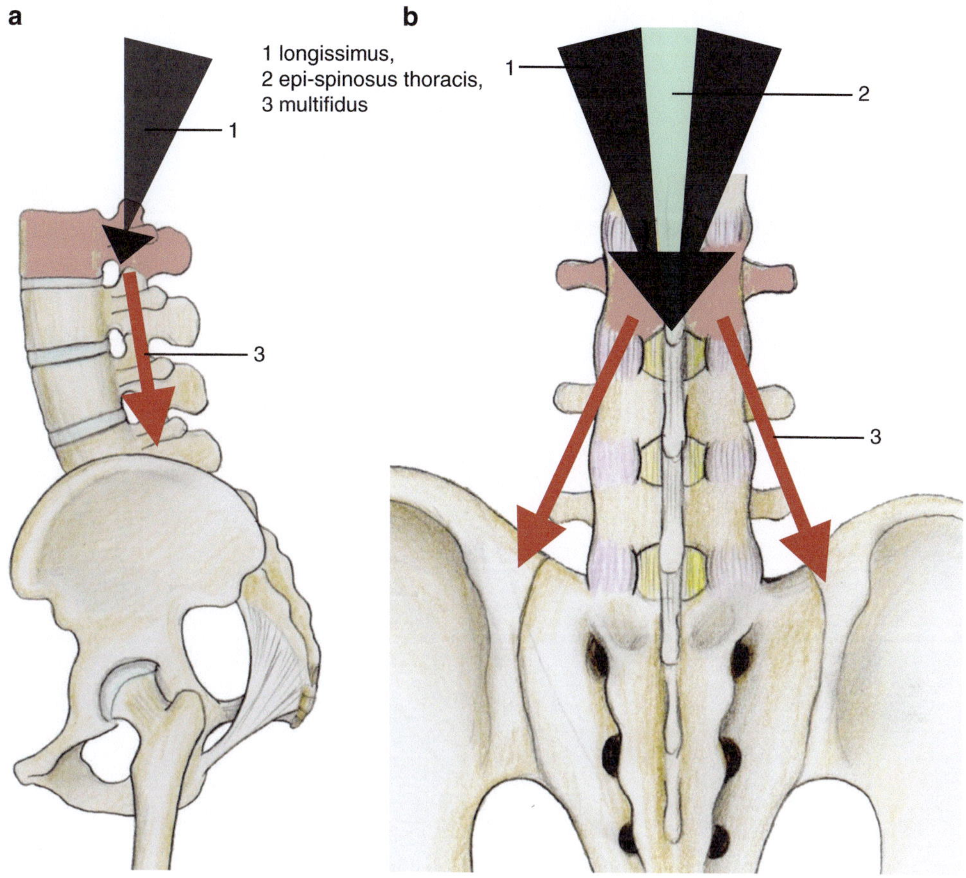

Fig. 14 Concentric termination of the muscles like a star on the spinous process of L3: (**a**) left lateral view, (**b**) posterior view

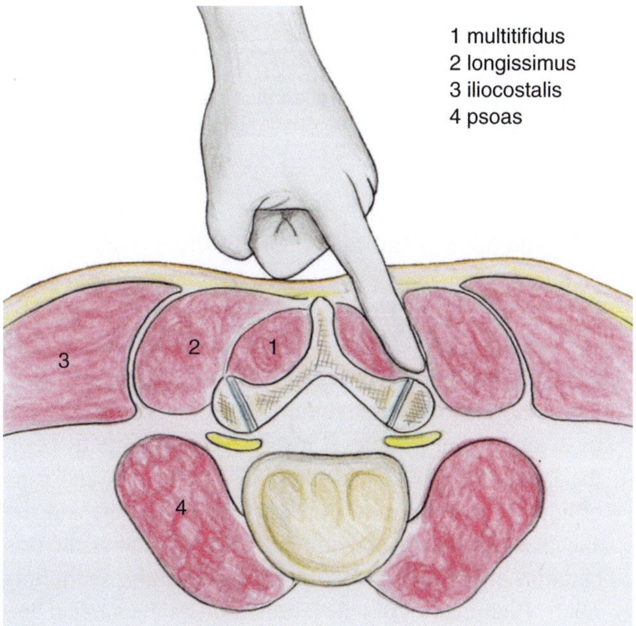

Fig. 15 Wiltse approach [6] between the multifidus and the longissimus

The serratus posterior inferior is inserted on the spinal processes of the last thoracic vertebrae and the first lumbar vertebrae and ends on the caudal margin of the last four ribs. These two muscles have a function in inspiration.

The Superficial Plane

It consists of the trapezius, the rhomboideus, the latissimus dorsi, which are mobilizers of both the spine and the scapular girdle.

Lateral Muscle Group

These lateral muscles are located in the lumbar spine (Fig. 17).

1. The ilio-psoas consists of three heads (small and large psoas and iliac). It is innervated by the femoral nerve and has an action of lateral bending-rotation of the hip. Its action on the vertebral column is discussed: its contraction causes a homolateral inclination and a contralateral rotation (Fig. 18). In the sagittal plane, it is a lordosing muscle with lumbo-sacral flexion, as shown in the diagram of Kapandji [3] (Fig. 19).
2. Quadratus lumborum occupies the costo-vertebral angle between the fascia transversalis posteriorly and the ilio-psoas anteriorly. It has a posterior head extending from the iliac crest to the tip of the transverse lumbar processes, with oblique fibers above and below, and an anterior head situated between the lower edge of the 12th rib and the

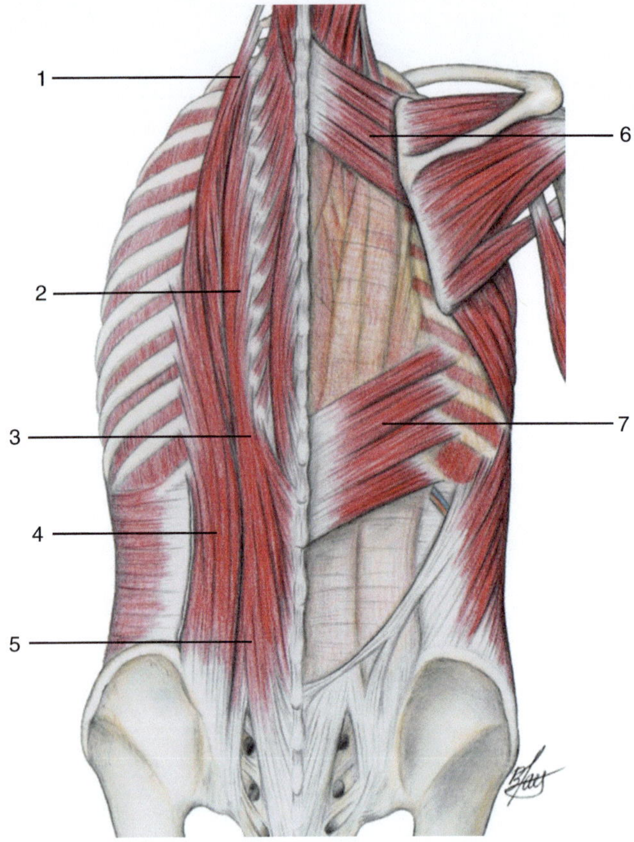

1 iliocostalis cervicis,
2 iliocostalis thoracis,
3 iliocostalis lumbaris,
4 longissimus,
5 common lumbo-sacral mass,
6 serratus posterior superior,
7 serratus posterior inferior.

Fig. 16 Posterior muscles of the medium plane

same transverse processes. Like the ilio-psoas, this muscle leads to a homolateral inclination and a slight controlateral rotation.

Anterior Muscle Group (Fig. 20)

It consists of the muscles of the abdominal wall including the rectus abdominis and the lateral muscles of the abdomen.

- The rectus abdominis is vertical and separated from the contralateral side by the linea alba. It inserts on the anterior arches of the fifth and sixth ribs, on the seventh rib cartilage, and on the xiphisternum. Along its path, it displays tendinous intersections characteristic of a polygastric muscle which ends on the pubic symphysis.
- The transversus abdominis is the deepest lateral muscle. It is inserted into the lateral cartilages and via the posterior aponeurosis on the lumbar transverse processes. The muscular fibers are transverse and extend to the anterior aponeurosis, which terminates in the inguinal ligament.

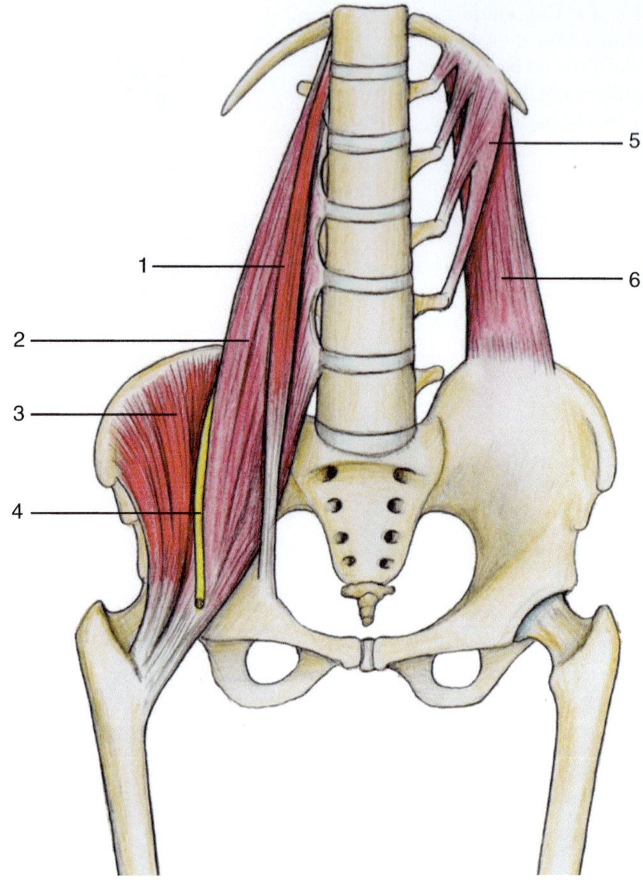

1) psoas minor,
2) psoas major,
3) iliacus,
4) femoral nerve,
5) anterior fascicle of the quadratus lumborum,
6) posterior fascicle of the quadratus lumborum.

Fig. 17 The lateral muscles

- The obliquus internus abdominis (internal oblique) is in an intermediate position. It inserts on the iliac crest and its oblique fibers superoanteriorly end on the floating ribs and nearby costal cartilages to the sternum. Anteriorly, it provides the aponeurosis of the internal oblique.
- The obliquus externus abdominis (external oblique) is the most superficial muscle. It inserts through digitations on the lateral arch of the last seven or eight ribs and runs obliquely anteroinferiorly to join the iliac crest and the sheath of the rectus abdominis. Figure 21 shows the orientation of the rectus abdominis and lateralis abdominis fibers. Figure 22 shows the termination on the median line of these abdominal muscles.

The other muscles act indirectly on the vertebral column but have an essential action on its physiology.

- The thoracic diaphragm and the pelvic diaphragm (levator ani), together with the abdominal muscles described

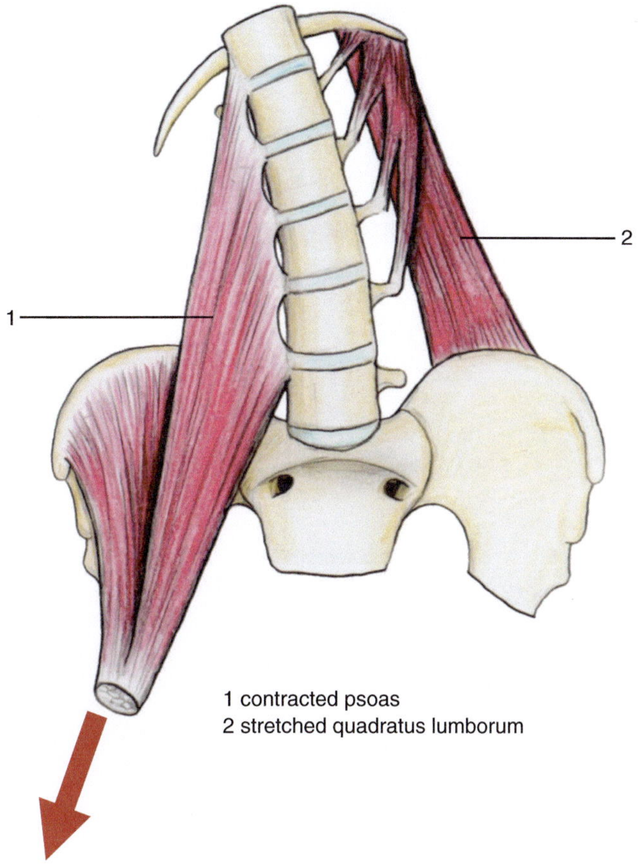

Fig. 18 Action of the psoas in the frontal and horizontal planes

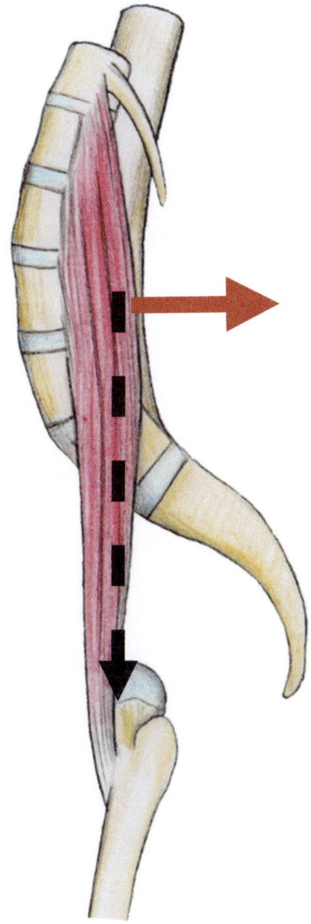

Fig. 19 Lordotic action of the psoas in the sagittal plane

Fig. 20 Abdominal muscles

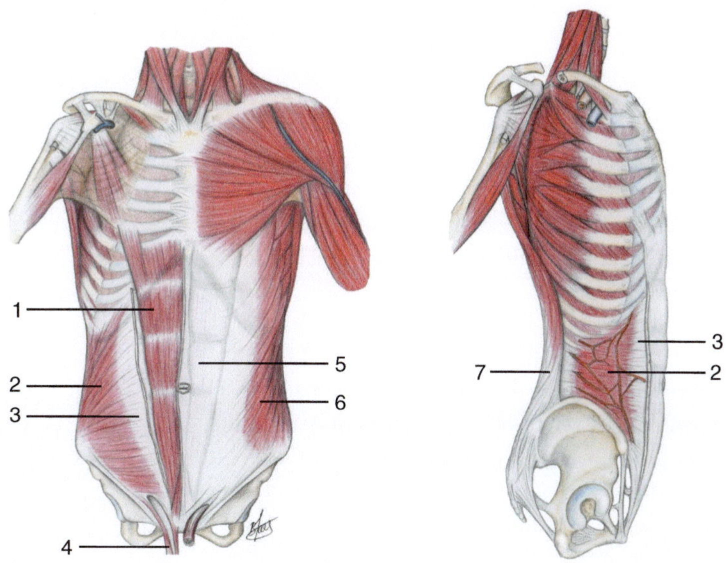

1 rectus abdominis,
2 transversus abdominis (obliquus externus abdominis and obliquus internus abdominis have been removed),
3 anterior fascia of the transversus abdominis,
4 cremaster
5 posterior fascia of the rectus abdominis,
6 obliquus externus abdominis,
7 common sacrolumbar mass.

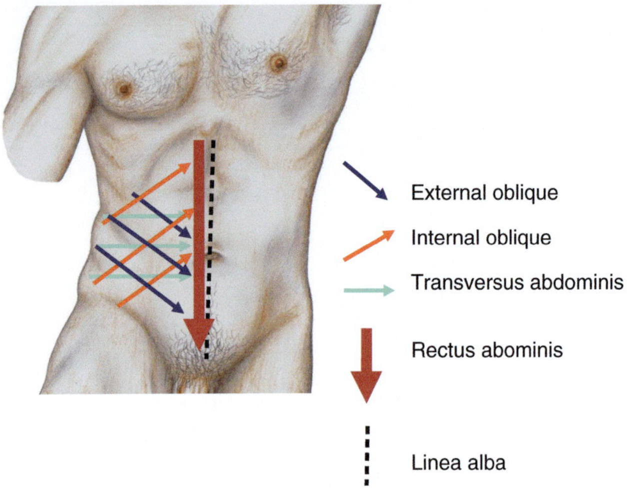

Fig. 21 The abdominal muscles schematized on an anterior view

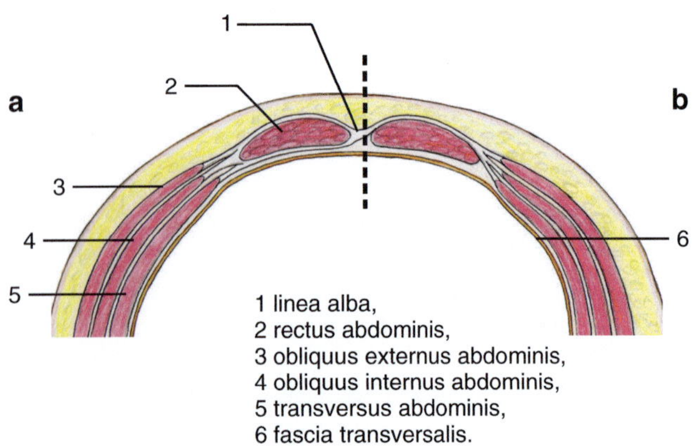

Fig. 22 Horizontal section showing the arrangement of the abdominal muscles: (A) section above the umbilicus, (B) section below the umbilicus

above, limit the abdominal cavity which can be compressed by their contraction and thus achieve an anterior pneumatic column (Fig. 23).

- The muscles connecting the pelvis to the femur (Fig. 24) may alter the position of the pelvic ring, which can be considered as a vertebra.

The tensor fasciae latae, the rectus femoris, and the ilio-psoas (not represented in the diagram) rotate the pelvis forwards, in anteversion. Conversely, the gluteus maximus, the adductors, and the hamstrings may cause the pelvis to tilt backwards, or retrovert, typically as a compensation during an anterior imbalance, especially when the subject is walking. The difference in the insertion surface of the gluteus maximus in the Homo sapiens, which can maintain a correct erect position and in the chimpanzee, which has great difficulty in maintaining itself, is demonstrated here (Fig. 25). Loss of lumbar lordosis will decrease the length of the lever arm of the extensors and hence their effectiveness (Fig. 26).

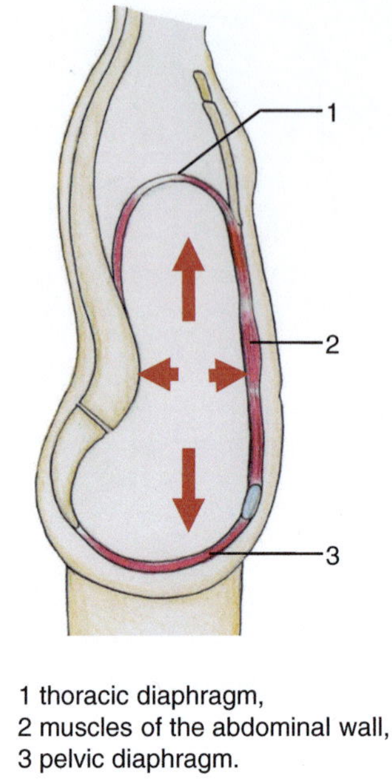

Fig. 23 Muscles participating in the anterior pneumatic support of the spine

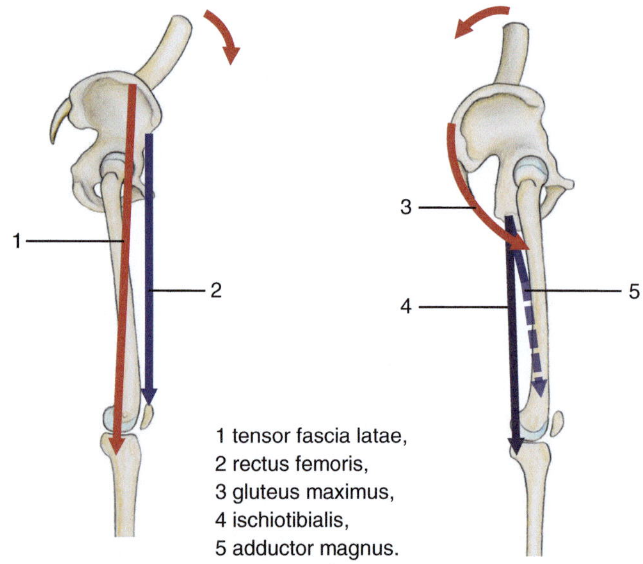

Fig. 24 Muscles of the pelvic limb acting on the position of the pelvis: (1) and (2) result in anteversion. (3), (4) and (5) result in retroversion

Anterior sagittal imbalance with retraction of the psoas and insufficiency of the extensors (the ilio-costalis, longissimus and multifidus and gluteus maximus) may not appear on static profile images, such as EOS or lateral full spine radio-

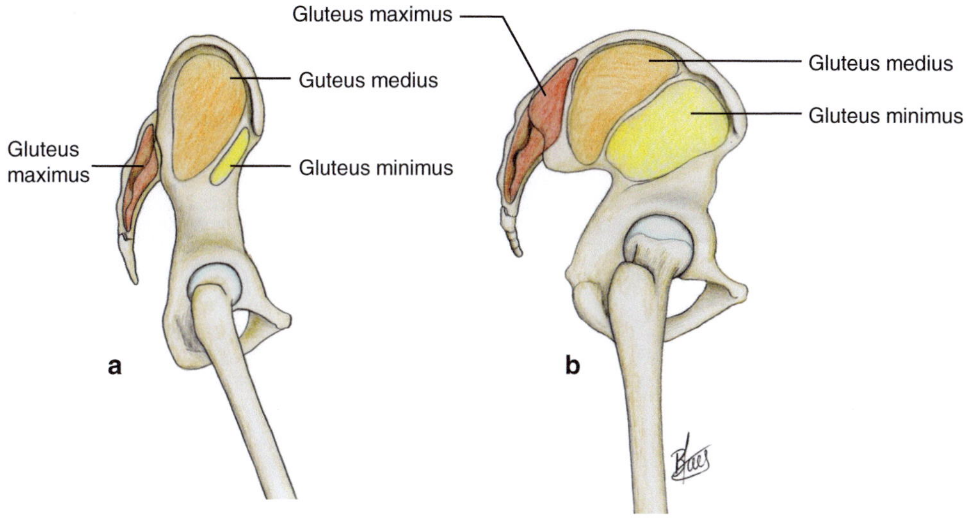

Fig. 25 Comparison of insertion surfaces of three gluteal muscles: in chimpanzee (**a**) and in man (**b**)

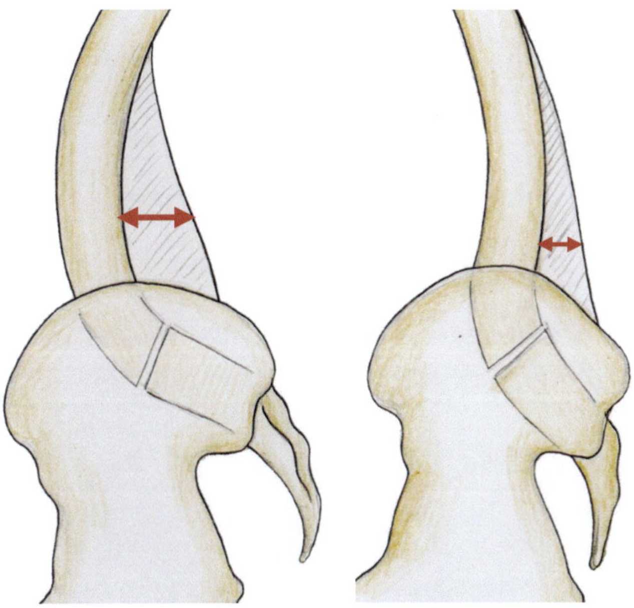

Fig. 26 Lumbar hypolordosis decreases the lever arm of the extensors

graphs, but is evident on walking, especially when the gluteus maximus cannot maintain a vertical sacrum or the pelvis in retroversion (Lee [7]) (Fig. 27).

The Aponeurosis

They will be studied schematically on horizontal cervical and thoraco-lumbar sections.

Three anterior cervical aponeuroses (Fig. 28)

- The superficial aponeurosis (fascia superficialis) enveloping the SCM.
- The intermediate aponeurosis (fascia pretrachealis) enveloping the omohyoid and which is a good landmark for anterior approach to the lower cervical spine.
- The deep aponeurosis (fascia prevertebralis) located in front of the longus colli and the cervical spine.

The Thoraco-Lumbar Aponeuroses

In Fig. 29, which shows the array of muscles in this region, it should be noted that there is a perfect continuity between the aponeuroses of the posterior muscles and that of the abdominal muscles [3].

- Anteriorly, we find the linea alba. The aponeurosis of the rectus abdominis is flanked by the two leaf-like formations of the internal oblique muscles superior to the umbilicus. On the deep aspect, the fascia transversalis is very adherent to the peritoneum.
- Posteriorly (Fig. 30), we find the thoraco-lumbar fascia as described by Bogduk [8] and which behaves like an inextensible envelope put under tension by the contraction of the posterior muscles to create another system of posterior pneumatic spinal support. According to Bogduk, therefore, there are three layers: the superficial layer consists of the extension of the fibers of the latissimus dorsi inferomedially; the intermediate layer is formed by transverse fibers from the middle aponeurosis of the posterior serratus superior and inferior; the deep arises from the aponeurosis of the ilio-costalis and longissimus. The ensemble gives a thick, pearly, triangular structure with fibers intersecting almost perpendicularly near the spinous midline.

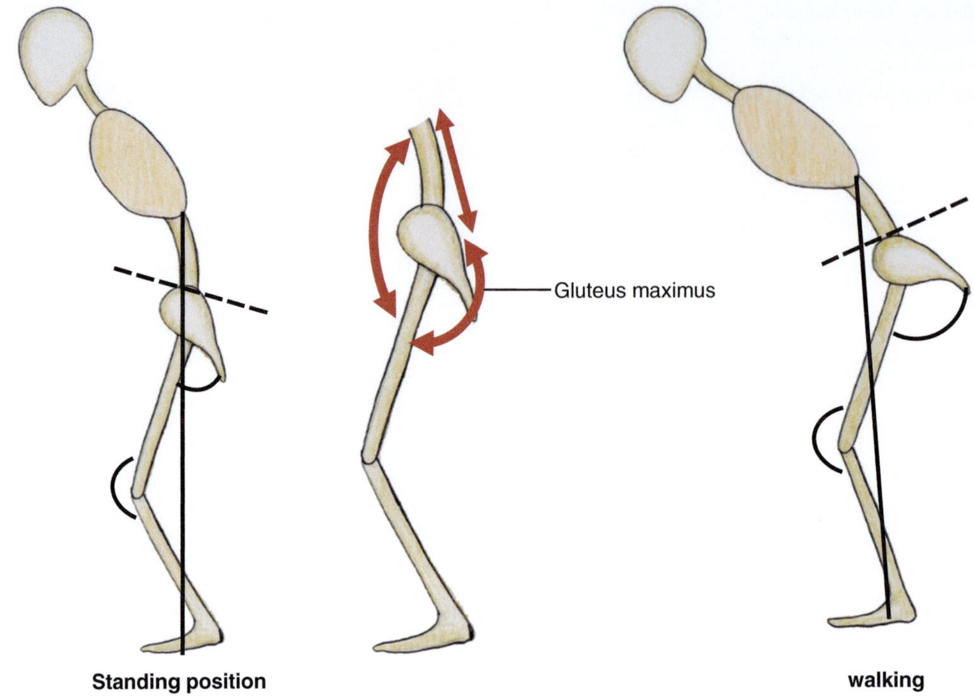

Fig. 27 Failure to stabilize the pelvis in retroversion, in particular by the worsening of gluteus maximus during walking. Anterior imbalance in standing position which worsens during walking

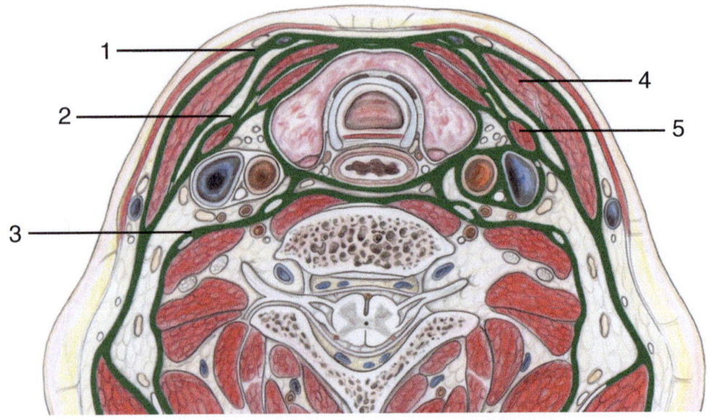

1 deep aponeurosis (lamina prevertebralis),
2 middle aponeurosis (lamina pretrachealis),
3 superficial aponeurosis (lamina superficialis),
4 sternocleidomastoid,
5 omohyoid.

Fig. 28 Anterior cervical aponeuroses

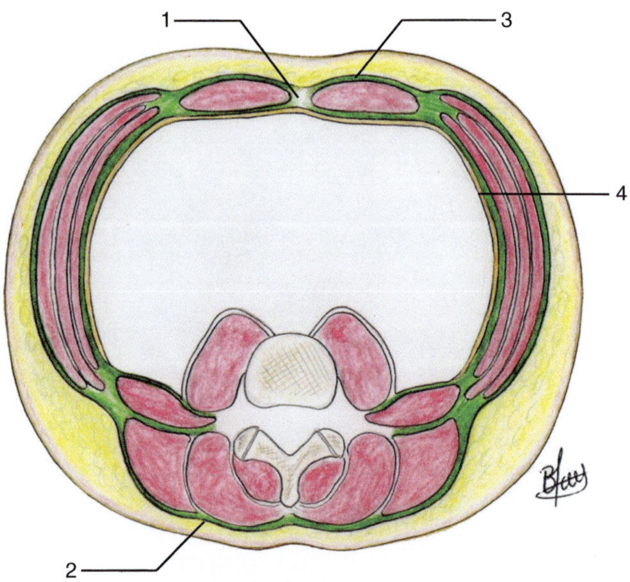

1 linea alba,
2 thoraco-lumbar fascia,
3 fascia of the rectus abdominis,
4 fascia transversalis.

Fig. 29 Muscles and aponeuroses of the trunk on a horizontal section

Action

As we have said, the spinal muscles have a double action—stabilizing and dynamic actions.

Stabilizing Action

In the stabilization of the spine, the muscles behave like active dampers as opposed to the passive dampers such as the discs and the articular facet joints.

- The ventral muscles (scaleni and longus colli at the cervical level, intercostalis and pectoralis at the thoracic level, lumbo-sacral mass, glutei, and hamstrings have a tightening or contractile effect that corrects the natural buckling of the spine (Fig. 31).
- Pneumatic abdominal support is achieved by contraction of the abdominal muscles, and thoracic and pelvic dia-

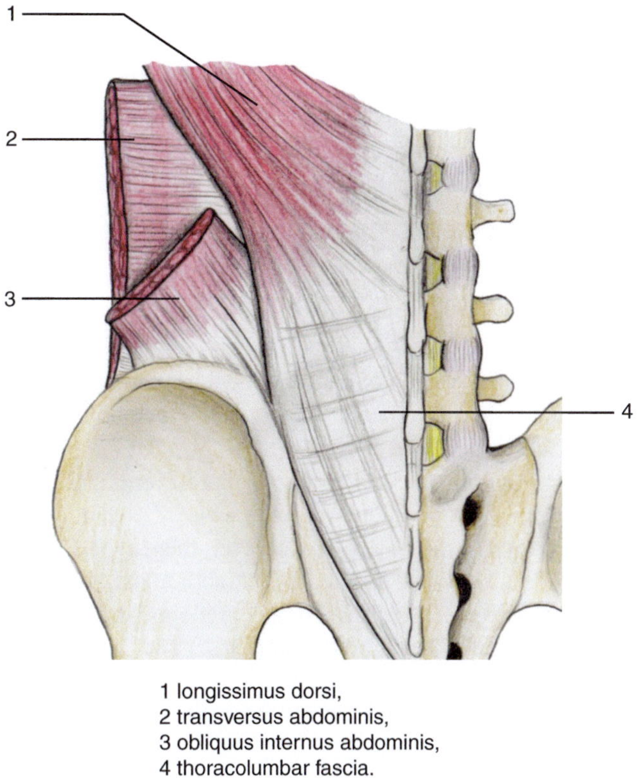

Fig. 30 Thoraco-lumbar fascia (Bogduk [8])

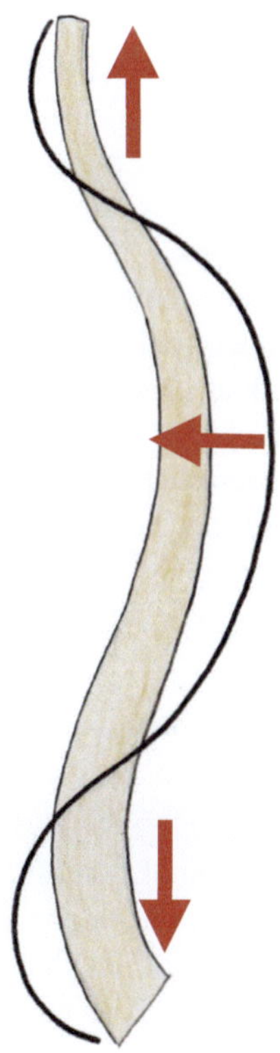

Fig. 31 Phenomenon of buckling (black line) and shrinking or tightening

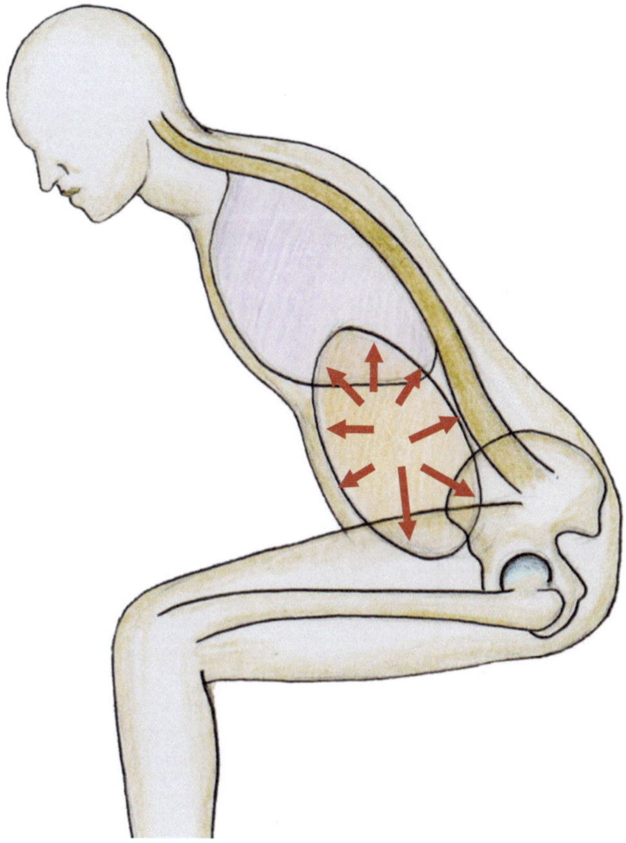

Fig. 32 Anterior pneumatic support

phragms on the abdominal cavity. Morris [9] has demonstrated that the presence of this abdominal box or column reduces the stresses on the spine by almost 1/3, particularly when lifting a weight (Fig. 32).

The muscles constituting the lumbo-sacral mass (iliocostalis, longissimus, and multifidus) enveloped by the inextensible thoraco-lumbar aponeurosis form a composite beam with the vertebral column (Blaimont [10]) (Fig. 33). A composite beam is a beam composed of two or more different materials, joined together, so that there is no sliding movement from one material to another; these materials share the stresses according to their modulus of elasticity: the muscles therefore discharge the stresses of the bone. This explains the importance of the repair and reinsertion of thoracolumbar fascia on spinous process in posterior lumbar surgery (Fig. 34).

Dynamic Action

There are two large movements in the spine: flexion-extension and inclination-rotation.

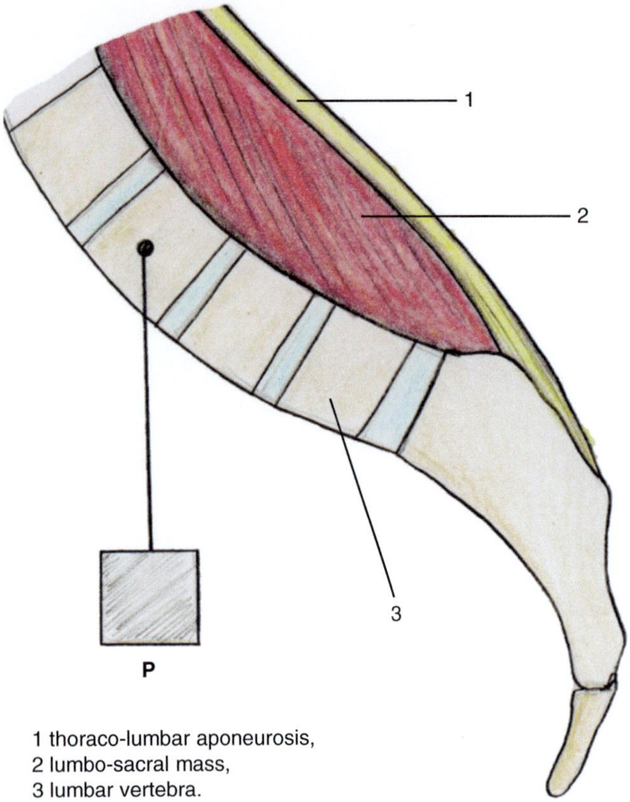

Fig. 33 Composite beam

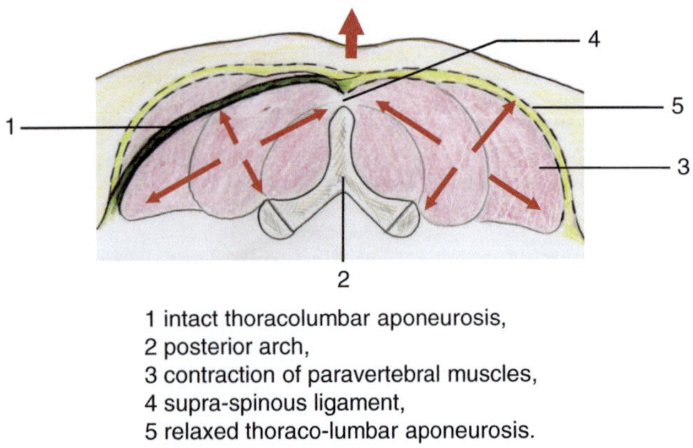

Fig. 34 The contraction of the lumbo-sacral mass under the inextensible thoracolumbar aponeurosis has a protective effect of the spine (schematic horizontal section)

- In flexion-extension, regardless of the spinal level considered, the muscles in front of the line of gravity are flexors and those behind the extensors.
- The inclination-rotation movement is controlled by muscles that intersect this axis of gravity such as SCM, trapezius, scaleni in the cervical region, and quadratus lumborum, and ilio-psoas in the lumbar area. All of these muscles induce an inclination on their same side and a rotation on the opposite side.

Histophysiology

Since 1678, Lorenzi has distinguished the white muscular fibers from red fibers in the animal. Ranvier, in 1874, differentiated white fibers with rapid contraction from red fibers with slow contraction. In the years 1950–1960, Dubowitz-Pearse, and then Kengel developed the histoenzymology which allows recognition of the different types of muscle fibers.

The different types of muscle fibers

- Type I (slow twitch oxidative) fibers are red, with high capillary density. They have an aerobic metabolism and are rich in oxidative enzymes (SDH, NADH) but poor in glycolytic enzymes. In electron microscopy, there is a richness of mitochondria and wide Z band striae (760 A°). On the physiological level, these type I fibers provide a slow and sustained contraction and are resistant to fatigue. They are found predominantly in the endurant and anti-gravity muscles. The force they develop is lower than that of type II fibers. Finally, the motor neuron which controls these fibers is small and the conduction is slow.
- The type IIb fibers (fast twitch glycolytic or fast fatigable) are white, of small size and of weak capillary richness. They have an anaerobic metabolism and are poor in oxidative enzymes but rich in glycolytic enzymes. In electron microscopy, there is a relative poverty of mitochondria and narrow Z striae (320 A°). On the physiological level, these fibers provide a rapid contraction and are not very resistant to fatigue. They are more numerous in the phasic muscles (in sprinters for example) and are innervated by large-sized motoneurons.
- Type IIa (fast twitch oxidative glycolytic or fast resistant) are intermediate fibers rich in oxidative and glycolytic enzymes; they provide less rapid contractions but are more resistant to fatigue.
- Type IIc fibers, present in very low amounts (<1%), are embryonic and can be seen in regenerating muscles. All these data are summarized in the table (Fig. 35).

Distribution of Muscle Fibers According to the Spinal Level

The percentage distribution of I and II fibers varies for each muscle as a function of its tonic or phasic action. In the paravertebral muscles, one might think that there is an equal distribution of fibers I, IIa, and IIb. In fact, at the thoracic level, 70% are type I fibers compared to 60% in the lumbar level (Slager [11]).

Fig. 35 Characteristics of the I, IIa, and IIb fibers

	Type I	Type II a	Type II b
Color	Red	Intermediate	White
Capillary density	High	High	Low
Metabolism	Aerobic	Aero and Anaerobic	Anaerobic
Oxidative enzymes	Rich	Rich	Poor
Glycolitic Enzymes	Poor	Rich	Rich
Anglo-saxon denomination	Slow twitch oxidative	Fast twitch oxidative / glycolytic	Fast twitch glycolytic
Mitochondria	+++	++	+
Z band	Intermediate	Wide	Narrow
Action	Tonic	Phasic	Phasic
Effort	Endurant		Resistant
Contraction	Slow	Fast resistant	Fast fatigable
Fatigability	Late	Late	Early
Motoneurone	Small size (low conduction speed)		Large size (high conduction speed)

In the transverse direction, the percentage of I fibers is variable (Jorgensen [4]).

- Multifidus: 50.7–57.4%
- Longissimus: 65.2–73.4%
- Ilio-costal 52.4–57.7%

In the antero-posterior direction, according to Jorgensen [4] and Bagnall [5], there are more type I fibers in the deep layers than superficially. Finally, to complicate the matter, Bagnall [5] demonstrated on 19 cases of discectomies that there was a difference in distribution of type I fibers between the right and left sides.

Morphological and Functional Variations of Muscle Fibers

The natural aging process leads to a loss of muscle mass (sarcopenia): at age 50 a sedentary subject has lost 10% of his muscle mass and a loss of 50% by 80 years. In other words, Buckwalter [12] says that we lose 10% of our remaining muscle mass with each decade. For some, there would be a decrease in the number of I and II fibers equally. For others, there is a preferential decrease in the size of the type II fibers. The oxidative (and globally enzymatic) action decreases. Classically, the lesions are of the neurogenic type with the presence of target cells or ragged red fibers (RRF), we will come back to this. Finally, fatty degeneration, especially of the deep part of the paravertebral muscles (multifidus), is classical and led Hadar [13] to describe three stages of gravity (Fig. 36).

During *exercise*, there is firstly a paradoxical recruitment of I fibers whose motoneurons are nevertheless of small caliber, then IIa and b fibers. While some believe that there is no change in the fibers through training, many believe that endurance exercises (such as the marathon) first solicit and then increase the number of I fibers, while in the high intensity exercises (as in sprinters), there is first solicitation and increase of II fibers. MacDougall estimates that working with heavy loads increases II fibers by 33% and I fibers by 23%. It is conventional to say that the appearance of muscular "bulking" is the hypertrophy of II fibers. In these modifications due to training, the dilemma is whether there is an increase in the number or size of the fibers, the second hypothesis being the most probable.

Electric stimulation recruits fast fibers, especially at low frequency.

The *immobilization* of 4 weeks results in a loss of strength of 30–50%. There is an atrophy of the I and II fibers but especially of the I fibers because they predominate in anti-gravity muscles.

Paravertebral Muscles in Spinal Pathology

This chapter will largely summarize the presentation made to the French Scoliosis Study Group (G.E.S.) in Nantes in 1994 [14] on morphological, histoenzymological, and ultrastructural aspects in 33 patients with various spinal pathologies on tests performed by Coquet, anatomopathologist.

We will analyze these results by comparing them with those of other authors for four pathological entities:

1. Lumbar instability with chronic low back pain for which a surgical procedure (flexible or rigid arthrodesis or hernia discectomy) was proposed. In parallel with standard anatomopathological examinations, the subjects underwent isometric tests,
2. Arthrogenic kyphosis, with severe and progressive forms of lumbar degeneration,
3. Idiopathic scoliosis (previously documented muscular histology and electromyography),
4. Iatrogenic effects on the muscles after posterior spinal surgery.

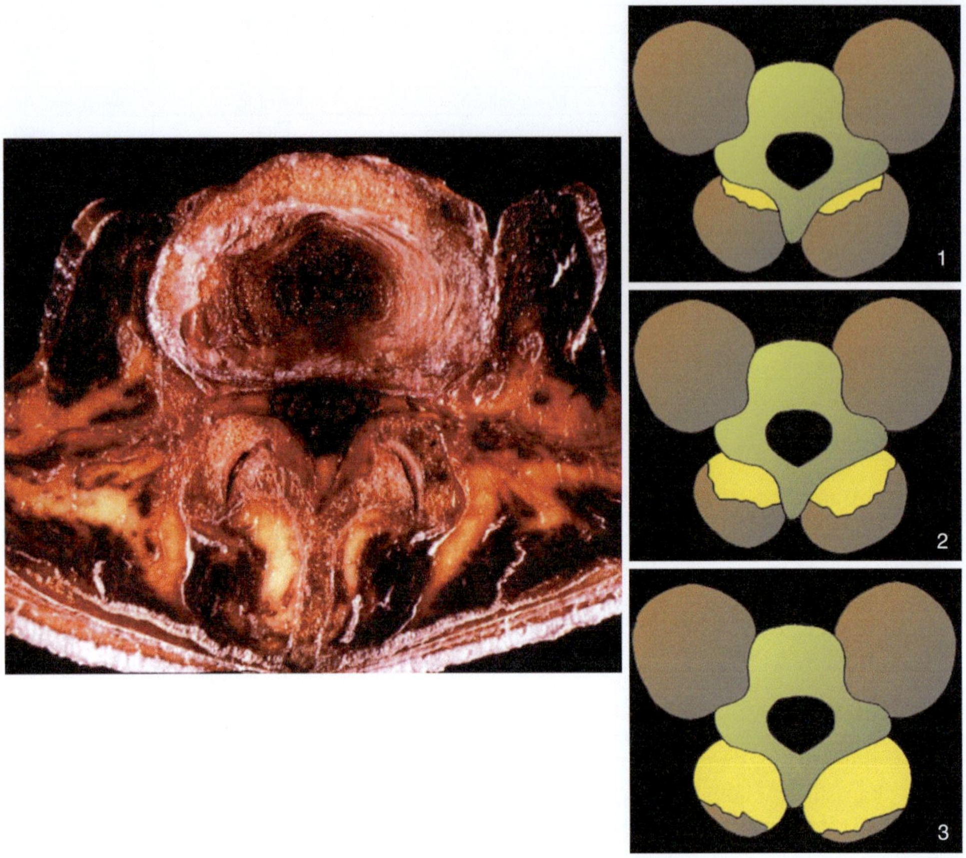

Fig. 36 The three stages of fatty degeneration of Hadar [13]

Technical Reminder: in all cases, the muscular specimen is surgical when approaching the paravertebral muscles (multifidus, longissimus, or more rarely ilio-costal). This sampling must be done carefully, without using the electric scalpel, without damaging the muscle piece which must have a length of 10 mm (long axis parallel to the fibers) and a width of 4–5 mm for the histo-enzymology study, 2 mm for electron microscopy with inclusion in glutaraldehyde. The pieces are sent as quickly as possible to the laboratory to be frozen in isopentane cooled to −160° by liquid nitrogen. These few elementary details avoid artifacts that complicate interpretation. Three types of examinations are carried out: optical microscopy with specific staining that provides 5–20% of the diagnosis [15], histoenzymology which is instructive in about 80% of cases, electron microscopy that complements information on constituents of the myocyte and interstitial tissue.

Elemental Lesions, Lesional Groups

This succession of exams allows one to describe:

1. Elemental lesions of the muscular fibers with some abnormal characteristics such as (Fig. 37):
   - Targeted cells (most often referred to as neurogenic lesions),
   - Targetoid cores (pseudocore fibers, central cores in myofibers) visible on the oxidative preparations in histoenzymology,
   - Ragged red fibers (RRF), visualized by a modified Gomori trichrome, confirmed by the ultrastructure; these RRF are found in certain myopathies, muscle ischemia and in the elderly,
   - The lipid overload highlighted by black Sudan staining (nonfluorescent, relatively thermostable lysochrome (fat-soluble dye) diazo dye) on freezing cut,
   - The fibroadiposis on paraffin cut.

2. Lesional groupings:
   - Neurogenic lesions with grouped involvement of the fibers since it is the motor unit that is affected (grouping phenomenon),
   - Myogenic lesions with irregular fiber involvement and variegated topography,
   - Dystrophy which is equivalent to a severe myogenic lesion with significant necrosis and fibroadiposis.

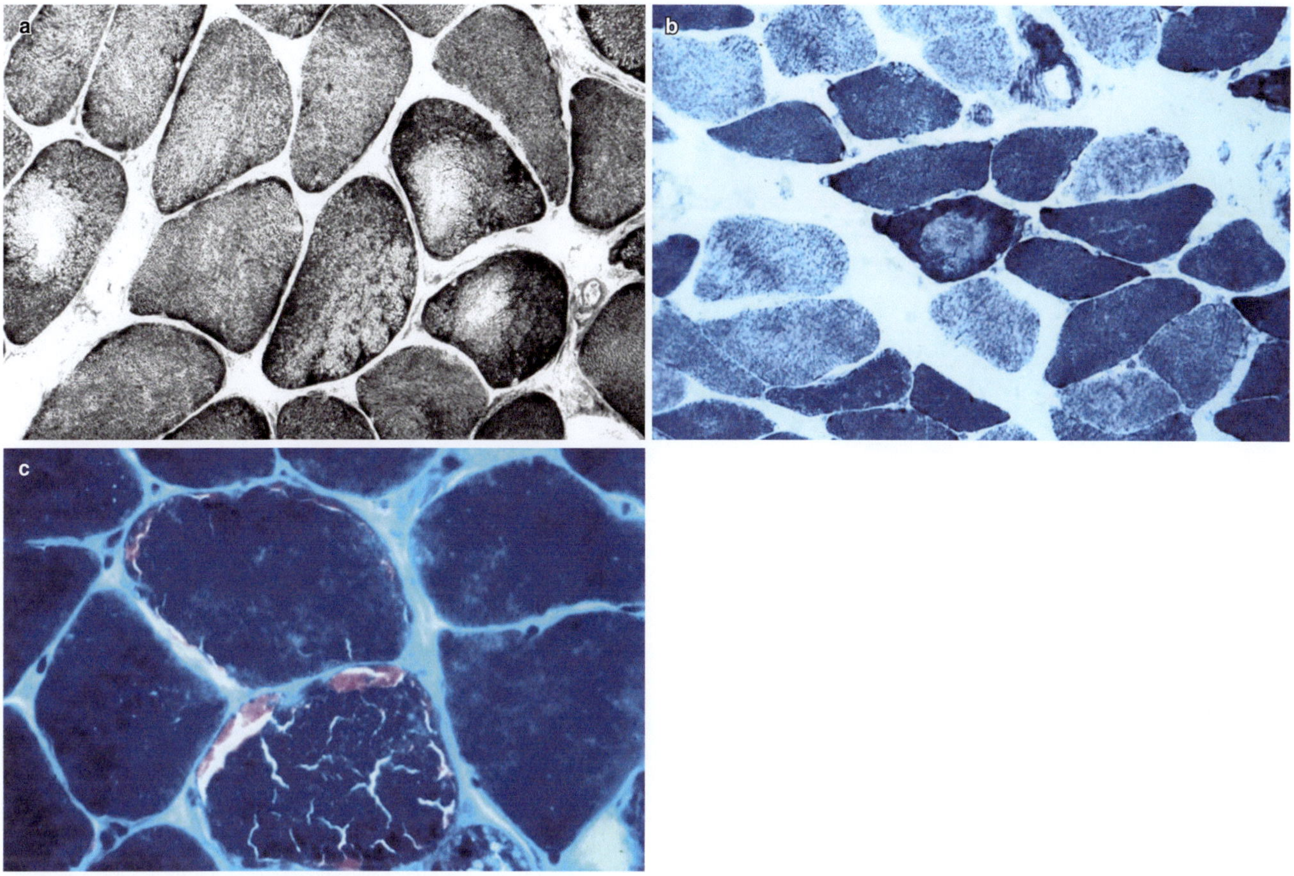

Fig. 37 Elementary histological lesions. (**a**) target cells of a neurogenic lesion. (**b**) core targetoid or pseudocore of a myogenic lesion. (**c**) ragged red fiber (RRF) of a myogenic lesion

Lumbar Instability Resulting in Chronic Low Back Pain

Twelve patients operated on for lumbar instability (discectomy or arthrodesis) underwent muscle sampling. Twice, there were no abnormalities. The most typical lesion is atrophy more than the decrease in the number of type II fibers, the predominance of type I fibers, and the presence of targetoids core and RRF. The presence of some RRF (3%) is significant in subjects of 40 years on average. Laroche [16] describes degenerative myopathy of the paravertebral muscles. The fibroadiposis is sometimes very marked and corresponds to the images of fatty degeneration found on CT (Hadar [13]) or MRI (Parkkola [17]) scan. Anderson [18], in a recent study, also found this decrease in the diameter of II fibers with the presence of targetoid cores. They carried out post-rehabilitation checks in operated patients: there was regular improvement in histological evidence demonstrating the reversible state of the lesions. Rantanen [19] on 18 discectomies recognizes a decrease in II fibers; at 5 years, this imbalance disappears and adiposis diminishes. Similarly, Larsson [20] found RRF eight times out of 11 in the trapezius and only four out of ten in normal subjects. Finally, all of these histological studies recognize, at the early stage of lumbar instability, an atrophy of the fast II fibers and, at a later stage, a fibroadiposis and the high presence of RRF. The subject, losing its potential in fast fibers, loses, in some way, its adaptation to inappropriate or wrong movements. This deficit of the extensors was confirmed by isometric and isokinetic investigations.

Arthrogenic Kyphosis

It is a nosological entity central to degenerative lumbar pathology. It affects patients at approximately 60 years having often worked extensively in a flexion position, with a loss of lumbar lordosis without major degenerative scoliosis. The inflection of the trunk is generally aggravated by walking and requires the aid of a stick. Radiologically, there are signs of severe lumbar degeneration with anterior narrowing of the lower lumbar discs (hence this very important loss of lordosis) and hypertrophy of the facet joints and the laminae limiting spinal extension. Lipomatous muscular degeneration in

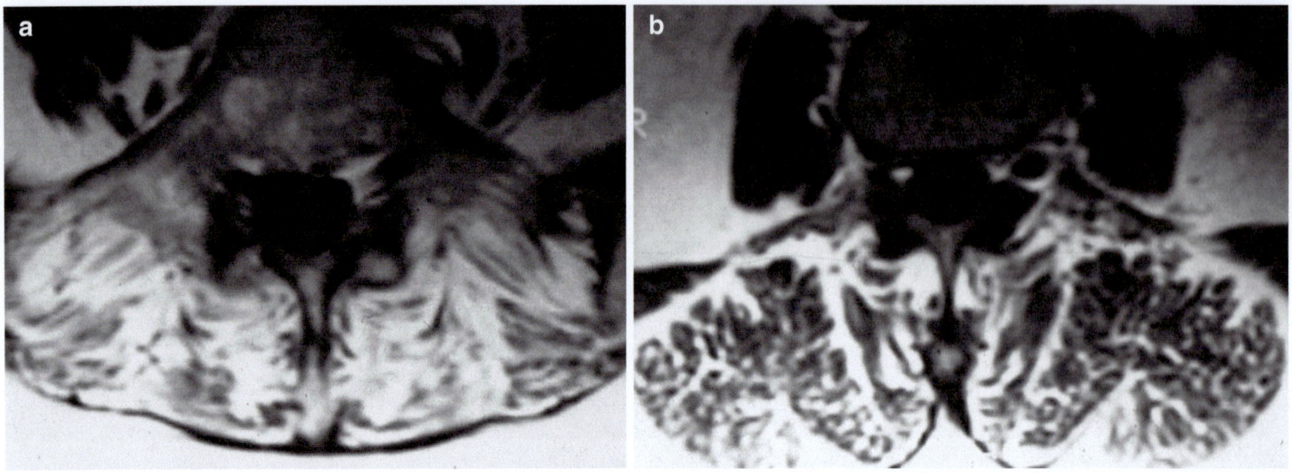

Fig. 38 M.R.I. of arthrogenic kyphosis with stage Hadar 3 in lumbo-sacral area (**a**) and stage Hadar 2 in thoraco-lumbar area (**b**)

CT/tomodensitometry and MRI is significant (stage 2 or 3 in the Hadar classification) near the lumbo-sacral junction and has the peculiarity of extending to the thoraco-lumbar area (Fig. 38). Numerous denominations have been proposed for this condition: camptocormia (truncal inclination) has rather a hysterical connotation (described during the First World War). Rénier [21] proposes instead the term of reducible kyphosis with myopathy.

We prefer most to speak of degenerative or arthrogenic kyphosis because in the five patients operated on for surgical correction, there appeared increased histopathological signs observed in the group of lumbar instabilities: almost complete disappearance of type II fibers, major fibroadiposis affecting both the lumbar and specifically thoracolumbar muscles, abnormal presence of targetoid cores and RRF. On bibliography, Takemitsu [22] described a homogeneous series of 105 cases with five stages of radiological progression of gravitation according to the prevalence of lumbar kyphosis and retroversion of the pelvis; the common factor predominant in this series is the prolonged bent forward labor, such as working in rice fields, and thus both the disuse of the extensors and their prolonged tension. The histological aspect of this has not been studied. Laroche [16] describes 14 cases of neighboring clinical cases with muscle samples showing the presence of targetoid cores and an abnormal distribution of the mitochondria. Revel [23] supports a neurogenic hypothesis, advocating compression of the posterior motor branches that fit into the framework of osteoarthritic neurological compressions.

Hilliquin [24] describes inflammatory lesions and speaks of myositis responding to anti-inflammatory treatment. Finally, Styf [25] raised the hypothesis of a syndrome of the muscular compartments. We will recall that Simmons [26], which studied the under-used paravertebral muscles of ankylosing spondylitis, showed that there was atrophy of I and II fibers and the presence of core targetoids. Our impression [27] is that there is usually a lack of use and thus a major degeneration that can progress as far as dystrophy.

Idiopathic Scoliosis

Seven patients were sampled during posterior arthrodesis surgery. These were adolescent scoliosis, severe thoracic lordoscoliosis, and infantile scoliosis over 100°. In a fairly regular manner, there were few abnormalities on the concave side and on the convex side, the reminiscent signs of lesions of the underused muscles of the lumbar instabilities: atrophy of the II fibers, predominance of the I fibers. In the case of infantile scoliosis, the signs suggest a neurogenic involvement with severe fibro-adiposis, somewhat as if the intercostal nerves, very compressed between the ribs, no longer transmitted the nerve impulses.

This chapter of idiopathic scoliosis is probably the one that has been the most studied: the results are also somewhat discordant. Bylund [28] studied 16 idiopathic scolioses and seven congenital: he found in idiopathic scoliosis an increase of I fibers on the convex side and a decrease of the same fibers on the concave side. The same findings are made in congenital scoliosis, which suggests that muscular lesions are the consequence of spinal asymmetry, whatever the cause. Zetterberg [29] also found an increase in I fibers on the convex side. Slager [11] studied 19 cases of non-idiopathic scoliosis and notes a preponderance of I fibers on the convex side as in an overtrained muscle. Yarom [30] out of 45 operated idiopathic scoliosis noted an atrophy of the I fibers on the concave side; suggesting a global neuromuscular disorder because the studied deltoids and quadriceps also present anomalies. Sangal [31] finds these same anomalies on the gluteus maximus. Chan [32] in an S.T.I.R. M.R.I.

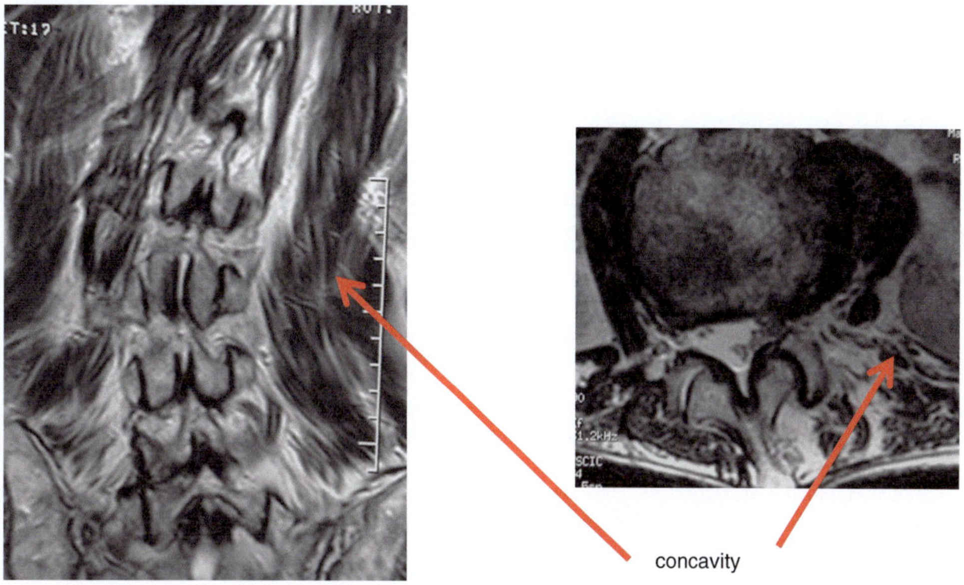

Fig. 39 M.R.I. of an adult scoliosis showing concave fatty degeneration

study found an increase in fatty hypersignals at the apex of the concavity, in proportion with the Cobb angle and curve evolution. For our part, we found fatty degeneration in the concavity (Fig. 39).

Muscle Integrity After Posterior Arthrodesis

We report the case of a 25-year-old woman who was operated on for post-traumatic spinal kyphosis, the initial fracture not being complicated by neurological deficit. A Dove frame fixation was applied and the material was removed 16 months later: the thoracic muscles near the graft and the underlying lumbar muscles were compared. In the arthrodesis, there are typical neurogenic signs of degeneration with phenomena of grouping in histoenzymology and mitochondrial abnormalities; we can judge here the consequences of the posterior approach—dissecting off the muscles from the median line to the transverse processes. Kawaguchi [33] studied the development of muscles in the rat after prolonged stretching; there is sometimes irreversible damage depending on the length of the distraction. Direct trauma, devascularization, and denervation have a reduced pejorative effect in minimally invasive approaches. More recently, Gille [34] published on the study of posterior lumbar muscles in M.R.I. with an evaluation of the axial sectional area (proportional to the force) and the contractile component (also proportional to the force). After posterior arthrodesis, the contractile component decreases more inferiorly than towards the superior aspect of the arthrodesis, probably due to the descending action of posterior nerves altered by dissection [35]; this unfavorable effect is not diminished by the use of curare (muscle relaxant) [36].

In conclusion, on these mainly histological findings concerning certain spinal pathologies, we will report that:

- In the lumbo-radiculalgia series, a consistent atrophy of type II rapid fibers, which means a certain loss of muscular reactivity due to lack of use or training,
- The increase of these signs with impairment of the mitochondrial function for the more advanced forms such as arthrogenic kyphosis,
- The involvement of convex muscles in idiopathic scoliosis with invasion by type II fibers while the concave side is a quasi-normal side except in severe cases of infantile scoliosis where there are neurogenic signs,
- Finally, the predictable repercussion of surgical dissection on the muscles near the arthrodesis and below the arthrodesis.

References

1. Martinez C. Le Rachis, Cahier d'Anatomie Vivante. Paris: Masson; 1982.
2. Poisson P. Protection intrabuccale: epidémiologie – evaluation biomécanique et physiologique [Thèse d'Université, mention Sciences Biologiques et Médicales, option Sciences Odontologiques]. Ecole Doctorale, Université Victor Segalen Bordeaux II; 2005; n° 1247.
3. Kapandji IA. Physiologie articulaire 3. Tronc et Rachis. Paris: Maloine; 1994.
4. Jorgensen K, Mag C, Nicholaïsen T, Kato M. Muscle fiber distribution, capillary density and enzymatic activities in the lumbar paravertebral muscles of young men: significance for isometric endurance. Spine. 1993;18:1439–50.

5. Bagnall KM, Ford DM, McFadden KD, et al. The histochemical composition of human vertebral muscle. Spine. 1984;9:470–3.
6. Wiltse LL, Spencer CW. New uses and refinements of the paraspinal approach to the lumbar spine. Spine. 1988;13:696–706.
7. Lee CS, Lee CK, Kim YT, Hong YM, Yoo JH. Dynamic sagittal imbalance of the spine in degenerative flat back. Significance of pelvic tilt in surgical treatment. Spine. 2001;26:2029–35.
8. Bogduk N. The applied anatomy of the thoracolumbar fascia. Spine. 1984;9:165–70.
9. Morris JM. Biomechanic of the spine. Arch Surg. 1975;107:418–24.
10. Blaimont P, Alameh M. Biomécanique de l'arthrodèse lombaire. Acta Orthop Belg. 1981;47:605–18.
11. Slager UT, Hsu JD, Swank SM. Pathology and morphometry of the paraspinous muscles in nonidiopathic scoliosis. J Pediatr Orthop. 1987;7:301–4.
12. Buckwalter JA, Golberg VM, Booth, et al. Current concepts review: soft tissue aging and musculoskeletal function. J Bone Joint Surg. 1993;75A:1533.
13. Hadar H, Godoth M, Heifetz M. Fatty replacement of lower paraspinal muscles normal and neuromuscular disorders. AJR Am J Roentgenol. 1983;141:895–8.
14. Vital JM, Coquet M, Cernier A, Pointillart V, Sénégas J. Les muscles paravertébraux en pathologie rachidienne: aspects morphologiques, histo-enzymologiques et ultrastructuraux. Communication au G.E.S. de Nantes. 1994.
15. Fardeau M, Tome FMS, Coquet M. Rôle diagnostic de la microscopie électronique en pathologie musculaire. Arch Anat Cytol Pathol. 1982;30:155–9.
16. Laroche M, Delisle MB, Mazières B, Rascol A, Cantagrel A, Arlet PH, Arlet J. Myopathie tardive localisée aux muscles spinaux: une cause de cyphose lombaire acquise. Rev Rhum Mal Ostéo-Artic. 1991;58:829–39.
17. Parkkola R, Rytokoski U, Kormano M. Magnetic renonance imaging of the discs and trunk muscles in patients with chronic low back pain and healthy control subjects. Spine. 1993;18:830–6.
18. Anderson GB. Evaluation of muscle function. In: Frymoyer JW, editor. The adult spine: principles and practice. New York: Raven Press; 1991.
19. Rantanen J, Hurme M, Falck B, et al. The lumbar multifidus muscle five years after surgery for a lumbar intervertebral disc herniation. Spine. 1993;18:568–74.
20. Larsson B, Libellius R, Ohlsson K. Trapezius muscle changes unrelated to static work load. Clinical and morphologic controlled studies of 22 woman with and without neck pain. Acta Orthop Scand. 1992;63:203–6.
21. Rénier JC. Cyphose réductible, camptocormie, proclinorachie. Rev Rhum Mal Ostéo-Artic. 1993;60:943.
22. Takemitsu Y, Harada Y, Iwahara T, Miyamoto M, Miyatake Y. Lumbar degenerative kyphosis: clinical, radiological and epidemiological studies. Spine. 1988;13:1317–26.
23. Revel M, Mayoux-Benhamou A. La cyphose acquise réductible du sujet âgé. In: Simon L, editor. Le Rachis Vieillissant. Paris: Masson; 1992.
24. Hilliquin P, Menkes CJ, Laoussadi S, et al. Camptocormie du sujet âgé: une nouvelle entité par atteinte des muscles paravertébraux. Rev Rhum Mal Ostéo-Artic. 1992;19:169–75.
25. Styf F, Lysell E. Chronic compartment syndrom in the erector spinae muscle. Spine. 1987;13:680–2.
26. Simmons EH, Graziano GP, Heffner R. Muscle disease as a cause of kyphotic deformity in ankylosing spondylitis. Spine. 1991;16(s):351–60.
27. Vital JM, Sénégas J, Pointillart V. Cyphoses dégénératives lombaires. In: Le Rachis Vieillissant, Simon L. éditeur. Paris: Masson; 1992.
28. Bylund P, Jansson F, Dahlberg E, Eriksson E. Muscle fiber type in thoracic erector spinae muscles. Fibers types in idiopathic and other forms of scoliosis. Clin Orthop Relat Res. 1987;(214):222–8.
29. Zetterberg C, Anisson A, Grimby G. Morphology of the paravertebral muscles in adolescent idiopathic scoliosis. Spine. 1983;8:457–64.
30. Yarom R, Robin GC. Studies on spinal and peripheral muscles from patients with scoliosis. Spine. 1979;4:12–21.
31. Sangal V, Shah A, Flanagan N, Schaefer M, Kane W, Subizami V, Singh H. Morphologic and morphometric studies of muscle in idiopathic scoliosis. Acta Orthop Scand. 1979;50:759–69.
32. Chan YL, Cheng JC, Guo X, King AD, Griffith JF, Metreweli C. MRI evaluation of multifidus muscles in adolescent idiopathic scoliosis. Pediatr Radiol. 1999;12:61–7.
33. Kawaguchi Y, Matsui H, Tsuji H. Back muscle injury after posterior lumbar spine surgery: histology and histochemical analysis in rats. Spine. 1994;19:2590–7.
34. Gille O, De Sèze MP, Guérin P, Jolivet E, Vital JM, Skalli W. Reliability of magnetic resonance imaging measurements of the cross-sectional area of the muscle contractile and non-contractile components. Surg Radiol Anat. 2011;33:735–41.
35. Gille O, Jolivet E, Dousset V, Degryse C, Obeid I, Vital JM, Skalli W. Erector spinae muscle changes on magnetic resonance imaging following lumbar surgery through a posterior approach. Spine. 2007;32:1236–41.
36. Gille O, Obeid I, Degryse C, Guérin P, Skalli W, Vital JM. The use of curare during anesthesia to prevent iatrogenic muscle damage caused by lumbar spinal surgery through a posterior approach. Spine. 2007;32:402–5.

Configuration of the Posterior Lumbar Muscles: Study of Lumbosacral Malformations and the Extraforaminal Approach (ELIF)

D. Recoules-Arche and T. Somon

Purpose

A correlation between the shape of the three posterior lumbar muscles (Multifidus, Longissimus pars lumborum and Iliocostalis pars lumborum) and the vertebral levels has been studied with application to lumbosacral malformations and the extraforaminal approach (ELIF).

Background

The extraforaminal approach [1, 2] to the lumbar spine makes it possible to treat a very lateral herniation or to perform an interbody fusion with cages (ELIF). The approach is made through a natural cleavage plane between the three posterior lumbar muscles (Multifidus (M), Longissimus pars lumborum (L) and Iliocostalis pars lumborum (IC)). The shape of these muscles varies with the level of the lumbar spine. To help the surgeon in this intermuscular approach, we have made, at every level, a correlation between the shape of these muscles and the level of the vertebral discs. A pattern has been found in the normal lumbar spine and in spines with lumbosacral malformations.

With lumbosacral malformations, the bony architecture is somewhat ambiguous and not always easily described despite a lot of classic markers [3–5]. The vertebral segmentation, from genetic origin, includes both muscular and bony structures. Every lumbar posterior muscle has its own shape that varies with each vertebral level. Every muscle belongs to a clearly defined vertebral segment. A global study can help the understanding of these malformations.

D. Recoules-Arche (✉) · T. Somon
Centre Hospitalier J.Monod, Le Havre Cedex, France

Anatomy [6]

Every lumbar vertebra gives insertion to five fascicles of the Multifidus. Every fascicle spans the underlying vertebrae. The belly of the Multifidus lies behind the vertebral lamina as far as the mamillary processes. The last mamillary process is the sacral one, near the ala sacra and the internal iliac aisle. The length of the posterior vertebral lamina increases from L1 to S1. So, the belly of the Multifidus is larger in S1 than in L1.

The Longissimus and Iliocostalis (pars lomborum) have one fascicle at each level. Each fascicle attaches to a transverse process. The muscular belly spans to the iliac crest and the postero-superior iliac spine. So, their bellies are the largest in the middle lumbar level and decrease towards the iliac crest where they attach and form a musculo-aponeurotic sheet.

The inversion of the muscular shapes, larger in the upper level, for the Iliocostalis and the Longissimus (pars lumborum), larger in L5S1 for the Multifidus, must be noted.

Patients and Method

A series of 90 lumbar spines have been analyzed by two experienced spine specialists, a neuroradiologist and a neurosurgeon. The results of each specialist were also repeated. The study was performed with X-ray and CT-scan with a specialized software (Fig. 1). Among the 90 studied lumbar spines, 59 presented a normal bony anatomy. Thirty one were recognized as having a lumbosacral malformation. A disc, above a vertebra that is attached to the pelvis is named "free or functional disc". The first "free disc" is usually L5S1. The upper discs, named second, third and fourth discs are usually L4L5, L3L4 and L2L3 (Table 1).

Instead, a disc, under a vertebra completely or partially attached to the pelvis is a false or non-functional disc. Usually, this disc is S1S2.

The surface of the posterior muscles has been measured at the level of the four last "free discs" and, if necessary, the

J. M. Vital, D. T. Cawley (eds.), *Spinal Anatomy*, https://doi.org/10.1007/978-3-030-20925-4_19

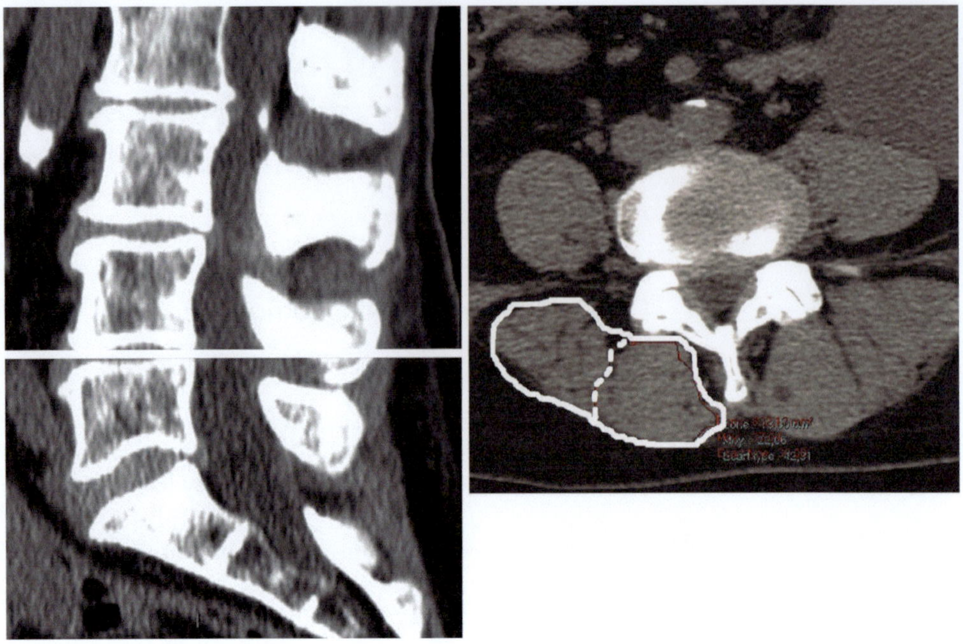

Fig. 1 CT-scan lateral and axial views L4–L5. Measurement of the surfaces of Multifidus and the three posterior muscles (M + L + IC) with horizontal cross-section

Table 1 True levels

		Normal lumbar spine	Lumbar spine with sacralization
False or non-functional disc		S1S2	L5S1
Free disc	First disc	L5–S1	L4–L5
	Second disc	L4–L5	L3–L4
	Third disc	L3–L4	L2–L3
	Fourth disc	L2–L3	

"non-functional disc", with horizontal cross-sections, that go through the posterior part of the inferior endplate.

These horizontal cross-sections are studied from native slides acquired during CT scan and not with cross-sections made in the axis of the disc.

The axis of the disc varies with lumbar lordosis. The cross-sections overlap and represent a shifting surface of the muscles. Instead, horizontal cross-sections, by definition, are parallel and represent a specific surface of the muscle.

Two muscular surfaces have been measured: the surface of the Multifidus (MS) alone and the global surface (GS) of the three muscles (M + L + IC). The ratio of the two surfaces (MS/GS) has been calculated.

The vertebrae have been named in accordance with classic data:

- Five free lumbar vertebrae
- The L3 transverse process is longer, larger and more horizontal than any other

Table 2 Surfaces ratio of the lumbar posterior muscles at every disc level

$$\text{Surfaces ratio} = \frac{\text{Multifidus}}{\text{Multifidus} + \text{Longissimus} + \text{Iliocostalis}}$$

		Normal lumbar spine	Sacralization
Number of spines		59	31
False or non-functional disc		–	–
Free disc	First disc	95% (80–100%)	64% (43–81%)
	Second disc	51% (43–66%)	37% (33–42%)
	Third disc	34% (27–39%)	20% (15–27%)
	Fourth disc	18% (15–21%)	15% (12–18%)

- Instead the L4 transverse process is short, slender with an oblique ascending slope
- The innominate line crosses the disc L5S1 in its posterior part, on the lateral X-ray
- The sacral slope (S1 endplate) is 38° (± 8°)
- The superior attachment of the psoas muscle is at T12L1 level

Results

The results are reported in Table 2.

- Those of a lumbar spine that has been seen as normal
- Those of lumbar spine with lumbosacral malformation

Discussion

At every level, the mean ratio between the surface of the Multifidus and the global surface of the three muscles is very precise, with a very narrow range.

To be the most precise, the extreme values, at every level, never overlap the values of the adjacent levels.

The smallest range is at L3L4 level. This can be explained by the lumbar lordosis. The L3L4 disc is usually in a horizontal plane. A horizontal cross-section is not affected by the lordosis. The cross-sections are nearly perpendicular to the muscles, that is, always with the same angle, as previously described.

At every level a precise pattern can be described at that specific segment.

Instead, if the figures do not match the presumed level, a malformation can be suspected. The true level must be identified in Table 1.

Other authors have studied the posterior lumbar muscles. Fortin et al. [7] have described a quantitative paraspinal measurement. Hoh et al. [8] have searched the anatomical features of the paramedian muscles with application to the splitting approach to the lumbar spine.

If we compare the results we have obtained with this method to the classic anatomical markers, we notice that all classic markers can be wrong but one: the superior attachment of the psoas muscle. In summary, it is the muscular system or myomer, that is, the anterior psoas muscle and the posterior lumbar muscles that mark the segmentation most precisely. The L3L4 disc, or the third "free disc", is the most reliable (MS/GS 34%). This disc is key to this research.

In our study, we find 31 sacralizations for 90 lumbar spines.

Two forms of sacralizations can be described:

- The first one (Fig. 2) is a lumbar spine with four free vertebrae and one vertebra which is attached to the pelvis. It is an obvious sacralization, usually well described radiologically. We named this form, 4FV + 1 (4 free vertebrae + 1 attached).
  The s, at every level (those of the free discs and the figure of the transitional disc), are those obtained for a normal lumbar spine from L2L3 to L5S1.
  Thirteen forms of this sacralization (4FV + 1) have been found on 31 various sacralizations.
- The second form of sacralization (Fig. 3) represents the other 18 sacralizations. This form, unlike the sacralization 4VF + 1, is far from obvious. The lumbar spine presents, at the first glance, five free lumbar vertebrae and one transitional vertebra. For this reason, we named this form 5FV + 1. At every level the ratios are different from those obtained in a normal lumbar spine. Or, as we have written, the ratios are very precise, specific for a level. The discrepancy has prompted a search for a hidden malformation.
  For these 18 lumbar spines, we studied the insertion of the psoas muscle, either with MRI or by coronal cross-sections. The thoracic vertebrae were also counted:
  - The first free vertebra, under the rib cage, is not L1 but T12.
  - The last free vertebra, at the lumbosacral junction, is not L5 but L4.

This form of sacralization (5FV + 1) presents also these particularities:

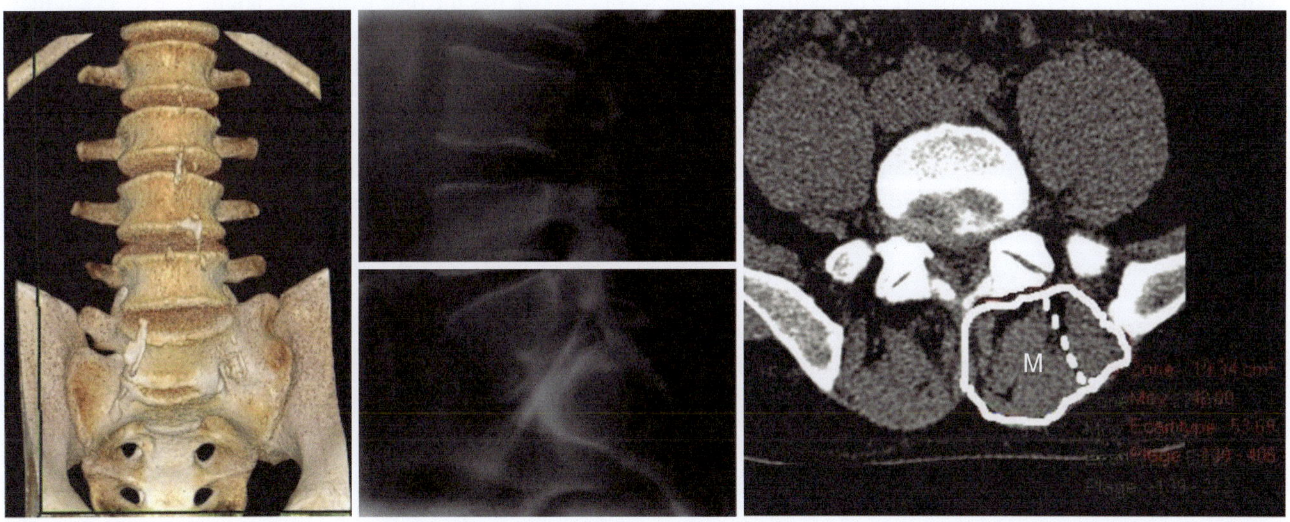

Fig. 2 Sacralization form 4 FV + 1. CT-scan volume 3D and axial view + X-ray lateral view: 12 thoracic vertebrae; four lumbar vertebrae; one transitional vertebra (L5)

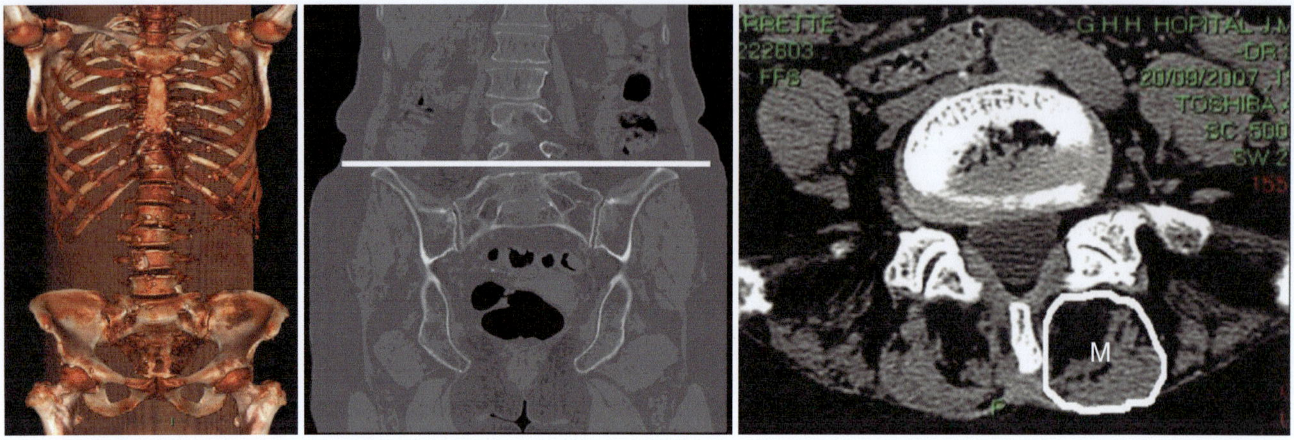

Fig. 3 Sacralization form 5 FV + 1. CT-scan volume 3D, axial and coronal views: 11 thoracic vertebrae; five free vertebrae (T12 + 4 lumbar vertebrae); one transitional vertebra (L5)

- The last free vertebra has a transverse process smaller than the next superior vertebra that is the second free vertebra. This last one often presents the longest transverse process (instead, usually, these particularities are respectively those of L4 and L3).
- The innominate line, on the lateral X-ray view, does not cross the last free disc but the non-functional disc (instead, usually, this particularity respectively belongs to L4L5 and L5S1).

This form of 5FV + 1 sacralization is obviously the most difficult to identify, commonly described by radiologists as a normal lumbar spine or as lumbarization.

Though, the lumbarization, in our study, is hardly identified. It seems to be a normal lumbar spine with few variations. Sometimes, there are a prominent ala sacra and a somewhat posterior innominate line.

Instead, the transverse processes (L3 larger than L4), the attachment of the psoas muscle and the figures of our study are those of a normal lumbar spine. No specific pattern has been used as a criterion.

Hox genes encode transcription factors essential for patterning the anterior to posterior animal body axis [9, 10]. During development, hox genes are activated in a time sequence. A slight time delay in expression leads to caudal transposition of the sacrum.

Concerning monkeys [11], the primitive monkeys (macaque, gibbon) have seven or eight free vertebrae (11 thoracic vertebrae, six or seven free lumbar vertebrae and one free sacral vertebra). The lumbar spine mobility between the thorax and the pelvis is important.

Instead, the great monkeys (gorilla, chimpanzee) stand up: this required a strong bony pelvic frame for sustaining the weight of the erect trunk. The chimpanzee has 12 or 13 thoracic vertebrae, three free lumbar vertebrae and six or seven fused sacral vertebrae.

The lumbar spine of homo sapiens seems to be placed between these two forms.

The lumbar spine flexibility may be linked to the persistence of either one free thoracic vertebra or one free sacral vertebra (Fig. 4).

Instead, the lumbar spine inflexibility may be linked to the complete dorsalization of 12 thoracic vertebrae and the thorax or the superior (sacralization) progression of the sacrum, including the fifth or even the fourth lumbar vertebrae.

Proponents of the lumbar interbody fusion surgery tend to increasingly prefer a more lateral approach in recent years.

The Extraforaminal Lumbar Interbody Fusion (ELIF) (Fig. 5) reaches the disc with a 45° angle, due to a skin incision 10 cm lateral to the midline. The approach reaches the plane between the Multifidus and the Longissimus pars lumborum [1, 2]. The surgeon is able to glide between the muscles, described by CT. The surgical approach is led, not by an ambiguous bony architecture due to vertebral distribution abnormalities but by the pattern of the muscle groups at the level of the foramen.

For example, at the L4L5 level the surgeon will find the plane between the Multifidus and the Longissimus pars lumborum midway between the midline medially and the iliac crest laterally.

At L3L4 level, the plane will be at one-third of the way from the midline to the iliac crest.

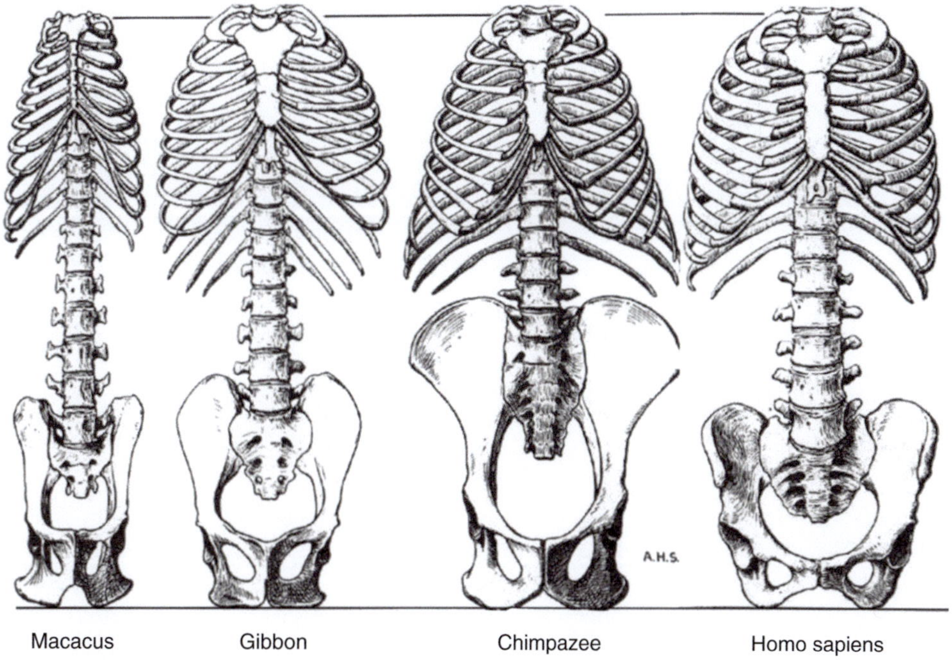

Fig. 4 Monkeys and human skeletons

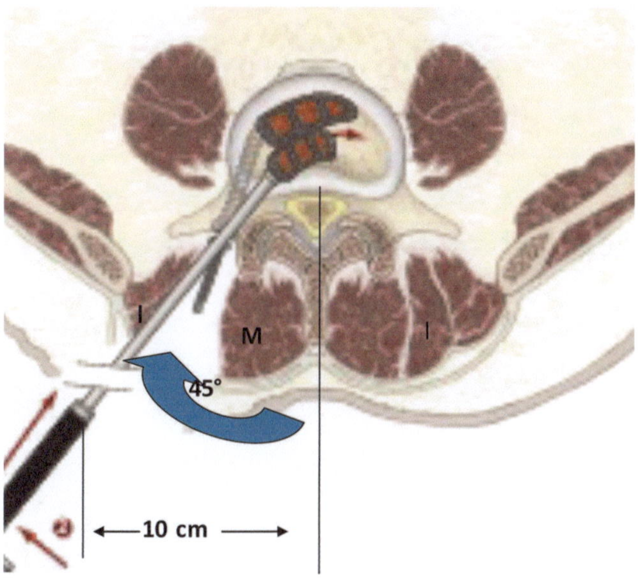

Fig. 5 Extraforaminal lumbar interbody fusion. The approach to the foramen through the intermuscular plane with a 45° angle

Conclusion

The muscle pattern, genetically controlled, is specific to each level of the lumbar spine. The figures of the three muscles (M, L and IC) surfaces, measured with CT horizontal cross-sections, match one vertebral level. That leads the clinician in the study of the lumbosacral malformation and the surgeon in the extraforaminal intermuscular discal surgery.

ELIF makes it possible to insert two cages in the disc with an approach between the muscles. This explains that this technique respects the muscles and can be called a really mini invasive technique.

References

1. Recoules-Arche D, Alcaix D. Fusion lombaire intersomatique par voie extraforaminale unilatérale (ELIF unilatérale). A propos de 75 cas. Rachis. 2006;2:4.
2. Recoules-Arche D, Alcaix D. Extraforaminal lumbar interbody fusion (ELIF) 30 degenerative lumbar dislocations. 1 year follow-up. Rachis. 2004;16:197–204.
3. Mahato NK. Morphometric analysis and identification of characteristic features in sacra bearing accessory articulations with L5 vertebrae. Spine J. 2010;10:616–21.
4. Konin GP, Walz DM. Lumbosacral transitional vertebrae: classification, imaging findings, and clinical relevance. AJNR Am J Neuroradiol. 2010;31(10):1778–86.
5. Hughes RJ, Saifuddin A. Imaging of lumbosacral transitional vertebrae. Clin Radiol. 2004;59:984–91.
6. Bogduk N. Clinical anatomy of the lumbar spine and sacrum. London: Churchill Livingstone; 1997.
7. Fortin M, Battie MC. Quantitative paraspinal measurements. Phys Ther. 1992;6:853–64.
8. Hoh DJ, Wang MY, Rithland SL. Anatomic features of the paramedian muscle – splitting approach to the lumbar spine. Neurosurgery. 2010;66:13–24.
9. Zákány J, Gérard M, Favier B, et al. Deletion of a HoxD enhancer induces transcriptional heterochrony leading to transposition of the sacrum. EMBO J. 1997;16:4393–402.
10. Soshmikova N, Duboule D. Epigenetic control of hox genes collinear activation during vertebrate development. Mech Dev. 2009;126:S6–7.
11. Abitbol MM. Evolution of the sacrum in hominoids. Am J Phys Anthropol. 1987;74:65–81.

Vertebral Column: Muscles, Aponeurosis, and Fascia

F. Bonnel and A. Dimeglio

The anatomical complexity of the muscles of the vertebral column is subtended by a concept based on a muscle–aponeurosis–tendon synergy. In 1989, Zajac [1] and Ettema-Huijing [2] contributed to a new concept on their morphology and behavior with the notion of pennate muscle and function of the aponeurosis. In 1936 Winkler [3] noted (in French) “The comparative study of the vertebral column muscles does not seem to have interested many researchers, if we judge by the minimal work carried out in this field. The great complexity of the muscle systems is difficult to study, thus the descriptions by the authors are various. Comparative anatomy confirmed the conceptual principles of the vertebral muscles according to the overall bone morphology in the analyzed species. For Gracovetsky [4], to understand its function was to evaluate the nature of the forces it must support. On an ontological plan, he suggested that the vertebral column of the fish and the surrounding tissues would have been the first “engine” which allowed motion and concluded that the column was a “mega muscle.” A knowledge of the morphology of the intrinsic constitution of the muscles of the thoracolumbar column allows modeling [5] in the context of low back pain in order to determine the factors responsible and its prevention.

> The model proposed in 2012 by Chrystophy [6] on the lumbar column involved 238 muscle fascicles and 5 intervertebral discs, from the vertical neutral position up to 50° of flexion.

F. Bonnel (✉)
Orthopedic Surgery, Clinique Beau Soleil, Montpellier, France

A. Dimeglio
Department of Pediatric Orthopedic Surgery, Polyclinique Saint Roch, Montpellier, France

History

The number of muscles, with the difficulty of dissection, has limited their study. Books of anatomy (“Dionis [7], Heister [8] Spigelius [9]) Fig. 1)” showed a difficulty and critical analysis based on a lot of dissections.

As early as 1685, Stenonis [10] described the geometry of the fasciculi: its diaphragm, although simplified, gave a clear picture of its organization at the tendon which becomes progressively thicker. Borelli [11] noted that “the length of a muscle was proportional to its degree of motion, which depends on the shortening” and admitted seven forms: *prismatic, rhomboidal, orbicular, crossed, penniforme, radiate, helical*. Stenonis noted [10] that the length of fascicles was constant for each type of muscle (Fig. 2).

In 1892, Trolard, describing the spinal muscles, noted that the transversospinalis was most often reduced to a few fascicles. “Despite its numerous dissections, it refused to allow a classification and adopted a topographic description from superficial to deep” [12].

The papers on the strength of the muscle were carried by the German anatomists Fick [13], von Lanz, and Wachsmuth [14] at the end of the nineteenth and twentieth centuries. Fick [13] noted the relations between size and power and characterized the importance of the notion of all fascicles in relation to their maximum strength (“Cross Section Area”).

The conventional descriptions were based on the complex muscle-tendon with 2 parts, a red central muscle and a tendinous terminal. The histological and physiological evaluation must be modified and has not been developed in anatomy textbooks. Dissections that we have done since 1985 have led to a macroscopic dissection on the disposition of the fascicles with the pennation, the aponeurosis, and the fascia to support innovative therapies [15].

J. M. Vital, D. T. Cawley (eds.), *Spinal Anatomy*, https://doi.org/10.1007/978-3-030-20925-4_20

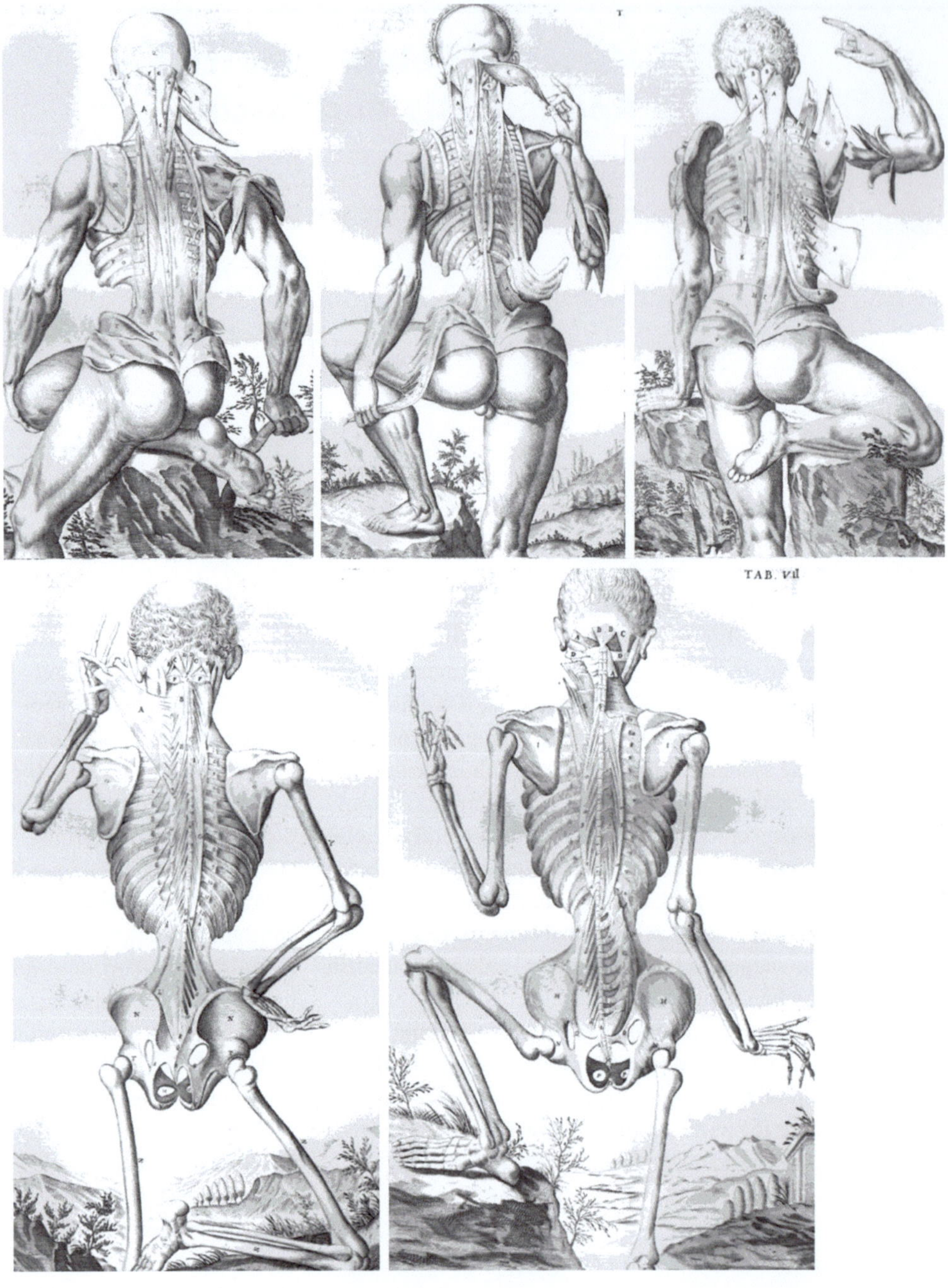

Fig. 1 Representations of the muscles of the vertebral column as per Spigelius (1685). Note the attention to detail in the presentation

Organogenesis

Embryologically, the skeletal muscles derive from the mesoderm, whose cells are organized into regular groups with anteroposterior distribution with the somites. There are several species of myoblasts during ontogenesis, those who remain in the somitic territory, at the origin of the trunk muscles, and those who migrate to the limb bud. The differentiation of mesoderm into myoblastic cells is dependent on four regulatory genes: myoD, myogenin, myf5, myf6, plus a fifth less well identified: myd [16]. They are organized into 42–44 somites.

Some (e.g., rectus abdominis) derive from the fusion of several myotomes. The muscular precursors of a myotome give rise to separate muscles in the horizontal plane (trapezius, sternocleidomastoid) or in the frontal plane (external oblique and transversus abdominis) and migrate at a distance from their original myotome (trapezius, latissimus dorsi). Before birth, the number of fascicles increases and between 2 and 16 years, according to a multiple of 14 with a regular rhythm up to 50 years, their size is greater in men than in women, measuring 3–10 cm long and less than 0.1 mm thick (Figs. 3, 4, and 5).

By the fifth week, the myotubes appear; at 8 weeks (30 mm vc), all the muscles have their mature form and change their orientation with the exception of the axial longitudinal muscles.

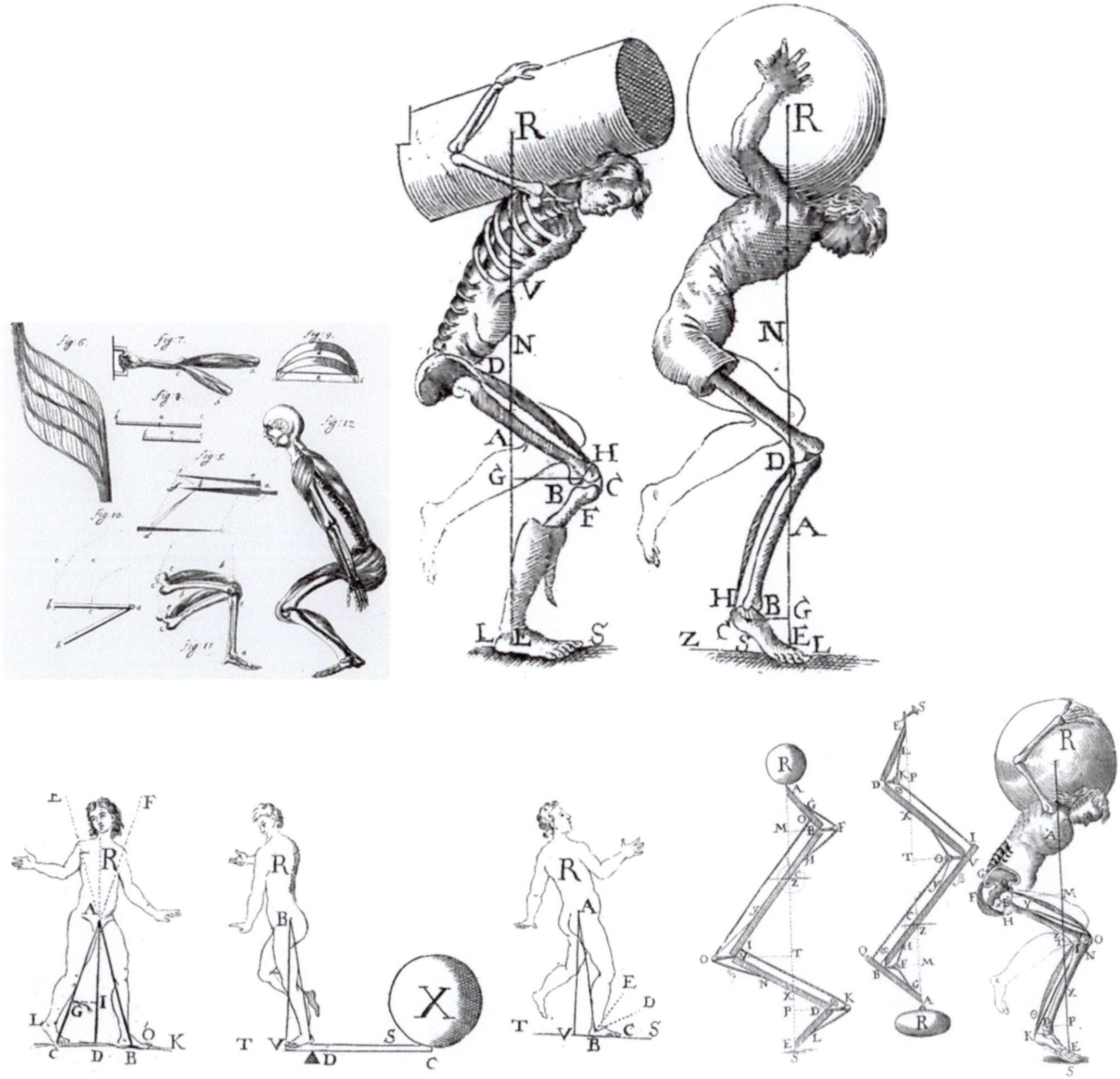

Fig. 2 Modeling of the vertebral column by Stenonis (1685) with integration of the globality of the load. In this representation, note the mechanical continuity between the column and the lower limb

General and Semantic Organization of the Muscle

Curvatures: Anatomical and Biomechanical Fundamentals

The human column has undergone a double evolution with adaptation for bipedal stance and recumbency. Throughout its height, it is unstable in the three planes of space, the regulation of which is ensured by all the structures constituting two essential mechanical principles with variable curvatures and the articular tripod. The notion of curvature is old, Fick [13] integrated the hip and pelvis entirely and the functional consequences of other types of curvature. At the end of growth, we consider that its morphology is stable. If it were straight and rigid, we would have difficulty maintaining our balance and in the face of mechanical stress, the deformation would be unpredictable (buckling).

> To adapt, each segment has a curvature that ensures a prestressed state of defined shape, organized to oppose precise predictive forces so as to avoid breakage.

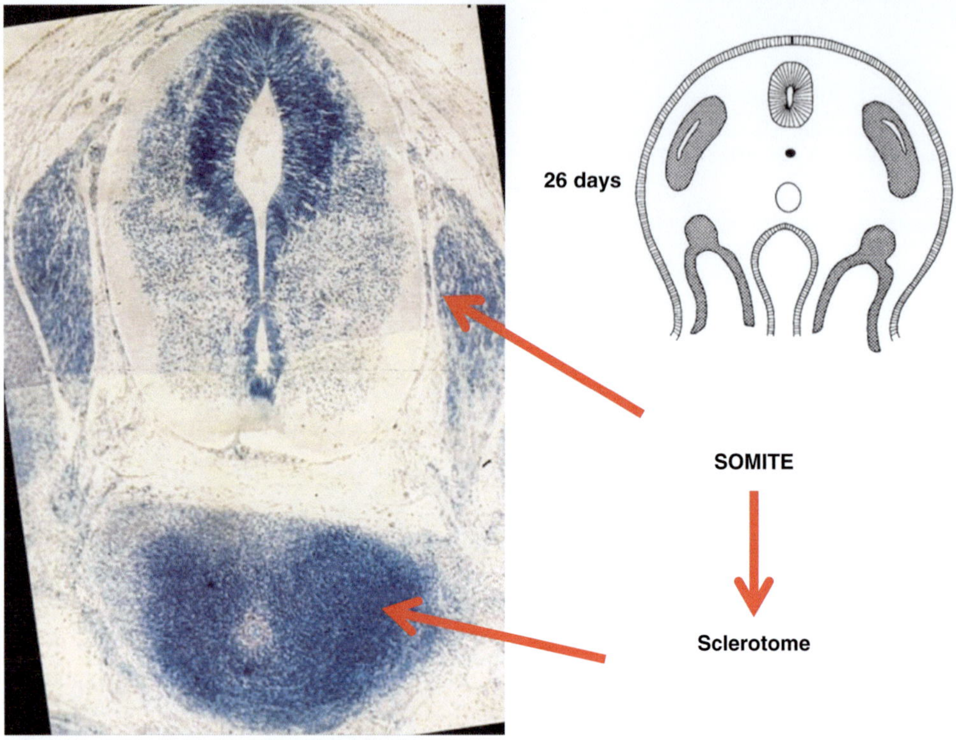

Fig. 3 Histological sections of a fetus with positioning of somites and neural tube

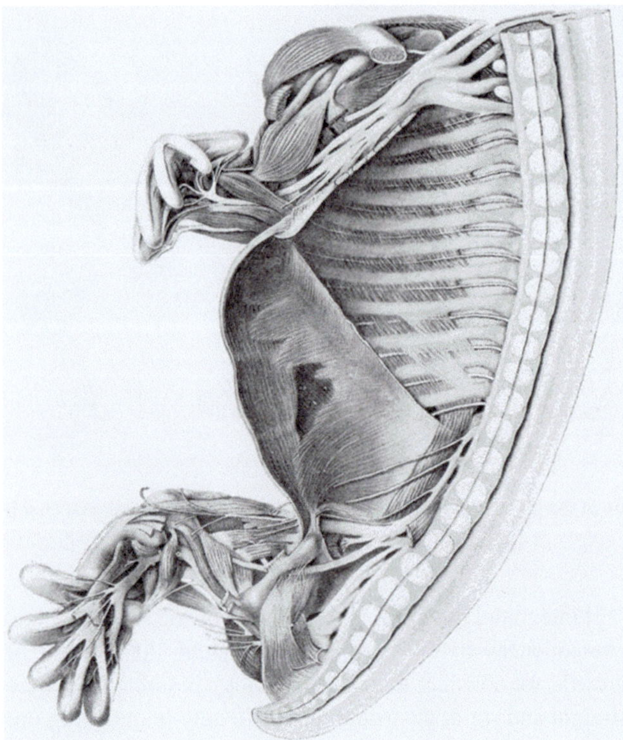

Fig. 4 At the 60th day of intrauterine life, all muscles are in their final position

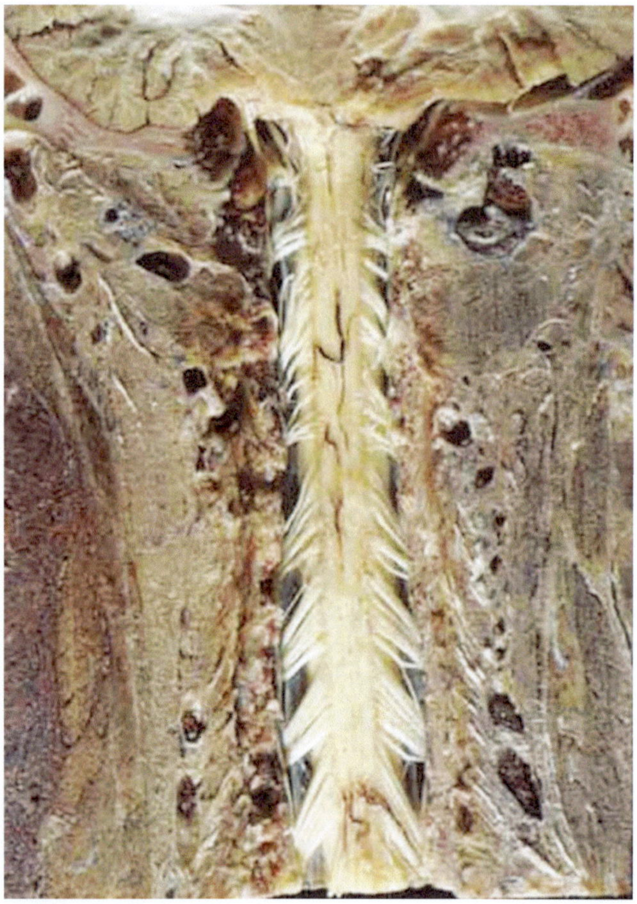

Fig. 5 During the same period, the neural tube will protect the spinal cord. Coronal section of the cervical spine: topographic relationships with the spinal cord

Thus, during loading, the deformation will occur by accentuating the curvature, and under such conditions, it is easier to resist the deformation by concentrating the muscular insertions into the concavity. The existence of curvatures and the flexibility of the intervertebral joints contribute to its stability in an erect position. There are so-called physiological curvatures which provide greater resistance according to the laws governing the elastic columns with alternating curvatures. For these, the resistance to the pressure is expressed by the relation $N2 + 1$, where N is the number of curvatures (4×4) and 1 the resistance of a rectilinear column of the same diameter. In the case of the column with 4 curvatures: cervical, thoracic, lumbar, and sacral, the resistance is 17 but it is not appropriate to consider the rigid sacral curvature thus resulting in 3 curvatures ($3 \times 3 + 1 = 10$) (Figs. 6 and 7). It is excessive to establish a strict relationship in a structure where

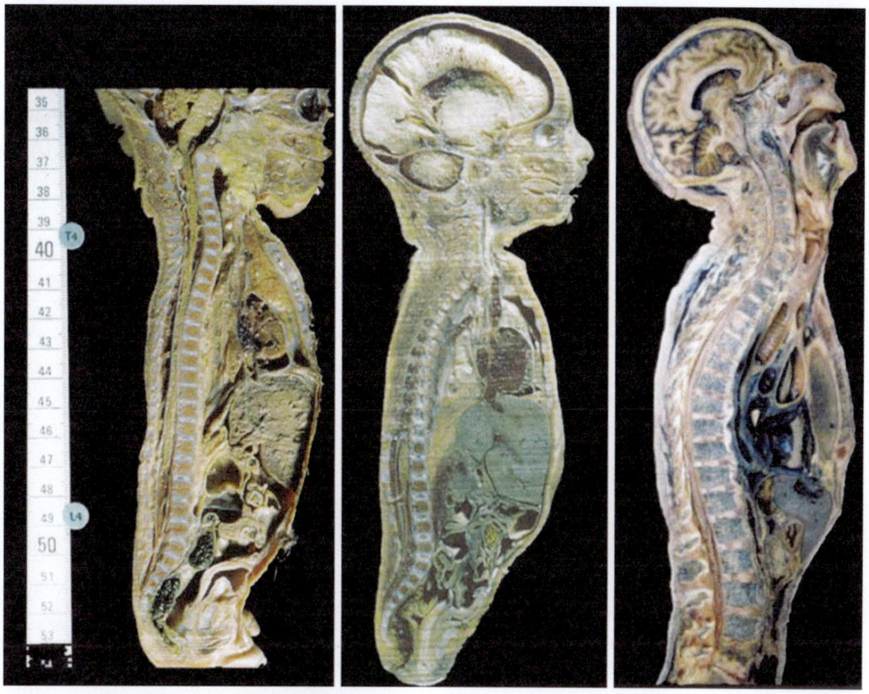

Fig. 6 Sagittal sections of 2 fetuses (**a**, **b**) and adult subjects (**c**) to show the configuration of curvatures of the spine. Progressive placement of column curvatures from the fetal period, from the newborn to the adult

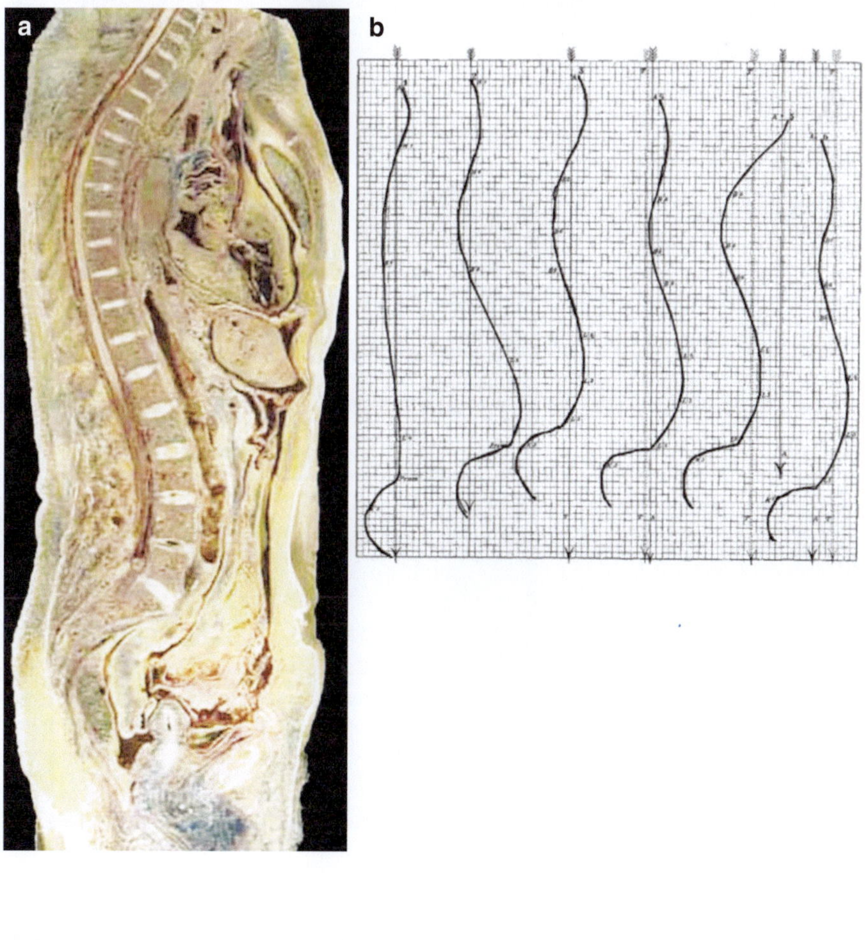

Fig. 7 Sagittal section of a vertebral column with its curvatures (**a**). Varieties of curvatures considered physiological according to Fick [13] (**b**)

bone density, power of muscles, and ligaments intervene in strength as much as the number of curvatures. Some vertebrae or "keystones" have a special position with respect to these curvatures, neutral, and passive vertebrae during movements. The keystone of the cervical spine is C5 or C6, the thoracic and lumbar spine in T7 and L3. The transition vertebrae T1, T12, and L5 are not very mobile during the movements between the different segments. The first and last are protected, but the thoracolumbar junction is not and forms the frequent traumatic focus that extends from T10 to L1. Cervical lordosis is in harmony with thoracic kyphosis and lumbar lordosis specific to humans. Standing exists only in part for semi-bipeds (semi-brachiators) and more fragile extent in other primates. It hardly exists in infants and only forms when the trunk is erect and then when walking.

The essential role in the maintenance of this attitude is devolved to the muscular tone of posture, in particular to small permanent contractions of the muscles of the paravertebral gutters and the pelvic girdle. The first biomechanical experiment on stability with incorporated muscles was presented by Bergmark [17] with an elastic function. In a histological study, Nitz [18] determined the number of neuromuscular spindles in the muscles of the lumbar portion with, in the interlamellar and interspinous muscles, where a much larger percentage of neuromuscular spindles exist than in multifidus and semispinalis.

Musculo-Aponeurotic Static and Dynamic Mechanical Imperatives

These intersegmental muscles, in addition to their mechanical role, are regulators of tension (Fig. 8).

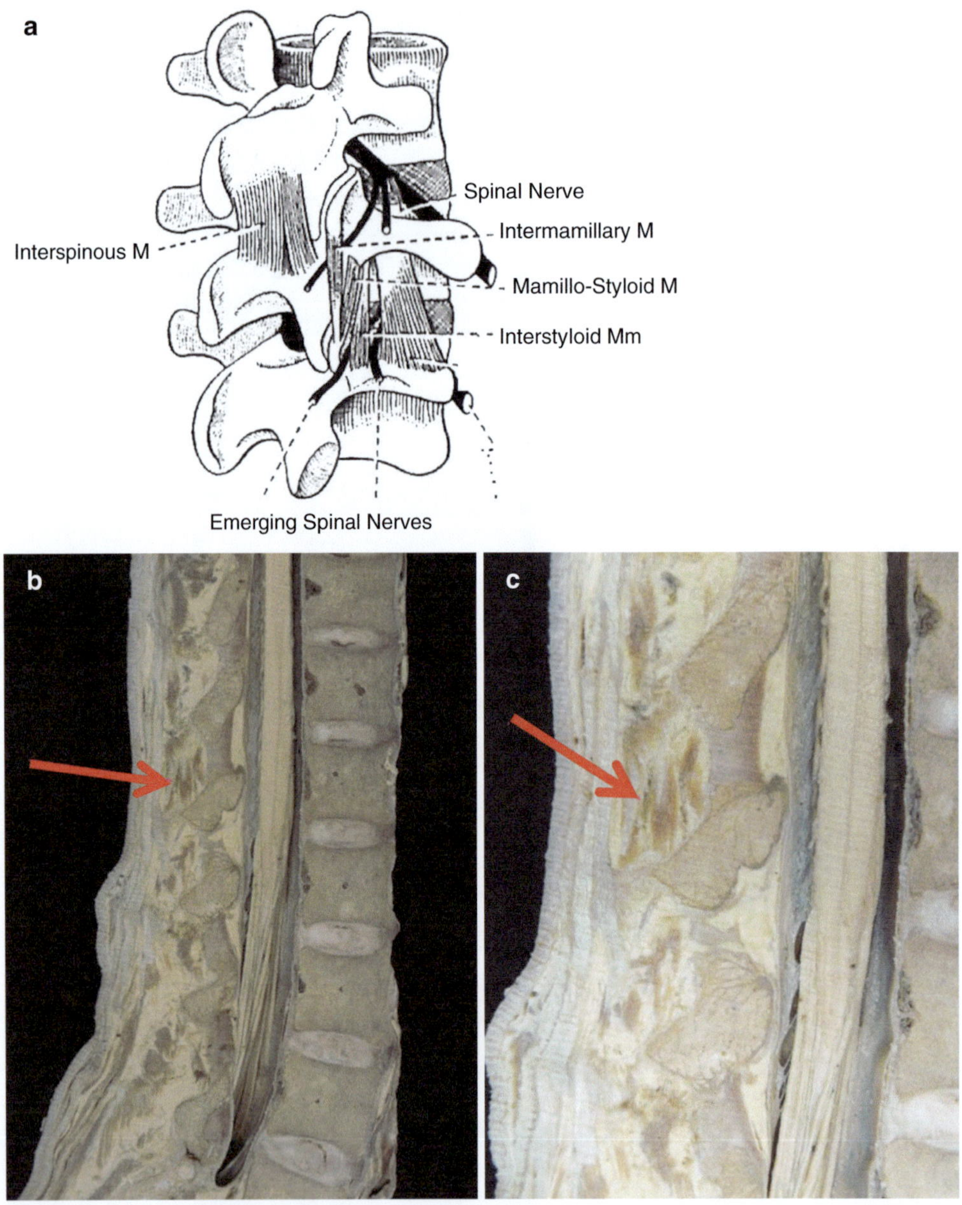

Fig. 8 (**a**) Diagram of the short muscles [3], (**b**) sagittal section centered on lumbar spinal processes and (**c**) close-up of unipennate muscles: interlamellar, interspinous, intertransverse

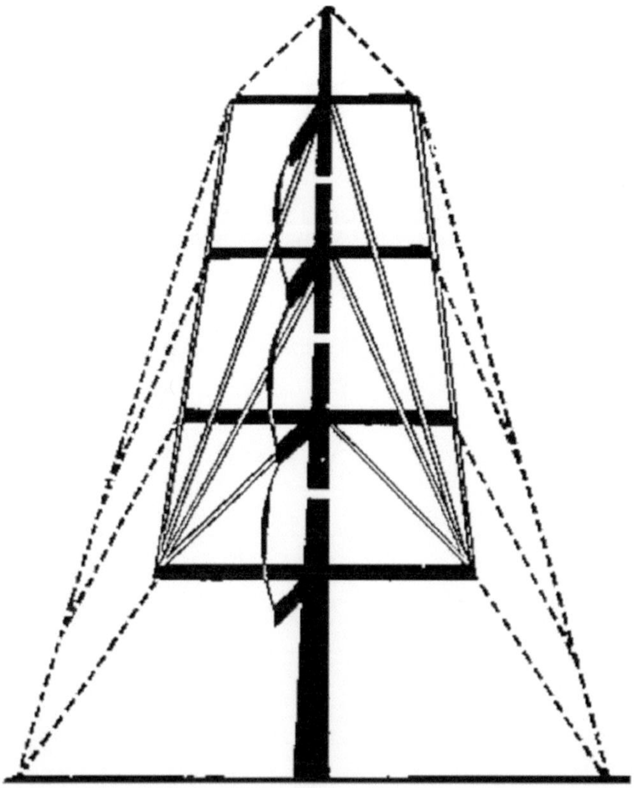

Fig. 9 Organization of the muscles according to the principle of the stays (akin to a guy rope or cable tethers) from the shortest to the longest

The muscles and their fascia provide stabilization in an automatic control mode via the extrapyramidal system. Each vertebral body is positioned statically and dynamically, not only in relation to its neighbors, by the play of the short intersegmentary muscles placed in the depth of the vertebral gutter, but also in relation to the whole of the spine by the action of the superficial long muscles, which supposes complex muscular attachments. The imperative is the maintenance of a symmetry, with a rigorous adjustment of ligamentary traction and tension with 3 muscular groups: posterior vertebral, oblique latero-vertebral (vertebral rotation) in case of deflection and anterior, so that any imbalance may cause a deviation (Fig. 9).

The general systematization of the posterior muscles is based on the direction of their bundles which comprise different groups, for example, at the lumbar level: a sacro-transverse group (ilio-costal and longissimus dorsi), transverso-spinal group (transverse spinous with several long lamellar chevrons, short and long spinous), interspinal group (7 pairs of interspinous muscle), and intertransverse group (7 pairs of intertransverse muscles). The laterovertebral muscles form 2 powerful muscular columns at the lateral lumbar part (quadratus lumborum and ilio-psoas). The anterior abdominal muscles counterbalance the action of the posterior muscles along with those at the cervical level (longis coli, rectus abdominis) and by a continuous superficial set from the head to the pelvis (sterno-cleidomastoid, sternum, rectus abdominis, and 3 lateral oblique muscles with, from surface to deep, the external oblique, internal oblique, and transversus of the abdomen, whence their importance in lumbar posture (Fig. 10).

Comparative Anatomy: Curves and Muscles

The studies of comparative anatomy by Winkler [3] were a response to the relationship between the notion of curvature and the anatomy of the muscles: "We did not hesitate to extrapolate this study in the field of comparative anatomy, knowing that it would be of great interest by observing simpler cases, less evolved than in humans." One of the main factors that oppose the thoracic vertebrae to the lumbar is the anticline with the orientation of their spinous processes in relation to the intermediate vertebra (approx. T12). Those of the thoracic vertebrae are inclined towards the intermediate vertebra, and they generally diminish in height as they approach it. At the level of the lumbar vertebrae, we find approximately these same features provided that they are observed in the caudal-cranial direction. The spinous processes gradually incline towards the limiting vertebra and diminish in value as we get closer to it. Those of the thoracic region are in retroversion, while the lumbar are in anteversion with respect to the intermediate vertebra. Anticlinia does not uniformly exist in the mammalian series, which is a function of the degree of mobilization of the trunk subdivided into two: cervico-thoracic or anterior and lumbosacral or posterior chains. In quadrupeds, the ilio-costal muscle is subdivided into two segments, one lumbar and the other thoraco-cervical. The lumbar part may be lacking (insectivores), while the other two still exist. The muscle is all the more flat and tendinous as the convexity of the column is accentuated. In the latter case, when the curvature is too strong, there is no muscle (insectivores), when it is neutral, neither convex nor concave, the muscle does not exist (ungulates). It is observed that, in quadrupeds, the ilio-costal muscle is generally weak and tending to its initial lumbar part, that it is more and more "strong and fleshy" at its thoraco-cervical terminal part. In semi-orthostatic simians, the ilio-costal muscle is consistent in size from one end to the other. In anthropoids and in man, on the other hand, it is highly developed and fleshy in the lumbar region and progressively weakens in the cranial direction (Figs. 11 and 12).

Numbers

The number of muscles presumed to be 400 varies: for Chaussier [19] 368, Theile [20] 346, Sappey [21] 501 distributed into 190 truncal, 63 head-neck, 98 upper limbs, 104 lower limbs, and 46 of the abdomino-pelvic system.

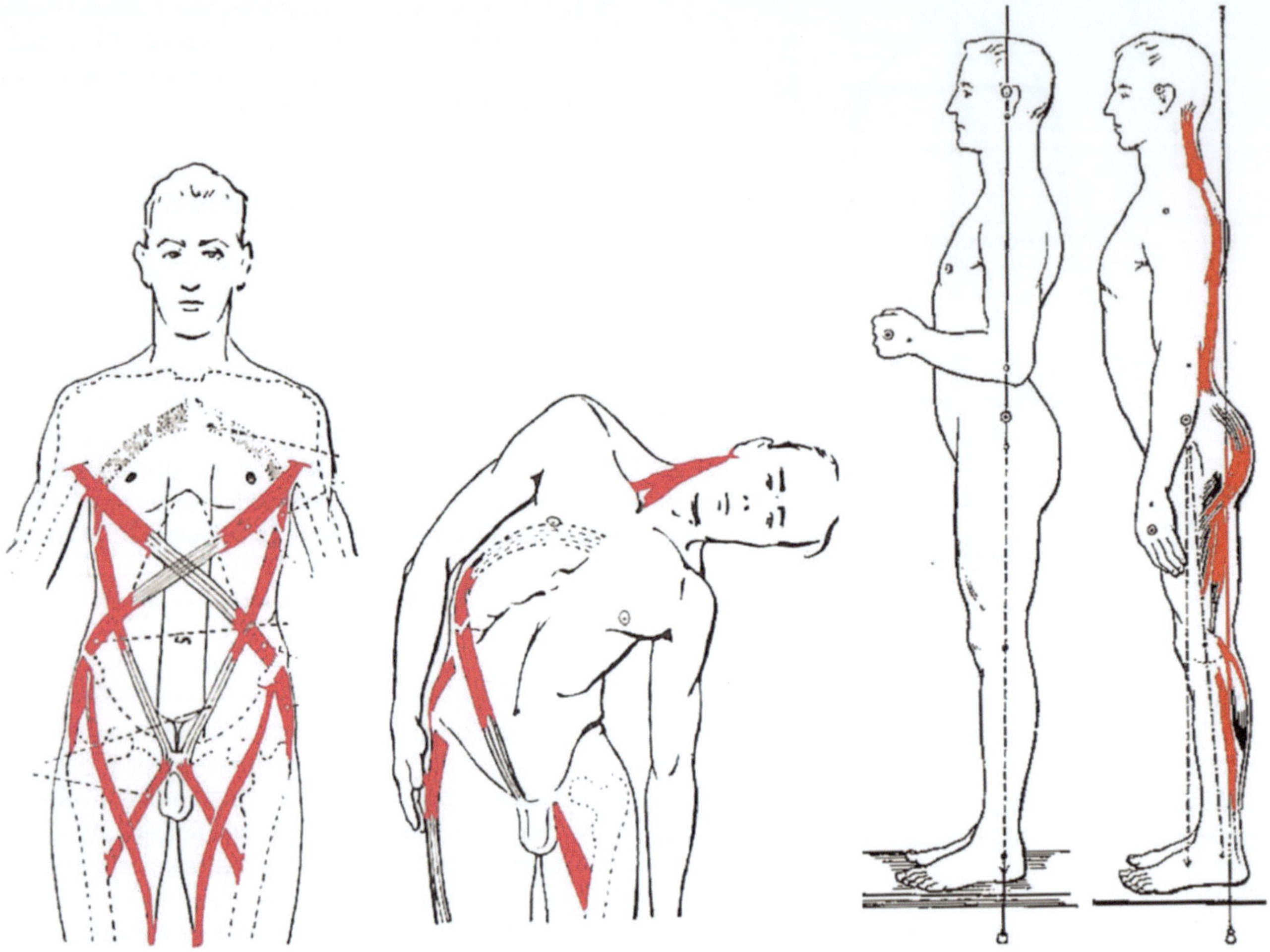

Fig. 10 Three-dimensional functional continuity of the pelvis, thoraco-lumbar and cervico-thoracic muscles

Old Nomenclature

Their denominations were based on a single principle. Before Sylvius [22], they were designated by the numerical names of first, the second, following the order of their superposition or their use. The order of Galen [23] was entirely topographical. Vésale [24] substituted a physiological order according to their use, true or supposed, and corrected many errors.

Modern Nomenclature

For Cruveilhier [25], their shape was determined: from their resemblance either with geometric forms, with generally known objects, according to their symmetry or their lack of symmetry. Under this last report, there was a very great difference between the osseous and muscular systems. "The topographical order was preferable in many respects, in that it was essentially anatomical and offered the advantage of appreciating the relations of the muscles between them and the various regions between them; it had, from the point of view of the economy of the subjects and the facility of the preparations, an incontestable advantage on the physiological order, with which, moreover, could be reconciled for a few regions. He adopted the topographical order with some modifications which made it possible to study all myology on the same subject."

Since the twentieth century, anatomists had wanted to use a vocabulary that is understood by everyone with a universal language with Latin, which was that of Nomina Anatomica. Since the adoption in principle of Nomina Anatomica at Oxford in 1950, they were recognized and legitimized, then recognized by the International Federation of Associations of Anatomists (IFAA).

Muscle Insertions

The modalities of their insertions are one of the characteristics that allow their distinction into several groups. Those

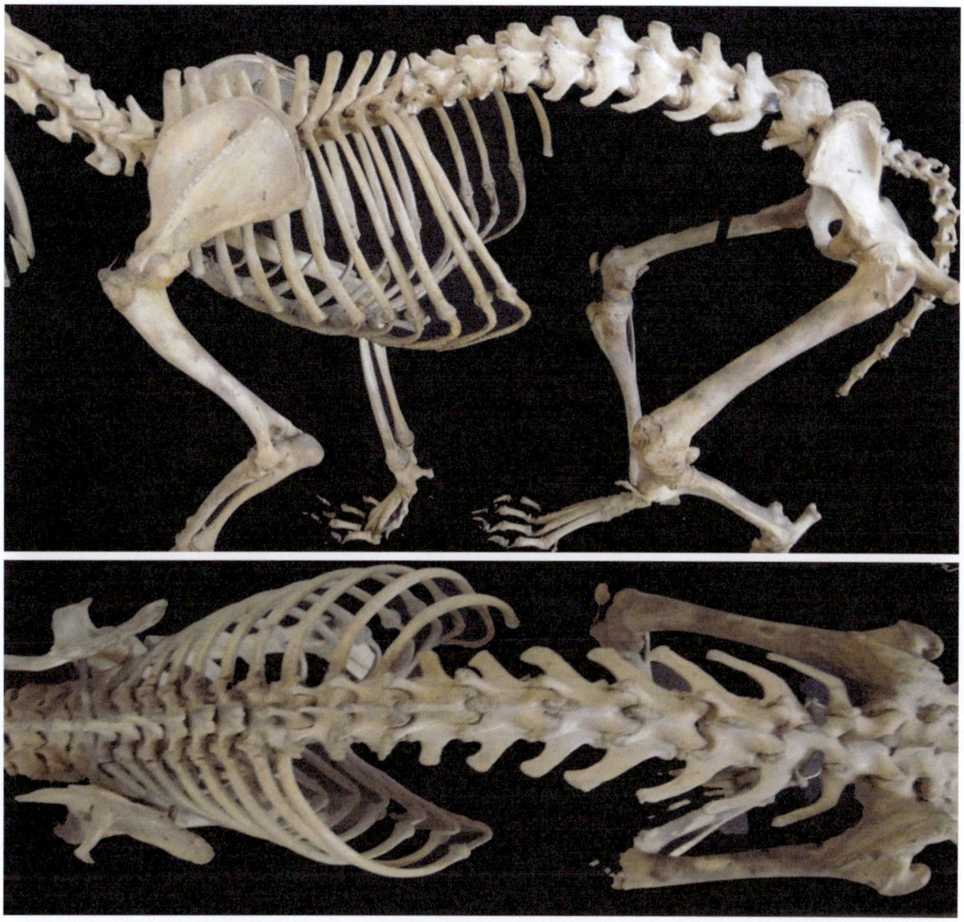

Fig. 11 Principle of anticlinism: arrangement of the spinous processes (**a**: side view) and transverse processes (**b**: dorsal view) in the dog (Anatomy museum, Montpellier)

with insertions of extended origin having variable shapes (rectilinear, curved) or with multiple digitations (levator scapulae) (Figs. 13, 14, and 15).

Another group is distinguished by the presence of the single or double origin tendon with two or more muscular bodies, with all of these musculo-aponeurotic complexes grouping together on a single tendon at its termination. The longissimus dorsi in its thoracic portion is detached from the sacral crest by a fascial layer which extends with the ilio-costal and ends with two chevrons: costal on the last five ribs and transverse on the transverse processes of T12–T7. Conversely, it may have insertions of osteo-periosteal origin as after constitution of the muscular body; it divides into several distinct tendons such as the two bundles of the dorsal part of the ilio-costal strand of the longissimus dorsi which consists of 6 tense strands of the posterior arch of the 1st and 2nd ribs towards the posterior arches of the ribs of the 5th to the 11th.

Intrinsic and Semantic Morphology

It is worth distinguishing the "anatomical muscle fascicles of the functional muscular fibers." The new anatomical approach benefits from details of anatomical architectural parameters with overall muscular length, length of anatomical fascicles, length of muscle fiber, and angle of pennation. Its actual length is defined as the distance between the proximal insertion of the muscle fiber and its distal insertion on the fascia. This measurement is variable according to the torsion of the fibers. Their length consisting of 500–10,000 parallel myofibrils can only be determined by micro-dissection after fixation. The fascicle is the sum of several muscle fibers, difficult to isolate by microdissection and which can contain from 5 to 50 fibers. Fundamentally, the anatomical fascicle is not necessarily representative of the real function of the muscle, which can only be identified histologically [26]. The determination of long or short fibers depends on the method of fixation, the measurement of the length of the sarcomere being difficult to interpret.

Sarcomere and Myofibrils

The sarcomere forms the histological functional unit and the fascicle the macroscopic functional unit. The universal organization consists of sarcomeres, which group together in the form of myofibrils, which in turn constitute the fascicles. The sarcomere consists of actin and myosin interconnected

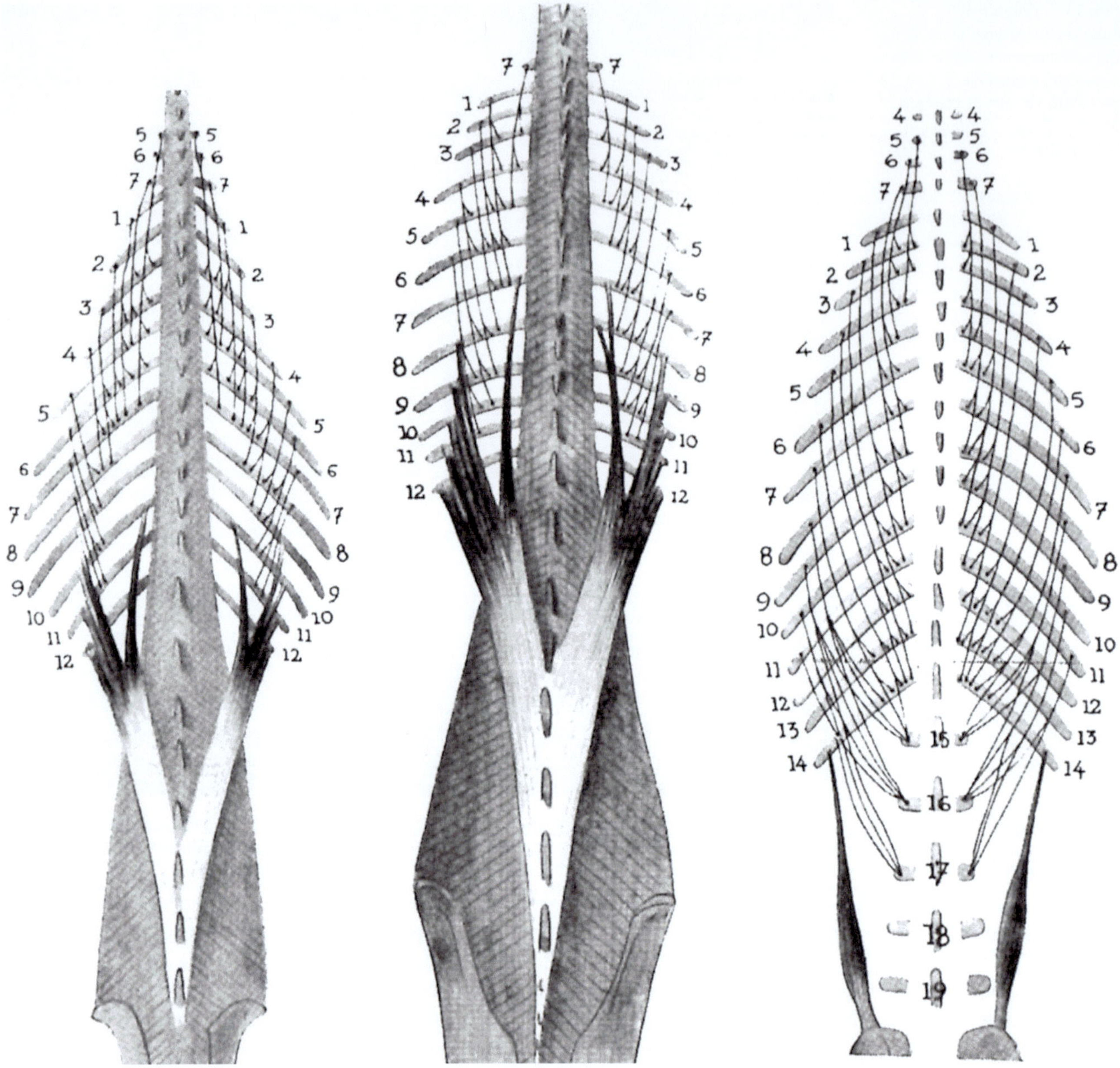

Fig. 12 Results of the arrangement of the vertebral column muscles by Winkler (1936) after dissection of several animal species (*Sciurus vulgaris, Lupus cuniculus, Scrofa domesticus*), the insertions are related to the principle of thoracolumbar vertebral anticlinism

contractile proteins arranged to slide relative to each other. The energy allowing their movement comes from the hydrolysis of the adenosine triphosphate fixed on the head of the myosin which can then tilt. This tilting pulls the action on the M band and causes shortening of up to 1 μm which can then create shortening of up to 10 cm [27].

> Each myofibril is composed of 1000 to 2 million sarcomeres in series, 2–3 μm in length and 1 μm in diameter.

The muscular fascicle of the brachial biceps contains more than 100,000 sarcomeres that can be arranged in parallel or in series to increase their power and movement. Its reactivity during growth or a period of immobilization can only be interpreted to the extent that one knows the type of fascicles and the disposition of the sarcomeres. Experimentally, Huijing [28] studied the degree of atrophy in rats (soleus, gastrocnemius) in these two situations. The results showed that their intrinsic structure was different. For the soleus, the sarcomeres were arranged in parallel and well adapted in their reactivity. Conversely for the gastrocnemius, only sarcomeres in parallel adapted to the circumstances. He concluded that the architecture had a considerable role in explaining these different behaviors without changing the length of the fascicles (Figs. 16 and 17).

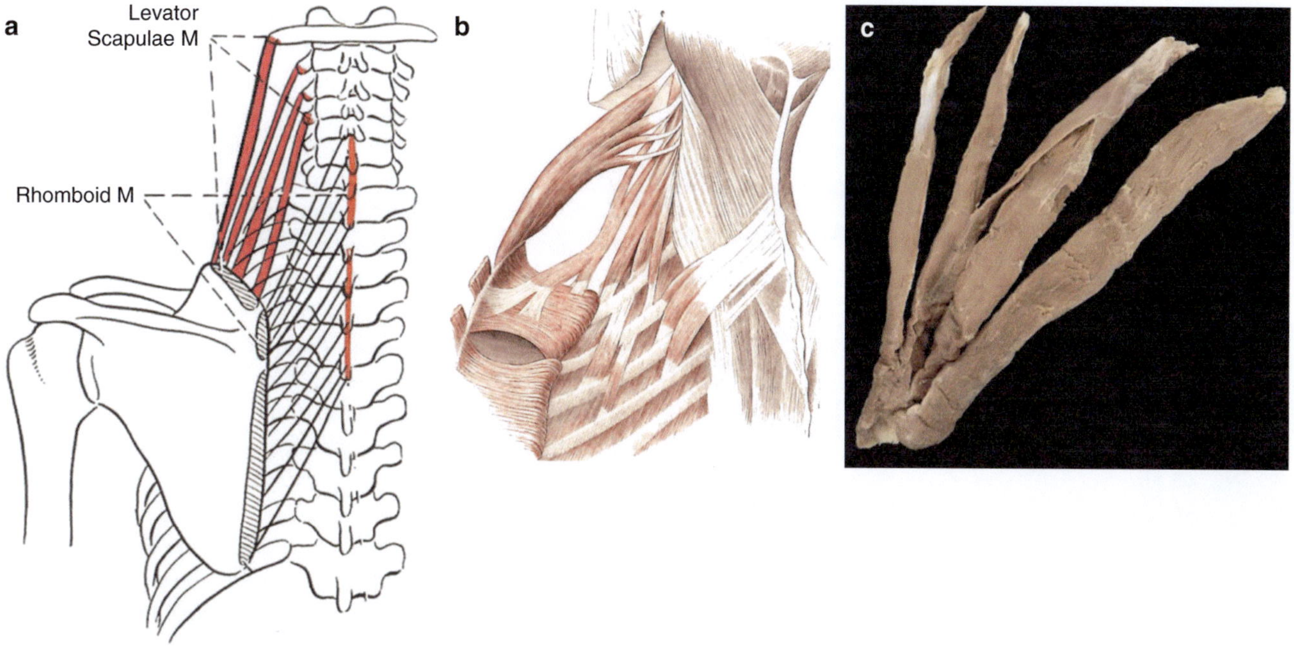

Fig. 13 Diagram of digitations of the levator scapulae muscle (**a**, **b**) and dissection with its four strands (**c**)

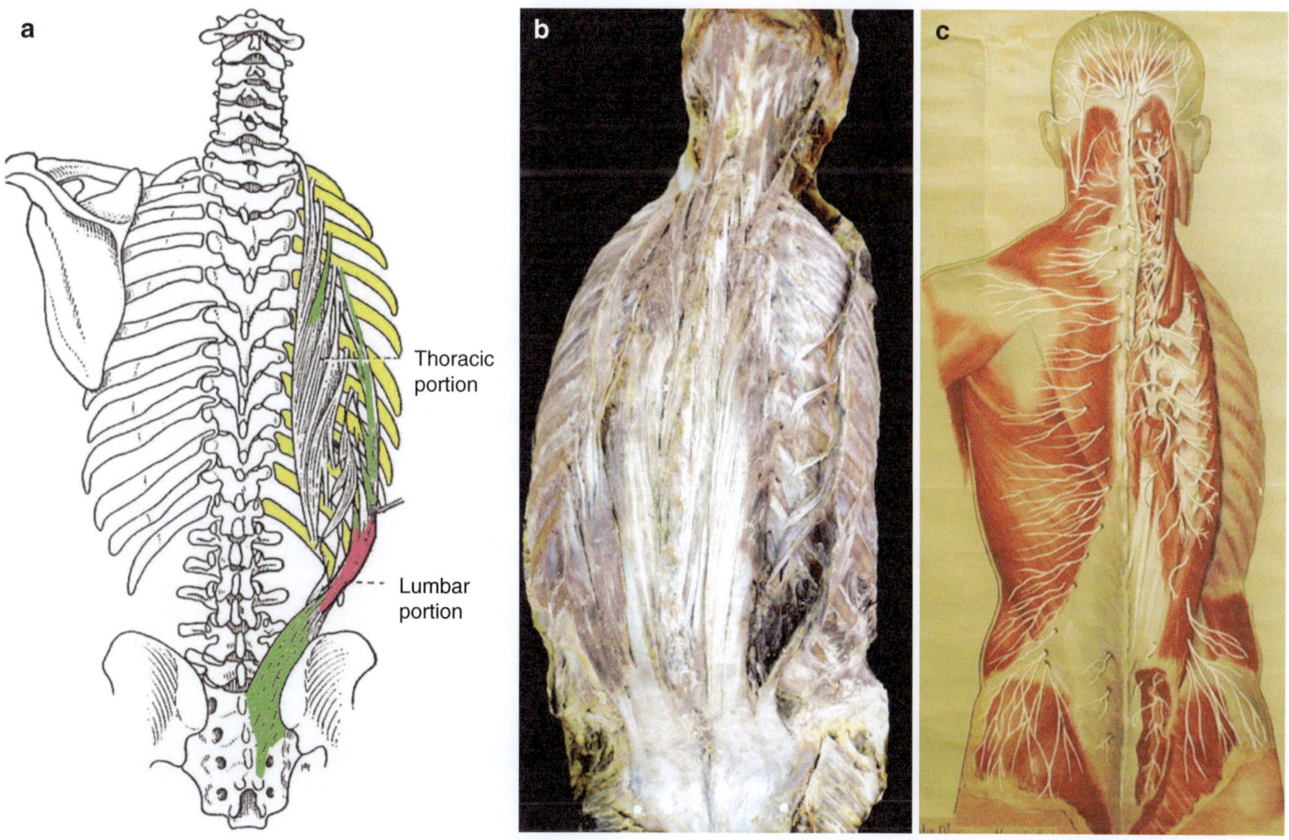

Fig. 14 Ilio-costal muscle with its lumbar and thoracic portions, schematic aspect according to Winkler (**a**), after dissection of an anatomical specimen (**b**) and representation of the emergence of the posterior branches of the spinal nerves (**c**). The muscular strands are very short in reference to the thoraco-lumbar aponeurosis. The thoraco-lumbar aponeurosis represents 90% of its total length, the principle of an antigravity muscle that stores energy to restore it in any circumstance

Titin: The Primary Elastic Protection of the Sarcomere

Titin is the most abundant "connective" protein in striated muscle, representing 10% of the myofibrillar mass, playing a role in the organization of sarcomere components essential for their growth.

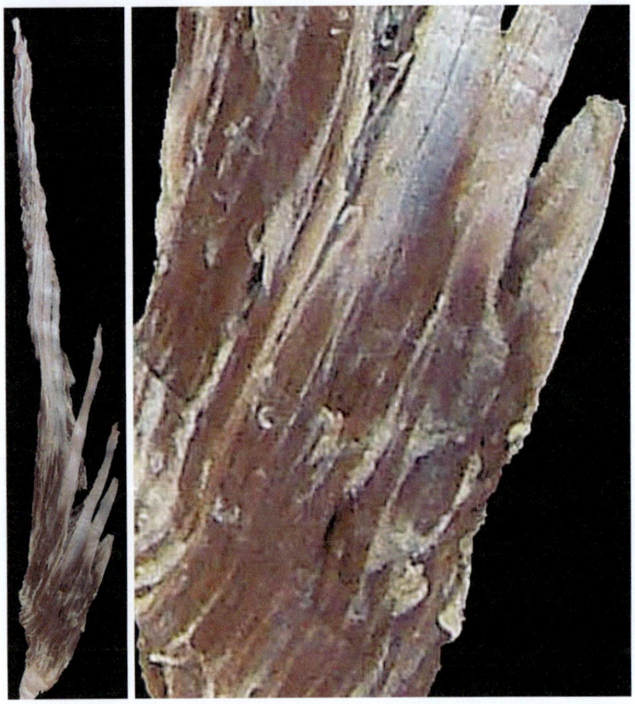

Fig. 15 Dissection and removal of the thoraco-lumbar portion of the ilio-costal mm (**a**) with, in close-up (**b**), the muscular strands which continue with a aponeurosis for each digitation. Note the reduced length of the strands (fascicles) compared to that of aponeuroses (aponeurosis)

It is involved in the control of the assembly of sarcomeric proteins regulating the elasticity of sarcomere related to thick myosin filaments and extends from the Z disc to the M band (almost half a sarcomere, i.e., more than a micron in length). With a length of 1 μm, about 30,000 amino acids and a molecular weight of 4000 kDa, it is the largest known polypeptide chain controlling integrity and ensuring the mechanical stability of the sarcomere. During traction, it generates a force sufficient to oppose the stretching tension of the sarcomere and plays a role in myofibrillogenesis, thus its degradation weakens the muscle. At its termination, it constitutes an element of information at the level of the Z and M bands as a factor of stabilization of passive stretching, a true spring of protection of the sarcomere during extension. Friden and Lieber [29] showed that passive stretching imposed strains equivalent to painful maximal muscle tension that degraded titin. By force or equivalent elongation, the extensibility of the elastic component of a rat soleus was about half that of a rat's rectus femoris. Such a difference would come from the existence of the different isoforms of titin and from its length of the extensible part. According to the type of muscle, it has different mechanical properties.

Its role is fundamental in the protection of sarcomeres during excessive traction, mainly in the vertebral column where its constraints are central to its stability.

The control of displacement during contraction is controlled by titin, which has a finely tuned passive tension setting (Fig. 18).

Fig. 16 Schematic organization of a sarcomere which is the fundamental motor of all muscles

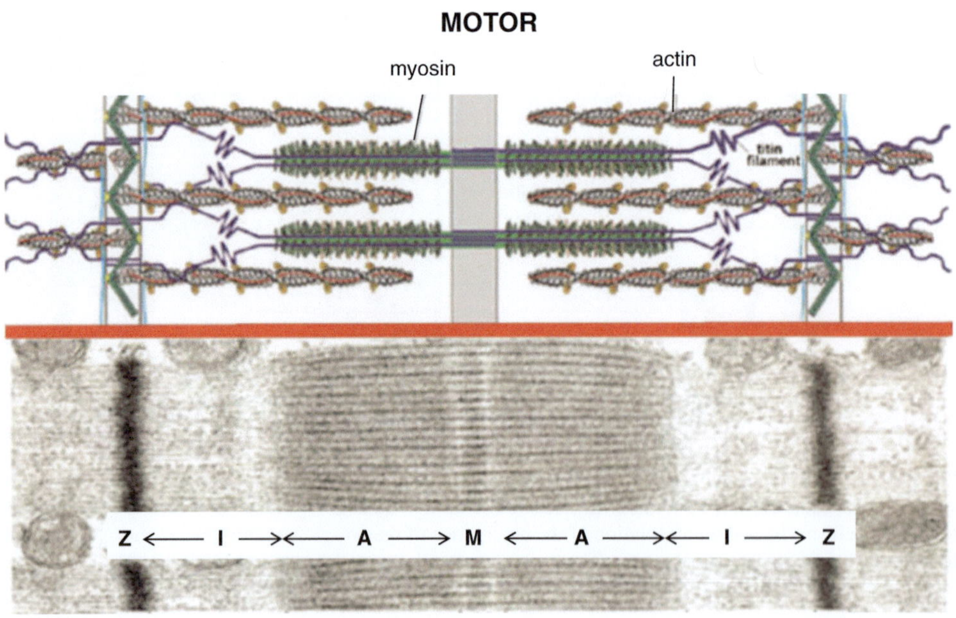

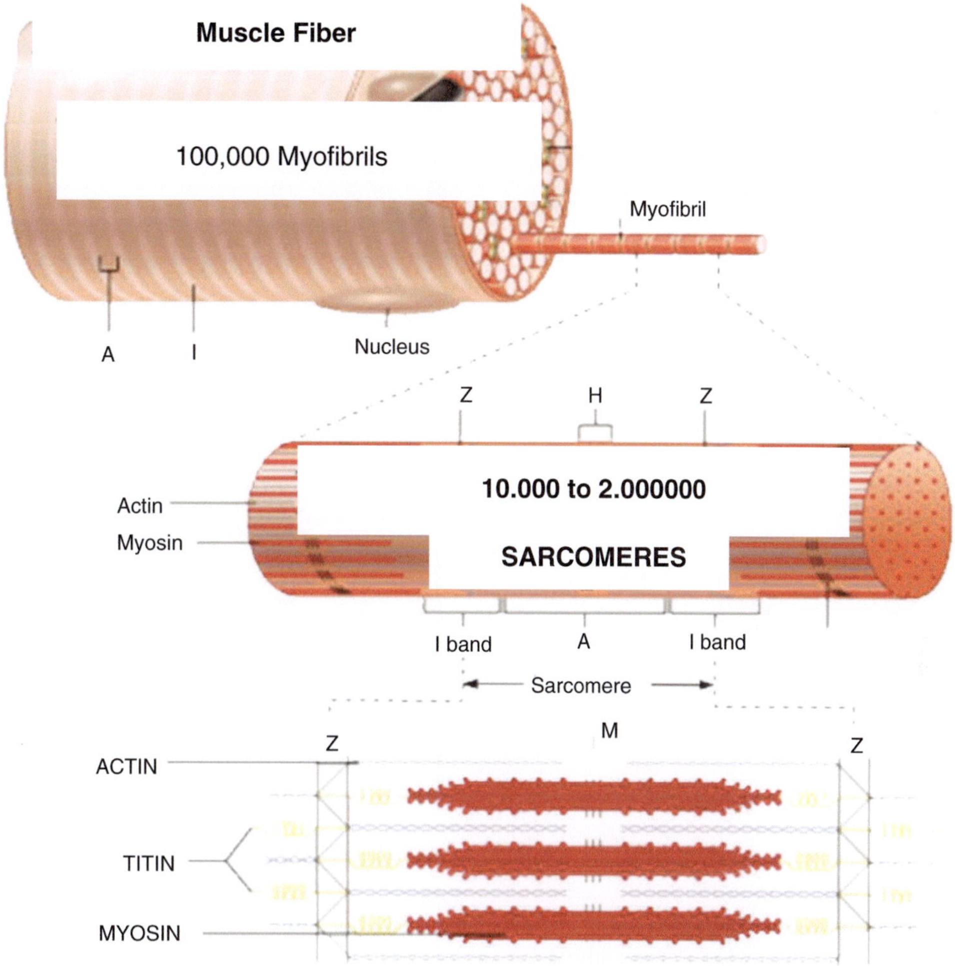

Fig. 17 Organization from the sarcomeres of the constitution of a muscular fiber

> When stretching the sarcomere, it generates a force capable of opposing the physiological tension of stretching. Exceeding this causes a rupture of the myosin actin bridge with trauma to the sarcomere [29]. The length of the sarcomeres varies according to the position of the joint.

Muscles and Aponeurosis

When these models join together, they result in a complex muscular organization of effective functionality. The length of fascicles of a long muscle should not be judged by that of the fleshy aspect but should encompass its associated fascial elements.

The generic term of fascicle is a functional set of sarcomeres as discussed by Huxley [30] and Alexander [31]. The particular fusiform shape of many muscles is a false image of the true length of the fascicles. The observation before dissection gives the impression that a fascicle extends from one end of the muscle to the other [32]. After a specific dissection, the particular disposition of each muscular fascicle whose muscular constitution is based on fundamental models adapted to their function with parallel fascicles, convergent with three-dimensional arrangements [13, 33–35]. In man, the length of fascicles is on average 4–5 cm, the longest being 10–15 cm. The axis of the muscle being not the same as that of the fascicles which compose it, we must study, for each, their direction with respect to the aponeuroses and the tendon.

Muscle Fasciculi and Aponeurosis

Muscle Fasciculi and Pennation: Topographical Economics

Muscles requiring considerable efforts have a large cross section with parallel fascicles, which would require an extensive and non-punctiform bone insertion. But there being no room for a muscle too large and thick, a solution has been found by an oblique arrangement of the fascicles (pennate) over the whole length of the bone and the

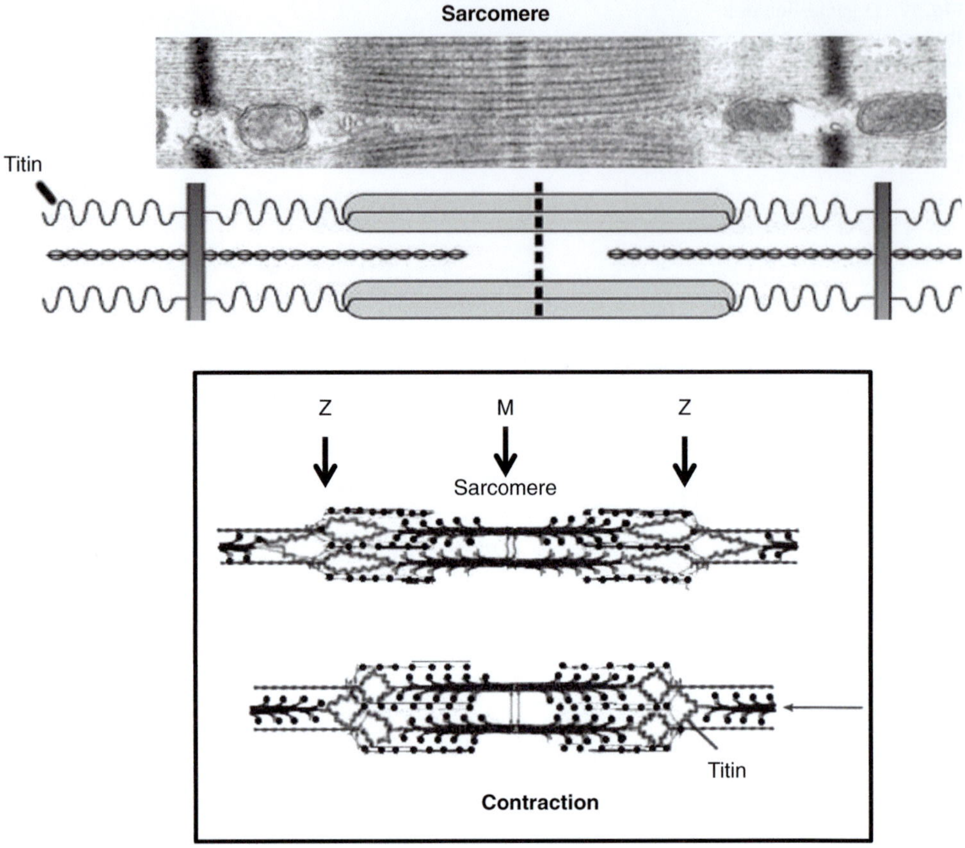

Fig. 18 Schematic representation of titin which is the protection factor of the sarcomere during excessive lengthening. During extension movements, titin, by its extension properties, protects the sarcomeres

fascia, which continues with a tendon, an organ of transmission.

The dissections show in all cases the presence of an aponeurosis with two types of fasciculi which are inserted into the main axis of the aponeurosis or alternatively, laterally according to the principle of a unipennate or bipennate muscle. On a global level, the insertions of the fascicles are arranged in the three planes of space (Fig. 19). The justification for this provision has two functions. The first is the constant development of a rotational movement with a certain amplitude according to the length of the fascicles. The second is based on the principle of permanently maintaining the tension of the aponeurosis which allows the fascicles to maintain a permanent tension for a maximum yield, whatever the position of the joint.

For the muscles of the pelvis, the central fascia is important and the fascicles which are involved are of the unipennate type. For the extensors, the aponeurosis are in the form of two resilient layers on which short fascicles fit into the category of unipennate antigravity muscles. In this case, the two fasciae are broad, flattened, and mirrored, are very powerful, less rapid, and have limited displacement. For the flexors, the constant central fascia occupies between 90 and 95% of the total length of the muscle, from its origin to its termination. In the case of the intrinsic ones, the arrangement is proportional to those of the girdles with a central fascia and a comparable arrangement of the fascicles (Fig. 20). Each muscle has two extremities, mostly with two tendons, one of origin, and the other of terminals with fascicles having a particular disposition, we can predict innumerable varieties in their constitution.

The fascicles are implanted directly or obliquely on the aponeurosis, like the barbs of a feather on their common stem: (penna: feather), as per Borelli [11] and Stenonis [10].

Aponeurosis: Fundamental Structure

The aponeurosis is the indissociable complementary element of the muscle. The fascicles are inserted either along the axis of the fascia or obliquely to distribute the mechanical stresses avoiding rupture during muscular contraction, all along its length.

Small posterior serrated muscles are often joined by a continuous fascia. This disposition is present in mammals (rodents), which plays a role in respiration (spino-costal muscle) (Figs. 21, 22, and 23).

A Historical Conceptual Error

For Cruveilhier [36] the term aponeurosis was used, a name whose etymology displayed a great anatomical error

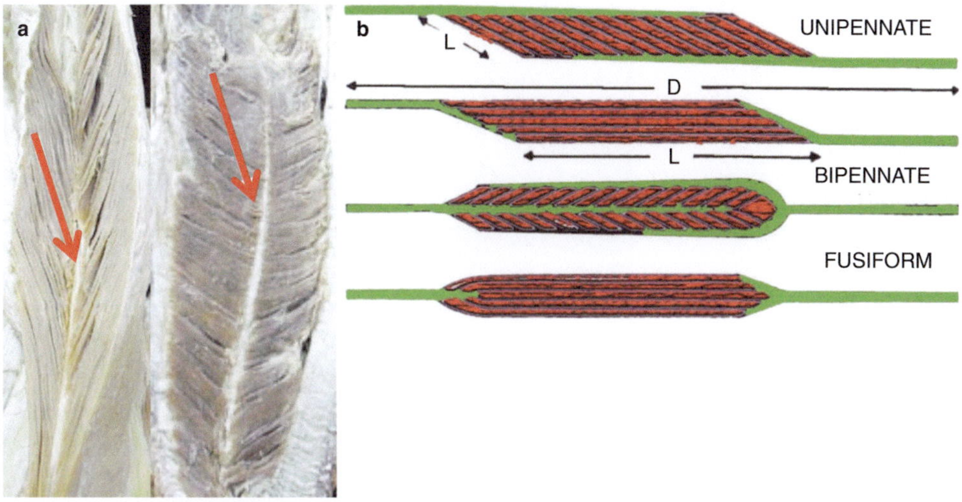

Fig. 19 Arrangement of the fascicles in a bipennate fashion with their insertion on a central fascia (white fibers) (**a**), and diagram of different modes of insertion of the fascicles with respect to the fascia (**b**)

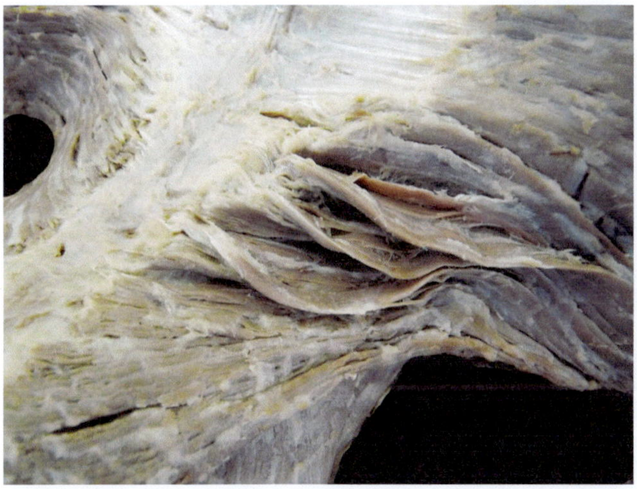

Fig. 20 Insertions of fascicles of the trapezius muscle at the level of the spinous processes of the cervico-thoracic vertebrae, lamellar aspect

(aponeurosis, from the Greek apo neuron as the ancients regarded the nerve as the white parts). Today they are referred to as fascia (fascia: band), applied by extension to all the aponeuroses as the dedicated name in the form of a broad band. In 1847, thanks to his observation [36] and his reflection, he gave a macroscopic description of a remarkable precision "the most general disposition is as follows:

> It is along the faces and edges of this aponeurosis that the fascicles are born (insert). It is again on a membranous surface or aponeurosis that they terminate. This aponeurosis, gathering on itself, constitutes a terminating tendon which the fleshy fibers (fascicles) leave at a more or less considerable distance from its extremity. It results from this provision: (1) a considerable development of surface for the insertion of the fascicles which the tendon collects, so to speak, in order to concentrate their efforts on the same point; (2) the obliquity of insertion or incidence of the fasciculi in relation to the tendon which represents the axis of the muscle, that is, the direction. It is conceivable that this obliquity is of the greatest relevance in the dynamic relation of the force of action of the muscles and leads necessarily to a great loss of forces. There is a great variety in these angles of insertion or incidence of fascicles on the aponeurosis. It is conceivable that the facility of multiplying the fascicles by arranging them in this way obliquely outweighs the disadvantage of their direction.

The original tendon extends as a form of membrane or aponeurosis in the thickness or surface of the muscle.

Intrinsic Structure of the Aponeurosis: Endomysium and Perimysium Aponeurosis

Electron microscopy of the fascicles shows that the endomysium is a continuous collagenous tissue that allows it to be individualized. It forms an important part of the isolation mechanism of the fascicles or constitutes the outer part or reticular leaflet of the sarcolemma. The epimysium sends fine septae of connective tissue called perimysium determining primary, secondary, and tertiary bundles. Within these fasciculi, each fascicle is surrounded by a thin layer of connective tissue consisting mainly of an outer lamina (basal lamina) and reticulin fibers, the endomysium. It is the whole of this connective tissue that transmits the constraints of the fascicles to the fascia (Fig. 24).

The different muscular fascicles are not randomly grouped, but constitute regular bundles surrounded by an outer layer of dense connective tissue, limiting the muscles as a whole called epimysium.

In 1989, Ettema and Huijing [2], on the physiological level, led to an interpretation and a comprehensive mechanical synthesis of the internal structures of the fascicle and aponeurosis. For the sarcolemma of isolated fibers, the endomysium contributes to the elastic static function as it can be stretched to 140–150% and contributes to the elasticity and viscosity of the muscular complex. The sum of the connective tissue increases the compliance of the muscle in addition to that of the fascicles and the tendon.

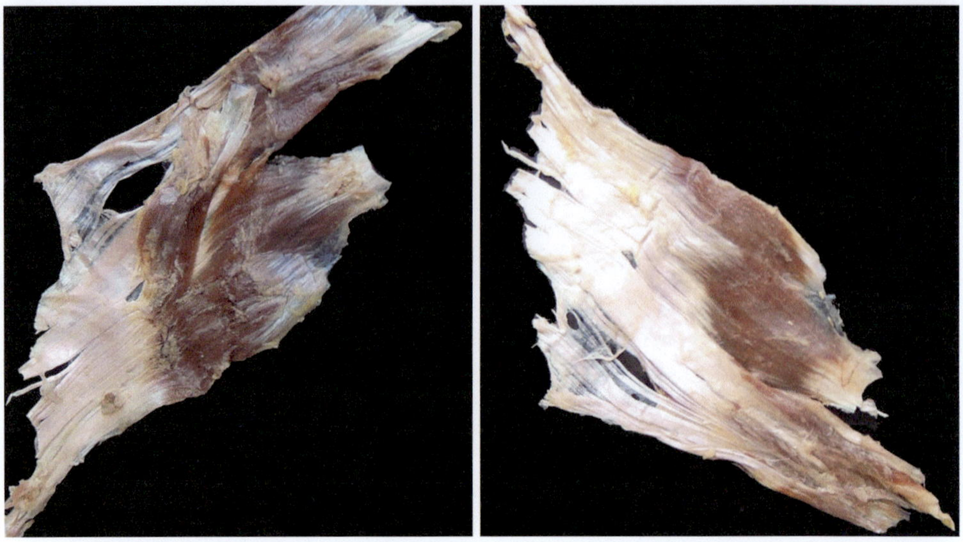

Fig. 21 Disposition of aponeuroses (aponeurosis) (whitish fibers) of superior serratus posterior intended to distribute the constraints of muscular fascicles. It is a unipennate muscle type, observe the disposition of these aponeuroses (aponeurosis) of the superficial (**a**) and deep (**b**) aspects. Most anatomical depictions represent only one aspect that does not make it possible to understand the essential role of the aponeuroses (aponeurosis)

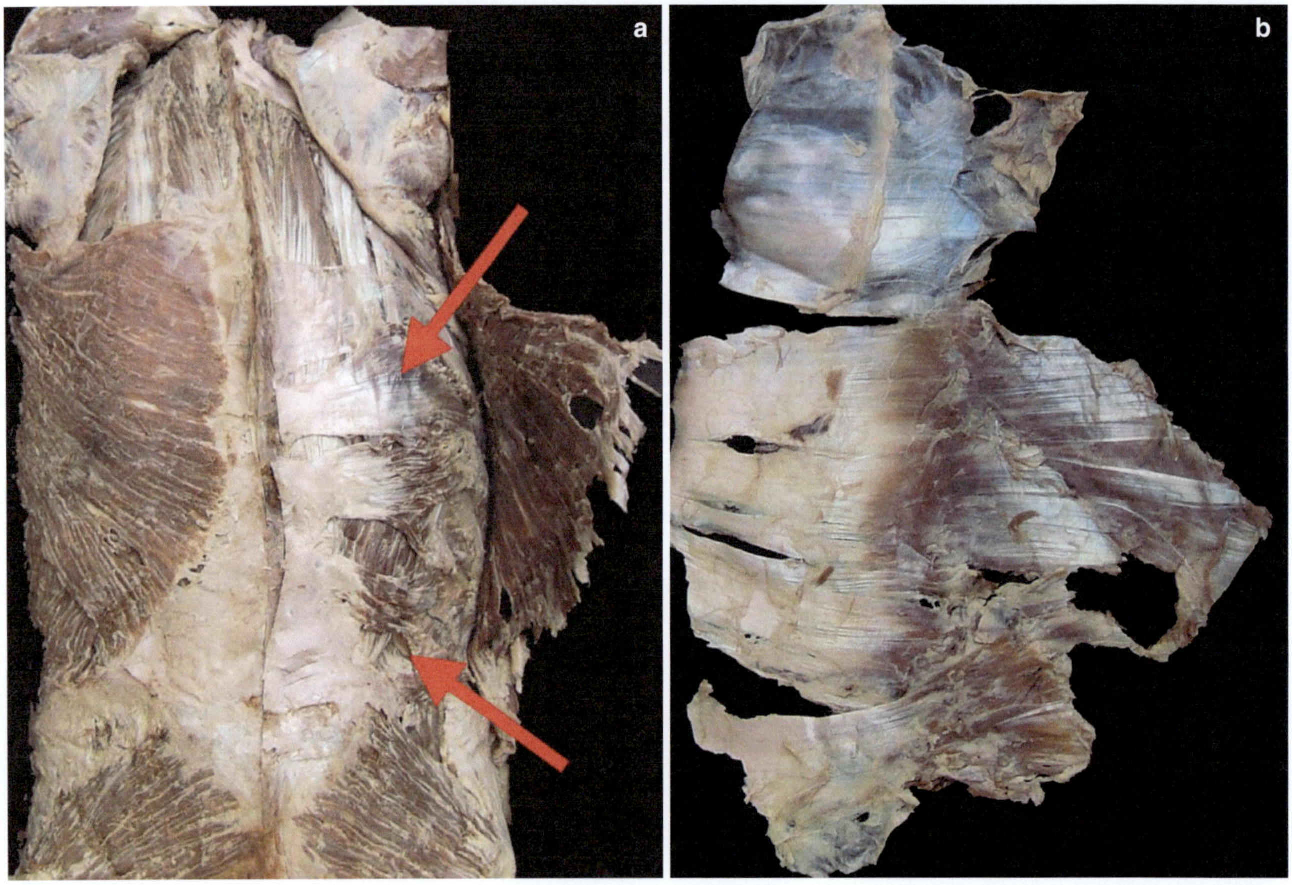

Fig. 22 Dissection of serratus posterior superior and inferior (**a**) joined by a continuous aponeurosis (**b**), in this case, muscular fascicles persist along its length with the aponeurosis

Due to the tension that is transmitted through the aponeurosis to the endomysium, the mechanical properties of this connective tissue are a factor contributing to improve the mechanical properties of the muscle, transferring the stresses between the discontinuous fascicles through transendomysial bundles. In contrast to the high tensile forces of the collagenous fibers on which the fascicles attach themselves, the translaminar leaflets undergo shear forces of the endomysium. Each muscle fiber is surrounded by a fibrous tissue (perimysium) which is organized into cells which, by

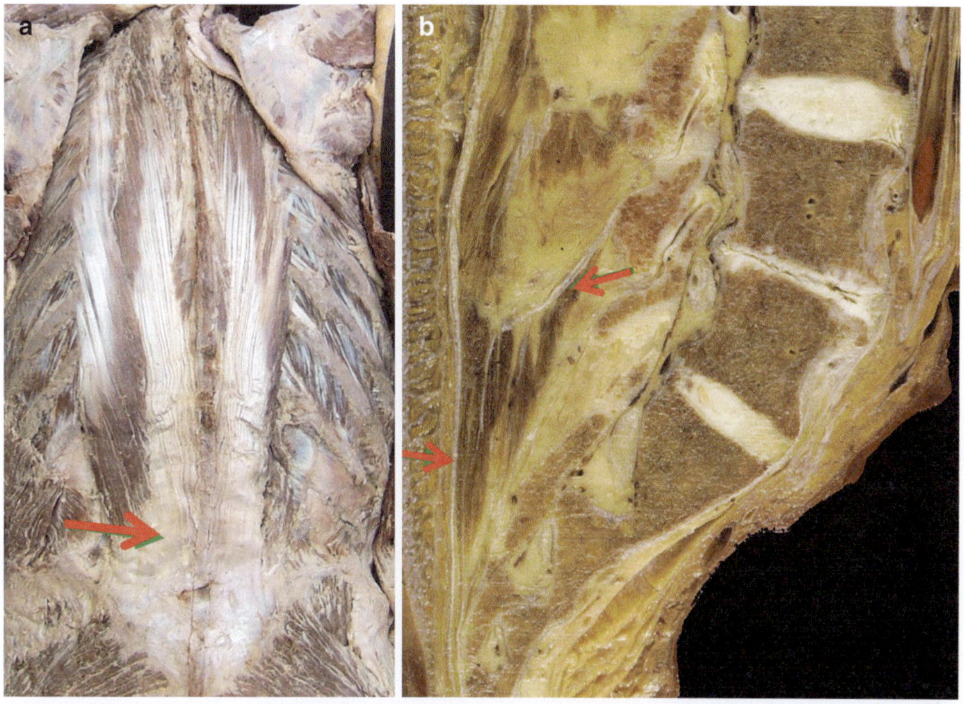

Fig. 23 Common aponeurosis (green arrow) for longissimus dorsi and ilio-costal: posterior view (**a**). Sagittal section (**b**) at the insertion on the sacrum, contrary to the overall appearance of the muscle, the muscular fascicles are very short, responding to the mechanical principle of maximum yield during contraction

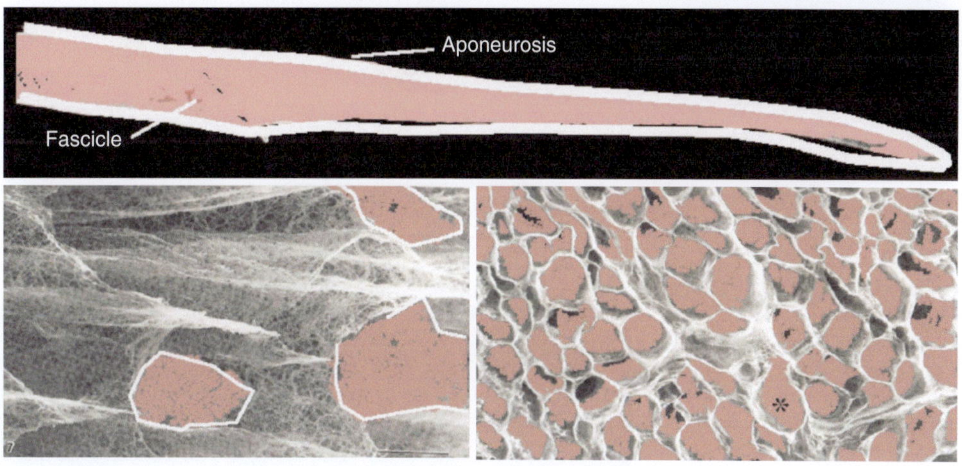

Fig. 24 Organization of the aponeurosis in the muscle which promotes the transmission of the stresses. Histological section at high magnification

their adhesion, undergo progressive elastic transmission of mechanical shear stresses.

In certain configurations, the intramuscular fascial segments may be subdivided into any number of small segments or grouped into a whole (law of commutativity and associativity) (Figs. 25 and 26). When bending the head, the muscle stretching is such that the sarcomeres may be destroyed. To combat this eventuality, there are multiple aponeuroses in the muscle to distribute the constraints and protect them. In addition, depending on the length of the lever arm, the muscle has a resistant and elastic aponeurosis structure giving it a "digastric" appearance. The semi-spinalis cervicis responds to these objectives (transverse processes of C3–T5 with two bundles, medial (T5–T3), lateral (T3–C3), terminating at the occipital nuchal line) with a fascial intersection.

Mechanism of the Aponeurosis

At the level of the aponeurosis, there is no uniform extension zone during passive or active movements [2]. These tension variations are according to the axial stresses that have already been observed for tendons, ligaments, and aponeurosis. For the aponeurosis, it appears that the tension forces are higher at the two extremities of the muscle than in the middle part. Its behavior varies between passive movements and active movements. In passive movement, it deforms more in the direction of the length and less in the direction of the width. Knowledge of its elastic properties is essential for understanding changes in fascicle length or of the sarcomere. When modeling the muscle–tendon complex, the variations in length, the difference observed in the changes between the

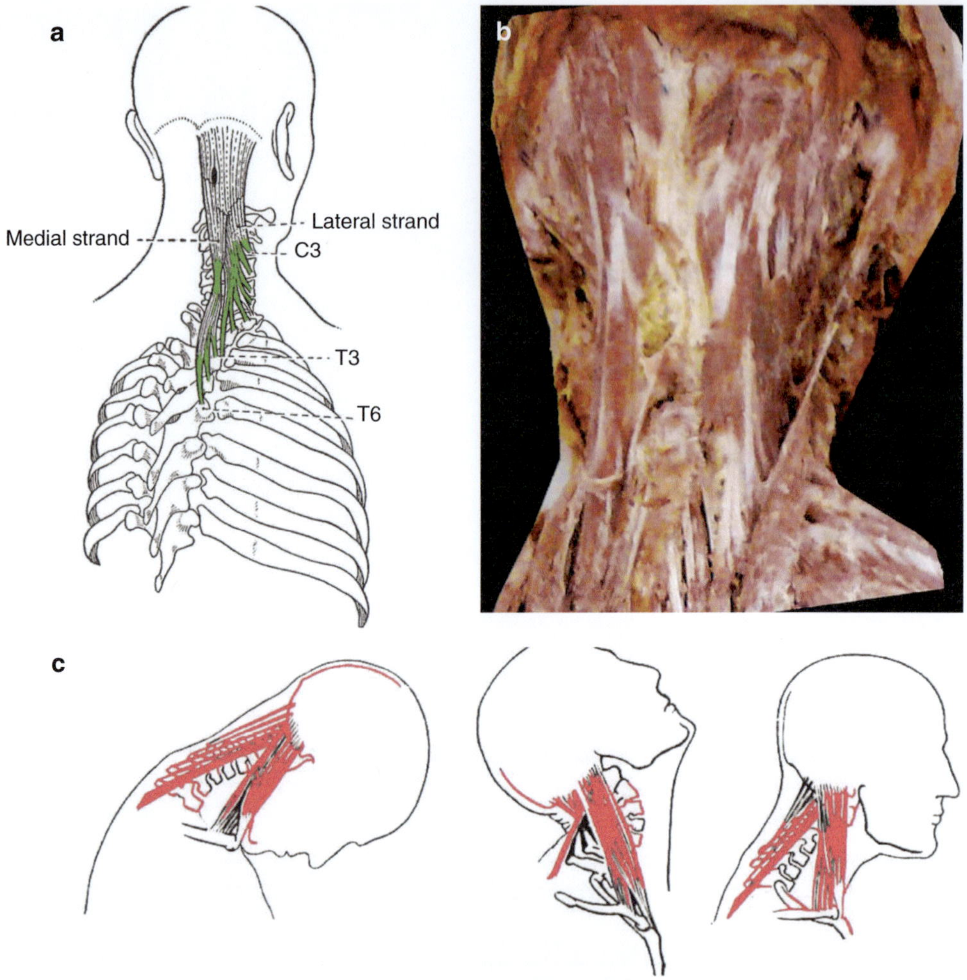

Fig. 25 Posterior view of the large posterior cervical complex according to Winkler (**a**) and after dissection with its fascial intersection and its two bundles (**b**). During the movements of anterior flexion of the head (**c**), it is essential that the muscles consist of an aponeurosis (**c**) which protects the tension of the sarcomeres

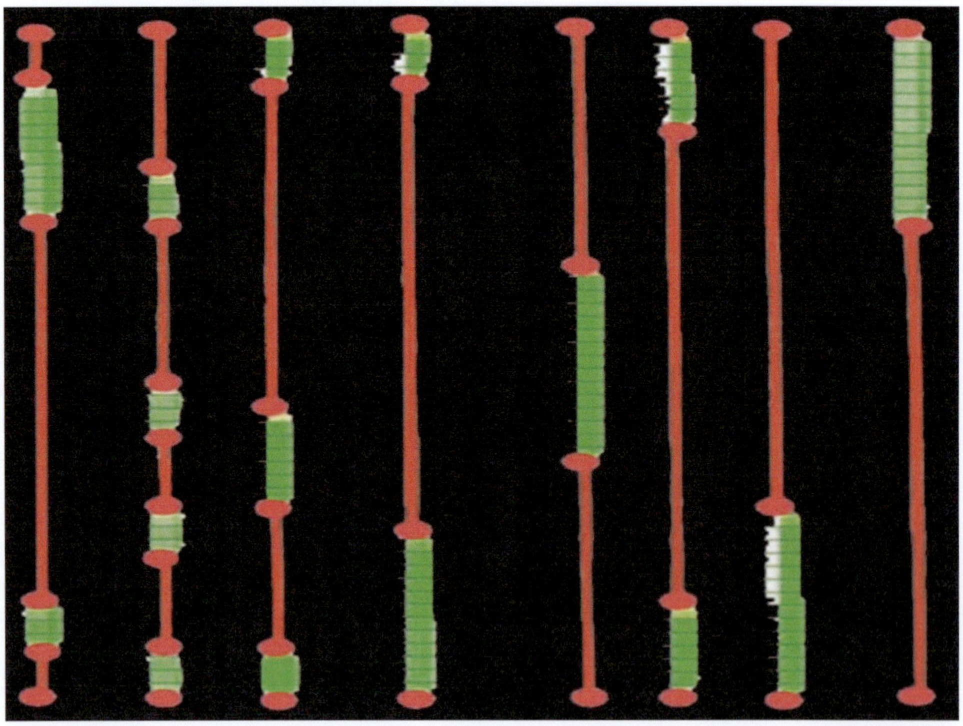

Fig. 26 Disposition of variable aponeuroses (aponeurosis) in the continuity of the muscles according to the law of association and commutativity intended to balance the transmission of stresses with identical contraction of all muscular fascicles

fascicles and the muscular length were attributed to the elastic compliance component of this fascia in the muscle according to Hill's conceptual model, created with contractile and elastic structures [2, 37]. This concept is reinforced by the junction between the aponeurosis and the tendon, which has a conical shape to distribute the harmonious transmission of the stresses (Fig. 27).

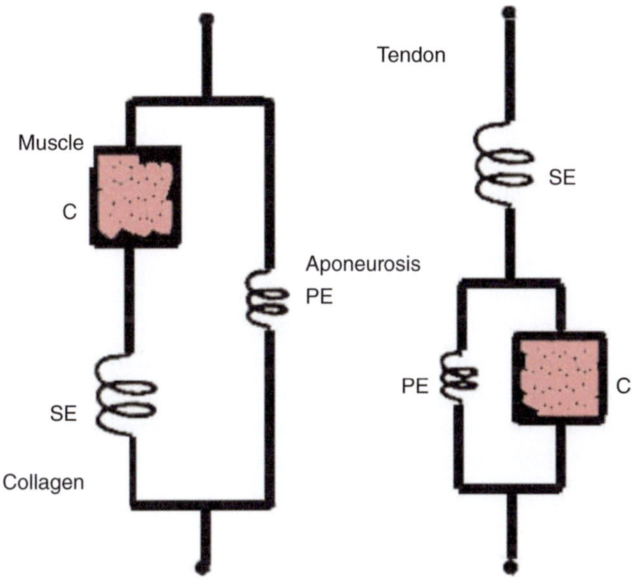

Fig. 27 Modeling of the muscle–aponeurosis–tendon complex according to the Hill principle with the contractile muscle component (C) and the elastic aponeurotic component (PE) and that of the tendon (SE) in series and in parallel

Mechanical tests on the elastic properties of a muscle focus on the tendinous structures isolated from the rest of the muscular element, ignoring the role of the aponeurosis [2, 37, 38]. Comparative studies of the reaction pattern during muscular contraction or passive stretching showed that fascial characteristics differ significantly: in passive movement, there is more fascial length involved in weak forces than comparatively for muscle contraction activities. The difference in length may be greater than 1.25 mm for approximately 6% of the length of aponeurosis. During an isometric contraction of a muscle, the contraction of the fascia is limited to about 3.5% of the total fascial length. During this isomeric contraction, the energy expenditure of the aponeurosis is evaluated at 2.8 microJoules (μJ). As a passive element, this finding may seem paradoxical. Although passive, any structure during a displacement is subject to an intimate cellular change that is accompanied by energy-releasing cellular metabolic variations, either in the form of a loss or a recovery. According to a more affordable model, the fascia can be compared to a piece of elastic which, when tensioned beyond its length, stores a force (requiring an energy expenditure for its tensioning) which, when stopped will regain its initial length and as a result, restore the energy stored during tensioning (e.g., archery and pole vaulting) (Fig. 28).

When the force decreases from the maximum force (optimum length) to a force equal to its passive resistance (initial state), the aponeurosis decreases in length by 9%, resulting in work of 4.8 μJ. Dissection of the lumbar portion of the longissimus dorsi (antigravitary) shows a aponeurosis that occupies 95% of its length. The aponeurosis mass occupies

Fig. 28 Representation of sporting activities based on the restitution of energy (archery, pole vault)

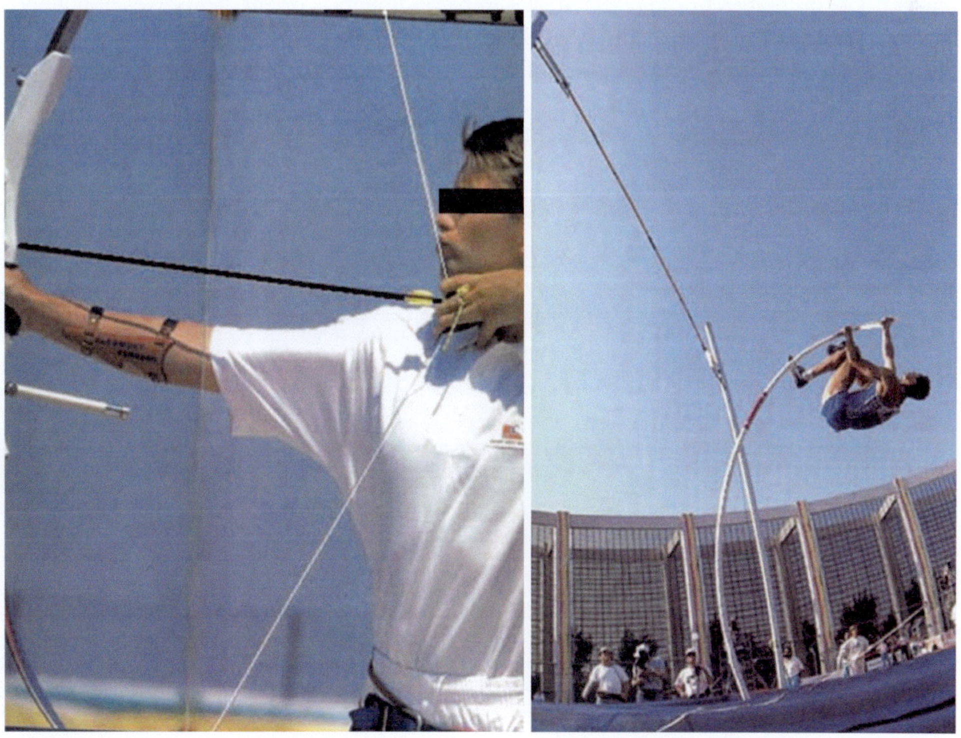

the lateral part of the lumbar curvature which inserts on the deep medial aspect of the rough surface of the iliac bone between the articular surface and the medial lip of the iliac crest. Each bundle ends with a lateral chevron on the costiform processes and a medial chevron on the accessory tubercles of the lumbar vertebrae.

When standing, the fascia behaves like a passive rope that maintains joint balance without involving muscular contraction resulting in a significant saving of energy expenditure.

During one movement, its length variation is considered an important factor in explaining the difference in muscle length changes. For Lieber [27], during passive movements in the frog, the elasticity of the aponeurosis was 8% and for the tendon of the semi-tendinosis it was 2%. Huijing [28] showed a greater extension of the aponeurosis of gastrocnemius in the rat when the muscle was in contraction. For the same mechanical effect, the tendon had a tension of 3 to 4%, which indicated that the compliance of the aponeurosis was different from that of the muscle. The lengthening of the muscle depends on the properties of the aponeurosis which is an important element as a factor of storage of energy and its release during muscle contraction. The elastic energy stored during the passive elongation is very low (about 0.04 μJ) because of the small levels of force, if the muscle is activated to a certain length, the aponeurosis is stretched by about 2% resulting in 0.56 μJ elastic energy storage. For an active muscle, if the muscular force decreases, the force exerted on the aponeurosis is also reduced; this results in a release of energy of 3.15 μJ. The consequence is that the relaunched energy of 3.5 μJ can be obtained if the fascia follows the force/length displacement curve during the isometric contraction of a muscle. The properties of the fascia appear to be an important field for architectural modeling applications of a muscle. For muscular modeling, therefore, the stiffness of the fascia must be incorporated for elongations of less than 10%. The origin of the restitution of energy is still obscure, but may be dependent on the aponeurosis-tendon junction. All these fundamental notions find their application in the structure of the posterior muscles of the vertebral column, where the aponeuroses occupy a prominent place.

Muscle with Parallel Fascicles: Pseudo-Penniform

The fascicles have the same direction between the two insertions with parallel fascicles. This arrangement is mechanically ideal and has maximum efficiency requiring simultaneous contraction of all sarcomeres in parallel or series. This anatomical arrangement is met for some muscles: rhomboid, serratus posterior (Fig. 29).

Unipennate Muscle (Fig. 30)

The muscle is semi-penniform or unipennate when the fascicles are arranged on one side of the fascia, the other side remaining free. The longus capitis is broad and thick above, narrow below, and arises by four tendinous slips, from the anterior tubercles of the transverse processes of the third, fourth, fifth, and sixth cervical vertebrae, and ascends, converging toward its fellow of the opposite side, to insert into the inferior surface of the basilar part of the occipital bone. It presents in its continuity an intermediate aponeurosis which strengthens its power and protects the sarcomeres in cephalic extension movements.

Bipennate Muscle

The aponeurosis extends a great distance, and the fascicles orient themselves obliquely on both sides of the aponeurosis. The longissimus cervicis, observed individually, consists of fusiform bundles but as a whole is functionally bipennate (Fig. 31). It is presented in three portions with rectilinear fascicles stretched from T1–T2–T3 to the anterior aspects of

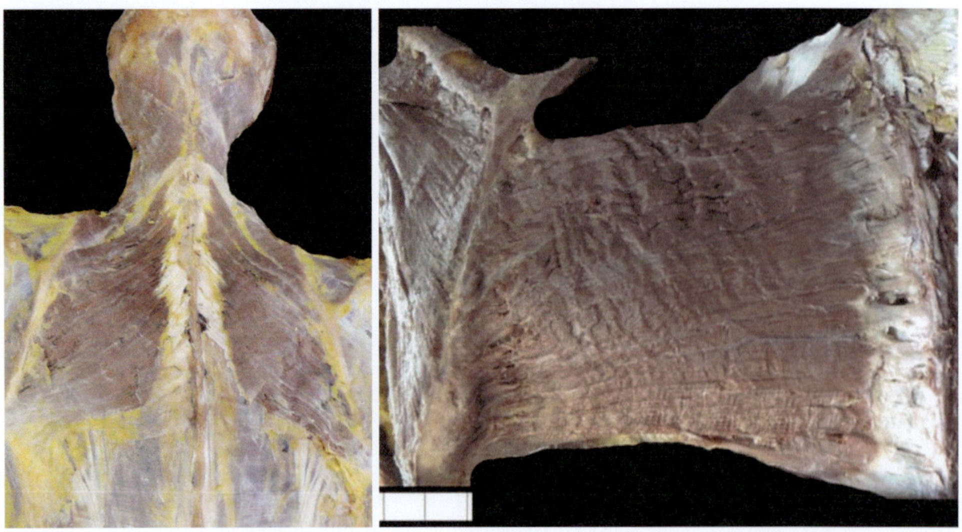

Fig. 29 Unipennate rhomboid muscle with direction of the muscular fascicles in the axis of the aponeuroses (aponeurosis) granting it increased power

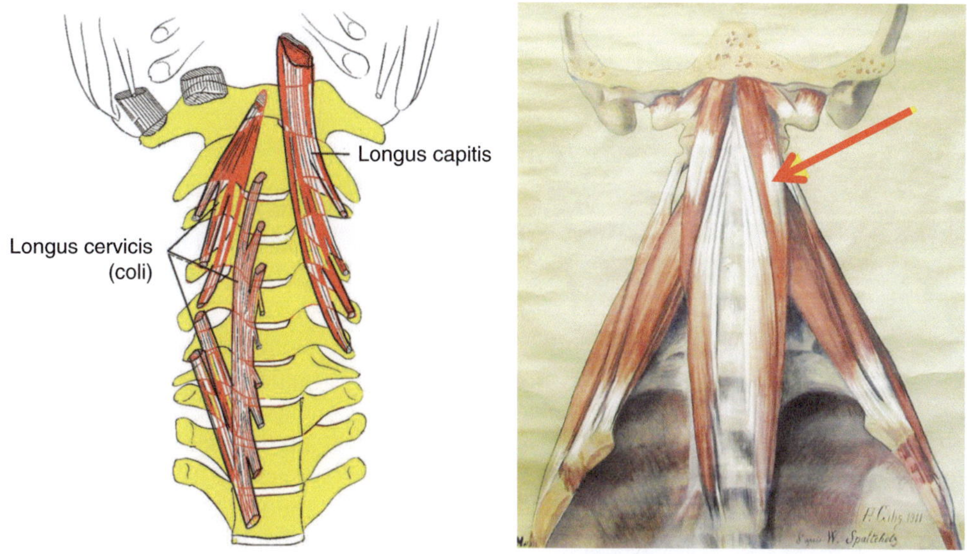

Fig. 30 Muscles along the head and neck, note the presence of aponeurosis at its medial part

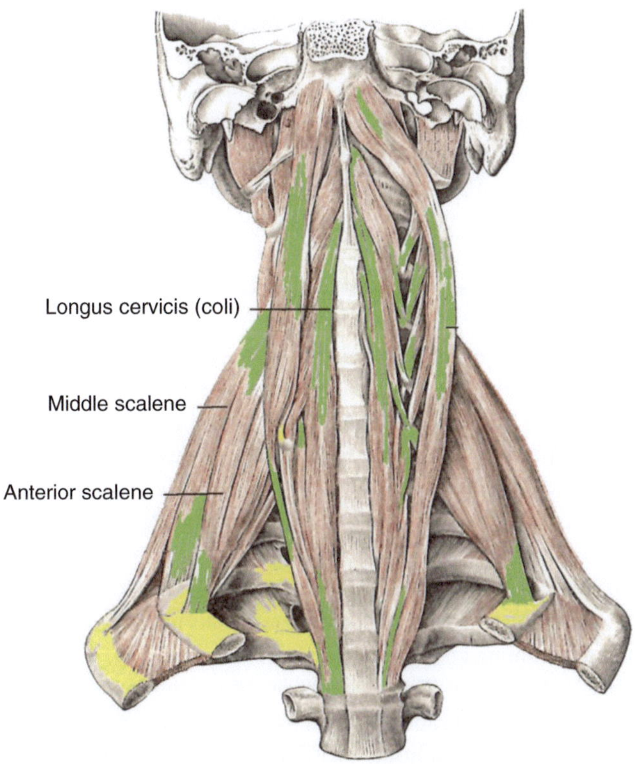

Fig. 31 Long neck muscles with its three types of vertical and oblique fascicles drawing a rhombus with permanent three-dimensional adaptation of the musculo-aponeurotic fascicles

C2–C3–C4. A cervico-cephalic oblique portion is detached from the anterior tubercles of the transverse processes of C45–C4–C3 to terminate on the anterior tubercle of the atlas and a stretched oblique cervico-thoracic portion of the anterior tubercles of the transverse processes of C5–C6–C7, the anterior surface of the vertebral bodies of T1–T2–T3. This inverted V arrangement with oblique fascicles is a factor of rotational stability of the cervical spine with cerebral-thoracic mechanical coupling.

The disposition of transversospinales (transversospinales) muscles (the deep layer of the intrinsic back muscles) at the thoracic level with its 23 bundles is comparable with the long and short erector spinae, long and short lamellar which act as multisegmental rotational and oblique limiters, simulating a bipennate muscle (Fig. 32).

The quadratus lumborum was modeled after dissection into three subgroups with anterior fascicles, intermediate lumbocostal fibers, and posterior fibers with variability in 50% of the subjects [39] (Fig. 33).

The insertion of the fascicles on the aponeurosis is the essential element of the organization of the muscle (Fig. 34). The pennate disposition of the fascicles allows an increase of the physiological Cross Sectional Area (PCSA) hence increased power. If the muscular hypertrophy causes an increase in the angle of pennation of the fascicles, this angle will be disadvantageous for the development of force. On the other hand, an increase in the angle of pennation with a greater number of fascicles attached to the tendon will increase muscle volume and power (PCSA) [40].

Angles of Pennation Articulation and Muscular Power

If all the fascicles were parallel and of the same length, they would have to contract at the same time to produce an articular displacement, thus limiting amplitude. The distribution of the fascicles over the entire length of the aponeurosis, which occupies 50–80% of the total length of the muscular complex, allows their progressive mechanical play during the movement of the joint with a variation of the pennation angle which has an influence on the speed of shortening. At identical sarcomere length, a pennate muscle has a lower rate of shortening than a muscle with parallel fascicles. The architecture of the muscle is essential if one wants, for example,

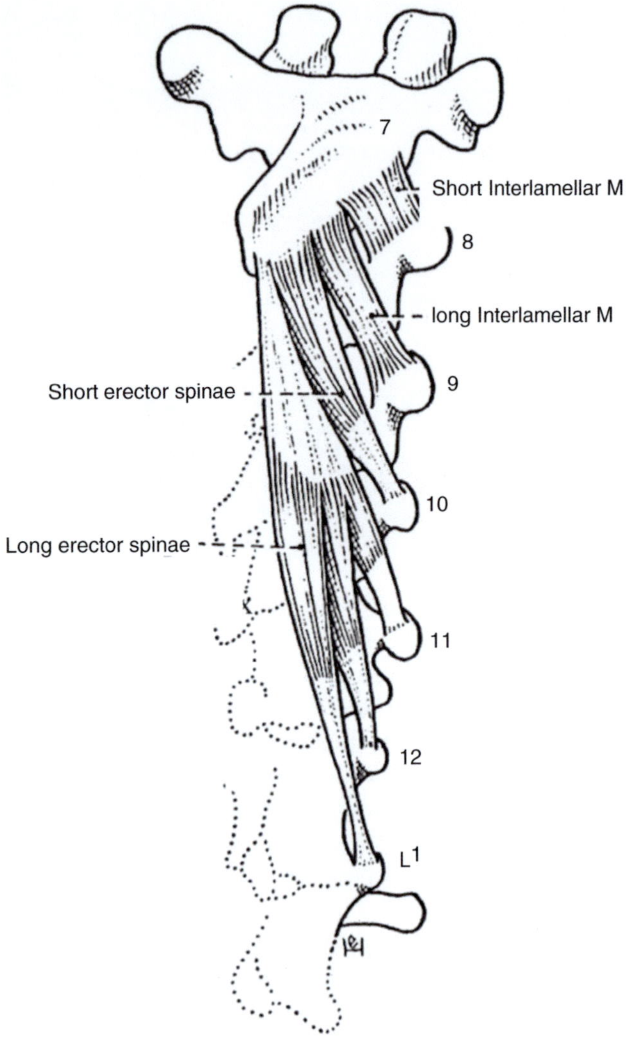

Fig. 32 Transversospinales Mm (Winkler)

to correlate mechanical data and biochemical data. The force transmitted by the muscle to the tendon is correlated with the angle of pennation. The greater the angle of pennation, the less the tension force and, conversely, an acute pennation angle increases its power.

The arrangement of fascicles during articular mobilization *with rotation* alters the pennation angle, increasing its power [40, 41]. In the extended position, an obturated pennation angle from the fascicles results in a reduction of the muscular force while in bending an acute angle increases the power. In all cases, the aponeurosis are under elastic tension. The morphology of the ilio-costalis in its lumbothoracic portion with its oblique bundles together with all other muscles can be schematized according to the principle of a game of "tug-of-war." This makes it possible to understand the essential role of the position of the athletes' inclination (pennation angle) for maximum performance. The angles of pennation of the anterior, lateral, and posterior muscles of the column have penultimate angles between 0° and 15° with aponeuroses of 90–95% of the total length of the muscle (Figs. 35, 36, 37, and 38).

Muscular Action and Topography

The deep muscles fit over the length of the bone they surround, and the superficial muscles correspond to the bones only by their extremities or by their tendons, which slide over the bones before they insert, and surround the articulations and contribute powerfully to ensure their stability. The appreciation of the strength of a muscle supposes the knowledge of the number of its fibers, of the quality, of the constitution of the fascicles, of the disposition of the lever on which it acts, of its angle on the lever and the angle of incidence of the fascicles with respect to the virtual axis of the muscle. Each fascicle being very distinct from the neighboring fascicles, and which may be considered as a small power, it is conceivable that the more fibers there are in a muscle, the more vigorous its contraction. The quality, the constitution of the fibers, the intensity of the stimulant, affect not so much the contraction force of a muscle but the number of its fibers. To be convinced of this, one only has to compare the movement energy of an individual during sporting activities.

Topography and Global Functionality

The longest muscles are the most superficial and pass in front of several articulations, resulting in compound or rather successive movements which simplify the mechanism of locomotion at the same time as they increase the energy of movements.

This considerable length of certain muscles is advantageous in that it enables them to take a fixed point of support on a less mobile part, on the trunk those which move the pelvic limbs take a point of support on the pelvis. As a result of the different mechanism of the shoulder and pelvis, it ensures the fixed insertion of all the muscles of the lower limb, while the spine of the scapula, the sternum, clavicle, column, and ribs serve as a fixed insertion to those of the upper limb.

The movements of the body segments spontaneously organize under mechanical conditions such that the muscle–fascia (apeurosis)–tendon complex yield is optimized and the energy expenditure required to perform a given task is at a minimal level. During walking, the subject chooses his speed at a comfortable level which corresponds to the minimum caloric expenditure to cover a unit distance of one meter. In the reference conditions, the muscles insert by their tendons on the skeleton so that their length is as close as possible to their optimal length. It is at this length that they develop the highest tension and speed when they begin to contract. Walking is a relatively inexpensive activity in

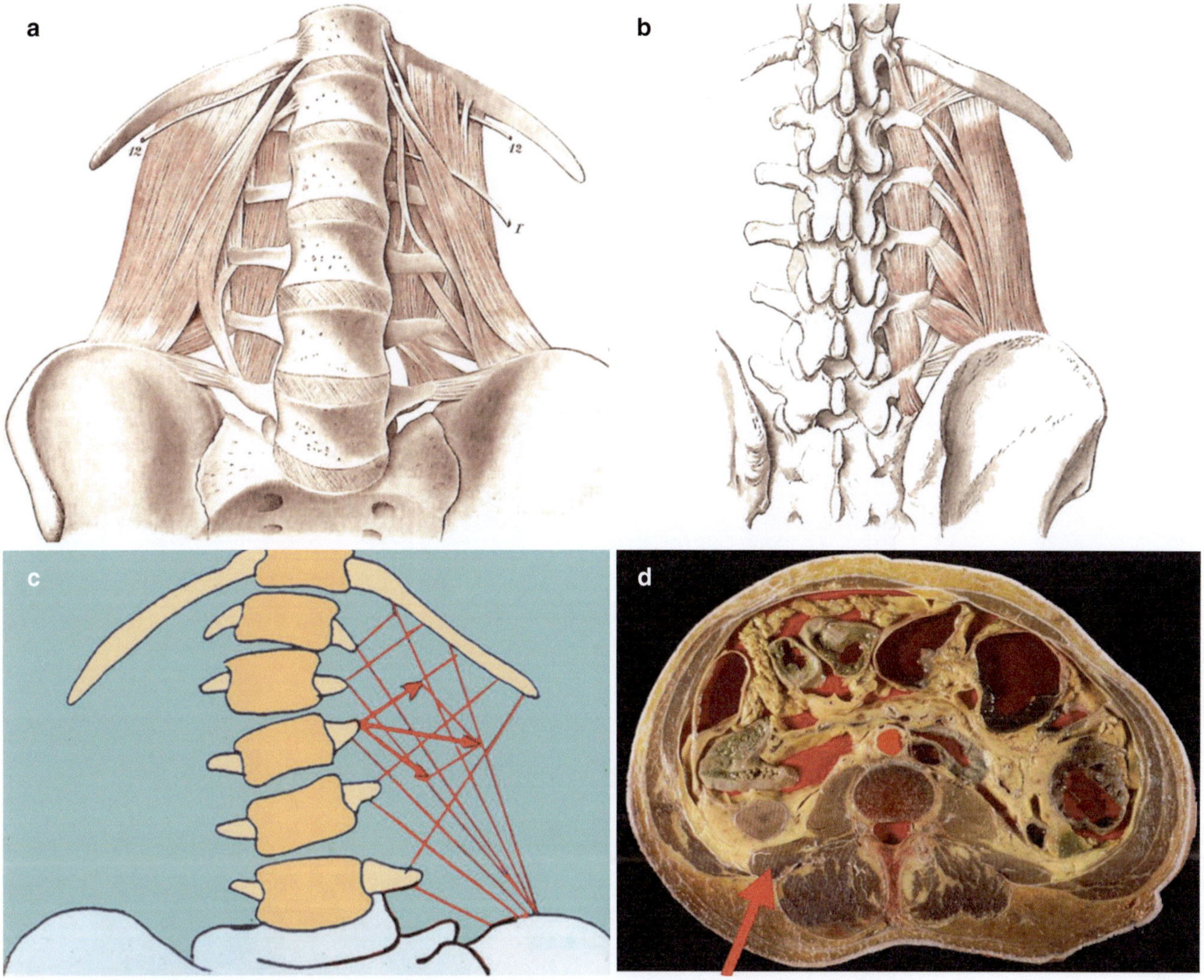

Fig. 33 The Quadratus lumborum (square muscle of the loins) in ventral and dorsal view (**a**, **b**) with its modeling (**c**). The set of insertions of the muscular fasciculi with its 45° pennation angles is similar to a bipennate muscle contributing to its lumbo-costo iliac rotation function compared to the 3 muscles of the anterolateral wall of the abdomen. Horizontal cut (**d**) at the lumbar level with all the posterior, anterolateral, and anterior muscles constituting the abdominal chamber

energy, since the kinematics of the displacements of the two lower limbs allow the best exploitation of quantitatively important inertial phenomena because of the mass of mobilized parts.

The broad muscles occupy the walls of the large cavities. Quadrilaterals go from one part of the trunk to another (quadratus lumborum), whereas they are triangular when they are extended from the trunk to the limbs. When there are several superimposed large muscles, their fascicles affect an opposite direction in such a way as to cut at an angle or to cross one another, an arrangement which singularly increases the resistance of the abdominal walls. In place of the three broad muscles of the abdomen, if this were a single muscle, three times thicker with a single direction, their purpose would be less well achieved (Fig. 39).

If, in order to characterize the short muscles, only the brevity of the fascicles was considered, there would be a very large number which deserve this name, but it is the brevity of the muscular body which serves artificially as a basis. Short muscles are everywhere where there are short bones to move (inter-transverse, interspinous). The muscles of the vertebral gutters are short, although they present as lengthy arrangements, as they are only a series of short muscles arranged following each other, so as to simulate a long muscle (longissimus dorsi: lumbar-thoracic-cervical-cephalic, ilio-costalis: lumbar-thoracic-cervical). Their modeling by Bogduk [42] was divided into four components with lumbar, thoracic, iliocostal thoracic, and ilio-costal lumbar portions. This type of systematization moves away from anatomical reality and limits conclusions of experiments. The functional interrelation-

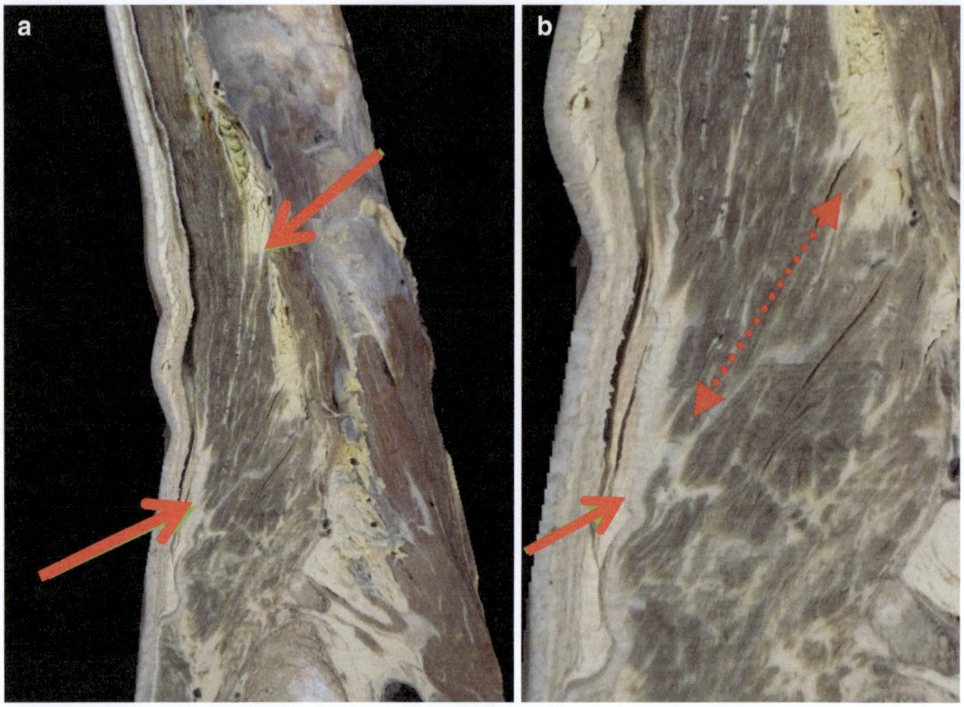

Fig. 34 Sagittal section (**a**) of aponeurosis (green arrow), and longissimus dorsi and ilio-costalis (common mass) at their insertion on the posterior aspect of the sacrum. The very short muscle fascicles (**b**) are oblique at 45° with pennation angles of 0–5° and proximal and distal insertions on aponeurosis. The angle of pennation varies according to the degree of flexion-extension of the lumbar spine. Whatever its position, the fascia is in permanent tension (anti-gravity) intended to protect the sarcomeres and to restore the energy

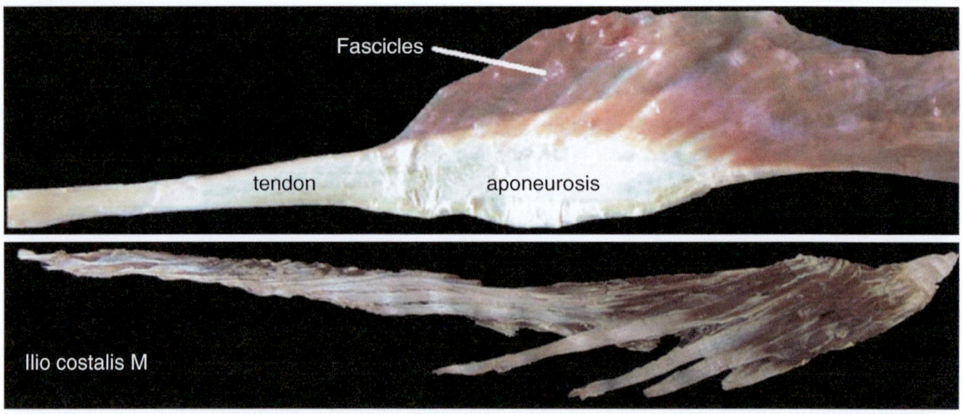

Fig. 35 Overall arrangement of the muscle–aponeurosis–tendon complex and the insertion of muscle fascicles according to a variable pennation angle (**a**). Organization as an example of ilio-costalis muscle (**b**)

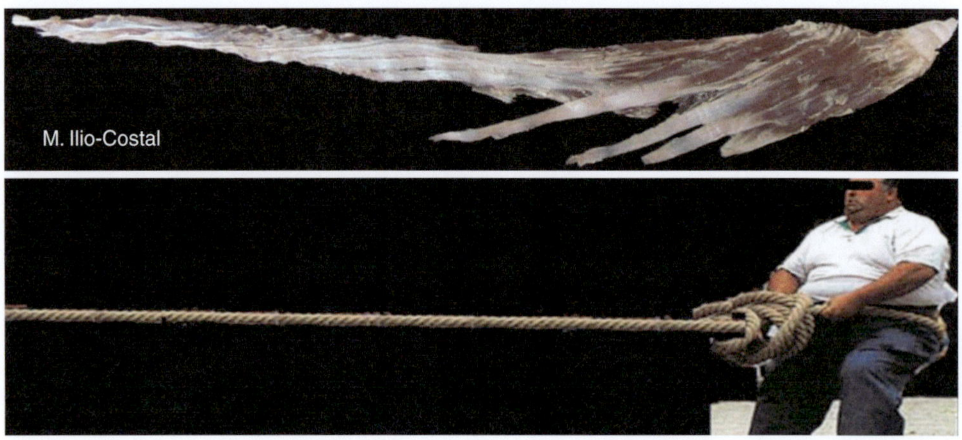

Fig. 36 The mode of action of this complex can be compared to the game of "tug of war" with, at one end, the permanent tensioning of the central aponeurosis materialized by a competitor endowed with a power proportional to its weight (PCSA)

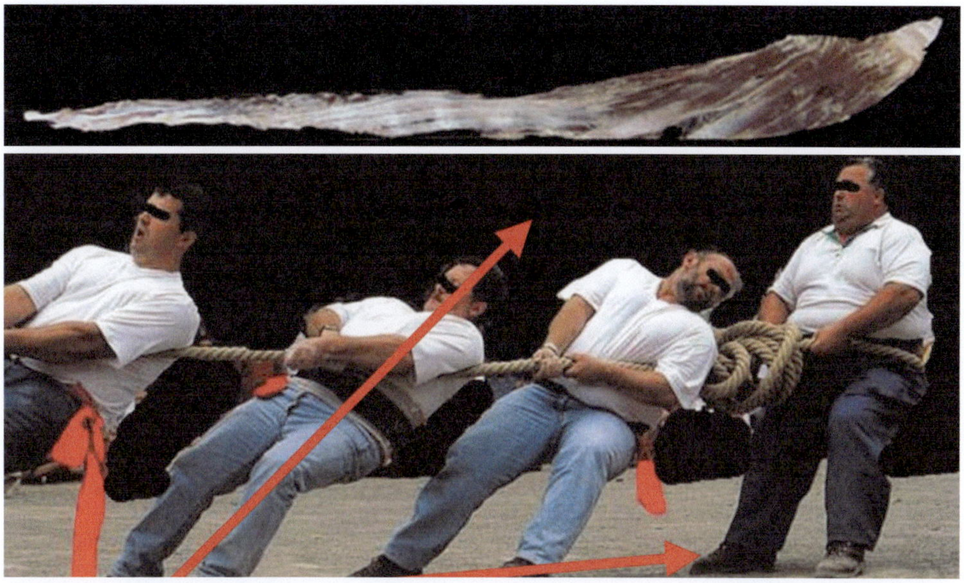

Fig. 37 To increase the traction power, we use teammates who by their position (acute angle of pennation) participate in maximum performance

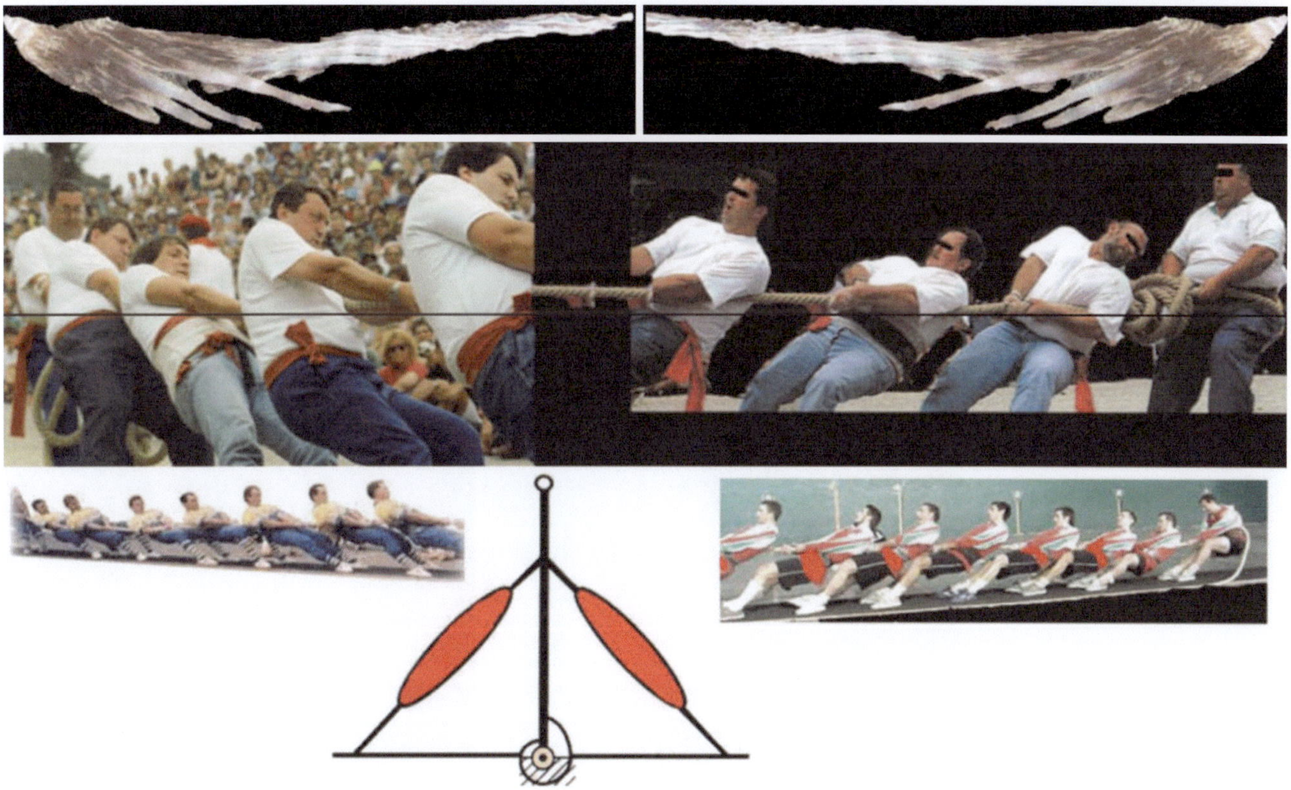

Fig. 38 The equilibrium between the competitors induces a resistant identical structure which responds to the global concept of the Euler column (agonist and antagonist muscles) underpinned by the permanent action of the aponeuroses with energy restitution

ships between the muscular-aponeurotic complexes of the spine and the lower limbs are numerous. An unequal length of the lower limbs induces an increase in the amplitude of the vertebral column and the oscillation of the pelvis. A loss of mobility of the vertebral column decreases the oscillation of the pelvis and the rate of walking. Blockage of the column by a brace or extended arthrodesis results in a considerable change in the stride. A loss of function of the ilio-psoas causes a lack of control of lumbar lordosis (Fig. 40).

Muscle Direction

This is one of the most important points. It is impossible to exactly evaluate their action, so the angles of pennation between the fascicles and (aponeurosis) must be evaluated much more than is usually done for the precise determination of this direction. The axis of the muscle being not the same as that of the fascicles which compose it, we must study both the direction of the muscular body and its tendon, and the direc-

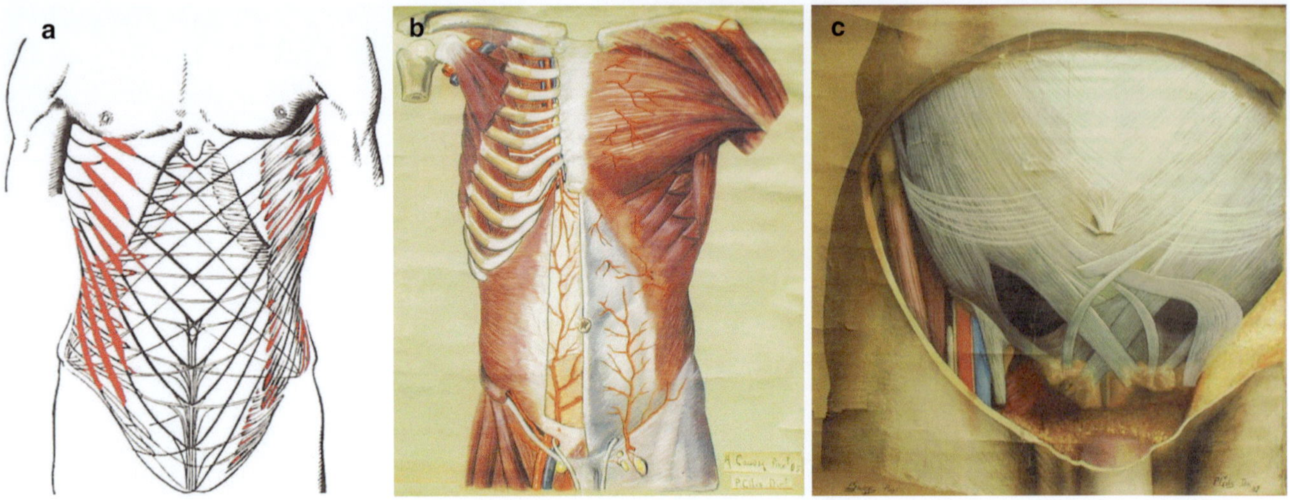

Fig. 39 Schematic representation of the three muscles of the anterolateral-lateral region of the abdomen (**a**), anterior view of the abdominal wall (**b**), the dissection reveals a fascial structure with crossing angles in the three planes of space (**c**)

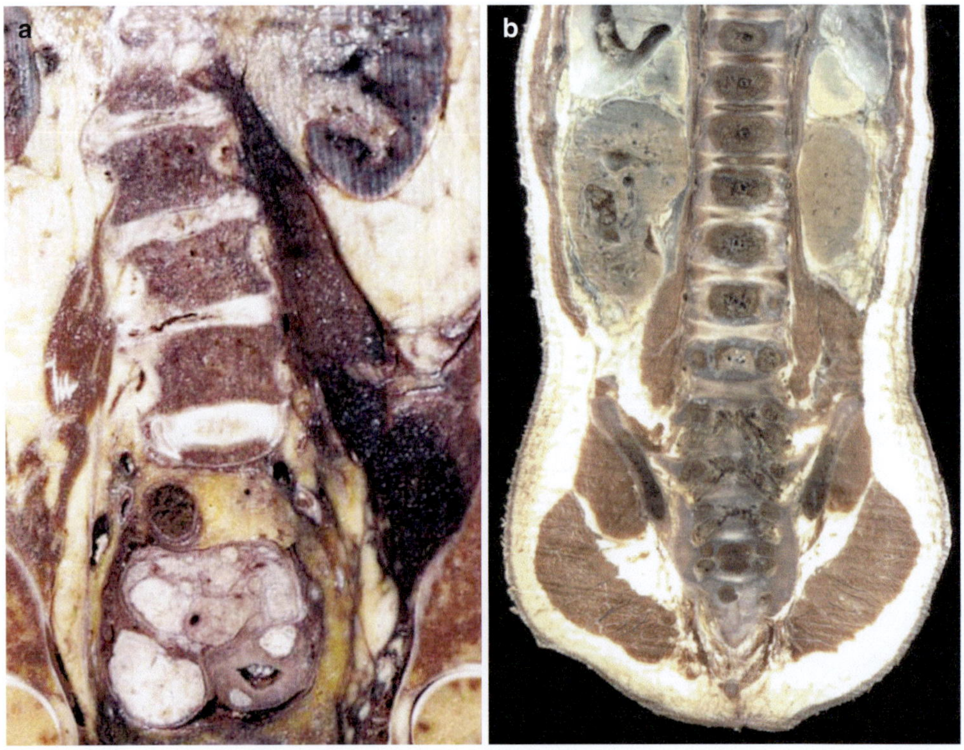

Fig. 40 Mode of insertion of the ilio-psoas muscles with their insertion on the lumbar vertebrae, a factor of stability of the lumbar lordosis: adult subject (**a**) and fetus (**b**)

tion of the muscle fascicles with respect to the fasciae. Sometimes the fascicles follow the same direction as the aponeurosis (e.g., rhomboid), sometimes they follow obliquely along the aponeurosis to form the penniform or semi-penniform, convergent or radiated muscles, as in the latissimus dorsi, trapezius, or extend obliquely between two aponeurotic planes, etc. (Figs. 41 and 42). Often, the different portions of a muscle have very different directions, so that, in order to know its action, it must be decomposed into as many portions as there are directions in the fascicles: longissimus dorsi, iliocostalis, trapezius, serratus anterior. It is the large muscles that offer examples of this complex arrangement, and the total effect is the result of all the partial actions.

Each muscle has an axis or a median line, to which we can relate the general effect of its fascicles. This line is well traced; it is only to shorten it in the various attitudes of the components to determine their action. There are muscles that have a curvilinear direction; the first effect of their contraction is to straighten their fascicles, and this effect produces, one may appreciate their uses as those of rectilinear muscles.

The direction of the muscles must be studied with respect to the axis of the body, and especially to the axis of the limb, the lever on which they act (functional globality). A very large number is almost parallel to the axis of the lever that they are moving, but in certain attitudes they move away from parallelism, forming pronounced angles with the levers on which they take their insertion, and even sometimes become perpendicular to these levers. In this respect, the direction of the muscles is not absolute; it is subordinate to the attitude of the levers, offering various incidents which are much closer to parallelism than to perpendicular incidence.

Muscle Torsion

The mechanical approach of the muscle is indissociable from the study of the aponeurosis and the tendon which constitute the elements of transmission and regulation of the power and articular displacement. There are several models concerning the functional organization of the muscular–aponeurosis–tendon complex. Rouvière [43] showed that in certain muscle groups fascicles in the macroscopic anatomical sense (to be distinguished from functional muscular fibers) spiral together (splenius capitis, splenius cervicis). The splenius capitis separates from the caudal part of the septum nuchae, from the C7 to T3 spinous processes and from the interspinous and supraspinous ligaments and terminates at the lateral end of the lower lip of the occipital nuchal line and on the lateral surface of the mastoid process. The splenius cervicis (spinous process of T3–T5 with transverse processes from C1 to C5) circumvents the lateral surface of the splenius capitis (Fig. 43).

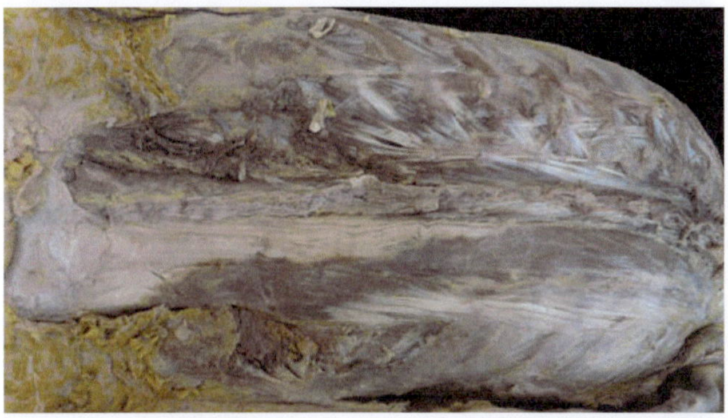

Fig. 41 Arrangement of beams of L. dorsi Mm and Ilio-costalis Mm on an anatomical subject with a thoracic kyphosis putting under tension the aponeuroses and fascicles modifying the bending moment

The organization of the small complexes of the longissimus cervicis (transverse processes from C4 to T4 ending on the mastoid), by their twisted disposition with an acute pennation angle, increases its power and stiffness in the context of its action in rotation torque of the cephalic segment (Fig. 43b).

The torsion of the fascicles of the latissimus dorsi is a factor for its increase in power according to a fixed point. Its description by Bogduk et al. [42] was 13 strands with 5 to the lumbar spinous processes, 6 to thoracic spinous process, and the 11th and 12th ribs (Fig. 44).

On an experimental basis, if we take a certain number of strands of any material and we attach them parallel to each other, we will have a beam whose resistance will be equal to the sum of the partial resistances of each strand, but also slightly more than each of these strands. If the spiral beam is twisted, its tensile strength will not change but if sudden traction occurs, the first effect is to lengthen the bottom of the helix, similar to that produced by a coil spring. The lengthening of the bottom of the helix, whose fascicles have a spiral arrangement, attenuates the effects of shocks and

Fig. 42 Trapezius muscles with their insertion on the cervico-thoracic spine. Note the importance of the aponeurosis which balances the stresses at the different levels, with the torsion of the fascicles of the cervical portion

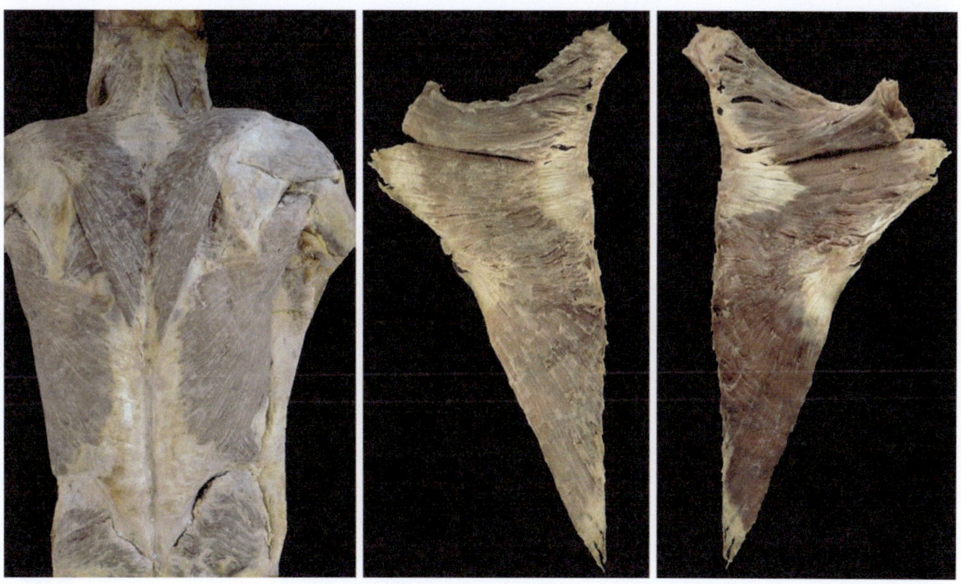

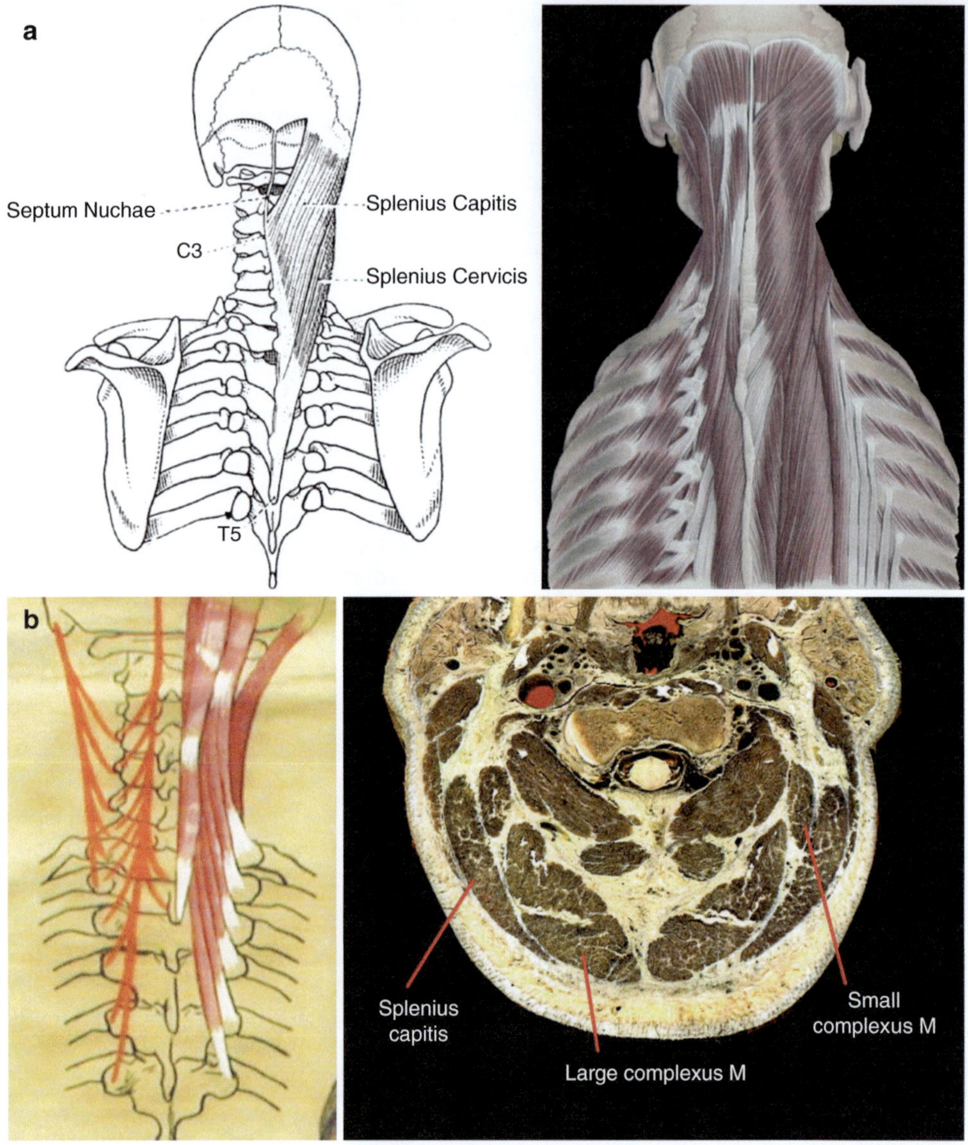

Fig. 43 (**a**) Posterior view of the cervical region with splenius capitis which is bypassed by the splenius cervicis increasing the overall power through the torsion of the fascicles. (**b**) Insertions of the small complexus (semispinalis capitis) characterized by an intermediate fascia and its twisted global axis (a). Horizontal section of the posterior muscles of the neck with the different muscular planes (b) which constitute dynamic elements according to the principle of the composite beam

the danger of breakage resulting from a sudden and violent pull. The angle of pennation between the aponeurosis and the axis of the muscle shows a torsion of the order of 10–15°. Morphological analysis in contraction shows that the arrangement of the fascicles with an angle of pennation in rotation increases its power.

Monoarticular Muscles and Mechanical Rotary Results

A monoarticular muscle crosses only one joint. Any muscular contraction causes two actions: one longitudinal and one rotational component. The longitudinal component has the effect of either applying the joint surfaces against each other (coaptation effect) or to separate the articular surfaces (dislocation effect). The rotational component causes a rotation about the mechanical axis of the joint and according to the articular type is called flexion.

The rotational movement, (Mf) the "moment" is the product of the muscular force (Fm: PCSA) by the distance (*d*) of this force to the axis of rotation: Mf = Fm × *d*. The distance (*d*) is equal to the sine of the angle defined by the insertion distance of the muscle at the center of the joint and its direction. The rotational force varies according to its place of insertion in relation to the center of the joint. The bending moment of the thoracic ilio-costal decreases in extension whereas that of the long thoracic remains unchanged. The weak bending moment of the abdominal obliques, psoas, and quadratus lumborum have little influence during anterior flexion [6] (Tables 1 and 2).

The monoarticular muscles are sufficiently long and extensible to allow complete extension and, during flexion, to completely flex the joint. The simultaneous presence of

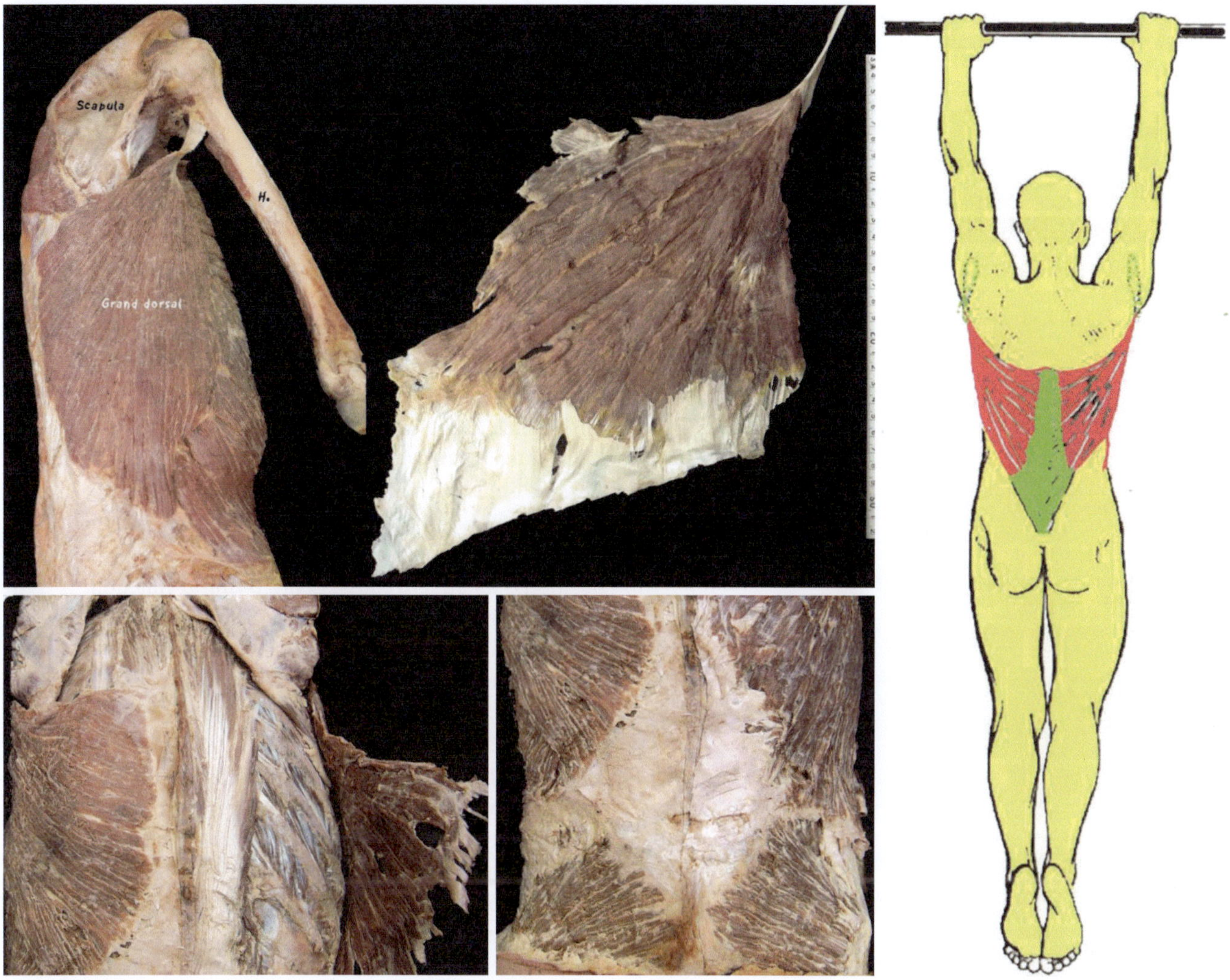

Fig. 44 Overall aspect of latissimus dorsi coursing the costal wall and its change of direction with the torsion according to the direction of its fascicules at the humeral tendon insertion. The thoraco-lumbar insertion zone is made by means of a very resistant aponeurosis plane designed to oppose excessive tension in certain pathological situations (e.g., hypertrophy of the muscle in the paraplegic, fixed bar traction). The progressive change of direction of the fascicles potentiates its power

monoarticular and polyarticular being constant, it is concluded that such a provision must have a mechanical advantage. The question is to know why these two types of muscles are present, since only the monoarticulars are sufficient, whereas the polyarticulars limit movement. The answer is provided by their distribution whose muscular masses are not evenly distributed between all segments. In its lumbar portion the muscles are bulky to respond to the important constraints of the entire column.

Polyarticular Muscles and Resultant Mechanical Rotators

A polyarticular muscle (bi-articular or multi-articular) bridging two or more articulations intervene in such a way that their shortening is minimal. Within this perspective, the displacement linked to the mobilization of a joint is compensated by a complementary displacement of another joint, which is observed at the level of the cervical spine. The conditions are not very different from the isometry, so that the developed tension remains as close as possible to the optimum value corresponding to the resting length.

The primary functional objective is essentially focused on the distal articulation, the positioning of the proximal articulation being intended to reinforce their main action. For example, the extension of the knee puts on tension the gastrocnemius and favors the impulse power of the triceps sural (triceps) on the foot whose actions are closely correlated with each other. The action of the trunk muscles is more important if the knees are bent, which has the effect of releasing the pelvis and allowing its anterior tilt. Their role is essential in the positioning of the joints, with improvement of the yield and equilibrium of the stresses at the level of the cartilage.

Table 1 Intrinsic biometry with: length of sarcomeres (ls), fascicle length (lf), pennation angle (a) and Physiological Cross Sectional Area (PCSA) (Christophy [6])

Muscle	Sarcomere Length, ls (μm)	Fascicle Length, lf (m)	Angle of Pennation (a) (°)	PCSA (mm^2)
Psoas: L3	3.11	0.14	10.7	101
Rectus abdominis	2.83	0.3	0	567
Erector spinae, L. dorsi, L. costal, lumbar portion	2.37	0.03	13.8	154
Erector spinae, L. dorsi, L. costal, thoracic portion	2.37	0.11	13.8	100
Quadratus lumborum	2.36	0.03	7.4	40
Latissimus dorsi	2.30	0.3	0	90
Internal oblique	2.83	0.04	0	185
External oblique	2.83	0.04	0	196

Table 2 Biometrics of morphological characteristics of major columnar muscles by Seireg [63]

Muscle	Muscle length (m)	PCSA (cm^2)	Angle pennation (°)
Longissimus capitis	0.12	1.22	10
Longissimus coli	0.08	0.82	10
Rectus capitis anterior	0.03	0.13	10
Rectus capitis lateralis	0.025	0.21	10
Semispinalis	0.1	1.89	10
Splenius cervicis	0.16	3.73	10
Sternocleidomastoid	0.2	2.08	10
Rhomboid major	0.11	3.87	
Interspinalis		5.68	
Longissimus dorsi multifidus		1.25	
Piriformis	0.08	20.54	9.5
Psoas	0.25	2.65	7.5
Latissimus dorsi	0.27	12.90	

Mechanical Properties

Muscular Work

Studies on the mechanical properties of isolated muscle fibers have shown the important role of the elastic components located in these fibers and particularly at the level of the intramuscular junction zones. However, the comparison of values with elongation as a consequence of the optimum force exerted obtained in the fibers or fascicles and in an intact muscle generally concludes that most of these components must be located outside the fascicules in the aponeurosis and tendon. The muscular fibers consist of elementary contractile units (sarcomeres placed in series or in parallel), and the result is that the speed of shortening of the muscle is all the greater because it is longer, because it has more sarcomeres. The relation $V_{max} = 10 \times LF\ s^{-1}$ for a contraction without resistance means that for long muscles with a large number of sarcomeres, the maximum speed of shortening is equal to 10 times the length of muscle fibers per second (a muscle having fibers of a length of 10 cm would have, in the absence of any resistance, a maximum speed of shortening of 100 cm/s).

Described in 1891 by Blix [44] on the isolated and tetanized muscle, the characteristic force/length relationship shows that up to a reference length the force increases with length. Beyond this reference length (limit length), breaks arise in the structure. The strength/length relationships of the contractive component differ according to the slow or fast percentage. On a frog gastrocnemius (slow muscle) the force does not diminish rapidly with length: the muscle thus has a fairly wide range of length for which its maximum force remains constant whereas a fast muscle like the flexor hallucis exhibits an optimum force for a relatively narrow range of length. This allows a postural muscle like the longissimus dorsi to develop maximum strength for a wide range of joint positions. Its effectiveness, being postural function, is reinforced by the development of a passive tension that does not consume biochemical energy for short lengths.

The components of the muscle are shortened on average in the ratio 2/3 of its length up to 50% of the total length. The muscles passing in front of a joint must have functional muscle fibers three times longer than the insertion distance on either side of this articulation correlated with the shortening during the complete realization of the movement. This length allows them to exert maximum force when the movement starts and stays with a certain force when the maximum movement is reached. The relationship between the length of muscle fibers (sarcomeres) and the extent of shortening is an important element.

Muscle Yield

The evaluation of the work shows that a muscle strand 2 cm long has the same output as two strands located in parallel of 1 cm each. The essential organization in the approach of the mechanical functioning and the performance of a muscle rests on the direction of the fascicles and the arrangement of the aponeuroses. The shortening of the fascicles results in an increase of the pennation angle. For example, for long fibers of 6.5 cm, contraction results in a shortening of 3.3 cm, but the overall shortening is 3.8 cm (Fig. 45).

Fascicle Mechanic Performance and Physiological Cross-Sectional Area (PCSA)

Muscle strength is proportional to the cross-sectional area of the muscle (5–10 kg/cm^2) but independent of its length

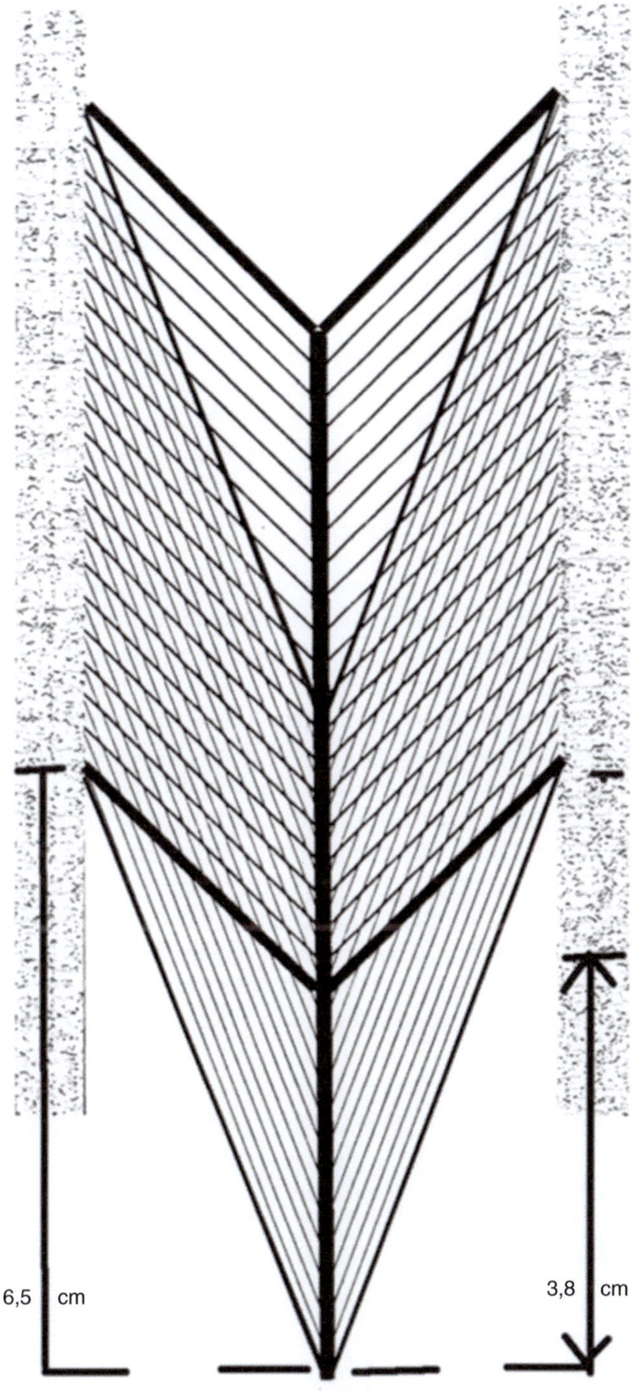

Fig. 45 Evaluation of the displacement of the fascicles for a bipennate muscle

[45–48]. The resistance of an elastic is not changed by increasing or decreasing its length, but the force is increased by increasing the number of fascicles of the muscle (Fig. 46).

The contractile properties of the muscle depend on the importance of the fascicles. The capacity of a muscle to produce a force is proportional to its PCSA (Physiological Cross Sectional Area) which can be translated as "physiological

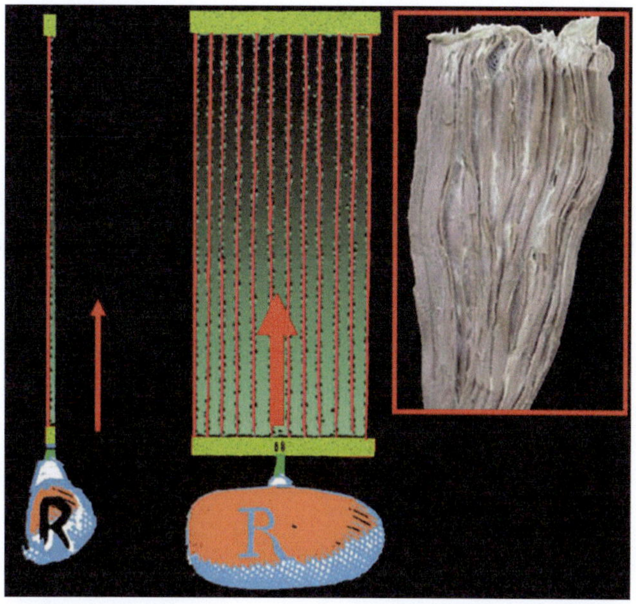

Fig. 46 Relationship between the number of muscle fibers and the overall muscle yield

surface of muscular cross-section" that is, say a theoretical sectional area if all the fascicles were placed in the longitudinal axis of the muscle (all the fascicles are found in the cut section), it is a reflection of the number of sarcomeres in parallel.

The PCSA described empirically by Fick [13], Haxton [49], computed mathematically, is maintained by the muscular volume divided by the average length of the muscle or the length of the fascicles with or without consideration of the pennation [1, 2] and is defined by the total area of the fascicles which induces the power and the number of sarcomeres leading to displacement. When the training is accompanied by a muscular hypertrophy, the maximum force developed, relative to the surface unit of the muscular section, remains minimally modified. A hypertrophied muscle due to muscle training is capable, for the same resistance, to distribute it to a larger surface, which leads to the force developed per unit area decreasing, conversely, for the same force developed per unit area, the total force developed by the whole muscle is greater.

The evaluation of the PCSA is based on data of the muscle–aponeurosis complex

$$\left\{ \begin{aligned} &\mathrm{PCSA}\left(\mathrm{m}^2\right) = \text{Muscle mass}\left(\mathrm{g}\right)\text{cosine}\,\theta\,/ \\ &\qquad\qquad p\left(\text{density}: \mathrm{g}/\mathrm{cm}^3\right)\text{fascicle length}\left(\mathrm{mm}\right) \end{aligned} \right\}.$$

The introduction in the Theta cosine measurement results from the fact that the loss of force with respect to a muscle or the angle of pennation is zero. This equation is based on a constant pennation angle while it is found that this angle varies with a rotation of 1–15°. This twisting arrangement of the fascicles has the effect of increasing the power of the muscle.

The maximum force F (kg/cm^2) is calculated from the formula: maximum tension (kg) mass (g)/density (1056 g/cm^3) length of fascicle (cm). Specific features of the PCSA have been proposed by Alexander [31].

A muscle with parallel fascicles (pseudo-fusiform) is shortened by the same amplitude as the shortening of its fascicles, the force potential produced by the muscle is calculated by the formula {PCSA (m^2) = MV/FL = m/pL (*MV* muscle volume, *FL* length of fascicles, p muscle density (1.05 gm/cm^3), L (muscle length)}.

For a pennate muscle, the direction of the fascicles moves away (increasing the angle of pennation) from the longitudinal axis of muscle during shortening while muscle thickness remains relatively constant. The result is a greater variation in muscular length compared with fascicles. The angle of pennation (for a given muscle) increases as the fascicle length decreases. For a pennate muscle, because of the obliquity of the fascicles, the theoretical sectional area is the reflection of the section of the muscle if all the fascicles were arranged in the longitudinal axis [44]. The surface (S) of the dissection of the muscle derives its physiological importance from the fact that the theoretical maximum force (FM) developed by the fasciculi (lf) is directly proportional to it (FM = lf × S) whose peak of maximum force developed is 25 or 35 N/cm^2.

The force transmitted to the tendon, (FT), depends on the angle α and involves the cosine of the angle "theta" of pennation which normalizes the angulation of the fascicles in the axis of work of the muscle.

$$\{\text{PCSA cm}^2 = m/2\,p\,l\cos\theta\,(m\text{ mass}, p\text{ density}\left(1.05\text{ g}/\text{cm}^3\right),$$
$$l\left(\text{fascicles length}\right),$$
$$\cos\left(\text{cosine of the pennation angle}\right),$$
$$a\left(\text{penetration angle}\right)\}$$

A pennate muscle has the capacity to generate a force transmitted by the tendon particularly when the pennation angle is high. This factor has a relative importance only for higher angles at 20° (the muscles of the forearm or the hand, muscular strength is not very different, in contrast to the triceps surae). As part of these measurements, the aponeurosis was not taken into consideration. In 1990, Zajac [1] led to a physiological interpretation and an understandable mechanical synthesis with modeling of the internal structures of the fascicle by introducing pennation angles and aponeurosis (Figs. 47 and 48).

The speed and amplitude of shortening measured at the end of the fascia or at the end of fascicles are related by a cos α (the less pennate the muscle, the quicker the speed and amplitude shortening for each of the muscular and aponeurotic structures). If all the fascicles of the same muscle had the same length, the speed of shortening of the whole muscle would be proportional to the length of its fascicles. The force/length relationship expresses the dependence of maximal isometric force production by the contractile component and of passive tension by the elastic component parallel to the length of the muscle. The relationship forces describe the dynamic behavior of the contractile component under constant load and velocity. The tension-extension relationship characterizes the elastic component in terms of stiffness and

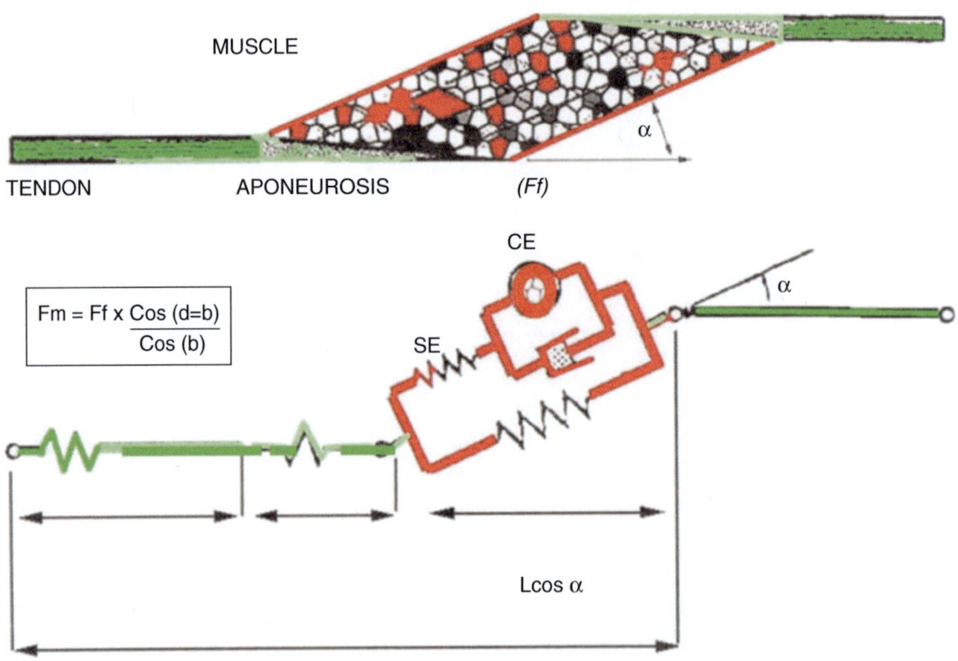

Fig. 47 Representation (Zajac [1]) of the mode of operation of the muscle–aponeurosis–tendon complex for the calculation of the force of a muscle

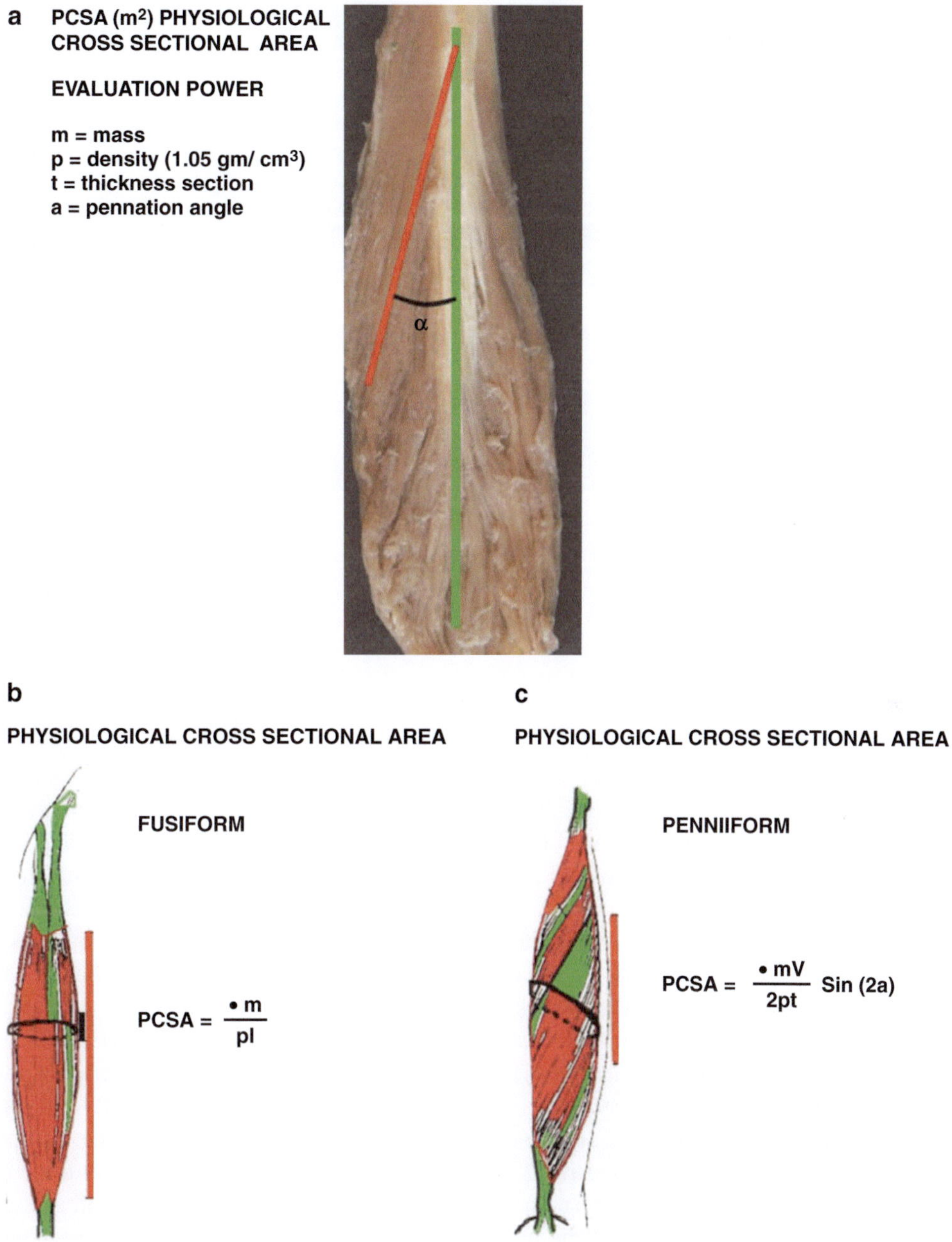

Fig. 48 (**a**) Data to measure the Physiological Cross Sectional Area (PCSA). (**b**) Principle of measurement of the Physiological Cross Sectional Area of a fusiform muscle. (**c**) Principle of measurement of the Physiological Cross Sectional Area of a penniform muscle

potential energy. All these notions bear witness to the extreme complexity of the muscle–aponeurosis–tendon complex.

Global Mechanical Properties of the Muscle–Aponeurosis–Tendon Complex

Muscle Functions and Composite Beam (Fig. 49)

A bone segment, isolated from its environment, subjected to a stress, may reach its fracture level very quickly whereas during the exercises of everyday life, this eventuality does not occur. The arrangement and insertion of the muscles are based on the principle of the composite beam with an anti-buckling stabilizing effect. The stresses developed at the bone are the result of bending actions. In reality, the moments of action generated by the bone because of its curvature exceed the loads which are exerted transversely at the ends. The muscles are provided by their mode of fixation at the level of the curvature to decrease the mechanical constraints of bending. Thanks to this arrangement, the muscular force will neutralize bone deformation. By its presence with its multiple bone insertions while increasing the moment of inertia of the whole bone-muscle, it increases in considerable proportions the mechanical strength of the bone. A concave curvature allows a larger muscle insertion area with an antigravity function. Jansen [50] enacts the "minimum-maximum" law which stipulates that the maximum

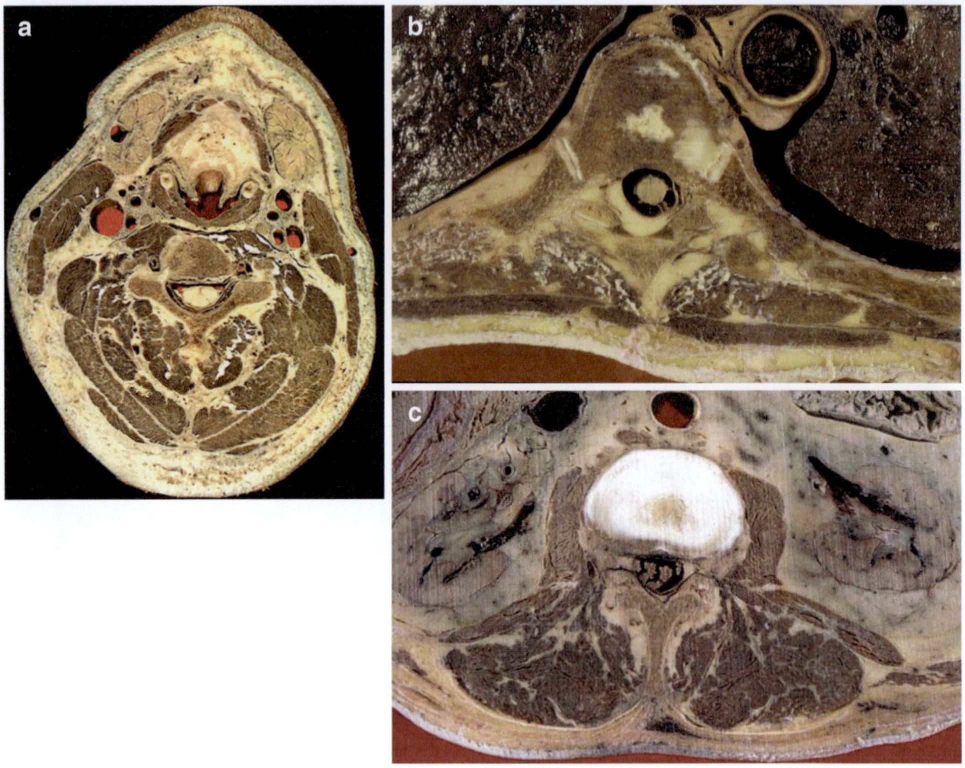

Fig. 49 Anatomical sections at three levels (cervical (**a**), thoracic (**b**), lumbar (**c**)) to determine the importance of the composite beam in relation to the curvature. At the thoracic level, the ribs with the sternum stabilize this portion and require reduced muscle mass. Note whitish fibers, evidence of aponeurotic tissue absorbing the mechanical stresses at the top of the thoracic curvature

mechanical resistance is achieved with the minimum cancellous bone material which has a well-defined architectural trajectory and compensates for the bone material. Adaptation processes are under the control of a feedback mechanism that is closely related to mechanical constraints. Throughout life, osteoblastic and osteoclastic action manifests itself in multiple circumstances such as the consolidation of fractures or the bone response to muscle insertions. Frost [51] defined the concept of the "minimum effective strain" whose values were between 0.08 and 0.2% of strain.

Above, the bone was adapting and the signs of remodeling appeared. Enlow [38] demonstrated that osteogenesis was induced by compressive forces and osteolysis by extensional stresses. This adaptation of the bone to mechanical stresses was possible thanks to its elastic and visco-elastic mechanical properties. "Negative feedback" is the essential process of regulating bone remodeling. The application of a force causes deformities that induce the remodeling process; a high stress causes osteoblast hypertrophy. This hypertrophy is followed by a decrease in deformities and osteoclasts, which leads to bone atrophy with rapid osteolysis and major calcium excretion.

Purpose, Symmetry, Variability

Of all the organic systems, the muscular system is the most important in terms of mass and volume; no system of organs presents greater differences from individual to individual, and even within the same individual. Anatomical symmetry derives functional symmetry. In the series of even muscles, each of them has an action identical to that of its counterpart and if it is the odd muscles, the two halves that constitute them contract together to contribute to a single effect. The scalene muscles are an example of symmetry of the tethers of the cervical spine (Fig. 50).

The study of various movements shows, between most homologous muscle regions, a complete dependence: the independency is the exception. The glottis, pharyngeal, labial muscles are all those on the right and left, associated together in a common action. What solidarity is closer than that which exists between the muscles of the two eyes? The right and left muscles of language combine their function in the complex act of phonation? This harmony of action between the symmetrical organs is less perfect. When it comes to limbs, the isolated movement of a left arm and right leg is not associated with the opposite side to achieve a parallel movement.

Why are the muscles on the right side more developed than those on the left? Is there a congenital difference in relation to the frequency of the left occipito-cotyloid position of the fetus? Would the number of left-handers be proportional to the number of children born by right occipito-cotyloid position, as has been suggested, or would this predominance on the right be the pure and simple effect of where we are to practice a lot more often the right side than the left? [25]. In

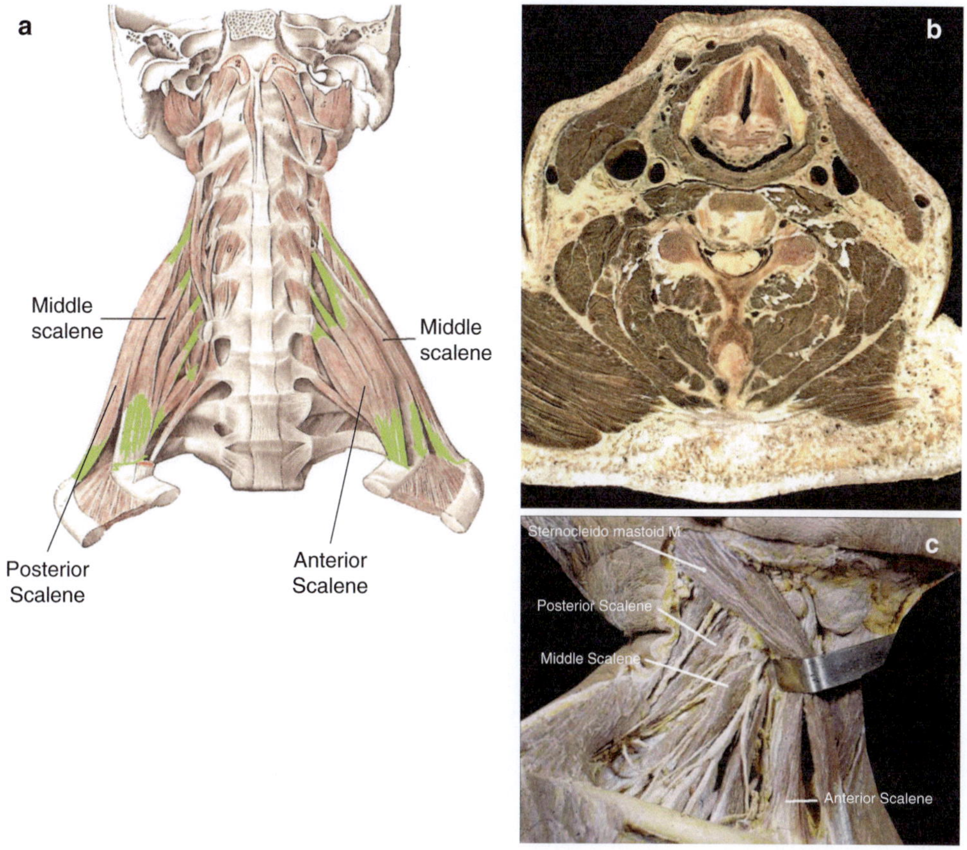

Fig. 50 Scalene muscles of stabilization of the overall vertebral column (**a**), horizontal anatomical section with their symmetrical insertions on the transverse processes of the cervical vertebra (**b**). Topographic reports of the 3 muscles during a dissection (**c**)

humans, the predominant muscles of the lower limbs and paravertebral gutters predesignate it to the bipedal attitude.

Volume and Strength of Muscles

Considered in relation to their volume and their own form, they have many varieties. The volume of a muscle is in direct relation to its strength, but it is not the only condition of force.

Two elements are to be considered: the force as measured by the volume (number of fascicles), and the energy of its contraction, which results from the cerebral influx. Muscular hypertrophy may result from hypertrophy of the fascicles or an increase in their number as a result of resistance training. In humans, the increase in muscle volume is quite slow with an average of 0.1% per day, with extreme values of 0.07–0.23% per day, to reach a maximum increase, on average of the order of 10–25% after 8–12 weeks. The increase of the muscular section results from the increase as represented by the fast fibers, whereas the slow fibers remain minimally modified. With the help of the temporal summation of nerve stimulation and the increasing recruitment of motor units (spatial summation), the force developed by a muscle can vary in important ranges. The highest values can be evaluated between 400 and 1000 kg for triceps sural or the gluteus maximus. An approximate calculation leads to a maximum value of 25 ton if all the muscles were active at the same time with maximum force! This phenomenon is based on an asynchronous activation of the fibers according to their capacity. A large high-threshold motor neuron that holds a large number of muscle fibers under its control is put into play after a small inverse-mode motor. The electromyogram is a reflection, during a muscular contraction with increasing load, of the activation of more and more numerous, efficient and asynchronous motor units [52].

Law of Third Dimensional Articular Dynamic Rotational Centering

The analytical study of the action of a muscle alone cannot solve the mechanical behavior of a joint. The harmonious movement of a joint requires the synchronous activation of all the muscular groups that surround it. The objective of this dynamic equilibrium ensures the distribution of stresses on the cartilage avoiding its wear (Euler column). This organization responds to the three-dimensional dynamic articular rotational centering law which is part of a principle of functional globality and takes into account other articulations [53]. In relation to the three planes of space, there is a movement of flexion extension, a movement of abduction adduction, and a movement of rotation. This terminology is specific to anatomy and does not correspond to that used in mechanics which uses only the term rotation. The extension component is always weaker than flexion and requires only one muscle. In certain positions of the articulation, gravity is sufficient to cause the extension movement.

Muscular Ambivalence: Articular Chains and Stato-Dynamic Effects of Muscles

In the context of an isotonic contraction, two situations are distinguished insofar as one of its extremities is kept fixed and the other connected to a load offering a resistance *R*: concentric contraction, i.e., its length decreases and its ends come closer to the extent that the developed tension is greater than *R*, or eccentric contraction where its length increases and its extremities move away to the extent that the tension is less than *R*. If the developed tension increases during the shortening, the first part of a muscular contraction can be performed in isotonic mode, then in isometric mode. Thus at the level of the masticatory muscles where they are shortened at first, then contract isometrically to overcome the resistance offered by food fragments. For the extension muscles, they function during contraction initially in isometric mode, then in a second one in isotonic mode.

The static effect (isometric force) of a muscle is defined as the state of equilibrium between power and resistance. The moment of resistance is proportional to the length of the lever arm and the angle between the two levers. For a 90° angle with a long lever arm, the articular stress is maximum. To reduce this constraint, it is necessary to shorten the point of application of the resistance and to make the angle and the levers tend towards 0°. The dynamic effect (isokinetic force) is the situation in which its power is greater than resistance and induces motion. The speed and amplitude of the displacement are greater when one of the insertions is close to the joint space. For this purpose, produced by a muscle, the indirect action must be added by modifying the position as a function of the center of gravity. In the pelvic limb, the flexion of the thigh on the pelvis is accompanied by a flexion on the leg by the action of gravity.

The mechanical stresses on the articulations are different according to the overall position of the body and the methods of application of the resistance. Three articular situations can be envisaged with the open articular chain, the closed articular chain and the semi-closed articular chain. The open articular chain is the succession of several joints whose distal is free, continuity between the chest, the shoulder girdles, the arm, the forearm and the free hand with isolated mobilization of a joint. The closed articular chain is characterized by a succession of articulations interposed between two extreme extremities: athlete in a horizontal position with support of the hands and feet performing a series of dynamic exercises, elevation, lowering. The semi-closed articular chain is the situation where one of the two fixed extremities is subjected to a determined vectorial resistance: cyclist with his lower limb whose foot is embedded in the pedal.

Muscle Force and Levers

The organization of the musculoskeletal system is based on the principle of the levers which are composed of 3 elements: a fulcrum, a power, and a resistance. The fixed point of support is the articulation, power is materialized by the muscle, and resistance is opposed to force. To improve the muscular quality with respect to a load, it is necessary to improve the speed of execution (*V*), which is a function of the ratio of the power of shortening (*P*) to the mass to be displaced and the resistances to be overcome (*M*): $V = \text{PM}$. To decrease the resistance (*M*), it is important to promote the flexibility of the articulation. There is a compromise between tone and suppleness, which requires a varied and alternating pace of training. Muscles that are intended for large displacement due to the length of fibers will not have the same performance if the moment of action is high. Similarly, if a muscle with a large Cross Sectional Area (CSA) is placed with a weak moment of action, it will produce only a large angular displacement and not a large force.

Compliance

Compliance is defined as the ability of a muscle to change shape (elongate or contract) for a given force while returning to the initial state when the deforming force is removed. This compliance is a reflection of the elastic energy that can be stored by the different elastic structures of the three-level complex: fascicles-aponeurosis-tendons. Scott [54] found a similarity in the mechanical properties of aponeuroses and tendons where the elasticity of these two components could reach 8% for the fascia and 2% for the tendon. The angular compliance is the consequence of the angle formed by fascicles with aponeurosis, the latter not being in the axis of work of the muscle. This angle forces a transformation of the length-changing forces of fascicles which are no longer in the axis of global muscle deformation. From this change of direction follows the appearance of a component perpendicular to the muscular action line which explains the loss of force necessary for this transformation. As a result, increasing the pennation angle increases the perpendicular component, decreases the effective muscular force transmitted but increases system compliance.

When increasing the pennation, one reduces its rigidity, the rule of the interdependence of the muscular work between the muscular complex and its elements appear perfectly realized if the elastic work is carried out perpendicular to the fascia and takes it into consideration. In order to keep the muscle volume constant when the fascia is stretched elastically, elastic deformation must occur on the surface of the fasciae. When the elastic energy is stored in the fascia at the same time, the energy will be stored in the surface of this fascial structure; its quantity is small but essential to obtain a good equilibrium during the work.

New Compliance Concepts: Muscular Fascicles and Fascia (aponeurosis)

The models that have so far been studied do not differentiate between the tendon structures and the aponeurotic features of a muscle. Jewel [55] reported that 50% of the change in the length of the elastic series (muscle-fascia-tendon) of the shortening of a frog muscle during isometric contraction reside in the collagen fibers. Morgan [56] found that eight times more movements were observed in the tendinous structures than in the aponeuroses (aponeurosis) of the kangaroo muscles. These results seemed to indicate that there are differences in elastic characteristics between different species and muscles. For a unipennate muscle, a wide angle of pennation results in another angular compliance. The behavior of the fascia does not only depend on the strength, but also depends on its length. It has been shown that the difference in length between the aponeurosis during the contraction of a short muscle subjected to a weak force and that of a muscle subjected to a great force exceeds the extension of the calculated elastic series. according to the compliance. It can be concluded that the length of the muscle determines the equilibrium length of the fascia (aponeurosis) which changes in the same way.

This mechanism shows that there is a plastic deformation induced by the forces developed during the movement. During the passive movement of a muscle, the fascia (aponeurosis) elongates easily and adapts at the same time as all fibrous structures. However, during muscle contraction, significant forces perpendicular to the fascia (aponeurosis) occur and this results in internal frictional forces between different structures that prevent excessive stretching. Fascicles opposing the extension of fibrous structures are still active in the aponeurosis even when large forces are exerted, this mechanism is not possible in experimental studies where the tendons are separated from one another and the muscles are not in contact. This hypothesis of plastic deformation of the aponeurosis induced by the loss of force was in contradiction with the plastic deformation proposed by Alexander [44] which determined that a certain level of force was necessary to cause deformation. It is essential to note that changes in the compliance of a muscular system due to the geometry of the muscle do not influence the amount of elastic energy stored in the series of the elastic element. In posture, three systems intervene: head-neck, thoracolumbar, and the global body—talo-crural joint (ankle).

Gregory [57] showed that rectus femoris and the gastrocnemius were energy transporting elements from the proximal to the distal lower limb. Functionally, it is found that during extension of the knee there is an associated plantar flexion—a strong power that is transmitted from the rectus femoris to gastrocnemius. These two muscles have important similarities in their anatomical morphology, the posterior surface of the rectus femoris is essentially aponeurotic, spreading over its entire length and for the gastrocnemius the presence of both superficial and intramuscular aponeurosis extends from proximal insertion to distal insertion. These muscles should be considered as antigravity muscles with a great energy saving and a return of energy in the phases of the walk which reverberate in the thigh and the pelvis with adaptation of the vertebral column. Stiffness is lower (higher compliance) in the cervical spine for all modes of inclination with the C1–C2 junction responsible for rotation and the distribution of flexion from C3 to C7. The thoracic column is compliant in rotation and the lumbar spine has a great potential of flexion and less in lateral flexion and in extension.

Fasciae

Fasciae are an important component of the musculoskeletal system and cannot be dissociated from the study of muscle. Long studied independently of each other and only in some of their main parts, they were, for the first time, considered in a general way by Bichat [58], who united them in its division of the membranous fibrous system. The fascia is an extended sheet of strong connective tissue that surrounds the whole muscle and gives it an anatomical unity. It has 2 other mechanical functions by realizing a counter-pressure factor towards the muscle during the contraction and by promoting their independence and their sliding.

The fasciatherapy that has developed describes a painful myofascial syndrome that is a reversible functional disturbance that originates in skeletal muscles or fasciae. It is highlighted as a Myofascial Trigger Point (point-relaxation) which is a painful area of a few mm, located in its fascia. These fasciae are intimately related to the skin, which presents a specific mechanical organization with traction zones described by Langer which are at the origin of the choice of cutaneous incisions.

Terminology: Fascia of Contention

Bichat [58] "had divided the aponeuroses (aponeurosis) into two classes: some (wrongly) serve as insertion to the true muscular aponeuroses (aponeurosis) and are only tendons: they are the aponeuroses (aponeurosis) of insertion, the others are used to these same muscles of means of contention: it is the fasciae (fascia) of envelope or contention." Thus, the muscles are situated between two fibrous laminae, one deep, the other superficial, which is the enveloping fascia; Multiple and varied partitions go from one to the other and divide them into a multitude of compartments designed to isolate, contain, protect the different muscles and promote their sliding and action. Bichat's analysis [9] was close to the modern concept of Ettema and Huijing [2], Winters [59] which determined the dominant role of fascia and fascicles.

The fasciae of contention sometimes envelop the totality of the limbs: they are generic; at once they are only one muscle or more: they are partial and meet not only in the limbs where they play an essential role, but also in the trunk (Fig. 51).

General rule: wherever there is a muscle that can move in its contraction, there is a aponeurosis, or sheath whose thickness is proportional to the length of the muscle, its strength, and especially its tendency to move. Each fascia is considered an outer surface, an inner surface, an edge, or circumference. By their pearly white outer surface, the superficial envelope fasciae respond to the skin, from which they are separated by the subclinical cellular tissue, enclosing the veins, the lymphatic vessels, and the superficial nerves.

The inner surface of the fascia is dull white. Through this surface, some give attachment to certain points in the fascicles: this is that of the forearm and the leg. But over most of its extent, this surface remains independent of the underlying muscles, to which it adheres only by a loose connective tissue. It follows that the skin is mobile on these fasciae; sometimes they adhere intimately by means of fibrous prolongations born from the deep aspect of the dermis.

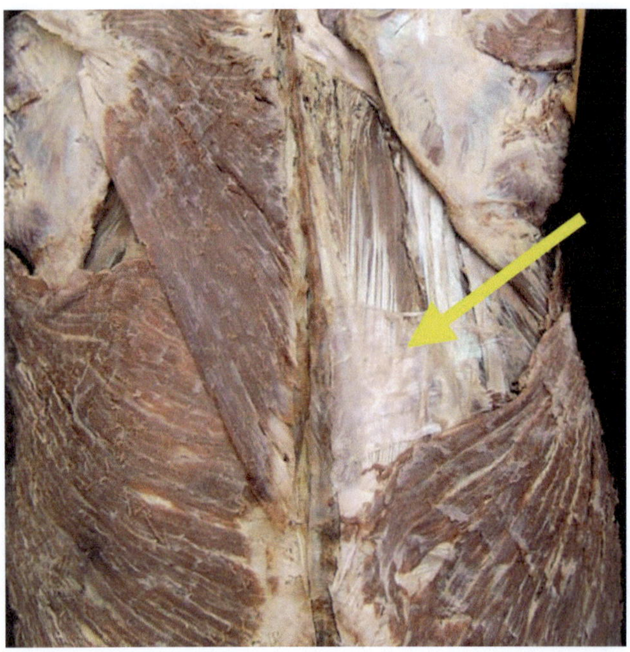

Fig. 51 Morphological aspect of a fascia in the thoracolumbar region, note the transverse direction of its fibers (yellow arrow)

Structure of the Fascia

The mobility of the skin on the fasciae takes place by the following mechanism: from the deep surface of the dermis, multiple fibrous prolongations leave, intercepting the areoles which are the reservoir of the adipose tissue; these united prolongations develop into a membrane which glides over the fascia, vessels, and superficial nerves, and is called fascia superficialis. It is only found in parts where superficial vessels and nerves are distributed between the skin and the fasciae.

The thin fasciae are composed of a single plane of parallel fibers, leaving between them considerable intervals; the thick fasciae are composed of several superimposed planes whose fibers intersect sometimes at right angles and sometimes at acute angles. It is rare that, in intertwined fasciae, the anatomical reason of the difference of direction of the fibers in that of the muscular fibers is not found. Sappey [21] has highlighted considerable evidence of neural tissue. Fascia of compression, which must be adapted to the changes of form which accompany the muscular contraction, contains a quantity of elastic fibers which perpendicularly traverse those of the muscle. Fascia of large muscles especially at trunk and neck levels differs from long muscles. They are thinner, less resistant, dull white and not pearly white. The specific arrangement of fasciae of the muscles of the column is related to long dorsal and ilio-costal delineating gutters. It is, however, difficult to make the precise distinction by dissection between the aponeuroses and the fasciae (Figs. 52 and 53).

Properties of Fascia

As an integral part of fibrous tissue, fascia shares physical, chemical, anatomical, physiological, and pathological properties. Because of their great cohesive strength, the fasciae resist the considerable traction or distensions exerted on them by the muscular fibers. They establish, among the different layers of organs, very precise limits which are of the highest importance to "know exactly if one wants to make an accurate account of a host of morbid phenomena"... Cruveilhier [25].

They are not very extensible, hence the resistance they oppose to the inflammation of the underlying parts (for example, compartment syndrome). They are not very elastic; when their distention has exceeded a certain extent, they never revert on themselves.

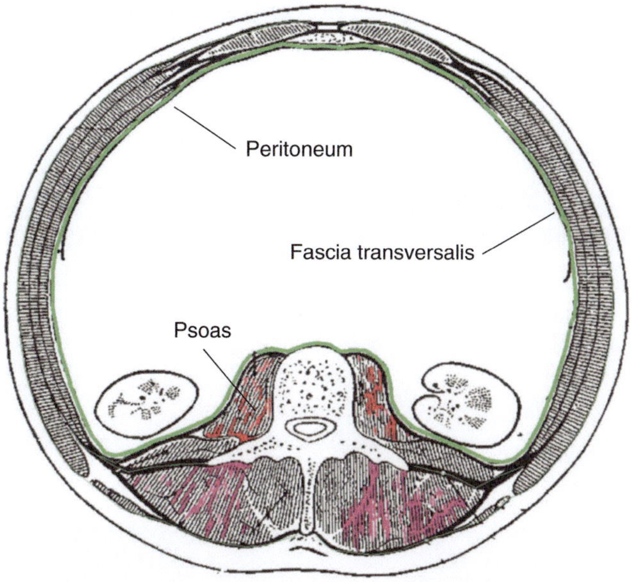

Fig. 52 Schematic horizontal section at the lumbar level delimiting spaces through the fasciae (green)

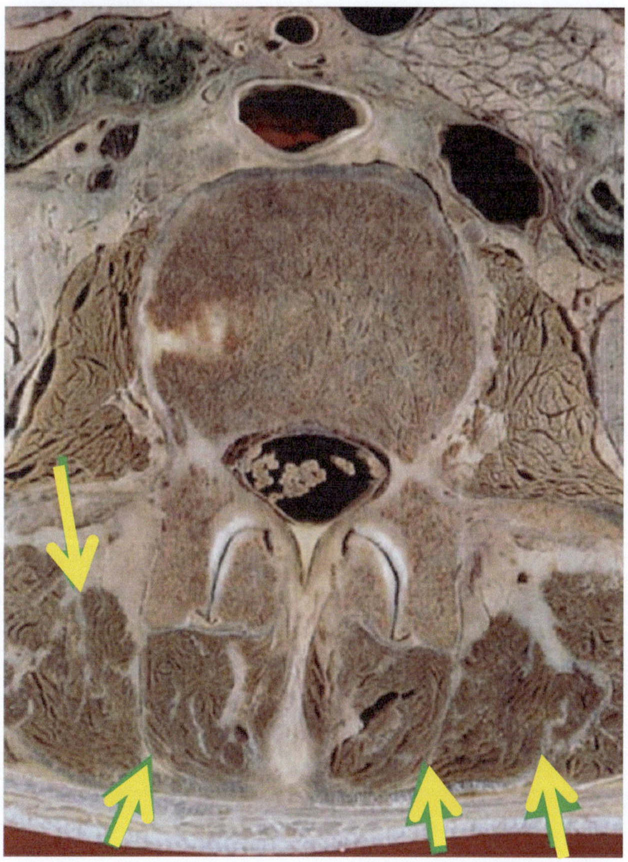

Fig. 53 Horizontal section of lumbar spine muscles with bony gutter boundaries specific to each muscle

This layer of dense connective tissue which covers the muscles delimits compartments or compartments by the septae, which provide a rigid compression of the muscle during their contraction. Among the other functions, they allow a sliding between the muscles making them functionally independent. The space induced between them is a factor of cooling and electrical insulation. The spaces are occupied by vascular arterial, venous, and lymphatic elements.

Clinical Implications

Epidemiological studies confirm the societal impact of low back pain, which is observed in 60% of an industrialized population. Every year, 5% of adults in the USA have a low back pain episode. Of five million patients with low back pain, two million are at out of work for a minimum of 6 months and only 20–40% return to work, Kelsey [60]. The concept of postural stability is at the root of the exploration and therapy of the vertebral column. The stability of overall body mass is proportional to the support represented by the feet, at a distance in the horizontal plane between the center of gravity and the edges of the support, inversely proportional to the height of the center of gravity but proportional to the weight from the body. Walking is a succession of unstable periods that are at the base of propulsion. To maintain stability, there must be dynamic modulation of the upper and lower limbs relative to the fulcrums. This system has to deal with variations in order to restore balance. To fulfill this contract, the neuromuscular system must behave in an elastic system with a certain amount of energy and restitution of the aponeurosis.

The zones of stiffness and their evaluation at different levels listed by Ashton-Miller [61] are six with compression, anteroposterior shear, lateral shear, flexion-extension inclination, lateral inclination, and torsion.

For Crisco [62], the polyarticular muscles are advantageous in terms of stability. These superficial muscles have high bending moments and are especially suitable for modulating stiffness. On the cervical level, the small suboccipital muscles are essential for maintaining the head (Fig. 54).

Muscle and Infiltration Fat: Aging

In the elderly, the adipose system reappears and the muscles become less bulky. The reliefs weaken; the forms tend to resemble their primitive roundness without being comparable to those of the young man. In the latter, they are rounded, but slender and firm; after middle age, they are sometimes rounded and firm, but thicker, which occurs if the adipose tissue predominates; sometimes rounded and slender, but softer, as a result of slimming or aging. They participate in the general atrophy manifested by the most sensitive effects. After their withdrawal, they no longer fill the boxes between the fasciae that surround them, with a

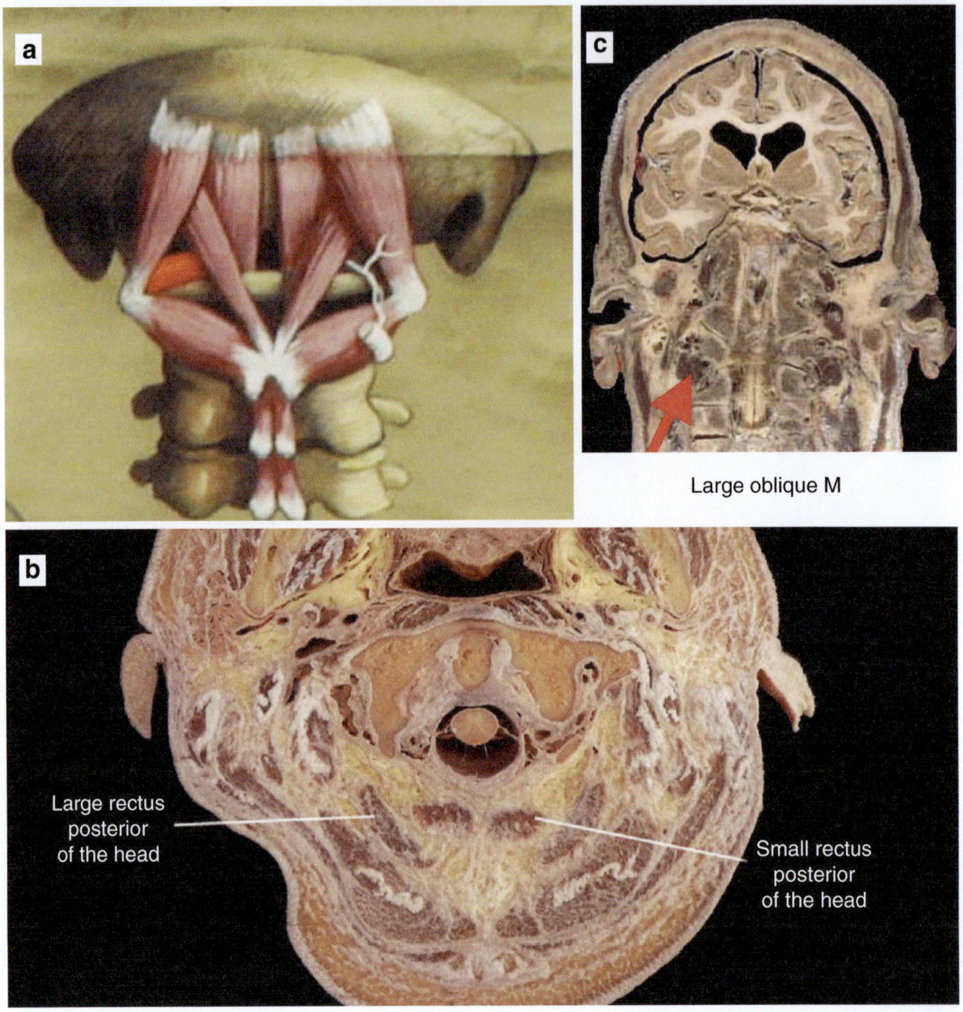

Fig. 54 Muscles of the cranio-cephalic junction with the four muscles (Rectus posterior of the head- large and small, large oblique of the head, small oblique of the head) which constitute the triangle of Tillaux (**a**). These muscles adjust the movements of the head and act as limits in large rotational movements. Anatomical cuts (**b**) horizontal plane (**c**) frontal section with large oblique

kind of flaccidity to which is added their greater softness. In extreme old age, the adipose tissue infiltrates in greater abundance between the various bundles of the muscular tissue, which very often takes a yellowish hue. Often, lobules of fat appear in the primitive bundles, and sometimes even fat cells (Fig. 55).

Conclusion

The normal operation of the vertebral column is still poorly known despite over 2 million references found in the literature. The difficulties lie in the actual evaluation of the structures and the current technical means available. The morphological bases since the work of Winkler [3] are an important achievement. The new concept associating the contractile and elastic components of Zajac [1] of the muscle (aponeurosis) complex is at the basis of modeling programmes in the dissection of pathology. Three-dimensional explorations should improve our knowledge provided that the column is integrated into a functional set with individual variability. Following advances in its understanding and applications in biology, the tensegrity model will represent one of the most relevant concepts for understanding the musculoskeletal system with two structure-function pairs associating "tension-cohesion" and "compression solidity."

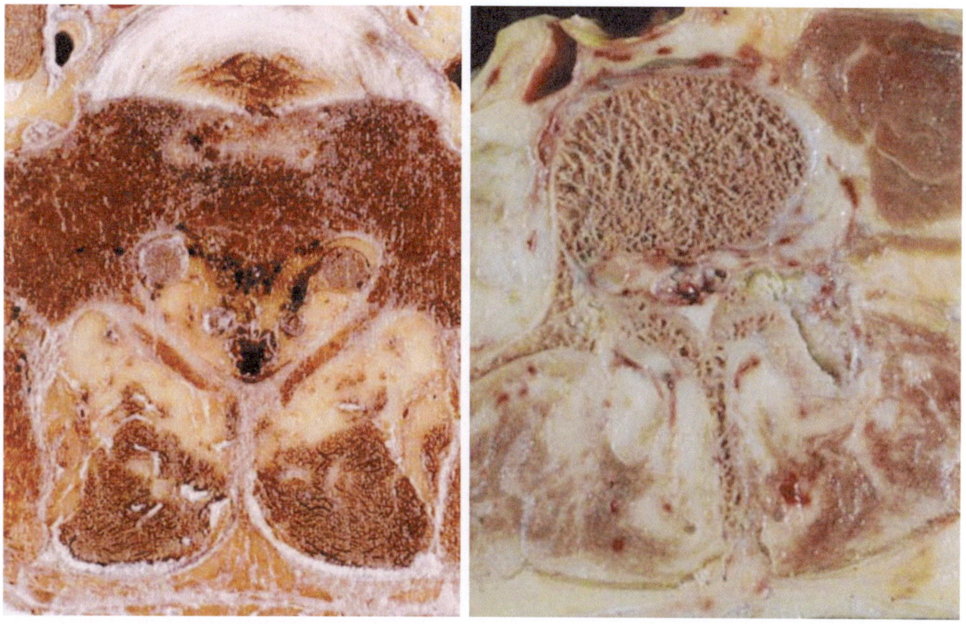

Fig. 55 Horizontal section of the lumbar portion of the column highlighting fatty infiltration of the muscles of the gutters at advanced stages

References

1. Zajac F, Winters J. Modelling musculoskeletal movement systems: joint and body segmental dynamics, musculoskeletal actuation, and neuromuscular control. In: Winters JM, Woo SLY, editors. Multiple muscle systems, biomechanics and movement organization. New York: Springer; 1990. p. 121–34.
2. Ettema GJC, Huijing PA. Properties of the tendinous structures and the elastic component of EDL muscle-tendon complex of the rat. J Biomech. 1989;22:1209–15.
3. Winkler G. The ilio-costal muscle. Study of its structure and its morphology according to the curvatures of the rachis. Arch Anat Histol Embryol. 1936;21:143–252.
4. Gracovetsky S. Musculoskeletal function of the spine. In: Winters JM, editor. Multiple muscle systems, vol. 25. New York: Springer; 1990. p. 411–37.
5. Delp SL, Anderson F, Arnold AS, et al. OpenSim: open source software to create and analyze dynamic simulation of movement. IEEE Trans Biomed Eng. 1990;37(8):757–67.
6. Chrystophy M, Wiemann K, Klee A. Die Bedeutung von dehnen und stretching in der aufwärmphase vor Hochsstleistungen. Leistungssport. 2000;4:5–9.
7. Dionis A. Demonstrations of anatomy. Paris: House of Saint Come; 1690.
8. Heister A. The anatomy of Heister with physical tests on the use of parts of the human body. In Paris at Vincent, 5 rue S. Severin at the Angel 1753; with approval and privilege of the King.
9. Spigelius A. De humani corporis fabrica. Brussels; 1578.
10. Stenonis N. From ossibus musculis, from motu animalium. Pars prima, Bibliotheca anatomica. Geneva: Joannis Anthonii Chovet; 1685. p. 527–52.
11. Borelli J. From motu animalium. From externis animal. Pars prima, Bibliotheca anatomica, Geneva: Joannis Anthonii Chovet; 1685. p. 817–910.
12. Trolard P. The spinal muscles and in particular the transverse spiny muscles. Algiers, Casabianca printing, rue du commerce; 1892.
13. Fick R. Handbuch der Anatomy und Mechanik der Gelenke unter Berucksichtigung der bewegenden Muskein. 1904–1911. Vol. 3. Specielle gelenk und muskelein Mechanik. Jena: Gustav Fischer; 1911.
14. Von Lanz T, Wachsmuth W. Praktische anatomy. Erxter Kand, Driter Teil: Arm. Berlin: Springer; 1935. p. 154–243.
15. Bonnel F. Muscles and joints (law of three-dimensional articular dynamic centering). In: Muscle and sport: Springer; 1992. p. 277–98.
16. Alonso S. Regulatory factors specific to myogenesis. Med Sci. 1990;6:635–44.
17. Bergmark A. Stability of the lumbar spine. A study in mechanical engineering. Acta Orthop Scand. 1989;230:581–10.
18. Nitz AJ, Pick D. Comparison of muscle spindle concentrations in large and small human epaxial muscle acting in parallel combinations. Am Surg. 1986;52:273–7.
19. Chaussier quoted by Sappey Ph. Descriptive anatomy. Paris: Delahaye & Cie; 1876. p. 52.
20. Theile P. Cited by Sappey Ph. Descriptive anatomy. Paris: Delahaye & Cie; 1876. p. 52.
21. Sappey PH. Descriptive anatomy treaty. Paris: Delahaye & Cie; 1876.
22. Sylvius A. Quoted by Sappey Ph. Descriptive anatomy. Paris: Delahaye & Cie; 1876. p. 52.
23. Galien (Galen). Anatomical, physiological, scientific, medical works, translated by Ch. Daremt, editors. Paris: Baillière; 1854.
24. Vésale A. De Humani corporis fabrica libri septem. Basileae: Joannis Oporinus; 1543.
25. Cruveilhier J. Anatomy treaty. 1st ed. Paris: Bechet Jeune; 1837.
26. Squire JM. The structural basis of muscular contraction. New York, NY: Plenum; 1981.
27. Lieber RL. Muscle fiber length and moment arm coordination during dorsi and plantar flexion in the mouse hindlimb. Acta Anat. 1997;159:84–9.
28. Huijing PA, Ettema JC. Inflammatory muscle contractions of the rat and the muscles of the gastrocnemius muscle. Acta Morphol Neerl Scand. 1989;26:51–62.
29. Friden J, Lieber RL. Eccentric exercise-induced injuries to contractile and cytoskeletal muscle fiber components. Acta Physiol Scand. 2001;171(3):321–6.
30. Huxley H. The mechanism of muscular contraction. Science. 1969;164:1356.
31. Alexander RM, Vernon A. The dimensions of knee and ankle muscles and the forces they exert. J Hum Mov Stud. 1975;1:115–23.

32. Bogduck N, Macintosh JE, Pearcy MJ. A universal model of the lumbar back in the upright position. Spine. 1992;17(8):897–913.
33. Boyer Cited by Chaussier Summary exposure of the muscles of the human body. Thesis n ° 507. Dijon; 1789.
34. Gauthier G, Padykulah A. Cytological studies of fiber types in skeletal muscle: a comparative study of mammalian diaphragm. J Cell Biol. 1966;28:333.
35. Jewel BR, Wilkie DR. The mechanical properties of relaxing muscle. J Physiol. 1960;152:30–47.
36. Cruveilhier J. Anatomy treaty. 3rd ed. Paris: Bechet Young; 1847.
37. Hill AV. First and last experiments in muscle mechanics. Cambridge: Cambridge University Press; 1970.
38. Enlow DH. Wolff's law and the factor of architectonic circumstance. Am J Orthod. 1968;54:803–22.
39. Philips S, Bogduk RV. Anatomy and biomechanics of lumborum quadrates. Proc Inst Mech Eng H. 2000;222(2):151–9.
40. Yamagushi GT, Sawa AGU, Moran DW, Fessler MJ, Winters JM. A survey of human musculotendon actuator parameters. In: Winters JM, Woo SLY, editors. Multiple muscle systems, biomechanics and movement organization. New York: Springer; 1990. p. 717–25.
41. Fukunaga T, Ichinose Y, Ito M, Kawakami Y, Fukashiro S. Determination of fascicle length and pennation in a contracting human muscle in vivo. J Appl Physiol. 1997;82(1):354–8.
42. Bogduk N, Johnson G, Spalding D. The morphology and biomechanics of latissimus dorsi. Clin Biomech. 1998;13(6):377–85.
43. Rouvière H. Architecture of striated muscles. Law of direction of fleshy fibers and tendinous fibers. Ann Anat Pathol. 1936;9:1–5.
44. Blix M. Die Lange und die Spannung of the Muskels. Skand Arch Physiol. 1891;3:295–318.
45. Cheney RA, Melaragno PG, Prayson MJ. Anatomic investigation of the deep posterior compartment of the leg. Foot Ankle Int. 1998;19(2):98–101.
46. Maughan RJ, Watson JS, Weir J. Strength and cross-sectional area of human skeletal muscle. J Physiol. 1983;338:37–49.
47. Wickiewicz TL, Roy RR, Powell PL, Edgerton VR. Muscle architecture of the human lower limb. Clin Orthop Res. 1983;179:275–83.
48. Scott S, Winter D. A comparison of three muscle pennants and their effect on isometric and isotonic force. J Biomech. 1991;24(2):163–7.
49. Haxton HA. Absolute muscle strength in the ankle flexors of man. J Physiol. 1944;103:267–73.
50. Jansen M. On bone formation: its relation to tension and pressure. London: Longmans; 1920.
51. Frost HM. Bone remodelling dynamics. Springfield, IL: C.C. Thomas; 1963.
52. Winters JM, Stark L. Estimated mechanical properties of synergistic muscles involved movements of a variety of human joints. J Biomech. 1988;21:1027–41.
53. Bonnel F, Marc TH. Muscle: new concepts, anatomy-biomechanics-surgery-reeducation. Montpellier: Medical Sauramps; 2009.
54. Scott SH, Engstrom CM, Loeb GE. Morphometry of human thigh muscles. Determination of fascicle architecture by magnetic resonance imaging. J Anat. 1993;182(2):249–57.
55. Jewel BR, Wilkie DR. An analysis of the mechanical components in frog's striated muscle. J Physiol. 1958;143:515–40.
56. Morgan DL, Proske U, Wamen D. Measurements of muscle stiffness and the mechanism of elastic storage of energy in hopping kangaroos. J Physiol. 1978;282:253–61.
57. Gregory L, Veeger HE, Huijing PA, Ingen Schenau GJ, et al. Int J Sports Med. 1984;5:301–5.
58. Bichat X. Treatise on descriptive anatomy. Paris: Gabon & Cie; 1801.
59. Winters JM, Stark L. Analysis of fundamental human movement patterns through the use of in-depth antagonistic muscle models. IEEE Trans Biomed Eng. 1985;32:826–39.
60. Kelsey JL, White AA. Epidemiology and the impact of low back pain. Spine. 1980;5:133–48.
61. Ashton-Miller JA, Schultz AB. Biomechanics of the human spine and trunk. Exerc Sport Sci Rev. 1988;16:169–204.
62. Crisco JJ, Panjabi MM. Postural biomechanical stability and gross muscular architecture in the spine. In: Multiple muscle systems. New York: Springer; 1990. p. 438–50.
63. Seireg A, Arvikar R. Biomechanical analysis of the musculoskeletal structure for medicine and sport. New York: Hemisphere Publishing Corporation; 1989.

Functional Anatomy of the Erector Spinae: Review

M. De Sèze and O. Gille

Introduction

The final decades of the twentieth century have seen a sharp rise in the prevalence of back pain in the western world [1]. From a purely osteoarticular perspective, this may seem paradoxical insofar as, at the same time, working and living conditions seem to have improved [1]. Recent animal and human studies have repeatedly advanced the importance of paraspinal muscle dysfunction in the pathogenesis of low back pain [2–4]. Similarly, the increase in disorders of sagittal balance of the spine, related to idiopathic paravertebral atrophy with increasing age underscores the functional importance of these muscles [5]. These muscles, because of their insertions, are extensors of the spine, that is to say that their concentric contraction tends to induce an extension of the spinal segments with respect to each other. This conception of their action is, not sufficient to account for their protective role of the spine. It also seems a little limited to account for their postural and dynamic actions. Is their action unambiguous? What synergistic action do they have with each other and with other muscles? What mechanisms can induce their dysfunction? What are the postural and dynamic consequences of their dysfunction? Are their lesions irreversible or can we resist the durability of these induced disorders? Technological advances have recently allowed us to conduct work aimed to address all of these issues. They are based on a fine analysis of the trunk movements and the simultaneous recording of the activity of many muscles, as well as on the magnetic resonance (MRI) of contractile components of paravertebral masses.

This is a synthesis of current knowledge based on a literature review. It aims to expose the recent functional anatomy data of the paraspinal muscles and emphasize the clinical implications that may arise.

In the first part, we will study the topographic and functional organization of the paravertebral muscles, including a recall of the descriptive anatomy of the paravertebral muscles and the different functional anatomy models that have been proposed to explain the postural role of lumbar and abdominal muscles and therapeutic prospects they offer. Then we will summarize the functional implication of the erector spinae during walking.

Secondly, we will recall the theories that tend to explain the muscular role in the perpetuation of chronic low back pain.

Descriptive Anatomy of the Paravertebral Gutter

It should be noted that, compared with the joints of the limbs which, when they are in one plane, have a relatively simple muscular control, the organization of the axial muscular system is more complex because of the high degree of freedom associated with stacked vertebrae. Most spinal muscles are housed in the paravertebral gutter, which is between the spinous and transverse processes of the vertebrae. The muscles in the paravertebral gutter are organized in four superimposed planes [6]. To emphasize this organization, we chose to report it, as a whole, at the cervical, thoracic, and lumbosacral level, starting with the deepest plane. They are covered by the muscles of the posterolateral wall of the trunk whose spinal insertions form the thoracolumbar fascia [7].

Plane of the Transverse—Spinous Process Muscles (Deepest)

It extends from the second cervical vertebra to the sacrum. It includes three muscles. Intertransverse muscles (intertransversarii) are small muscles from transverse process to transverse process. They are even, symmetrical, and located

M. De Sèze (✉)
Orthopedic Medicine, University Hospital, Bordeaux, France

O. Gille
Spinal Unit, University Hospital, Bordeaux, France

J. M. Vital, D. T. Cawley (eds.), *Spinal Anatomy*, https://doi.org/10.1007/978-3-030-20925-4_21

laterally all along the spine. Their unilateral concentric contractions provoke homolateral inclination of the spine. The 11 rotatores muscles are small symmetrical muscles that fill the base of the paravertebral gutters inserting on the transverse process to the lamina of the superjacent vertebra. Their concentric contraction induces an extension and a contralateral rotation of the superjacent vertebra. The multifidus muscle is composed of muscle bundles that medially fill the paravertebral gutter, inserting on a transverse process and which send muscular extensions to each of the superjacent lumbar spinous processes. Its contraction, concentric, causes an extension and a contralateral rotation of the vertebrae of termination with respect to the vertebra of insertion.

Plane of the Spinalis and Semispinalis Muscles

It covers the multifidus muscle. It consists of two groups of muscles called spinalis (spinalis dorsi, spinalis cervicis, and spinalis capitis) and semispinalis (semispinalis capitis, semispinalis cervicis, and semispinalis dorsi/thoracis), which span from top to bottom. The spinalis muscles are located nearest to the midline, spanning from top to bottom in the paravertebral gutter and have an action of extension of the spine.

The spinalis cervicis is stretched between the lateral surfaces of the C2–C7 spinous processes. The spinalis dorsi extends between the lateral surfaces of the spinous processes of T1 to L3. The semispinalis muscles are more lateral and extend laterally and obliquely downward. The semispinalis capitis extends from the superior nuchal line of the occiput to the transverse processes of T1–T6. It covers the spinalis cervicis. The semispinalis thoracis is stretched from spinous processes of C2 to T4 to transverse processes from T2 to T11. It is covered at the top by the semispinalis capitis and at the bottom by the spinalis dorsi.

Plane of Longissimus and Iliocostal Muscles

The muscles of this plane (longissimus capitis, longissimus cervicis, longissimus thoracis, and iliocostalis) overlap partially and laterally, over the spinalis and semispinalis muscles. They are extensors of the spine, extending downwards towards the midline. The fibers of the longissimus muscles are the most medial and intertwine from top to bottom. The longissimus capitis muscle extends laterally to the semispinalis cervicis. It inserts itself on the mastoid process and ends on the transverse processes from C3 to T1. The longissimus muscle of the thorax inserts on the transverse processes of the 12 thoracic vertebrae, on the upper edge of the posterior arches of the last eight ribs and unites inferiorly with the iliocostalis muscle to form the lumbosacral mass, largely encompassing the spinous processes of the last 4 lumbar vertebrae, the posterior third of the iliac crests, and posterosuperior iliac spines. The iliocostalis muscle, more lateral than the longissimus muscle, inserts on the transverse processes of the last four cervical vertebrae, arising as flattened tendons from the posterior arch of the last ten ribs. It is then further reconstituted by fascicles laterally inserting on the posterior arches of the last six ribs, culminating in a larger volume. It ends by providing the lateral fibers of the lumbosacral mass.

Plane of the Splenius Muscles

It partially covers the semispinalis muscles. It is limited to the upper cervical and thoracic regions and includes two muscles: splenius capitis and cervicis. The splenius capitis inserts on the mastoid and superior nuchal line and ends on the cervical spinous processes. It is an extensor of the head and ipsilateral rotator. The splenius cervicis wraps laterally and caudally around the splenius capitis. It inserts on the transverse processes from C1 to C3 and ends on the spinous processes of the first five thoracic vertebrae. It is an extensor of the neck.

The thoracolumbar fascia that covers the paravertebral muscles seems particularly interesting to study. The dimensions and nature of this electrically inactive fascia allow electromyographic recording of the activity of the erector spinae muscles (longissimus and iliocostalis) by surface electrodes over almost the entire height of the vertebral column [8]. Moreover, it is perforated by vessels from the paravertebral muscles in relation to a fascial zone that accompanies their neurovascular bundle and separates the multifidus and longissimus muscles [9] and seems to be a natural pathway for the surgical approaches of the lumbar spine (Wiltse) [10].

Anatomical Models (Figs. 1 and 2)

The oldest model of functional anatomy of the spinal muscles is based on the observation of the effect of the concentric contraction of the muscles. The paravertebral muscles (dorsal to the spinal axis) oppose the abdominal (ventral) muscles. Thus, truncal extension movements are related to a contraction of the paravertebral muscles, while the flexion movements are related to the contraction of the abdominal muscles [11]. The vertebral column is then considered as a guyed mast (with radiating cable stays) by the anterior and posterior muscles of the pelvis and whose inclinations respond to alternating shortening of antagonistic muscles (Fig. 1). However, this model did not respond to the alternation of activity of the paravertebral muscles observed during anterior flexion movements of the trunk [12]. Thus, some authors have explored the activity of all the muscles surrounding the spine during flexion-extension of the trunk [12]. The observation of simultaneous contractions of the

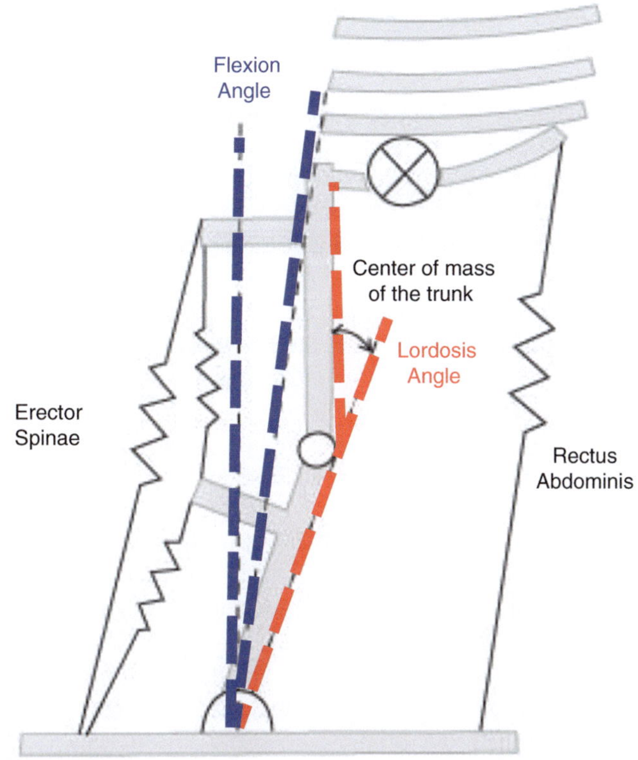

Fig. 1 Traditional anatomical model (modified from Granata and Wilson [11])

paravertebral and psoas muscles led these authors to propose the notion of a composite beam that is actively constituted by contractions of the deep muscles that stabilize the lumbar spine by adhering to the vertebrae during trunk movements. The latest model based on the different conditions of stabilization and mobilization of the trunk tends to oppose the action of the central qualified muscles: multifidus (M), internal oblique (IO), transversus abdominis (TA), psoas (P), and rectus abdominis (RA); to the action of so-called peripheral muscles: external oblique (OE), erector spinae (ES) including longissimus (L) and iliocostalis (IC) but also divided into ES pars lumborum (LES) and ES pars thoracis (TES), gluteus maximus (GM) and rectus femoris (RF). In the latter model, the core muscles are considered protective muscles of the spine, while the peripheral muscles are seen as stabilizing and mobilizing muscles (Fig. 2).

In addition to histological arguments clearly differentiating paraspinal deep muscles from the superficial muscles, the construction of the latter model is based primarily on information provided by the analysis of dynamic multichannel EMG tracings from trunk muscles recorded synchronously with data kinematics and dynamics. Three categories of muscle behavior can be studied by these electromyographic techniques: the study of the muscular synchronization during voluntary movement, the analysis of the

Fig. 2 Conventional anatomical model

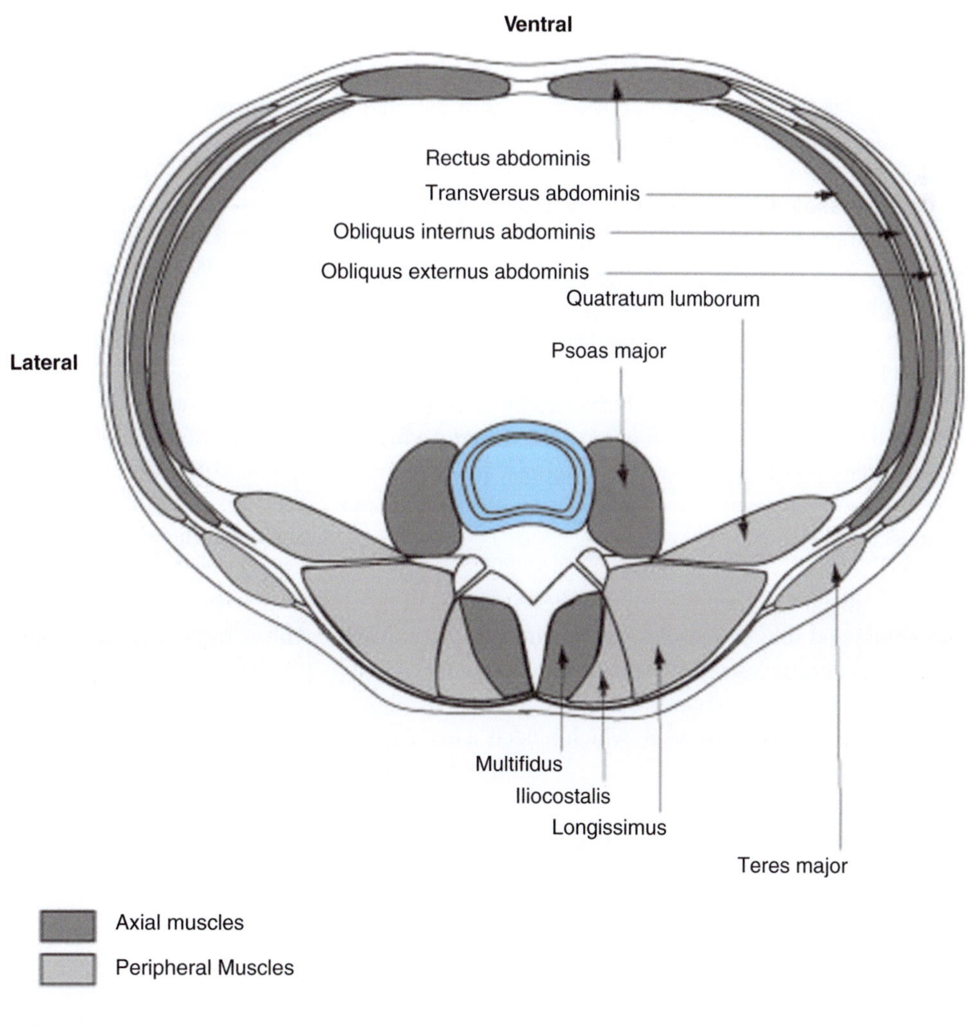

reaction times of the spinal muscles reacting to an environmental stimulus, and the measurement of the strength and endurance for each muscle based on the analysis of the frequency of the action potentials and the surface markers. All of these behaviors have been studied in healthy subjects and compared to those observed in patients with low back pain during standardized flexion-extension movements with the pelvis held stationary, free movement, or in response to disturbances of balance.

The study of the synchronization of the spinal muscles during movement and their reaction times in response to a disruption of sagittal balance reveals, in healthy subjects, a stereotyped muscular organization of the abdominal and lumbar muscles. Thus, in subjects without low back pain we find:

- during standardized movements, a symmetrical co-contraction of P and MF or RA and MF [11, 13], to protect the lumbar spine during movement,
- during free movements, a symmetrical initial and protective co-contraction of MF, OI, and RF, then a mobilizing and independent contractions of ICT, OE, GM [14],
- during postural reactions induced by a sudden disturbance of sagittal balance, a co-contraction of MF and TA [15], followed by alternating anti-phase contractions of the agonist and antagonist muscles accompanying stabilization oscillations around the new sagittal balance position [3].

On the other hand, in chronic low back pain, we find a certain desynchronization resulting in:

- during standardized movements, by a loss of symmetric co-contraction of MF and RA [16],
- during free movements, by a loss of the specificity of peripheral movement-inducing muscles associated with LES hypoactivity compensated by hyperactivity of TES [17],
- during the reactions to a disturbance, by a delay of the stabilizer reaction of central muscle [15, 18] and a loss of secondary phase opposition of the agonist and antagonist muscles [3] in favor of a co-contraction of disseminated muscles [19].

The clinical consequence of the desynchronization of abdominal and lumbar muscles can be advanced to explain the clinical lumbar instability defined as the presence of lumbalgic (low back pain) recurrences starting abruptly following an inappropriate movement, which reflects a decrease of muscular vigilance as well as the dysfunction of the corrective programs [20].

The estimation of muscular strength and endurance also reveals changes occurring in low back pain relative to a subject free from spinal pathology. Thus, in those without low back pain we find:

- a symmetry of force and EMG activity of RA and MF [17, 21, 22],
- EMG activity of extensors proportional to the applied force [22],
- a decrease in EMG activity of RA and OE during heavy lifting,
- and during endurance exercises, the effort is initially provided by the axial muscles then relayed by the peripheral muscles [23]. Fatigability predominates at the MF at the level of L5 [24].

In contrast, we find in low back pain:

- an asymmetry of force and activity for EMG and MF [17, 21, 22],
- an initial overuse of OE and underuse of axial muscles [19, 23],
- EMG over-activity for extensors for the applied force [22],
- an absence of a decrease in EMG activity of RA and OE [19] during heavy lifting,
- in endurance, effort is initially provided by the OE muscles then relayed by the TES muscles and fatigue prevails at the thoracolumbar level [17, 23].

This lack of strength and endurance is to be related to low back pain secondary to sustained efforts, due to the muscle weakness and poor management of the muscular forces that expose the bone and joint structures to harmful stresses.

Control and Genesis of Trunk Movements During Walking

Understanding the activity of ES during locomotion requires understanding of the genesis of trunk movements in rhythmic locomotor activities. Many authors consider that the main role of the trunk is to limit accelerations suffered by the head during locomotion, particularly in the anteroposterior direction, to optimize the work of equilibration of the ocular and vestibular sensory centers integrated into the skull [25, 26]. During walking, accelerations and curvatures of the trunk being weak, Thorstensson et al. [27] equate the trunk with a rigid segment whose different inclinations make it possible to maintain its equilibrium. For some, spinal functioning during walking helps to regulate the movements of the head despite acceleration imposed by changes in direction of the pelvic floor [28, 29]. During running, while undergoing greater accelerations, there is an anticipation of accelerations, an increase of the flexion of the trunk, and a phase shift between the movements of the different segments of the trunk which participate in the increase of its capacities of absorption of the accelerations [25, 30]. The theory that the trunk is passively displaced on the pelvic floor is conceptualized on the model of the inverted double pendulum. In the latter, the upper part of the body associating the trunk, the arms, and the head whose mechanical representation is reduced to a rigid segment [31] articulates at the level of the pelvis with two rigid segments which represent the lower limbs [32]. This theory seems robust since the truncal movements observed during walking are quite predictable in a theoretical manner, from accelerations imposed by the lower limbs [32]. Nevertheless, other authors take into account the intrinsic movements of the trunk such as lateral flexion and rotation, and give them a stabilizing role of kinetic energy of the trunk [33] or stabilizer of the head [30, 34].

Some authors support the hypothesis of Gracovetsky [35] that the intrinsic movements of the trunk are involved in the genesis of forward movement during human walking [36, 37]. Other authors noting preponderant trunk stability compared to sub- and super-jacent segments [38, 39], giving two predominant functions in locomotion; would be to foster the stability of the head during motion, the other is to serve as an inertial base facilitating movements of the pelvis and lower limbs during walking. In both cases, the erector muscles spinae seem to be heavily involved in the work done by the trunk.

Erector Spinae Muscle Activity During Locomotion

During walking and running, studies have reported the presence of two bursts of activity during walking by ES lumbar muscles at L4 levels [25, 27], L2 or L3 and L5 [30, 40, 41]. Other studies have reported the existence of ES muscle activity all along the vertebral column in walking [42, 43]. These flushes of activity vary in terms of organization, amplitude, and duration depending on the locomotion conditions [8]. The intensity of the electromyographic activity of ES seems to increase with walking speed [8, 43–45]. These bursts of activities occur at the lumbar level, synchronously with an anteversion movement of the pelvis at the moment of contact of each heel on the ground [25, 30, 45] and after the burst of activity of lateralis gastrocnemius muscle [43, 46]. During walking, ES activity begins at the C7 level significantly earlier than that at the lumbar level [8]. This eliminates an organization of the activity of purely reaction order mediated by a reflex arc of proprioceptive origin [47] and suggests the proactive nature of their contraction, whether it is related to postural anticipation phenomena [25, 48] or to the spinal interneurons of locomotion [8, 49–51]. Thus, at the biomechanical level, the ES muscles seem to participate in both the anteversion of the pelvis observed at each step, which allows an appropriate attitude to resist the stresses induced by the laying of the foot on the ground but also to participate in the transformation of the regular movement of the thorax in phasic movements of anteversion of the pelvis which favor the propulsion of the body forward by the lower limbs [8, 52, 53].

Theory of Chronic Lumbago of Muscular Origin

A cascade of reactions seems to be implicated in the transition to chronic low back pain. An initial disc lesion appears to be the origin of lumbago [54, 55]. The neural reaction that follows, carried by the sinuvertebral nerve induces muscle contraction of the ES muscles, responsible for muscle contractions and antalgic postural attitude classically described in lumbago. As the relief arrives, the plasticity of the nervous system seems to favor the persistence of the new functional schema induced by the pain. The patient's mainly neuromuscular static or dynamic abnormalities are induced by persistence of the functional pattern caused by pain.

Thus, there is an early and persistent dysfunction of the spinal muscles after an episode of lumbago, resulting simultaneously in an inhibition of multifidus muscles and a permanent and inappropriate contraction of the erector spinae muscles which persist beyond the acute episode of pain [56].

This dysfunction is manifested in chronic low back pain by a collective deficit of the extensors and by postural abnormalities related to a spinal proprioception disruption originating in the spinal muscular type Ia neuromuscular spindles [18]. MRI demonstrates in low back pain the occurrence of early atrophy of MF [56] and histochemical analysis demonstrates alterations of this muscle whose aerobic metabolism is disturbed in chronic low back pain [57].

All in all, all these arguments have led some authors to choose muscle as a therapeutic target in low back pain. Some, like Mayer [58], propose a repackaging of intensive therapy of 5 weeks. This kind of support appears to have significant efficacy in reducing the inability to work especially young motivated patients, with improving compensatory mechanisms and cardiovascular functional restoration which go beyond an exclusively spinal problem.

Others propose a targeted action against the atrophy and endurance of MF [4]. In this context, Danneels shows that among the 3 exercises usually proposed (stabilization, isometric work, and dynamic work), only the isometric and dynamic exercises allow after a program of 6 weeks at the rate of 3 sessions per week, correction of atrophy and MF endurance in CLBP. Finally, Hides [20] applied the same procedure as Danneels [4], showing in the immediate aftermath of lumbago, a major reduction in low back pain recurrence over the 3 years following the initial episode. Indeed, if the percentage of recurrence of a lumbago outside rehabilitation is 80% each year, the introduction of a physiotherapy program reduces this rate to 30% [20].

Finally, some propose acting on reflex contractures. Thus, vertebral manipulations in sub- acute low back pain result in stretching, a measurable secondary relaxation in electromyography [59] which is certainly responsible for the proven analgesic efficacy of vertebral manipulations in this indication [60]. Another way to lift reflex contractures is to paralyze the contracted erector muscles spinae. This was proposed by Foster et al. as part of a randomized placebo-controlled double-blind study, with spectacular results showing a relief rate of 72% among subjects treated against 16% among subjects treated with placebo [61].

Conclusion

The new models of functional anatomy proposed in the literature have therefore made it possible to propose new therapeutic approaches that seem effective in the secondary prevention of low back pain.

References

1. Beaudreuil J. Les lombalgies et leur traitement. Impact Médecin. 2000;508(27):6–22.
2. Solomonow M, Zhou BH, Baratta RV, et al. Biomechanics and electromyography of a cumulative lumbar disorder: response to static flexion. Clin Biomech (Bristol, Avon). 2003;18(10):890–8.
3. Radebold A, Cholewicki J, Panjabi MM, et al. Muscle response pattern to sudden trunk loading in healthy individuals and in patients with chronic low back pain. Spine. 2000;25(8):947–54.
4. Danneels LA, Vanderstraeten GG, Cam Bier DC, et al. Effects of three different training modalities on the cross-sectional area of the lumbar multifidus muscle in patients with chronic low back pain. Br J Sports Med. 2001;35(3):186–91.
5. Delcey V, Hachulla E, Michon-Pasturel U, et al. Camptocormia: a sign of axial myopathy. Report of 7 cases. Rev Med Interne. 2002;23(2):144–54.
6. Drake R, Wayne Vogl A, Mitchell A. Musculature du dos. In: Gray's anatomie pour les étudiants. Ed française. Issy-les-Moulineaux: Elsevier Masson SAS; 2006. p. 45–65.
7. Bogduk N. Les muscles lombaux et leurs fascias. In: Anatomie du rachis lombal et sacré. Paris: Elsevier; 2005. p. 131–67.
8. De Seze M, Falgairolle M, Viel S, et al. Sequential activation of axial muscles during different forms of rhythmic behavior in man. Exp Brain Res. 2008;185(2):237–47.
9. Vialle R, Court C, Khouri N, et al. Anatomical study of the paraspinal approach to the lumbar spine. Eur Spine J. 2005;14(4):366–71.
10. Olivier E, Beldame J, Slimane MO, et al. Comparison between one midline cutaneous incision and two lateral incisions in the lumbar paraspinal approach by Wiltse: a cadaver study. Surg Radiol Anat. 2006;28(5):494–7.
11. Granata KP, Wilson SE. Trunk posture and spinal stability. Clin Biomech (Bristol, Avon). 2001;16(8):650–9.
12. Samuel J, Revel M, Andres JC, et al. An electrokinesiologic study of the lumbar paravertebral muscles. Rev Rhum Mal Osteoartic. 1988;55(5):389–94.
13. Huang QM, Andersson E, Thorstensson A. Intramuscular myoelectric activity and selective coactivation of trunk muscles during lateral flexion with and without load. Spine. 2001;26(13):1465–72.
14. Danneels LA, Vanderstraeten GG, Cambier DC, et al. A functional subdivision of hip, abdominal, and back muscles during asymmetric lifting. Spine. 2001;26(6):E114–21.
15. Hodges PW. Changes in motor planning of feed- forward postural responses of the trunk muscles in low back pain. Exp Brain Res. 2001;141(2):261–6.
16. Ng JK, Richardson CA, Parnianpour M, et al. EMG activity of trunk muscles and torque output during isometric axial rotation exertion: a comparison between back pain patients and matched controls. J Orthop Res. 2002;20(1):112–21.
17. Lariviere C, Gagnon D, Loisel P. A biomechanical comparison of lifting techniques between subjects with and without chronic low back pain during freestyle lifting and lowering tasks. Clin Biomech (Bristol, Avon). 2002;17(2):89–98.
18. Radebold A, Cholewicki J, Polzhofer GK, et al. Impaired postural control of the lumbar spine is associated with delayed muscle response times in patients with chronic idiopathic low back pain. Spine. 2001;26(7):724–30.
19. Chen WJ, Chiou WK, Lee YH, et al. Myo-electric behavior of the trunk muscles during static load holding in healthy subjects and low back pain patients. Clin Biomech (Bristol, Avon). 1998;13(Suppl 1):S9–S15.
20. Hides JA, Jull GA, Richardson CA. Long-term effects of specific stabilizing exercises for first-episode low back pain. Spine. 2001;26(11):E243–8.
21. Ng JK, Parnianpour M, Richardson CA, et al. Functional roles of abdominal and back muscles during isometric axial rotation of the trunk. J Orthop Res. 2001;19(3):463–71.
22. Alexiev AR. Some differences of the electromyographic erector spinae activity between normal subjects and low back pain patients during the generation of isometric trunk torque. Electromyogr Clin Neurophysiol. 1994;34(8):495–9.
23. Ng JK, Richardson CA, Parnianpour M, et al. Fatigue-related changes in torque output and electromyographic parameters of trunk muscles during isometric axial rotation exertion: an investigation in patients with back pain and in healthy subjects. Spine. 2002;27(6):637–46.
24. Lee RG, Tonolli I, Viallet F, et al. Preparatory postural adjustments in parkinsonian patients with postural instability. Can J Neurol Sci. 1995;22(2):126–35.
25. Thorstensson A, Carlson H, Zomlefer MR, et al. Lumbar back muscle activity in relation to trunk movements during locomotion in man. Acta Physiol Scand. 1982;116(1):13–20.
26. Cappozzo A. Analysis of the linear displacement of the head and trunk during walking at different speeds. J Biomech. 1981;14(6):411.
27. Thorstensson A, Nilsson J, Carlson H, et al. Trunk movements in human locomotion. Acta Physiol Scand. 1984;121(1):9–22.
28. Sun LW, Lee RY, Lu W, et al. Modelling and simulation of the intervertebral movements of the lumbar spine using an inverse kinematic algorithm. Med Biol Eng Comput. 2004;42(6):740–6.
29. Schache AG, Bennell KL, Blanch PD, et al. The coordinated movement of the lumbo-pelvic-hip complex during running: a literature review. Gait Posture. 1999;10(1):30–47.
30. Cromwell RL, Aadland-Monahan TK, Nelson AT, et al. Sagittal plane analysis of head, neck, and trunk kinematics and electromyographic activity during locomotion. J Orthop Sports Phys Ther. 2001;31(5):255–62.
31. Winter DA, Mackinnon CD, Ruder GK, et al. An integrated EMG/biomechanical model of upper body balance and posture during human gait. Prog Brain Res. 1993;97:359–67.
32. Ziljistra W, Hof AL. Displacement of the pelvis during human walking: experimental data and model predictions. Gait Posture. 1997;6(3):249.

33. Stokes IA. Axis for dynamic measurement of flexion and extension torques about the lumbar spine. A computer simulation. Phys Ther. 1987;67(8):1230–3.
34. Nadeau S, Amblard B, Mesure S, et al. Head and trunk stabilization strategies during forward and backward walking in healthy adults. Gait Posture. 2003;18(3):134–42.
35. Gracovetsky S. An hypothesis for the role of the spine in human locomotion: a challenge to current thinking. J Biomed Eng. 1985;7(3):205–16.
36. Syczewska M, Oberg T, Karlsson D. Segmental movements of the spine during treadmill walking with normal speed. Clin Biomech (Bristol, Avon). 1999;14(6):384–8.
37. Breniere Y, Ribreau C. A double-inverted pendulum model for studying the adaptability of postural control to frequency during human stepping in place. Biol Cybern. 1998;79(4): 337–45.
38. Kubo M, Holt KG, Saltzman E, et al. Changes in axial stiffness of the trunk as a function of walking speed. J Biomech. 2006;39(4):750–7.
39. Kavanagh J, Barrett R, Morrison S. The role of the neck and trunk in facilitating head stability during walking. Exp Brain Res. 2006;172(4):454–63.
40. Lamoth CJ, Daffertshofer A, Meijer OG, et al. Effects of experimentally induced pain and fear of pain on trunk coordination and back muscle activity during walking. Clin Biomech (Bristol, Avon). 2004;19(6):551–63.
41. Bird AR, Bendrups AP, Payne CB. The effect of foot wedging on electromyographic activity in the erector spinae and gluteus medius muscles during walking. Gait Posture. 2003;18(2):81–91.
42. Prince F, Winter D, Stergiou P, et al. Anticipatory control of upper body balance during human locomotion. Gait Posture. 1994;2:19–25.
43. Ivanenko YP, Poppele RE, Lacquaniti F. Spinal cord maps of spatiotemporal alpha-motoneuron activation in humans walking at different speeds. J Neurophysiol. 2006;95(2):602–18.
44. Callaghan JP, Patla AE, McGill SM. Low back three-dimensional joint forces, kinematics, and kinetics during walking. Clin Biomech (Bristol, Avon). 1999;14(3):203–16.
45. Anders C, Wagner H, Puta C, et al. Trunk muscle activation patterns during walking at different speeds. J Electromyogr Kinesiol. 2006;17:245–52.
46. Cappellini G, Ivanenko YP, Poppele RE, et al. Motor patterns in human walking and running. J Neurophysiol. 2006;95(6): 3426–37.
47. Zedka M, Prochazka A, Knight B, et al. Voluntary and reflex control of human back muscles during induced pain. J Physiol. 1999; 520(Pt 2):591–604.
48. Yamazaki Y, Suzuki M, Ohkuwa T, et al. Maintenance of upright standing posture during trunk rotation elicited by rapid and asymmetrical movements of the arms. Brain Res Bull. 2005;67(1–2):30–9.
49. Juvin L, Simmers J, Morin D. Propriospinal circuitry underlying interlimb coordination in mammalian quadrupedal locomotion. J Neurosci. 2005;25(25):6025–35.
50. Falgairolle M, De Seze M, Juvin L, et al. Coordinated network functioning in the spinal cord: an evolutionary perspective. J Physiol Paris. 2006;100(5–6):304–16.
51. Ballion B, Morin D, Viala D. Forelimb locomotor generators and quadrupedal locomotion in the neonatal rat. Eur J Neurosci. 2001;14(10):1727–38.
52. Gracovetsky SA, Iacono S. Energy transfers in the spinal engine. J Biomed Eng. 1987;9(2):99–114.
53. Gracovetsky S. The spinal engine. New York: Springer; 1988.
54. Indahl A, Kaigle AM, Reikeras O, et al. Interaction between the porcine lumbar intervertebral disc, zygapophysial joints, and paraspinal muscles. Spine. 1997;22(24):2834–40.
55. Indahl A, Kaigle A, Reikeras O, et al. Electromyographic response of the porcine multifidus musculature after nerve stimulation. Spine. 1995;20(24):2652–8.
56. Danneels LA, Vanderstraeten GG, Cambier DC, et al. CT imaging of trunk muscles in chronic low back pain patients and healthy control subjects. Eur Spine J. 2000;9(4):266–72.
57. Zhao WP, Kawaguchi Y, Matsui H, et al. Histochemistry and morphology of the multifidus muscle in lumbar disc herniation: comparative study between diseased and normal sides. Spine. 2000;25(17):2191–9.
58. Mayer TG, Gatchel RJ, Kishino N. A prospective short-term study of chronic low back pain patients utilizing novel objective functional measurement. Pain. 1986;25(1):53–68.
59. Dishman JD, Ball KA, Burke J. First Prize: Central motor excitability changes after spinal manipulation: a transcranial magnetic stimulation study. J Manip Physiol Ther. 2002;25(1):1–9.
60. Abenhaim L, Rossignol M, Valat JP, et al. The role of activity in the therapeutic management of back pain. Report of the International Paris Task Force on Back Pain. Spine. 2000; 25(4 Suppl):1S–33S.
61. Foster L, Clapp L, Erickson M, et al. Botulinum toxin A and chronic low back pain: a randomized, double-blind study. Neurology. 2001;56(10):1290–3.

Connective Tissues of the Posterior Aspect of the Trunk

Martin Seyres and Philippe Seyres

Abbreviations

DAT	Deep adipose tissue
dPLF	Deep lamina of the posterior layer of the fascia profundis
FS	Fascia superficialis
GM	Gluteus maximus muscle
IC	Iliocostalis muscle
L	Longissimus muscle
Lcap	Longus capitis muscle
Lcol	Longus colli muscle
LD	Latissimus dorsi muscle
LS	Levator scapulae muscle
M	Multifidus muscle
EO	External oblique muscle
IO	Internal oblique muscle
P	Psoas muscle
PLF	Posterior layer of the fascia profundis
QL	Quadratus lumborum muscle
R	Rotatores muscle
R1	1st rib
R12	12th rib
Rh	Rhomboidus muscle
S	Spinalis muscle
SAT	Superficial adipose tissue
Sc	Scalene muscles
Scap	Splenius capitis muscle
Scerv	Splenius cervicis muscle
SCM	Sternocleidomastoid muscle
Sp	Splenius muscles
SPi	Serratus posterior inferior muscle
SPs	Serratus posterior superior muscle
sPLF	Superficial lamina of the posterior layer of the fascia profundis
SSp	Semispinalis muscle
T	Trapezius muscle
Ti	Inferior fibres of the trapezius muscle
Tra	Transversus abdominis muscle

M. Seyres (✉)
Institute for Science and Technology in Medicine, The Guy Hilton Research Centre, Keele University, Keele, UK
e-mail: m.a.seyres@keele.ac.uk

P. Seyres (✉)
INCIA - UMR 5287 CNRS-Université de Bordeaux, Bordeaux, France
e-mail: philippe.seyres@u-bordeaux.fr

Introduction

The difficulty in approaching the description of the connective tissues of the back or of any other area of the body lies in the diversity of aspects of these tissues.

Even though the histology of these structures shows several aspects and properties depending on their locations, they all share a common base: a dense gel (the ground substance) in which cells and fibres are suspended, providing colloidal properties to the tissue [1].

The interlinking and overlapping of different connective structures with different aspects, the difficulty to differentiate them due to the lack of literature on their mechanical properties, as well as the fact that the different types of tissues are linked by transitional forms [2], adds to the difficulty to describe the connective tissues.

There are as many variations in the types of connective tissues as there are in the vocabulary used to describe them. Aponeurosis, fascia, tendon, membrane: all describe connective tissues. They are used indifferently and interchangeably based on the appreciation of the authors, and therefore do not allow an exact identification of the type of connective tissue by the reader.

Fascia is a term that is commonly used. It is a connective tissue, although its exact definition diverges depending on the author [3, 4]. The Latin etymology of the word "fascia" means band, bandage or ribbon, and illustrates the notion of wrapping.

J. M. Vital, D. T. Cawley (eds.), *Spinal Anatomy*, https://doi.org/10.1007/978-3-030-20925-4_22

Liptan[1] refers to this etymology defining the fascia as a "dense connective tissue that envelopes muscles grossly, and also surrounds every bundle of muscle fibres and each individual muscle cell". This connective tissue appears intimately and inextricably linked to the muscle and is continuous with the tendon and with the periosteum. The word "fascia" is not only used in the sense of enfolding. It is also indifferently used to refer to a variety of structures that all belong to the family of connective tissues.

Bonnel [5] mentions Cruveilhier and Bichat who tried, amongst others, to define these structures, concluding that their classification was complex and imprecise. This ambiguousness and complexity was already highlighted by Hyrtl [6], one of their contemporaries, who claimed that: "nobody needs an explanation of the word fascia". The organisations in charge of the harmonisation of the anatomical terminology as well as numerous authors (FCAT - Federative Committee on Anatomical Terminology) [3, 4, 7–16] discussed this definition which resulted in the elaboration of definitions.

However, three main terminologies remain in use to define the word fascia: Gray's Anatomy [17], FCAT and FRC (Fascia Research Congress). They diverge in how they integrate the different anatomical and connective structures, and therefore in their definition of the word "fascia", and they are oriented towards specific applications [3].

The organisation and definition of the connective tissues can be based on several factors:

(1) Based on their mechanical properties

Leeson [2], amongst others, distinguishes loose and dense connective tissues. The loose connective tissues are characterised by their high degree of deformability compared to the dense connective tissues. The dense connective tissues include tissue the fibers of which are regular and parallel to one another (tendons, ligaments and aponeuroses). This organisation relies particularly on mechanical forces experienced from the embryonic development [2, 17–19]. The dense connective tissues also include some tissues the fibres of which are irregular, such as the fasciae and the fibrous capsules of some organs, or the dermis of the skin.

We will use the description of Leeson in this chapter, and differentiate regular and parallel fibres (aponeurosis, tendons and ligaments) from irregular fibres (fasciae, fibrous capsules). In addition, the epimysium is considered as a fascia.

(2) Based on their anatomical position

The term "plane" [20], which originates from dissections, is often used in the anatomical language to present the different layers. However, other terms have been employed to define the disposal of the anatomical elements:

- "Layers" as per Bourgery and Jacob [17, 21]
- "Groups" as per Drake [22]: posterior, middle, anterior

We will use the "layer" denomination to describe the connective tissues of the back.

Traditionally, the connective structures of the back are described in two layers: a superficial layer (fascia superficialis) and a deep layer (fascia profundis). These terms will be used in this description. The superficial layer, under the dermis, is surrounded by layers of fat. The deep layer (fascia profundis) is directly linked to the muscular and bony structures, and is itself divided in sub-layers.

Several authors describe the fascia profundis in the lumbar region with three sub-layers separating (1) the posterior layer: the latissimus dorsi (LD) from (2) the middle layer: the iliocostalis (IC) and longissimus (L) from (3) the anterior layer: the quadratus lumborum (QL). Some authors only describe two layers (posterior and anterior layers) and omit the fascial band that passes between the paraspinal muscles (iliocostalis and longissimus) and the QL [23]. In order to be thorough, we will include this band and therefore describe three sub-parts to the fascia profundis on the cervical, thoracic and lumbar region: posterior layer, middle layer and anterior layer.

Furthermore, in the thoracic and cranio-cervical regions of the fascia profundis, we will add an additional "intermediate layer" between the vertebral gutters and the deep aspect of the posterior layer.

Additionally, the structures appear in various aspects throughout the dorsum of the trunk. It is therefore necessary to describe the fascia profundis in layers while distinguishing the lumbosacral, thoracic and cervico-cranial portions in order to better understand their layout.

Following the description of the fasciae of the back, their innervation as well as their mechanical properties will be presented.

Fascia Superficialis (FS)

Introduction and definition

The FS does not only concern the dorsal region of the trunk it also surrounds the body [23]. According to Cunningham [24] and Godman [25], the FS doubles the skin of the whole body to the exception of some rare regions. A century later, Langevin [15] still describes it as being a layer directly beneath the skin, hence the appellation of subcutaneous fascia or tissue by some authors [13, 26, 27] (Fig. 1).

Numerous authors describe it as comprising "fatty lobules" [28] or being "more or less impregnated with fat" [15, 24], while the most common nomenclature define the FS as including all the adipose which accompanies it [14].

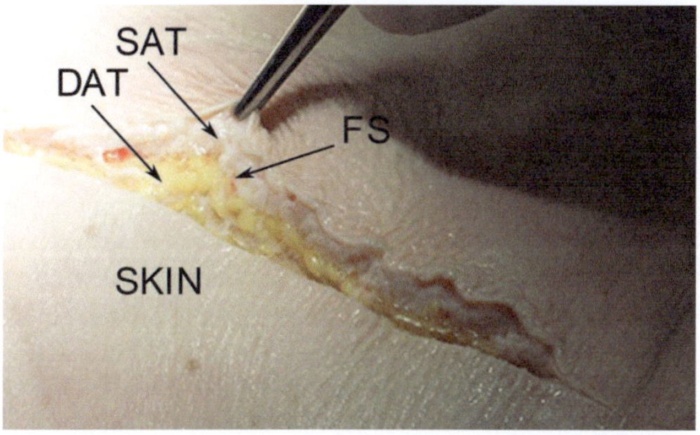

Fig. 1 Once the epidermis removed (SKIN), the superficial adipose tissue (SAT) and deep adipose tissue (DAT) appear, separated by the fascia superficialis (FS)

Lockwood [29] proposed to include the adipose layers in the term superficial fascial system (SFS). We will use Lancerotto's [28] and Stecco's [30] definition of the FS, that is to say, the FS refers to the membranous layer within the SFS only.

Composition and Location of the FS

The FS is surrounded by fat and separates the superficial layer of adipose tissue (SAT) from the deep layer of adipose tissue (DAT). Compared to the superficial layer of adipose tissue, the deep layer has smaller fatty lobules, and the transversal liaisons of its septae are more obliquely oriented. Their size varies depending on the location in the body, the sex, as well as the adiposity of the subjects ("thin in the thoracic region, it can reach several centimetres in the lumbar region") [28] (Fig. 2).

Several authors and anatomists [14, 27, 28] describe that this membranous layer (the FS) can be made of one to several fine and horizontal membranous sheets. It is made of areolar connective tissue [27] and does not have clearly identified cranial or caudal borders [28]. In cases where there is more than one membranous sheet, they are separated by variable quantities of fat (Fig. 3).

Additional fibrous septums arise from the FS and form a three-dimensional mesh of transversal or oblique interlinking through the SAT and DAT. This network forms a honeycomb-like structure [28, 85] on which are attached the fatty lobules of the SAT and DAT. In the SAT, this network of septae is called retinacula cutis superficialis.

The collagen fibres of the FS are associated with elastin fibres that provide a great deformability to the fibro-elastic structure [21, 27]. The FS appears as well-defined, continuous and well-organised membrane or layer, of aspect predominantly membranous, with irregular islands of fat cells. Microscopically, it appears lamellar [4] or honey-comb-like [28, 85].

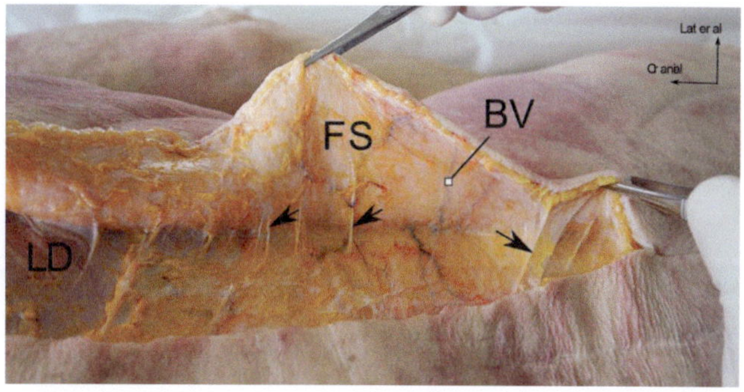

Fig. 2 The fascia superficialis (FS) is attached to the latissimus dorsi (LD) via connective fibres (ARROWS) that protect the nervous fibres and blood vessels (BV) by limiting the sliding motion

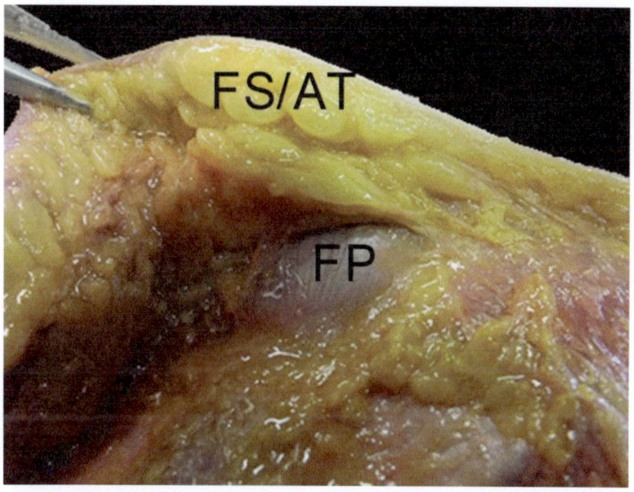

Fig. 3 In the lumbar region, the fascia superficialis (FS) is merged with the adipose tissue (FS/AT) and remains closely linked to the fascia profundis (FP). The FS is made up of fat lobules embedded in a connective mesh transversally linking and unifying different layers, while ensuring an important degree of deformability

Function

The mechanical roles of the FS are to cover, maintain and shape the fat of the trunk, and to connect the skin to the underlying structures while allowing sliding motion of soft tissues to occur with movement.

Furthermore, the fatty lobules of the FS ensure a mechanical protection to compression. The fatty lobules provide a resilience to compression that guaranties the protection of the underlying structures and the restitution of the initial form [27, 28].

In addition, some skeletal muscles attach only to the superficial fascia, such as the platysma muscle or the muscles of facial expressions that enable humans to smile, frown and cry [15].

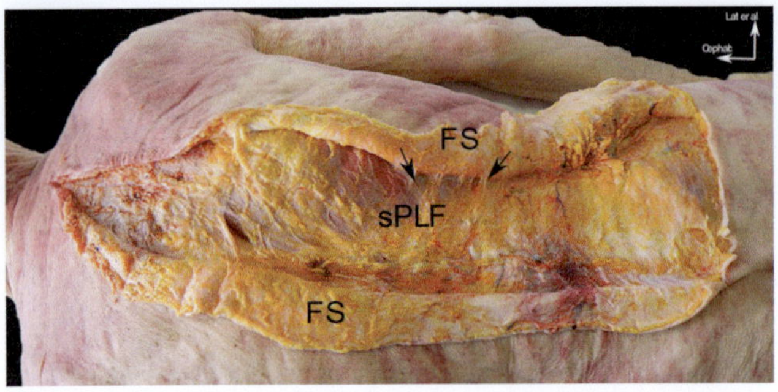

Fig. 4 Removal of the epidermis and of the fascia superficialis (FS) exposes the superficial lamina of the posterior layer of the fascia profundis (sPLF). The fascia superficialis (FS) and the sPLF are connected by connective fibres that protect nerves and blood vessels by limiting the sliding motion

Fascia Profundis (FP)

The fascia profundis is situated deeper than the fascia superficialis and is directly in contact with the bones and muscles (Fig. 4).

It is found in the literature by the name of deep fascia, thoracolumbar fascia [23, 31, 32], lumbodorsal fascia [24], tendon of the latissimus dorsi [33], or lumbar aponeurosis or fascia [26, 33–35]. It is described by Gray [36] as being made up of the lumbodorsal fascia, the lumbar aponeurosis and the vertebral fascia. Its close relationship with the muscles and the bones justifies that it is described as a "false aponeurosis" or "tendinous membrane" by Rouviere [20] and of "aponeurosis of the latissimus dorsi" by Cunningham [24].

Depending on the nature of its constitution and on where it is situated on the trunk, it will act as a means of docking for the contractile fibres on the bones, or act like a flexible sheath or like a rigid shell. The posterior layer and the middle layer, together with the postero-lateral region of the vertebral column, constitute an "osteofascial" compartment [17] that encloses the muscle group called erector spinae.

Lumbosacral Region

In the sacral region, below the level of L5, the fascia profundis, or thoracolumbar fascia, is a thick aponeurotic structure which attaches to the sacrum and laterally to the posterior iliac spines.

It comprises the aponeurosis of the Multifidus (M), L and IC muscles, as well as the aponeurosis of the latissimus dorsi. It is called by some authors the thoracolumbar composite (TLC).

Cranially to L5, the fascia profundis splits into three layers: the posterior layer (PLF), the middle layer (MLF) and the anterior layer (ALF).

Posterior Layer of the Fascia Profundis, Lumbosacral Region

The posterior layer of the fascia profundis (PLF) appears as a large, pearly white membranous sheet—a colour that is characteristic of this tissue. It is a dense, fibrous connective tissue. The fibres are parallel to one another within the matrix. Their orientation is oblique, cephalic or lateral.

The PLF is made up of the aponeurosis of the latissimus dorsi (LD), the aponeurosis of the serratus posterior inferior (SPi) and the posterior aponeurosis of the extensors (L+IC).

The aponeurosis of the latissimus dorsi (LD) and of some of the extensors (L+IC) emerge from the thoracolumbar composite (TLC) of the sacral region, and they define two layers or laminae:

The posterior aponeurosis of the LD and the aponeurosis of the SPi become the superior lamina of the PLF (sPLF). It allows the insertion of the contractile fibres of the latissimus dorsi. The insertion roughly follows a line, starting between the median third, the posterior third of the iliac crest and the spinous process of T7.

The anterior aponeurosis of the LD and of the aponeurosis of the SPi, as well as the posterior part of the retinacular sheath that surrounds the paraspinal muscles (L+IC) becomes the deep lamina of the PLF (dPLF).

Middle Layer of the Fascia Profundis, Lumbosacral Region

The aponeurosis of the QL and of the M, L and IC muscles separate from the thoracolumbar composite (TLC) of the sacral region. The middle layer of the PLF is made up of the anterior fascia of the M muscle, the posterior fascia of the QL, and the aponeurosis of the transversus abdominis (Tra) and internal oblique (IO).

The middle layer of the PLF is located in the plane of the costiform processes of the lumbar vertebrae.

Cephalically, it inserts on the inferior edge of the 12th rib and on the lumbo-costal ligament [22]; however this information varies depending on the authors.

At the L2 level, the middle layer will merge with the anterior layer. We will refer to the resulting layer as the anterior layer. The term "middle layer" therefore only exists in the lower lumbar region and in the cervical region.

Anterior Layer of the Fascia Profundis, Lumbosacral Region

From its differentiation with the TLC and up to the level of L2, the anterior layer of the PLF is made up of the anterior sheath of the QL muscle and extends laterally with the sheath of the psoas muscle (*P*), [33]. Going cranially from L2, the middle layer merges with the anterior layer that is then made up of the anterior fascia of the multifidus muscles (*M*), and the surrounding sheath (anterior and posterior) of the QL [24, 36, 37].

The anterior layer is not taken into account identically by all the authors that can describe two or three layers to the fascia profundis in the lumbar region. Authors describing two layers do not include this anterior layer and refer to it as the transversalis fascia [23].

It inserts caudally on the superior edge of the iliolumbar ligament and on the iliac crest [22]. The cephalic insertion of the deep layer varies according to authors. It is described as being on the arcuate ligament [22] or the lateral arcuate ligament (lateral lumbocostal arch) or medial arcuate ligament (medial lumbocostal arch) [20]. Medially, it merges with the fascia iliaca, and with the sheath of the psoas muscle [20, 24] and inserts on the costiform processes of the lumbar vertebrae, laterally and posteriorly to the fascia iliaca [22]. Its lateral insertion is on the lateral raphe.

The Lateral Raphe

The lateral raphe is made up of the merging of the posterior, middle and anterior layers, laterally to the QL muscle. It extends antero-laterally via the connective sheaths of the transversus abdominis (TA) and internal oblique (IO) abdominal muscles.

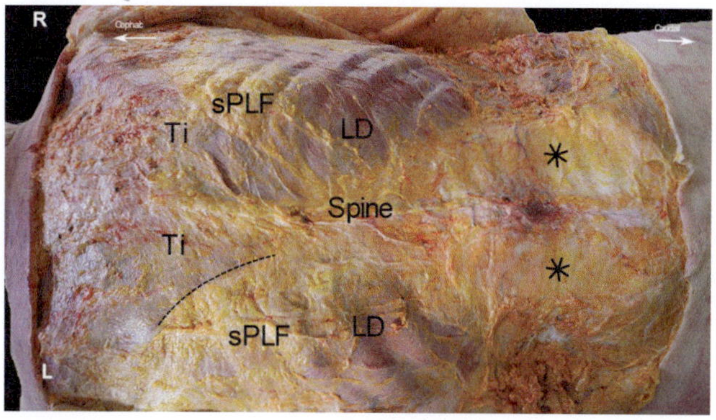

Fig. 5 Bilateral removal of the skin reveals the posterior layer of the fascia profundis (sPLF). It covers, on both sides of the vertebral column (Spine), the latissimus dorsi (LD), its aponeurosis ("asterisk"), and the inferior fibres of the trapezius (Ti—dashed line)

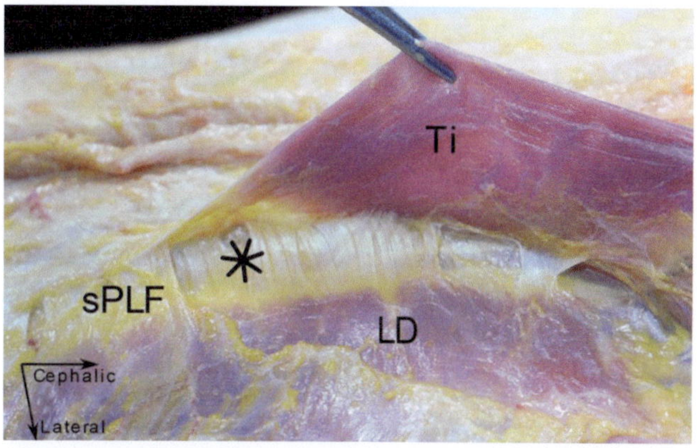

Fig. 6 The opening of the superficial lamina (sPLF) reveals the aponeurotic fibres of the LD ("asterisk") connecting the latissimus dorsi (LD) and Trapezius (Ti) muscles

Thoracic Region

In the thoracic region, the fascia profundis consists of the posterior and anterior layers of the lumbosacral region. In between them, an additional fibrous element separates the extensors (L+IC+S) from (M+R): the intermediate layer.

Posterior Layer of the Fascia Profundis, Thoracic Region

In the thoracic region, the superficial lamina of the posterior layer (sPLF) covers the inferior fibres of the trapezius muscle (*T*). It is made up of the posterior aspect of the sheath of the trapezius muscle and therefore inserts on the spinous processes of the lower vertebrae (Fig. 5).

In the thoracic region, the deep lamina of the posterior layer (dPLF) is made up of:

- the anterior sheath of the rhomboid muscle (Rh), then also includes the anterior sheath of the levator scapulae (LS) and of the serratus posterior inferior (SPi) and superior (SPs) (in continuity with this of the LD and SPi).
- the posterior sheath of the spinalis muscle (in addition to this of the L+IC) then also includes this of the splenius muscle (Sp).

The Deep Lamina of the Posterior Layer of the Facia Profundis in the Thoracic Region

This connective layer is visible underneath the DL in the thoracic region. It contains thin and spaced-out pearl white fibres, the density of which varies according to the spinal level and the individual.

The fibres, parallel to one another, are arranged transversally from the spinous processes of T10 to C7 and do not reach the ribs. They provide aponeurotic properties to this structure. However, since they do not serve the purpose of docking of the contractile fibres as the superficial lamina does with the trapezius muscle, Loukas [32] does not consider this layer as an aponeurosis (Fig. 6).

Laterally, the deep lamina extends with the sheath of the splenius, subscapularis, teres major and teres minor muscles.

Its large side is on the spinous processes of T10 to T2. According to Rouviere [20], its large side has a common spinal origin with the aponeurosis of the LD and a part of the Trapezius muscle. The two layers merge near the median axis. The smaller side is located at the costal angles of the 4th to 9th ribs, and varies of one to two rib levels according to authors (Fig. 7).

Cunningham [24] considers that it continues laterally in the intercostal area through the intercostal aponeurosis. This sheet is named differently according to the authors and to the level on the trunk:

- Intermediate aponeurosis of the serratus muscle [33, 38, 39].
- Vertebral aponeurosis [26, 35, 40, 41]
- Aponeurosis of the serratus posterior muscle [42]
- Lumbodorsal fascia (posterior layer) [17, 36, 43]
- Dorsal fascia [34]
- Lumbar fascia [24, 44]
- Thoracolumbar fascia (TLF) [17, 24, 44–48] (Figs. 8 and 9)

The generally admitted inferior spinal insertions globally correspond to the insertion of the serratus posterior inferior (SPi). Its superior insertion is controversial. According to some authors [20, 21, 39, 42] it links the superior edge of the SPi to the inferior edge of the serratus posterior superior (SPs), which justifies the denomination of (intermediary) aponeurosis of the serratus.

For others, [35, 38, 44, 46, 48] it goes underneath the SPs to extend through the connective sheath of the splenius muscles (Sp) and therefore is part of the deep cervical fascia. According to Drake [22], it goes in front of the SPs before merging with the superficial layer of the deep cervical fascia (Fig. 10).

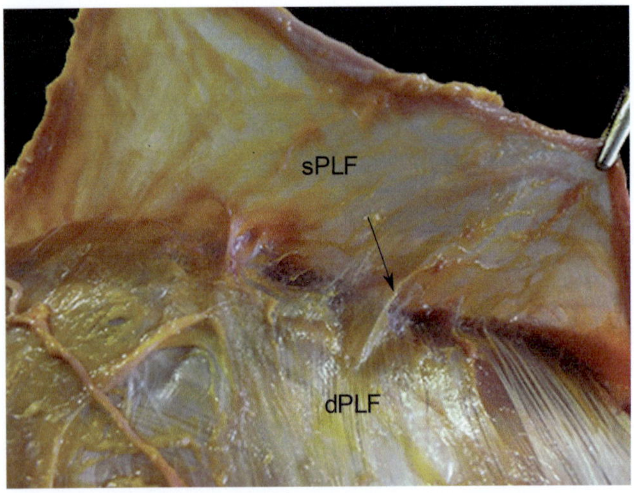

Fig. 7 Strong connective fibres (arrow) accompanying nerves and blood vessels between the deep lamina (dPLF) and the superficial lamina (sPLF)

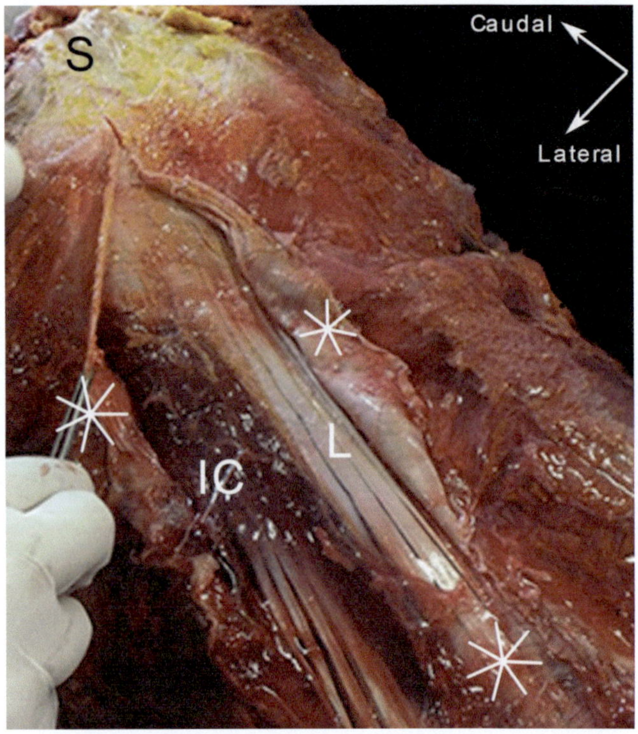

Fig. 9 The opening of the deep lamina ("asterisk") reveals the longissimus (*L*) and iliocostalis (IC) muscles. The sacral region (*S*) is covered by the thoracolumbar composite, the superficial part of which is represented by the aponeuroses of the latissimus dorsi (white part)

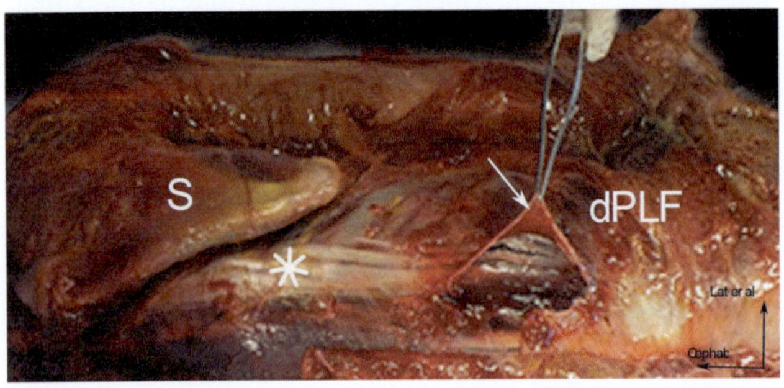

Fig. 8 Removal of the latissimus dorsi, Trapezius and Rhomoidus muscles show the deep lamina dPLF. A window in the dPLF shows the iliocostalis (IC) and longissimus (*L*) muscles, the aponeurotic fibres of which are visible below the transparent dPLF. *S* scapula, aponeurotic fibres ("asterisk")

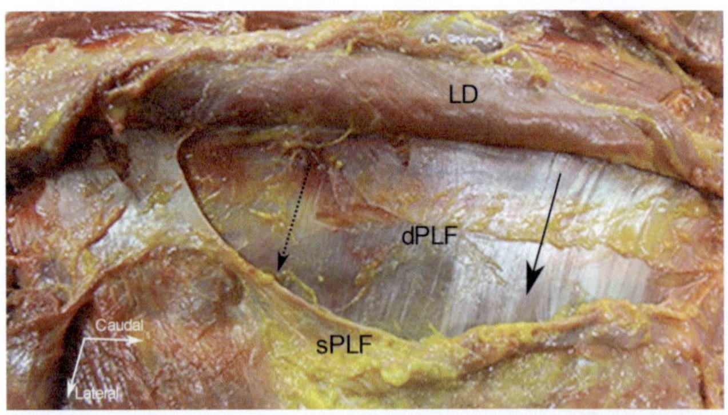

Fig. 10 The fibres of the deep lamina (dPLF) are situated deeper than the superficial lamina (sPLF) and the latissimus dorsi (LD). The fibres of the dPLF are parallel to one another, and the dPLF is denser caudally (plain arrow) than cranially (dashed arrow)

The dPLF follows the shape of the costal arc. It forms the arch of the vertebral grooves, separating the superficial longitudinal spinal muscles from the transverse and oblique muscles [26, 41]. Embryologically, this connective sheet is the separation between the dorsal epimere that gives rise to the epaxial muscles, which form the deep muscles of the back (spinalis, longissimus, iliocostalis, rotatores (R) and multifidi), and the ventral hypomere that gives rise to the hypaxial muscles of the lateral and ventral body wall in the thorax and abdomen and extending to the shoulder girdle (latissimus dorsi, trapezius, rhomboidi, levator scapulae) (Figs. 11 and 12).

Its close links with the abdominal muscles internal oblique and transversus seem to allow the transmission of the force that they develop to participate in the extension of the spine [49].

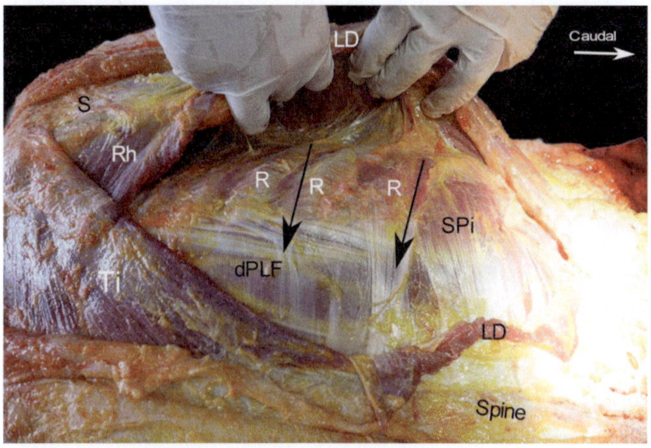

Fig. 11 The removal of the superficial lamina (sPLF) and of the latissimus dorsi (LD) reveals the serratus posterior inferior muscle (Spi) and the deep lamina (dPLF). The fibres of the dPLF cover the iliocostalis (IC) and longissimus (*L*) muscles in the costal region (*R*). It also shows the trapezius (Ti) and rhomboidus (Rh) muscles that insert on the scapula (*S*)

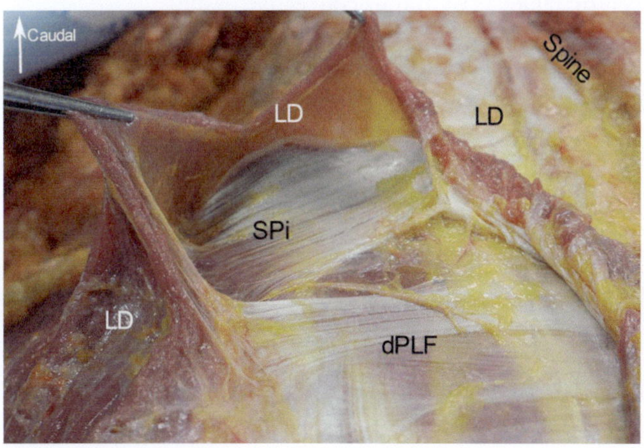

Fig. 12 The latissimus dorsi (LD) is closely linked to the serratus posterior inferior (Spi) muscle via its aponeurotic fibres that extend to the spine (Spine). The fibres of the dPLF are oriented in the same direction

Intermediate Layer of the Fascia Profundis, Thoracic Region

Within the erector spinae or paraspinal muscles compartment, the intermediate layer is not a perfectly identified real layer but a sliding plane between more superficial longitudinal muscles (L + IC + E) and deepest muscles (M + R + Ssp).

Anterior Layer of the Fascia Profundis, Thoracic Region

The anterior layer of the fascia profundis does not have major changes in the thoracic region compared to the lumbosacral region. In the thoracic region, the anterior layer is in continuity with the extension of the sheath of the QL.

Cervico-Cranial Region

Posterior Layer of the Fascia Profundis, Cervico-Cranial Region

In the cervico-cranial region, the superficial lamina of the posterior layer (sPLF) is in continuity with the thoracic region and is therefore made up of the posterior aspect of the sheath of the trapezius muscle.

Cranially, from the upper nuchal line, it merges with the connective sheath of the skull.

LD wraps the latissimus dorsi in the thoracic region. In the cervico-cranial region, this same layer wraps the trapezius. It forms the superficial blade of the nuchal fascia and merges, from the superior nuchal line, with the connective sheath of the skull.

Intermediate Layer of the Fascia Profundis, Cranio-Cervical Region

The sheaths of the iliocostalis cervicis and longissimus cervicis muscles reach the transverse processes of the cervical vertebrae from C2.

The sheath of the longissimus capitis muscle becomes one with the connective sheaths of the skull from the mastoid process.

Middle Layer of the Fascia Profundis, Cranio-Cervical Region

At the T4 level, the middle layer emerges from the anterior layer. It is made up of the anterior fascia of the M+SSp and the posterior fascia of the Lcol+Lcap.

Anterior Layer of the Fascia Profundis, Cranio-Cervical Region

The sheaths of the scalene musles (Sc) insert on the superior edge of the first two ribs, and on the cervical vertebrae on their costiform process (anterior tubercle) and transverse process (posterior tubercle).

The sheaths of the suboccipital muscles reach the connective sheath of the skull from the inferior nuchal line.

Innervation

The connective tissues of the back compose an envelope that individualises anatomical structures. Being continuous, this envelope homogenises and links the different anatomical structures. It has therefore a fundamental role in providing nervous information. Each of the layers that composes the connective tissues of the back has a specific organisation, constitution, appearance, function and relation. In consequence, their innervation is also variable and specific [13].

This informative function is insured by the sensitive information which remains not well-known in its distribution and function. It appears difficult to study with precision the sensitive innervation of the connective tissues, since they can have ramifications in the tissue as well as in the muscles or the skin. There are four types of sensory fibres in the connective tissues of the back that originate from different sensory receptors. These receptors differ in size, configuration, organisation, form and density. They are not specific to this region and are found throughout the whole body.

Sensory innervation is essential from the first weeks of the embryological development [50], and connective tissues have an essential role in the organisation and formation of the nerve fibres and of the muscles [51].

We will consider the sheath of the muscles as being part of their aponeurosis. All these aponeuroses compose the thoracolumbar fascia described above. This part will focus on the sensory innervation of the thoracolumbar fascia, the nervous endings of which are located within the muscle sheaths and aponeurosis. This description is not limited to the TLF and is applicable to the connective tissues in general.

Fibres and Receptors

The thoracolumbar fascia is innervated by the dorsal ramus of the spinal nerve [52–54]. The dorsal ramus has myelinated motor fibres (Aα, Aβ and Aγ), unmyelinated vasomotor fibres (*C*) and sensory fibres.

There are 4 types of sensory fibres, carrying information from the endings located in the muscle sheaths and aponeuroses to the dorsal horn of the spinal cord.

Sensory Fibre Types Found in the Connective Tissues of the Back

Type I sensory fibres have the largest diameter (12–20 μm) and are distributed in two sub-groups: type Ia sensory fibres that originate as annulospiral endings in muscle spindles, and type Ib sensory fibres that originate as Golgi tendon organs, Meissner corpuscles or Merkel corpuscles. They have the thickest myelin sheath and have therefore the highest conduction velocity (79–114 m/s) [55].

Type II sensory fibres transmit the information from secondary sensory endings, intrafusal fibres located within the muscle spindles, Pacinian, Ruffini or Golgi-Mazzoni corpuscles. They are thinner of diameter (6–12 μm) and their thin myelin sheath allows for a conduction velocity of 30–65 m/s [55, 56].

Type III sensory fibres convey information from secondary endings of muscle spindles and paciniform corpuscles in a small (~1 μm of diameter), not well myelinated and slow fibre. They can be considered as pressure-pain receptors since they are stimulated by local pressures of high intensity [57]. Most endings are free nerve endings within the muscle or in the surrounding tissues.

Type IV sensory fibres have a higher threshold. They have no myelin sheath, a small diameter (1–6 μm of diameter) and a slow conduction velocity. All of their endings are free nerve endings, and they are stimulated by prolonged contractions under ischemic conditions. Therefore, they provide information on the mechanical, thermal and chemical changes that happen during dangerous contractions of the muscle.

Sensory Receptors Found in the Connective Tissues of the Back

Pacinian corpuscles (or lamellar corpuscles) are oval-shaped, encapsulated sensors. Their capsule is made of 20–60 concentric lamellae of fibrous connective tissue.

They detect rapid vibrations (200–300 Hz) and are found in the deep layers of the fascia superficialis (dermis). Stilwell [58, 59] highlighted their presence in fibrous connective tissues (such as fasciae, aponeuroses and tendons). They transmit their information via type II fibres, have a low threshold and act as rapidly adapting mechanoreceptors.

Paciniform corpuscules, also called Pacinian-like corpuscle, or modified Pacinian corpuscles, have been described by several authors as nerve II type endings [55, 60].

Golgi-Mazzoni sensors have a similar composition to that of Pacinian corpuscles. They are found in several connective tissues and have been studies more specifically along the inside surface of articular capsules. They are type II fibres endings and respond to compression applied perpendicularly to the plane of the capsule, and not to tensional loading [58–62].

Golgi tendon organs are located at the junction between the contractile and the fibrous part of muscles. They are considered as major proprioceptive organs and act as slowly adapting mechanoreceptors with a low threshold [53, 63, 64]. They continuously transmit information on the active forces that are being produced in the muscle [64]. They have been long considered as having a high threshold and acting as a protective mechanism against overload, becoming active towards the end of range of motion [56].

Ruffini corpuscles (or bulbous corpuscles) are characterised by elongated, fibrous capsules and splayed endings. Their capsules are thinner (only one to two lamellae) than those of Golgi tendon organs. They are distributed in three-dimensional clusters of up to six corpuscles [56] and are located mainly in the deep layers of the skin, but also within the fasciae, tendons, tendon sheaths and retinacula [58, 65]. Unlike Golgi tendon organs, that are connected in series, Ruffini corpuscles are in-between the collagen fibres. They have a low threshold, very little adaptation and respond to skin stretch (skin deformation) as well as sustained pressure [66].

Meissner's corpuscles (or tactile corpuscles) are mechanoreceptors that respond to light touch. They have a low threshold and are rapidly adapting. They are primarily located in the fascia superficialis, under the epidermis, mostly in regions of hairless skin and at the finger pads. The fibrous capsule has a length of 30–140 μm and a diameter of 40–60 μm.

Merkel nerve endings are mechanoreceptors found in the basal epidermis. Like Meissner's corpuscles, they are located in regions of hairless skin, but they are also in hairy skin and are mostly found in the fingertips. They are slowly adapting, and respond to low frequencies (5–15 Hz), to very small displacements of less than 1 μm and to sustained pressure.

Free nerve endings represent 75% of all the endings: they are unencapsulated [83] and are mainly type III and type IV fibre endings. In some rare occasions, large sensory axons, even of type I, have been described as ending in free nerve terminals within muscles. They are mostly type IV non-myelinated, but have be found with myelinated fibres of type II, III, and on some occasions in type I [65]. They express polymodality as some endings work as thermoreceptors, and others work as mechanoreceptors or nociceptors. Free endings are not specific to the type of tissue of fascia they innervate.

Sympathetic innervations are unmyelinated fibres with a small diameter and a low conduction velocity (~2 m/s). They are part of the group C nerve fibres. The thoracolumbar fascia has a rich innervation with sympathetic fibres (fibres being immunoreactive to enzymes characteristic of postganglionic sympathetic fibres have been found in the superficial layer) [52, 55].

Thermic Effects on Fibre Activity

A general slowing of the fibre activity can be observed by cooling the muscles, where a considerable activation is observed by warming the muscles. More specifically, Ia units, and type II units when the muscle is stretched, are the most sensible to this change of temperature. When the muscle is relaxed, group II units exhibit an opposite pattern: they appear to increase their discharge rate on cooling and decrease it on warming [67, 68].

Conclusion of Innervation

The sensory information delivered by the sensory fibres of the fascia (and more specifically the TLF) plays an important role as inputs for the dorsal horn of the spinal cord.

The TLF has a dense network of nerve fibres [23, 28, 85] with different endings, in variable quantities and distributions amongst its different layers.

The sensors are mostly located in the fascia superficialis. Amongst them are nociceptive fibres, which could be an important source for low back pain, as well as for the general proprioceptive function of the TFL [69].

In general, the sensory fibres respond to compression and tension. The fascia superficialis, together with the other areolar structures, has a particular role. Its innervation responds to the translation of the different layers that it links from an anatomical point of view.

The TLF being a continuous connective tissue linking different anatomical structures, the sensitive information it conveys is part of a vast innervation network. This network provides information on the mechanical forces delivered by all the different muscles to which the TLF is linked.

Biomechanics

The orientation and alignment of the fibres of the fibrous connective tissue is the consequence of the mechanical tensions and tensile mechanical stress applied during the embryological stage [2, 22, 70–72, 84]. These connective tissues are the link between bone segments and muscles (aponeurosis and tendons), or between two bone segments (ligaments).

Embryologically, connective tissues develop autonomously and independently from the muscle belly. Muscles fibres develop within the connective network and are under the control of connective tissue cells. Therefore, the connective tissue has an organising role and is responsible for the muscular pattern formation and architecture [19, 73–76].

The diversity and non-specificity of the orientation of the fibres of the fasciae provide them with isotropic properties that allow them to withstand deformations in different directions, being in tension or compression.

Fasciae transmit forces, either directly (tendons and aponeurosis) or indirectly (the peripheral, fibrous sheath of the thoracolumbar fascia is in continuity with the muscles [77]). This transmission of force is involved in providing sensory information (via the sensory innervation network described in the previous section), or in transmitting mechanical force. Cruveilhier [38] already expressed that, when there was a need for a localised application of force, the aponeurosis of the muscle formed a tendon.

Bogduk [78] found that the latissimus dorsi applies a force estimated between 162 N and 529 N on the upper limb, while applying only 30 N on the sacroiliac joint. Barker [79] showed that tension is transmitted from the transversus abdominis and the latissimus dorsi, to the posterior and middle layers of the thoracolumbar fascia. Ultimately, this force is applied to the lumbar column (T12-S1). Tensions from the gluteus maximus (GM) and the internal oblique are applied to the lower lumbar region (below L3). Barker [80] later demonstrated, in experimental conditions, that the middle layer of the lumbar fascia "can transmit substantial tensile forces" and is even capable of "transverse process fracture".

The TLF is a link between the upper limb and the lower limb (Fig. 13).

Functionally, the posterior layer of the TLF (PLF) is in continuity with the fascia that covers the epimysium of:

- (caudally) the gluteus maximus,
- (infero-laterally) the gluteus medius,
- (laterally) the external oblique (EO) and the lateral raphe,
- (supero-laterally) the latissimus dorsi,
- (cranially) the trapezius inferior.

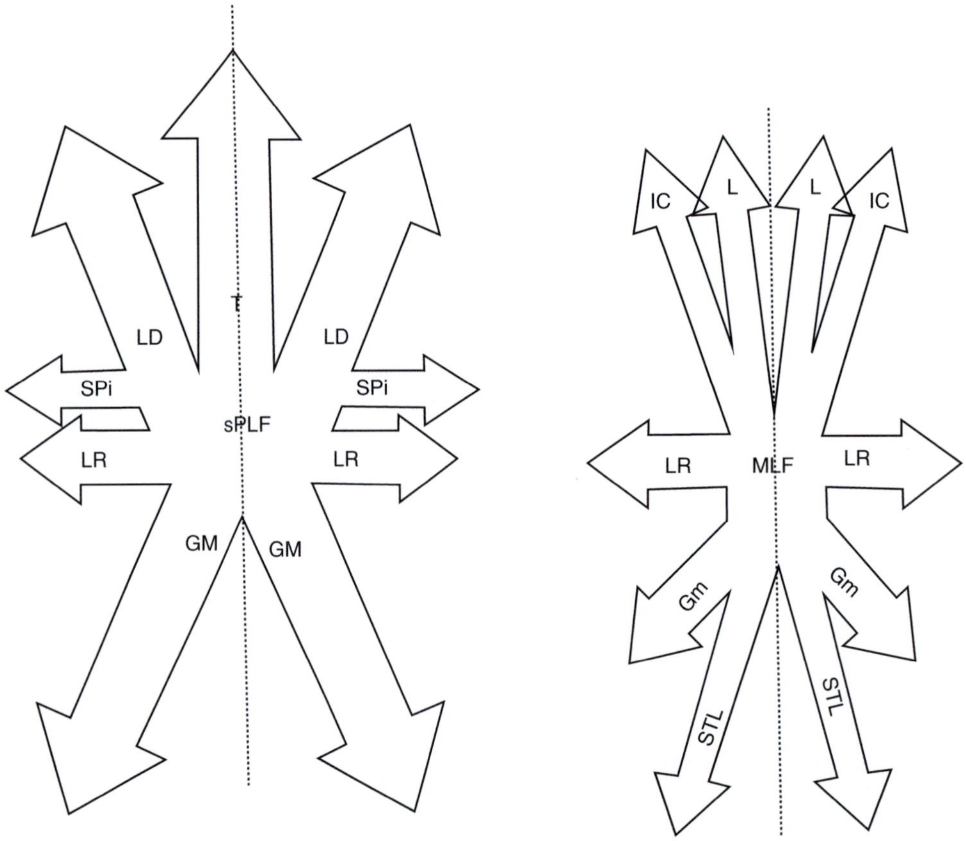

Fig. 13 The thoracolumbar fascia is an anatomical and mechanical crossroad. The superficial lamina of the posterior layer (sPLF) is the link between the superficial, cranial muscles (latissimus dorsi (LD) and trapezius (*T*)), the superficial, caudal muscles (gluteus maximus (GM)) and the lateral muscles (serratus posterior inferior (Spi) and connective structures (LD))

Functionally, the middle layer of the TFL is in continuity with:

- (caudally) the sacro-tuberal ligament,
- (laterally) the lateral raphe,

And in continuity with the fascia that covers the epimysium of:

- (infero-laterally) the gluteus medius,
- (supero-laterally) the internal oblique,
- (cephalically and laterally) the serratus posterior inferior.

Functionally, the intermediate layer inserts on:

- (cranially) the occiput,
- (caudally) the lower lumbar region,
- (laterally) the transverse processes and the costal necks.

Functionally, the anterior layer

- (medially) is in continuity with the fascia that covers the epimysium of the psoas,
- (cranially) inserts on the 12th rib,
- (on its whole length) inserts on the transverse processes,
- (caudally) inserts on the iliac crests.

The mechanical force is transmitted throughout the entire connective network. Barker [79] showed that traction forces on the latissimus dorsi and transversus abdominis diffuse in the ipsilateral and contralateral posterior layer of the thoracolumbar fascia.

Fasciae and Contractile Abilities

Connective tissues and fasciae do not have contractile abilities as such. However, Hinz [81] showed that myofibroblasts, present in the fasciae, are activated by fibroblasts and generate mechanical tensions (they contract the extracellular matrix) as part of the healing process and restore mechanical stability. Schleip [82] reported an increase in stiffness due to changes in matrix hydration following repeated stretching, and smooth muscle-like contractions induced pharmacologically. However, there was no response to electrostimulation. This capacity of the fasciae to increase their stiffness could have implications in stability and pain management.

General Conclusion

Amongst the connective tissues of the back, fasciae remain poorly researched and poorly understood. This is illustrated by difficulties in describing their properties, and by the fact that several terminologies remain in use today. The inaccuracy of the vocabulary used works against a clear, understandable and precise description of the role of this tissue in human function.

However, careful anatomical and functional analyses, as well as the studying of the embryology and recent evidence, show the importance of the fascia and more specifically of the thoracolumbar fascia. They compose a continuous network of sheaths that individualise and link different anatomical structures. Each fascia layer has a complex, unique organisation and a specific role, and each region is a tangle of several types.

From the first weeks of embryological development, fasciae play an important role as they "give birth" to the majority of the musculoskeletal tissues and guide the general organisation of the embryo. Any disruption in its development will consequently have a snowball effect on the various anatomical elements it is correlated to.

They have a fundamental role in providing proprioceptive and nociceptive information, and have a key role in spreading the mechanical forces of the muscles, avoiding localised stresses on bony segments.

From a functional point of view, the TLF can be considered as a crossroad, with force transmission axis arranged on different overlapping layers, and unified within a common sheath.

Further anatomical, neurological, mechanical and functional research on the thoracolumbar fascia, and on the connective tissues in general, could help harmonising the terminologies and could have several applications in orthopaedics and traumatology in general.

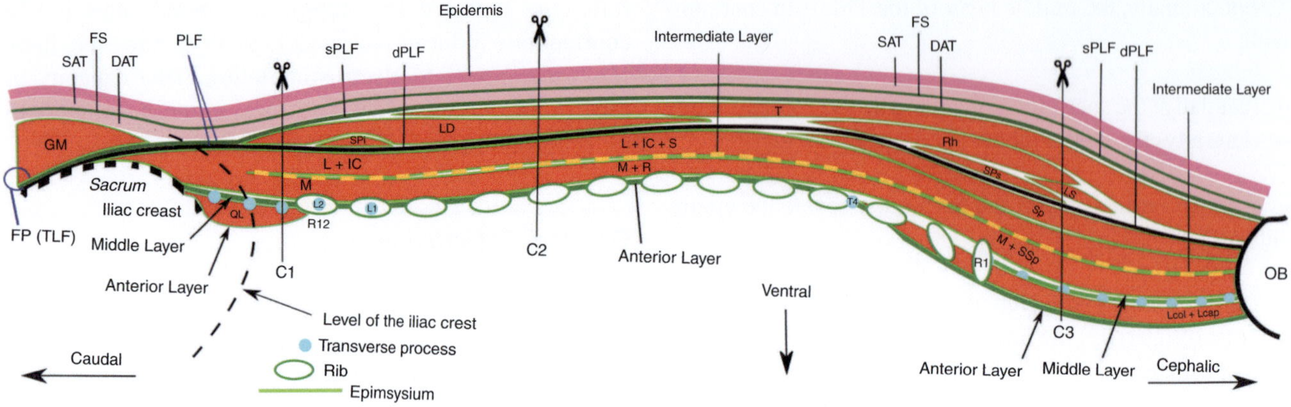

Epidermis
FS
SAT
DAT
PLF
sPLF
dPLF
Intermediate Layer
SAT
FS
DAT
sPLF dPLF
Intermediate Layer
GM
Sacrum
Iliac creast
FP (TLF)
Middle Layer
Anterior Layer
QL
R12
L2
L1
M
L + IC
LD
T
L + IC + S
M + R
Rh
C1
C2
C3
Anterior Layer
Ventral
R1
OB
Level of the iliac crest
Transverse process
Rib
Epimsysium
Caudal
Anterior Layer
Middle Layer
Cephalic

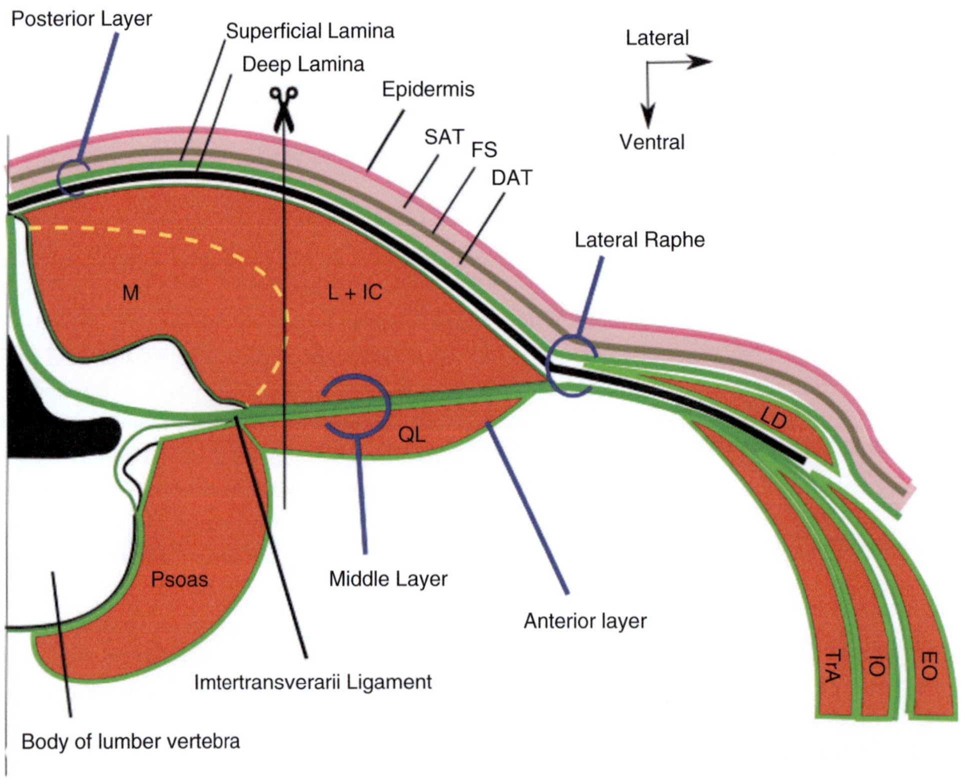

Posterior Layer
Superficial Lamina
Deep Lamina
Epidermis
SAT
FS
DAT
Lateral
Ventral
Lateral Raphe
M
L + IC
QL
LD
Psoas
Middle Layer
Anterior layer
Imtertransverarii Ligament
Body of lumber vertebra
TrA
IO
EO

C1

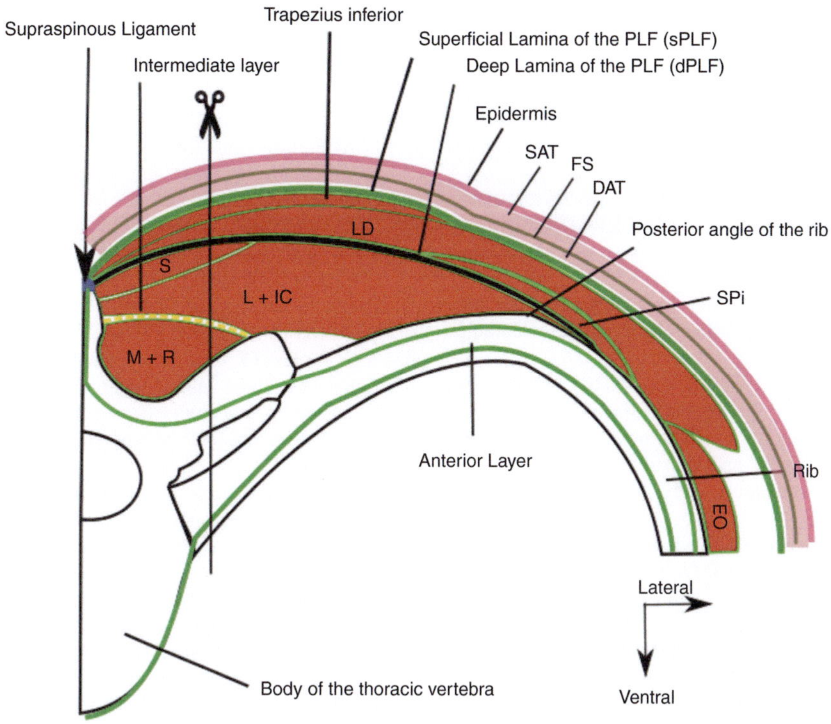
Supraspinous Ligament
Trapezius inferior
Intermediate layer
Superficial Lamina of the PLF (sPLF)
Deep Lamina of the PLF (dPLF)
Epidermis
SAT
FS
DAT
LD
Posterior angle of the rib
S
L + IC
SPi
M + R
Anterior Layer
Rib
EO
Lateral
Ventral
Body of the thoracic vertebra

C2

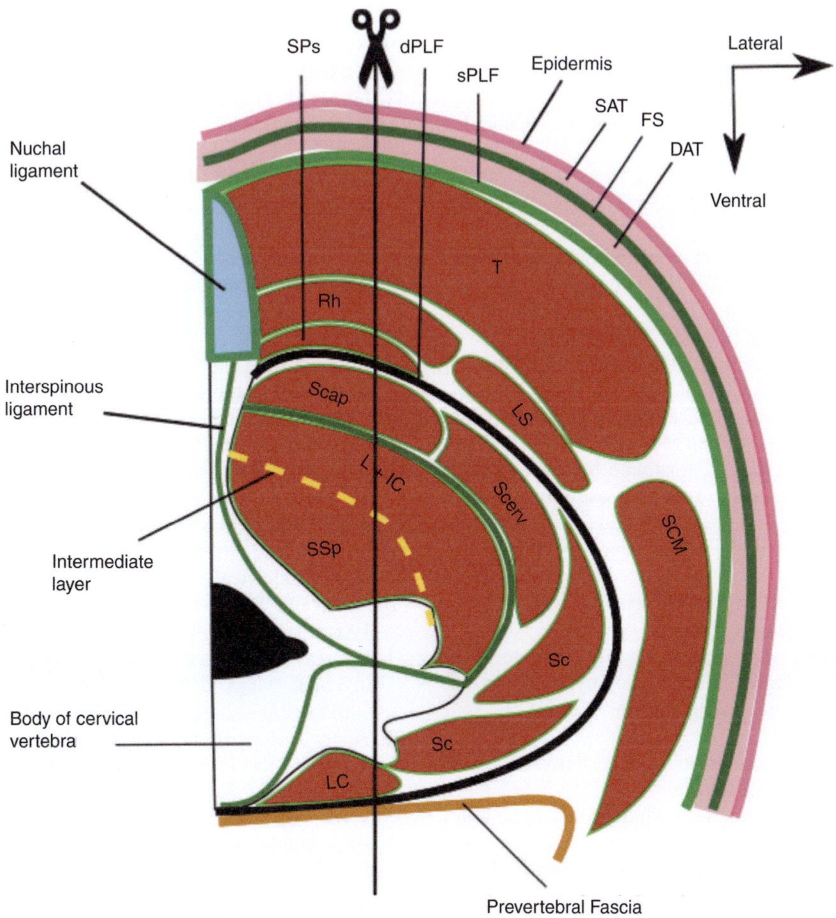
SPs
dPLF
sPLF
Epidermis
Lateral
SAT
FS
DAT
Ventral
Nuchal ligament
T
Rh
Interspinous ligament
Scap
LS
L + IC
Scerv
SCM
Intermediate layer
SSp
Sc
Body of cervical vertebra
Sc
LC
Prevertebral Fascia

C3

References

1. Liptan GL. Fascia: a missing link in our understanding of the pathology of fibromyalgia. J Bodyw Mov Ther. 2010;14(1):3–12.
2. Leeson CR, Leeson TS. Histology. 3rd ed. Philadelphia: Saunders; 1976. p. 605.
3. Schleip R, Jäger H, Klingler W. What is 'fascia'? A review of different nomenclatures. J Bodyw Mov Ther. 2012;16(4):496–502.
4. Findley T, Chaudhry H, Stecco A, Roman M. Fascia research – a narrative review. J Bodyw Mov Ther. 2012;16(1):67–75.
5. Bonnel F. Les muscles, membre supérieur: nouvelle anatomie, biomécanique, chirurgie, rééducation. Montpellier: Sauramps Médical; 2011.
6. Hyrtl J. Onomatologia anatomica. Vienna: Wien W. Braumüller; 1880.
7. Ercoli A, Delmas V, Fanfani F, Gadonneix P, Ceccaroni M, Fagotti A, et al. Terminologia anatomica versus unofficial descriptions and nomenclature of the fasciae and ligaments of the female pelvis: a dissection-based comparative study. Am J Obstet Gynecol. 2005;193(4):1565–73.
8. Kachlik D, Baca V, Bozdechova I, Cech P, Musil V. Anatomical terminology and nomenclature: past, present and highlights. Surg Radiol Anat. 2008;30(6):459–66.
9. Kachlik D, Bozdechova I, Cech P, Musil V, Baca V. Mistakes in the usage of anatomical terminology in clinical practice. Biomed Pap. 2009;153(2):157–61.
10. Stecco C. Why are there so many discussions about the nomenclature of fasciae? J Bodyw Mov Ther. 2014;18(3):441–2.
11. Bove GM. Weaving a mat of fascia research. J Bodyw Mov Ther. 2012;16(2):132–3.
12. Chaitow L. Learning about fascia. J Bodyw Mov Ther. 2011;15(1):1–2.
13. Kumka M, Bonar J. Fascia: a morphological description and classification system based on a literature review. J Can Chiropr Assoc. 2012;56(3):179–91.
14. Hedley G. Fascia science and clinical applications: editorial. J Bodyw Mov Ther. 2012;16(4):494–5.
15. Langevin HM, Huijing PA. Communicating about fascia: history, pitfalls, and recommendations. Int J Ther Massage Bodywork. 2009;2(4):3–8.
16. Wendell-Smith. Fascia: an illustrative problem in international terminology. Surg Radiol Anat. 1997;19:173–277.
17. Standring S, editor. Gray's anatomy: the anatomical basis of clinical practice. 41st ed. New York: Elsevier; 2016. p. 1562.
18. Kardon G. Development of the musculoskeletal system: meeting the neighbors. Development. 2011;138(14):2855–9.
19. Kieny M, Chevallier A. Autonomy of tendon development in the embryonic chick wing. J Embryol Exp Morphol. 1979;49:153–65.
20. Rouvière H, Delmas A, Delmas V. Anatomie humaine, descriptive, topographique et fonctionnelle: Tome 2, Tronc. Paris: Masson; 1940.
21. Bourgery M, Jacob AM. Anatomie élémentaire en 20 planches. Paris: Crochard; 1843.
22. Drake RL, Vogl W, Mitchell AWM, Paulsen F. Gray's anatomie pour les étudiants. Paris: Elsevier; 2006.
23. Willard FH, Vleeming A, Schuenke MD, Danneels L, Schleip R. The thoracolumbar fascia: anatomy, function and clinical considerations: the thoracolumbar fascia. J Anat. 2012;221(6):507–36.
24. Robinson A, editor. Cunningam's text-book of anatomy. New York: William Wood and Company; 1918.
25. Godman JD. Anatomical investigations. Philadelphia: H.C. Carey & I. Lea; 1824.
26. Thomson A, Schafer EA, Thane GD. Quain's - elements of anatomy. London: Longman, Green & Co.; 1882.
27. Abu-Hijleh MF, Roshier AL, Al-Shboul Q, Dharap AS, Harris PF. The membranous layer of superficial fascia: evidence for its widespread distribution in the body. Surg Radiol Anat. 2006;28(6):606–19.
28. Lancerotto L, Stecco C, Macchi V, Porzionato A, Stecco A, De Caro R. Layers of the abdominal wall: anatomical investigation of subcutaneous tissue and superficial fascia. Surg Radiol Anat. 2011;33(10):835–42.
29. Lockwood TE. Superficial fascial system (SFS) of the trunk and extremities: a new concept. Plast Reconstr Surg. 1991;87(6):1009–18.
30. Stecco L, Basmanjian JV, Day JA. Fascial manipulation for musculoskeletal pain. Padova: Piccin; 2004. p. 251.
31. Tank P, Gest TR. Atlas d'anatomie. Bruxelles: De Boeck; 2010.
32. Loukas M, Shoja MM, Thurston T, Jones VL, Linganna S, Tubbs RS. Anatomy and biomechanics of the vertebral aponeurosis part of the posterior layer of the thoracolumbar fascia. Surg Radiol Anat. 2008;30(2):125–9.
33. Testut L. Traité d'anatomie humaine: anatomie descriptive, histologie, développement. Paris: O. Doin; 1896. p. 1212.
34. Macalister A. A text-book of human anatomy. London: Griffin; 1889.
35. Buchanan AM. Manual of anatomy, systematic and practical, including embryology. Toronto: Macmillan; 1916.
36. Gray H, Lewis WH. Anatomy of the human body. 20th ed. Philadelphia: Lea & Febiger; 1918.
37. Bogduk N, Twomey LT. Clinical anatomy of the lumbar spine. 2nd ed. Melbourne/New York: Churchill Livingstone; 1986. p. 197.
38. Cruveilhier J. Traité d'anatomie descriptive. Tome 1. 5th ed. Paris: P. Asselin; 1871.
39. Kamina P. Précis d'anatomie clinique. Tome II. Paris: Maloine; 2002.
40. Holmes T, Carter HV, Gray H, Guise WJ. Anatomy, descriptive and surgical. London: Longmans, Green; 1875.
41. Luther H. Holden's anatomy: a manual of the dissection of the human body. Philadelphia: P. Blakiston's Son; 1901.
42. Sappey PC. Traité d'anatomie descriptive T2. Paris: Medical Heritage Library; 1876.
43. Spalteholz W. Hand-atlas of human anatomy. 7th ed. Philadelphia: Lippincott Williams & Wilkins; 1861.
44. Agur AMR, Lee MJ, Anderson JE. Grant's atlas of anatomy. 9th ed. Baltimore: Lippincott Williams & Wilkins; 1991. p. 650.
45. Hansen JT, Weber EC. Netter's atlas of human anatomy. Basel: Novartis; 2014.
46. Schünke M, Schulte E, Schumacher U, Rude J, Voll M, Wesker K. Atlas d'anatomie Prométhée. Paris: Maloine; 2006.
47. Cleland J. Examen clinique de l'appareil locomoteur. Amsterdam: Elsevier Masson; 2007.
48. Clemente CD. Anatomy - a regional atlas of the human body. 6th ed. Baltimore: Lippincott Williams & Wilkins; 2011.
49. Gatton ML, Pearcy MJ, Pettet GJ, Evans JH. A three-dimensional mathematical model of the thoracolumbar fascia and an estimate of its biomechanical effect. J Biomech. 2010;43(14):2792–7.
50. Hewer EE. The development of nerve endings in the human foetus. J Anat. 1935;69:369–79.
51. Lewis J, Chevallier A. Muscle nerve branches do not develop in chick wings devoid of muscle. J Embryol Exp Morphol. 1981;64:211–32.
52. Tesarz J, Hoheisel U, Wiedenhöfer B, Mense S. Sensory innervation of the thoracolumbar fascia in rats and humans. Neuroscience. 2011;194:302–8.
53. Wyke B. Articular neurology - a review. Physiotherapy. 1972;58:94–9.
54. Bove GM, Light AR. Unmyelinated nociceptors of rat paraspinal tissues. J Neurophysiol. 1995;73(5):1752–62.

55. Mitchell JH, Schmidt RF. Cardiovascular reflex control by afferent fibers from skeletal muscle receptors. In: Terjung R, editor. Comprehensive physiology. Hoboken: Wiley; 1983.
56. Wyke B. The neurology of joints. Ann R Coll Surg Engl. 1967;41(1):25–50.
57. Paintal AS. Functional analysis of Group III afferent fibres of mammalian muscles. J Physiol. 1960;152(2):250–70.
58. Stilwell DL. Regional variations in the innervation of deep fasciae and aponeuroses. Anat Rec. 1957;127(4):635–53.
59. Stilwell DL. The innervation of tendons and aponeuroses. Am J Anat. 1957;100(3):289–317.
60. Freeman MAR, Wyke B. The innervation of the knee joint. An anatomical and histological study in the cat. J Anat. 1967;101:505–32.
61. Yahia L, Rhalmi S, Newman N, Isler M. Sensory innervation of human thoracolumbar fascia: an immunohistochemical study. Acta Orthop Scand. 1992;63(2):195–7.
62. Grigg A, Hoffman AH, Fogarty KE. Properties of Golgi-Mazzoni afferents in cat knee joint capsule, as revealed by mechanical studies of isolated joint capsule. J Neurophysiol. 1982;47(1):31–40.
63. Kiter E, Karaboyun T, Tufan AC, Acar K. Immunohistochemical demonstration of nerve endings in iliolumbar ligament. Spine. 2010;35(4):E101–4.
64. Houk J, Henneman E. Responses of Golgi tendon organs to active contractions of the soleus muscle of the cat. J Neurophysiol. 1967;30(3):466–81.
65. Barker D, Hunt CC, McIntyre AK. Muscle receptors. Berlin: Springer; 1974.
66. Barrett KE, Ganong WF. Ganong's review of medical physiology. New York: McGraw-Hill Medical; 2010.
67. Mense S. Effects of temperature on the discharges of muscle spindles and tendon organs. Pflugers Arch - Eur J Physiol. 1978;374(2):159–66.
68. Eldred E, Lindsley DF, Buchwald JS. The effect of cooling on mammalian muscle spindles. Exp Neurol. 1960;2(2):144–57.
69. Schleip R. Possibilities and limitations of fascia oriented concepts in research and treatment of low back and pelvic pain. In: 8th Interdisciplinary World Congress on Low Back & Pelvic Pain, Dubai, 2013; 2013. Available from https://www.fasciaresearch.com/literature/wc-low-back-and-pelvic-pain/Schleip2013_PossibilitiesandLimitations.pdf.
70. Nowlan NC, Sharpe J, Roddy KA, Prendergast PJ, Murphy P. Mechanobiology of embryonic skeletal development: insights from animal models. Birth Defects Res Pt C. 2010;90(3):203–13.
71. Blechschmidt E, Gasser RF. Biokinetics and biodynamics of human differentiation: principles and applications. Berkeley: North Atlantic Books; 2014.
72. Blechschmidt E, Freeman B. The ontogenetic basis of human anatomy: a biodynamic approach to development from conception to birth. Murrieta: Pacific Distributing/North Atlantic Books; 2004. p. 255.
73. Chevallier A, Kieny M. On the role of the connective tissue in the patterning of the chick limb musculature. Wilhelm Roux's Arch Dev Biol. 1982;191(4):277–80.
74. Kieny M, Mauger A, Chevallier A, Pautou M-P. Origin and development of avian skeletal musculature. Reprod Nutr Dev. 1988;28(3B):673–86.
75. Charvet B, Ruggiero F, Guellec DL. The development of the myotendinous junction. A review. Muscles Ligaments Tendons J. 2012;2(2):53–63.
76. Stopak D, Harris AK. Connective tissue morphogenesis by fibroblast traction. Dev Biol. 1982;90(2):383–98.
77. Monti RJ, Roy RR, Hodgson JA, Reggie Edgerton V. Transmission of forces within mammalian skeletal muscles. J Biomech. 1999;32(4):371–80.
78. Bogduk N, Johnson G, Spalding D. The morphology and biomechanics of latissimus dorsi. Clin Biomech. 1998;13(6):377–85.
79. Barker PJ, Briggs CA, Bogeski G. Tensile transmission across the lumbar fasciae in unembalmed cadavers: effects of tension to various muscular attachments. Spine. 2004;29(2):129–38.
80. Barker PJ, Freeman AD, Urquhart DM, Anderson CR, Briggs CA. The middle layer of lumbar fascia can transmit tensile forces capable of fracturing the lumbar transverse processes: an experimental study. Clin Biomech. 2010;25(6):505–9.
81. Hinz B. The myofibroblast: paradigm for a mechanically active cell. J Biomech. 2010;43(1):146–55.
82. Schleip R, Klingler W, Lehmann-Horn F. Fascia is able to contract in a smooth muscle-like manner and thereby influence musculoskeletal mechanics. J Biomech. 2006;39:S488.
83. Fishman SM, Ballantyne JC, Rathmell JP. Bonica's management of pain. 4th ed. Philadelphia: Lippincott Williams & Wilkins; 2010. p. 1698.
84. Nowlan NC, Murphy P, Prendergast PJ. Mechanobiology of embryonic limb development. Ann N Y Acad Sci. 2007;1101(1):389–411.
85. Stecco C, Veronica M, Andrea P, Fabrice D, Raffaele DC. The fascia: the forgotten structure, vol. 116; 2011. p. 127–38.

The Spinal Canal

Jean Marc Vital

The vertebrae, the discs, and the ligaments delineate spinal canals in which the cord and the roots, the arteries, and the intraspinal veins will circulate. These channels include:

- The central canal (or vertebral foramen) that surrounds and protects the cord and the cauda equina
- The root canals that surround and protect the roots, each including the lateral recess, the intervertebral foramen
- The transverse canals which surround and protect the vertebral arteries.

The Central Spinal Canal (Vertebral Foramen)

More than the dimensions of this canal, it is the reserve volume around the dura mater which one must take into account.

Limits (Fig. 1) **Superior and Inferior**

It opens into the cranial cavity through the occipital foramen, or foramen magnum, and ends caudally, in a flute-like beak, at the sacrococcygeal hiatus, at the distal end of the sacral canal.

Peripherals (in the Horizontal Plane)

These are osteofibrous:

- Anteriorly the canal is limited by the posterior aspect of the vertebral bodies, of the discs and the posterior longitudinal ligament (PLL). It is the posterior wall that can recoil under the effect of an axial compression (vertebral fracture) or of a vertebral tumor and compress the neural structures
- Posteriorly by the laminae and the yellow ligaments (ligamentum flavum). These structures are stacked like roof tiles at the thoracic level but allow a gap between them at the cervical and lumbar level thus providing access for needle puncture under the occiput or lumbar level
- Laterally by the pedicles separated by intervertebral foramina.

Diameter—Internal Surface

The spinal canal follows the spinal curvatures, but its diameter varies widely depending on the segment. There are two diameters:

- anteroposterior median (or fixed medial sagittal diameter, FMSD) between the posterior wall and the union of the laminae and the spinous process (spinolaminar line)
- transverse between the pedicles.

In reality, it is more interesting to determine the surface of the canal.

The latter is wide at the cervical and lumbar level and less at the thoracic level, especially at T9. Dimeglio [1] (Fig. 2) reminds us that the high cervical vertebra can fit the thumb, whereas the lumbar vertebra can fit the index and the thoracic vertebra the little finger.

We admit that the minimum anteroposterior diameter is:

- Average 20 mm upper cervical, 12 mm lower cervical,
- Average 10 mm thoracic,
- Average 15 mm in lumbar.

J. M. Vital (✉)
Spinal Unit, University Hospital, Bordeaux, France

J. M. Vital, D. T. Cawley (eds.), *Spinal Anatomy*, https://doi.org/10.1007/978-3-030-20925-4_23

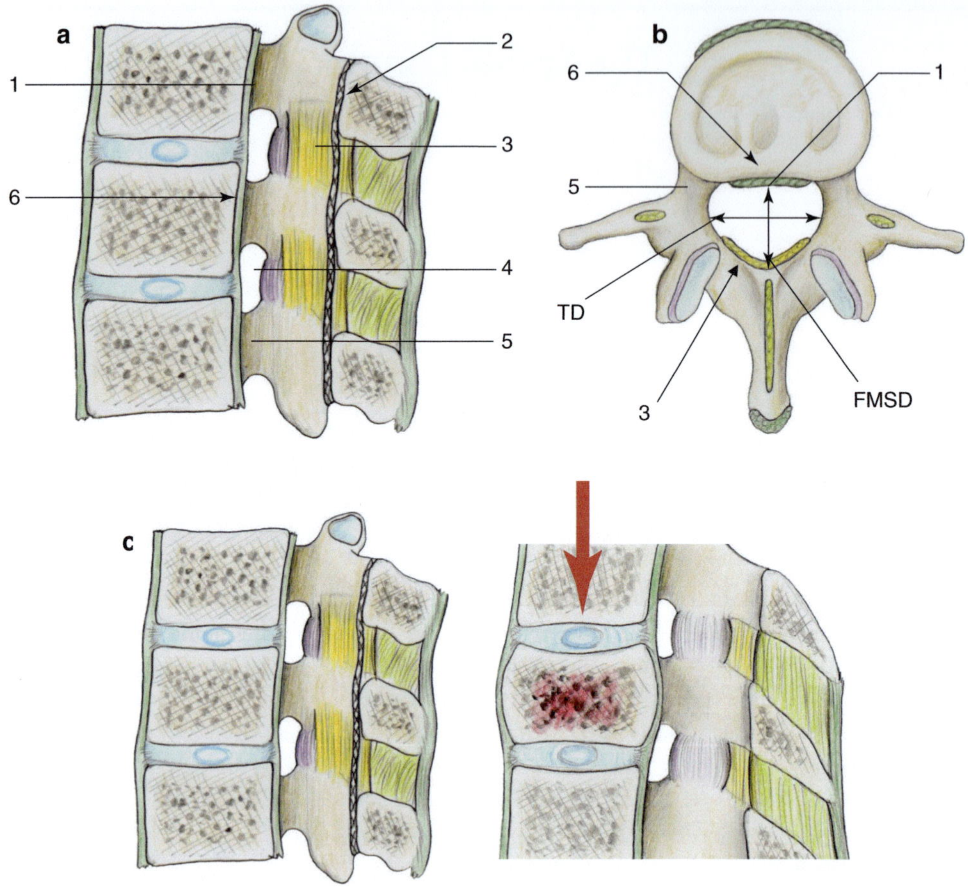

Fig. 1 Central spinal canal (or vertebral foramen). (**a**) Sagittal section (**b**) Superior view. 1. Dorsal longitudinal ligament; 2. Spinolaminar line; 3. Yellow ligament; 4. Intervertebral foramen; 5. Pedicle; 6. Posterior wall; TD transverse diameter; FMSD fixed medial sagittal diameter, (**c**) expansion of the posterior wall by fracture or tumor

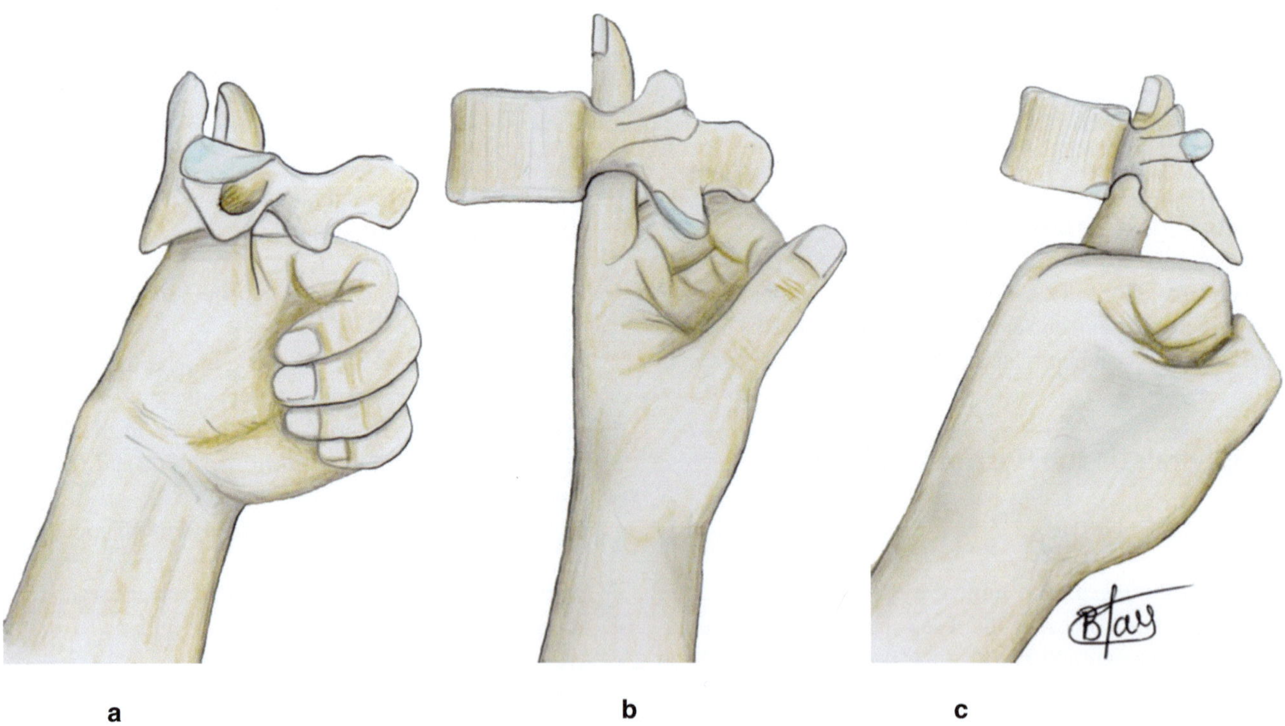

Fig. 2 Respective dimensions of the central spinal canal (Dimeglio [1]). (**a**) The axis admits the thumb, (**b**) The lumbar vertebra admits the index, (**c**) The thoracic vertebra admits the little finger

The Reserve Volume (RV)

In reality, more than the anteroposterior or transverse diameter, the reserve volume (RV) around the dura mater is most important: it is defined in the lumbar region by Lee [2] but can be used at all levels (Fig. 3). This RV is relatively important in the cervical and lumbar spine and is lower in the thoracic area despite the small diameter of the thoracic spinal cord (Fig. 4). The most classic example is that of the C1C2 region where the spinal cord occupies one-third of the canal, the odontoid process (peg) another third, the last third corresponding to free space for the cord, the RV (rule of thirds): spinal trauma lesions, having survived the trauma, are rare at this level sometimes despite large traumatic osteoarticular movements (Fig. 5).

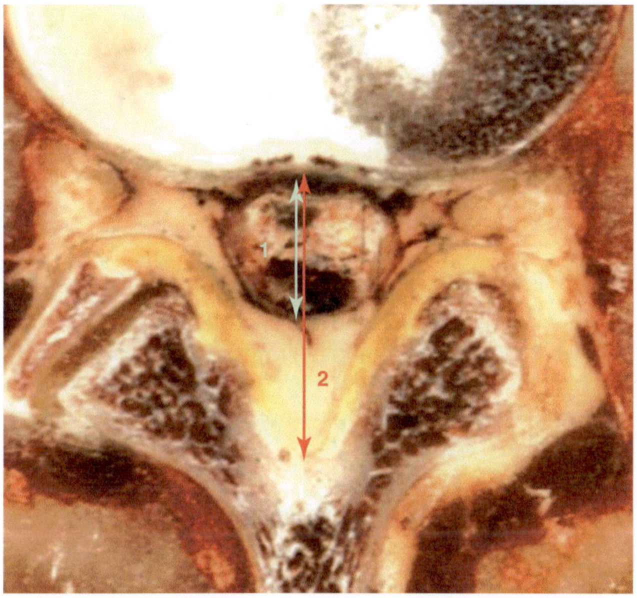

Fig. 3 The reserve volume (RV). 1. Sagittal diameter of the dura mater; 2. sagittal diameter of the canal. RV = 2 − 1

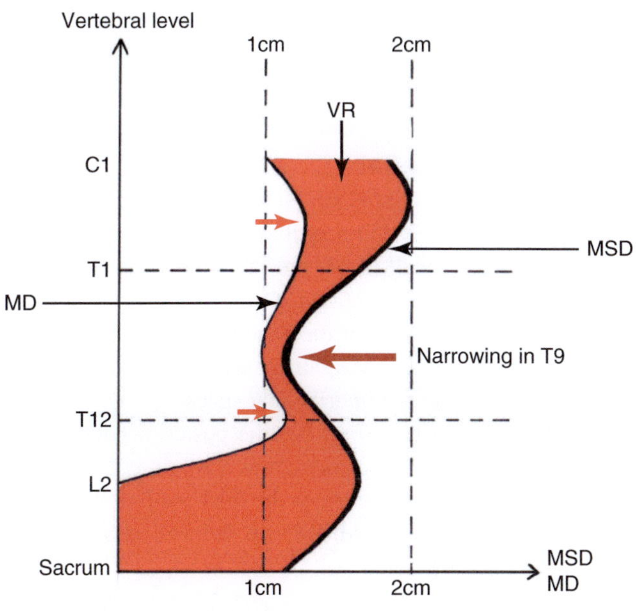

Fig. 4 Variations of the volume of reserve (VR) according to the spinal level. *MSD* median sagittal diameter, *MD* diameter of the cord with cervical and lumbar prominences

The Cervical Spinal Canal

It is the widest; in fact, its median sagittal diameter decreases from top to bottom since it is on average 22 mm in relation to C1, 20 mm in relation to C2, and 14–17 mm in the lower cervical level (Fig. 6).

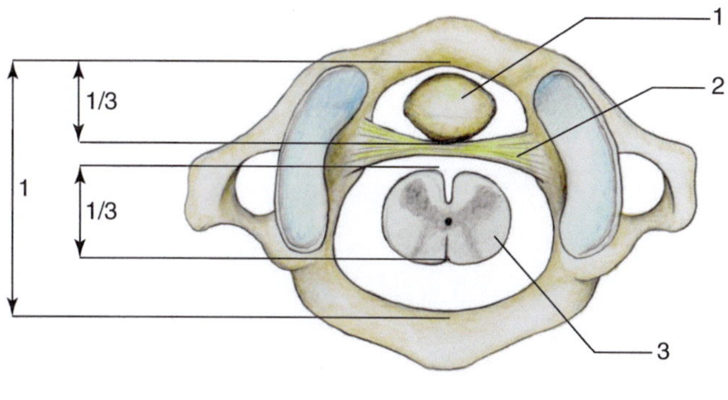

Fig. 5 The spinal cord in the spinal canal at the level of the atlas. 1. Odontoid; 2. Transverse ligament; 3. Spinal cord

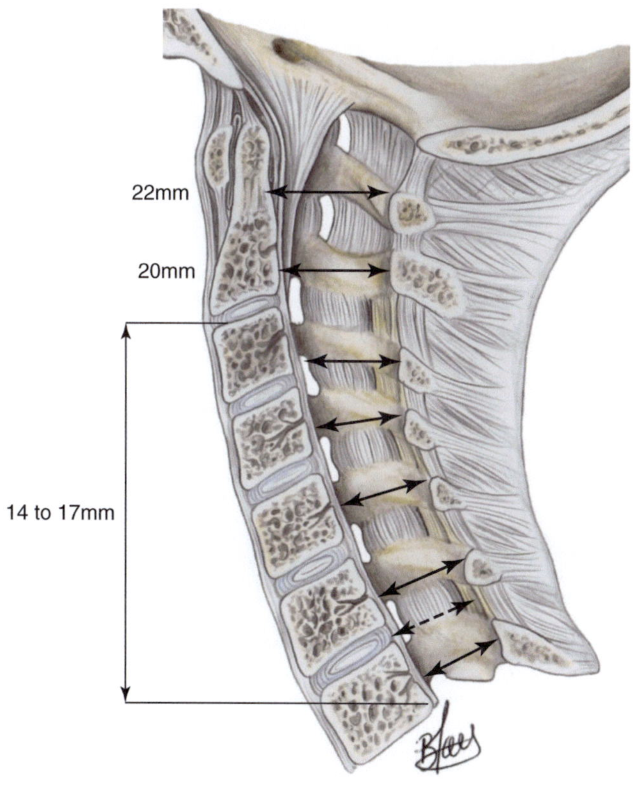

Fig. 6 Median sagittal diameters (MSD) at the cervical level. Solid arrows: FMSD or bone; Dotted arrow at C6C7: MMSD

The fixed medial sagittal diameter (FMSD) corresponds to the solid arrows in Fig. 6 drawn between the middle of the posterior vertebral body and the upper part of the lamina: this bone diameter is fixed and said to be "constitutional" since in principle its size does not vary after the closure of the neurocentral cartilage, around 5–6 years. The dotted arrow joining the yellow ligament at disc C6C7 is called the mobile medial sagittal diameter (MMSD) since it corresponds to the Junghanns mobile segment; in degenerative cervical (or lumbar) pathology, this segment is the most affected. Classically, a cervical spinal canal of normal size is the sagittal diameter of a cervical vertebral body (Wackenheim [3]) (Fig. 7).

Specifically, Pavlov et al. [4] provide an index which is the ratio of A (FMSD) and B (anteroposterior diameter of vertebral body). If this index is less than 0.8, there is canal narrowing (Fig. 8).

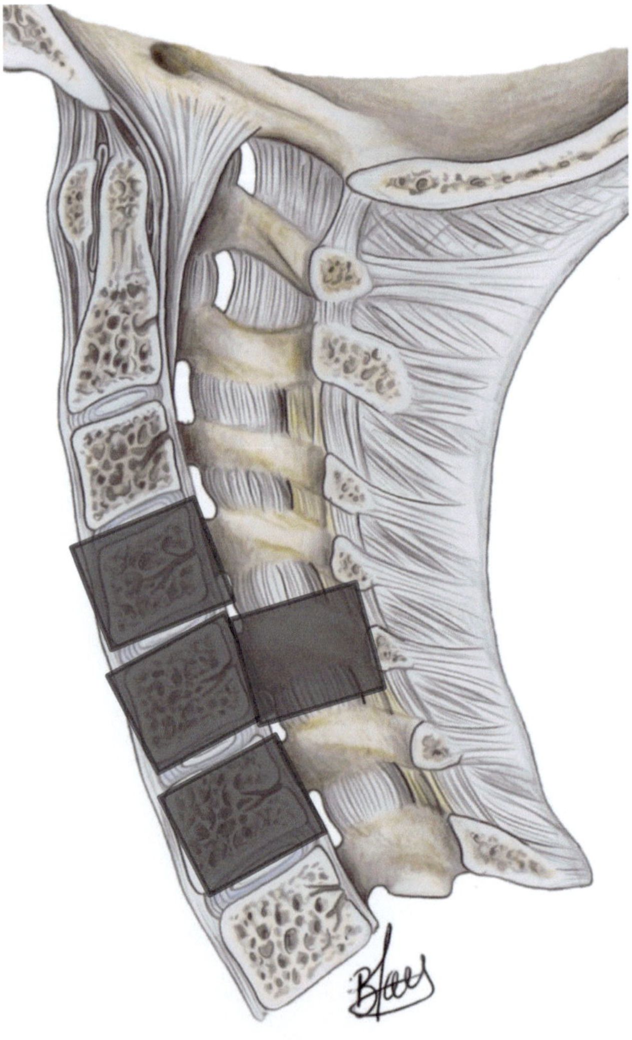

Fig. 7 Normal cervical canal admitting the projection of a normal vertebral body [3]

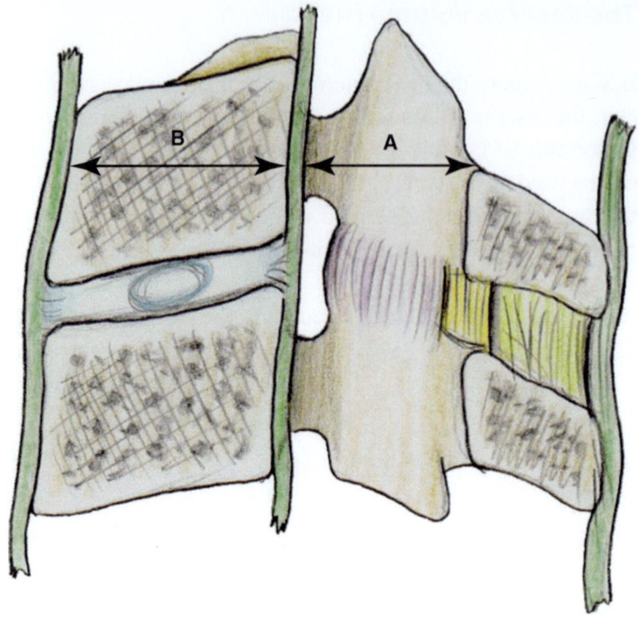

Fig. 8 Torg and Pavlov index [4] = A/B (normally greater than 0.8)

Finally, on a lateral radiograph, we can distinguish 3 portions of 5 in the lateral projection of the cervical canal which is located between the body (portion 1) and the spinous process (portion 5) (Fig. 9).

- portion 2 is the pedicle (transverse),
- portion 3 is articular,
- portion 4 is lamina; it is often considered a safe space.

Thoracic Spinal Canal

It is oval as at the cervical level but much smaller (FMSD 10 to 12 mm).

Lumbar Spinal Canal

It also represents a FMSD drawn between the middle of the posterior vertebral wall (more precisely the posterior longitudinal ligament) and the cranial part of the spinous process which is more ventral than the caudal part; on this caudal part is inserted the yellow ligament which goes up high on the cranial lamina in the interlaminar space.

The MMSD is traced between the posterior edge of the annulus and the yellow ligament: thus a bulging disc, hypertrophy of the yellow ligament or the thickened joint capsule frequently reduces the MMSD in lumbar degenerative pathology (Fig. 10).

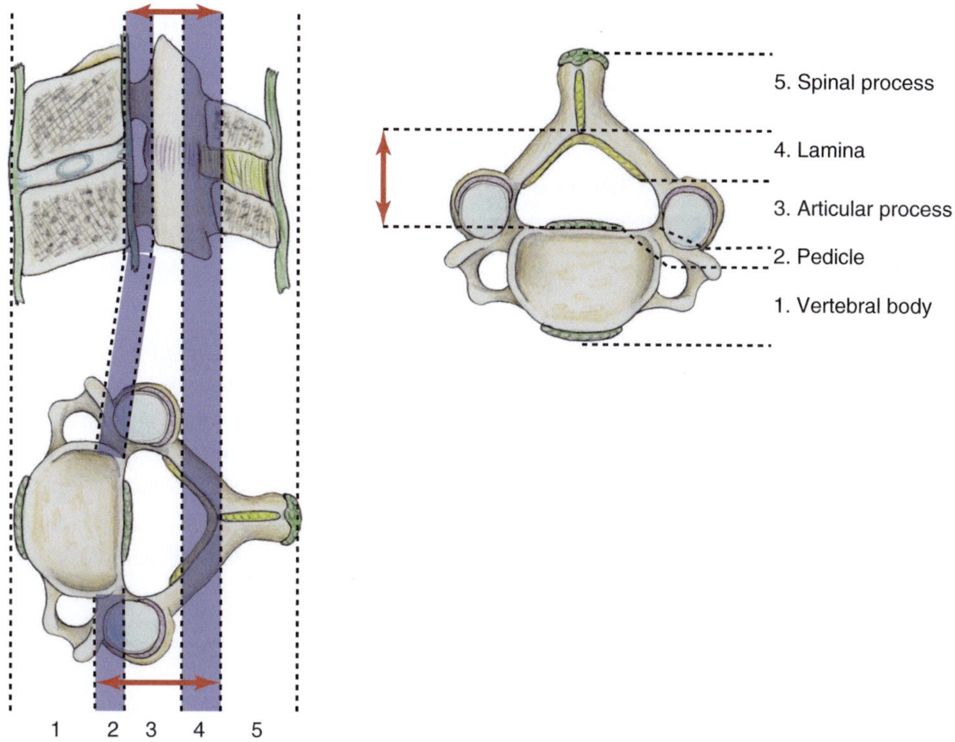

Fig. 9 The 3 portions of the cervical spinal canal which is marked by the red arrow with the portions 2, 3, and 4. 1. Vertebral body; 2. Pedicle; 3. Articular; 4. Lamina; 5. Spinous process

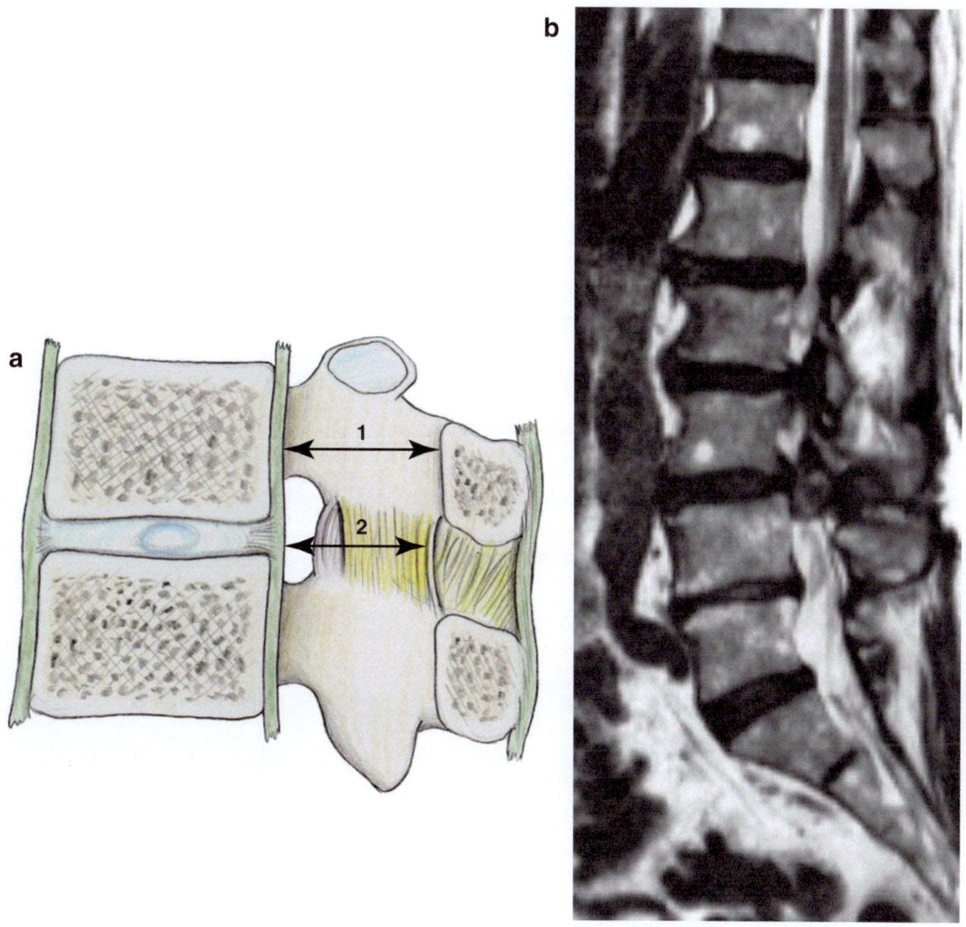

Fig. 10 The 2 median sagittal diameters: (**a**) Normal anatomy (1. FMSD, 2. MMSD); (**b**) Stenotic osteoarthritis at the MMSD

For Verbiest [5], there is absolute stenosis if the measurement (which at the time was performed intraoperatively) is less than 10 mm and relative stenosis if this measurement is between 10 and 12 mm. If the measurement is radiological, the canal is said to be wide if the FMSD is greater than 14 mm and narrow if it is less than 12 mm. Ullrich [6] sets the limit at 11.5 mm for the anteroposterior diameter, 16 mm for the interpedicular diameter, and 145 mm^2 for the surface area.

The shape of the lumbar spinal canal changes from L1 to L5; it is rather predominantly ovoid at its upper part (as at the cervical and thoracic levels). Due to the imprint of the articular processes which are becoming increasingly coronal, there appears a side portion of the spinal canal which is called lateral recess as described later. The lumbar canal thus becomes triangular (or deltoid, or trefoil), if the impression of the articular is more marked [2] (Fig. 11). It is as if the lumbar spinal canal tends to extend transversely and to shrink from front to back.

Beside the spinal canal, we can describe:

- the lateral recess which are a lateral expansion of the spinal canal,
- the intervertebral foramina, lateral openings towards the outside of the spinal canal,
- the transverse foramina that exists only at the cervical level and contains the vertebral artery.

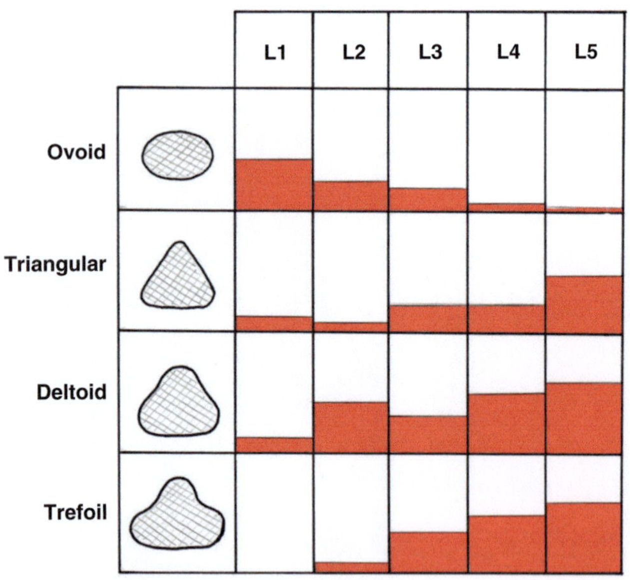

Fig. 11 Morphology of the central spinal canal according to the lumbar level [2]

The Lateral Recess

Described by Crock [7], *Lassale* [8], *and Vital* [9], *this is only an expansion of the vertebral foramen but which is very exposed to crowding in the case of osteoarthritis and thus to radicular compression in the lumbar region.*

It is defined as a lateral expansion of the spinal canal limited laterally by the pedicle and posteriorly by the articular facets; it is not entirely integral at the cervical and thoracic levels where the spinal canal is oval. It becomes increasingly marked as one descends the lumbar spine towards the lumbosacral junction where the impression of the S1 articular facet, oriented coronally, is marked in the lumbar spinal canal (Fig. 12).

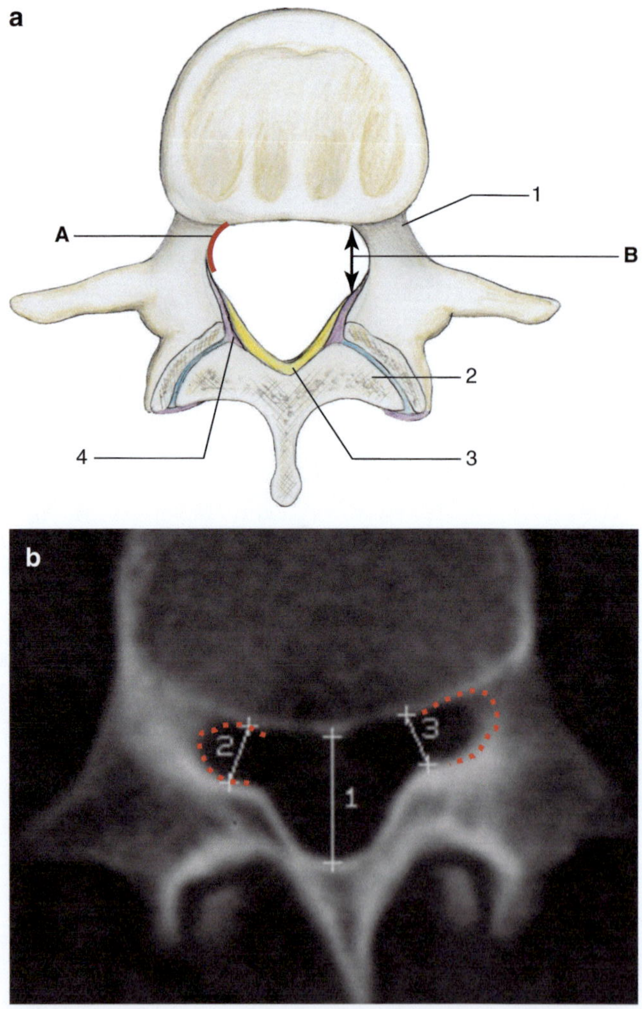

Fig. 12 (**a**) The lateral recess (horizontal section): A. pedicular and articular limits; B: Anteroposterior diameter; 1. Pedicle; 2. Lower articular process of the superjacent vertebra; 3. Yellow ligament; 4. Joint capsule. (**b**) The lateral recess (horizontal section in CT scan). 1. Central canal; 2. and 3. lateral recess

Considering the osseous morphology, the lateral recess is therefore limited laterally by the pedicle, anteriorly by the vertebral body directly within the pedicle, posteriorly by the superior articular facet, and inferiorly by the isthmus. We can thus oppose the lateral recess superior to the superior articular (pediculoarticular portion in tomodensimetry) and the lateral recess to the isthmus (pediculolamary portion) (Fig. 13).

The caudal edge of the transverse process corresponds to the limit of these two portions. According to Scoles [10], the anteroposterior diameter of the lateral recess which corresponds to the length of the pedicle decreases from L1 to L5 from 10 mm to 7.5 mm. The study by Lee [2] CT scan shows slightly higher values (12 mm and 8 mm from L1 to L5). In reality, the presence of the capsule and the yellow ligament, lining the articular facet, reduces this diameter to 8 mm on average.

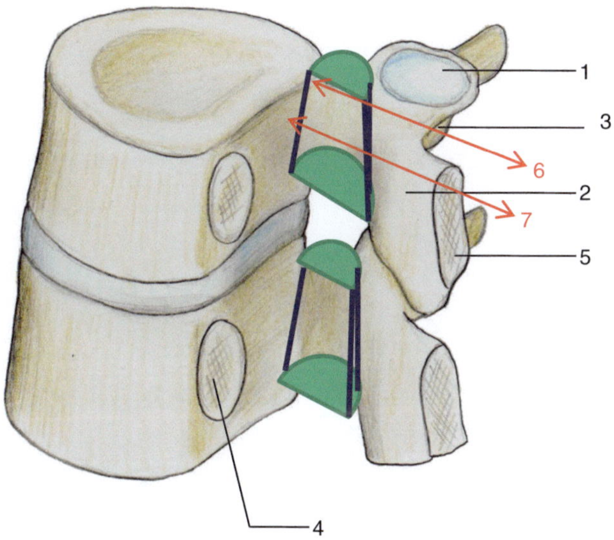

Fig. 13 The 2 parts of the posterior wall of the right lateral recess (intracanal view with removal of the left half of the neural arch after section at the level of the left pedicle (4) and the right lamina (5)): 1. Upper articular surface; 2. Isthmus; 3. Caudal edge of the transverse process; 4. Left pedicle; 5. Right lamina; 6. pediculoarticular; 7. pediculolamary portions of the lateral recess

In 3D, the recess is open-ended towards the midline and spinal canal and continues at the inferior border of the pedicle through the intervertebral foramina (Fig. 14).

The lumbar root after its departure from the dura, will first traverse posterior to the disc, then in the recess and finally in the intervertebral foramen.

From its exit from the dura mater to that of the spinal canal, the lumbar root traverses the root canal, which therefore comprises 3 portions from top to bottom (Fig. 15):

- Sub-pedicular (retro-discal)
- Para-pedicular (in the lateral recess)
- Infra-pedicular (in the intervertebral foramen).

The Intervertebral Foramen

In the lumbar region, it is the hidden area of MacNab, posterior surgical access is difficult.

Form and Orientation

It has a variable shape and orientation depending on the spinal level (Fig. 16).

- at the cervical level: it is a concave upwardly directed trough directed obliquely forwards and outwards with respect to the anteroposterior axis of the spine
- at the thoracic level: the foramen has a comma shape and faces directly outwards
- at the lumbar level: the foramen has an ear shape and also faces directly outwards.

Fig. 14 Schematic 3D the right lateral recess

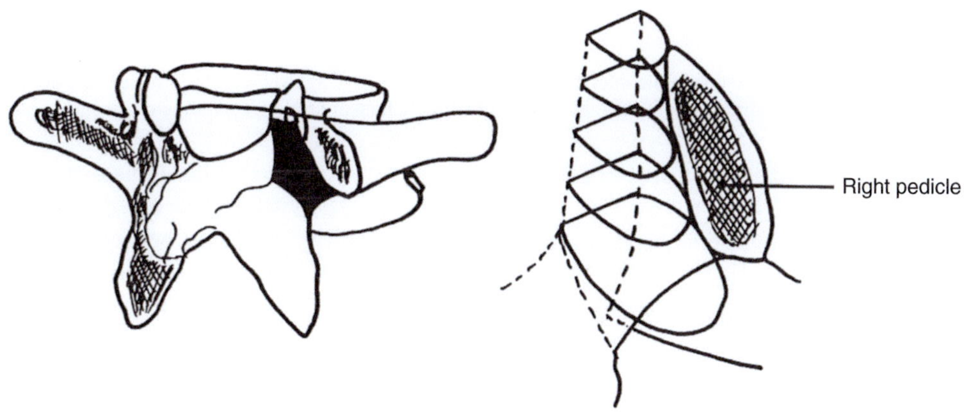

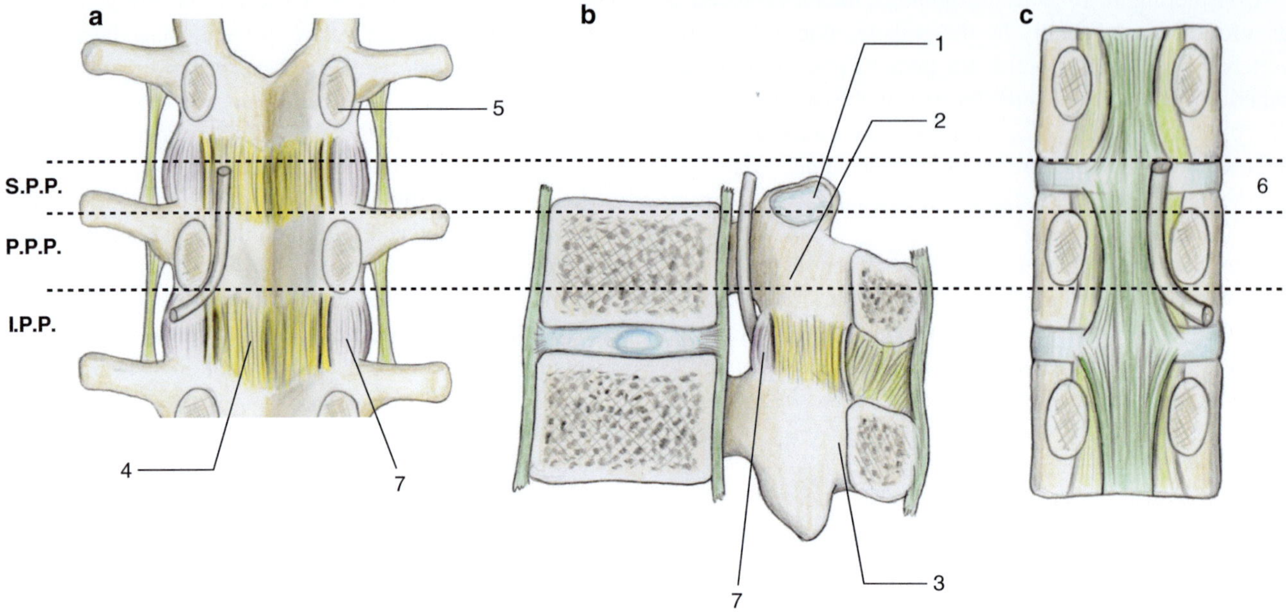

Fig. 15 The root canal: (**a**) Anterior view after removal of the vertebral body. (**b**) Intracanal view. (**c**) Rear view after removal of the neural arch: 1. Upper articular; 2. Isthmus; 3. Lamina; 4. Yellow ligament; 5. Pedicle; 6. Disc space. 7. articular capsule. *SPP* subpedicular portion, *PPP* parapedicular portion, *IPP* infrapedicular portion

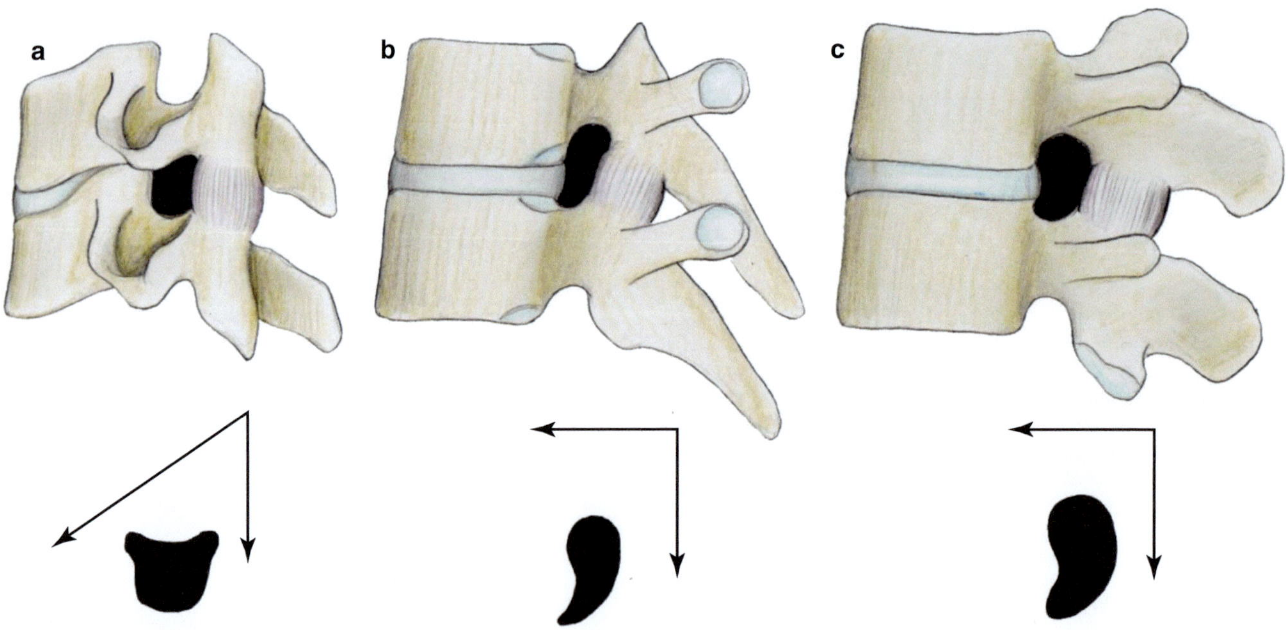

Fig. 16 Shape and orientation of the intervertebral foramina: (**a**) Cervical level = gutter directed forward and outward (3/4 view). (**b**) At the thoracic level = "comma" directed outward (lateral view). (**c**) In the lumbar level = "ear" directed outward (lateral view)

The Cervical Intervertebral Foramen

It is actually a conjugation canal directed 60° forward and outward with respect to the anteroposterior axis; a true root gutter, it has an average length of 7 mm and has three portions from within outwards:

- pedicular: limited anteromedially by the uncus and containing the anterior and posterior roots
- articular: between the articular process posteriorly and the transverse foramen anteriorly and containing the spinal ganglion

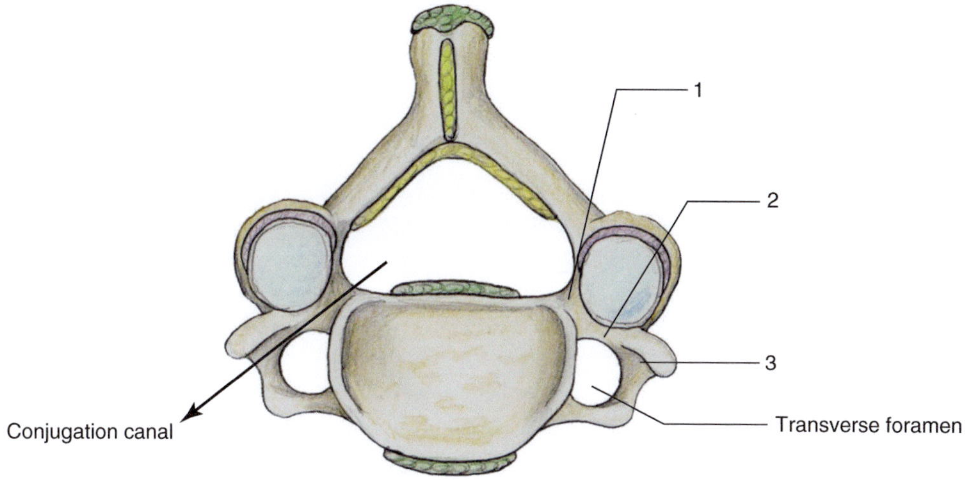

Fig. 17 The 3 portions of the cervical intervertebral foramen: 1. Pedicle; 2. Articular; 3. Transverse

- transverse: corresponding to the process of the same name with its two anterior and posterior tubercles (Fig. 17) and containing the spinal nerve which is divided into its two ventral and dorsal branches.

The Lumbar Intervertebral Foramen

This foramen may also be considered as a canal especially in the lower lumbar area because the pedicles of the lower lumbar vertebrae are not vertical but oblique inferolaterally (Fig. 18). In reality, this oblique portion of the inner surface of the pedicle is rather part of the lateral recess and one can consider that the foramen begins at the inferior border of the pedicle.

Figure 19 shows the limits: pedicles upper and lower at the top and bottom, lateral part of the disc in front, superior articular process of the vertebra underlying, and isthmus of the vertebra overlying covered by capsule and ligamentum yellow, posteriorly. On this sagittal section, with its fat content, we find the root at the top of the foramen that wraps around the superior pedicle with the spinal artery, sinuvertebral nerve, root, and foraminal veins. The anterior and posterior limits of the foramena must be distinguished in 2 portions:

- the first is superior and it is fixed anteriorly by the lateral vertebral body covered by the lateral part of the dorsal longitudinal ligament (epidural membrane or periosteum of Wiltse), behind the isthmus (pars interarticularis), and the anterior part of the lamina.
- the second is inferior and mobile; it is limited by the underlying disc anteriorly and posteriorly through the articular mass, mainly by the superior articular process of the underlying vertebra, in its medial part, covered by the articular capsule and the yellow ligament which are in continuity.

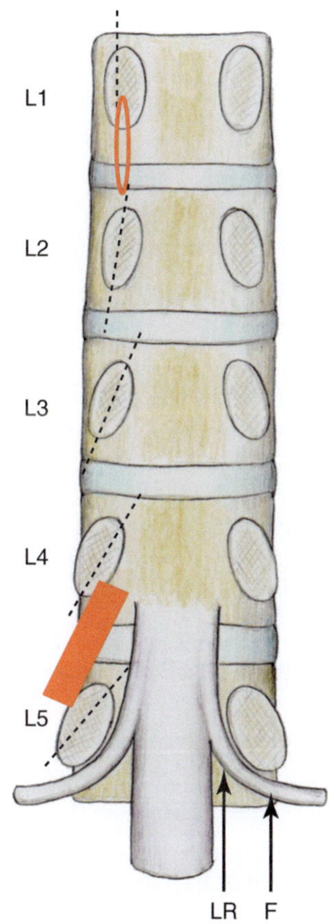

Fig. 18 Variable orientation of pedicles L1–L5 transforming the foramen, with a true hole at L1L2 but a canal at L4L5; thus, the position of the Lateral Recess (LR) and Foramen (F) at the inferior border of the pedicle regardless of its orientation

So, like the vertebral foramen presents 2 sagittal diameters, fixed opposite the vertebral body and mobile opposite the disc, the intervertebral foramen also presents 2 sagittal diameters, opposite the vertebral body below the pedicle and opposite the underlying disc; the fixed part is generally wider than the moving part, giving a general shape in inverted pear or auricular.

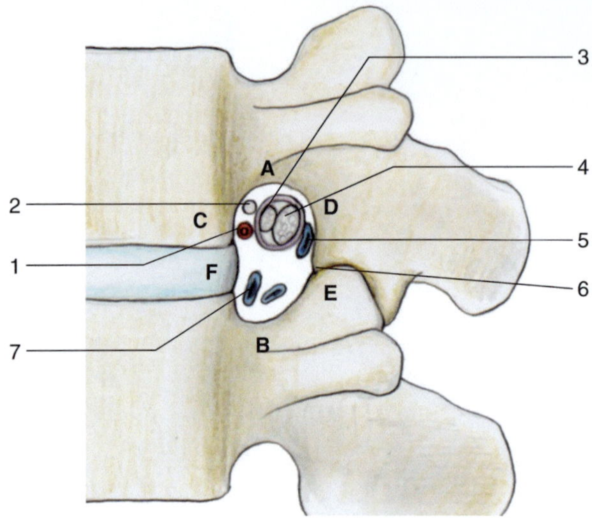

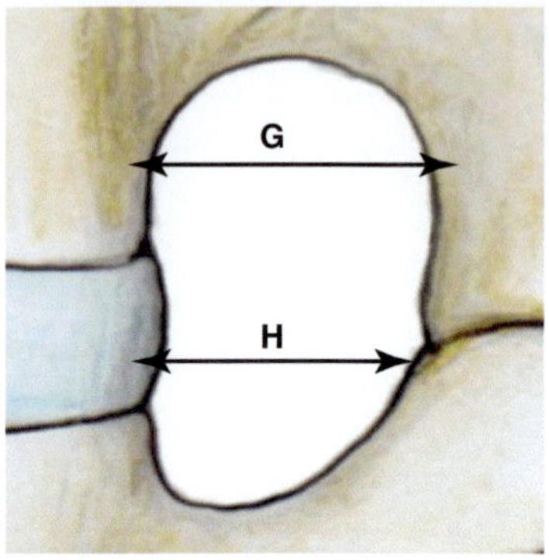

Fig. 19 The lumbar intervertebral foramen. Limits: A. Superior pedicle; B. Inferior pedicle; C. Superior vertebral body; D. Isthmus; E. Superior Articular Process of the lower vertebra; F. Disc; G. Fixed portion of the foramen; H. Mobile portion of the foramen. Contents: 1. Root artery; 2. Sinuvertebral nerve; 3. Anterior root; 4. Posterior root; 5. Radicular vein; 6. Joint capsule; 7. Foraminal venous plexus

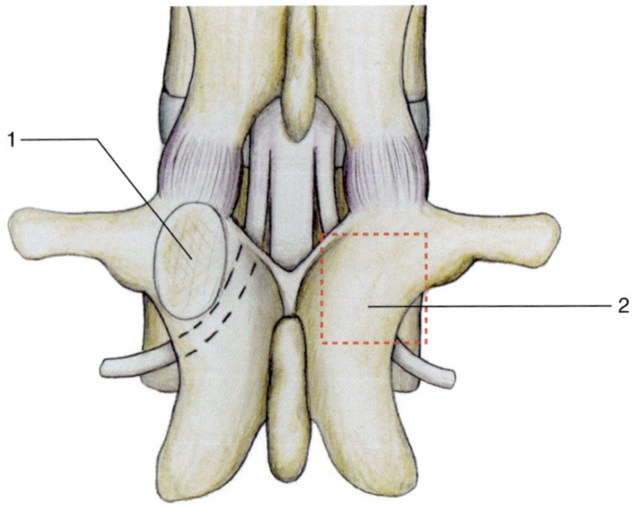

Fig. 20 The roof of the foramen (back view), "hidden zone" of MacNab. 1. Projection of the pedicle; 2. Hidden area

The roof (or posterior wall of the intervertebral foramina) is mainly composed of the lamina and the isthmus, which make it the "hidden zone" of MacNab (Fig. 20) [11], difficult to access surgically (Fig. 21a).

The vertical ridge that laterally limit the lamina and the isthmus is more or less lateral with respect to the pedicle and thus the roof covering more or less to the intervertebral foramen: this ridge extends in fact increasingly laterally as and has as one descends to the L5S1 hinge (Fig. 21b, c).

The area of the intervertebral foramen ranges from 41.5 mm^2 to 164 mm^2. The L5S1 foramen has the largest area, then L2L3 foramen, then L3L4, L4L5, and finally L1L2. The height varies from 10.3 to 19.5 mm, the L1L2 foramen having the smallest height. Finally, the anteroposterior diameter is 8 mm on average.

De Peretti [12] has studied, at all spinal levels, the percentage of occupation of the structures, particularly the nervous structures, in the intervertebral foramen: it is 34.4% at C6, 29.5% at T1, 23% at T6, 26.9% at L1, 18.9% at L3, and 19.3% at L5. Overall, the nerve elements do not exceed 1/3 of the intervertebral foramen surface.

The Transverse Canal

The transverse canal is constituted by foramena situated at the middle part of the transverse processes of C7–C1 (Fig. 17): the transverse canal is where the vertebral arteries pass, starting at C6. In C7, only the vertebral vein passes through the transverse foramen (Fig. 22).

Between transverse processes, the canal is closed by intertransverse muscles anteriorly and posteriorly (Fig. 23). The artery progresses with the vertebral venous plexus and the vegetative nerve of François Franck. The spinal nerve passes behind the artery and gives anterior and posterior branches.

The Spinal Canals and the Movements of the Column

All spinal canals, regardless of the level, have an anteroposterior diameter which decreases in extension and increases in flexion

At the same time, according to a well-known radiculomedullary dynamic, the rootlets, and nerves advance towards the column of bodies and discs in flexion and retreat towards the posterior arc in extension (Fig. 24).

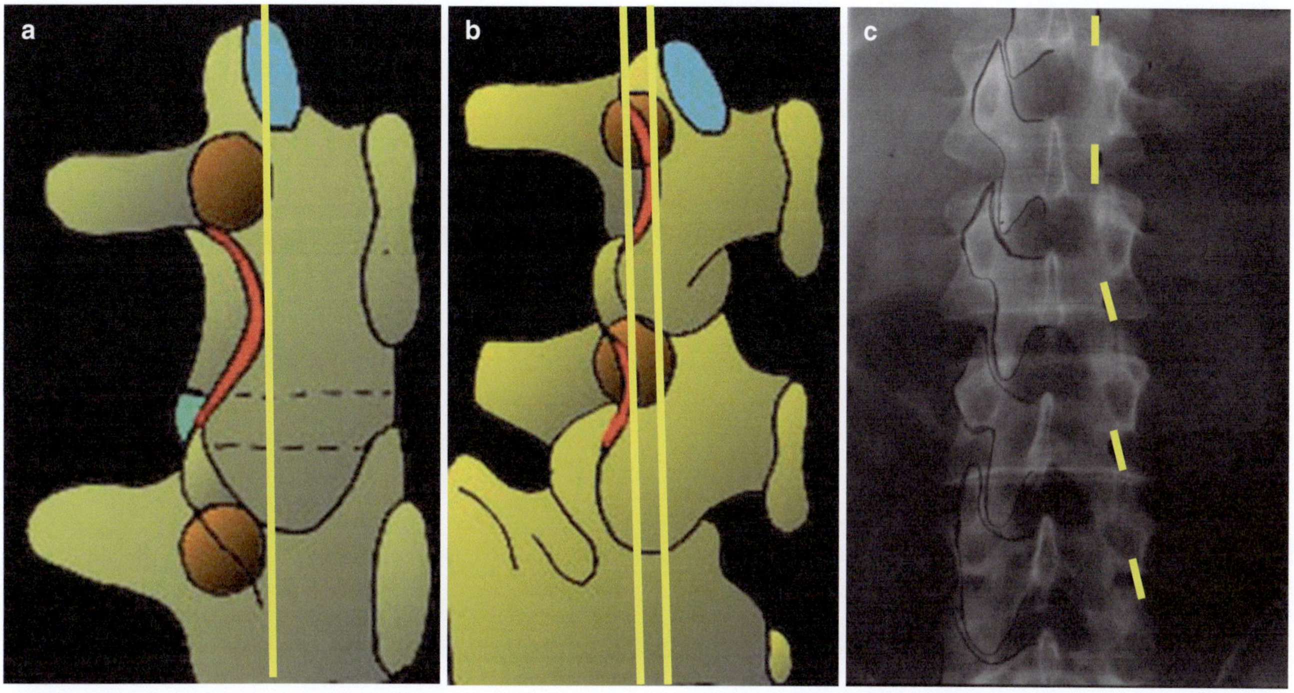

Fig. 21 The roof of the foramen (dorsal view) (Sénégas). (**a**) high lumbar, the lamina is not very overlapping (the lateral crest, in red, of the lamina is in medial position relative to the pedicle). (**b**) at L5 the lamina extends more laterally. (**c**) Yellow boundary of the lateral roofs of the intervertebral foramina L1 to L5

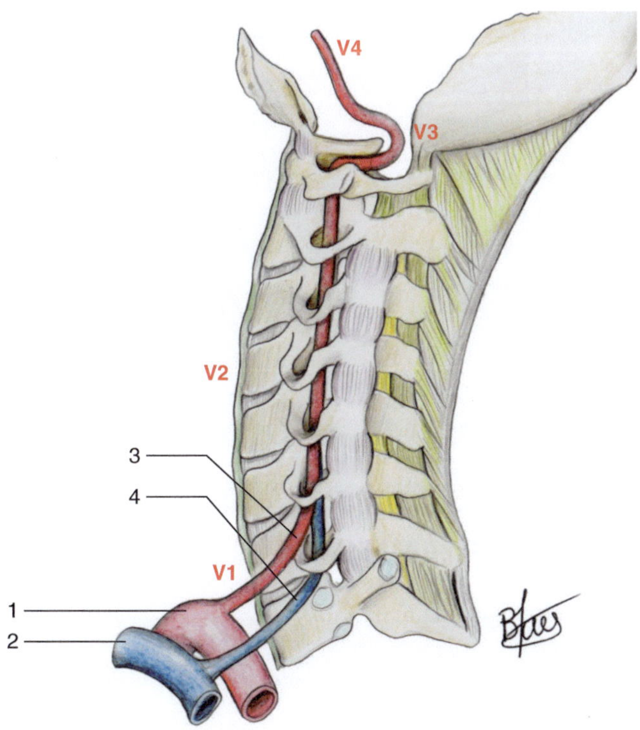

Fig. 22 The transverse canal (left side view): 1. Subclavian artery; 2. Subclavian vein; 3. Vertebral artery with the 4 portions V1, V2, V3, and V4; 4. Vertebral vein

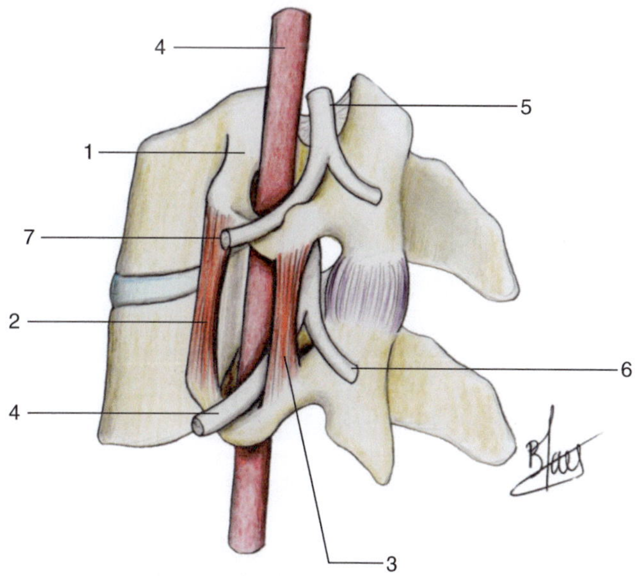

Fig. 23 The transverse canal (left lateral view, enlarged). 1. Transverse process; 2. Ventral intertransverse muscle; 3. Intertransverse dorsal muscle; 4. Vertebral artery; 5. Spinal nerve; 6. Posterior branch; 7. Anterior branch

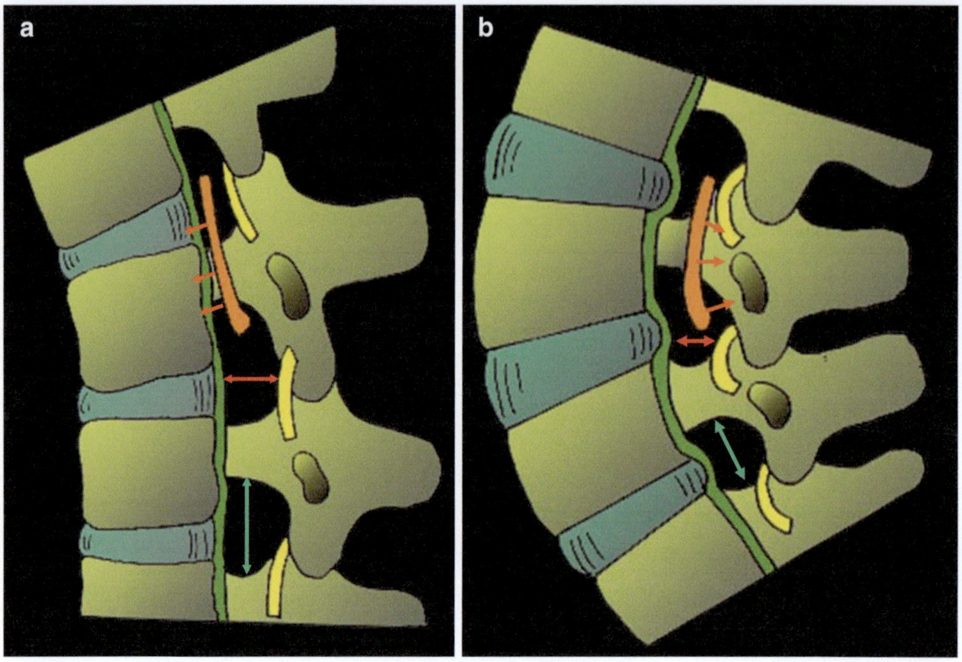

Fig. 24 Root displacement and spinal canal size variation in flexion (**a**) and extension (**b**)

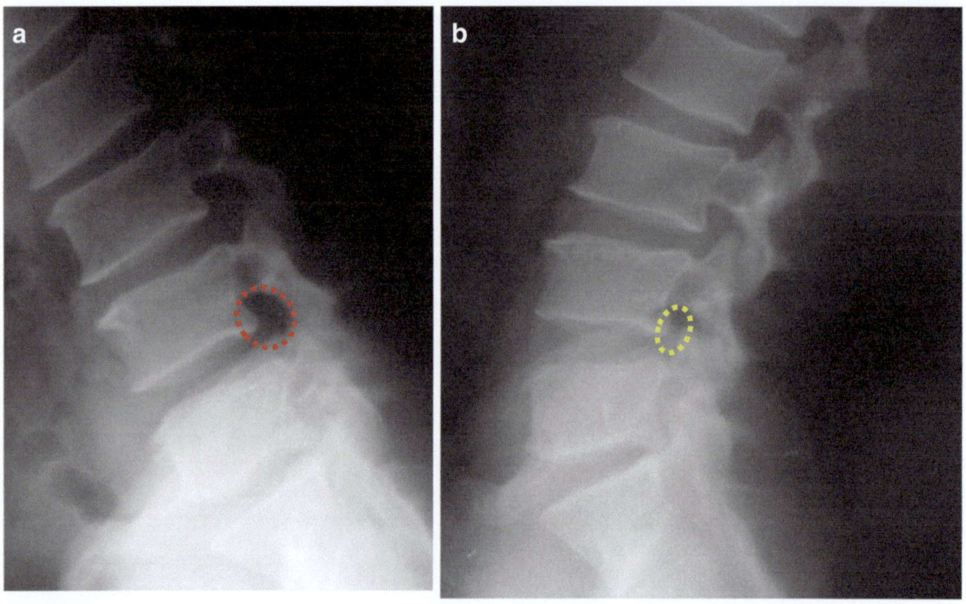

Fig. 25 Comparison of the size of the intervertebral foramina in flexion (**a**) and extension (**b**)

This explains the aggravation of cervicobrachial compressive osteoarthritic neuralgia with neck extension and improvement of lower limb claudication in the narrow lumbar canal in flexion or lumbar kyphosis. Radiographic images standing in extension with (Fig. 25) or without opaque product injection (saccoradiculography or myelography, Fig. 26) allow visualization of this dynamic compression.

Degenerative Pathology and the Effects on the Spinal Canals

In degenerative pathology, especially lumbar pathology, we can observe:

Herniated discs (already described with the intervertebral disc)

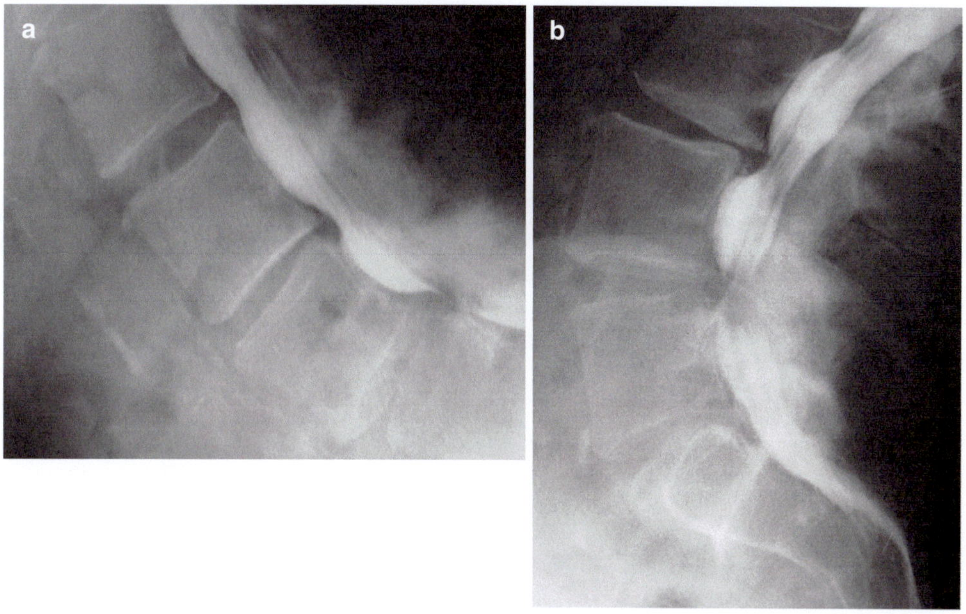

Fig. 26 Reduction of the central canal size in L3L4 and L4L5 on a saccoradiculography image in extension (**b**) with respect to flexion (**a**)

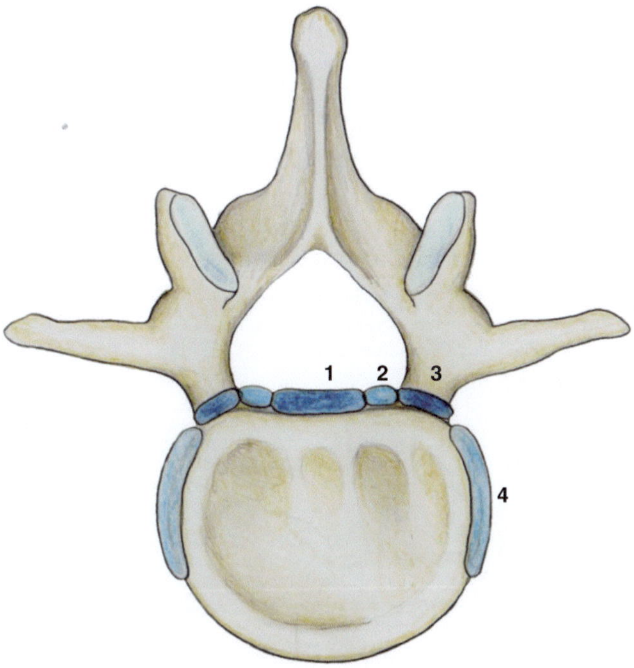

Fig. 27 Possible location of herniated discs in the horizontal plane. 1. Median; 2. Posterolateral (in the lateral recess or intraforaminal, within the pedicle); 3. Foraminal (above the pedicle); 4. Extraforaminal (outside the pedicle)

Figures 27 and 28 represent their location, in the horizontal plane (Fig. 27) and on a posterior view (Fig. 28): which are rarely median since the posterior longitudinal ligament has a protective role in the midline, are most often posterolateral (compared to the lateral recess, within the pedicles, and therefore in the intraforaminal position), less often foraminal (perpendicular to the pedicles), and more rarely extraforaminal (outside the pedicles).

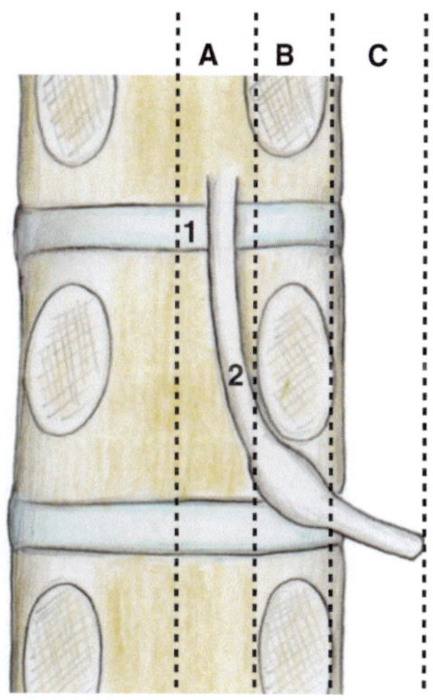

Fig. 28 Possible location of herniated discs on a posterior view taking into account the intervertebral foramen: A: Intraforaminal (1. Retrodiscal space 2. Lateral recess). B: Foraminal. C: Extraforaminal

Spinal Canal and Lateral Recess

This can be reduced in size by (Fig. 29):

- a hypertrophy of the articular facets
- a hypertrophy of the articular facets and disc herniation
- a congenital narrowing including short pedicles.

The Intervertebral Foramen

Tanaka [13] has described the anatomical relationships of the spinal roots and nerves in spinal intervertebral foramina and their consequences in degenerative pathology. The disc collapse associated with joint hypertrophy leads, in the osteoarthritic process, to a closure of the intervertebral foramen (Fig. 30). Any process leading to disc kyphosis will open the foramen, while an extensional retrolisthesis will close it (Fig. 31). In lumbar spondylolisthesis (SPL), the intervertebral foramen is more horizontalized than collapsed if the SPL is degenerative (the main compression being in the central canal and the lateral recesses) (Figs. 32 and 33). Alternatively the foramen is clearly narrowed in the lytic SPL (Figs. 34 and 35), the root of the level of the cephalad olisthetic vertebra that can be compressed by the isthmic hook, the cartilaginous nodule (Gill), and very exceptionally by the L5S1 disc which is more stretched than herniated. Finally, asymmetric disc disease is a characteristic cause of foraminal compression (Figs. 36 and 37); it can be primitive, secondary to a discectomy or ipsilateral lumbar scoliosis: it is then in the lumbosacral concavity (the side of the convexity of the main lumbar curvature) and can be expected with significant intervertebral displacement and subluxation (Vital [14]).

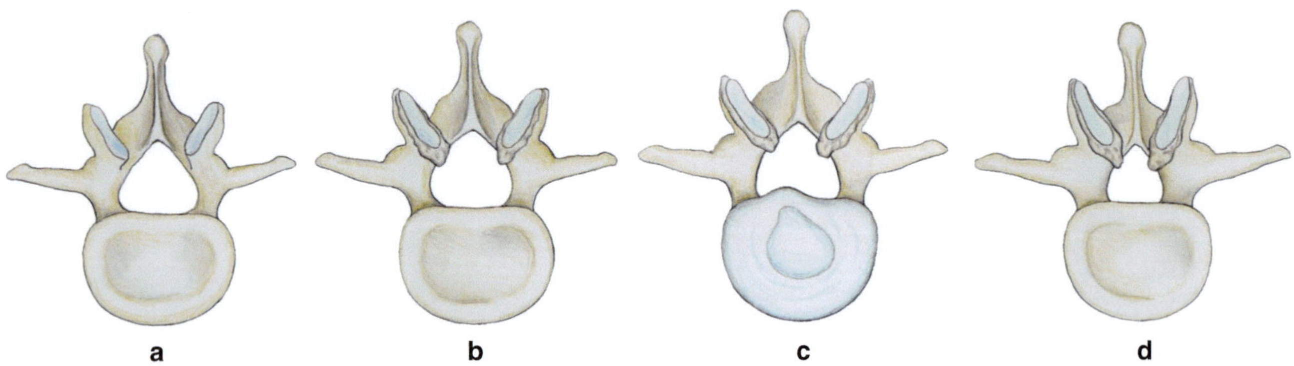

Fig. 29 Reductions in the central spinal canal and lateral recess in degenerative lumbar pathology. (**a**) Normal anatomy; (**b**) Articular arthrosis; (**c**) Osteoarthritis and hernia; (**d**) Congenital narrowing and osteoarthritis

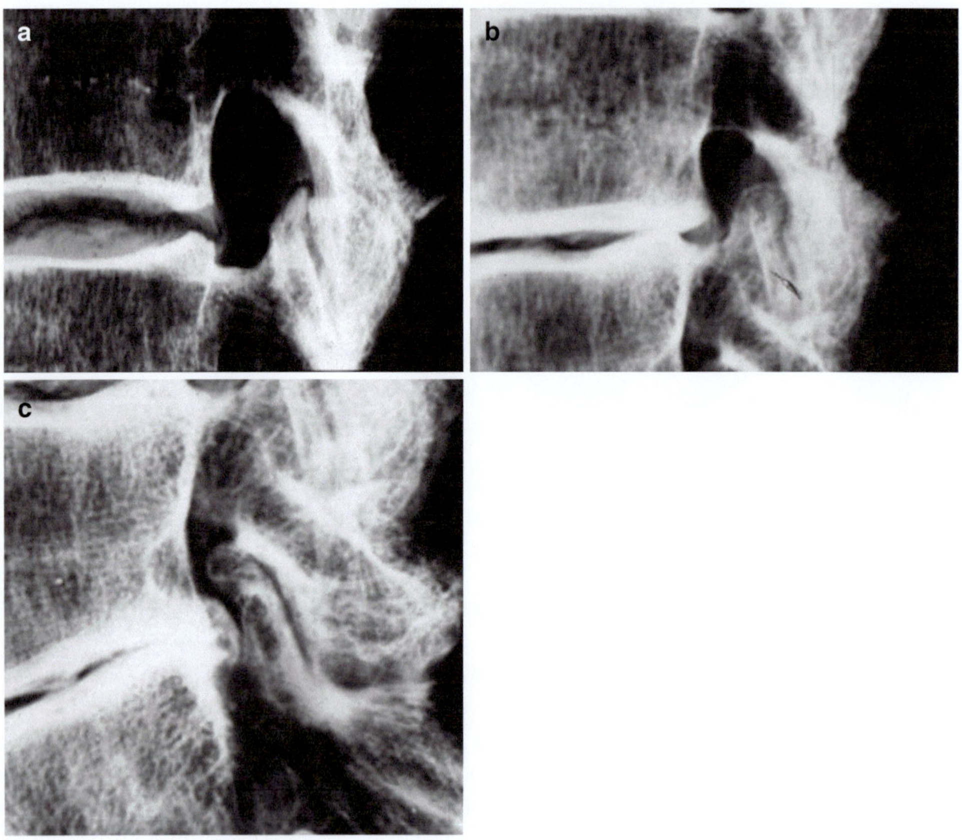

Fig. 30 Progressive reduction from (**a**) to (**c**), the size of the intervertebral foramen parallel to the disc collapse

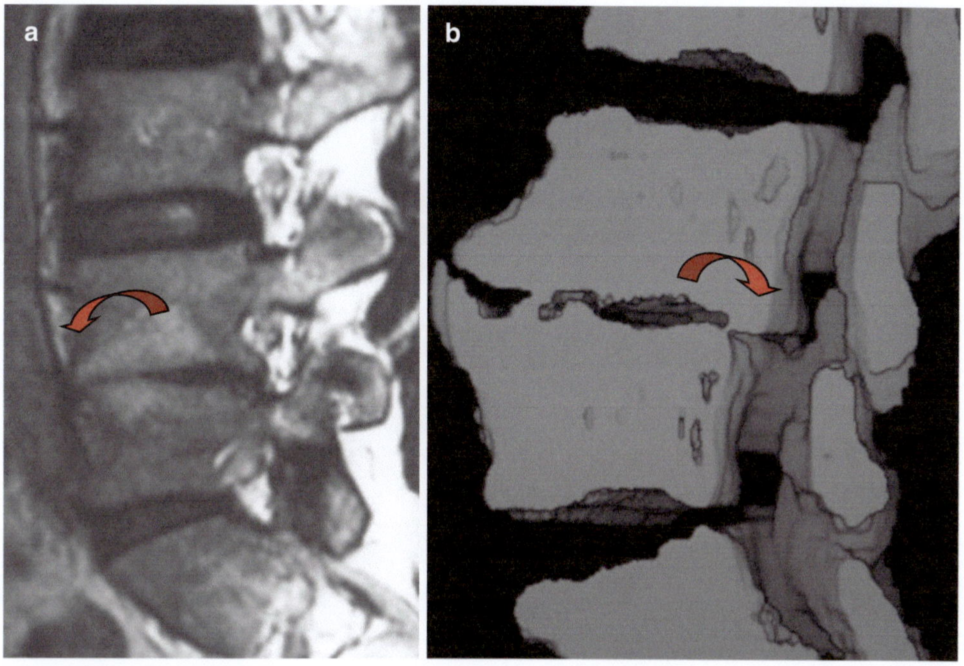

Fig. 31 Intervertebral foramen enlarged by disc kyphosis (**a**) and reduced in size by retrolisthesis in extension (**b**)

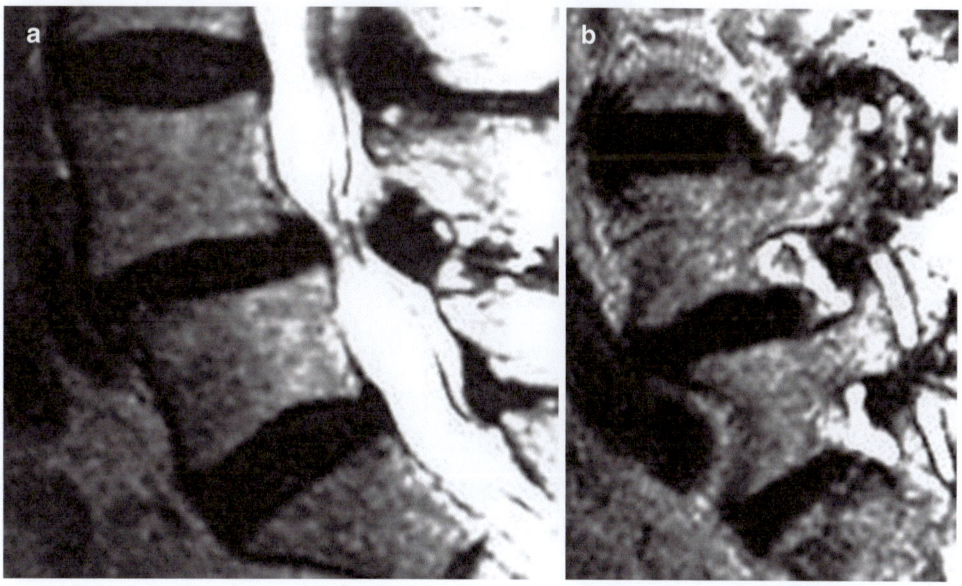

Fig. 32 Intervertebral foramen and degenerative spondylolisthesis on sagittal sections: (**a**) central stenosis; (**b**) horizontalized intervertebral foramen

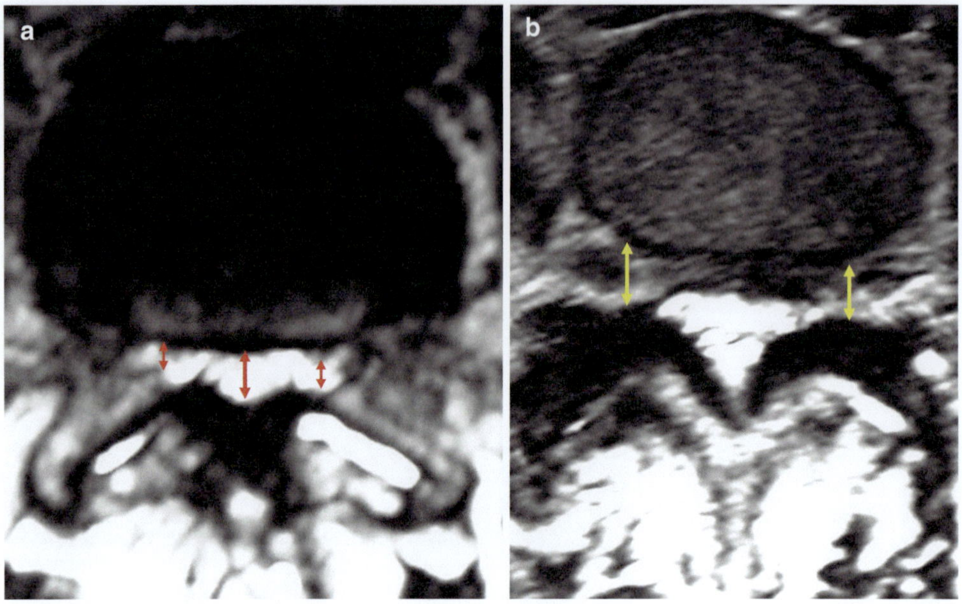

Fig. 33 Intervertebral foramen and degenerative spondylolisthesis on axial sections: (**a**) central stenosis and in the lateral recess; (**b**) intervertebral foramen not shrunk

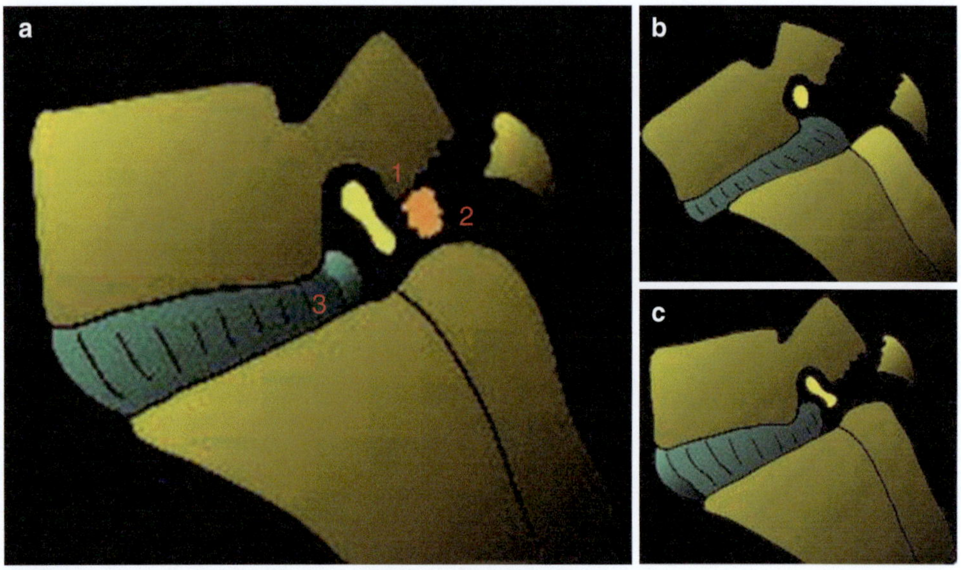

Fig. 34 Intervertebral foramen and spondylolisthesis by isthmic lysis. (**a**) the 3 possible compressive elements—the isthmic hook (1), the nodule of Gill (2), more rarely the disc (3); (**b**) flexion displacement; (**c**) extension displacement, more compressive

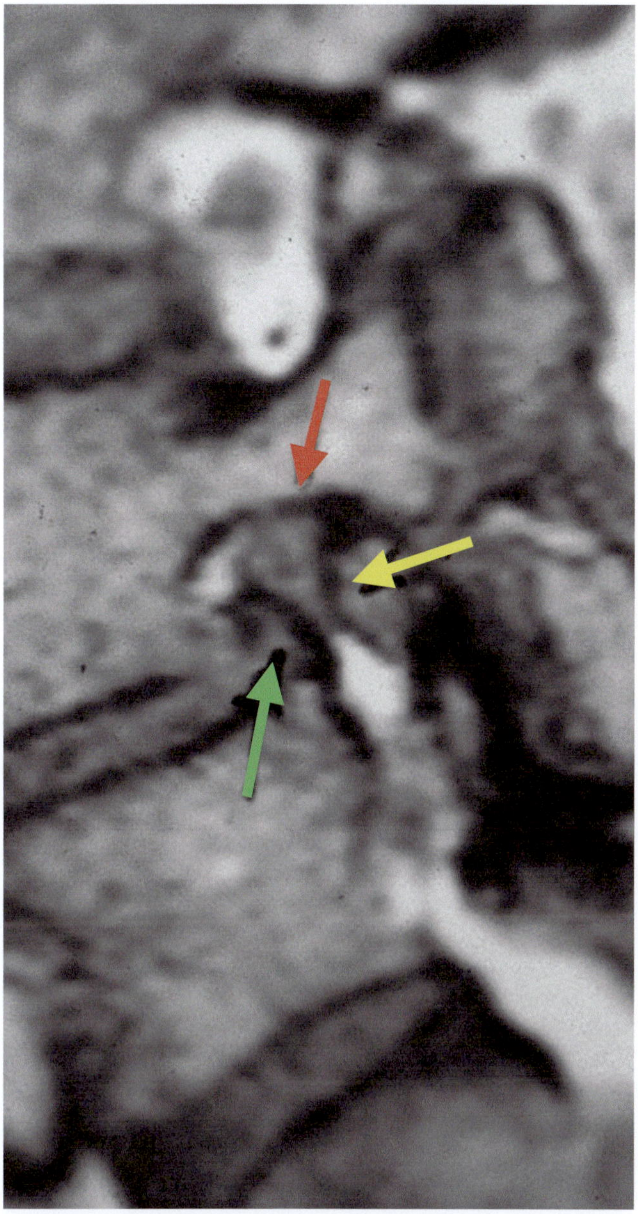

Fig. 35 Intervertebral foramen and spondylolisthesis by isthmic lysis on a sagittal section on MRI

Fig. 36 Asymmetrical discopathy on an anteroposterior radiograph (**a**) and its consequence on the nerve structures (**b**)

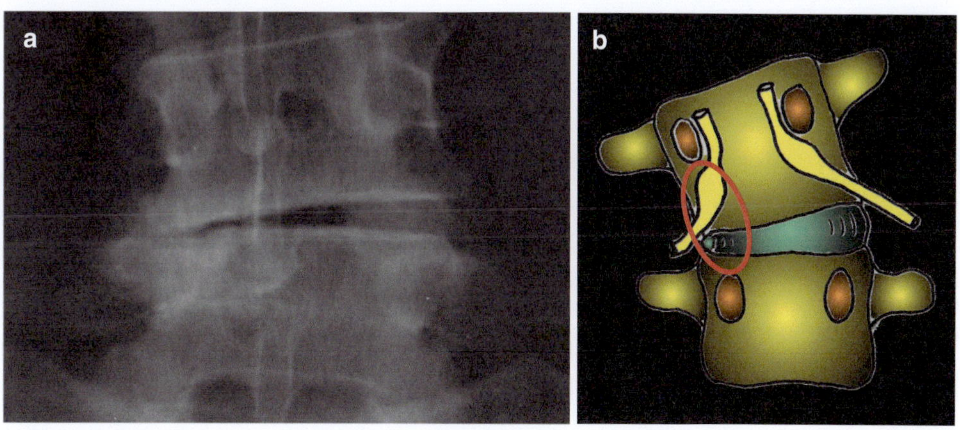

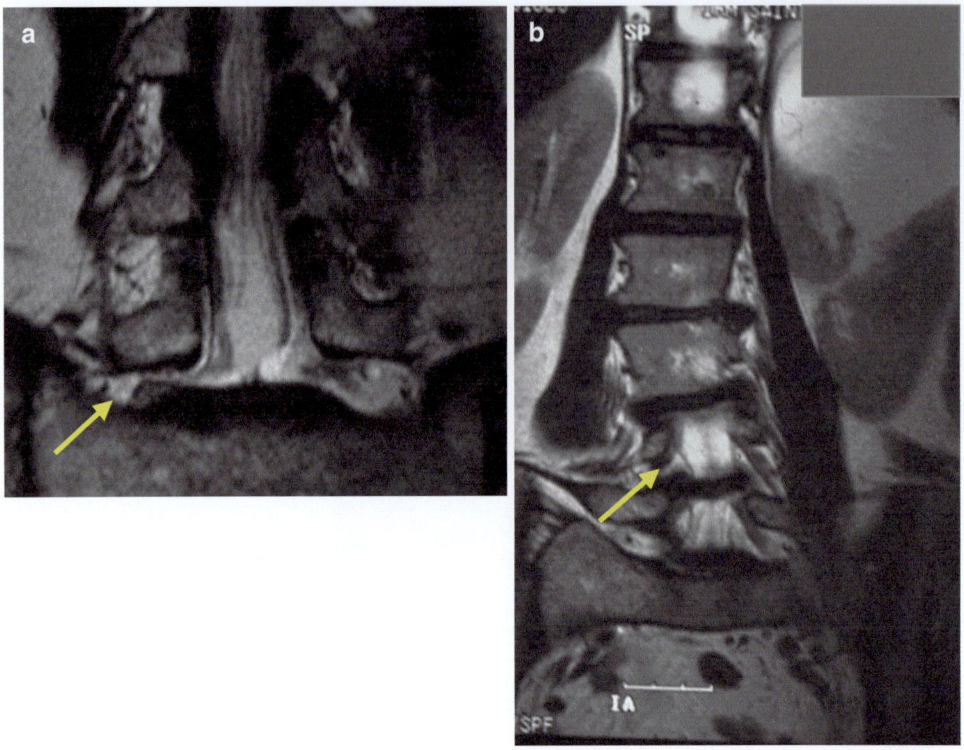

Fig. 37 Primary asymmetric disc disease in MRI (**a**) and at the base of the scoliosis (**b**)

References

1. Dimeglio A, Bonnel F. Le rachis en croissance. Paris: Springer; 1990.
2. Lee BCP, Kazam E, Newman AD. Computed tomography of spine and spinal cord. Radiology. 1978;128:95–102.
3. Wackenheim A. Roentgen diagnosis of the cranio-vertebral region. Berlin: Springer; 1994.
4. Pavlov H, Torg JS, Robie B, Jahre C. Cervical spinal stenosis: determination with vertebral ratio method. Radiology. 1987;164:771–5.
5. Verbiest M. A radicular syndrome from developmental narrowing of the lumbar vertebral canal. J Bone Joint Surg. 1954;36B:230–7.
6. Ullrich CG, Binet EF, Sanecki MG, Kieffer SA. Quantitative assessment of the lumbar spinal canal by the computed tomography. Radiology. 1980;134:137–43.
7. Crock HV. Normal and pathological anatomy of the lumbar spinal nerve roots canal. J Bone Joint Surg. 1981;63B:487–90.
8. Lassale B, Morvan G, Gottin M. Anatomy and radiological anatomy of the lumbar radicular canals. Anat Clin. 1984;6:195–201.
9. Vital JM, Lavignolle B, Grenier N, Rouais F, Malgat R, Senegas J. Anatomy of the lumbar radicular canal. Anat Clin. 1983;5:141–51.
10. Scoles PV, Linton AE, Latimer B, Levy ME, Digio-Vanni BF. Vertebral body and posterior element morphology; the normal spine in middle life. Spine. 1988;13:1082–6.
11. MacNab J, Mac Culloch J. Bachache. 2nd ed. Baltimore: Williams & Wilkins; 1990.
12. De Peretti F, Hovorka I, Ganansia P, Puch JM, Bourgeon A, Argenson C. The vertebral foramen: a report concerning its contents. Surg Radiol Anat. 1993;15:287–94.
13. Tanaka N, Fujimoto Y, An HS, Ikuta Y, Yasuda M. The anatomic relation among the nerve roots, intervertebral foramina and intervertebral disc of the cervical spine. Spine. 2000;25:286–91.
14. Vital JM. Foramen lumbar intervertebral. Anatomy, exploration and pathology. In: Teaching conference. SOFCOT 2000. Paris: Elsevier; 2000. p. 139–63.

The Spinal Cord

J. Guérin

The spinal cord is the part of the neuraxis contained in the spinal canal. It extends from the foramen magnum where it follows the medulla oblonga to the L1L2 vertebrae forming the conus medullaris (Fig. 1).

It has a cylindrical appearance, slightly flattened from front to back. Its average diameter is 1 cm, less than that of the spinal canal, which gives it a relative freedom in the axial plane. It is about 45 cm long and occupies 2/3 of the spinal canal, anchored at its lower end by a fibrous structure, the filum terminale to the coccygeal vertebra and laterally by the denticulate ligament. It comprises two fusiform swellings: the cervical enlargement, corresponding to the nervous structures involved in the innervation of the upper limbs, and the lumbar enlargement, corresponding to the lower limbs.

It is protected by the meningeal envelopes that form a continuous sheath (Fig. 2). The dura mater is the outermost, fibrous in nature, it terminates next to S3 and engages the spinal nerves up to the intervertebral foramen. The arachnoid represents the intermediate covering. It delineates the subarachnoid space filled with cerebrospinal fluid and in anatomical continuity with the peri-cerebral meningeal spaces. Thus CSF analysis by simple lumbar puncture makes it possible to detect the presence of an inflammatory or hemorrhagic pathology and to analyze the pressure of the entire fluid compartment. The pia mater adheres to the surface of nerve structures; it is a vascular membrane.

The spinal cord is connected to the peripheral nervous system by the spinal nerve roots whose regular emission marks a metameric organization mode in superimposed segments. There are 31 pairs of spinal nerves born from the union of ventral motor roots and dorsal sensory roots: 8 cervical, 12 thoracic, 5 lumbar, 5 sacral, 1 coccygeal.

During fetal life, the spine elongates more than the spinal cord which remains fixed at its cranial extremity so that if the cervical nerves lie in the same plane as the corresponding vertebra, as one goes down, they incline more and more to reach the corresponding intervertebral foramen, resulting in a vertebra-medullary shift of two levels for the thoracic roots

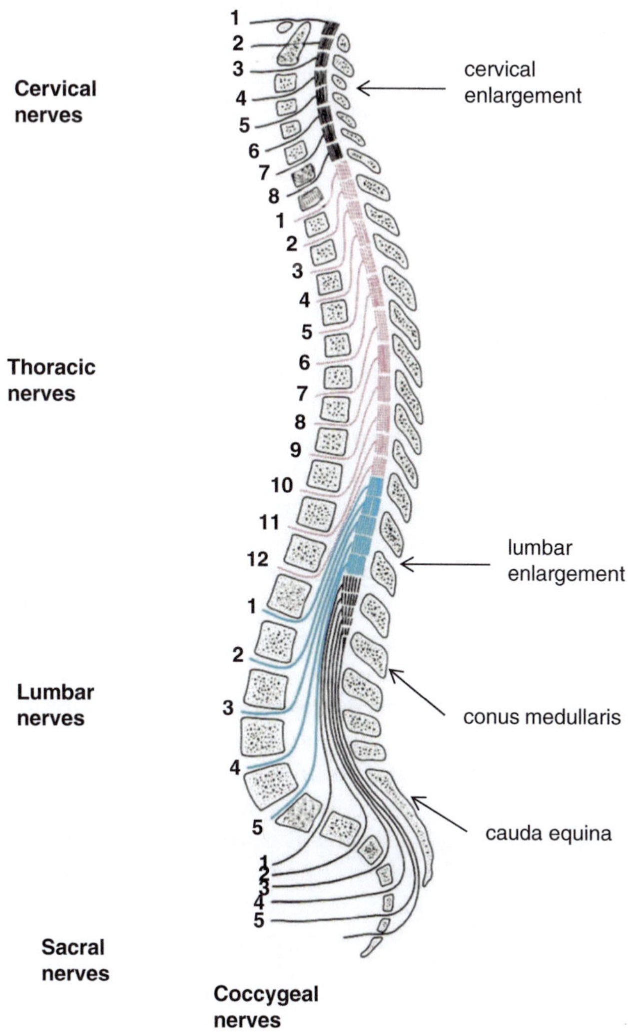

Fig. 1 Organization of the spinal cord in metameric segments. Relationships with vertebrae and spinal nerves

J. Guérin (✉)
Department of Neurosurgery, CHU Bordeaux, Bordeaux, France

J. M. Vital, D. T. Cawley (eds.), *Spinal Anatomy*, https://doi.org/10.1007/978-3-030-20925-4_24

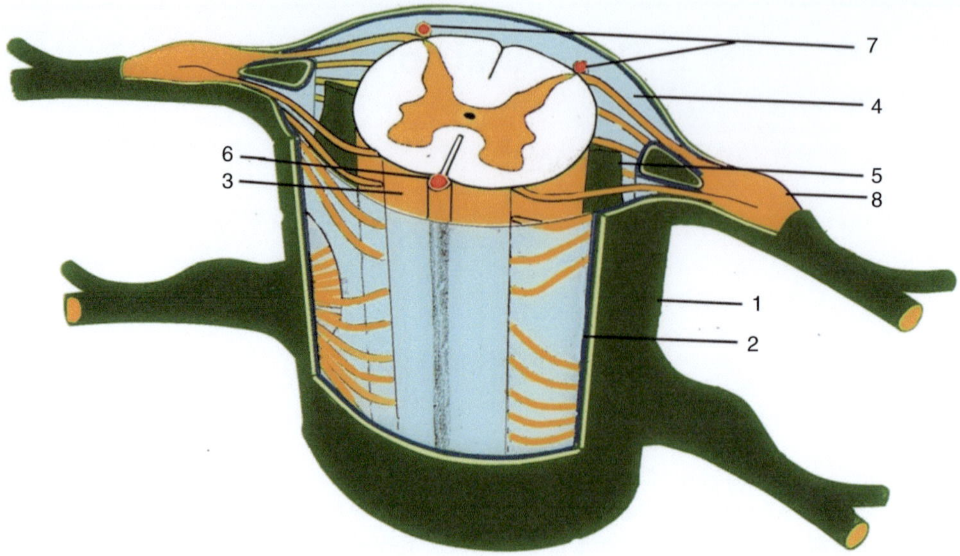

Fig. 2 The spinal cord and meningeal envelopes: (1) dura mater, (2) arachnoid, (3) pia mater, (4) subarachnoid space, (5) denticulate ligament, (6) anterior spinal artery, (7) posterior spinal arteries, (8) spinal ganglion

and more than three levels in the lumbosacral section, the conus medullaris projecting opposite T12L1. Below, the roots gather to form the cauda equina that occupies the lumbosacral space, thus allowing lumbar puncture without risk of causing spinal cord injury.

Description

The spinal cord is constituted (Fig. 3) by a peripheral white matter and a central gray matter:

- The white matter contains the ascending and descending nerve fibers that form tracts that connect the spinal cord to the other sections of the neuraxis. It is organized along an axis of sagittal symmetry which is marked on the surface, anteriorly by the medial anterior sulcus (ventral medial fissure) and posteriorly by the posterior medial sulcus (dorsal medial fissure), narrower and in contact with the gray matter. On both sides of this midline plane, the ventrolateral sulcus corresponds to the emergence of the ventral roots of the spinal nerves and the dorsolateral sulcus to that of the dorsal roots. These sulci delineate funiculi or columns of white matter: the dorsal (or posterior) column is located between the posterior medial sulcus and the posterior collateral sulcus. It is subdivided at the level of the cervical segments by an intermediate dorsal sulcus into a lateral tract, inserted as a wedge, the cuneatus fasciculus (Burdach) and an inner tract, the gracilis fasciculus (Goll). The lateral column is delimited by the ventral and dorsal collateral sulci. The anterior columns are located on both sides of the median fissure and communicate with each other by the ventral white commissure.
- The gray matter contains the cells and the nerve centers. It is also arranged along an axis of sagittal symmetry which gives it the shape of an "X" or a "butterfly with spread wings."
- It is described (Figs. 4 and 5) as:
  1. Dorsal or posterior horns do not reach the circumferential edge of the cord where the sensory fibers contained in the dorsal roots of the spinal nerves arrive by the collateral dorsal sulcus. They are separated in the dorsolateral fasciculus of Lissauer that lies in the interval between the surface of the cord and the apex of the dorsal horn. The nucleus proprius occupies most of it, covered by the clearer gelatinous substance (substantia gelatinosa) and the more distal marginal zone (or substantia spongiosa) which forms as a hood. The nucleus dorsalis (Clarke's column) is recognizable on the posterior edge of the base of the dorsal horns, only at segments C8 to L2.
  2. Ventral or anterior horns are larger. Their jagged edges remain at a distance from the circumferential edge and correspond to the passage of nerve fibers for motor purposes which exit through the ventral collateral sulcus and will constitute the ventral roots of the spinal nerves. They are characterized by the presence of motor neurons grouped in nuclei which are arranged in juxtaposed columns (Fig. 6):
- The medial nuclei are present throughout the cord. They correspond to the innervation of the cervical, thoracic, and abdominal axial musculature.
- The lateral nuclei are mainly developed at the level of the cervical and lumbar swellings. They correspond to the innervation of the limbs and are arranged according to a double plan of organization: one is functional and corresponds to the ventral nuclei for the extensor muscles and to the dorsal nuclei for the flexor muscles, the

other is somatotopic: the medial columns correspond to the axial musculature of the limb roots, the lateral columns to the proximal musculature of the elbow and

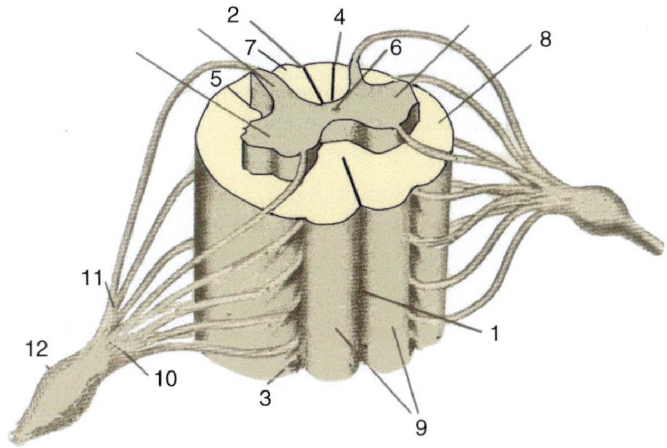

Fig. 3 Configuration of the spinal cord: (1) medial ventral sulcus; (2) medial dorsal sulcus; (3) ventral collateral sulcus; (4) dorsal intermediate septum; (5) dorsal collateral sulcus; (6) ependymal canal; (7) dorsal funiculus; (8) anterolateral funiculus; (9) Ventral funiculi; (10) ventral spinal roots; (11) dorsal spinal roots; (12) spinal ganglion

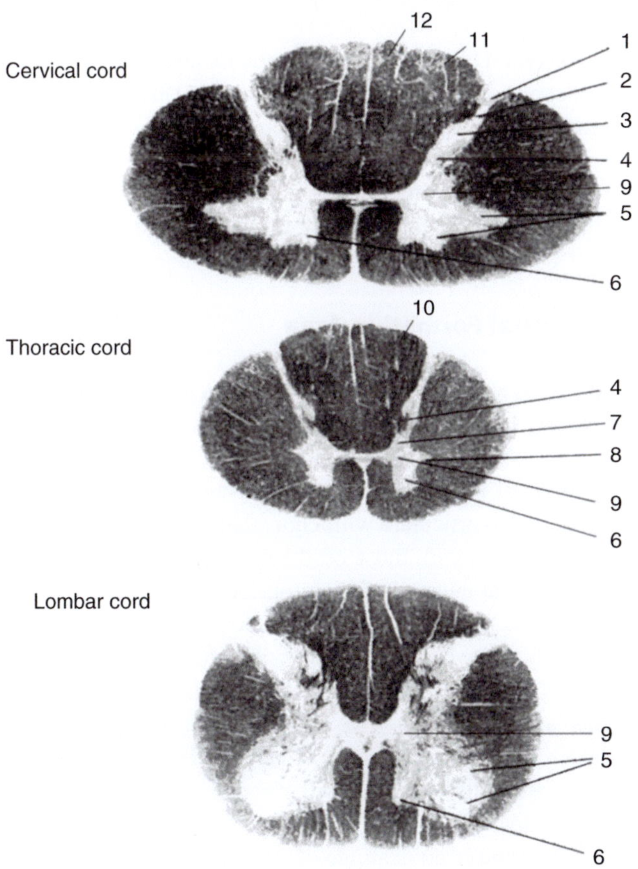

Fig. 4 Internal structure of the spinal cord: (1) dorsolateral fasciculus of Lissauer; (2) Waldeyer's marginal nucleus; (3) substantia gelatinosa of Rolando; (4) nucleus proprius; (5) lateral and retrolateral nuclei; (6) medial nuclei; (7) Clarke's column dorsalis nucleus; (8) nucleus intermediolateralis; (9) nucleus intermediomedialis; (10) dorsal column; (11) cuneatus fasciculus; (12) gracilis fasciculus

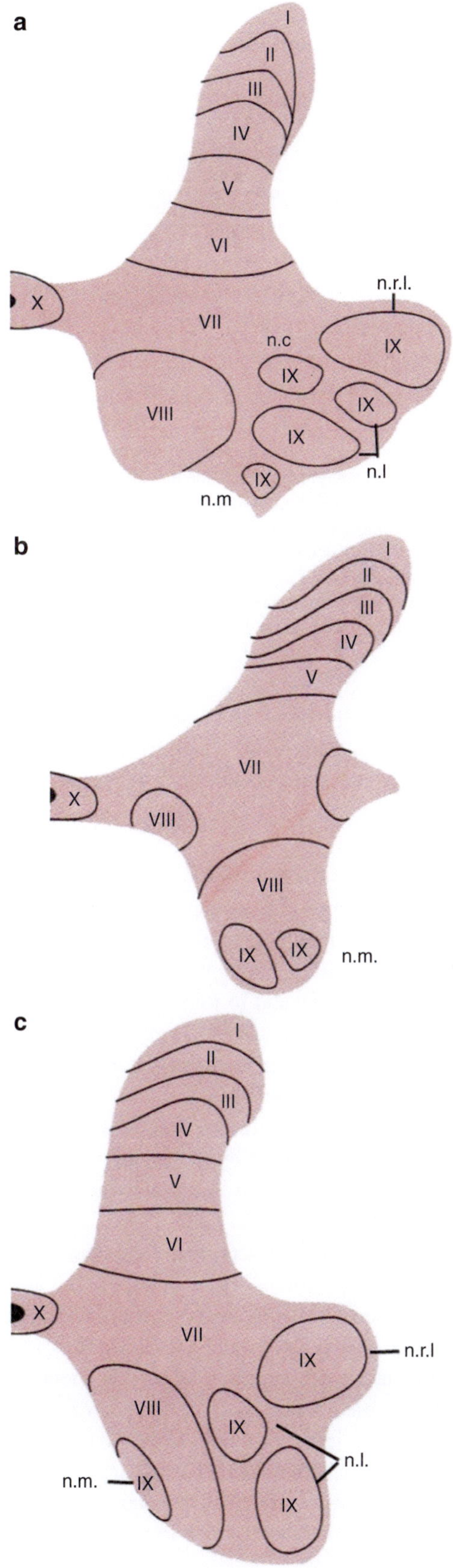

Fig. 5 Cytoarchitecture of the gray matter of the spinal cord in cross section [1]: (**a**) cervical spinal cord; (**b**) thoracic spinal cord; (**c**) lumbar spinal cord; *nl* lateral nuclei, *nrl* retrolateral nuclei, *nc* central nuclei, *nm* medial nuclei

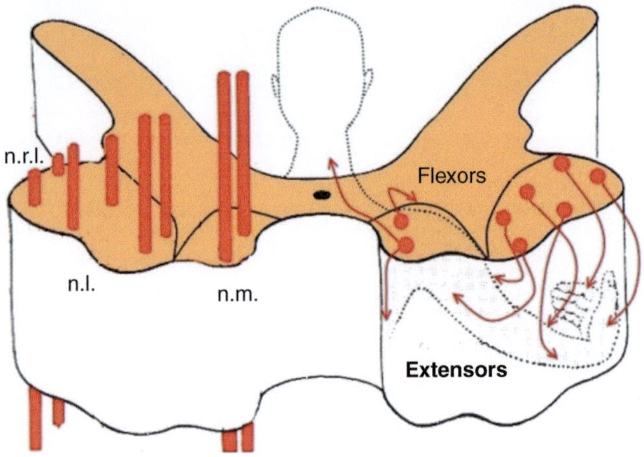

Fig. 6 Organization in juxtaposed columns of ventral horns. Somatotopic correspondences: (nm) medial nuclei present along the entire cord corresponding to the axial musculature; (nl) lateral nuclei present in the enlargements, corresponding to the proximal musculature; (nrl) retrolateral nuclei present at the level of the enlargements and corresponding to the distal musculature. The columns are arranged in two planes: the ventral plane corresponds to the musculature of the extensors, the dorsal plane to the musculature of the flexors

knees, the retrolateral columns to the distal musculature of the extremities (hand and feet).

- At the level of the cervical cord, the central nuclei correspond to the nucleus of the phrenic nerve which extends from C3 to C7. Its fibers borrow the anterior roots of C4 to form the phrenic nerve that descends to innervate the diaphragm. The fibers of the spinal accessory nerve (nerve XI) occupy segments C1–C6. Its fibers, after having emerged along the lateral cord, go up towards the foramen magnum to penetrate into the posterior cerebral fossa and to join the fibers of the medullary root of accessory nerve (XI) to leave posterior fossa by the jugular foramen to innervate the trapezius and sternocleidomastoid muscles.

3. An intermediate central area between the ventral and dorsal horns, centered by the ependymal canal which is usually obstructed. It is characterized by its reticular organization forming rich networks of interneurons articulating between them and also includes the intermediate columns which belong to the autonomic nervous system involved in vegetative life: the intermediomedial cell column is located along the ependymal canal, is present along all of the spinal cord and the intermediolateral cell column which occupies only the thoracic segments from T1 to L2, where it corresponds to the lateral horn. They both belong to the sympathetic system. The intermedioventral column corresponds to the pelvic parasympathetic system. It is present only at the level of the sacral segments of S2–S4 and specifically intended for the innervation of the viscera of the pelvic cavity.

Anatomofunctional Organization of the Neural Centers of the Gray Matter

The gray matter of the spinal cord is organized according to a cytoarchitectonic model with 10 laminae (Rexed) numbered starting from the dorsal expansions (Fig. 5). They can be grouped into three zones which correspond to different organizational and functional arrangements and which would be like the superposition of three successive layers in the evolution of the animal species.

1. A central formation or fundamental zone is the oldest in the phylogenetic scale and corresponds to the intermediate zone and to laminae VII and VIII. It is characterized by a network organization of interneurons in charge of the basic motor and vegetative programs essential to the survival of the individual.
2. The dorsal horns correspond to laminae I–VI. Their radial organization corresponds to the complex systems in charge of the specific treatment of pain and temperature messages essential for survival by alerting for the environment danger by the information brought to each metameric level by the dorsal roots of the spinal nerves.
3. The ventral horns correspond to the IX layer and the motor functions from which the orders coming from the spinal and the supraspinal structures converge to form the common final motor pathway. The axons of the motoneurons which constitute them correspond to the ventral roots of the spinal nerves intended for the somatic musculature.

The Central Formation Area

- It is organized into networks of interneurons that support programmed motor activities (Fig. 7) [3].

The small interneurons are largely anastomosed to each other and also articulate with equivalent cells of the contralateral cord and with those on the neighboring levels by the intersegmental neurons of the proprioceptive spinal system. They form networks of varying complexity that reproduce on the spinal level what has been described for the reticular substance of the brainstem and where elementary somatic programs are developed. These are present from birth but intended to be refined when they are then invested by supraspinal afferents which will widen their functional potentialities.

Locomotion is an example of such an autonomous mode of activity, just like swimming or birds flying [4].

Its reality is easily attested by the example of the chicken where its head has been cut off and who is able to continue to run for a few moments, that is, to realize a rhythmic and

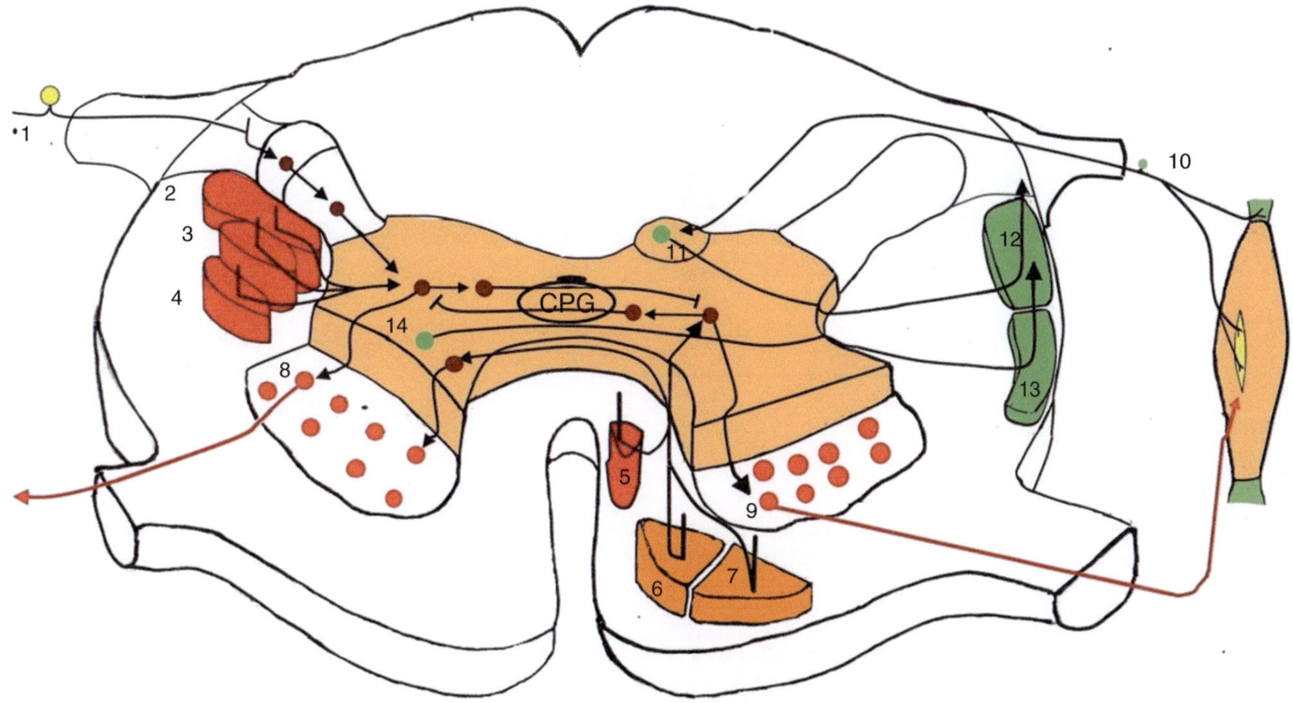

Fig. 7 Organization of the central zone into networks of central pattern generator interneurons (*CPG* central pattern generators) [2]. Afferents: (1) peripheral sensory segmental afferents; (2) lateral corticospinal tract; (3) rubrospinal tract; (4) medullary reticulospinal tract; (5) ventral corticospinal tract; (6) pontine reticulospinal tract; (7) vestibulospinal tract. Efferents: (8) flexor motoneurons; (9) extensor motoneurons; (10) segmental proprioceptive fibers; (11) Clarke's dorsal nucleus; (12) spinocerebellar dorsal tract; (13) ventral spinocerebellar tract: (14) pericornual zone

alternating activation of the flexor and extensor muscles of the two legs.

It has been studied experimentally in lamprey [5], the spinal cord of which can be easily isolated. The recording of its swimming by a ripple shows a rostrocaudal sequential activation in the form of rhythmic pulses, responsible for contractions of the longitudinal paravertebral muscles. This activity is not reflexive but reflects the intervention of central generators [6], CPG (central pattern generators), right and left segmentaries connected by commissural interneurons responsible for rhythmicity and alternation (Diagram 1). The functional plan is that of oscillatory systems based on the interaction of commissural inhibitory interneurons.

In mammals, the pattern is identical according to a cycle of increasing complexity to ensure the synchronization of the different limb segments. The stance phase is when the limb touches the ground. It solicits the extensor muscles and it is from there that depend on the variations of the duration of the locomotive cycle. The swing phase, conversely, varies little and involves the flexor muscles.

In newborns, these patterns can be effectively observed in the form of automatic swimming or the cyclical motion of the legs akin to walking. They then disappear with myelination of supraspinal tracts. However, they are likely to reappear clinically, in the form of automatisms (mass reflex, triple withdrawal, crossed synkinesis, and Babinski's sign) when cord lesions prohibit supraspinal downward influences.

It is not a reflex activity because experimentally division of sensory roots does not abolish the operation of these generators whose expression remains however basic and stereotyped requiring afferents to modulate their use.

1. The afferents are segmental, of a proprio- and exteroceptive sensory (external stimuli) nature, adapting to the conditions of the environment. A cat with transected spinal cord is thus able to experimentally adapt its speed of unwinding of the carpet from the proprioceptive information provided by the spinal sensory endings. Similarly, electrical or mechanical stimulation of the cutaneous receptors of the cat's foot, applied during the swing phase, leads to a considerable increase in the activity of flexor motoneurons and a greater elevation of the limb as to avoid a hypothetical obstacle whereas if it intervenes in the stance phase, it causes on the contrary a reinforcement of the activity of the extensors of the limb so as to compensate a possible unexpected load, or during a misstep creating the sudden failure of the limb (Diagram 1).

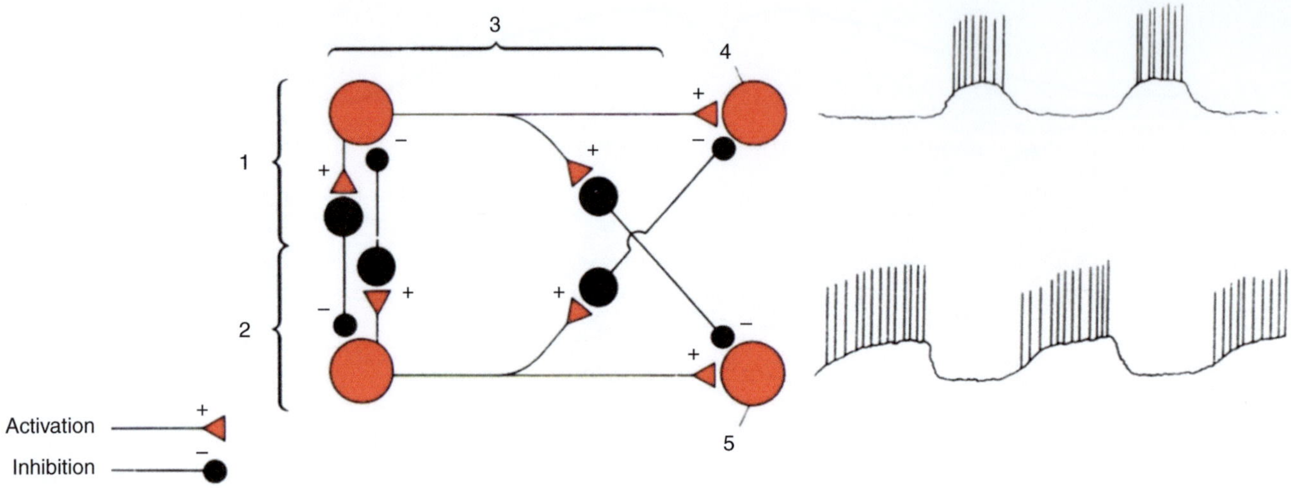

Diagram 1 Model of organization by semicenters of central rhythmic activities in locomotion [4]: (1) flexor hemicenter; (2) extensor hemicenter; (3) inhibitory interneurons (in blue) and activators (in red); (4) flexor motor neuron; (5) extensor motor neuron

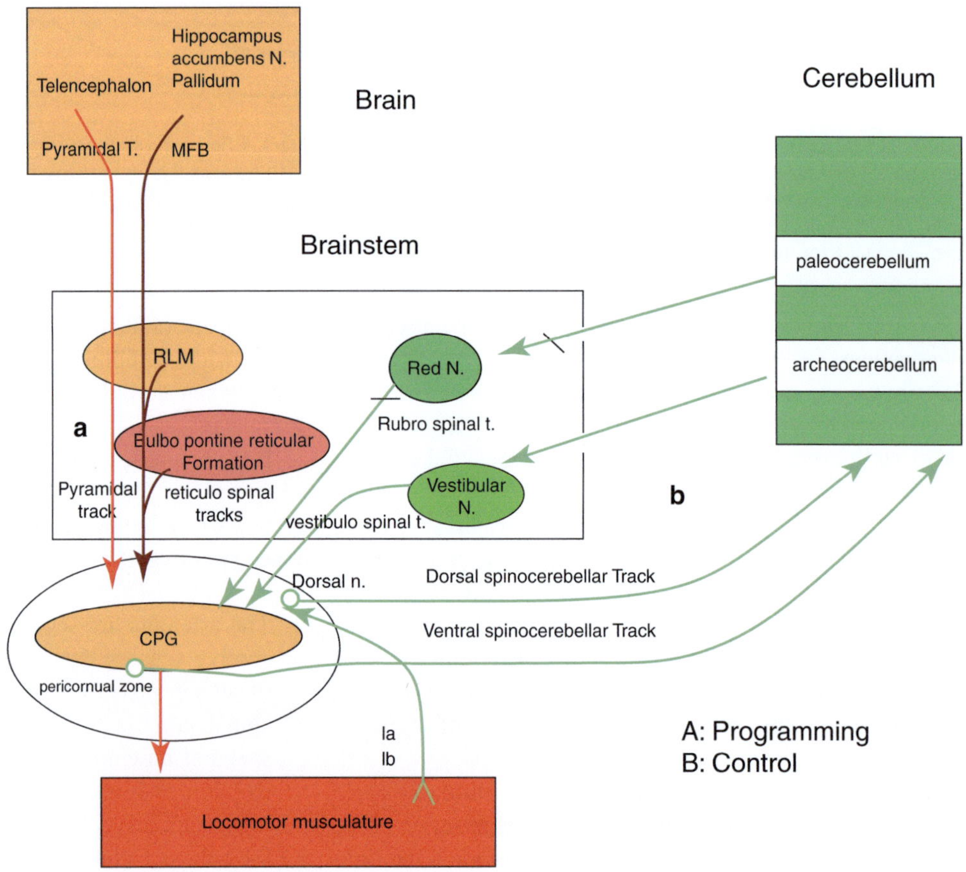

Diagram 2 Structures involved in the triggering (A) and control (B) of locomotion [3]. Locomotor command is sent to the spinal cord CPGs (central pattern generators). It comes from the brain by the pyramidal tract and the medial forebrain bundle (FMB), passes through the mesencephalic reticular nuclei (*RLM* mesencephalic locomotor region) and the medullopontine reticular nuclei. The copy of the pattern is sent to the cerebellum by the ventral spinocerebellar tract and its adjustment is achieved by the spinocerebellar feedback loops

2. The supraspinal afferents intervene to trigger and modulate these motor patterns (Diagram 2)
   a. The corticospinal tracts come from the cerebral cortex investing these interneuronal networks so as to widen the range of possibilities and place them under voluntary control. Babinski's sign, which is physiological in the newborn, disappears thus when the pyramidal tract imposes its regulating influence so that clinically, when it is found, it is a pathognomonic sign of a pyramidal lesion.
   b. At the level of the brainstem, the nuclei of the mesencephalic reticular formation and the pedunculopontine nucleus have been identified as a locomotor region. Its stimulation in the cat triggers perfectly organized

locomotor sequences whose speed follows the intensity of the stimulation. It intervenes as a trigger for spinal patterns. It receives the median forebrain bundle (FMB) which places it in relation with the ventral pallidum, the nucleus accumbens, and the hippocampus. It projects on the pontine reticular formation that activates central pattern generators by reticulospinal tracts. Thus, starting from an initial impulse and because of this central connectivity, the rhythmic generators of the cord enter into activity, with longitudinal and transverse logical coordination and by a harmonious combination of the upper and lower limbs more complex locomotive modules can afterward be acquired such as trotting, galloping, jumping, etc.

c. The cerebellum intervenes to achieve the necessary locomotor adjustments that occur through the spinocerebellar pathways organized into feedback loops where rapid conduction velocity (120 m/s) allows almost an instantaneous response:
   - The ventral spinocerebellar tract originates in the pericornual zone near the ventral motor horns and therefore informs the cerebellum directly of the activity of the central pattern generators (CPG) as soon as they come into play and as a reference copy.
   - The dorsal spinocerebellar tract originates in the Clarke dorsal nucleus, which is based on the dorsal horn that receives proprioceptive information from muscle and the neuromuscular spindle during movement and relates to the motor function of the lower limbs. Its equivalent for the upper limbs is represented by the cuneocerebellar tract. These bundles are projected on the somatotopically organized spinocerebellum (paleocerebellum) and on the corresponding intermediate nuclei (globulus and emboliform nuclei).
     - This double cerebellar device thus allows the cerebellum to compare the copy of the schedulated spinal pattern and its effective realization at the level of the muscular effectors and to make the necessary adjustments by acting on the spinal networks. They are explored clinically for the lower limb by the "sensibilisated" Romberg test and the Stewart-Holmes maneuver for the upper extremity.
     - The spinocerebellospinal feedback loops involve brainstem structures:
       - The rubrospinal tract originates from the mesencephalic red nucleus, which receives cross afferents from the paleo (or spino) cerebellum. It controls the activity of the flexor muscles of the limb thus involved during the swing phase in locomotion.
       - The ventromedial reticulospinal tract that originates from the pontine reticular nuclei alternatively intervenes during the stance phase during locomotion being a facilitator of the extensor muscles.
       - The vestibulospinal tract provides postural balance essential for locomotion that requires constant adjustments due to the imbalance created by bipodal and alternating walking in humans. Its facilitating action is bilateral and is exerted on the extensors of the anti-gravity axial muscle chains on which the verticalization depends.

- The central formation also contains the intermediate columns that belong to the autonomic system [7].

It is responsible for the functional control of the viscera and the maintenance of homeostasis by the combined intervention of two systems: the parasympathetic system and the sympathetic system, the common feature of which is a peripheral organization comprising two neurons, a preganglionic cholinergic connector, and a postganglionic effector, articulated on a ganglion relay near peripheral effectors, some of which already have a functional autonomy (enteric system). Thus, it is a functional control that is exerted on these autonomous systems so as to integrate them with the conditions of the internal or external environment.

1. The parasympathetic system has a trophotropic function and predominates under physiological conditions. Its action is local and relies on short postganglionic cholinergic neurons, located near and in the wall of the viscera. At the level of the digestive tract, it captures the intrinsic enteric system consisting of networks of interneurons located in the submucosal and myenteric plexuses that already reflexively provide intestinal peristalsis. This function is largely controlled by the vagus nerve (*X*). Only the viscera contained in the pelvic cavity receive parasympathetic innervation of spinal origin. It corresponds to the parasympathetic sacral or pelvic contingent that comes from the intermedioventral column present on the sacral segments S2–S4 (Fig. 8). Preganglionic fibers are the pelvic splanchnic nerves that accompany the spinal nerves and directly enter the external genitalia, bladder, distal portion of the colon and rectum, as well as the internal vesical and anal sphincters. The relay ganglia are located in contact with or even in the wall of these viscera making the postganglionic effector neurons very short.
2. The sympathetic system, on contrary, has an ergotropic purpose. It is involved in emergency or warning situations where energy reserves must be mobilized to respond to threats from the external environment. The relay ganglia are therefore remote from the effector so as to cover a large functional area. Its nerve centers are all located at

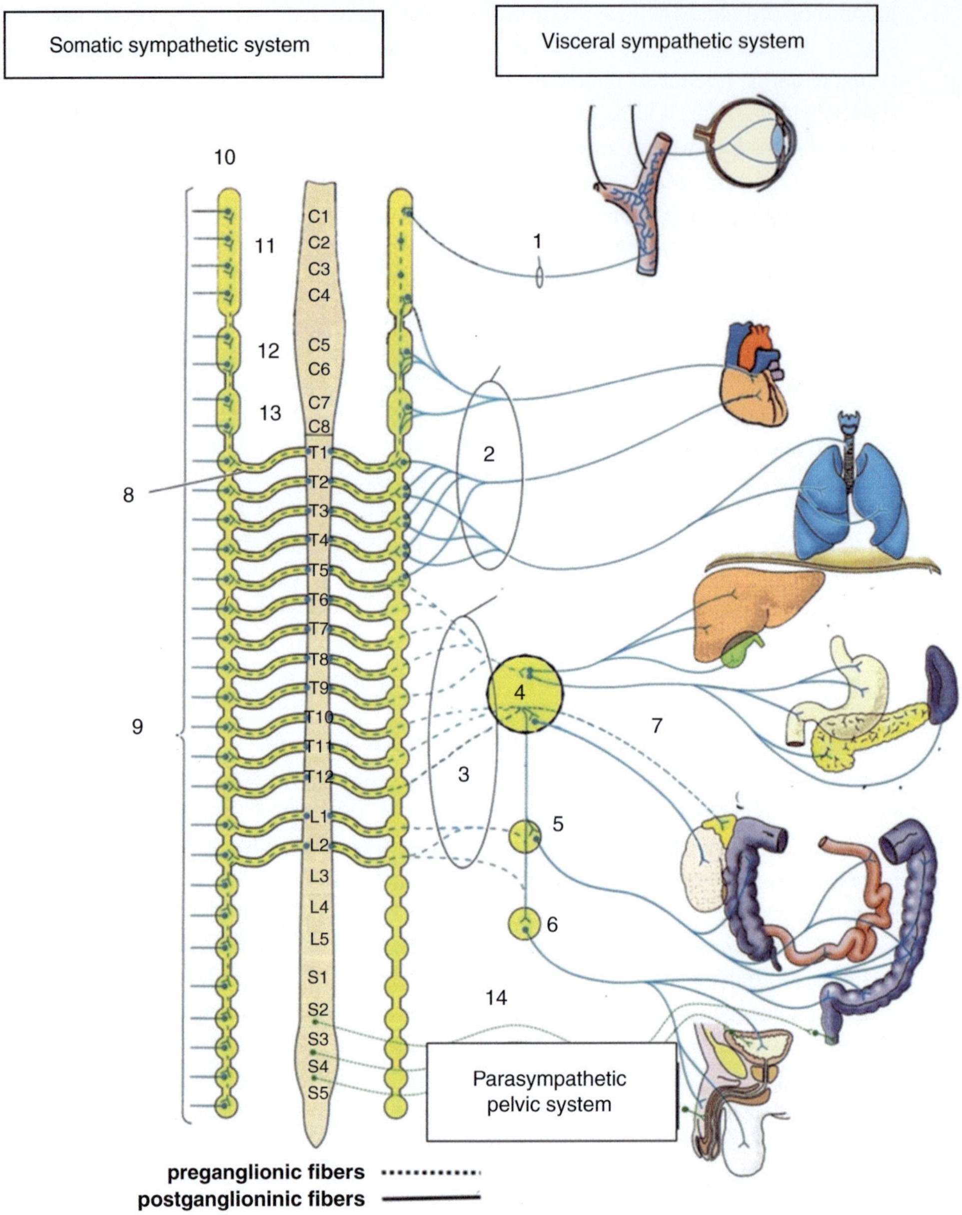

Fig. 8 Distribution of the somatic and visceral sympathetic systems and the parasympathetic pelvic system: (1) periarterial cephalic branch; (2) cardiopulmonary splanchnic nerves; (3) abdominopelvic splanchnic nerves; (4) celiac ganglion; (5) superior mesenteric ganglion; (6) inferior mesenteric ganglion; (7) adrenal branch; (8) white ramus communicans; (9) gray ramus communicans; (10) sympathetic chain; (11) superior cervical ganglion; (12) middle cervical ganglion; (13) stellate ganglion; (14) pelvic splanchnic nerves

the level of the spinal cord and correspond to two modes of organization, one visceral, the other somatic [8]

- The visceral sympathetic contingent (Fig. 9) is intended for the innervation of the viscera itself, and its action is most often in opposition to that of the parasympathetic system. The nerve centers are contained in the intermediolateral columns that occupy the lateral horns of segments T8 to L2. The preganglionic fibers accompany the ventral roots of the spinal nerves for a short distance, then follow the white communicating branches and pass directly through the ganglia of the paravertebral chains, without any synaptic articulation. They constitute the splanchnic nerves that join the prevertebral and preaortic relay ganglias, celiac ganglia, and superior and inferior mesenteric ganglias. The postganglionic fibers are noradrenergic and are distributed to the viscera of the abdominal and pelvic cavities, forming with the visceral arteries neurovascular pedicles. The adrenal gland, which is a chromaffin organ and secretes adrenaline, directly receives preganglionic fibers. For the organs contained in the thoracic cavity (heart, lungs, trachea, esophagus) and those of the cephalic extremity (head and neck), the relay ganglia are represented by the three cervical ganglias and the first four ganglias of the paravertebral chain. Postganglionic fibers join their target by forming periarterial plexuses surrounding the carotid and subclavian vessels and cardiac plexuses (Fig. 8).

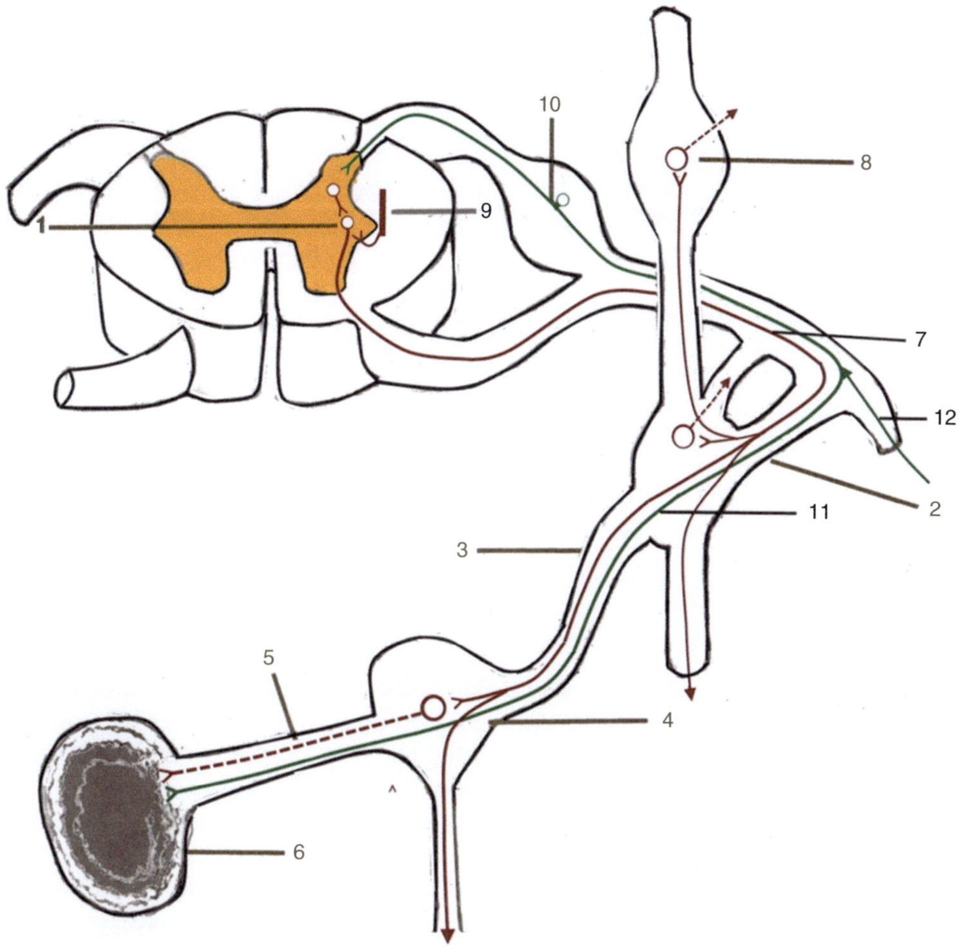

Fig. 9 Organization of the visceral sympathetic system: (1) nucleus intermediolateralis; (2) white ramus communicans; (3) splanchnic nerve; (4) pre-aortic relay ganglion; (5) postganglionic neuron; (6) viscera; (7) preganglionic neuron; (8) sympathetic laterovertebral chain; (9) supraspinal afferents; (10) dorsal sensory roots; (11) interoceptive nociceptive sensory fibers; (12) fibers of nociceptive sensitivity extero- and proprioceptive (referred pain)

The somatic sympathetic contingent (Fig. 10) ensures the innervation of the sweat glands, the pilomotor muscles, and the cutaneous vessels. It innervates these alone as the parasympathetic system is absent (although for the sweat glands the postganglionic fibers are cholinergic). Its anatomical organization is modeled on the metameric distribution of the spinal nerves. The spinal cord nerve centers are located at the level of the intermediolateral columns or are more likely to correspond to the intermediomedial columns which extend over the entire length of the cord. Preganglionic fibers are short. They follow the ventral roots of the spinal nerves from T1 to L2 and follow the white ramus communicans to join their paravertebral relay ganglia, which form the sympathetic chain from C1 to S5. The postganglionic fibers join the path of the corresponding spinal nerves by borrowing the gray ramus communicans and are distributed on the smooth muscles of the vascular walls and the pilomotor muscles by their adrenergic endings and the sweat glands by their cholinergic fibers.

The control of vegetative centers can be reflexive, but most often under the influence of supraspinal influences that integrate them into behavioral patterns with both somatic and vegetative components [9]:

- Vegetative reflexes are produced by various sensory afferents stimuli coming from the viscera or the skin. Thus, the thermal information conveyed by the Aδ and C sensory fibers from their exteroceptive origin allows local thermoregulation so that the application of cold causes arterial vasoconstriction with paleness of the limb and piloerection whereas, conversely, an increase in temperature leads to vasodilation and sweating to create heat loss.
- This mode of reflex functioning is particular to the parasympathetic pelvic system and responsible for the physiological control of urination, defecation, and sexual reflexes.
- The supraspinal afferents come from the nuclei of the medullopontine lateral reticular zone (superficial reticular area and nuclei of the pontine tegmentum) where the pneumotaxic, inspiratory and expiratory respiratory centers, the cardioregulatory and vasomotor centers, and the micturition center have been located. The noradrenergic fibers visible in histofluorescence (Fig. 26) descend into the lateral spinal cord and terminate on the intermediolateral and intermedioventral nuclei and on the phrenic and intercostal nuclei. They correspond to the control exerted by the hypothalamus where the ergotropic and

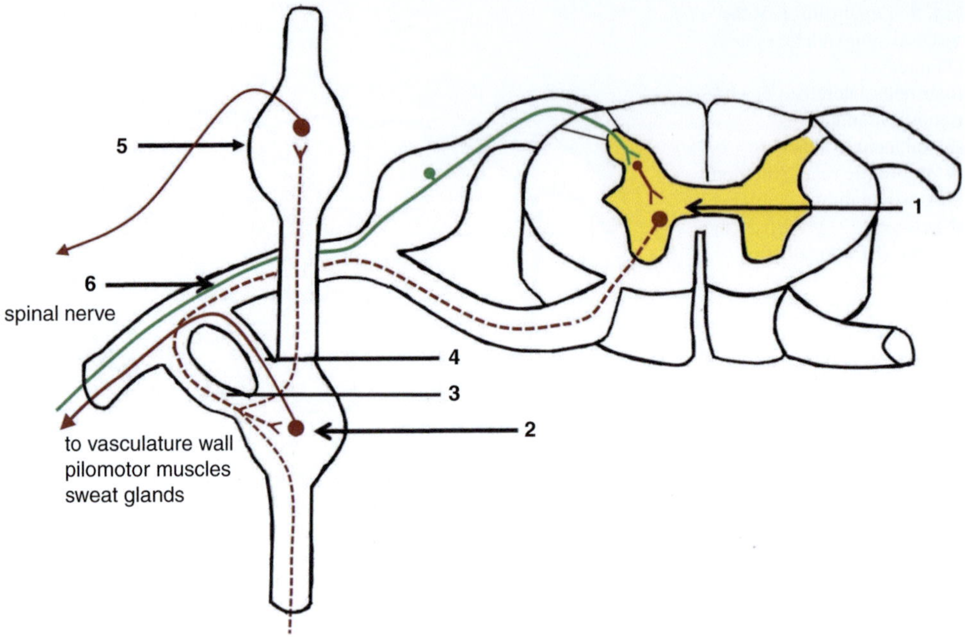

Fig. 10 Organization of the somatic sympathetic system: (1) nucleus intermediomedialis; (2) paravertebral ganglion; (3) white ramus communicans; (4) gray ramus communicans; (5) sympathetic chain; (6) Aδ and C sensory fibers from the skin

trophotropic regulatory centers are located in relation to the limbic system. They integrate them into behavioral patterns of an emotional nature, for example, but also dietary, sexual, or thermoregulatory factors involved in homeostasis.

Dorsal Horns

The dorsal horns correspond to the first six layers of Rexed, at which the abilities responsible for treating the dolorothermal (pain & temperature) information are located. It is brought to each metameric level by the dorsal roots of the spinal nerves. They contain several types of fibers that differ in their size and conduction velocity as well as in their functional significance; myelinated large fibers, with fast conduction velocity belonging to the exteroceptive sensitivity (Aβ (30–70 m/s)) and to proprioceptive sensitivity coming from the muscle (Ia and Ib fibers) (70–110 m/s) and the small, non-myelinated fibers (C fibers) (0.5–2 m/s) or poorly myelinated (Aδ fibers) (10–30 m/s), at slow conduction velocity. At entry into the cord, a separation into two contingents takes place: the large fibers form the median contingent which corresponds to the tactile epicritic (fine touch) and kinesthetic proprioceptive sensitivity is directed towards the dorsal column, the Clarke's dorsal nucleus, and the motor neurons of the ventral horns. The small fibers that carry the dolorothermal sensitivity constitute the lateral contingent that ends in the dorsal horns. It travels in the dorsolateral tract of Lissauer where the fibers bifurcate to give ascending and descending branches on 2–3 segments before ending at the extremities of the dorsal horns (Fig. 12).

1. The Aδ fibers terminate on the I and II layers and on the deep V layer. The amyelinic C fibers terminate on II layer only. Many substances are involved in the transmission of the nociceptive transmission: substance P in the superficial layers I and II but also other peptides: somatostatin, vasoactive intestinal peptide, cholecystokinin, CGRP (calcitonin gene related peptide), and excitatory amino acids (glutamate).
2. The relay neurons occupying the superficial layers I and II and the more central layers IV, V, and VI are of two types. Specific nociceptive neurons respond to mechanical or thermal stimulation, which is only nociceptive. They are localized in layer I. The nonspecific neurons (*wide dynamic range*) located at the level of the layers I, II, IV, V, and VI respond to mechanical or light thermal stimulations, non-nociceptive but capable of becoming nociceptive with the intensity of the stimulus. They are convergence cells whose stimulus can be located at the level of the cutaneous layer but also of the muscles and the viscera. This convergence makes it possible to account for referred pain (Fig. 11), which sometimes expresses the visceral pain felt on a superficial cutaneous territory other than its real deep origin. The classic example is that of myocardial pain (infarction or angina pectoris) which projects up the chest and at the level of the left arm and hand, gallbladder pain that projects into the scapular region, and appendicular pain felt in the abdominal wall in the para-umbilical area. Indeed, the visceral and somatic afferents fibers converge on the same relay neuron, thus creating the illusion of a superficial pain projected on the corresponding dermatome. These two types of cells allow a discriminative coding of the dolorothermal message with regard to its intensity and its topography. Their axons cross the median line at each metameric level and move towards the ventrolateral (Déjerine) quadrant where they form the spinothalamic tracts responsible for transmitting this information to supraspinal structures (Fig. 12):

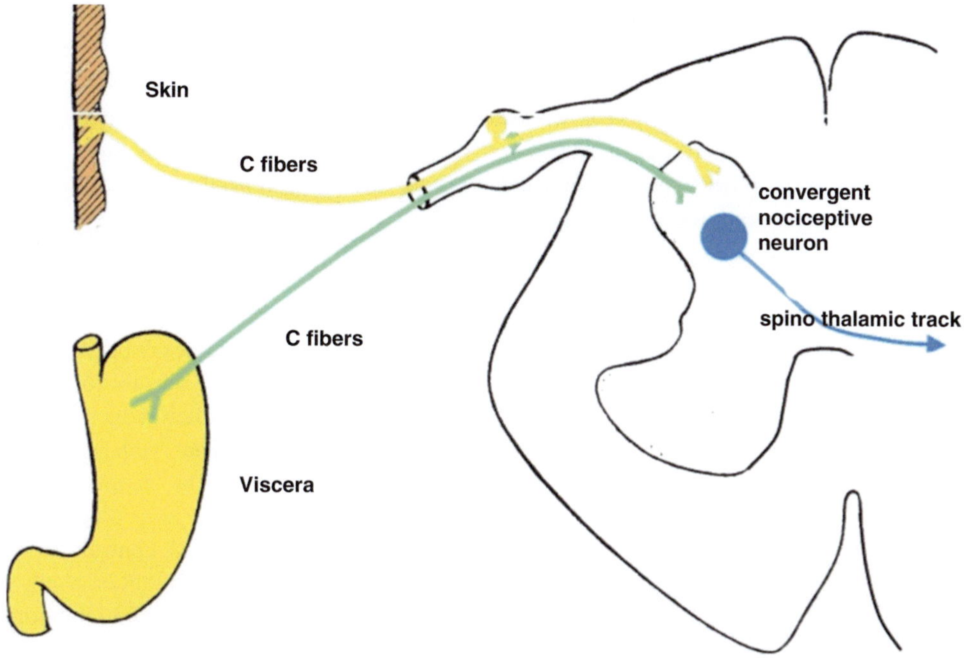

Fig. 11 Referred pain. The visceral pain is perceived at a distance from the lesion due to a viscero-somatic convergence at the level of the same metamere

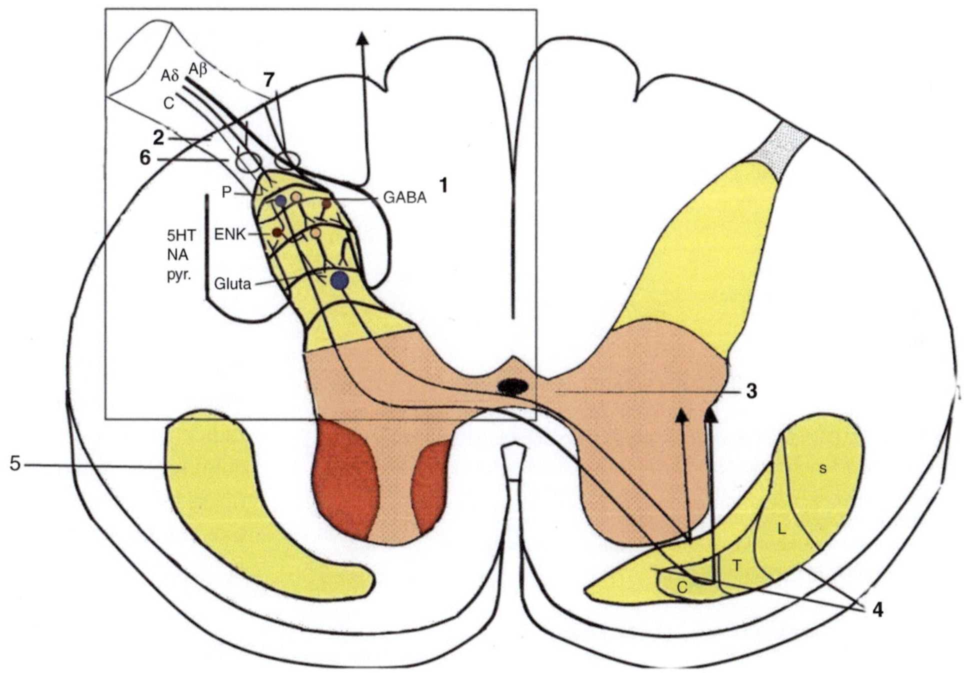

Fig. 12 General organization of the dorsal horns. (1) dorsal column; (2) Lissauer tract; (3) white commissure; (4) spinothalamic tracts; (5) ventrolateral tract; (6) lateral contingent; (7) median contingent

The neospinothalamic tract intended for specific thalamic relay nuclei has a somatotopic organization which depends on the origin of the fibers, whose lumbosacral component is posterior and thus more surgically accessible to interruption by anterolateral cordotomy in the treatment of pelvic pain.

The paleospinothalamic tract lies within the previous one in the anterolateral cord; it is intended for the nonspecific nuclei of the thalamus and gives, during its course in the brainstem, collaterals for the medial reticular (gigantocellular nucleus), involved in the awakening reactions triggered by painful stimulations, as well as for the reticular mesencephalic periaqueductal gray matter (PAG) by its spinomesencephalic contingent, involved in the diffuse inhibitory control of pain (see below). Other fibers also reach the hypothalamus, amygdaloid nucleus, nucleus accumbens, and septal nuclei and contribute to the development of affective and emotional expressions that accompany pain. The syringomyelic syndrome corresponds to the involvement of these spinothalamic tracts at their crossing, at each metameric level at the level of the white commissure; it is expressed at the level of the corresponding dermatome by a loss of the pain and temperature informations sensitivity which contrasts with the conservation of epicritic and kinesthetic sensitivities.

Onto this system that transmits the nociceptive and thermal messages and occupies the radial axis of the dorsal horn, come various control systems that modulate the signal so that pain that represents a punctual alarm signal does not extend and become permanent and intolerable.

The control systems are segmental and supraspinal (Fig. 13):

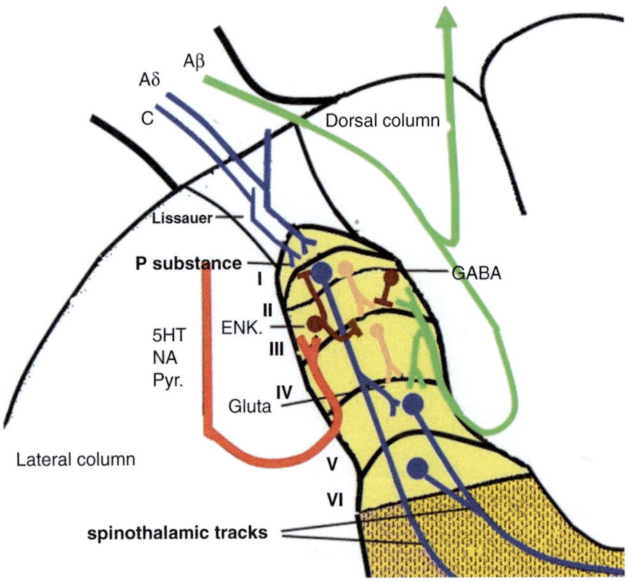

Fig. 13 Organization of the dorsal horns of the spinal cord [10] Aδ and C: afferent fibers constituting the dorsolateral contingent (protopathic sensitivity). Aβ afferent fibers constituting the dorsomedian contingent (epicritic and kinesthetic sensitivity). *Lis* Lissauer's tract, *P* substance P, *Gluta* excitatory glutaminergic interneurons, *Gaba* GABAergic inhibitory interneurons (gamma amino butyric acid), *Enk* enkephalinergic inhibitory interneuron, *5HT* serotoninergic afferents, *NA* noradrenergic afferents; *Pyr* pyramidal tract

1. In the gelatinous substance (layers II and III), interneurons (islet cells) exert a pre- and postsynaptic inhibitory action on the passage of the nociceptive message. They are enkephalinergic and GABAergic. This influence is confirmed by the analgesia obtained with the administration of intrathecal or epidural morphine in the treatment of pain in anesthesiology. Other interneurons secrete opposite excitatory amino acids (aspartate and glutamate) which are amenable to pharmacological neutralization (anti-epileptics).
2. The large caliber Aβ fibers which form the medial contingent of dorsal roots emit collaterals which penetrate the dorsal horn edges at the level of the IV and V layers and articulate with these interneurons or with convergent cells. The competition between these two types of fibers whose conduction velocity is not equivalent is the origin of the gate control theory of Wall and Melzach (Diagram 3). Large-caliber fibers with a fast conduction velocity stimulating the inhibitory interneurons close the gate to the passage of the nociceptive message conveyed by the smaller and slower fibers. In fact, the uncomfortable sensation of pruritus attenuates at least transiently if the pruritic area is scratched; in the clinic, transcutaneous neurostimulation makes it possible to treat certain types of pain. We can indeed distinguish:
   – Pain by nociceptive excess which reflects the predominance of the influences carried by the Aδ and C fibers: it is the usual pain due to traumatic or inflammatory lesions which release at the level of the periphery algogenic substances (histamine, serotonin, substance P) which are potentiating and sensitizing. In addition to the usual analgesics, they are indications of techniques that neutralize the nociception pathways by local anesthesia (novocaine), or surgically by selective posterior radicellectomy at the Lissauer tract level of the lateral contingent, commissural myelotomies (section of the fibers at the level of the white commissure), or selective ventrolateral cordotomy (section of the spinothalamic pathways in the ventrolateral cord).

Diagram 3 Modulation of nociceptive information by segmental pathways. Theory of "gate control" [11]. The large-diameter Aβ fibers with fast conduction velocity close the "gate" and block the passage of the nociceptive information provided by the small-caliber and slower conduction velocity Aδ and C fibers using interneuron inhibitors

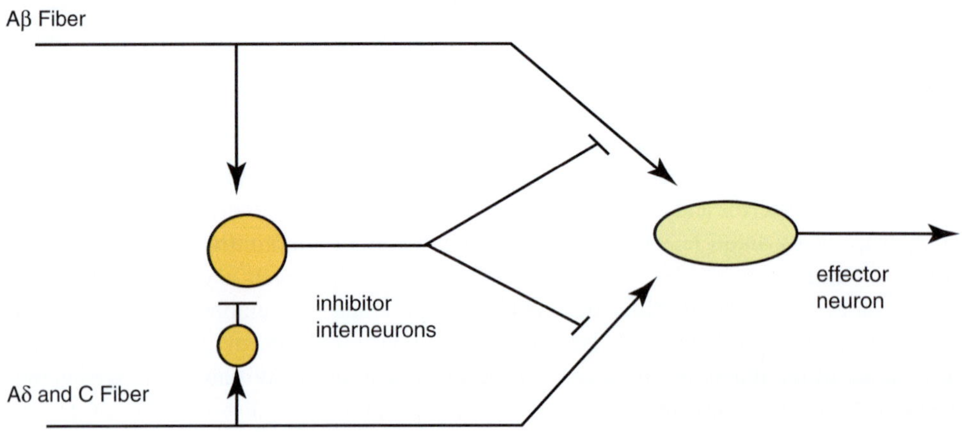

– Pain by deafferentation corresponds to a lack of inhibitory influence of the Aβ fibers. It is a neuropathic pain, during polyneuritis and other peripheral neuropathies, the pain of amputees or Zosterian pain where the pain is felt at the level of the dermatome which paradoxically is insensitive to touch. The treatment should aim to reinforce the "gate control" by percutaneous stimulation, posterior cord neurostimulation, antiepileptic drugs or by local intrathecal morphine administration so as to reinforce the action of the inhibitory interneurons.

Supraspinal control systems come from the reticular formation of the brainstem (Diagram 4).

The best studied circuit involves the mesencephalic reticular zone whose descending fibers constitute the endogenous control system of pain [12] and involves the descending serotonergic pathways (Fig. 25). It comprises the periaqueductal gray matter (PAG) and the nucleus raphe dorsalis, rich in opioid receptors (dynorphin). They emit fibers for the reticular nuclei of the pontine raphe (nucleus raphe magnus) and for the adjacent nucleus reticularis magnocellularis whose fibers descend sparingly into the lateral cord and terminate on the I and V layers. They exert a presynaptic inhibitory action on the primary endings that antagonizes substance P and postsynaptic via enkephalinergic interneurons. This device is verified by the analgesia obtained by stereotaxic stimulation of the PAG.

Another downward path is noradrenergic. It comes from the medial pontobulbar reticular nuclei (nucleus paragigantocellularis) and the pontine locus coeruleus. This would explain the lack of perception of pain during intense stress or strong emotion. Finally, other afferents come from the cerebral sensorimotor cortex. They are represented by collaterals of the pyramidal tract and also possess an inhibitory effect which is reflected in the absence of perceived injuries during intense physical engagement in combatants or athletes.

These descending analgesia systems correspond to the diffuse nociceptive inhibitory control function that are triggered by the ascending pathways of pain thus providing feedback loops from the spinoreticular tract fibers that articulate with the magnocellular reticular nuclei and the periaqueductal gray matter from which these descending serotoninergic and noradrenergic analgesic systems originate.

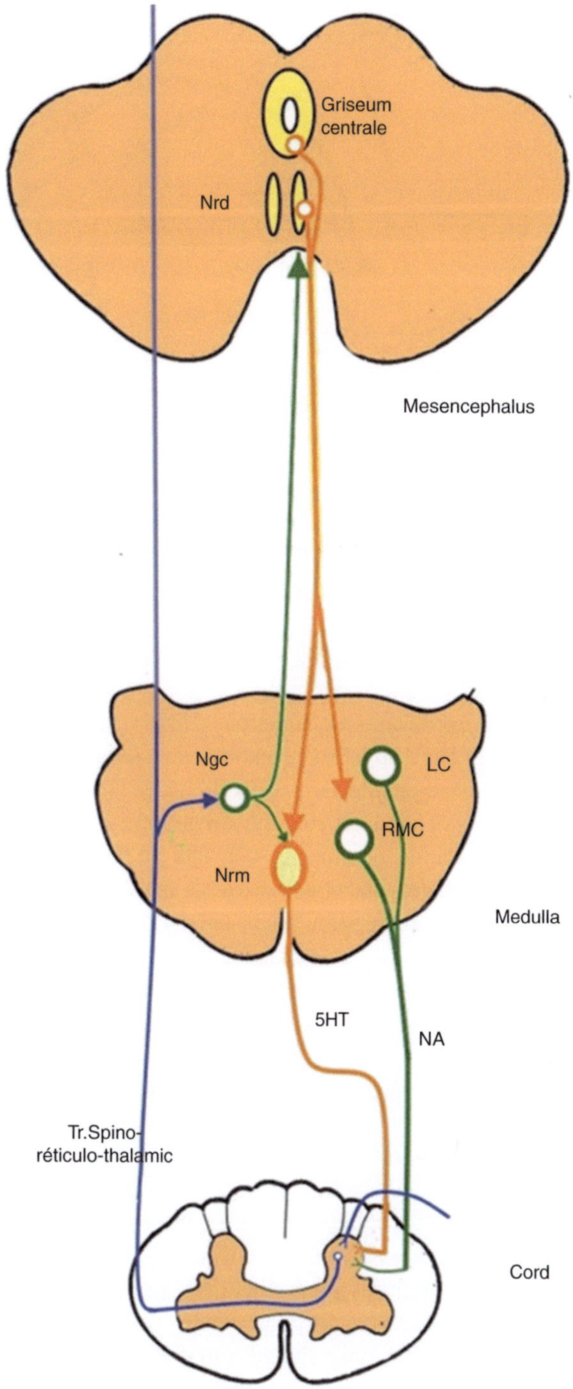

Diagram 4 Supraspinal function for pain control [13]. At the mesencephalic level, PAG: periaqueductal gray matter contains endogenous enkephalin and opioid receptors. It sends serotoninergic efferents to the reticular nuclei of the medullary raphe (*Nrm* nucleus raphe magnus) and the nucleus reticularis magnocellularis: RMC. At the spinal level, the serotoninergic fibers from the raphe nuclei project onto the dorsal horn layers II and III. Noradrenergic fibers from the locus coeruleus (LC) and the RMC also terminate on the interneurons of II and III layers where they exert an inhibitory effect on the neurons included in the dorsal horns whose axons form the spinothalamic tracts and send projections to the supraspinal sites of the medullary reticular formation (*Ngc* nucleus reticularis gigantocellularis) and relate to the descending analgesia devices forming an inhibitory feedback device

The Ventral Horns

The ventral horns contain the layers IX (Fig. 14). They are organized into cellular islets containing motor neurons whose axons are intended for skeletal musculature. They contain two types of neurons.

1. The large α motor neurons (10–17 μm) innervate the skeletal muscle fibers which then cause contraction. Their

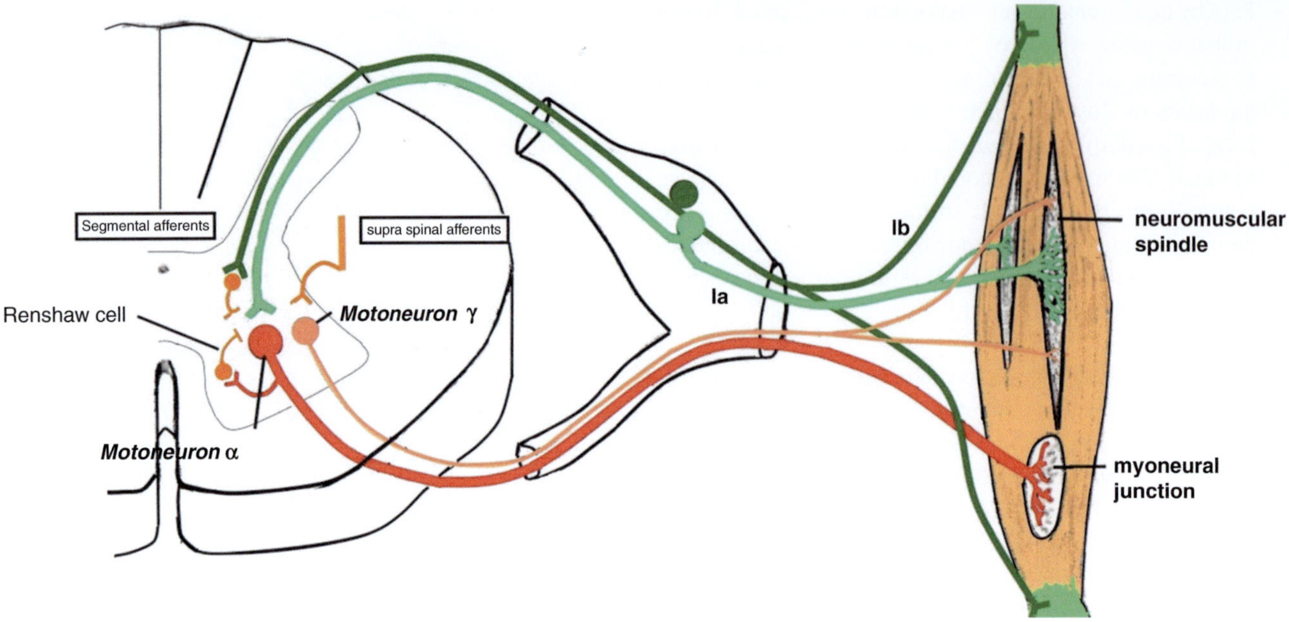

Fig. 14 Organization of the ventral horns of the spinal cord

dendritic expansions are numerous and form a vast receiving field. Their myelinated axons correspond to the Aα fibers whose conduction velocity is of the order of 60–90 m/s. They innervate the striated muscle by establishing synaptic cholinergic contacts at the myoneural junction (motor plate) with several muscle fibers. The α-motor neuron, its nerve fibers and the muscle fibers that it innervates constitute a motor unit. Their number for a muscle depends on its contractile force. However, the average number of muscle fibers per motor unit varies greatly depending on the location and functional value of the innervated muscle. Thus the extrinsic muscles of the fingers are richly innervated as opposed to the antigravity muscles of the trunk where the innervation is of the order of 1000 muscular fibers innervated by a single neuron. The precision and the ability to modulate the intensity of a contraction thus depend on the richness of the innervation.

2. The γ motor neurons are smaller (2–8 μm). Their myelinated axon whose conduction velocity is of the order of 10–45 m/s accompanies that of α-motor neurons and constitute the fusimotor fibers that will innervate the intrafusal myofibrils (proprioception) located at the polar end of muscle spindles, arranged in parallel with striated extrafusal muscular fibers. The neuromuscular spindles also have at their equatorial part, elongation-sensitive receptor organs, which enable them to measure the length of the muscle and to transmit this information to the α motor neurons to the spinal cord by the Ia fibers thus connecting the two types of motoneurons in a functional coupling.

The axons of the α-motor neurons terminate at the level of the myoneural junction (neural plate) and innervate the striated muscle fibers which they cause the contraction

γ-motor neurons innervate the muscular part of the neuromuscular spindles (intrafusal fibers), the contraction of which causes the stimulation of the intrafusal receptors and the Ia fibers which terminate directly on the α-motor neurons. γ-motor neurons receive descending supraspinal afferents involved in the control of muscle tone.

The ventral horn also presents small interneuronal, multipolar cells whose action is exerted on these motor neurons: Ia and Ib interneurons are inhibitory and located on reflex circuits. The Renshaw cell also represents a particular recurrent inhibitor function intended to limit the motoneuron activity over time. It is represented by a short collateral which takes a recurrent path and establishes a cholinergic excitatory contact with the inhibitory Renshaw cell which in turn articulates with the cell body of the emitting cell and the synergistic motor neurons. This recurrent inhibition loop of which the mediator is glycinergic or GABAergic thus renders the motor neuron temporarily inexcitable. Strychnine which blocks glycinergic receptors causes tetanic contracture at high doses.

This effector function, thus marked by a spatial and temporal coding, represents the common final pathway responsible for executing all motor orders of segmental or supraspinal origin.

1. Segmental sensory afferents are the basis for reflex activity which represents the functional originality of the spinal cord. The intrinsic mono- or oligosynaptic reflexes control the length and strength of muscle contraction and the extrinsic polysynaptic reflexes have a protective role.
   – Intrinsic reflexes involve muscle proprioceptive apparatus

The muscle stretch reflex (myotatic reflex) is monosynaptic (Fig. 15). Its afferents are constituted by the Ia fibers which convey proprioceptive information coming from the neuromuscular spindle and collected at the annulospiral endings wound helically at its equatorial zone.

Their stimulation is related to the lengthening of the muscle which distracts the spirals. Its efferents end directly on the α-motor neurons, provoke the contraction of the extrafusal muscle fibers, and diminish their length. This stretch reflex thus controls the length of the muscle in response to its own stretching and tends to bring it back to its original length. Clinically, its corresponding topographic value is helpful insofar as it is strictly metameric and monosynaptic. It is especially directly involved in the reflex adjustment of tonic and postural activity. The weight of the body continually tends to flex the joints and consequently stretch the antigravific extensor muscles which oppose the influence of gravity. This reflex thus ensures a postural tone that maintains the standing position.

A second means of putting this reflex into action is indirect and involves the γ-motor neuron (Fig. 16). It realizes the device of the γ-loop of Granit which establishes a functional coupling between the α- and γ-motor neurons. The stimulation of the γ-motor neurons causes the contraction of the intrafusal fibers from which Ia fibers come into play and by the muscle stretch reflex pathway elicits the stimulation of the corresponding α motor neuron. Many descending pathways of supraspinal origin terminate directly on the γ-motor neurons (reticulo and rubrospinal tracts) and thus allow static adaptations. Moreover, the supraspinal afferents simultaneously reach the α- and γ-motor neurons so that the neuromuscular spindle then behaves as an error detector by comparing the effective length of the muscle and the length that it had to reach, between the reality and the set-point. The muscle

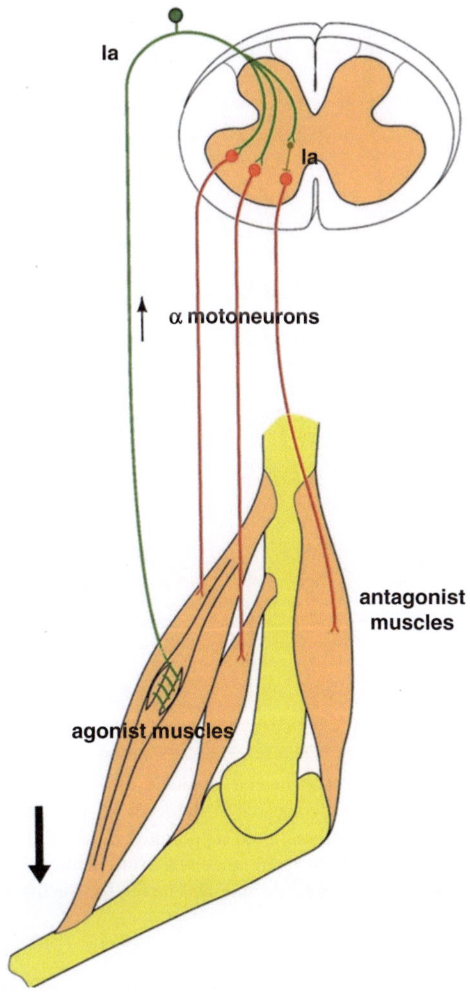

Fig. 15 Muscle stretch reflex. Activation by muscle stretching: the excitation of the receptors causes a stimulation of the Ia fibers which articulate monosynaptically with the α-motor neurons and leads to the reflex contraction of the agonist muscles aiming to maintain them at their initial position and disynaptical inhibition of antagonistic muscles (interneuron Ia)

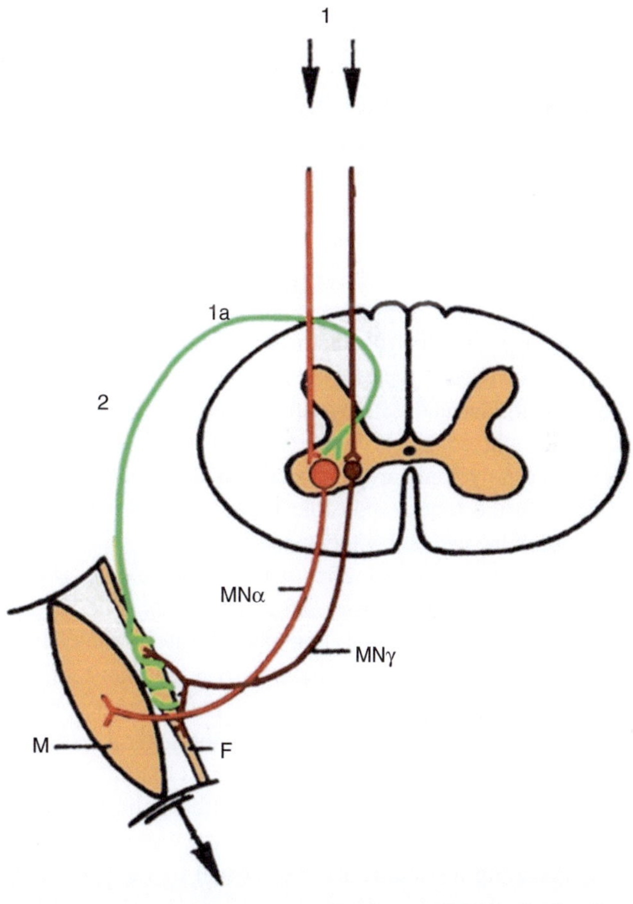

Fig. 16 γ-Loop. Concept of servo-assistance of the movements [14]. Involvement of the muscle stretch reflex indirectly by intervention of the γ-motor neurons (γ-loop) which receive a supraspinal command, a copy of that intended for the α-motoneurons. The neuromuscular spindle is an error detector comparing the length of the extrafusal muscle with the control message sent to γ-efferents. (1) Command coupled to α- and γ-motor neurons. (2) Error detector. Any deviation between extra and intrafusal muscle fibers induces an "error" signal and a stretch reflex response to bring the extrafusal fibers back to the desired value stretch reflex then corresponds to a servo-assistance device where any deviation between the intrafusal and extrafusal muscle fibers induces an error signal and triggers a reflex response which tends to bring the muscle back to the desired length and thus improves the precision of the movement.

The reciprocal inhibition reflex (Fig. 15) is disynaptic and connected to the stretch reflex device. It involves an inhibitory Ia interneuron, articulated on a collateral of the Ia fibers and intended for the motor neurons of the antagonist muscle, thus facilitating the action of the agonist.

The inverse myotatic reflex or autogenic inhibition (Figs. 5 and 17) is also disynaptic. The afferent path is represented by the Ib fibers whose receptors are represented by the Golgi tendon organs located on the tendons at the ends of the muscle itself. Unlike neuromuscular spindles placed in parallel, these mechanoreceptors are placed in series with respect to the muscular fibers and are thus sensitive to the state of tension of muscle during contraction. They are articulated with the agonist α motor neuron via the inhibitory Ib interneuron. Its role is to protect the muscle during its contraction as a damping system of the intensity of a muscular contraction. When the subject has to resist a force tending to mobilize a joint at a level of tension, the muscle suddenly relaxes like a penknife that closes suddenly (Clasp knife reflex).

Spinal inhibitory interneurons therefore appear important for balancing the influence of powerful myotatic reflexes. They receive, therefore, supraspinal afferents to balance the muscle tone and thus facilitate the achievement of motor control. However, in the case of spinal cord injuries affecting these pyramidal and extrapyramidal descending pathways, myotatic reflexes that become exaggerated, vivid, disseminated, and polyclonic are produced and accompanied by an increase in the tone responsible for spasticity in the paralyzed areas located below the lesion.

The flexor withdrawal reflex is polysynaptic (Fig. 18). It involves the afferent sensory Aδ and C fibers. The trigger threshold of the movement is that of a painful stimulus. Their stimulation causes flexion of the limb so as to remove it from the stimulus. This ipsilateral flexion reflex is also accompanied by a crossed activation of the contralateral extensor muscles. This reciprocal innervation serves to enhance postural support during withdrawal of the affected limb.

2. Descending influences are represented by the pyramidal and non-pyramidal pathways.
   - Non-pyramidal pathways (Diagram 5)

Non-pyramidal pathways are originated from suprasegmental formations located in the brainstem. They intervene on tone that accompanies movement.

1. The medial and lateral vestibulospinal tracts are involved in postural tone (Fig. 24). They originate in the vestibular nuclei of the medulla that relay the sensory information provided by the vestibular nerve (VIII) and collected at the vestibular receptors of the inner ear, sensitive to gravity and linear or circular movements of the head. They occupy the anterior funiculus and terminate on the motor neurons of the medial column, intended for the

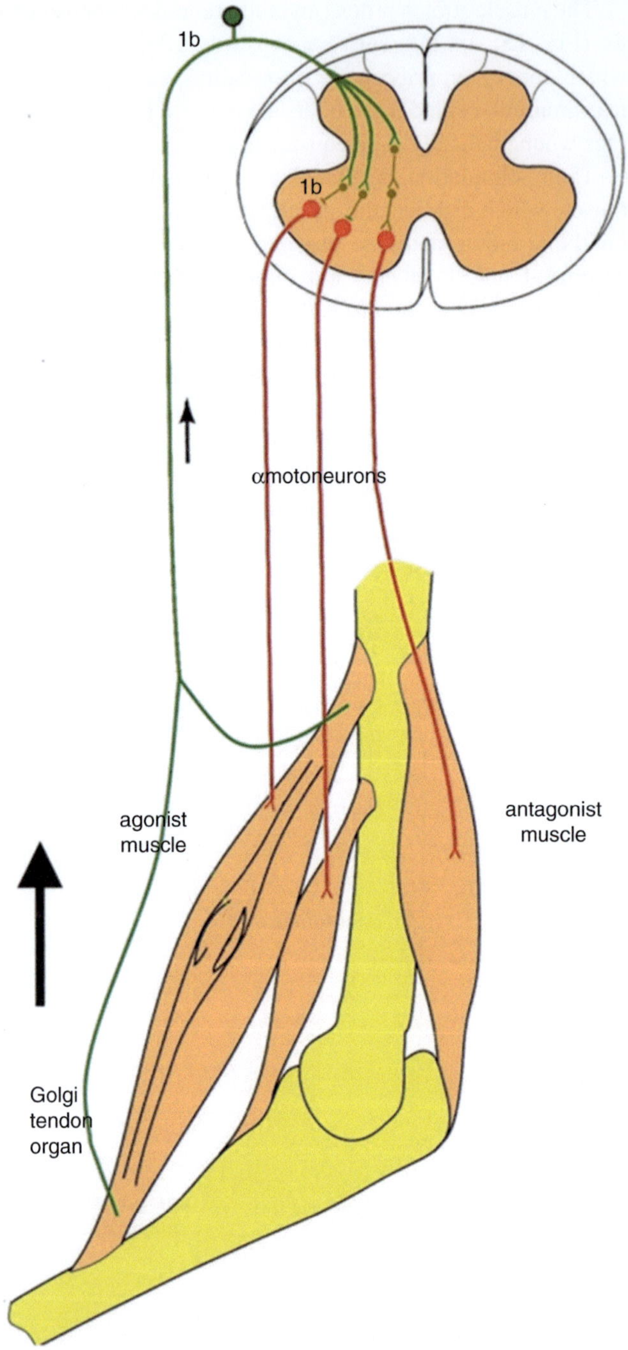

Fig. 17 Clasp knife reflex (inverse myotatic reflex). It is disynaptic. The receptors involved are located at the level of the tendons (Golgi tendon organ) and the afferent path represented by the Ib fibers which articulate after interneuronal inhibitory relay (interneuron Ib) with the motor neurons of the agonist muscle and facilitator for the antagonist motor neuron

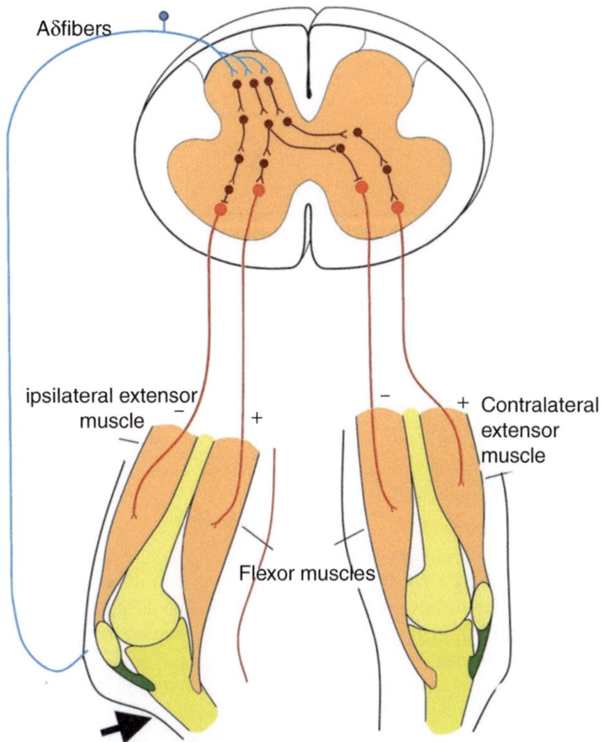

Fig. 18 Flexion reflex produces an ipsilateral flexion and contralateral extension of the entire limb. Nociceptive stimulation produces a polysynaptic reflex contraction of all the flexor muscles of this limb so as to subtract it from the stimulus and the mutual inhibition of ipsilateral extensors. It is accompanied by a contraction of the contralateral extensor muscles by activation of commissural interneuron facilitators with reciprocal inhibition of the flexor muscles on the same side, thus compensating for the lack of support due to the ipsilateral bending and thus contributing to the maintenance of the upright position

antigravific musculature. They provide a permanent muscle tone that aims to maintain the erect position and the axis of the body in a supportive polygon and also allow postural adjustments created by sudden and unpredictable imbalances occurring during locomotion.

2. The reticulospinal tracts come from the medullary and pontomesencephalic reticular formation. They end on the α and γ motor neurons. They are involved in programming muscle tone of the flexor and extensor muscles which must be balanced to allow movement.

The lateral reticulospinal tract represents the large descending inhibitory system. It is composed of axons whose cell bodies are located in the medial nuclei of the medullary reticular formation (nucleus reticularis gigantocellularis) (Fig. 23). It descends into the lateral aspect of the cord. It exerts an inhibitory action on the motor neurons of the extensors of the limbs and facilitator on those of the antagonistic flexors. It thus regulates the tone of muscle chains in flexion of the proximal segments of the limbs (elbows and knees) and in locomotion, intervening in programming for swing phase.

Alternatively, the medial reticulospinal tract represents the main descending activating tract. It arises from the medial nuclei of the pontine reticular formation (nuclei reticularis pontis caudalis and oralis) and descends into the ventral medial funiculus (Fig. 24). It ends bilaterally on layers VII and VIII and intervenes as a facilitator of the tone of the extensor muscles of the axial and proximal musculature and in the stance phase in the locomotion

The tectospinal tracts come from the upper and lower colliculi located on the visual and auditory pathways. They are crossed from their mesencephalic origin and do not exceed the level of the cervical cord. They intervene in the control of the orientation of the head in response to a visual or auditory stimulus.

- Pyramidal tracts are responsible for the strength and direction of movement (Fig. 22)

Pathology of these tracts causes paralysis. They are characterized by their origin located at the level of primary motor cortical areas (area 4), somatotopically organized and at premotor and supplemental motor areas (areas 6) for the planning of complex motor sequences. At the caudal end of the medulla, at the level of the pyramidal decussation, the fibers are divided into a crossed or lateral tract for 3/4 of them and a direct tract for the remaining quarter.

1. The direct pyramidal tract remains in the ventral column and does not extend beyond the cervical and thoracic segments. Its fibers are projected bilaterally on the interneurons and the motoneurons of the medial nuclei corresponding to the axial musculature of the trunk.
2. The lateral pyramidal crossed tract is organized somatotopically and occupies the lateral column. It ends in the interneuronal networks of the central zone from which it intervenes indirectly on the motoneurons except at the level of the cervical enlargement where the articulation can be direct with the retrolateral nuclei charged with the realization of fine and voluntary gestures of the hand and fingers.

It may be associated with the rubrospinal tract, the influence of which is less in man. It was formed from the red nucleus to the mesencephalic level and receives collaterals from the pyramidal tract so that it can be considered as a corticorubrospinal tract. Similarly, its fibers are crossed from their origin and they accompany it in the lateral column of the spinal cord and end by projecting on the lateral part of VII layers from where they exert a facilitating influence on the flexors of the proximal musculature.

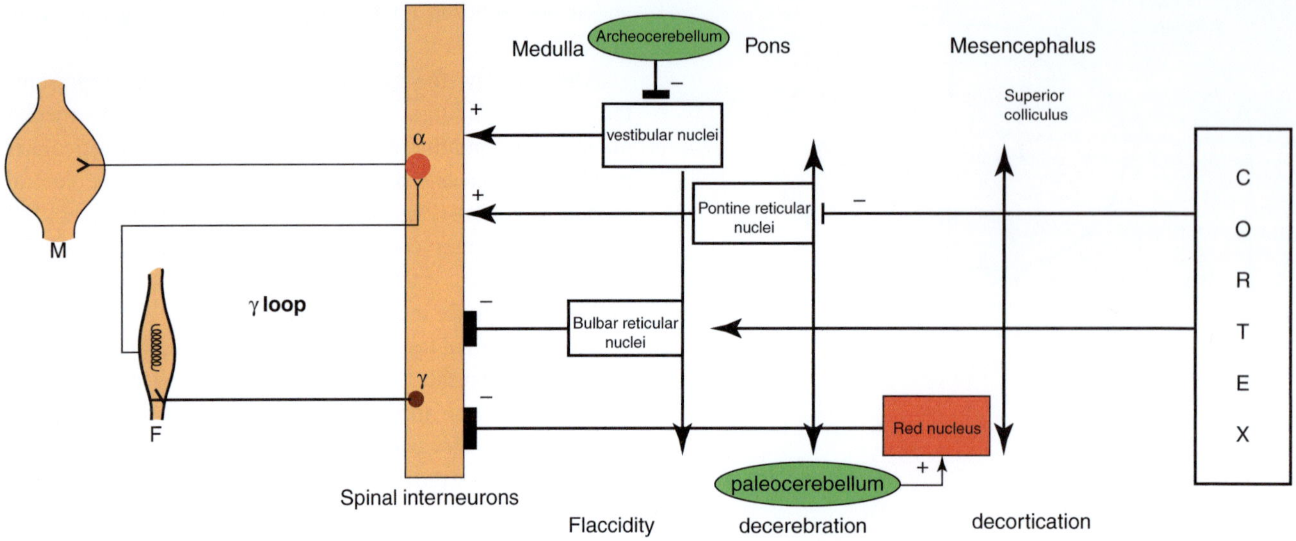

Diagram 5 Supportive and inhibiting supraspinal afferents involved in the muscle stretch reflex (myotatic reflex) and the tone of the extensor muscles. The pyramidal path is not represented. The vertical lines indicate the level of the brainstem lesions responsible for different hypertonic syndromes by disruption of functional balance. (1) Hypertonia of decortication in flexion by a sub-cortical lesion releasing the rubrospinal influence; (2) hypertonia of decerebration releasing the vestibulospinal and reticulospinal pontine influence; (3) medullary lesion releasing the reticulospinal medullar influences. *M* extrafusal muscle fibers, *F* neuromuscular spindles, *SC(TQS)* superior colliculi. γ-loop with Ia fiber and myotatic reflex

The syndrome of the anterior horn of the spinal cord demonstrates a clinical picture observed in acute anterior poliomyelitis expressed on the metameric segment, the combined involvement of the α- and γ-motoneurons responsible for paralysis with amyotrophy and the abolition of reflexes without affecting sensation.

Anatomofunctional Organization of the White Matter

It represents the place of passage of the fibers from or destined for the cord, organized in ascending or descending tracts that occupy well-defined territories to which specific functions correspond (Fig. 19).

Somatosensory Ascending Pathways (Fig. 20)

- The dorsal column carries epicritic and kinesthetic information

The epicritic sensitivity corresponds to fine tactile sensations recorded at the mechanoreceptors of the skin and the kinesthetic sensations collected at the level of the neuromuscular spindles and tendons. They correspond to qualitative information about the size and consistency of objects as well as the position and movement of limbs. It is conveyed in the dorsal roots of spinal nerves by myelinated fibers of large caliber (Aβ) that will join the ipsilateral cord in a somatotopic manner according to their somatic origin: The most medial fibers correspond to those that come from the sacral, then lumbar and thoracic segments and constitute the fasciculus gracilis. Those of cervical origin are arranged more laterally and constitute the fasciculus cuneatus. They join, respectively, the corresponding relay nuclei, gracilis, and cuneatus, located at the dorsal colon nuclei of the medulla. The fibers they emit are the medial lemniscus. It crosses the median line at the level of the medullary sensory decussation, ascends the entire brainstem behind the pyramidal tract and ends on the specific sensory relay nuclei of the thalamus (posterolateral ventral nucleus), from which the thalamocortical fibers borrowing the superior thalamic pedicle joins the primary somatosensory area (S1) located at the postcentral gyrus of the parietal lobe (areas 3, 1, 2) in the brain.

The Von Monakov's accessory cuneate nucleus receives also directly from the fasciculus cuneatus proprioceptive afferents of the upper limb but has a particular organization that links it to the cerebellar system. It emits the cuneocerebellar tract which borrows the lower cerebellar pedicle (restiform body) and ends on the interposed cerebellar nuclei and on the paleocerebellar cortical areas corresponding to the ipsilateral upper limb. So it is for the upper limb the equivalent of the spinocerebellar dorsal tract for the lower limb. It acts on spatiotemporal control of movement and its achievement creates a dyssynergy with hypermetry and dysmetry.

- The anterolateral funiculus contains spinothalamic tracts that convey the protopathic sensitivity which corresponds to painful and thermal sensation as well as to the immediate

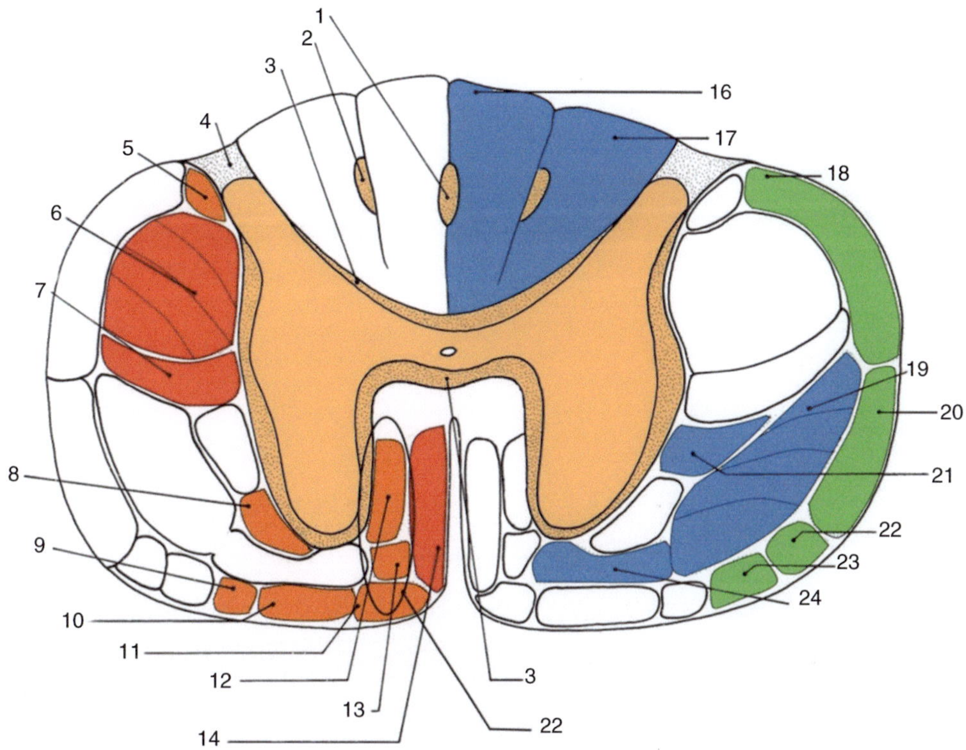

Fig. 19 General organization of the white matter. The descending tracts are on the left and marked in red. The ascending tracts on the right are blue for information systems and green for programming systems

1 Tractus septo-marginalis
2 Tractus Interfascicularis
3 Fasciculus proprius
4 Fasciculus dorso lateralis (of Lissauer)
5 Tractus raphe-spinalis
6 Tractus pyramidalis lateralis
7 Tractus rubrospinalis
8 Tractus bulboreticulospinalis
9 Tractus olivospinalis
10 Tractus vestibulospinalis
11 Tractus tectospinalis
12 Tractus Pontoreticulospinalis
13 Tractus Interstitio- and solitary spinalis
14 Tractus pyramidalis anterior
15 Funiculus posterior
16 Fasciculus gracilis
17 Fasciculus cuneatus
18 Tractus spinocerebellaris posterior
19 Fasciculus anterolateralis
20 Tractus spinocerebellaris anterior
21 Tractus paleospinothalamic
22 Tractus spino olivaris
23 Tractus spinotectal
24 Ventral spino-halamic track
25 Fasciculus longitudinalis medialis

touch and to the Aδ and C, nerve fibers of dorsal roots and whose origin may be exteroceptive, proprioceptive, or interoceptive. They end on the dorsal horns where they synapse. The spinothalamic tracts correspond to the axons of the relay neurons located at the level of the laminae I, III, and IV–V, which cross the median line in the ventral white commissure. On the contralateral side they constitute the anterolateral tract (of Dejerine).

Its contains two contingents

- The neospinothalamic contingent is organized somatotopically. The fibers corresponding to the sacral segments are in the dorsolateral position, those of cervical origin in a ventromedial position. Its fibers constitute the extralemniscal tract which rises in the brainstem and will join the medial lemniscal tract which it then shares the path to the lateral thalamic relay nuclei, from which the thalamocortical fibers will be projected on the parietal cortex at the somesthetic areas, SI and SII. Nociceptive and thermal information is included as a conscious sensation of pain, heat, and cold that can be assessed for location, intensity, and nature.
- The paleospinoreticulothalamic contingent is located in its deep aspect. It remains in the lateral position in the brainstem and ends in the nonspecific nuclei of the thalamus (intralaminar nuclei) involved in cortical awakening. It gives collaterals for the medial reticular nuclei (nucleus gigantocellularis) and lateral reticular nuclei (superficialis and pontine tegmentum) involved in the somatovegetative expression of pain as well as in the nuclei of the medullary raphe (nucleus raphe magnus) and mesencephalic raphe (nucleus raphe dorsalis) and periaqueductal gray matter and in the locus coeruleus that correspond to the supraspinal analgesic apparatus delivered by serotonergic and noradrenergic pathways. A spinopontoamygdalian pathway also projects on the amygdaloid nucleus after

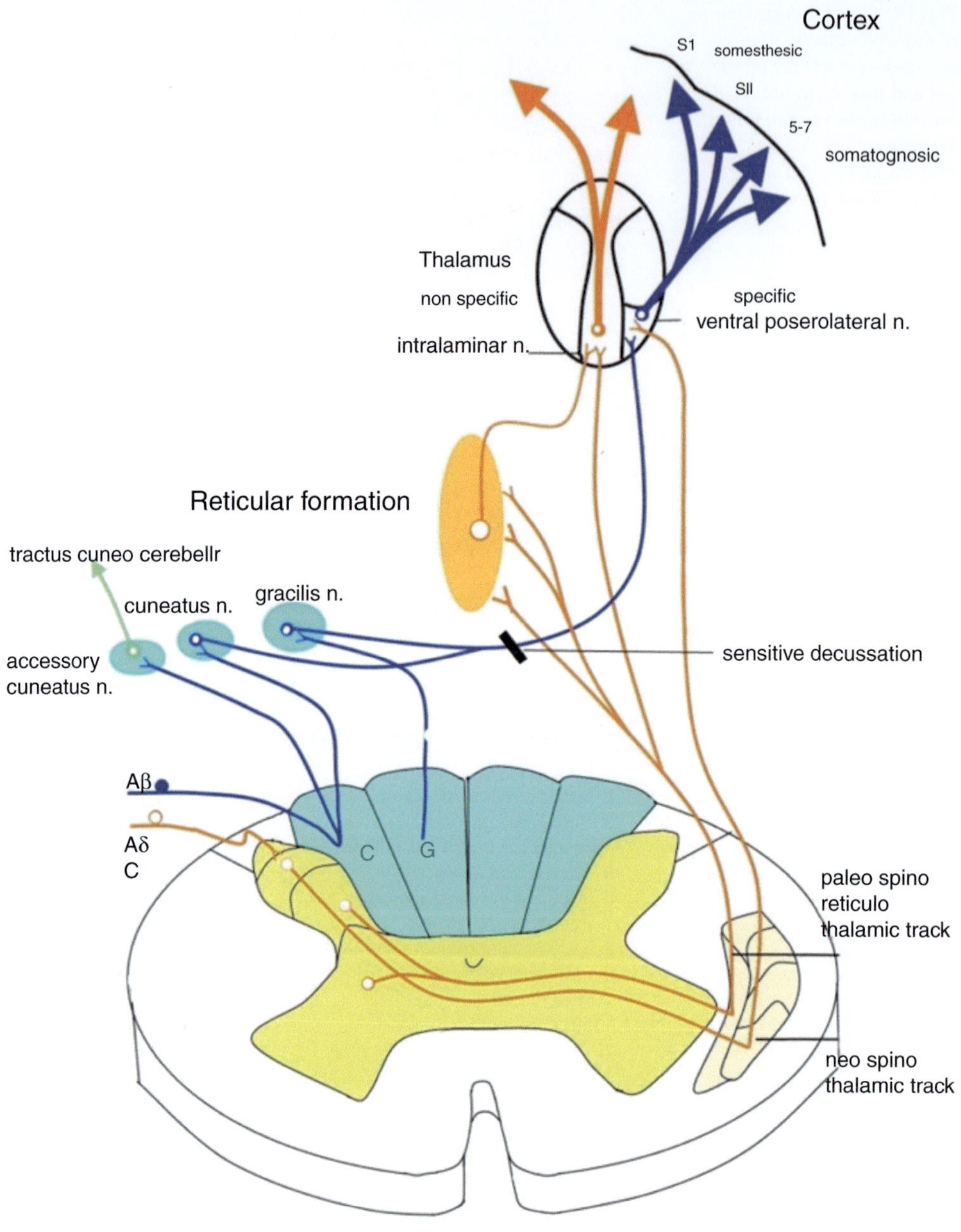

Fig. 20 Dorsal and spinothalamic ascending tracts

relaying at the level of the parabrachial area of the pons and intervenes in the manifestations of anxiety, apprehension, and fear related to the memorization of painful experiences.

– The spinocerebellar tracts (Fig. 21) occupy the lateral column along the circumferential edge of the cord. They provide the paleocerebellum (or spinocerebellum) with information necessary for the control and coordination of movement by spinocerebellospinal feedback loops.

- The dorsal (direct) spinocerebellar tract is composed of fibers originating at Clarke's dorsal nucleus which is present only from T8 to L3 and thus receives proprioceptive information from the myelinated Ia and Ib fibers from muscles and neuromuscular spindles of the lower limbs and lower body. It occupies the dorsal portion of the lateral cord and joins the cerebellum by borrowing the restiform body (inferior cerebellar peduncle). It ends by projecting on the interposed cerebellar nuclei (N. globulus and emboliform) and on the cerebellar cortex, in the areas representing the lower limbs. This spinocerebellar device thus allows the necessary motor adjustments from proprioceptive information collected directly at the level of the muscles performing the movement. It is the rubrospinal tract that represents the descending path of the spinocerebellar regulation loop.
- The ventral spinocerebellar tract (Gower's tract) is more complex. Its origin is in the VII layer, in the pericornual

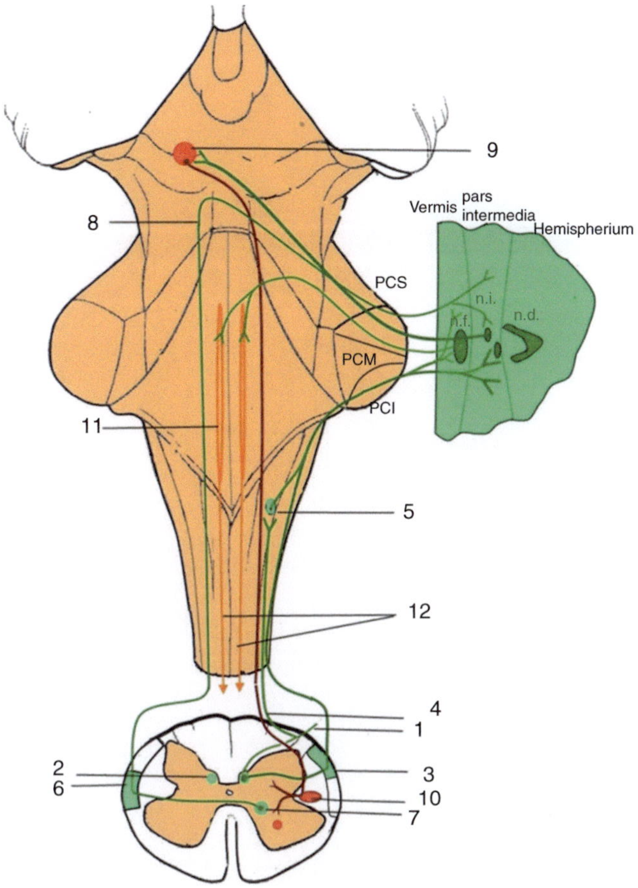

Fig. 21 Spinocerebellar pathways: (1) proprioceptive afferents Ia and Ib; (2) Clarke's dorsal nucleus (thoracolumbar spinal cord); (3) spinocerebellar direct dorsal tract; (4) cuneocerebellar tract (cervical cord); (5) accessory cuneatus nucleus; (6) crossed ventral spinocerebellar tract; (7) pericornual zone in the vicinity of the motor neurons of the ventral horns; (8) tractus uncinatus (Russell's hook); (9) red nucleus; (10) rubrospinal tract; (11) reticular nuclei; (12) reticulospinal tracts

zone located near motoneurons of IX lamina, which is directly informed before the muscle moves. Its fibers cross the median line at each metameric level and join the ventral side of the lateral column, in front of the spinocerebellar dorsal tract. It is present throughout the spinal cord and ascends the entire brainstem constituting the tractus uncinatus (Russell's hook), most of whose fibers cross the median line again to use the brachium conjunctivum (superior cerebellar peduncle) and project on the respective areas of the cerebellar cortex corresponding to their original metameres. This tract thus brings to the cerebellum the copy of the selected motor programme even before its actual realization.

Other ascending bundles are located in the ventral cord. They correspond to indirect spinocerebellar pathways through the bulbar olive (spinoolivary tract) and the vestibular nuclei (spinovestibular tract).

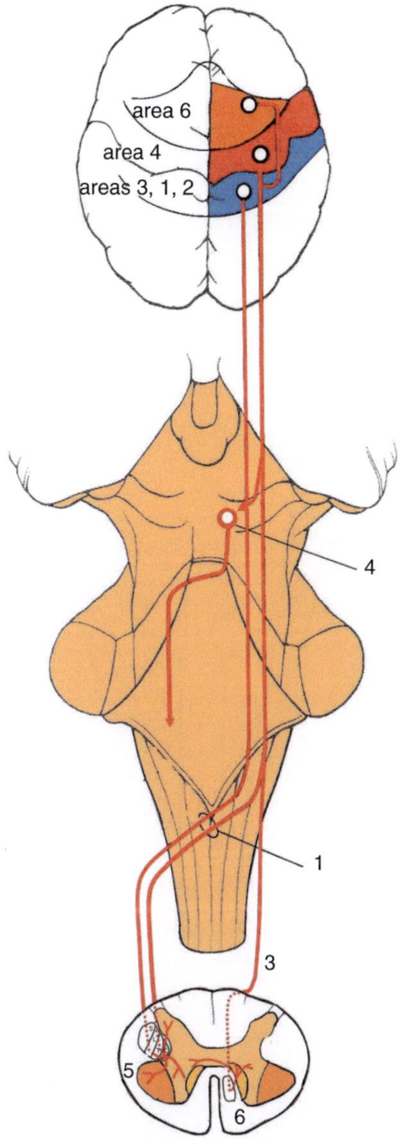

Fig. 22 Pyramidal tracts: (1) pyramidal decussation; (2) crossed pyramidal tract; (3) direct pyramidal tract; (4) red nucleus and rubrospinal tract; (5) lateral and retrolateral nuclei; (6) medial nuclei

In total, the ascending tracts of the white matter can therefore be grouped into three systems:

- An information system that includes the dorsal cord tract and the neospinothalamic tract that are characterized by their somatotopic organization. They carry information intended for the cerebral cortex where it becomes conscious and can be analyzed, identified, and localized. It corresponds to tactile, kinesthetic, and dolorothermal sensation. During progressive compressions of the spinal cord (Fig. 27), the sublesional syndrome is due to the white matter involvement whose level corresponds to the upper limit of insensitivity. The Brown-Sequard syndrome, which corresponds to the compression of a hemispinal

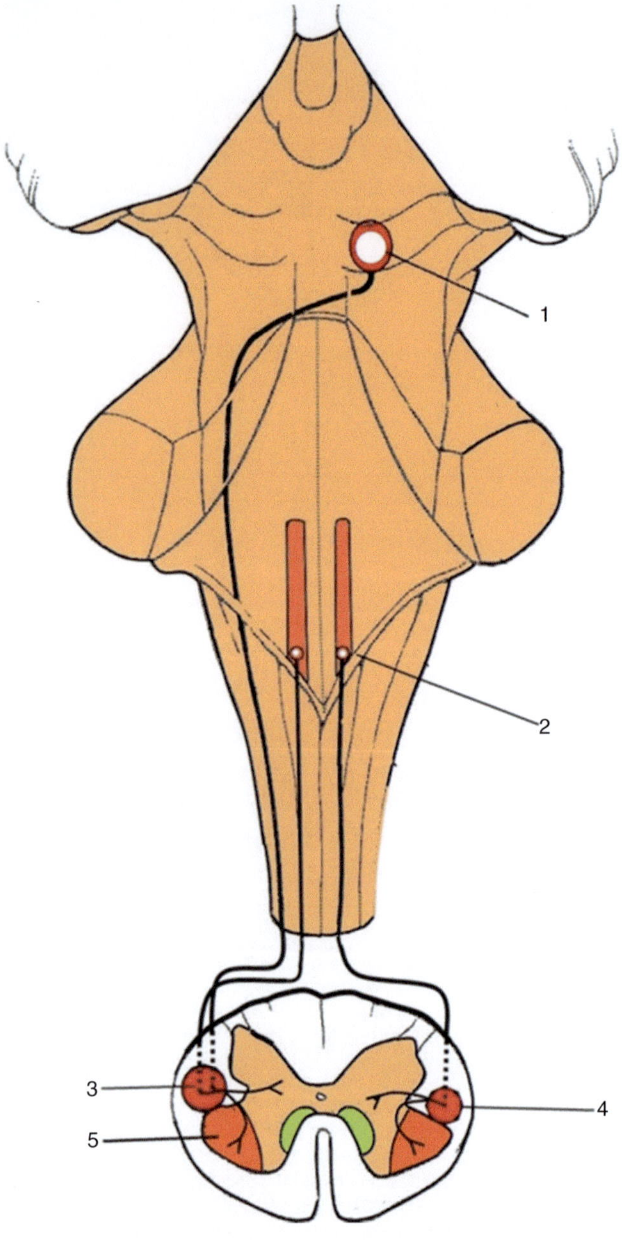

Fig. 23 Dorsolateral spinal contingent: (1) red nucleus; (2) reticular formation; (3) rubrospinal tract; (4) medullary reticulospinal tract; (5) lateral nuclei (flexors)

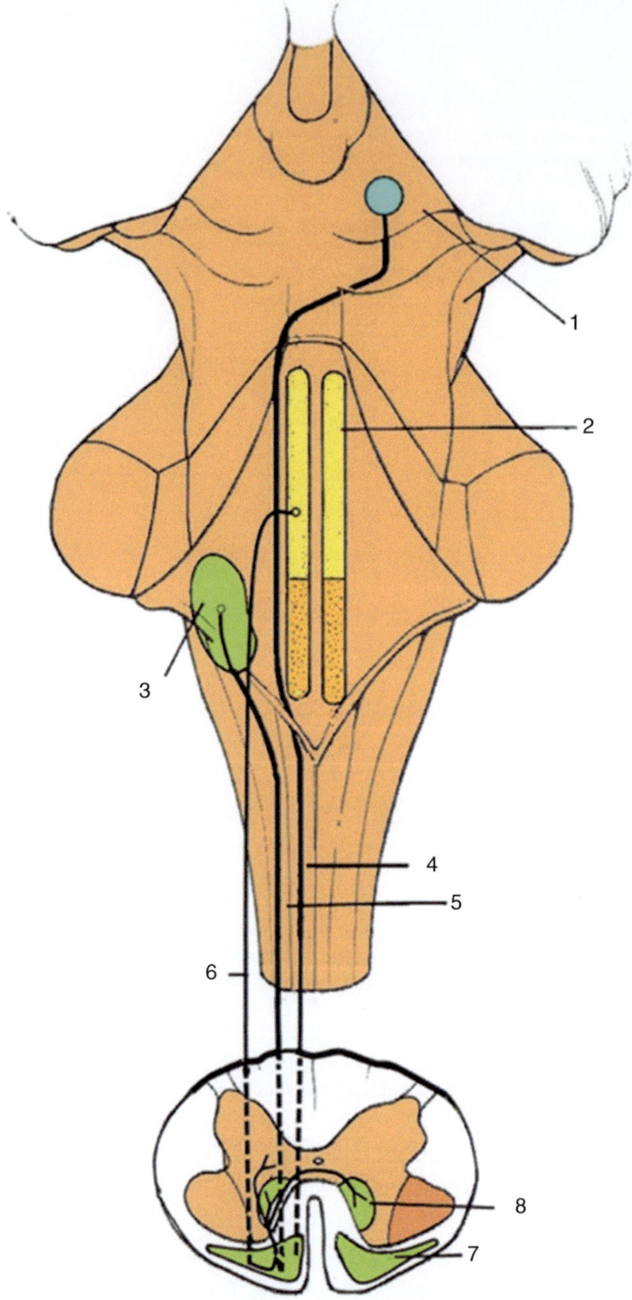

Fig. 24 Anteromedial spinal contingent, facilitator on the ton of extensors: (1) tectum; (2) pontine reticular formation; (3) lateral vestibular nucleus; (4) tectospinal tract; (5) vestibulospinal tract; (6) pontine reticulospinal tract; (7) anterior contingent; (8) medial nuclei

cord, dissociates the sensitivities at the level of the segments underlying the lesion, associating tactile and kinesthetic anesthesia on the same side as the lesion (dorsal funiculus) and a thermoalgesic sensitivity loss in the contralateral segments to this one (crossed spinothalamic tracts).

- A cerebellar programming system that includes the spinocerebellar dorsal tract for the lower limbs and cuneocerebellar tract for the upper limbs, the ventral spinocerebellar tracts, and the spinoolivary and spinovestibular systems. They provide proprioceptive information essential to motor programming through the play of spinocerebellar feedback systems and outside of any conscious perception. In hereditary degenerative spino cerebellar diseases (Friedreich disease and Charcot-Marie-Tooth heredoataxia), the clinical expression is essentially motor and is manifested by ataxia when walking without any sensory deficit.
- A non-specific system corresponds to the paleospinothalamic, spinoreticular, and spinotectal tracts. They do not provide specific information but lead to more global reactions. They activate systems represented by

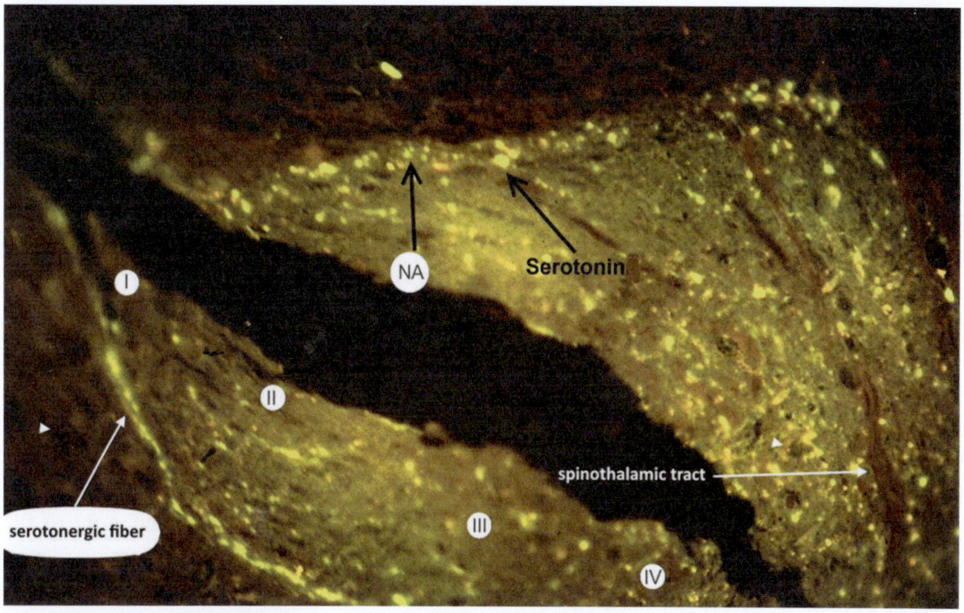

Fig. 25 Terminations of monoaminergic, serotoninergic, and noradrenergic fibers at the superficial layers of the dorsal horns

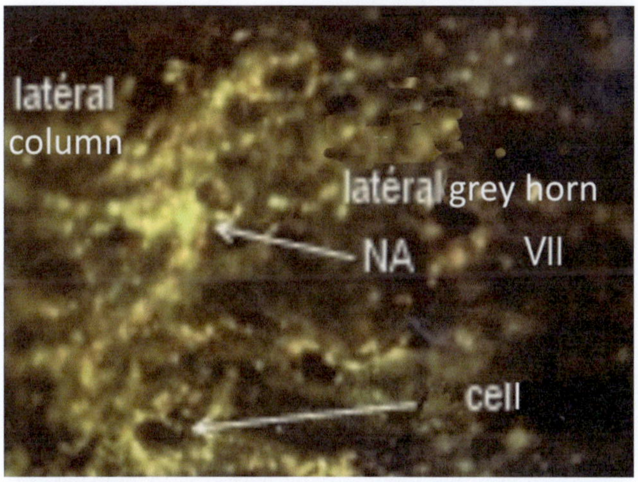

Fig. 26 Projections of noradrenergic fibers (NA) on intermediolateralis nucleus cells (vegetative cells). Fluorescence histochemistry

the reticular brainstem formation and nonspecific nuclei of the thalamus. These regulate levels of alertness, and the emotional and vegetative states that accompany pain and trigger the use of supraspinal analgesic systems that modulate the associated thought process. It is this system which is, therefore, the pharmacological target of surgical anesthesia and resuscitation techniques.

Descending Pathways

The descending pathways have in common their supraspinal origin and direct or, most often, indirect medullary termination on the common final path constituted by the motor neurons located in the ventral horns of the cord.

They convey the motor order that responds to two functional modalities: one is conscious, finalized and oriented towards a fine, precise, and often voluntary gesture, it is the idiokinetic motricity that solicits the distal musculature of the limbs. The other, automatic and more global, requires preprogrammed and synergistic muscle chains: it is the holokinetic motricity.

Two modalities correspond systems that differ in their organization:

1. The corticospinal pyramidal systems establish a direct connection between cerebral cortex and medullary gray matter;
2. Non-pyramidal systems perform an indirect connection between the cerebral cortex and the spinal cord by articulating with suprasegmental formations of the brainstem.

The Pyramidal Tract or Corticospinal Tract (Fig. 22)

The pyramidal tract, or corticospinal tract, comes from the motor (area 4) and premotor (area 6) cortices and descends into the ventromedial part of the brainstem to the medullary level stage, where it divides at the pyramidal decussation in two parts:

- The direct pyramidal tract represents the 20% of fibers that have not undergone decussation. It occupies the ventral cord in contact with the anterior medial fissure and does not extend beyond the cervical segments. It terminates bilaterally on VII and VIII laminae and articulates by interneurons with the medial nuclei of the IX laminae intended for the axial musculature of the neck.

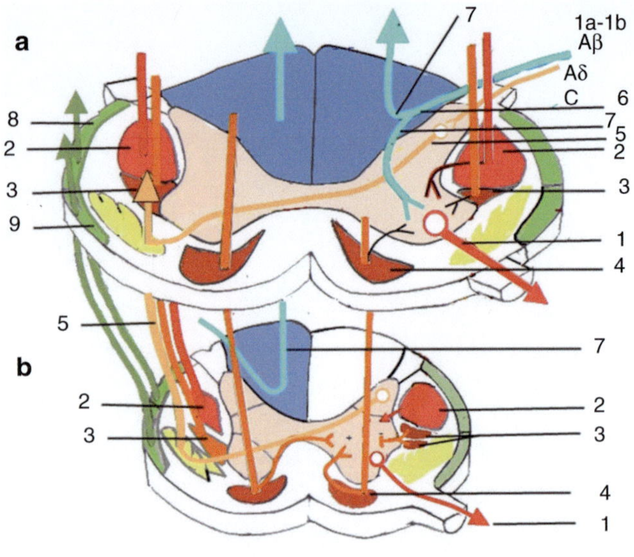

Fig. 27 Anatomical bases of medullary compression syndromes: (1) ventral horn motoneuron; (2) crossed lateral pyramidal tract; (3) dorsolateral contingent of extrapyramidal tracts; (4) ventromedial contingent of extrapyramidal tracts; (5) spinothalamic tract carrying dolorothermal sensation; (6) dorsal cord column; (7) myotatic reflex afferents; (8) dorsal spinocerebellar tract; (9) ventral spinocerebellar tract

- The crossed pyramidal tract is the most important and represents 80% of the fibers. It descends into the lateral column, of which it occupies the posterior part. Its fibers are organized somatotopically so that the most medial are intended for the innervation of the cervical metameres, the most lateral for the sacral segments. They end most often on the interneuronal networks of the VII laminae but, at the level of the cervical enlargement, articulate directly with the retrolateral nuclei of the IX laminae. Their action is to facilitate flexor motor neurons muscle chains mostly on proximal but both flexor and extensor motor neurons supplying the distal muscles are facilitated by this tract. It is exerted on the α-motoneurons. It thus allows fine and precise gestures which solicit especially the distal musculature of the hands and fingers. But this is only possible on the double condition that posture is stabilized in the axial plane and that in the transverse plane the attitude tone stabilizes the proximal segments as necessary support for the release of fine and precise gestures by distal segments of the hands and fingers.
- These conditions are fulfilled by the extrapyramidal systems (see below).

Other fibers use the pyramidal tract but originate in the parietal cortex. They terminate on the dorsal horns where they exert an inhibitory action on the passage of segmental nociceptive information. This would be the explanation of the current observation of the transient insensitivity to pain observed during intense physical engagement during a fight or match as if, in a situation of danger, priority is given to action for the survival of the individual.

Extra Non-pyramidal Tracts

The non-pyramidal tracts come from supra segmental formations of the brainstem where cortical or cerebellar influences are relayed.

The rubrospinal tract (Fig. 23) originates in the red nucleus in the mesencephalic tegmentum. It is crossed from its origin and descends laterally into the brainstem and cord, in front of the crossed pyramidal tract and like it, gives collaterals which terminate on the lateral part of the central zone and the lateral nuclei of the ventral horn corresponding to the proximal musculature of the intermediate segments (elbow and knees). Its action is exerted on the γ-motoneurons. The red nucleus receives collaterals from the pyramidal tract, but especially cross-cerebellar afferents that come from the intermediate lobe of the cerebellum and the corresponding cerebellar central nuclei (interposed nuclei). It is thus situated on the feedback loop of the spinocerebellar system whose afferent pathways are the spinocerebellar and cuneocerebellar pathways. It intervenes on the tone of attitude, which solicits the flexors of the intermediate segments of the limbs (elbows). A decorticate rigidity is characterized by hypertonia in flexion of the arms, thus expresses an impairment of the brainstem above the red nucleus, thus relinquishing its influence on the flexor muscles of the upper limbs (Diagram 4).

The vestibulospinal tracts originate in the lateral and medial vestibular nuclei. They descend into the ventral column and at each metameric level give collaterals that project bilaterally onto the interneuronal networks of lamellae VII and VIII. Their action is exerted on the α- and γ-motoneurons and on the medial nuclei intended for the axial, musculature in such a way to facilitate extensor muscles. They intervene in the control of postural tone and balance from the information which comes from the vestibular nerve (VIII), the spinal cord (by the spinovestibular tract), and the vestibulocerebellum (flocculonodular lobe) which converge towards the vestibular nuclei.

The reticulospinal tracts come from the medial reticular zone, the lateral reticular formation, the bulbar raphe nuclei, and the parvocellular reticular area formation [15].

- The medial reticulospinal tract is of pontine origin. It comes from the medial nuclei (pontis oralis and pontis caudalis) which are already involved in vigilance by their ascending efferents which constitute the ascending activator reticular system. On the other hand, they receive descending afferents of the cerebral cortex, mainly of the premotor area by collaterals of the pyramidal tract and by the medial telencephalon tract influences coming from the hypothalamus, limbic system, and pallidum which cross the cholinergic pedunculopontine reticular nucleus where the mesencephalic locomotor area is located. This reticulospinal tract is medial and descends into the ventral funiculus of the spinal cord. It ends on VII and VIII layers where it exerts a facilitating action on the tone of the axial and proximal extensor muscles of the limbs. The activity of this pontine facilitator system is related to the systems involved in vigilance. In the waking state, it is this facilitator system that is the most active and maintains the muscle tone to prepare the muscle for action. Conversely, during sleep or deep anesthesia, the muscle tone gradually decreases to reach flaccidity (Fig. 24).

- The lateral reticulospinal tract is of medullary origin and comes from the nucleus gigantocellularis. It receives excitatory afferents of cortical origin from the supplementary motor area, the caudate nucleus as well as the anterior lobe of the cerebellum (the destruction of which causes increased muscle tone); it descends into the lateral column of the spinal cord and terminates in the interneurons of the lateral part of the VII lamellae, where it exerts its action on the α- and γ-motoneurons of the lateral nuclei and on the proximal musculature. It is inhibitory for the musculature of the extensors and, on the contrary, facilitates the tone of the flexors. The activity of this bulbar inhibitor system is permanent and balances the strong influence of the myotatic reflex which tends to exaggerate tone.
- The fibers of bulbar raphe nuclei (raphe magnus, obscurus, and pallidus nuclei) are essentially serotoninergic and only identifiable by fluorescence histochemistry techniques. They descend into the lateral cord and constitute three parts:
  - the dorsal contingent terminates on the superficial dorsal horn layers (Fig. 25) and is one of the endogenous devices of supraspinal analgesia (descending pain control),
  - the intermediate contingent projects onto the intermediolateral columns at the level of the thoracic segments and has an inhibitory effect in the control of cardiovascular functions (Fig. 26),
  - the ventral contingent exerts an excitatory effect on both the motoneurons of the flexors and extensors. All these systems solicit these serotoninergic pathways seem to work together in a context of vital emergency combat or defense associating a suppression of the sensation of pain to an increase in the reaction capabilities of motor neurons directly involved in the action.
- Fibers from the parvocellular lateral reticular area nuclei are noradrenergic and involved in the control of vegetative functions. They are organized into a network and give scattered fibers that descend into the lateral and ventral cords identified by fluorescence histochemistry. At the medullary level (area superficialis ventrolateralis) the respiratory, inspiratory, and expiratory centers connected to the Kolliker-Fuse pneumotaxic nucleus articulate with the central motor neurons of the phrenic and intercostal nerves. They also emit fibers for the intermediolateral column of the thoracic spinal cord for blood pressure and heart rate control. At the pontine level, the reticular nucleus of the pontine tegmentum receives afferents from insular cortex, amygdala, and hypothalamus. It contains the mictionnal nuclei of Holstege that emits efferents towards the motoneurons and the cells of the intermedioventral columns of the sacral component of the cord, ensuring a vesicosphincteric synergy where the contraction of the detrusor is accompanied by the inhibition of the striated sphincter. At the mesencephalic level, the locus coeruleus gives descending fibers that terminate on the superficial lamellae of the dorsal horn (Fig. 25) and is one of the supraspinal analgesic functions, blocking the passage of nociceptive impulses. These noradrenergic fibers are also distributed (Fig. 26) on the intermediate columns of the spinal cord for the control of vasomotricity. These catecholaminergic pathways have thus been implicated in the pathophysiology of traumatic myelopathies. Experimentally, in cats [16] during spinal cord contusions respecting the white matter, they are intensely visualized at their endings in the gray matter creating the initial intramedullary ischemia lesions which then extend secondarily to the white matter by action on local vasomotricity.

Other tracts of supraspinal origin pass through the ventral column. They are mainly intended for the cervical segments of the cord. The tectospinal tracts come from the nuclei of the mesencephalic tectum, which receive visual afferents (upper contingent) and auditory afferents (lower contingent). They are crossed from their origin and occupy the ventral column to terminate bilaterally on the VII layers. They intervene in the control of the tone of cervical muscles with relation to visual and auditory information. The olivospinal tract originates from the olive located on the ventral surface of the medulla and presents the same systematization as the previous ones. It is part of the olivo-dentato-rubric triangle, a functional loop whose disruption causes myoclonic jerks in the limbs.

In Total

The extrapyramidal descending tracts can be grouped into two contingents organized into individual bundles (Kuypers):

1. The anteromedial contingent corresponds to the medial longitudinal tract. It comprises pontine reticulospinal

tracts, tectospinal, vestibulospinal, and olivospinal tracts. These bundles have in common their position in the ventral column of the cord, their mode of termination on the VII and VIII layers in an ipsi- and contralateral way, and finally their facilitating influence on the tone of the axial, extensor, and antigravific muscles. It thus intervenes in the control of the postural tone and during the stance phase of locomotion.

2. The posterolateral contingent includes rubrospinal and medullary reticulospinal tracts. It is located in the lateral column and ends on the interneurons of the lateral zone of the VII lamellae from which it intervenes on the lateral nuclei of the ventral horn; its influence is inhibitory for the tone of the extensors and facilitatory for that of the flexors of the proximal intermediate segments of the limbs. It thus intervenes in the control of the tone of attitude which facilitates the flexion the segments of limbs, bringing them closer to the visual control and then helps to increase the precision of gestures realized by the distal segments of the limbs.

This functional balance thus achieved in controlling the tone of the flexors and extensors by these extrapyramidal pathways can, in a pathological situation, be unbalanced and then create different states of rigidity depending on the level of impairment. The decortication rigidity is thus characterized by flexion hypertonia of the proximo-distal segments of the limbs and corresponds to an attack located above the upper colliculi, thus releasing the influence of the red nucleus and the rubrospinal tract from the tone of the flexors. The decerebration rigidity is characterized by a hypertonia in extension with rigidity of the axial musculature and winding movements in extension of the proximo-axial muscles of the limbs. It reflects a pontomesencephalic level brainstem involvement, located below the colliculi, which liberates the facilitating influence of the pontine reticular zone on the tone of extensor muscles of the axial and proximal musculature. If the lesion is at the medullary level, the only dominant influence is that of the bulbar reticulospinal inhibitory tract on the extensors so that a coma would be flaccid (Fig. 4).

The involvement of these different fascicles in the white matter corresponds to (Fig. 27) the clinically observed central sublesional syndrome. It is associated with the territories situated below the lesion and on the same side:

- a paralysis of all the muscles by involvement of pyramidal tracts,
- spastic hypertonia after the initial insult, when the influence of the myotatic reflex predominates over that of inhibitory interneurons deprived of the modulatory influence of the extrapyramidal descending tracts. The Babinski sign (inverted plantar reflex) reflects the resurgence of archaic reflexes and of medullary automatisms.
- a release of vegetative reflexes that reflects the recovery of autonomy of sympathetic and parasympathetic spinal cord centers.

On contrary, the lesional syndrome is metameric and pseudoradicular reflecting the involvement of the gray matter and thus affecting motor and sensitive functions at the same level.

(A) Metameric lesional syndrome (pseudoradicular) resulting in involvement of the gray matter: flaccid paralysis in the myotome, areflexia, anesthesia in the dermatome. If the lesion is centromedullary (syringomyelic syndrome), only the dolorothermal sensation is affected (and theoretically bilaterally) as well as the vegetative reflexes, but the tactile and kinesthetic sensation is preserved in the dermatome.

(B) Sublesional syndrome resulting to involvement of the white matter tracts
   - paralysis of all underlying segments and ipsilateral pyramidal lesion and Babinski sign (by release of the elementary motor programmes of pyramidal influence),
   - hyperreflexia with spasticity—tactile and kinesthetic anesthesia of all the underlying segments and dolorothermic analgesia of the subjacent and contralateral side to the lesion.

References

1. Rexed B. A cytoarchitectonic atlas of the spinal cord in the cat. J Comp Neurol. 1952;96(3):41595.
2. Defebre L, Kemoun G. Organisation neuroanatomique et physiologique de la marche. Presse Med. 2001;30(9):44551.
3. Buchanan JT, McPherson DR. The neural network for locomotion lamprey spinal cord. Evidence for involvement of commissural interneurons. J Physiol. 1995;89:22133.
4. Kiehn O. Locomotor circuits in the mammalian spinal cord. Annu Rev Neurosci. 2006;29:279306.
5. Stein PSG. Central pattern generator in the spinal cord. In: Davidoff R, editor. Handbook of the spinal cord, vol. 24. New York: Marcel Dekker; 1984. p. 64772.
6. Frigon A. Central pattern generators of the mammalian spinal cord. Neuroscientist. 2012;18(1):5669.
7. Pearson K. The control of walking. Sci Am. 1976;33:7286.
8. Purves D, Augustine GJ, Fitzpatrick D, Katz LC, Lamantia AS, McNamara WM. Lower motor neuron circuits and motor control. Spinal cord circuitry and locomotion. In: Neuroscience. Sunderland: Sinauer Associates; 2001. p. 36168.
9. Guerin J, Bioulac B. Organisation anatomique et physiologique de la moelle épinière. Anat Clin. 1979;1:26789.

10. Richard D, Orsal D. La moelle épinière est le siège d'activités automatiques. In: Neurophysiologie. Motricité et grandes fonctions du système nerveux central. Paris: Nathan; 1994. p. 7194.
11. Delmas A, Laux G. Systeme nerveux sympathique. Etude macroscopique et systématique. Paris: Masson; 1952.
12. Guerin J, Bioulac B, Henry P, Loiseau P. Le système nerveux végétatif. Anatomie, physiologie, pathologie. Paris: Sandoz; 1979.
13. Guerin J. Voies et centres du système nerveux autonome. In: Bossy J, editor. Anatomie clinique neuroanatomie. Paris: Springer; 1990. p. 291303.
14. Price DD. Dorsal horn mechanisms of pain. In: Davidoff R, editor. Handbook of the spinal cord, vol. 24. New York: Marcel Dekker; 1984. p. 75177.
15. Melzack R, Wall PD. Pain mechanism. A new theory. Science. 1965;15:97179.
16. Basbaum AL, Fields HL. Endogenous pain control systems. Brainstem spinal pathways and endorphin circuitry. Annu Rev Neurosci. 1984;7:309–38.

Spinal Nerves (Innervation of the Spine)

B. Lavignolle

General and Nomenclature

The nerves that emerge from the spine are mixed nerves (Fig. 1). They innervate the whole body, except the face. They provide somatic and autonomic (vegetative) innervation through common branches. There are 8 cervical nerves (C), 12 thoracic nerves (T), 5 lumbar nerves (L), 5 sacral nerves (S), and 1 coccygeal nerve (CO). The spinal nerves are located in the intervertebral or sacral foramina and are numbered as described: Until the seventh cervical vertebra (C7), the spinal nerves have the number of the underlying vertebra and from the T1 vertebra, the nerves carry the name and number of the overlying vertebra; the eighth cervical nerve represents the root that emerges between C7 and T1 (Figs. 2 and 3).

Descriptive Anatomy of Spinal Nerves

Each spinal nerve is connected to the spinal cord via two roots, ventral and dorsal, a few millimeters long, which unite to form the trunk of the spinal nerve:

- the ventral or motor root emerges opposite the ventral horn of the spinal cord;
- the dorsal or sensitive root penetrates opposite the dorsal horn of the spinal cord.

The dorsal root gives rise to the spinal ganglion.

The spinal nerve roots form the trunk of the spinal nerve in the intervertebral foramen where it is surrounded by the dura mater. Each spinal nerve gives a spinal meningeal branch or sinuvertebral nerve of Luschka (Figs. 4 and 5).

The spinal nerves have a variable course, horizontal in the cervical region, and increasingly oblique in an inferolateral fashion as the spinal cord descends because of the growth discordance between the spinal cord and the spine.

B. Lavignolle (✉)
Anatomy Laboratory, Bordeaux University Hospital, Bordeaux, France

Each spinal nerve is a mixed nerve that contains afferent and efferent, somatic and autonomic fibers:

- somatic fibers with centrifugal motor fibers of axons in the ventral horn of the spinal cord and sensory centripetal fiber sensory neurons of the spinal ganglion.
- autonomic fibers belong to the sympathetic and parasympathetic systems.

The autonomic efferent (away from) fibers travel in the anterior root and then in the spinal nerve, which they leave by the communicating white branches to make synapses in the paravertebral sympathetic ganglia.

Autonomic afferent (towards) fibers have their cell bodies at the level of the spinal ganglia that they join either directly by the peripheral nerves, or by the communicating gray branches and the paravertebral sympathetic ganglionic chain of visceral origin.

The spinal nerve divides into two terminal branches just outside the foramen and therefore the spinal nerves are sometimes very short (less than 7 mm) (Fig. 6).

- a small dorsal branch for the muscles and skin of the dorsal wall of the neck and trunk;
- a larger ventral branch for the ventral wall of the trunk and limbs. It forms the different cervical (C1C4), brachial (C5T1), and lumbosacral (T12S5) plexuses by multiple and complex anastomoses.

Relations of the Nerve Roots

At the Lumbar Level [1–6]

The spinal ganglion in L1 measures 7 mm by 5 mm and the size increases to S1 where it reaches a maximum of 13 × 6 mm.

The distance from the axilla of the root to the proximal part of the ganglion varies from 6 mm for L1 to 15 mm for S1. The ganglion is under the pedicle in 90% of cases, in 2% it is medial and in 8% inferolateral.

J. M. Vital, D. T. Cawley (eds.), *Spinal Anatomy*, https://doi.org/10.1007/978-3-030-20925-4_25

Fig. 1 Posterior general view

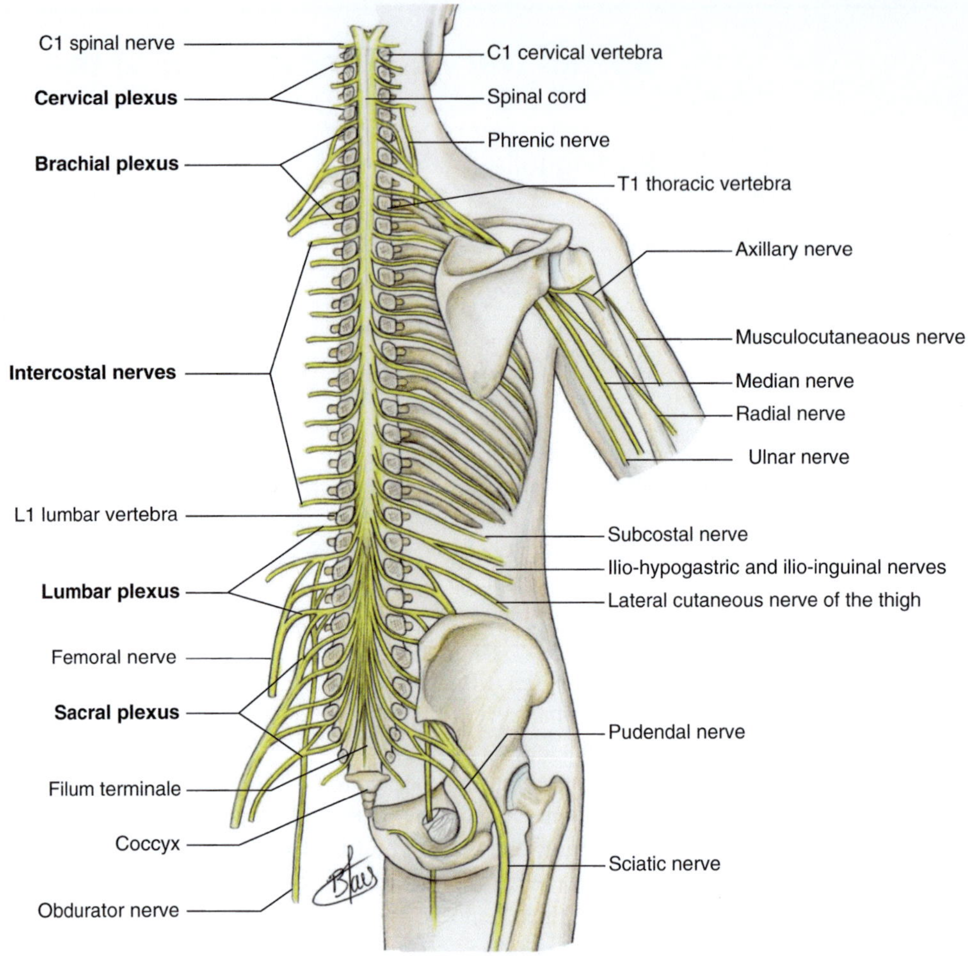

The meninges are in close relationship with the nerve roots.

Beyond the dural sac, the roots are enveloped by the pia mater, the arachnoid, and the dura mater. The arteries and root veins are transmitted within these sheaths. The dural sac rests on the posterior longitudinal ligament covering vertebral bodies and discs. Posteriorly, the dural sac is in relation with the laminae and yellow ligaments. The epidural space is relatively narrow because the dural sac is in very close contact with the osteoligamentary structures.

This connective space is filled by the epidural membrane that surrounds the dural sac and lines the laminae and pedicles. Anteriorly, the membrane lines the back of the vertebral bodies and attaches to the anterior surface of the deep portion of the posterior longitudinal ligament. The membrane does not cover the posterior portion of the annulus fibrosus because of the posterior longitudinal ligament that extends laterally over the posterior portion of the annulus fibrosus.

In front of the intervertebral foramen, the epidural membrane extends laterally to form a perineural envelope around the dural sheath of the roots and spinal nerve. The anterior and posterior vertebral venous plexuses are transmitted in the areolar tissue of the epidural membrane [7].

In the vertebral canal, the dural sac and the sheaths of the nerve roots are attached to the spine by thickening of the epidural fascia or meningovertebral ligament of Hoffmann. These ligaments pass from the anterior dural surface to the posterior longitudinal ligament, from the lateral surface of the dural sac to the periosteum of the pedicles, and to the ceiling of the vertebral canal by fine and fragile dorsal bundles.

At the cervical level, there are 8 pairs of cervical spinal nerves. The cervical spinal nerve is very short (7 mm) and the volume is greater for the last 4 cervical nerves of the upper limb than the first 4 cervical nerves for the neck.

The cervical spinal nerves are formed by the union of the anterior and posterior roots.

The ganglion of C1, when it exists, is located in the vertebral canal and that of C2, behind the C1C2 articulation.

The anterior root is three times smaller than the posterior root. The path in the intradural portion is horizontal from C1 to C4 and the obliquity increases as one descends to the tho-

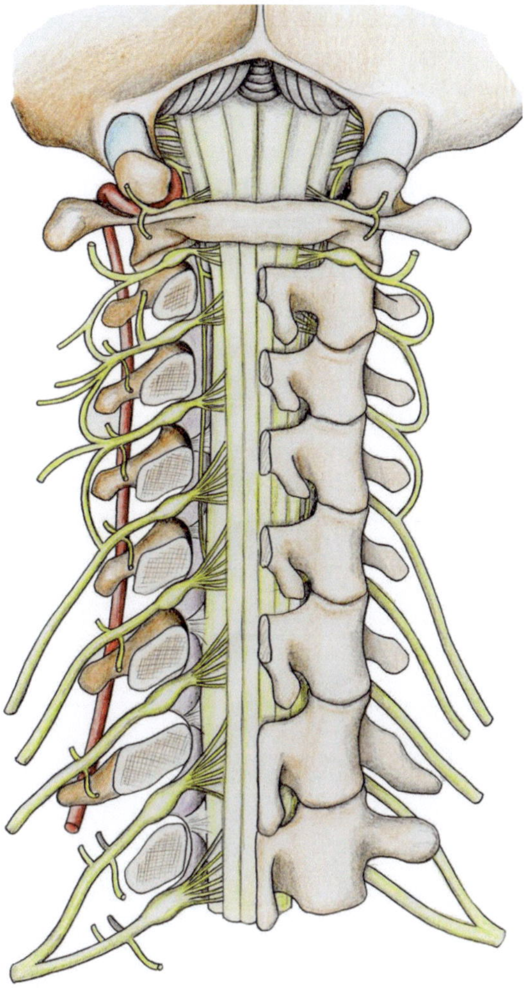

Fig. 2 Posterior view of cervical spinal nerves

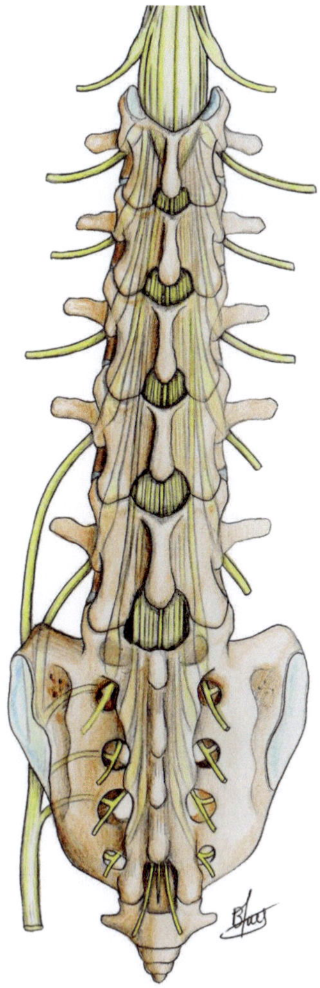

Fig. 3 Posterior view of lumbosacral spinal nerves

racic region. The roots leave the dural sheath by two orifices separated by a vertical septum.

The two roots pass behind the uncinate apophysis and the anterior motor root is anteroinferior to the posterior root and thus protected from disc compression.

The two roots form the spinal nerve at the outer pole of the spinal ganglion which is always in the foramen, behind the vertebral artery.

The cervical spinal nerve occupies only 20–50% of the foramen surface.

The remaining surface is occupied by the fat, the venous plexuses in continuity with those of the epidural space, and by the means of fixity of the spinal nerve, the epidural tissue condenses and constitutes a sheath which does not adhere to the wall of the foramen nor to the dura mater of the roots but only to the posterior longitudinal ligament in front and to the capsule of the interapophyseal joints behind. This sheath becomes adherent more laterally to the spinal nerve.

The fibrous bundles described by Sunderland [8–12] fix the epidural sheath to the sheath of the transverse process and to the transverse and supranuclear process for the nerves C5, C6, and C7. The dissection under a microscope [13] does not allow retention of a true tethering ligament, but connective attachments on the periphery of the nerve.

An experimental study of 50 cervical roots [13] to determine the tensile strength of the roots shows that tearing occurs by forces of 3–15 kg and is always preceded by rupture of the dura mater.

The spinal nerve crosses, with the root artery, the fibrous operculum of the central external orifice of the foramen and loses its dural sheath on the internal face of the operculum.

The sinuvertebral nerve penetrates with the venous plexuses into the foramina from outside inwards through a peripheral orifice distinct from that of the spine nerve which is situated in front of the latter [14, 15].

Arnold's nerve is the posterior branch of the second cervical nerve with its occipital ascending course. The posterior ganglion of C2 is extradural and located at the posterior aspect of the inferior articular facet of the lateral mass of the atlas. It is adherent to the capsule of the lateral atlantoaxial joint, 6–12 mm inside the vertebral artery. The large occipital nerve has a sinusoidal course and has been studied in detail [14].

It bypasses the inferior oblique muscle, traversing the semi-spinalis and trapezius to become subcutaneous and gives off its sensory terminal branches. The motor collaterals innervate the posterior intertransversarii cervicis muscles, the semi-spinalis capitis, the splenius, and the inferior oblique. The nerve is vulnerable in its passage under the inferior oblique during cervical flexion. Arnold's nerve anastomoses with the posterior branches of the mastoid branch of the cervical plexus, the articular branch of the facial nerve, and with the posterior cervical branches of C1 and C3.

1.1.1 Anomalies of the Lumbar Roots [16–18] (Fig. 7)

Type 1 abnormalities have an abnormal path (type 1A where two pairs of roots can emerge from a single dural sheath or the lower part of the dural sac). In type 2, the number of roots may vary in a foramen (type 2 B) or the foramen may be empty (2A). For type 3, these are extradural anomalies.

Abnormalities are infrequent (8%) and symptomatic, with atypical neurologic distribution and identification by the myelogram.

Innervation of the Spine

Luschka (1850) demonstrated the existence of a dorsal innervation different from the ventral innervation of the spinal nerve.

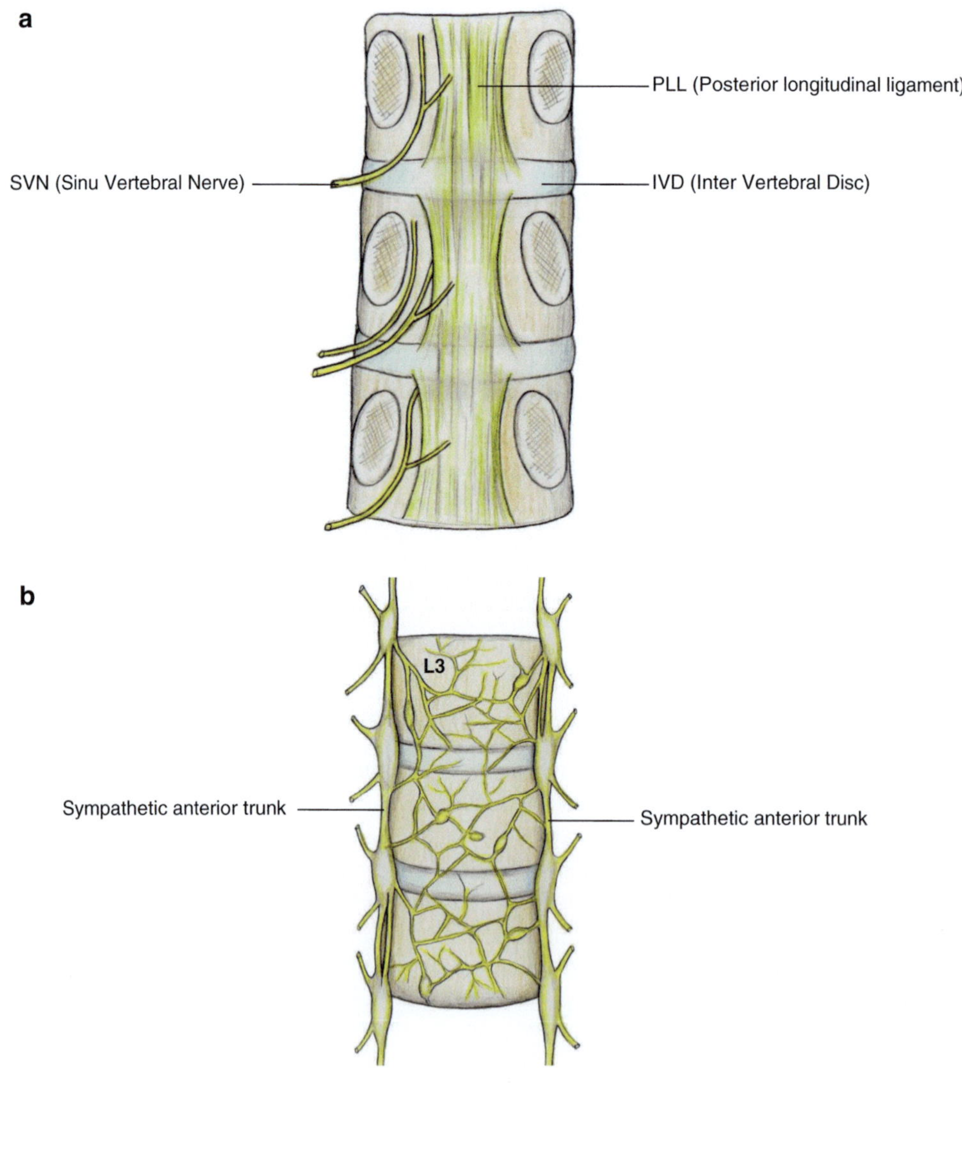

Fig. 4 Sinuvertebral nerve of Luschka and anterior and posterior plexus (according to Groen); sinuvertebral nerve on posterior view (**a**), anterior plexus on anterior view (**b**), posterior plexus on posterior view (**c**)

c

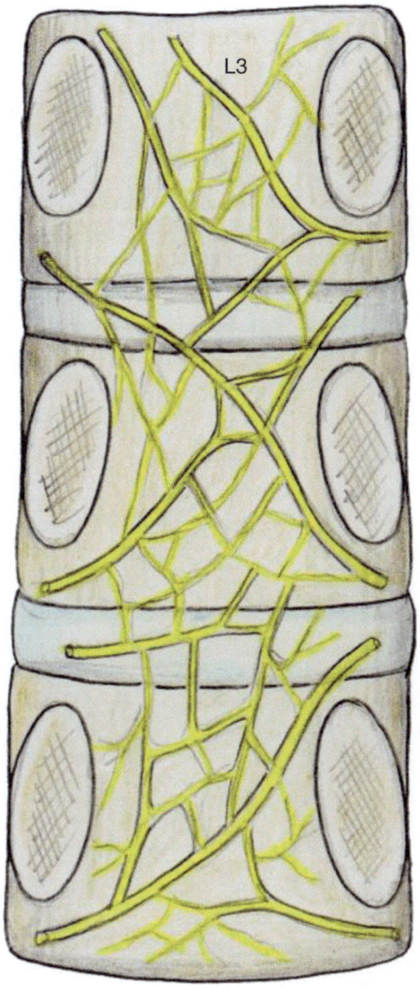

Fig. 4 (continued)

This distinction between hypomere (or ventral territory of the myotome) and epimer (or dorsal territory) was confirmed by Lazorthes [19, 20] which defines the innervation of the posterior vertebral arch and the anastomoses between the somatic and autonomic systems at the level of sinuvertebral nerve.

Bogduk [21] resumed the vertebral anatomical study under optical magnification and proposes a new diagram of the innervation of the spine.

There are two functional territories, ventral and dorsal, separated by a frontal or coronal theoretical plane passing through the transverse processes with the two ventral and dorsal territories (Fig. 8).

Innervation of the Ventral Territory [22–24]

It includes the ventral part of the dura mater and the dural sac, the intervertebral disc, the anterior and posterior longitudinal ligaments, and the prevertebral muscles.

The ventral branch of the spinal nerves innervates:

- at lumbar level, the two portions of the psoas muscle, quadratus lumborum, and intertransversarii muscles. The lumbosacral plexus consists of the ventral branches of the spinal nerves from T12 to S5;
- at the thoracic level, the intercostal muscles by the intercostal nerves which extend from the spinal nerves;
- at the cervical level, the cervical plexus formed from the ventral branches of the C1 to C4 cervical spinal nerves innervates the anterolateral muscles of the neck, the diaphragm (C4), and the skin of the cervical and superolateral regions of the thorax.

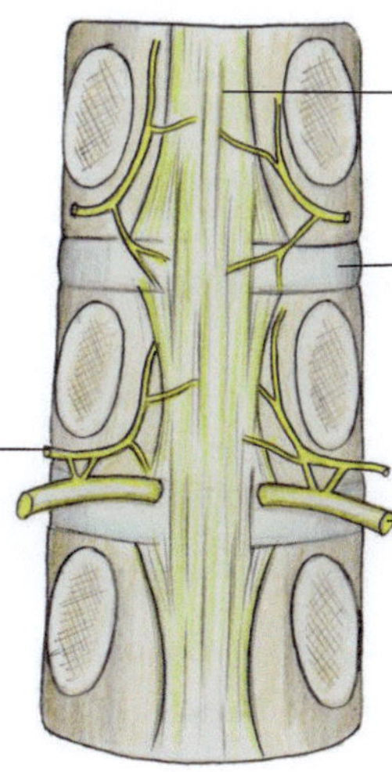

Fig. 5 Anterior ramus of the root on posterior view (according to Groen)

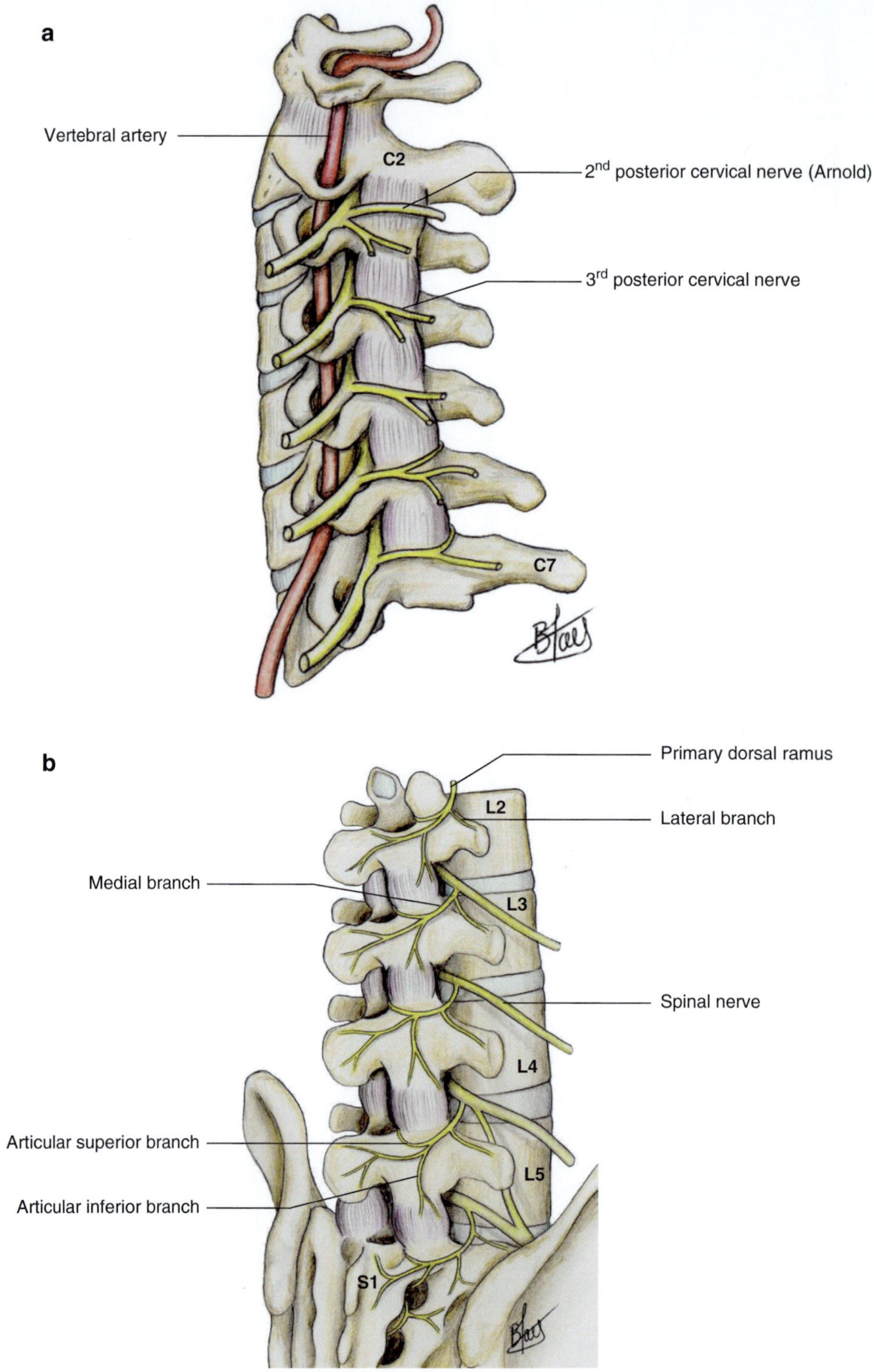

Fig. 6 Spinal nerve division in cervical area (**a**) and lumbar area (**b**)

The brachial plexus, formed by the ventral branches of cervical spinal nerves (C5T1), innervates the muscles of the scapular, ventral thoracic and thoracic limb muscles.

The sinuvertebral nerve (NSV) or meningeal branch is formed by the union of a somatic branch coming from the ventral root and an autonomic branch coming from the sym-

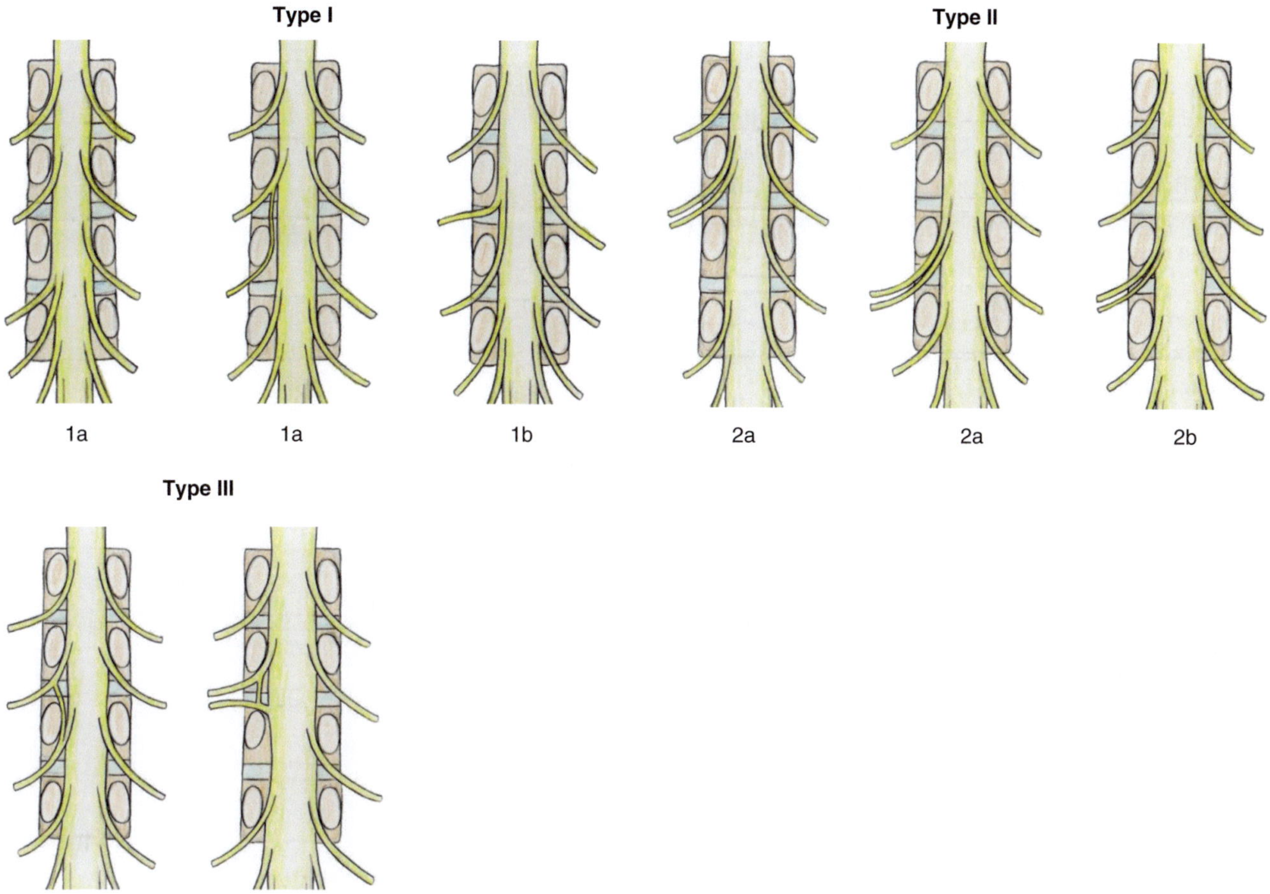

Fig. 7 Anomalies of the lumbar roots

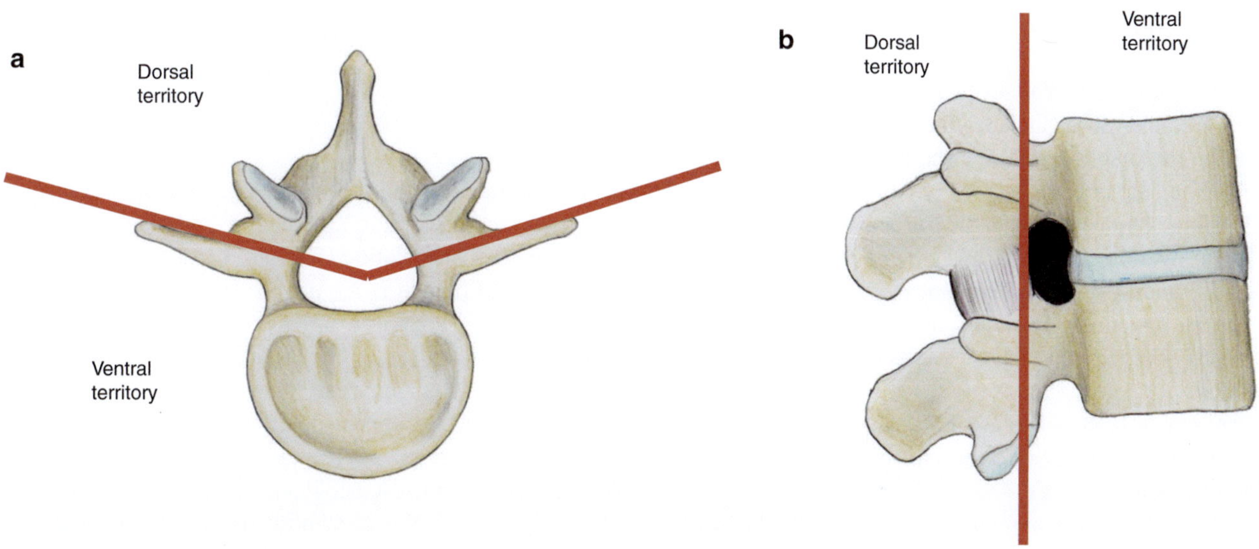

Fig. 8 Dorsal and ventral territories. (**a**) upper view; (**b**) lateral view

pathetic side chain, via the exclusively communicating gray branch.

These gray communicating branches are evident in all the spinal nerves and consist of postganglionic amyelinic (lacking a myelin sheath) neurofibers. The axons of the sympathetic cells of the branches take the ventral root of the spinal nerves from T1 to L2, leaving the nerves by the communicating white myelinated branches and connect the spinal nerve to the paravertebral ganglionic chain.

The territory of the NSV (Figs. 4 and 5) includes dura mater, epidural and intrasomatic vessels, and the dorsal longitudinal ligament.

Systematization makes it possible to describe:

- a descending branch for the dura mater to the same level and the underlying segment;
- a segmental transverse branch for the annulus fibrosus and the dorsal longitudinal ligament in the segmental posterolateral zone;
- an ascending limb for the LCV and the overlying retrocorporeal area.

Innervation of the Dorsal Territory [1, 21, 25, 26]

The dorsal territory includes the posterior vertebral arch and the deep intrinsic spinal muscles. Innervation is by the posterior branches of the spinal nerves by three distinct branches: lateral, intermediate, and median (Fig. 9).

Rickenbacher reports 61% of cervical posterior branch anastomoses, 7% at the thoracic level, and 22% at the lumbar level.

At the thoracolumbar level, muscular innervation: the common lumbar mass includes the longissimus dorsi innervated by the lateral branch and the iliocostal innervated by the intermediate branch.

The lateral branches of L1–L3 traverse the iliocostal muscle, cross over the iliac crest, and are distributed on the cutaneous aspect of the greater trochanter.

The intermediate branches of L1–L3 form a plexus inside the longissimus dorsi. There is no lateral branch for L5.

The medial branches of L1–L5 innervate the multifidus, interspinous, intertransverse muscles behind the intertransverse ligament.

The spinal innervation is entirely supported by the medial branch, which bypasses the base of the superior articular process from beneath and behind the mamilloaccessory ligament, which especially if calcified can create a compression for the medial branch. Lower down, the medial branch gives 4 branches: to the ligament and interspinous muscle, the posterior vertebral arch and the yellow ligament, the segmental interapophyseal posterior articulation and the underlying interapophyseal articulation.

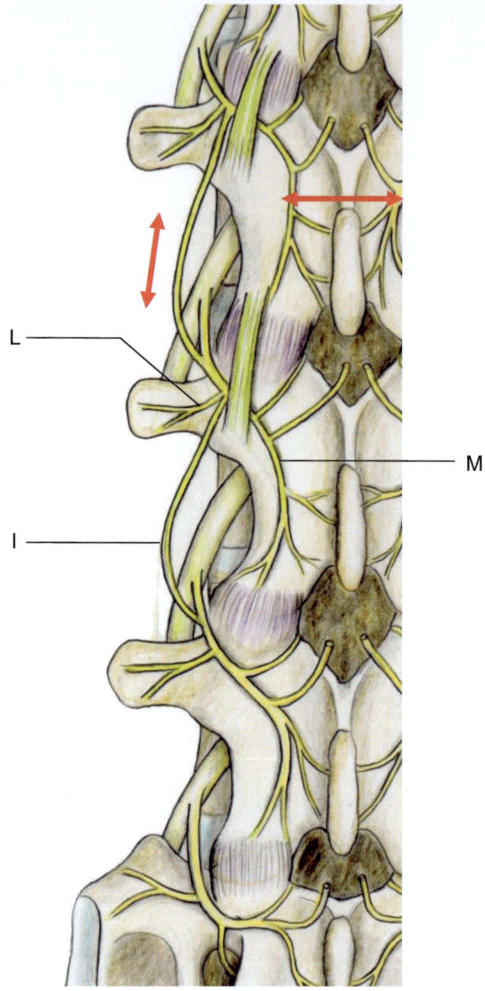

Fig. 9 *L* lateral branch of the posterior ramus, *I* intermediate branch, *M* medial branch. (Red arrows: vertical and transversal anastomosis, according to Bogduk)

This medial branch is the precise target of percutaneous radiofrequency rhizotomy in the arthrotransverse zone (Bogduk) [27] (Fig. 10).

Receptors: Zygapophyseal joint capsules [28, 29] are richly innervated by encapsulated and free nerve endings that transmit proprioceptive and nociceptive information. The nerves contain substance P and CGRP (calcitonin gene-related peptide) and Y neuropeptide frequently. The majority of zygapophyseal joint nerves are efferent sympathetic fibers and not sensory fibers.

Nerve endings are also found in the subchondral bone, interspinous and supraspinal ligaments, and thoracolumbar fascia in the form of mechanoreceptors.

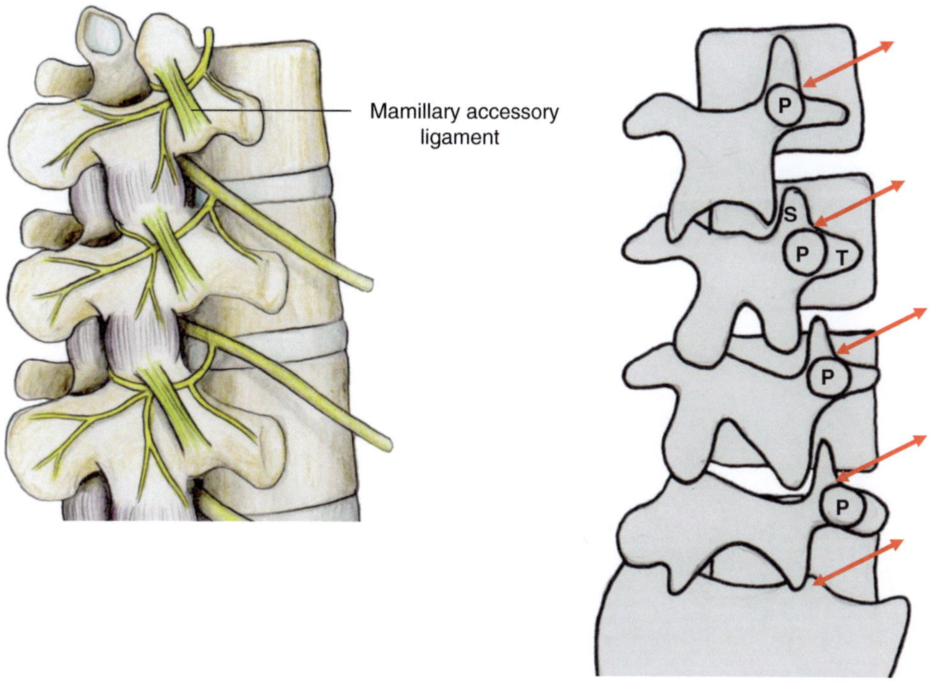

Fig. 10 Oblique view of the lumbar spine for needle position: *S* superior articular, *P* pedicle, *T* transverse process (red arrows: targets of the rhizotomy RF)

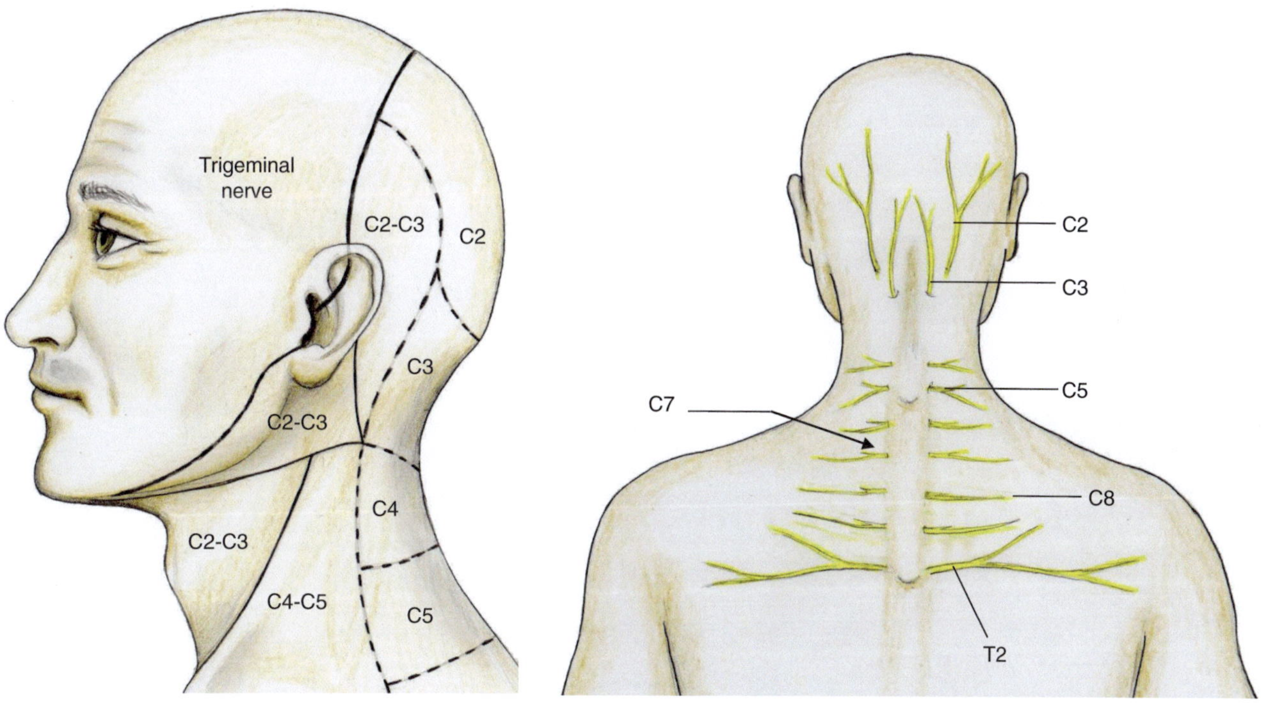

Fig. 11 Posterior cervical dermatomes

The advent of local anesthetic blocks of the lumbar and cervicothoracic spine nerves which are guided by fluoroscopy allow the evaluation of cutaneous distribution of dermatomes in individuals without any neurological pathology [30].

Applications

Pain syndromes of articular origin at the cervical and thoracolumbar level have a spinal topography that corresponds to the epimeric dermatome of the dorsal ramus (Fig. 11).

The triggering of pain by mechanical stimulation makes it possible to recognize these syndromes (Lazorthe G.) with physical treatment of muscle spasm to break the algogenic (pain causing) reflex loop and involve inhibitory mechanoreceptors (Fig. 12).

However, the recovery of the medial branches at the articular level makes it possible to explain certain failures of hyperselective infiltration and thermolysis performed at a single level.

Pseudoradiculalgia (cervico-brachial neuralgia, calf pain, sciatica) has a non-radicular referred topography with cellulo-tenomyalgic (e.g., Maigne) syndrome of the dorsal spinal ramus, compressed by ossification of the mamillary ligament or intertransverse ligament that may justify a surgical neurolysis of the dorsal ramus.

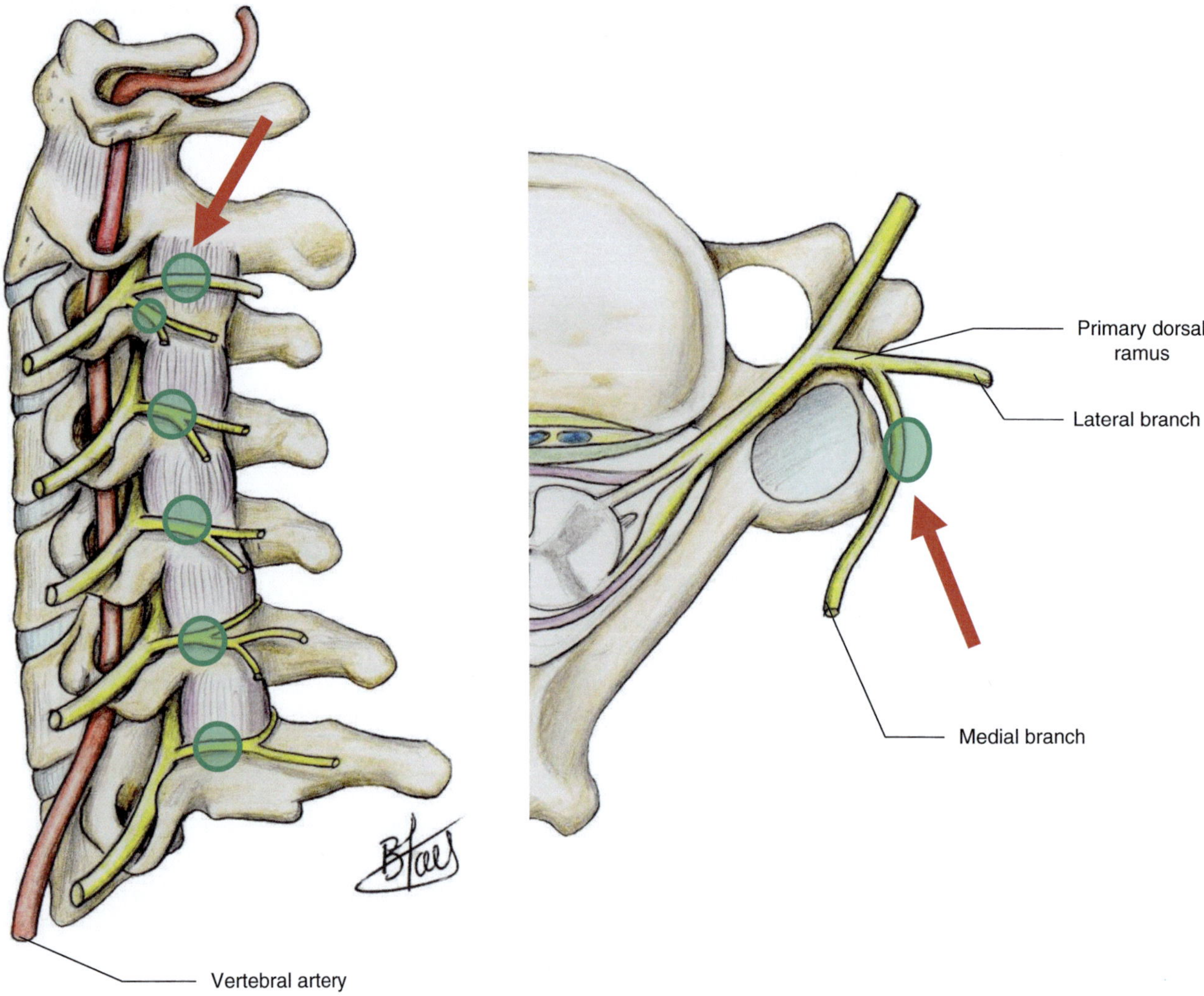

Fig. 12 Lateral and superior views of the cervical spine for needle position (green zones and red arrows)

References

1. Auteroche P. Innervation of the zygapophyseal joints of the lumbar spine. Anat Clin. 1983;5:17–28.
2. D'avella D, et al. Microsurgical anatomy of lumbosacral roots. J Neuro-Oncol. 1979;51:819–23.
3. Hasue M, et al. Anatomic study of the interrelation between lumbosacral nerve roots and their surrounding tissues. Spine. 1983;8(1):50–8.
4. Lazennec JY. Anatomie du rachis. In: Roy Camille R, Saillant G, et al., editors. Le Rachis. Paris: Masson Édit; 1995.
5. Penning L, et al. Biomechanics of lumbodural sac. Spine. 1981;6:4.
6. Rolland J, et al. Les veines lombaires épidurales. J Radiol. 1977;58(1):35–8.
7. Crock HV. The blood supply of the vertebral column and spinal cord in man. New York: Springer; 1977.
8. Scapinelli R. Anatomical and radiological studies of the lumbosacral meningovertebral ligaments of humans. J Spinal Disord. 1990;3:6–15.
9. Suntherland S. Meningo-neural relations in the intervertebral foramen. J Neurosurg. 1974;40:756–33.
10. Wadhwani S, et al. The anterior dural (Hofmann) ligaments. Spine. 2004;29:623–7.
11. Wiltse LL, et al. Relationship of the dura, Hofmann's ligaments, Batson's plexus, and a fibrovascular membrane lying on the posterior surface of the vertebral bodies and attaching to the deep layer of the posterior longitudinal ligament. An anatomical, radiologic, and clinical study. Spine. 1993;18:1030–43.
12. Yahia LH. Neurohistology of lumbar spine ligaments. Acta Orthop Scand. 1988;59:508–1.
13. Destandau J, Dautheribes M, Guerin J. La moelle épinière, les racines et leurs méninges dans la région cervicale. In les cervicalgies, la cervicarthrose, Senegas J. In congrès de pathologie rachidienne: les cervicalgies, la cervicarthrose, Bordeaux: Bergeret Édit; 1986.
14. Grenier F. Anatomie du nerf d'Arnold (applications cliniques et thérapeutiques). Thèse Médecine Bordeaux II; 1985. p. 327.
15. Grenier F, Senegas J, Lavignolle B. Les nerfs rachidiens cervicaux et leur distribution, la douleur cervicale in congrès de pathologie rachidienne: les cervicalgies. Bordeaux: Bergeret Édit; 1986.
16. Bouchard JM, et al. Preoperative diagnosis of conjoined root anomaly with herniated disks. Surg Neurol. 1978;10:229–31.
17. Neidre A, Mac Nab I. Anomalies of the lumbosacral nerve roots. Spine. 1983;8:61–4.
18. Postacchini F, et al. Lumbar nerve root anomalies. J Bone Joint Surg Am. 1982;64A(5):721–9.
19. Juskiewenski S. Les branches postérieures des nerfs rachidiens et articulations inter-apophysaires vertébrales. Bases anatomiques de certaines douleurs rachidiennes. Thèse Toulouse 1963; n° 60.
20. Lazorthes G, et al. L'innervation des articulations interapophysaires vertébrales. Presse Med. 1956;87:2002.
21. Bogduk N, et al. The human lumbar dorsal rami. J Anat. 1982;134:383–39.
22. Senegas J, et al. Rapports du foureau dural et des racines lombaires et sacrées avec les vertèbres et les disques intervertébraux. In Congrès International d'Anatomie Manchester; 1974.
23. Sicard JA, et al. Etude de la traversée méningo-radiculaire au niveau du trou de conjugaison. Le nerf de conjugaison (nerf radiculaire spinal). Bull Mem Soc Med Hop. Paris. 1904;21:715–25.
24. Vital JM, Lavignolle B, Grenier N, et al. Anatomy of the lumbar radicular canal. Anat Clin. 1983;5:141–51.
25. Bogduk N. The innervation of the lumbar spine. Spine. 1983;8:286–93.
26. Bogduk N. Anatomie clinique du rachis lombar et sacré, 4e Édit. Paris: Elsevier; 2005, 340p.
27. Bogduk N. Practices guidelines for spinal diagnostic and treatment procedures, Library of congress cataloging in publication data. San Francisco: International Spine Intervention Society; 2004.
28. Ashton IK, et al. The demonstration of nerve fibers and neuropeptides in the lumbar facet joint capsule but not in ligamentum flavum. J Orthop Res. 1992;10:72–8.
29. Beaman DN. Substance P innervation of lumbar spine facet joints. Spine. 1993;18:1044–9.
30. Bogduk N. Local anesthetic blocks of the second cervical ganglion: a technique with application in occipital headache. Cephalalgia. 1981;1:41–50.

Anatomy of the Spinal Meninges

Laurent Sakka

Introduction

The spinal meninges constitute a set of concentric envelopes wrapping the neuraxis and the nerve roots of all vertebrates. Classically described as providing a mechanical and hydrodynamical protection of underlying structures, recent experiments suggest their involvement in the development, homeostasis, and immune defenses of the central nervous system.

Phyllogenesis

In all vertebrates, the central nervous system is surrounded by meningeal structures. The three meningeal layers of higher mammals, the dura mater, the arachnoid, and the pia mater, gradually take place along the phyllogenesis. Restricted to a thin meninx primitiva surrounded by a thick spongy perimeninx in lampreys, they appear in large teleostei as a pia mater surrounded by a reticular tissue, a fibrous layer, and an adipose tissue that respectively prefigure arachnoid mater, dura mater, and epidural fat. The three layers are more differentiated in amphibians where subarachnoid cavities begin to develop. In reptiles subarachnoid cavities fill with cerebrospinal fluid and in birds arachnoid villi differentiate along veins and participate in cerebrospinal fluid absorption [1]. In mammals, epidural fat regresses as subarachnoid spaces develop in parallel, especially at the lumbar level [2, 3].

L. Sakka (✉)
Department of Neurosurgery, University Hospital of Clermont-Ferrand, Clermont-Ferrand, France

Faculty of Medicine, Department of Anatomy and Organogenesis, University of Clermont Auvergne, Clermont-Ferrand, France
e-mail: laurent.sakka@uca.fr

Ontogenesis

The embryologic origin of the spinal meninges has remained controversial for quite a century. Experiments using bird chimeras [4, 5] and more recent data provided by molecular biology techniques finally demonstrated that the three meningeal layers shared a common mesodermal origin in birds and mammals [6–10].

The chronology of the spinal meninges ontogenesis is not fully understood in humans because the date of conception and thus the age of human fetuses are difficult to determine precisely. Nevertheless several landmarks can be described. At day 27 post-conception, the neural tube surface is still surrounded by a non-differentiated mesenchyme (Fig. 1). At around day 33 the spinal pia mater begins to differentiate [11]. At day 37, a distinct cell layer similar to the pia mater is closely applied to the spinal cord especially at its ventral aspect. At the same time, a loose reticular tissue that might be related to a developing arachnoid layer expands all around and more particularly at the ventral aspect of the spinal cord (Fig. 2). The subarachnoid space that first differentiates at the ventral aspect of the brainstem at day 32 [12] might not extend to the spinal level before the 3rd trimester of gestation [13]. At day 48, in a specimen of our collection the subarachnoid space seems to develop all around the spinal cord (Fig. 3). Around day 44 the dura differentiates and between day 56 and day 60 the whole vertebral canal is lined by the dura mater [13]. In embryos of 48-day, 50-day, and 54-day post conception, the dura mater, the subarachnoid space, and the pia mater are well individualized (Figs. 3, 4, and 5). In embryos of 6 months of gestation, the arrangement of the three layers resembles that observed in adults (Fig. 6).

Before the 11th week of gestation the spinal cord fills the full width of the vertebral canal and extends caudally to the coccygeal region (Figs. 3 and 4). Thereafter tail structures regress progressively and the spinal cord within its meningeal sheath contracts into the *filum terminale* and the coccygeal ligament. The spine growing more rapidly than the spinal cord, the caudal end of the *conus terminalis* lies at the base of

J. M. Vital, D. T. Cawley (eds.), *Spinal Anatomy*, https://doi.org/10.1007/978-3-030-20925-4_26

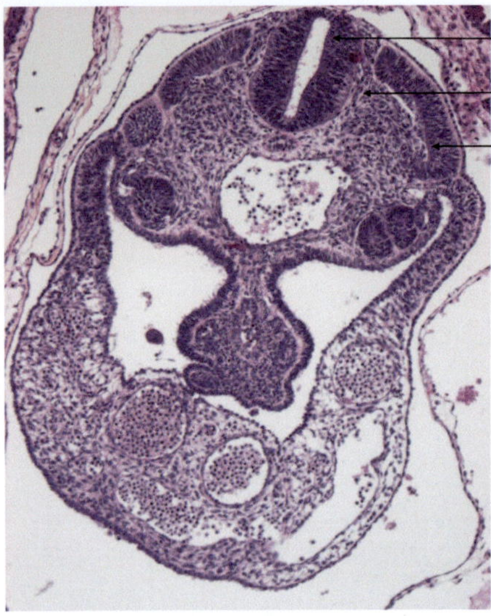

Fig. 1 Embryo at 27 days post-conception, stage 12, transverse section, hematoxylin and eosin staining. The neural tube is surrounded by a mesenchyme without meningeal differentiation. Courtesy of Pr P. Dechelotte

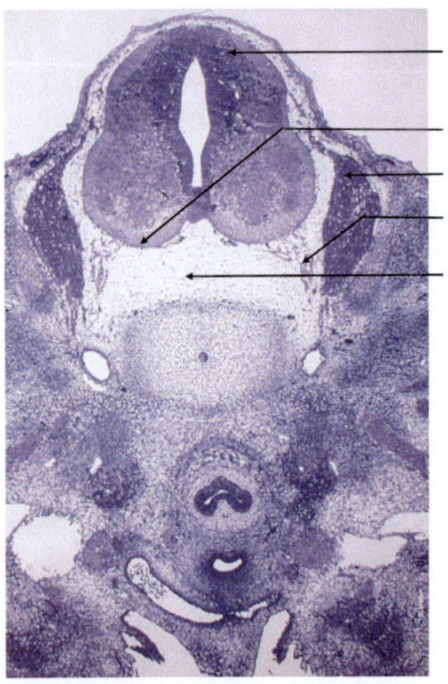

Fig. 2 Embryo at 37 days post-conception, stage 16, transverse section at thoracic level, toluidine blue. The pia mater has differentiated in the form of a thin cell layer particularly at the ventral aspect of the spinal cord. All around this, the mesenchyme has transformed into a loose reticular tissue evoking the arachnoid mater. The dura mater is still absent. Courtesy of Pr P. Dechelotte

the sacrum (S1) by the end of the 5th month of gestation and at the level of the 3rd lumbar vertebra (L3) by full term [14]. About 2 months after birth the *conus terminalis* takes its place at the adult level between L1 and L2 [15]. Then the dural sac below the *conus terminalis* contains lumbosacral nerves forming the *cauda equina*, the *filum terminale,* and their vascular supply in their leptomeningeal coating. Outside, the epidural adipose tissue separates the dural sac from the walls of

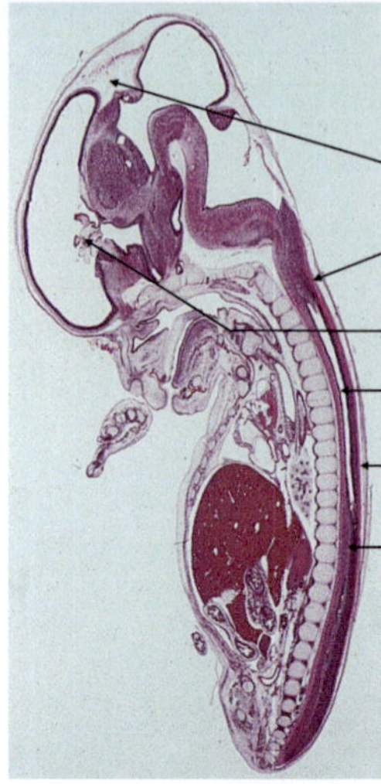

Fig. 3 Embryo at 48 days post-conception, stage 19, sagittal section, hematoxylin and eosin. The choroid plexuses have differentiated, the subarachnoid spaces surround the neuraxis particularly at its cranial part. The spinal cord, coated by the dura mater, occupies the whole length of the vertebral canal. Courtesy of Pr P. Dechelotte

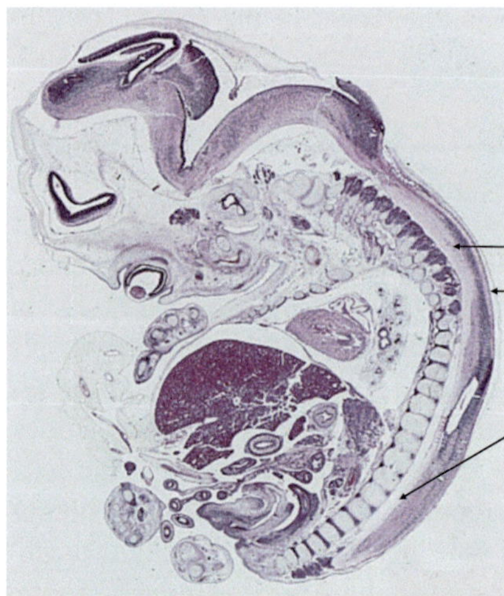

Fig. 4 Embryo at 50 days post-conception, stage 20, sagittal section, hematoxylin and eosin. The spinal cord still occupies the whole length of the vertebral canal. The subarachnoid spaces develop ventrally while the dura mater thickens. Courtesy of Pr P. Dechelotte

the vertebral canal. Laterally the meninges encase spinal nerve roots by two separate sheaths (Fig. 7).

Descriptive and Topographical Anatomy of the Spinal Meninges in Adults

The spinal meninges consist of three concentric layers that envelop the spinal cord, the *filum terminale,* and nerve roots.

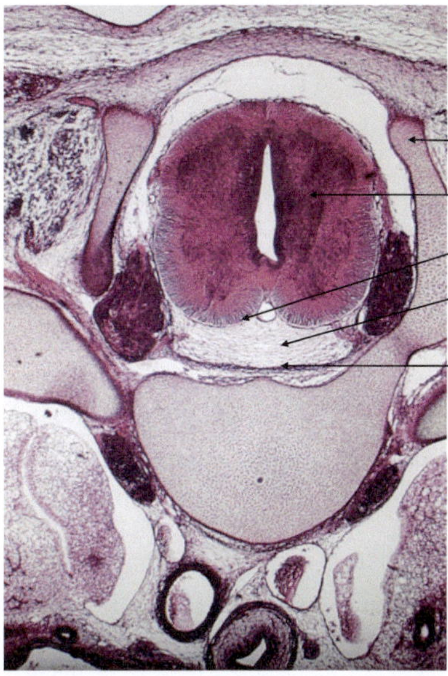

Fig. 5 Embryo at 54 days post-conception, sagittal section, hematoxylin and eosin. The pia mater and the subarachnoid spaces are now clearly individualized. The dura mater lines the arachnoid mater of the spinal cord and the nerve roots, but still cannot be distinguished laterally from the perichondrium of the vertebra. Courtesy of Pr P. Dechelotte

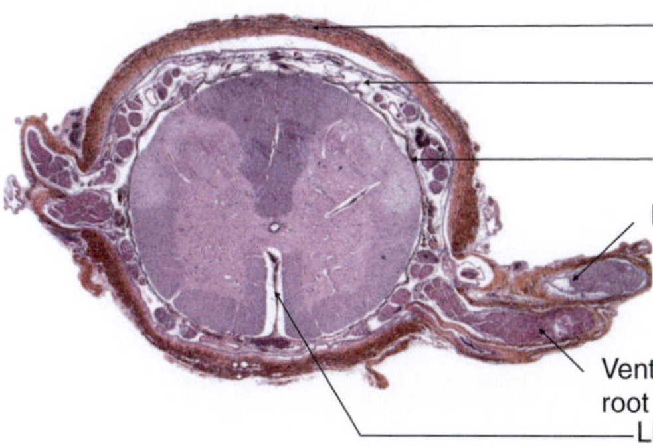

Fig. 6 Embryo at 27 weeks post-conception. Transverse section of the spinal cord with its meningeal coverings, hematoxylin and eosin. Meningeal structures are present in a form similar to their adult presentation, but subarachnoid spaces are still not fully developed. The *linea splendens* has differentiated. Courtesy of Pr P. Dechelotte

The Dura Mater

Morphology

The dura mater is the thick superficial meningeal layer or pachymeninx. It forms a white, inelastic but deformable sheath that grossly follows the contour of the spinal cord, the *filum terminale,* and nerve roots. Its thickness varies with individuals and decreases over a lifetime ranging from a thin transparent membrane to a thick pearly wall. The spinal dura corresponds to the inner, meningeal layer of the cranial dura with which it is continuous at the *foramen magnum*. Ventrally, the meningeal layer separates from the periosteal layer at the 3rd cervical vertebral body.

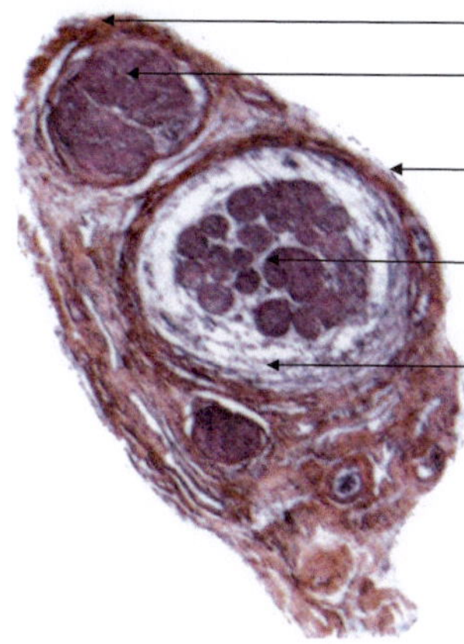

Fig. 7 Embryo at 27 weeks post-conception. Cross section of spinal nerve roots. Hematoxylin and eosin. Ventral and dorsal nerve roots are clothed by separate dural coverings. Note the large subarachnoid sleeve around ventral nerve root. Courtesy of Pr P. Dechelotte

The dural sac begins cranially at the *foramen magnum* (Fig. 8) and contracts caudally at the junction between first and second sacral vertebral bodies by a cul-de-sac which extends caudally into the filum of the dura mater or coccygeal ligament. The filum of the dura mater is a thin tubular formation 5 cm long that encases the *filum terminale* and terminates through fibrous processes at the periosteum of the dorsal aspect of the coccyx (Figs. 9 and 10). At both its cranial and caudal ends the spinal dura fuses with the periosteum of the vertebral canal. Laterally, the dura encases dorsal and ventral nerve roots in separate tubular sheaths (Figs. 11 and 12).

Dural ultrastructure is made of three distinct layers: an outermost fibroelastic layer, a middle fibrous layer, and an innermost cellular layer. The abundance of elastic fibers and the helicoidal arrangement of collagen bundles provide the flexibility and the resistance of the dural sheath that protect the spinal cord during movements [16].

The Fixation-Points of the Spinal Dura Mater

Cranially, the spinal dura tightly adheres to the periosteum of the *foramen magnum* where it continues the outer layer of the cranial dura. *Laterally*, the spinal dura covers the nerve roots by two separate sheaths that blend into one at the lateral side of the spinal ganglion, where it gives rise to the epineurium (Fig. 11). The dura is attached to the periosteum of the intervertebral foramina by the fibrous opercula of Forestier that constitute its lateral fixation-points. *Dorsally*, the spinal dura adheres to the posterior arch of the atlas and the axis and to the posterior atlanto-occipital membrane. *Ventrally*, the dura adheres to the 2nd and 3rd cervical bodies and to the dorsal longitudinal ligament, more particularly at cervical and lumbar segments. At these levels, both dorsally concave and mobile, ventral attachments hold the spinal cord at the inside of the spine curve during movements. Dural attachments to the dorsal longitudinal ligament are provided by

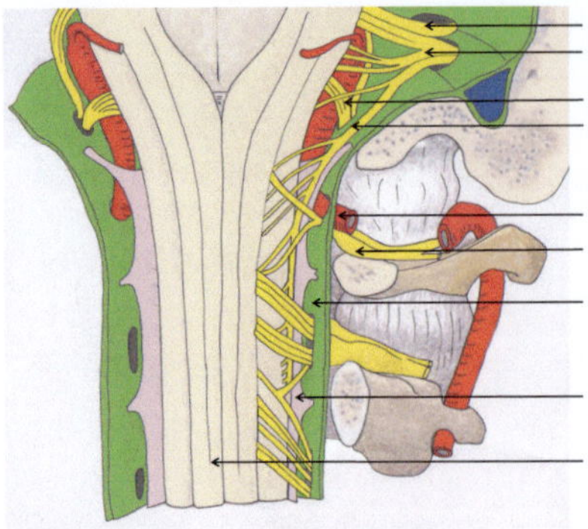

Fig. 8 Upper part of spinal meninges after opening of the *foramen magnum* and the posterior cranial fossa, and laminectomy of C1 C2, schematic drawing. Apices of *ligamenta denticulata* are inserted on the dura mater in the intervals between nerve root exits. The first *ligamentum denticulatum* is interposed between the first cervical nerve and the accessory nerve dorsally, and the vertebral artery ventrally. M. Chalus and L Sakka

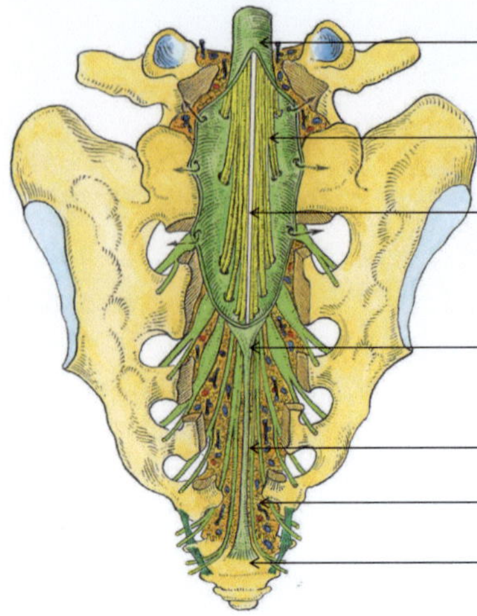

Fig. 9 *Cauda equina* and *filum terminale* after opening of the dura mater, dorsal view, schematic drawing. The dural cul-de-sac is located at the level of S1–S2, the filum of the dura mater is inserted on the first coccygeal piece, epidural space. JP Monnet

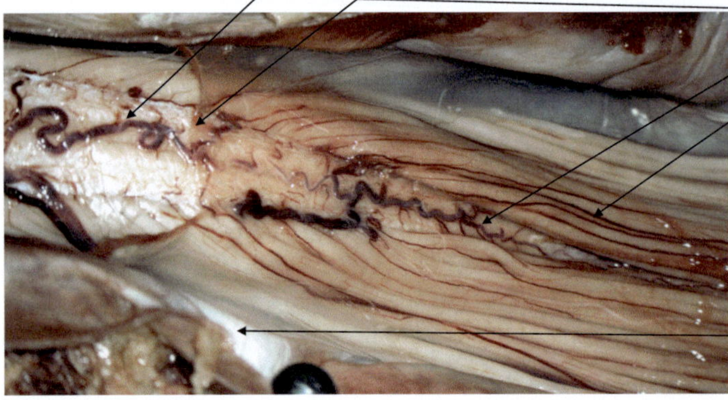

Fig. 10 Leptomeningeal coverings of the *conus terminalis* and the *cauda equina,* dorsal view after laminectomy of L1–L2 and opening of the dura mater. Cranially (left) the arachnoid mater has been opened to display perimedullary vessels. Perimedullary vessels are covered by the pia mater. The superficial arachnoid layer can be easily dissected from the dura mater

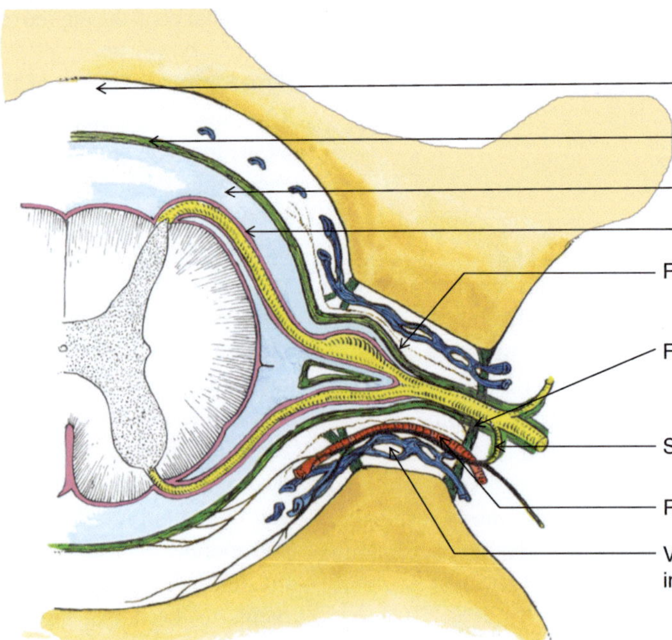

Fig. 11 Nerve roots in their meningeal sheath in the intervertebral foramen, schematic drawing. JP Monnet

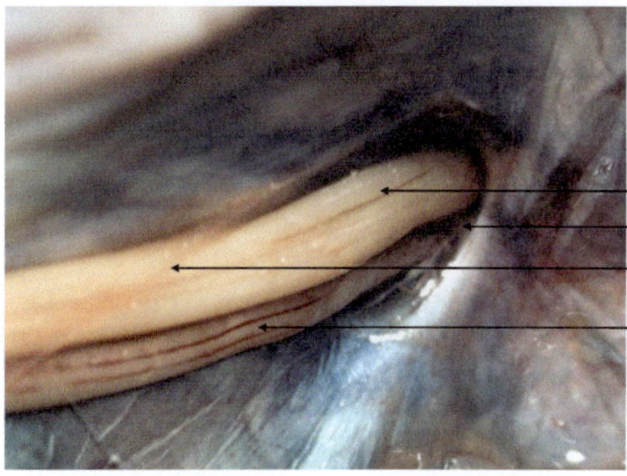

Fig. 12 Lumbar nerve root exit through opening of the dura mater

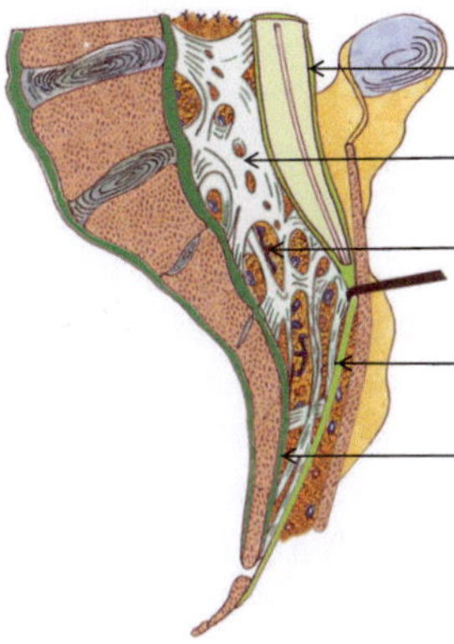

Fig. 13 Attachment of the dural sac and the filum of the dura mater to the ventral wall of the vertebral canal by the ligament of Trolard after sagittal section of the lumbosacral junction, schematic drawing. M Chalus and L Sakka

fibrous strands which constitute the ventral ligament of the spinal dura mater. They strengthen caudally from the intervertebral disc L4–L5 to the vertebral body of S5 to form the sacrodural ligament of Trolard. At this level, dural attachments are made of arcuate fibrous formations spanning adjacent vertebral bodies by their endings and adhering to the dural sac by their convexity. *Caudally*, the filum of the dura mater is attached to the periosteum of the dorsal aspect of the first coccygeal segment (Fig. 13).

Vascularization

Arteries

The spinal dura is poorly vascularized. Arterial supply is performed by thin branches of radicular arteries whose diameter does not exceed 0.5 mm. Dorsally a dense anastomotic network supplied by two cranio-caudal arterial axes contrasts with a loose ventral anastomotic network supplied by a ventro-median arterial axis. This disposition resembles the spinal cord arterial supply. This arterial network displays a metameric disposition with numerous anastomoses. At the dorsal aspect of the thoracic segment, spiral arteries and tufts of capillaries bulge into the epidural space. The significance of these formations is not understood [17].

Veins

The physiology of the connections between dural and spinal cord venous drainages remains unclear, anatomic observations and interventional neuroradiology providing conflicting data. There are generally two veins for one dural artery. At the cervical level they form a meshwork of large venous sinuses that communicate cranially with the basilar plexus and take part in the encephalic venous drainage. Anatomic studies describe radicular veins that collect from both the veins of the dura and the veins of the spinal cord, leave the vertebral canal by intervertebral foramina and drain into the internal vertebral plexus of the epidural space. Valves in radicular veins located just before they pass through the dura may prevent the blood from flowing back to the spinal cord. These can be regarded as a protective mechanism of the spinal cord in situations of hypertension in the vertebral venous system [17]. Reversely, angiographic procedures do not show communications between perimedullary and epidural veins. Perimedullary veins are described as draining upwards through the foramen magnum into the inferior cerebellar veins and the dural sinuses of the posterior cranial fossa. These reports are provided by procedures requiring the patient to be in a supine position. One can assume that the distribution of the venous return may be different in upright positions or during exercise.

Lymphatics

The lymphatic drainage of the spinal dura remains poorly understood. Lymphatic vessels were first described following experiments of ink injections into the ventricular or subarachnoid spaces of mammals. They were described as arising near the lateral points of attachment of the *ligamenta denticulata*, near lumbar vertebral bodies or around subarachnoid recesses [18]. They drain into paravertebral lymph nodes, the thoracic lymphatics into the nodes of the posterior mediastinum, and the lumbo-sacral lymphatics into the nodes of the posterior abdominal wall between psoas major muscles [19].

In animal models the lymphatic system has been demonstrated to take part in the absorption of cerebrospinal fluid [20]. In humans the participation of the spinal lymphatic pathway remains unknown under physiological conditions but might be significant in the upright position and during exercise. This function could be especially active in neonates whose arachnoid villi become fully functional only after the age of 18 months, and in the elderly where absorptive capacity of cranial arachnoid granulations gradually decreases.

Innervation

The ventral aspect of the spinal dura is innervated by a dense plexus supplied by sinu-vertebral nerves, the nerve plexus of the posterior longitudinal ligament and the perivascular plexus of radicular arteries. The sinu-vertebral nerve is a ventral branch of the spinal nerve (Fig. 11). It runs cranially and medially between the dorsal longitudinal ligament and the *annulus fibrosus* ventrally and the ventral aspect of the dura dorsally. These three structures are innervated by the sinu-vertebral nerve [21–24].

The dorsal aspect of the spinal dura is poorly innervated by nerves coming from the ventral dural nerve plexus in the intervals between nerve roots. They do not reach the median part of the dorsal dura. The lack of innervation of the median dorsal dura explains why lumbar punctures are not painful while traversing the dura mater [22].

Dural nerves are non-myelinated fibers involved in vasomotricity and nociception [22, 25]. The efficacy of epidural blocks performed in anesthesiology could be at least partially related to an action on dural nerves. The innervation of the dorsal longitudinal ligament and the dorsal part of the annulus fibrosus by sinu-vertebral nerves through free endings has suggested their involvement in low back pain syndromes [26, 27] and might explain the efficiency of periradicular infiltrations with anti-inflammatory drugs in this indication.

The Relationships of the Dura Mater with the Leptomeninges and the Spinal Nerves

The inner aspect of the spinal dura is covered by the outer arachnoid layer. Laterally, as the nerve roots pass through the dura mater, the arachnoid mater constitutes subarachnoid recesses around spinal nerves (Figs. 7 and 11). Ventral and dorsal nerve roots traverse the dura by two distinct openings and run toward the intervertebral foramen within two distinct dural sheaths. The roots of the first cervical nerve and the vertebral artery traverse the dura through the same opening (Fig. 8). In the intervertebral foramen nerve roots merge into a spinal nerve covered by a unique dural sheath. The sinu-vertebral nerve runs at the ventral aspect of the spinal nerve, outside the dural sheath, among the venous plexus of the intervertebral foramen (Fig. 11). The spinal nerve and the radicular artery running at its ventral aspect are disposed centrally in the cellulo-adipose tissue of the foramen surrounded by the epidural intervertebral venous plexus. The intervertebral foramen is closed laterally by the fibrous operculum of Forestier (Fig. 11). The area between the fibrous operculum and the nerve dural sheath is the *epidural space of the foramen*.

The Arachnoid Mater

The arachnoid mater is a thin transparent membrane enveloping the spinal cord, nerve roots, perimedullary vessels, and the intradural segment of radicular vessels (Figs. 6, 10, 14, 15, and 16). The arachnoid is usually described as a unique thick layer lining the inner aspect of the dura mater and connected to the pia mater by a network of delicate connective trabeculae. Ultrastructural studies using electron microscope rather describe a two-layer structure with a *superficial barrier cell layer* lining the dura mater and a *deep reticular cell layer* made of interweaved trabecular cells connected to the pia mater [16]. The superficial layer is composed of tightly packed cells connected with one another by numerous tight junctions suggesting a role as a meningeal barrier between the cerebrospinal fluid of the subarachnoid space and the blood circulation of the dura [16, 29]. The superficial barrier cell layer is attached to the dura mater by collagenous fibers so that there is no subdural space, but it can be easily dissected from it without opening the subarachnoid space.

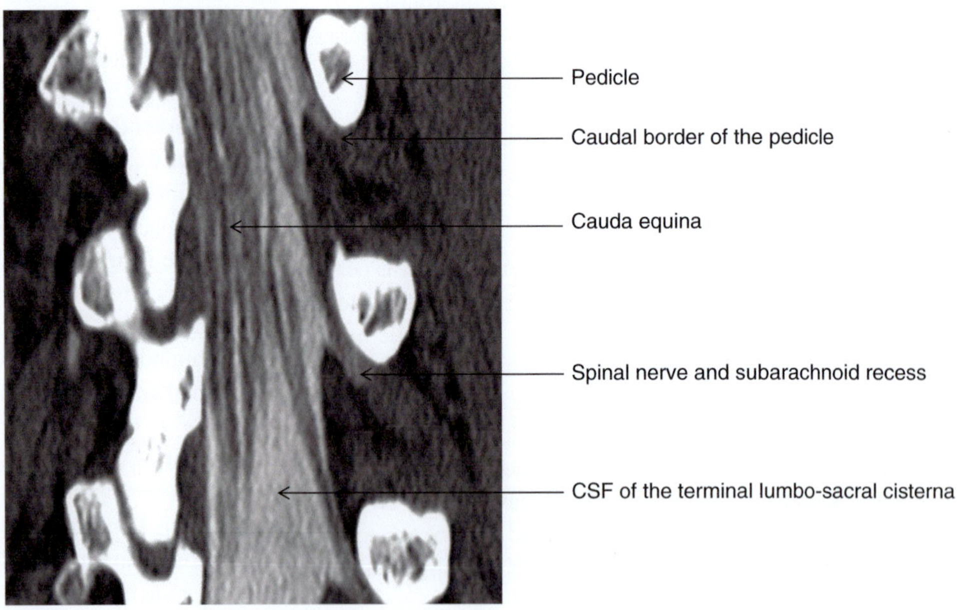

Fig. 14 *Cauda equina*, CT-scan after intrathecal injection of iodine contrast, oblique section. Arachnoid recesses are usually located medially from the caudal border of the pedicles. Courtesy of Dr J Gabrillargues

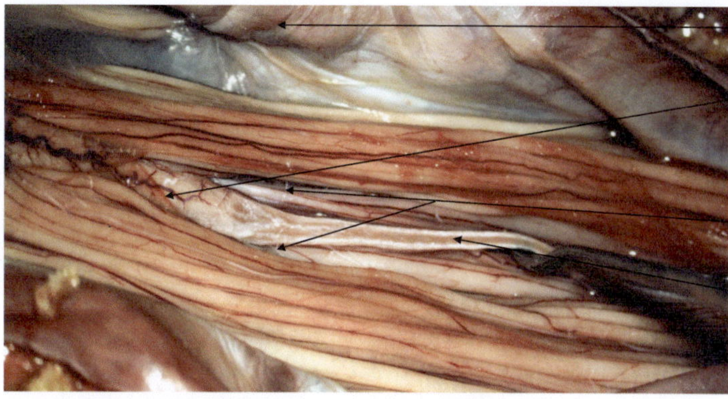

Fig. 15 Subarachnoid space of the *cauda equina* after opening of the superficial layer of the arachnoid. *Filum terminale* and nerve roots are connected to one another by fine arachnoid trabeculae

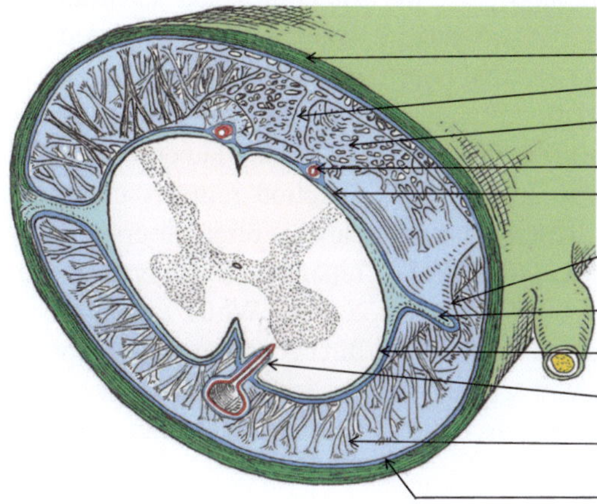

Fig. 16 Spinal leptomeninges. The arachnoid mater and the pia mater are continuous with each other as well as subarachnoid and parenchymal perivascular spaces. The collagenous core of *ligamentum denticulatum* merges with the subpial space medially and the inner aspect of the dura mater laterally (Modified after Nicholas and Weller [28])

According to this description, the subarachnoid space, filled with the extra-axial cerebrospinal fluid, takes the room between the superficial barrier cell layer and the pia mater, traversed by the arachnoid trabeculae of the reticular cell layer. On traversing the arachnoid mater blood vessels and nerve roots are sheathed by extensions of the reticular cell layer. Cranially, the subarachnoid space is continuous with the cranial subarachnoid space at the *foramen magnum.* Around the spinal cord it constitutes the perimedullary space, divided into ventral and dorsal chambers by the *ligamenta denticulata* (Figs. 8 and 20). In the dorsal chamber, arachnoid trabeculae form a dense network that firmly applies blood vessels against the spinal cord and constitutes medially a sagittal septum, the *septum posticum* of Schwalbe. An intermediate cell layer interposed between the superficial arachnoid layer and the pia mater to which it is tightly connected, might contribute to this septum [28]. Most developed at the lower cervical and thoracic levels, the *septum posticum* of Schwalbe connects dorsally to a thickening of the superficial arachnoid layer: the median raphe of Magendie (Fig. 16).

Caudally the subarachnoid space widens into the large lumbosacral terminal cistern that encloses the *cauda equina* and terminates between the 1st and the 2nd sacral vertebrae. Laterally it follows the nerve roots from the spinal cord to the intervertebral foramina. The two arachnoid layers merge to limit subarachnoid recesses around spinal nerves at the lateral limit of spinal ganglia just before they traverse the fibrous opercula. The abundance of cell debris and activated macrophages in arachnoid recesses [30] where fine lymph vessels have been described to drain into paravertebral lymph nodes [19] suggest the subarachnoid recess as an interface between the central nervous system, the cerebrospinal fluid, and CSF immune defense. There is no specific arachnoid vascularization; the vessels are those of the spinal cord.

Subarachnoid spaces can be precisely explored using CT-scan after intrathecal injection of iodinated contrast medium. MRI visualizes the subarachnoid space by the hypersignal of the cerebrospinal fluid in T2-weighted sequences.

Subarachnoid recesses have relationships with bone structures that constitute the safety landmarks of periradicular infiltrations, procedures commonly performed in anesthesiology and rheumatology (Fig. 14). Inadequate site of puncture can lead to CSF leak, nerve-root damage, or intra-arterial administration. Lateral limits of subarachnoid recesses vary according to vertebral segments and subjects. At cervical levels subarachnoid recesses usually stop at the anterior border of the pedicles. At thoracic and lumbar levels they usually do not extend laterally beyond the caudal border of the upper pedicle. To be safe, the tip of the trocar should remain extraforaminal, that is, outside the lateral recess to avoid intrathecal injection, puncture of a radiculomedullary artery, or a vertebral artery in the cervical segment.

In healthy subjects, the perimedullary space occupies about a third of the cervical vertebral canal in sagittal MRI sections (Fig. 17a, b). In a study including 140 healthy volunteers, the part of the subarachnoid space in the vertebral cervical canal was shown to vary according to sex, body height, and vertebral segment. Its relative anteroposterior diameter decreased from C1 to C6, confirming the lower cervical segments as more specifically exposed to compressive myelopathy. Its relative anteroposterior diameter increased with body height suggesting a lower susceptibility of taller subjects to the risk of cervical cord compression [31]. In clinical practice, the presence of hypersignal on T2-weighted sequence at the ventral or dorsal aspect of the cervical cord is a valuable sign for cervical stenosis (Fig. 17c).

Below the 2nd lumbar vertebra the subarachnoid space constitutes the lumbosacral terminal cistern around the *cauda equina* visualized by MRI as a large hypersignal on T2-weighted sequences. At this level the particularly developed epidural fat gives a hypersignal on both T1 and T2-weighted sequences (Fig. 18). Assessment of both subarachnoid space and epidural fat on T2-weighted sequences are essential in the diagnosis of lumbar canal stenosis, either congenital or acquired (Fig. 19). In the acquired syndrome, the stenosis of the vertebral canal and/or lateral recesses occurs secondary to degenerative changes involving intervertebral disc bulging, spondylolisthesis, hypertrophy of facet joints, and/or hypertrophy of the *ligamentum flavum*. Patients usually complain with low back pain, radicular pain, and a typical neurogenic claudication. The symptoms of neurogenic claudication typically described by patients consist of fatigue, heaviness or weakness in the legs without radicular topography, generated by standing upright or walking and relieved by sitting or flexion of the spine. The postural nature of symptoms is related to the variations in the size of the vertebral canal according to spine curvature changes. The symptoms are triggered by extension of the spine which decreases the anteroposterior diameter of the canal and relieved by flexion of the spine which increases the anteroposterior diameter [32, 33]. The pathophysiology of this affection remains unclear since anatomic stenosis of the canal is often observed in asymptomatic subjects. The signs reported by patients evoke a global effect on the *cauda equina*. While radicular symptoms can be explained by a direct compression of nerve roots or their vascular supply by degenerative changes, the impact of postural changes on neurogenic claudication favors a disturbance in the cerebro-

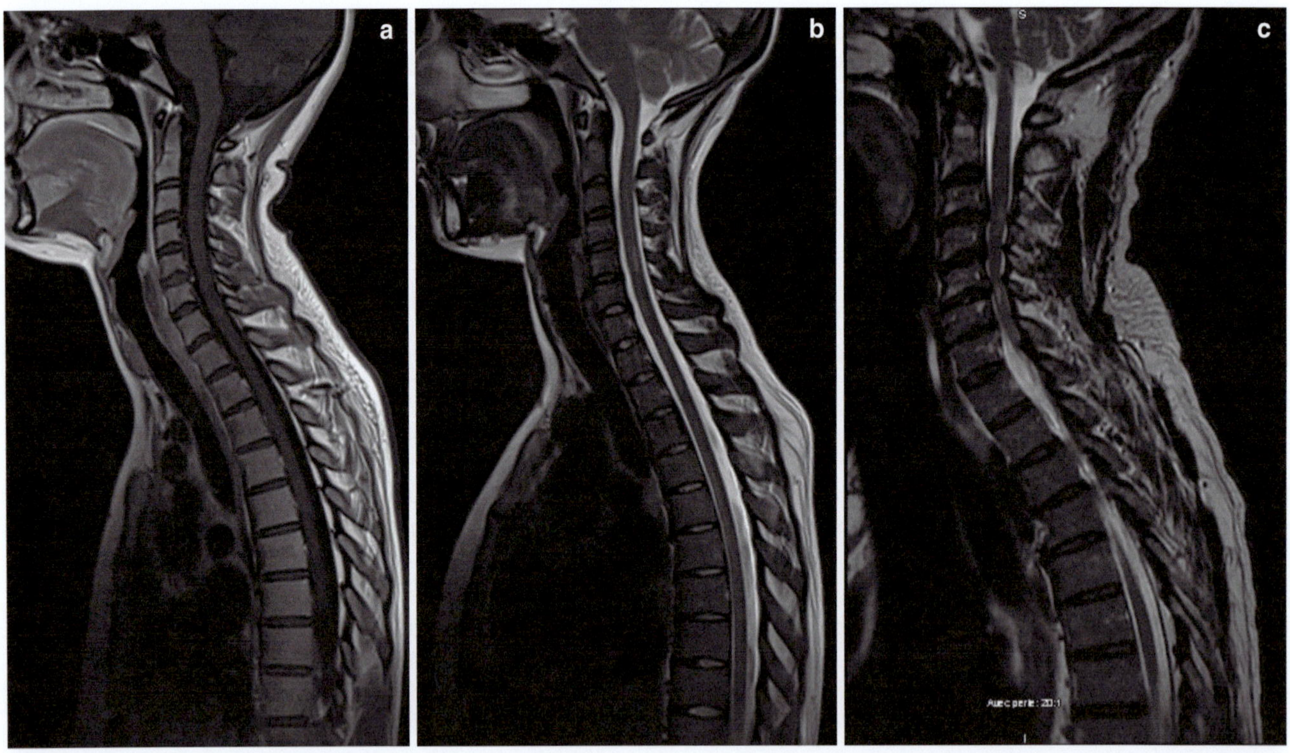

Fig. 17 Sagittal section of the cervico-thoracic spinal cord; (**a**) healthy subject, T1 weighted sequence; (**b**) healthy subject, T2 weighted sequence; (**c**) cervical canal stenosis with myelopathy, T2 weighted sequence. Perimedullary space appears as a hypersignal in T2-weighted sequence and hyposignal in T1-weighted sequence. Epidural fat appears as a hypersignal in T1 and T2-weighted sequences. Note the position of the spinal cord at the concavity of spine curves. Courtesy of Dr E. Chabert

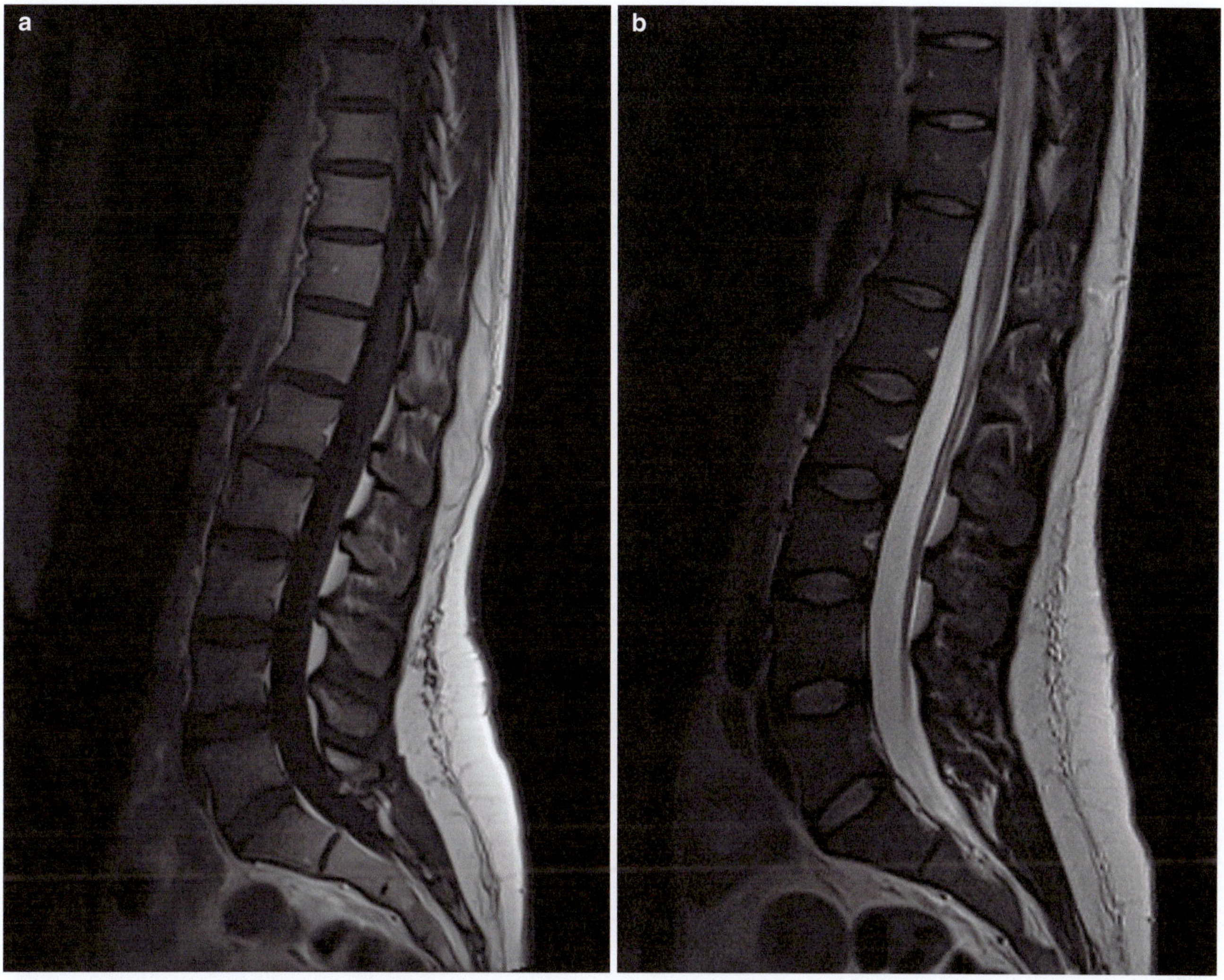

Fig. 18 Lumbosacral terminal cistern in a healthy subject; (**a**) T1 weighted sequence; (**b**) T2 weighted sequence. The cerebrospinal fluid of the lumbosacral terminal cistern appears as a hypersignal in T2-weighted sequence and a hyposignal in T1-weighted sequence. Epidural fat appears as a hypersignal in T1 and T2-weighted sequences. In this healthy subject, the conus terminalis is located at the caudal part of L1. Courtesy of Dr E. Chabert

spinal fluid dynamics. One can assume that symptoms settle when CSF and venous pressures overcome the blood pressure in the *cauda equina* arterial supply.

Around spinal nerve roots the arachnoid mater has been described to differentiate into arachnoid villi. Morphological similarities with cranial granulations and their relationships with epidural veins have suggested their involvement in CSF reabsorption [34, 35]. Usually located at or medially to subarachnoid recesses, they could be more frequent in thoracic or lumbar regions. In animal models, spinal arachnoid villi have been assessed to be responsible for about 25% of CSF drainage [36, 37]. In humans, their contribution in CSF absorption has never been assessed but might be effective in the first year of life and later on in upright posture or during exercise [38].

The Pia Mater

The spinal pia mater is a thin areolar tissue closely adhering to the *glia limitans* (Figs. 6 and 16). Cranially the spinal pia mater continues as the cranial pia mater at the *foramen magnum*. Caudally it encases the *filum terminale* below the *conus terminalis.* Classically considered a pial formation, the *filum terminale* was demonstrated to originate from apoptotic degeneration of the caudal spinal cord [39]. In human fetuses, the *filum terminale* is constituted of a connective tissue rich in type III collagen with nerve fascicles, blood vessels, ganglion cells, ependymal, glial, and adipose tissues [40]. The same components are found in adults, but connectives fibers are mostly type I collagen, elastin and elaunin fibers longitudinally arranged in a network of transversal type III collagen

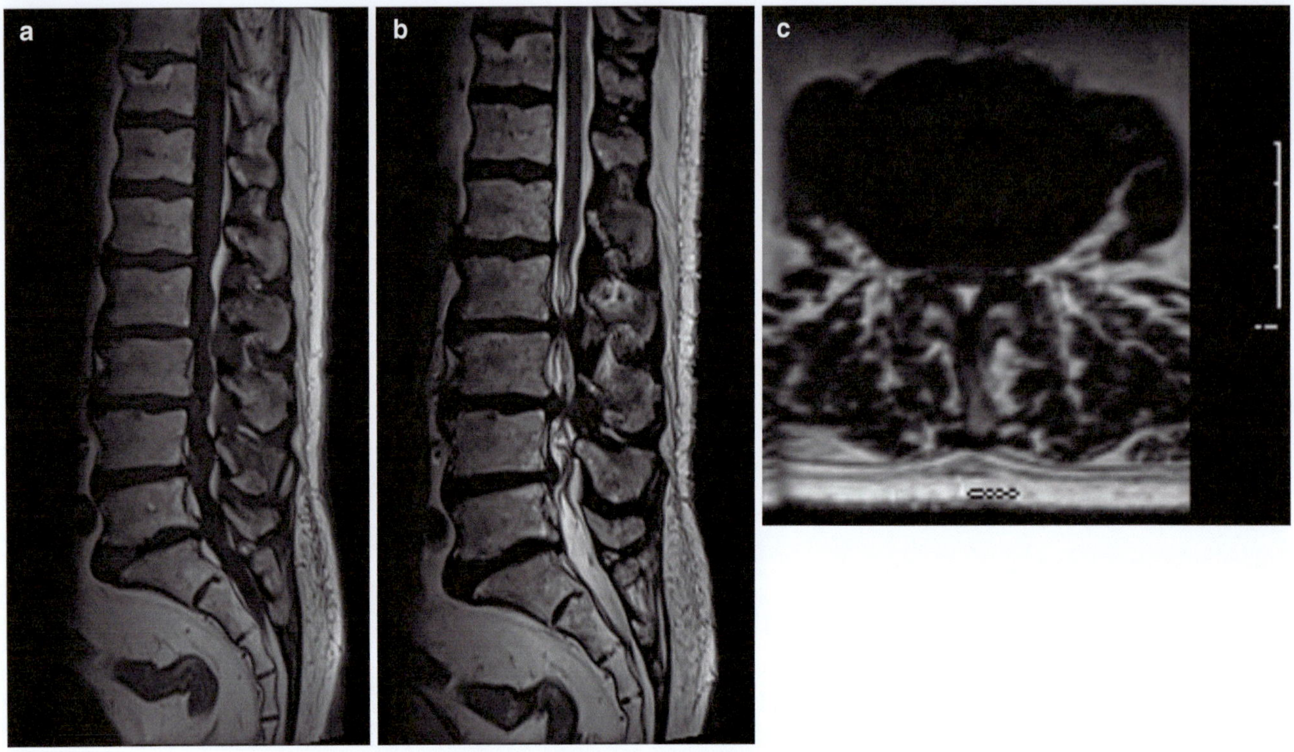

Fig. 19 Acquired lumbar canal stenosis; (**a**) T1 weighted sequence, sagittal section; (**b**) T2 weighted sequence, sagittal section; (**c**) T2 weighted sequence, transverse section. In this case, the canal stenosis is related to intervertebral disc bulging and hypertrophy of facet joints. The stenosis affects both the lumbosacral terminal cistern and epidural fat. Courtesy of Dr E. Chabert

fibers [41]. The *filum terminale* appears a bluish, white formation of about 20 cm long and less than 2 mm wide. Its upper part, located inside the dural sac *(filum terminale internum),* runs down along the lumbosacral terminal cistern among the roots of the *cauda equina*. Its lower part, located beyond the dural sac (*filum terminale externum*), is encased by the filum of the dura mater from the lower border of the first sacral vertebra to the dorsal aspect of the first coccygeal piece. Laterally the pia mater follows nerve roots and spinal nerves, fusing with the arachnoid before commencement of the perineurium.

In the ventral fissure of the spinal cord, the pia mater forms the *linea splendens,* a dense network of fibrous strands that bridge the two walls of the fissure and wrap the ventral spinal artery (Fig. 6).

Laterally the pia mater forms on each side of the spinal cord 20–22 *ligamenta denticulata* that anchor the spinal cord to the dural sac. Each *ligamentum denticulatum* is a triangular formation extending from the lateral side of the spinal cord by its base to the inner aspect of the dural sac by its apex, in the intervals between nerve roots (Fig. 20). The first *ligamentum denticulatum,* located above the first cervical roots, is inserted onto the dura of the medial aspect of the condylar part of the occipital bone (Fig. 8). The vertebral artery runs ventrally and the spinal root of the accessory nerve runs dorsally. The last *ligamentum denticulatum* is located above the first lumbar nerve. The *ligamentum denticulatum* is made of a collagenous core which fuses with the inner aspect of the dura mater laterally and merges with the subpial layer medially (Fig. 16). *Ligamenta denticulata* form incomplete septa that separate the subarachnoid space in ventral and dorsal compartments where the cerebrospinal fluid flows in opposite directions. It probably stabilizes the spinal cord within the subarachnoid space along the movements of the vertebral column [42].

The vessels of the pia mater are those of the spinal cord. They are less numerous than the vessels of the cranial pia mater, that is why the spinal pia mater is often described as a fibrous layer more than a vascular layer.

Innervation of the pia mater is made of a loose plexus, the plexus of Purkinje, constituted by vasomotor and sensory nerves. The plexus of Purkinje is supplied by sino-vertebral nerves, the perivascular plexus of the anterior spinal artery and perivascular plexuses of radicular arteries.

The spinal pia mater fuses with the arachnoid coating of the arteries that dive into the parenchyma. It follows that the perivascular space of the parenchyma is continuous with the perivascular space of the subarachnoid space. The perivascular spaces of the subarachnoid space and the perivascular spaces the parenchyma are separated from the subpial com-

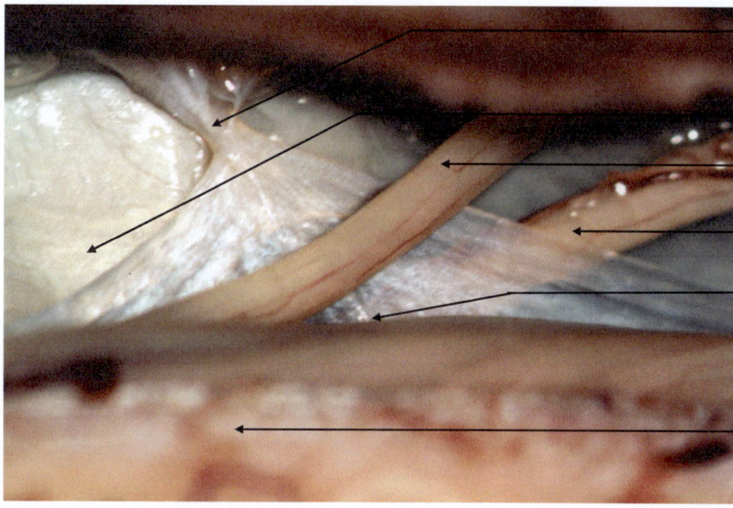

Fig. 20 Dorsal view of right *ligamentum denticulatum*, interposed between ventral and dorsal nerve roots. Note the translucent aspect of the ligament, attached by its base to the lateral aspect of the cord and by its apex to the dural sac

partment by the pia mater. In other words, the pia mater separates the subarachnoid space from the perivascular spaces which do not communicate with each other. In the depth of the parenchyma, the pial coating of arteries becomes gradually discontinuous and disappears around capillaries. No comparable pial sheath is observed around veins which are partially surrounded by a discontinuous pial layer [28, 42–45].

The pia mater fusing with the arachnoid sheath of perforating arteries, there is a continuum between the arachnoid and the pia mater at the points where arachnoid trabeculae anchor to the pia and around vessels. Both the pia and the arachnoid mater are made of the same morphological cell type and share the same immunohistochemical markers, vimentin, and epithelial membrane antigen. These morphological observations combined with their common mesodermal origin probably make artificial the conception of the pia and the arachnoid as separate structures and should strengthen the consensus that the pia and the arachnoid are the inner and outer parts of the same leptomeningeal layer.

Meningeal and Perineurial Cysts

Spinal cystic formations refer to distinct histological and anatomic entities often confused in clinical practice. They were first classified by Tarlov according to their histological nature, their location in relation to the dura, and their communication with the subarachnoid space [46] and later on by Nabors et al. who distinguished extradural cysts without spinal nerve root involvement (type I), extradural cysts with spinal nerve root involvement (type II), and intradural cysts (type III) [47].

Meningeal cysts are extradural or intradural evaginations of the arachnoid mater. Therefore they are located medial to the arachnoid/perineurium junction, around the spinal cord or nerve roots. *Extradural meningeal cysts* (Type I) are arachnoid expansions through a congenital defect of the radicular dura that communicate with the subarachnoid space [48]. Their wall is made of arachnoid mater lined by a superficial fibrous layer. They could result from a defect in the closure of embryonic mesenchymal structures surrounding the neural tube. In the sacral region they are more commonly called “sacral meningoceles” or “diverticula.” Periodic self-emptying generates fluctuating symptoms [46] and their puncture may result in CSF leak and intracranial hypotension. *Intradural meningeal cysts* (Type III) are less common anomalies that occur at any level of the vertebral canal. Their wall is made of an arachnoid epithelium. They communicate with the subarachnoid space and could develop in a one-way valve mechanism. Some authors consider these formations as resulting from the action of CSF pressure on a weak point of the meningeal sheath [46, 47].

Perineurial cysts (cysts of Tarlov) (Type II) develop between the endoneurium and the perineurium of spinal nerves (Fig. 21). Multiple or multiloculated, they usually occur along sacral nerves, generally S2 or S3, in the epidural space of the sacral canal. They are theoretically located beyond the spinal ganglion or at its lateral side where the arachnoid is replaced by the perineurium. Perineurial cyst wall contains nerve fibers and ganglion cells in a connective tissue. Evidence suggests a degenerative or inflammatory process taking place on a congenital defect [49]. Tarlov didn’t find a communication with the subarachnoid space. In some cases the pressure in the subarachnoid space could make the cerebrospinal fluid enter the cyst through microconnections between the cavity and the subarachnoid space. By a valve-like mechanism favored by the upright position, the cyst could progressively fill with CSF, gradually develop

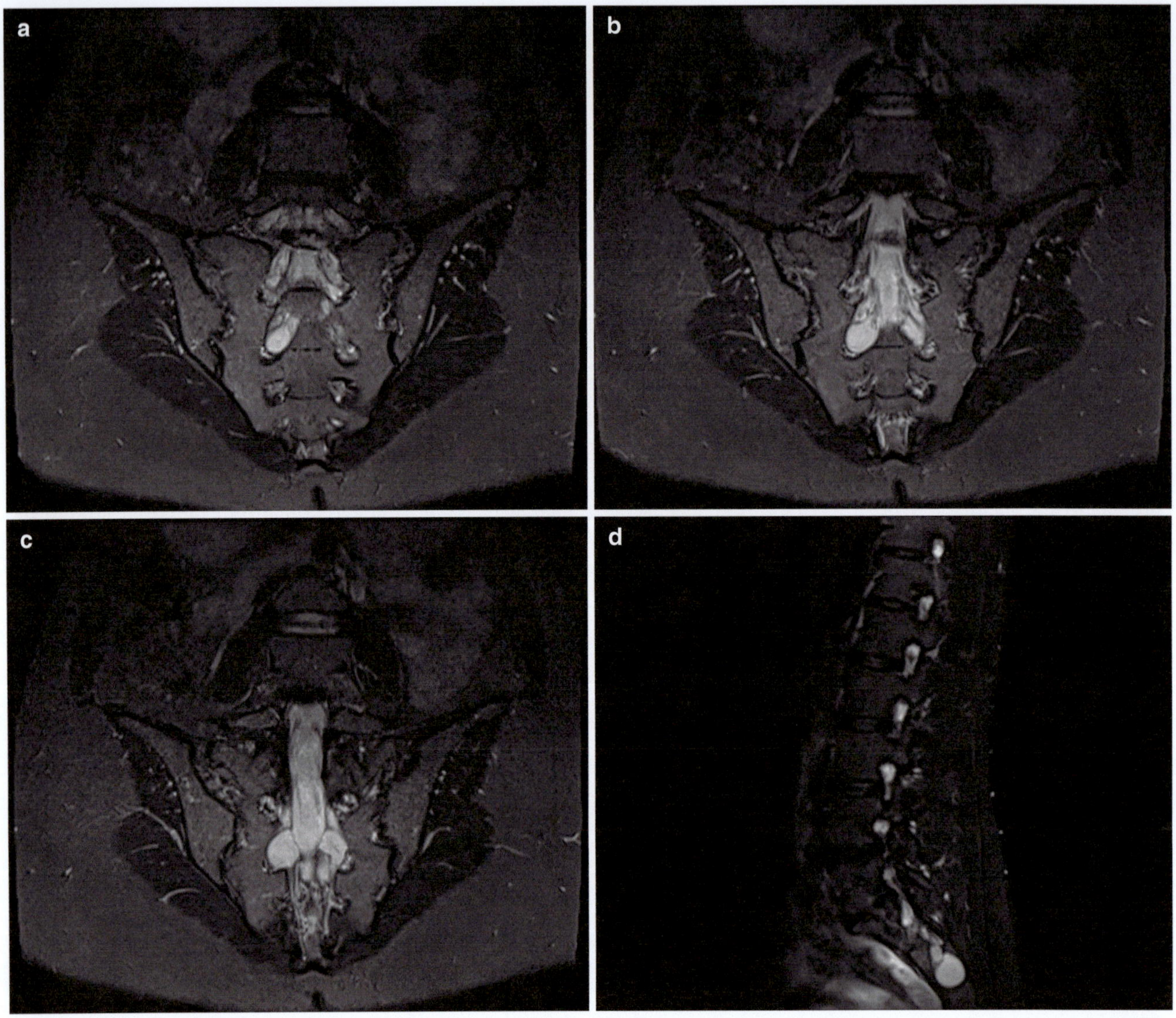

Fig. 21 Perineurial cysts of Tarlov. MRI, T2-weighted sequence. (**a–c**) coronal sections; (**d**) parasagittal section, right side. Courtesy of Dr E. Chabert

and compress neighboring nerve roots, and resulting in neurological symptoms [50].

The Epidural Space

The epidural space is interposed between the dura mater and the wall of the vertebral canal. It is limited cranially by the adherence of the spinal dura mater to the *foramen magnum* margin and the posterior aspect of the third vertebral body. It extends caudally to the sacro-coccygeal hiatus closed by the posterior sacro-coccygeal ligaments and the coccygeal insertion of the filum of the dura mater. Laterally it is limited by the pedicles and the intervertebral foramina closed by their fibrous opercula.

The epidural space is filled with adipose tissue traversed by connective fibers that secure the dural sac to the vertebral canal. Its size varies according to the vertebral segment. Maximal at the lumbar segment where its ventro-dorsal diameter ranges between 5 and 6 mm, it is almost absent at the cervical segment and ventrally (Figs. 17 and 18). The epidural space is partitioned by the ventral ligament of the spinal dura mater especially at the lumbosacral segment where it constitutes the ligament of Trolard. It is interrupted dorsally by local adhesions of the dura mater to the vertebral canal that may interfere with epidural catheter placement. The amount of epidural fat is an important factor because it influences the diffusion of molecules after epidural injection. Its variations according to body weight remain controversial. Several studies report that the body mass index or the body

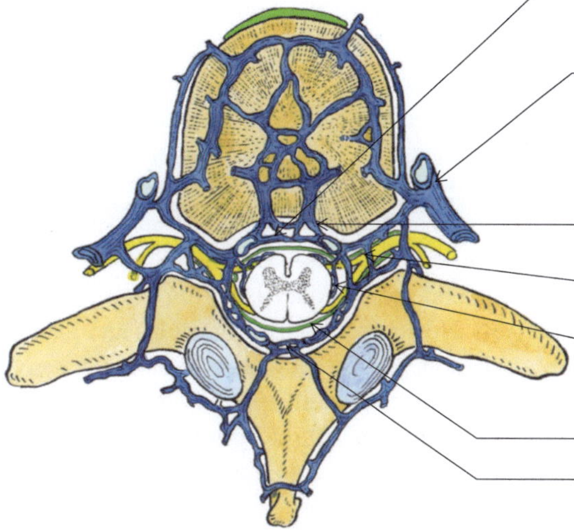

Fig. 22 Venous anastomoses between intradural and epidural systems. Schematic drawing. JP Monnet

habitus might not condition the global amount of epidural, adipose tissue but influence its repartition, posterior epidural fat increasing with the body weight [51, 52]. Reversely, epidural lipomatosis, a condition characterized by hypertrophy of epidural adipose tissue has been reported to occur in relation to obesity. In these cases, compressive symptoms and epidural fat have been both reported to regress with weight loss therapy suggesting a correlation between epidural adipose tissue and body weight [53–55].

Ventral and dorsal epidural venous plexuses extend from the *foramen magnum* to the coccyx and connect to each other by transverse anastomoses. They receive tributaries from the vertebrae, the dura, and the spinal cord and drain into the external vertebral plexus (Fig. 22). Cranially epidural plexuses connect with sub-occipital and lateral sinuses by anastomoses that could ensure most of the encephalic venous drainage in upright position [56] and the whole encephalic drainage in several patients [57].

The Subdural Space

The subdural space classically described between dura and arachnoid maters should actually be considered as an artefactual cavity produced by surgical manipulation or histological preparations. Thin trabeculae connect the outer surface of the arachnoid to the dura mater. Transmission electron microscopy studies have identified a *dura-arachnoid interface* filled with neurothelial cells and amorphous material [58]. The low resistance of this amorphous material easily permits the formation of subdural hematomas. In surgical practice, the dura mater can be safely opened without harm to the underlying arachnoid (Figs. 10 and 15). When post-mortem manipulations are avoided, the dura mater remains attached to the arachnoid layer. Therefore, there is no virtual space such as the pleural cavity.

Functional Anatomy

Mechanical Functions

The position of the spinal cord inside the vertebral canal follows the movements of the spine. The spinal cord is displaced laterally in lateral inclinations of the spine and its lower extremity is drawn upward when the spine is flexed. The attachments of the dura to the vertebral canal and the mooring of the spinal cord to the dural sac through leptomeningeal formations maintain without tension the stability of the spinal cord along these movements. Notably, the *ligamenta denticulata* might restrict cephalo-caudal movements of the spinal cord [59] and maintain its lateral diameter along spinal movements.

The stability of the spinal cord without tension along movements is an essential condition for the spinal cord to exert its physiological functions. Congenital abnormalities related to its elements of stability generate pathological conditions. Notably, low positioning of the *conus medullaris* following defects in the involution of tail structures is associated with the neurological, musculoskeletal, gastrointestinal or urological disorders of the tethered cord syndrome [60, 61]. Clinical evidences relate the symptoms to the caudal traction of the spinal cord, or anomalies in the elasticity of the *filum terminale* [62], some patients complaining with incontinence at the flexion of the vertebral column while others improve after section of the *filum terminale* [63].

Subarachnoid spaces, epidural venous plexuses and adipose tissue might behave as a hydromechanical cushion that protects the neuraxis. Unlike their cranial counterpart in the skull, the spinal meninges are separated from the bony walls of the vertebral canal by epidural fat that equally protects the spinal cord from potential injuries along movements. In asymptomatic cervical canal stenosis, these hydromechanical cushions no longer exist and severe decompensation can be induced by mild cervical trauma.

The mechanical properties of the pia mater on the spinal cord surface has raised considerably less attention than the dura mater and the subarachnoid space. In addition, its role in the protection of the spinal cord has probably been underestimated because of its apparent fragility and lightness. However, animal models of spinal cord compression show that its presence modifies the mechanical properties of the spinal cord and conditions its behavior in traumatic circumstances. In experiments performed on rabbits, spinal cord segments were excised alone or within their pial covering and submitted to compression forces. The spinal cord alone showed extremely low viscoelasticity that did not allow the restoration of its shape after compression. In the same experiments, the elastic modulus of the pia mater was measured to be 460 times higher than that of the spinal cord. These results suggest that the presence of the pia mater provides a constraint on the spinal cord surface that increases its stiffness and favors shape restoration after experimental compression. One could assume that the pial sheathing around the spinal cord combined with the anchorage of the dentate ligament might partially prevent deformation of the spinal cord in traumatic compressive injury. Conversely, in the case of intramedullary tumor, ischemia, or hemorrhage, the presence of the pia mater may be harmful by maintaining excessive parenchymal pressure and leading to further aggravation [64].

The Spinal Meninges in the CSF Dynamic System

Meningeal structures are involved in cerebrospinal fluid secretion, circulation and absorption. The cerebrospinal fluid turn-over is probably crucial in central nervous system homeostasis and the neuronal environment to ensure electrolyte balance, active molecule circulation and catabolite elimination.

Historical anatomic literature classically assessed the cerebrospinal fluid volume to be around 150 mL, 25 mL in the ventricles and 125 mL in the subarachnoid space. More recent studies using MRI updated the cranial cerebrospinal fluid volume to be around 250 mL [65] and the spinal subarachnoid space volume around 80 mL [66].

About a half of the spinal cerebrospinal fluid volume is located in the lumbosacral terminal cistern. This volume is far from being constant. It varies considerably in physiologic or pathologic conditions according to the content and the container. In the lumbosacral cistern the volume of the *cauda equina* varies expectedly at the expense of the CSF volume. In lumbar spinal stenosis the CSF volume decreases, falling below 20 mL [67]. Abdominal compression in relation to obesity or pregnancy might also decrease the CSF volume in the lumbosacral cistern [68]. CSF volume variations in the lumbosacral terminal cistern have therapeutic consequences. They condition the pharmacokinetics of drugs after intrathecal administration, smaller CSF volume resulting in less dilution, higher concentration and larger diffusion of drugs [69].

About 500 mL of cerebrospinal fluid are secreted every day [70, 71]. Sixty to seventy-five percent are actively produced by the choroid plexuses of the lateral, third, and fourth ventricles and the rest is produced by extrachoroidal sources such as the ependymal epithelium and the interstitial space. A leptomeningeal participation to cerebrospinal fluid production is suggested by reports of noncommunicating arachnoid cysts that develop against the pressure of the brain and the surrounding subarachnoid space.

Based on a CSF volume of 160 mL, historical studies assessed the CSF to renew about 4–5 times daily in young adults. If one considers the measures provided by more recent MRI studies the CSF turn over could not exceed 2 or 3 times daily.

Several models have been proposed to explain cerebrospinal fluid circulation. The bulk flow model, which might be both the simplest and the one that probably best matches current clinical situations, describes the cerebrospinal fluid to circulate from its sites of secretion to its sites of absorption along pressure gradients. The CSF secreted in the ventricles drains through the median opening of the fourth ventricle into the *cisterna magma*. Then, it circulates caudally into the spinal subarachnoid space where it is partially absorbed by spinal arachnoid villi. The remaining volume circulates back towards the cranial subarachnoid space where it is passively absorbed by arachnoid granulations along cranial venous sinuses. Global CSF flow results from active choroidal secretion and passive reabsorption into the venous system through arachnoid granulations or villi. Cerebrospinal fluid absorption by cranial arachnoid granulations or spinal villi follows the gradient between the CSF pressure in the subarachnoid space and the blood pressure in veins or sinuses [72, 73]. Systolic waves generate the pulsatility of the CSF flow as demonstrated by Cine-MR. The flow in the ventral subarachnoid space is caudal during the heart systole and cephalad during diastole [74]. The CSF in ventral and dorsal perimedullary spaces circulate in opposite directions. Intrathecal injections of radioactive tracers have suggested that 160–330 mL of CSF could be reabsorbed daily by the venous system through the spinal outflow system [66] via arachnoid villi [35] or via lymphatic vessels [75]. In clinical conditions, substantial contribution of the spinal outflow system to CSF reabsorption is suggested by the occurrence of hydrocephalus in tumors located in the lumbosacral cistern of the *cauda equina*.

The CSF System in the Immune Defense of the CNS

Until recently anatomic connections between the cerebrospinal fluid and the lymph system were supposed to be exclusively involved in the drainage of CSF and the regulation of CSF pressure in animal models. Lymphatic vessels have been identified in the cranial dura mater along venous sinuses [76] and around spinal subarachnoid recesses in humans. Their role in the immune defense of the CNS has been recently documented in humans by immunohistochemical studies suggesting a cooperation between the CSF, the leptomeninges, and the lymph system [77]. Immune cells could be transported by lymph vessels lining the dural sinuses from the subarachnoid space to cervical lymph nodes [78]. Apart from these lymph vessels, a fluid route along perivascular spaces could ensure soluble antigen delivery from the brain interstitium [79] to antigen presenting cells of the subarachnoid space. Soluble antigens could be then transported by the CSF flow to dural lymph vessels, cervical lymphatics, and cervical lymph nodes where they could accumulate. In other words, the cerebrospinal fluid compartment should be described as a functional equivalents of afferent lymphatics of the brain.

The Meninges in the CNS Development and Injury

The meninges have been experimentally proved to be involved in central nervous system development. More importantly, they participate in the formation and the maintenance of the *glia limitans*. Interposed between the central nervous system parenchyma and the pia mater, the *glia limitans* is a dynamic structure produced by both astrocyte end-feet and meningeal cells that serves as anchorage sites for radial glial cells in the course of development. Its experimental removal leads to the detachment of radial glial cell fibers and abnormal neuronal migration [80, 81]. The leptomeninges induce neuroblast proliferation, differentiation, and axonal growth in the underlying tissue [82] by the secretion of neurotrophic factors such as insulin growth factor [83], stromal cell-derived factor 1 [84], and retinoic acid [45]. Experimental destruction of fetal meninges over the cerebellum induced cerebellar hypoplasia, neuronal ectopia, and glial tissue formation in the subarachnoid space[85, 86].

The role of the leptomeninges as a source of neural stem cells in adults has been demonstrated by immunohistochemical studies [87]. Cells expressing neural stem markers nestin and doublecortin have been found in the spinal cord meninges of adult rats. Following injury, they proliferate and migrate toward the site of injury to form the glial scar. Their differentiation into functional neurons or mature oligodendrocytes under specific *in vitro* conditions places the spinal meninges as a potent target of regenerative medicine in spinal cord injury [88].

References

1. Kelkenberg U, von Rautenfeld DB, Brinker T, Hans VH. Chicken arachnoid granulations: a new model for cerebrospinal fluid absorption in man. Neuroreport. 2001;12(3):553–7.
2. Ariëns Kappers CU. Anatomie comparée du système nerveux, particulièrement de celui des Mammifères et de l'Homme. Paris: Masson et Cie Inc.; 1947.
3. Heisey SR. Cerebrospinal and extracellular fluid spaces in turtle brain. Am J Phys. 1970;219:1564–7.
4. Bagnall KM, Higgins SJ, Sanders EJ. The contribution made by cells from a single somite to tissues within a body segment and assessment of their integration with similar cells from adjacent segments. Development. 1989;107:931–43.
5. Halata Z, Grim M, Christ B. Origin of spinal cord meninges, sheaths of peripheral nerves, and cutaneous receptors including Merkel cells. An experimental and ultrastructural study with avian chimeras. Anat Embryol. 1990;82:529–37.
6. Aoto K, Sandell LL, Butler Tjaden NE, Yuen KC, Watt KE, Black BL, Durnin M, Trainor PA. Mef2c-F10N enhancer driven β-galactosidase (LacZ) and Cre recombinase mice facilitate analyses of gene function and lineage fate in neural crest cells. Dev Biol. 2015;402(1):3–16.
7. Catala M. Embryonic and fetal development of structures associated with the cerebro-spinal fluid in man and other species. Part I: The ventricular system, meninges and choroid plexuses. Arch Anat Cytol Pathol. 1998;46:153–69.
8. Pietri T, Eder O, Blanche M, Thiery JP, Dufour S. The human tissue plasminogen activator-Cre mouse: a new tool for targeting specifically neural crest cells and their derivatives in vivo. Dev Biol. 2003;259(1):176–87.
9. Shibata S, Yasuda A, Renault-Mihara F, Suyama S, Katoh H, Inoue T, Inoue YU, Nagoshi N, Sato M, Nakamura M, Akazawa C, Okano H. Sox10-Venus mice: a new tool for real-time labeling of neural crest lineage cells and oligodendrocytes. Mol Brain. 2010;3:31.
10. Yamauchi Y, Abe K, Mantani A, Hitoshi Y, Suzuki M, Osuzu F, Kuratani S, Yamamura K. A novel transgenic technique that allows specific marking of the neural crest cell lineage in mice. Dev Biol. 1999;212:191–203.
11. Sensenig EC. The early development of the meninges of the spinal cord in human embryos. Contr Embryol Carneg Instn. 1951;34:145–57.
12. Osaka K, Handad H, Matsumoto S, Yasuda M. Development of the cerebrospinal fluid pathway in the normal and abnormal human development. Childs Brain. 1980;6:26–38.
13. O'Rahilly R, Müller F. The meninges in human development. J Neuropathol Exp Neurol. 1986;45(5):588–608.
14. Streeter GF. Factors involved in the formation of the filum terminale. Am J Anat. 1919;25:1–11.
15. Barson AJ. The vertebral level of termination of the spinal cord during normal and abnormal development. J Anat. 1970;3:489–97.
16. Vandenabeele F, Creemers J, Lambrichts I. Ultrastructure of the human spinal arachnoid mater and dura mater. J Anat. 1996;189(Pt 2):417–30.
17. Lazorthes G, Gouazé A, Djindjian R. Vascularisation et circulation de la moelle épinière, anatomie, physiologie, pathologie, angiographie. Paris: Masson Inc.; 1973.
18. Ivanow G, Romodanowsky K. Uber den anatomischen Zusammenhang der cerebralenund spinalen submeningealen Raume mit den Lymphsystem. Z Gee Exp Med. 1928;58:596–607.
19. Brierley JB, Field EJ. The connexions of the spinal sub-arachnoid space with the lymphatic. J Anat. 1948;82:153–66.
20. Foldi M, Csillik B, Zoltan OT. Lymphatic drainage of the brain. Experientia. 1968;24:1283–7.

21. Edgar MA, Nundy S. Innervation of the spinal dura mater. J Neurol Neurosurg Psychiatry. 1966;29:530–4.
22. Groen J, Baljet B, Drukker J. The innervation of the spinal dura mater: anatomy and clinical implications. Acta Neurochir. 1988;92:39–46.
23. Massiat MH. Bases anatomiques de l'infiltration du nerf sinu-vertébral de Luschka en L2. Nantes: Université de Nantes, Faculté de Médecine; 2002.
24. Raoul S. Etude anatomique du nerf sinu-vertébral, Thèse de Médecine, Université de Nantes, Faculté de Médecine. 1999.
25. Jackson HC, Winkelmann RK, Bickel WH. Nerve endings in the human lumbar spinal column and related structures. J Bone Joint Surg. 1966;48:1272–81.
26. Kuslich SD, Ulstrom CL, Michael CJ. The tissue origin of low back pain and sciatica: a report of pain response to tissue stimulation during operations on the lumbar spine using local anesthesia. Orthop Clin North Am. 1991;22:181–7.
27. Wiberg G. Back pain in relation to the nerve supply of the intervertebral disc. Acta Orthop Scand. 1949;19:211–21.
28. Nicholas DS, Weller RO. The fine anatomy of the human spinal meninges. A light and scanning electron microscopy study. J Neurosurg. 1988;69:276–82.
29. Nabeshima S, Reese TS, Landis DM, Brightman MW. Junctions in the meninges and marginal glia. J Comp Neurol. 1975;164(2):127–69.
30. Himango WA, Low FN. The fine structure of a lateral recess of the subarachnoid space in the rat. Anat Rec. 1971;171:1–19.
31. Ulbrich EJ, Schraner C, Boesch C, Hodler J, Busato A, Anderson SE, Eigenheer S, Zimmermann H, Sturzenegger M. Normative MR cervical spinal canal dimensions. Radiology. 2014;271(1):172–82. https://doi.org/10.1148/radiol.13120370.
32. Genevay S, Atlas SJ. Lumbar spinal stenosis. Best Pract Res Clin Rheumatol. 2010;24(2):253–65.
33. Katz JN, Harris MB. Lumbar spinal stenosis. N Engl J Med. 2008;358:818–25.
34. Kido DK, Gomez DG, Pavese AM Jr, Potts DG. Human spinal arachnoid villi and granulations. Neuroradiology. 1976;11:221–8.
35. Welch K, Pollay M. The spinal arachnoid villi of the monkeys Cercopithecus aethiops and Macaca irus. Anat Rec. 1963;145:43–8.
36. Marmarou A, Shulman K, LaMorgese J. Compartmental analysis of compliance and outflow resistance of the cerebrospinal fluid system. J Neurosurg. 1975;43:523–34.
37. Pollay M. The function and structure of the cerebrospinal fluid outflow system. Cerebrospinal Fluid Res. 2010;7:9.
38. Voelz K, Kondziella D, von Rautenfeld DB, Brinker T, Ludemann W. A ferritin tracer study of compensatory spinal CSF outflow pathways in kaolin-induced hydrocephalus. Acta Neuropathol. 2007;113:569–75.
39. Fukushi J, Makagiansar IT, Stallcup WB. NG2 proteoglycan promotes endothelial cell motility and angiogenesis via engagement of galectin-3 and alpha3beta1 integrin. Mol Biol Cell. 2004;15:3580–90.
40. Kural C, Guresci S, Simsek GG, Arslan E, Tehli O, Solmaz I, Izci Y. Histological structure of filum terminale in human fetuses. J Neurosurg Pediatr. 2014;13(4):362–7.
41. Fontes RB, Saad F, Soares MS, de Oliveira F, Pinto FC, Liberti EA. Ultrastructural study of the filum terminale and its elastic fibers. Neurosurgery. 2006;58(5):978–84.
42. Weller RO. Microscopic morphology and histology of the human meninges. Morphologie. 2005;89:22–34.
43. Krahn V. The pia mater at the site of the entry of blood vessels into the central nervous system. Anat Embryol. 1982;164(2):257–63.
44. Krisch B, Leonhardt H, Oksche A. Compartments and perivascular arrangement of the meninges covering the cerebral cortex of the rat. Cell Tissue Res. 1984;238(3):459–74.
45. Zhang ET, Inman CB, Weller RO. Interrelationships of the pia mater and the perivascular (Virchow-Robin) spaces in the human cerebrum. J Anat. 1990;170:111–23.
46. Tarlov IM. Spinal perineurial and meningeal cysts. J Neurol Neurosurg Psychiatry. 1970;33:833–43.
47. Nabors MW, Pait TG, Byrd EB, Karim NO, Davis DO, Kobrine AI, Rizzoli HV. Updated assessment and current classification of spinal meningeal cysts. J Neurosurg. 1988;68(3):366–77.
48. Schreiber F, Haddad B. Lumbar and sacral cysts causing pain. J Neurosurg. 1951;8:504–9.
49. Rexed BA, Wennstrom KG. Arachnoidal proliferation and cystic formation in the spinal nerve-root pouches of man. J Neurosurg. 1959;16:73–84.
50. Lucantoni C, Than KD, Wang AC, Valdivia-Valdivia JM, Maher CO, La Marca F, Park P. Tarlov cysts: a controversial lesion of the sacral spine. Neurosurg Focus. 2011;31(6):E14.
51. Alicioglu B, Sarac A, Tokuc B. Does abdominal obesity cause increase in the amount of epidural fat? Eur Spine J. 2008;17(10):1324–8. https://doi.org/10.1007/s00586-008-0724-8.
52. Wu HT, Schweitzer ME, Parker L. Is epidural fat associated with body habitus? J Comput Assist Tomogr. 2005;29(1):99–102.
53. Beges C, Rousselin B, Chevrot A, et al. Epidural lipomatosis. Interest of magnetic resonance imaging in a weight-reduction treated case. Spine. 1994;19:251–4.
54. Fassett DR, Schmidt MH. Spinal epidural lipomatosis: a review of its causes and recommendations for treatment. Neurosurg Focus. 2004;16(4):E11.
55. Kumar K, Nath RK, Nair CP, et al. Symptomatic epidural lipomatosis secondary to obesity. Case report. J Neurosurg. 1996;85:348–50.
56. Clarot F, Callonnec F, Douvrin F, Hannequin D, Simonet J, Proust B, Thiébot J. Giant cervical epidural veins after lumbar puncture in a case of intracranial hypotension. AJNR Am J Neuroradiol. 2000;21:787–9.
57. Stoquart-Elsankari S, Lehmann P, Villette A, Czosnyka M, Meyer ME, Deramond H, Balédent O. A phase-contrast MRI study of physiologic cerebral venous flow. J Cereb Blood Flow Metab. 2009;29(6):1208–15.
58. Reina MA, De Leon CO, Lopez A, Andre JA, Mora M, Fernandez A. The origin of the spinal subdural space: ultrastructure findings. Anesth Analg. 2002;94:991–5.
59. Stoltmann HF, Blackwood W. An anatomical study of the role of the dentate ligaments in the cervical spinal canal. J Neurosurg. 1966;24:43–6.
60. Garceau GJ. The filum terminale syndrome (the cord traction syndrome). J Bone Joint Surg Am. 1953;35:711–6.
61. Hoffman HJ, Hendrick EB, Humphreys R. The tethered spinal cord: its protean manifestations, diagnosis and surgical correction. Childs Brain. 1976;2:145–55.
62. Selçuki M, Vatansever S, Inan S, Erdemli E, Bağdatoğlu C, Polat A. Is a filum terminale with a normal appearance really normal? Childs Nerv Syst. 2003;19(1):3–10.
63. Hendrick EB, Hoffman HJ, Humphreys RP. The tethered spinal cord. Clin Neurosurg. 1983;30:457–63.
64. Ozawa H, Matsumoto T, Ohashi T, Sato M, Kokubun S. Mechanical properties and function of the spinal pia mater. J Neurosurg Spine. 2004;1(1):122–7.
65. Courchesne E, Chisum HJ, Townsend J, Cowles A, Covington J, Egaas B, Harwood M, Hinds S, Press GA. Normal brain development and aging: quantitative analysis at in vivo MR imaging in healthy volunteers. Radiology. 2000;216(3):672–82.
66. Edsbagge M, Tisell M, Jacobsson L, Wikkelso C. Spinal CSF absorption in healthy individuals. Am J Physiol Regul Integr Comp Physiol. 2004;287:R1450–5.
67. Sullivan JT, Grouper S, Walker MT, Parrish TB, McCarthy RJ, Wong CA. Lumbosacral cerebrospinal fluid volume in humans

using three-dimensional magnetic resonance imaging. Anesth Analg. 2006;103:1306–10.
68. Hogan QH, Prost R, Kulier A, Taylor ML, Liu S, Mark L. Magnetic resonance imaging of cerebrospinal fluid volume and the influence of body habitus and abdominal pressure. Anesthesiology. 1996;84(6):1341–9.
69. Martyr JW, Song SJ, Hua J, Burrows S. The correlation between cauda equina nerve root volume and sensory block height after spinal anaesthesia with glucose-free bupivacaine. Anaesthesia. 2011;66(7):590–4.
70. Masserman JH. Cerebrospinal hydrodynamics: IV. Clinical experimental studies. Arch Neurol Psychiatr. 1934;32:523–53.
71. Rubin RC, Henderson ES, Ommaya AK, Walker MD, Rall DP. The production of cerebrospinal fluid in man and its modification by acetazolamide. J Neurosurg. 1966;25(4):430–6.
72. Welch K, Friedman V. The cerebrospinal fluid valves. Brain. 1960;83:454–69.
73. Di Chiro G. Observations on the circulation of the cerebrospinal fluid. Acta Radiol Diagn (Stockh). 1966;5:988–1002.
74. Quencer RM, Donovan Post MJ, Hinks RS. Cine MR in the evaluation of normal and abnormal CSF flow: intracranial and intraspinal studies. Neuroradiology. 1990;32:371–91.
75. Kida S, Pentazis A, Weller RO. Cerebrospinal fluid drains directly from the subarachnoid space into nasal lymphatics in the rat. Anatomy, histology and immunological significance. Neuropathol Appl Neurobiol. 1993;19:480–8.
76. Bucchieri F, Farina F, Zummo G, Cappello F. Lymphatic vessels of the dura mater: a new discovery? J Anat. 2015;227(5):702–3.
77. Aspelund A, Antila S, Proulx ST, Karlsen TV, Karaman S, Detmar M, Wiig H, Alitalo K. A dural lymphatic vascular system that drains brain interstitial fluid and macromolecules. J Exp Med. 2015;212(7):991–9.
78. Louveau A, Smirnov I, Keyes TJ, Eccles JD, Rouhani SJ, Peske JD, Derecki NC, Castle D, Mandell JW, Lee KS, Harris TH, Kipnis J. Structural and functional features of central nervous system lymphatic vessels. Nature. 2015;523(7560):337–41.
79. Ransohoff RM, Engelhardt B. The anatomical and cellular basis of immune surveillance in the central nervous system. Nat Rev Immunol. 2012;12(9):623–35.
80. Sievers J, Pehlemann FW, Gude S, Berry M. A time course study of the alterations in the development of the hamster cerebellar cortex after destruction of the overlying meningeal cells with 6-hydroxydopamine on the day of birth. J Neurocytol. 1994;23:117–34.
81. Sievers J, Pehlemann FW, Gude S, Berry M. Meningeal cells organize the superficial glia limitans of the cerebellum and produce components of both the interstitial matrix and the basement membrane. J Neurocytol. 1994;23:135–49.
82. Struckhoff G. Coculture of meningeal and astrocytic cells – a model for the formation of the glial limiting membrane. Int J Devl Neurosci. 1995;13:595–606.
83. Stylianopoulou F, Herbert J, Soares MB, Efstratiadis A. Expression of the insulin-like growth factor II gene in the choroid plexus and the leptomeninges of the adult rat central nervous system. Proc Natl Acad Sci USA. 1988;85:141–5.
84. Reiss K, Mentlein R, Sievers J, Hartmann D. Stromal cell-derived factor 1 is secreted by meningeal cells and acts as chemotactic factor on neuronal stem cells of the cerebellar external granular layer. Neuroscience. 2002;115:295–305.
85. Allen C, Sievers J, Berrety M, Jenner S. Experimental studies on cerebellar foliation. II. A morphometric analysis of cerebellar fissuration defects and growth retardation after neonatal treatment with 6-OHDA in the rat. J Comp Neurol. 1981;203:771–83.
86. Sievers J, Von Knebel Doeberitz C, Pehlmann FW, Berry M. Meningeal cells influence cerebellar development over a critical period. Anat Embryol. 1986;175:91–100.
87. Nakagomi T, Nakano-Doi A, Matsuyama T. Leptomeninges: a novel stem cell niche harboring ischemia-induced neural progenitors. Histol Histopathol. 2015;30:391–9.
88. Decimo I, Bifari F, Rodriguez FJ, et al. Nestin- and doublecortin-positive cells reside in adult spinal cord meninges and participate in injury-induced parenchymal reaction. Stem Cells. 2011;29:2062–76.

Intrinsic Innervation of the Spine

R. Robert and O. Hamel

From a biomechanical point of view, the spine is constituted of an anterior column, corresponding to a disco-corporeal compound, and two posterior columns, corresponding to facet joints. Intrinsic innervation must be divided in the same way:

- *Intervertebral discs and vertebral bodies* for which nerve pathways depend on the sympathetic chain ganglia and on its preferential connections with certain spinal roots. Its innervation is essentially an autonomic and transmetameric one;
- *Zygapophyseal joints*, possessing a metameric and somatic innervation regarding its dependence of the dorsal ramus of the spinal roots.

This specific nervous organization may explain some of the semiological characteristics of pain bound to the degeneration of the intervertebral disc or the facet joints, provided that these are isolated.

The lumbar spine will be of use as a model for the description of innervation, considering the main clinical and medico-economical interest of the treatment of low back pain. Specific findings concerning cervical and thoracic levels will be mentioned. Description of these sensitive pathways will follow the path of the signal: from the periphery to the spinal cord.

R. Robert
Department of Neurosurgery, Hôpital privé du Confluent, Nantes, France
e-mail: pr.robert@ncn.fr

O. Hamel (✉)
Department of Neurosurgery, Clinique des Cèdres, Cornebarrieu, France

Intervertebral Disc and Vertebral Body (Figs. 1, 2, and 3)

Which Receptors?

The InterVertebral Disc (IVD) is usually described, in the wrong way, as a non-innervated and a non-vascular tissue. This concept is not exactly correct, but we have to consider the scarcity of nervous fibers, as we have to for the vessels, within the IVD. This scarcity is linked to the huge intra-discal pressure which does not allow the existence of small fibers, especially within the normal nucleus pulposus (NP) [2].

However, some free nerve endings within a few peripheral millimeters of outer annulus fibrosus (AF), and especially within lateral parts of IVD [3], have been described. Ventral and dorsal portions of the IVD are associated with a powerful ligamentous system, crucial structures in this intrinsic innervation of the anterior column of the spine. Indeed, the anterior longitudinal ligament (ALL or VLL) and especially the posterior longitudinal ligament (PLL or DLL) contain many free nerve endings.

There are only few encapsulated endings evocating mechanosensitive afferent units. These rare mechanoreceptors which inform about pressure and tension are located between the layers of AF [4, 5]. This main articular system of the spine transmits little proprioceptive information but is dedicated to a real nociceptive function [6].

Finally, some receptors have been described within the vertebral end plates, mainly free nerve endings. These fibers reach the vessels of the vertebral body (basivertebral vein and artery) which carry these nerve fibers toward the center of the vertebral body and then to the PLL [7].

Which Pathways to the Spinal Root?

Sensory pathways coming from AF, ALL, and PLL converge toward lumbar ganglia of the sympathetic chain. Autonomic

J. M. Vital, D. T. Cawley (eds.), *Spinal Anatomy*, https://doi.org/10.1007/978-3-030-20925-4_27

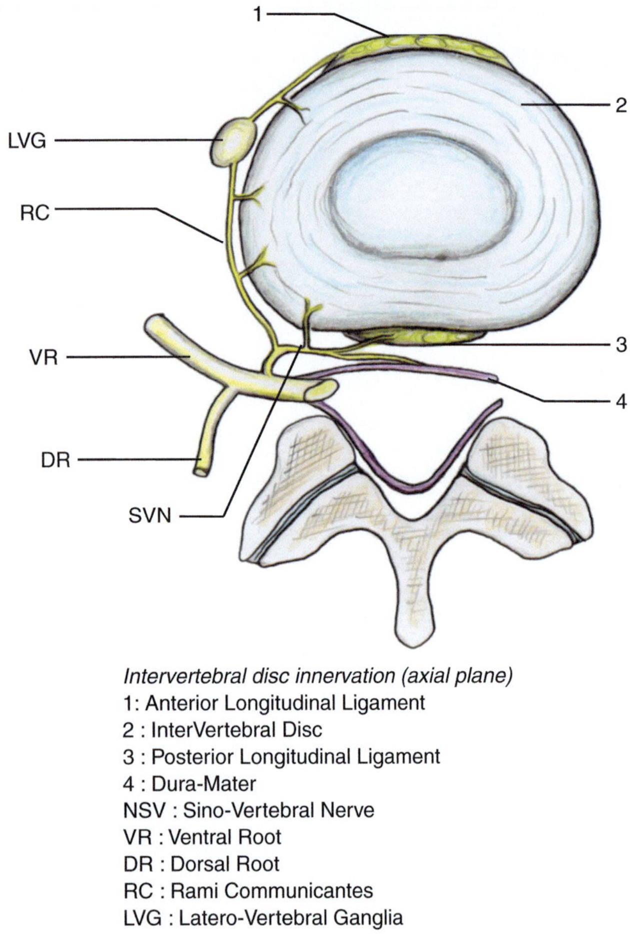

Fig. 1 Intervertebral disc innervation (axial plane). 1. Anterior longitudinal ligament. 2. Intervertebral disc. 3. Posterior longitudinal ligament. 4. Dura mater. *NSV* sinu-vertebral nerve, *VR* ventral root, *DR* dorsal root, *RC* rami communicantes, *LVG* latero-vertebral ganglia

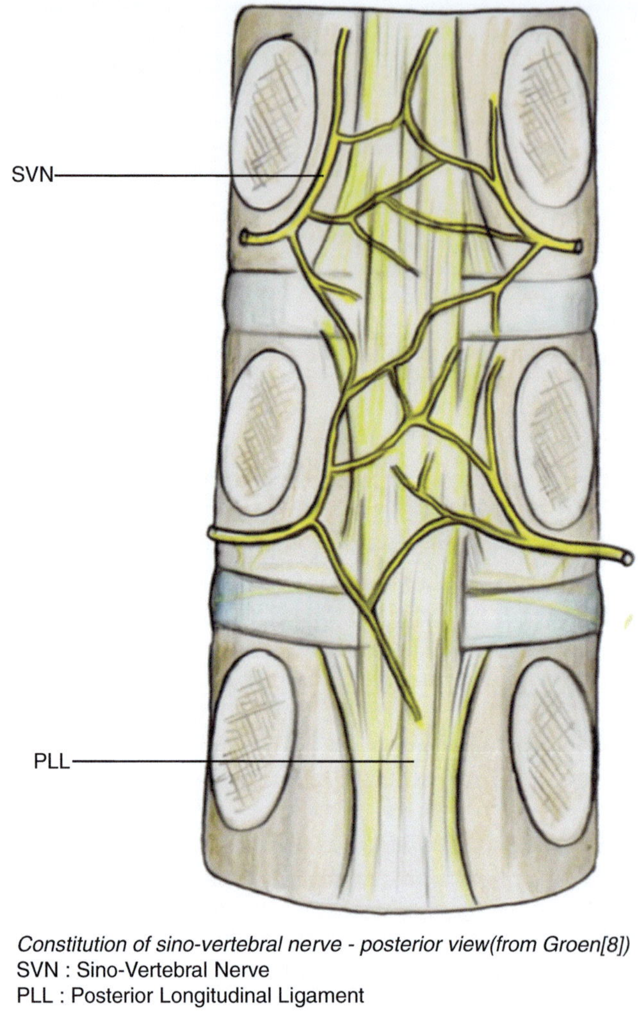

Fig. 2 Constitution of sinu-vertebral nerve—posterior view (from Groen et al. [1]). *SVN* sinu-vertebral nerve, *PLL* posterior longitudinal ligament

sensitive fibers coming from those peridiscal ligaments may transfer nociceptive messages. Presence of neurotransmitters like CGRP, VIP, and NPY, within these nervous structures, demonstrates their role in low back pain [5, 8]. The sympathetic nature of these nerves implies some specific features including numerous nervous and inter-nervous structures, therefore numerous ways to restore function in case of injury [9]. In addition, connections between the sympathetic nervous system and somatic nervous system imply that nociceptive messages may lead to somatic paravertebral muscular contractures [10].

Fibers coming from ALL and from the ventral part of the IVD form a ventral plexus which connects the two, right and left, latero-vertebral sympathetic chains. Each chain is constituted by four or five ganglia.

The largest contingent of sensitive fibers comes from PLL and dorsal part of AF. These fibers lead to the formation of the sinu-vertebral nerve. In addition to discal and ligamentous origins, fibers coming from the ventral part of the dura mater are associated with the constitution of the sinu-vertebral nerve. The real anatomical territory of this nerve is perfectly described by the clinical work of Kuslich [11], based on nearly 200 lumbar microdiscectomy procedures under local anesthesia. The sharing of neural pathways between IVD and dura mater, also demonstrated in dogs [8], can be explained by a common mesenchymal origin with the PLL. Otherwise, the sinu-vertebral nerve also engages with the few fibers coming from the basivertebral vessels [1].

The sinu-vertebral nerve, millimetric structure, has been first described by Luschka in 1850 [12].

The territory of each sinu-vertebral nerve partly overlaps that of the others. Indeed, connections between sinu-vertebral nerves exist on the midline and on at least one vertebral level above and below [1, 4].

Each sinu-vertebral nerve is formed at the ventral and cranial part of the intervertebral foramen, constituted by an

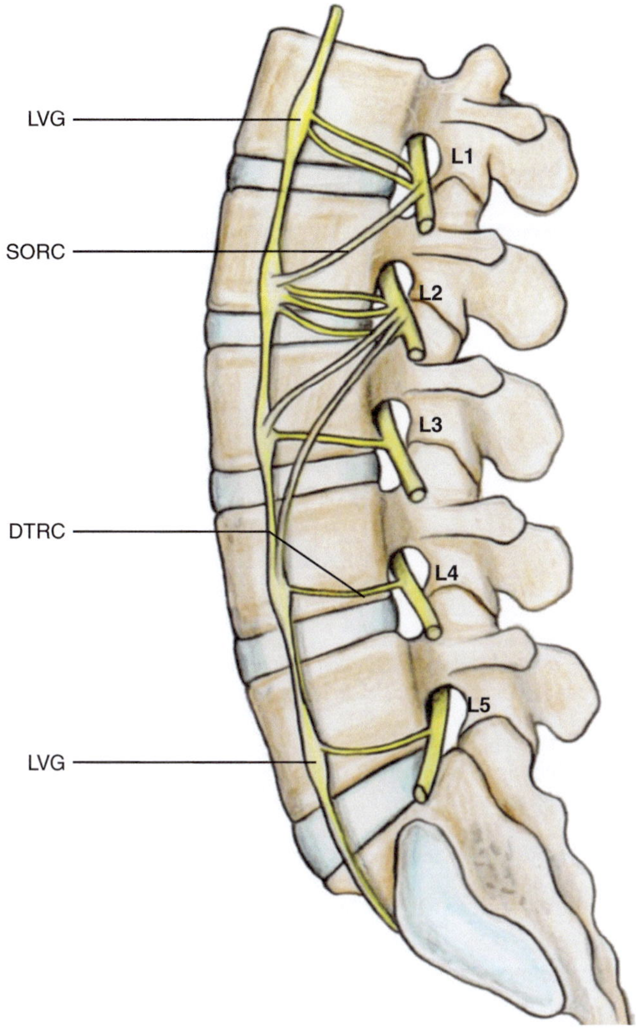

Fig. 3 Lumbar rami communicantes (left side view). *LVG* latero-vertebral ganglia, *DTRC* deep transverse rami communicantes, *SORC* superficial oblique rami communicantes

ascending branch and a descending branch. This sinu-vertebral nerve is located just ahead of the spinal root. It continues to the extraforaminal part of the spinal root while recovering fibers from the lateral portion of the AF. Some fibers of the sinu-vertebral nerve are connected to this part of the root. It is therefore considered, from a morphological point of view, as a recurrent branch of the spinal root. From a functional point of view, most of its fibers extend through the rami communicantes, connecting the spinal root to the latero-vertebral chain.

Few of the sinu-vertebral nerve fibers go directly into the spinal root and thus into the somatic nervous system [13]. These certainly have a role in acute pain which is often better localized and lateralized.

The specific element of this pathway of disco-corporeal innervation consists of the passage of this nociceptive corporeal and discal information in the latero-vertebral ganglia. This is done by the multiple connections (rami communicantes) between the gangliae of the latero-vertebral chain and the spinal roots [14]. These rami communicantes bring all of the sympathetic sensory information to the intra-axial centers, from spinal metameres C8 to L2.

Considering intrinsic innervation of the lumbar spine, it is important to be aware that there are two types of rami communicantes: direct ones and oblique ones [15]. Direct rami communicantes are similar to those found on all vertebral levels, located on a transverse plane next to the middle of the vertebral body. Higuchi [15] more specifically names them as transverse deep rami as they pass, with the segmental vessels, under the arches of the psoas muscle. But the most interesting rami communicantes are probably those called oblique superficial rami also passing under the psoas but externally to the previous ones. They are called oblique as they ascend toward L1 and L2 spinal roots. Therefore, the L2 root receives 4–5 rami communicantes while the underlying roots receive only one or two each [15].

L2 roots, which are not so important from a motor point of view, thus take the lead role in lumbar innervation, well beyond the innervation of the IVD since this root is also predominant on the cutaneous territory of the lumbar region. Indeed, L2 roots cover the sensory territory of the underlying roots whose dorsal branches have, in part, "aborted." The skin of the lumbar region is almost exclusively innervated by these roots. This phenomenon is called the "innervation hole" by Lazorthes and Zadeh [16].

As a brief summary, innervation of IVD and PLL depends on the sinu-vertebral nerve, characterized by minimal lateralization and metamerization. The fibers originating from the various sinu-vertebral nerves, via the complexity of the sympathetic nervous system, preferentially join some specific roots.

We have seen the case of lumbar innervation where fibers originating from IVD essentially go to the most cranial lumbar roots.

At the thoracic level, the vegetative organization is much more closely modeled on the metamerization.

At the cervical level, rami communicantes preferentially move toward the cervico-thoracic or cervical superior ganglia and therefore either to metameres C8 to Th1 or to metameres C2–C4. The concept of the "innervation hole" may also be used at the cervical level [16]. Concerning the first cervical metamere, it is important to remember that the cervical gray matter is closely related to the nociceptive part of the trigeminal nucleus. This interpenetration of gray matter is usually called "trigemino-occipital complex" [17].

Evolution

It is now essential to consider modifications that may exist over time, not with regard to the transmission pathways, but the receptors within the ligamentous structures. The description of the receptors within IVD is that of a healthy and mature disc, which is only a transient state. After the age of 20, the IVD evolves, most often toward a physiological senescence, sometimes toward a pathological degeneration.

During these processes, a neoinnervation develops [18], at the same time as a neovascularization [19]. This nerve sprouting, related to inflammatory phenomena, is also described in the vertebral end plates [20].

Clinical Anatomy

Discogenic low back pain has some particular semiological characteristics, even troubling for problems limited to a single disc. Patients usually describe all the peculiarities of pain mediated by the sympathetic nervous system, including deep and diffuse pain, sensitivity of the skin (healthy skin but reflective of the organ it covers) and reflex muscular reactions. Classical inguinal irradiation of low back pain, including L4–L5 and L5–S1 discopathies, may be explained by the convergence of nociceptive information transmitted by the sympathetic system preferentially to the L1 and L2 roots. We can recall that the cutaneous territory of these roots corresponds to this zone immediately under the inguinal fold [21].

This concept of nociceptive convergence toward L1 and mostly L2 roots has resulted in some clinical trials such as L2 root infiltration which has a well-proven temporary antalgic effect, rather specific of discogenic low back pain [22, 23]. In the same way, L2 rami communicantes infiltration also provides pain relief [10, 24]. However, we remain disappointed by the relative ineffectiveness of the surgical division of these rami communicantes [25]. The idea of suppressing this pathway was promising; its failure probably reflects the existence of the many compensatory mechanisms of the autonomic nervous system [9].

This type of referred pain is also described with neck pain that radiate either in the interscapular space, the skin territory of upper thoracic roots, or to the head, called "cervicogenic headaches" [17] linked to the trigemino-occipital system.

Neural Arch (Fig. 4)

Which Receptors?

The capsules of the zygapophyseal joints possess numerous free and encapsulated nerve endings, proprioceptive and nociceptive. Like the disco-corporeal system, there are free endings in the subchondral bone of the articular processes [26].

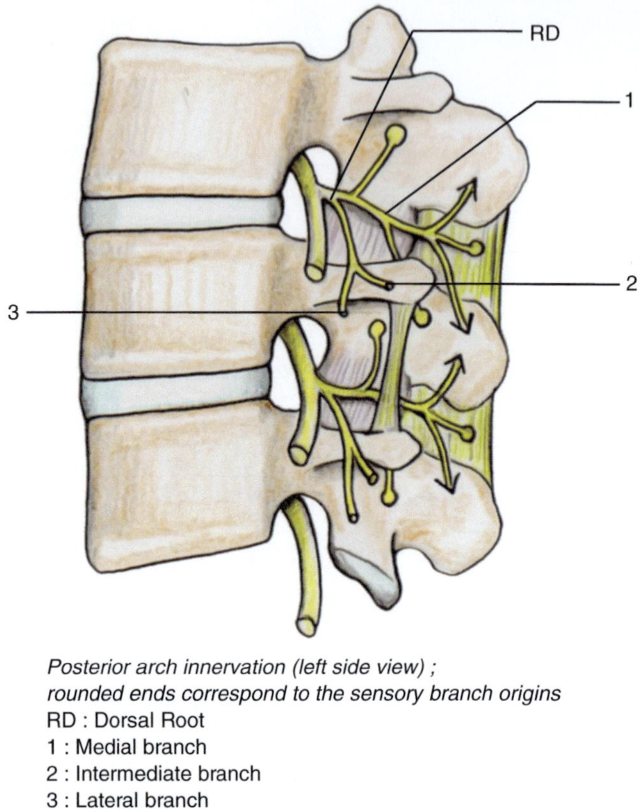

Fig. 4 Posterior arch innervation (side view); rounds correspond to the sensitive branch origins. *RD* Dorsal root. 1. Medial branch. 2. Intermediate branch. 3. Lateral branch

At the medial aspect of the zygapophyseal joint capsules, the ligamentum flavum does not have receptors and therefore no fibers come from it. Kuslich's experiment demonstrates this by the absence of pain during the incision of this structure [11].

Conversely, the interspinous ligament contains numerous encapsulated endings evocative of the corpuscles of Pacini and Ruffini [27]. Therefore, some mechanoreceptors sensitive to pressure can be linked to a sensitivity to extension. There are also free nerve endings in contact with its insertions on the spinous processes [27], linked to a sensitivity to flexion.

Which Pathways to the Spinal Root?

All these fibers will constitute the medial part of the dorsal branch of the spinal root. This medial branch also has a motor role, dedicated to a segmental innervation for the multifidus muscles inserted on the overlying vertebral lamina [26].

Each medial branch receives two articular branches, one called "ascending" from the overlying zygapophyseal joint, the other "descending" from the underlying zygapophyseal joint [28]. These branches join the medial branch of the dorsal root just before it passes beneath the mamillo-accessory ligament [26, 28]. The medial root then travels through the intertransverse ligament to the upper edge of the transverse process base. It joins the lateral root and sometimes an intermediate root [26], both of which have an essentially motor role.

In order to better understand the referred pains of spinal column injuries, whether disco-corporeal or neural arch, one must be interested in the skin territories of these spinal roots. Of course, the ventral branch has sensory cutaneous fibers, which are evident from the description of the radiculalgia presented by patients as described by Déjerine. With regard to the dorsal roots, we have already reported the existence of these "innervation holes." The work of Lazorthes and Zadeh demonstrated a cervico-thoracic hiatus between the C4 and Th2 roots and a lumbosacral hiatus between L3 and S3 [16]. On the other hand, all the dorsal roots between Th3 and L2 reach the skin, which implies that the C4, Th3, and L2 roots have a very developed cutaneous territory, on the dorsal part of the neck and trunk.

Clinical Anatomy

The "facet syndrome" has been well demonstrated; it has even been overexploited for the use of thermoablation treatments for innervation pathways of the capsules of these zygapophyseal joints.

Although the characteristics of zygapophyseal pain are as unspecific as discogenic pain, they have some specificities, particularly in their projections, explained by the progression of the innervation pathways. The most important is related to the somatic nature of this innervation: it is much more precise, even "punctual" in case of unilateral lesions. The patient can sometimes point to painful localization with one finger, while both hands are not sufficient to describe discogenic pain. In addition, each zygapophyseal joint being dependent of nerves that join two spinal roots, above and below, the painful projection will occur in the dermal territory of these two roots. Zygapophyseal pain is therefore very frequently marked by pseudo-radiculalgia, most often truncated in the proximal territory of the root [29]. However, this painful irradiation is much less precise than a true monoradiculalgia since it occurs in two root territories.

Conclusion

The vertebral column presents a substantial intrinsic somatic and autonomic innervation, segmental and transsegmental, with obvious nociceptive capacities. It is essential to understand this innervation in order to perceive the numerous semiological traps constituted by spinal pain and radicular pain. One may be surprised at the lack of description of proprioceptive structures for so many joints. This lack is largely filled by the innervation of the many powerful paravertebral muscles that play an obvious role as proprioceptors.

References

1. Groen GJ, Baljet B, Drukker J. The nerves and nerve plexuses of the human vertebral column. Am J Anat. 1990;188(3):282–96.
2. Rabishong P, Louis R, Vignaud J, Massare C. Le disque intervertébral. Anat Clin. 1978;1(5):55–64.
3. Malinsky J. The ontogenetic development of nerve terminations in the intervertebral discs of man. Acta Anat. 1959;38:96–113.
4. Bogduk N, Tynan W, Wilson AS. The nerve supply to the human lumbar intervertebral discs. J Anat. 1981;132(1):39–56.
5. Roberts S, Johnson E. Innervation du disque intervertébral et lombalgie discale. Rev Rhum. 2000;67(Suppl 4):225–31.
6. Sekine M, Yamashita T, Takebayashi T, Sakamoto N, Minaki Y, Ishii S. Mechanosensitive afferent units in the lumbar posterior longitudinal ligament. Spine. 2001;26(14):1516–21.
7. Antonacci MD, Mody DR, Heggeness MH. Innervation of the human vertebral body: a histologic study. J Spinal Disord. 1998;11(6):526–31.
8. Waber-Wenger B, Forterre F, Kuehni-Boghenbor K, Danuser R, Stein JV, Stoffel MH. Sensory innervation of the dorsal longitudinal ligament and the meninges in the lumbar spine of the dog. Histochem Cell Biol. 2014;142(4):433–47.
9. de Ribet RM. Le système nerveux de la vie végétative. Paris: Doin; 1955. 487p.
10. Robert R, Raoul S, Hamel O, Doe K, Lanoiselée JM, Berthelot JM, Caillon F, Bord E. Lombalgies chroniques. Une autre approche thérapeutique. Neurochirurgie. 2004;50(2-3):117–22.
11. Kuslich SD, Ulstrom CI, Michael CJ. The tissue origin of low back pain and sciatica: a report of pain response to tissue stimulation during operation of the lumbar spine using local anesthesia. Orthop Clin North Am. 1991;22(2):181–7.
12. Hovelacque A. Le nerf sinu-vertébral. Ann Anat Pathol. 1925;2(5):435–43.
13. Edgar MA. The nerve supply of the lumbar intervertebral disc. J Bone Joint Surg Br. 2007;89:1135–9.
14. Suseki K, Takahashi Y, Takahashi K, Chiba T, Yamagata M, Moriya H. Sensory nerve fibers from lumbar intervertebral discs pass through rami communicantes. J Bone Joint Surg Br. 1998;80(4):737–42.
15. Higuchi K, Sato T. Anatomical study of lumbar spine innervation. Folia Morphol (Warsz). 2002;61(2):71–9.
16. Lazorthes G, Zadeh J, Galy E, Roux P. Le territoire cutané des branches postérieures des nerfs rachidiens. Neurochirurgie. 1987;33:386–90.
17. Bogduk N. The anatomy and pathophysiology of neck pain. Phys Med Rehabil Clin N Am. 2011;22(3):367–82.
18. Freemont AJ, Peacock TE, Goupille P, Hoyland JA, O'Brien J, Jayson MIV. Nerve ingrowth into diseased intervertebral disc in chronic back pain. Lancet. 1997;350(9072):178–81.
19. Pai RR, D'sa B, Raghuveer CV, Kamath A. Neovascularization of the nucleus pulposus. A diagnostic feature of intervertebral disc prolapse. Spine. 1999;24(8):739–41.
20. Brown MF, Hukkanen MV, McCarthy ID, Redfern DR, Batten JJ, Crock HV, Hughes SP, Polak JM. Sensory and sympathetic innervation of the vertebral endplate in patients with degenerative disc disease. J Bone Joint Surg Br. 1997;79(1):147–53.
21. Oikawa Y, Ohtori S, Koshi T, Takaso M, Inoue G, Orita S, Eguchi Y, Ochiai N, Kishida S, Kuniyoshi K, Nakamura J, Aoki Y, Ishikawa T, Miyagi M, Arai G, Kamoda H, Suzuki M, Sainoh T, Toyone T, Takahashi K. Lumbar disc degeneration induces persistent groin pain. Spine. 2012;37(2):114–8.

22. Nakamura S, Takahashi K, Takahashi Y, Yamagata M, Moriya H. The afferent pathway of discogenic low back pain. Evaluation of L2 spinal nerve infiltration. J Bone Joint Surg Br. 1996;78(4):606–12.
23. Ohtori S, Nakamura S, Koshi T, Yamashita M, Yamauchi K, Inoue G, Orita S, Eguchi Y, Suzuki M, Ochiai N, Kishida S, Takaso M, Aoki Y, Kuniyoshi K, Nakamura J, Ishikawa T, Arai G, Miyagi M, Kamoda H, Suzuki M, Takahashi Y, Toyone T, Yamagata M, Takahashi K. Effectiveness of L2 spinal nerve infiltration for selective discogenic low back pain patients. J Orthop Sci. 2010;15(6):731–6.
24. Sluitjer ME. The role of radiofrequency in failed back surgery patients. Curr Rev Pain. 2000;4(1):49–53.
25. Rigaud J, Riant T, Labat JJ, Guerineau M, Robert R. Is section of sympathetic rami communicantes by laparoscopy in patients with refractory low back pain efficient? Eur Spine J. 2013;22(4):775–81.
26. Bogduk N, Wilson AS, Tynan W. The human lumbar dorsal rami. J Anat. 1982;134(2):383–97.
27. Yahia LH, Newman N, Rivard CH. Neurohistology of lumbar spine ligaments. Acta Orthop Scand. 1988;59(5):508–12.
28. Louis R. Chirurgie du rachis: anatomie chirurgicale et voies d'abord. Berlin: Springer; 1982. 325p.
29. Mooney V, Robertson J. The facet syndrome. Clin Orthop Relat Res. 1976;115:149–56.

Spinal Vascularization

D. Liguoro and X. Barreau

The vascular anatomy of the spine and spinal cord provides the basis for understanding the vascular, traumatic and tumoural lesions involving this area. Understanding this anatomy is crucial to the treatment of lesions from both a surgical and an endovascular approach [1, 2].

If the arterial vascularization of the osseous and muscular envelopes of the spinal cord is rich since it comes from multiple metameric arteries, it is not the case for spinal cord arteries.

Embryology [3, 4]

Early in gestation, 31 pairs of segmental vessels grow dorsally from the aorta to supply the developmental precursors of bone, muscle and nerve (Fig. 1).

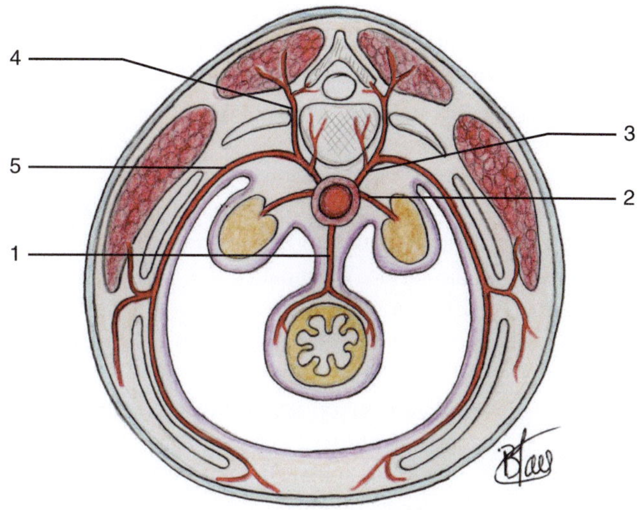

Fig. 1 Week 7, the branches of the dorsal aorta are evident in the thoracic region. (1) Visceral ventral segmental branch, (2) visceral lateral segmental branch, (3) intersegmental dorso-lateral branch, (4) dorsal branch of the intersegmental artery, (5) ventral branch of the intersegmental artery (intersegmental arteries from the aortic arch in the cervical region and intercostal and lumbar arteries in the thoracolumbar region)

Spine

Embryological modifications occur at the different regions of the spine. The blood supply to each vertebra is similar at all spinal levels. It is divided to supply the vertebral body, pedicle, transverse process and spinous process.

In the cervical region, extraspinal anastomoses from between segments form the vertebral artery, the ascending cervical artery and the deep cervical artery. These vessels are located within ventral and dorsal to the transverse processes of the cervical vertebrae. Additional contributions from the ascending pharyngeal artery or occipital artery may be present at the craniocervical junction.

In the thoracolumbar region, the constant origin of radicular arteries from intercostal and lumbar arteries reflects the persistence of the segmental embryological arrangement. The vertebrae receive blood supply from lumbar arteries.

In the sacral region, the regression of the dorsal aorta forms the median sacral artery. This region is also supplied by the internal iliac vessels.

Spinal Cord

The primitive arterial vascularization of the spinal cord relies on the dorsal aorta which gives off intersegmental arteries supplying the somites. Each intersegmental artery reaches the ventrolateral aspect of the developing spinal cord and

D. Liguoro (✉)
Neurosurgical Department A, University Hospital of Pellegrin, Bordeaux, France
e-mail: dominique.liguoro@chu-bordeaux.fr

X. Barreau
Department of Neuroradiology, University Hospital of Pellegrin, Bordeaux, France
e-mail: xavier.barreau@chu-bordeaux.fr

J. M. Vital, D. T. Cawley (eds.), *Spinal Anatomy*, https://doi.org/10.1007/978-3-030-20925-4_28

establishes longitudinal anastomoses at the capillary level with intersegmental arteries from the levels above and below.

During development, each radicular artery initially contributes to both the ventral and dorsal spinal arteries. They also supply the spinal roots, dura mater, bony structures, and paraspinal musculature at each level. Then most of the segmental branches regress.

Finally, 6–8 ventral branches of the radicular arteries continue to supply the entire axis of the ventral spinal artery; 10–20 dorsal branches of the radicular arteries provide the blood supply to the dorsal spinal arteries. Of the 62 radicular branches, at the most 7 or 8 truly participate on the vascularization of the spinal cord.

At the end of the third week, one can thus distinguish a fine longitudinal capillary network along each ventrolateral aspect of the spinal cord. The ventral aspect of the cord situated between the capillary network and the dorsal part of the spinal cord are still avascular at this stage.

Radicular arteries form by the division of the primitive intersegmental arteries into a ventral and a dorsal branch. The dorsal branches reach the dorsal aspect of the cord and, like their ventral homologues, form longitudinal anastomotic networks along the surface of spinal cord.

The dorsal radicular arteries give rise to two dorsal longitudinal axes on each side. The larger one courses dorsal to the dorsal root. The other one, which is finer, forms laterally, between the dorsal and ventral nerve roots, in proximity to the dentate ligament. With time, the capillary bed over the ventrolateral surface of the spinal cord progressively extends to its ventromedial aspect.

Between the sixth and tenth weeks of gestation, a single ventral spinal artery forms. Whether this occurs by fusion of the two parallel ventral axes or by a process of partial obliteration and remodelling of the primitive plexiform ventral axis is not clear. Incomplete fusion could explain why the ventral spinal axis is often fenestrated and sometimes duplicated, whereas obliteration and remodelling might account for the commonly tortuous course of the ventral spinal artery.

By the tenth week, the vasculature of the spinal cord essentially corresponds to its postnatal configuration. After this period, only a few significant changes occur. The dorsal anastomotic chains are remodelled into two distinct dorsal spinal arteries. There is a significant reduction in the number of radiculomedullary arteries supplying the spinal cord, with a transition from a regular, symmetric and ubiquitous distribution to an irregular and asymmetric distribution, a transformation that is particularly marked at the level of the inferior third of the spinal cord.

The course of radiculomedullary arteries is modified: during embryological development, the unequal growth of the spinal cord and the spinal column results in an apparent ascension of the cord relative to the column, a phenomenon that continues into postnatal life until about the age of 12 months. Consequently, the radiculomedullary arteries assume an ascending course, which becomes more and more marked as one progresses in a caudal direction.

The number of ventral and dorsal spinal contributors detectable by macroscopic anatomy and angiography decreases with age, until the spinal vascularization seems to be derived from a few branches only, including the artery of the lumbar enlargement or artery of Adamkiewicz. It has been clearly shown, however, that at the macroscopic and microscopic levels, the ventral and dorsal spinal contributors are present at every single level throughout life. The apparent vascular distribution observed in the adult human results from the combination of functional adaptation (largest branches at the level of the largest neuronal masses) and senescence. These observations are clinically important, as they imply that each radicular artery has the potential to become a feeding branch for a vascular malformation.

The definitive adult vascular pattern forms in a cranial-to-caudal direction: fusion and medial displacement of the paired ventrolateral channels form the midline ventral spinal artery; dorsally, two channels coalescence from a pial network on the lateral and dorsal surfaces to form the dorsal spinal arteries.

So, from early embryonic stages, these two intrinsic arterial supplies to the spinal cord remain separated anatomically and functionally.

Blood Supply of the Spinal Structures

Prespinal Vessels

Thoracic Aorta (Figs. 2 and 3)

The thoracic aorta extends from the termination of the aortic arch at the lower border of T4 to the lower border of T12. At T12, the thoracic aorta passes between the crura of the diaphragm and continues as the abdominal aorta. The first part of the thoracic aorta is situated to the left of the vertebral column. As the aorta descends, it approaches the front of the bony structures. At the diaphragm, it is almost in the midline. Initially the oesophagus is to the right of the aorta, then in front and finally near the termination of the oesophagus, slightly to the left.

The branches of the thoracic aorta are divided into visceral (pericardial, bronchial and oesophageal arteries) and parietal vessels (intercostal, superior phrenic and mediastinal arteries) [5].

The intercostal vessels are located in the centre of the vertebral bodies. Both right and left branches of the aorta supply each thoracic vertebra. There are 11 intercostal arteries and one subcostal artery arising from the aorta. But usually there are 10 pairs of intercostal arteries. The upper two interspaces are supplied by branches of the subclavian artery. The lowest

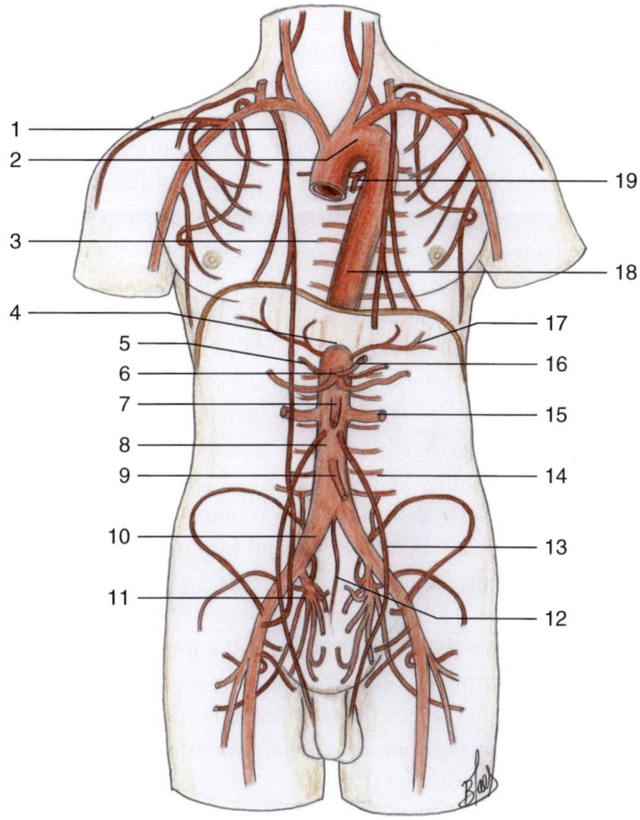

Fig. 2 (1) Right internal thoracic artery, (2) thoracic arch, (3) intercostal artery, (4) aortic hiatus, (5) right middle adrenal artery, (6) celiac trunk, (7) superior mesenteric artery, (8) abdominal aorta, (9) inferior mesenteric artery, (10) common right iliac artery, (11) right internal iliac artery, (12) medial sacral artery, (13) left gonadal artery, (14) lumbar artery, (15) left renal artery, (16) left gastric artery, (17) lower left phrenic artery, (18) thoracic aorta and (19) right bronchial artery

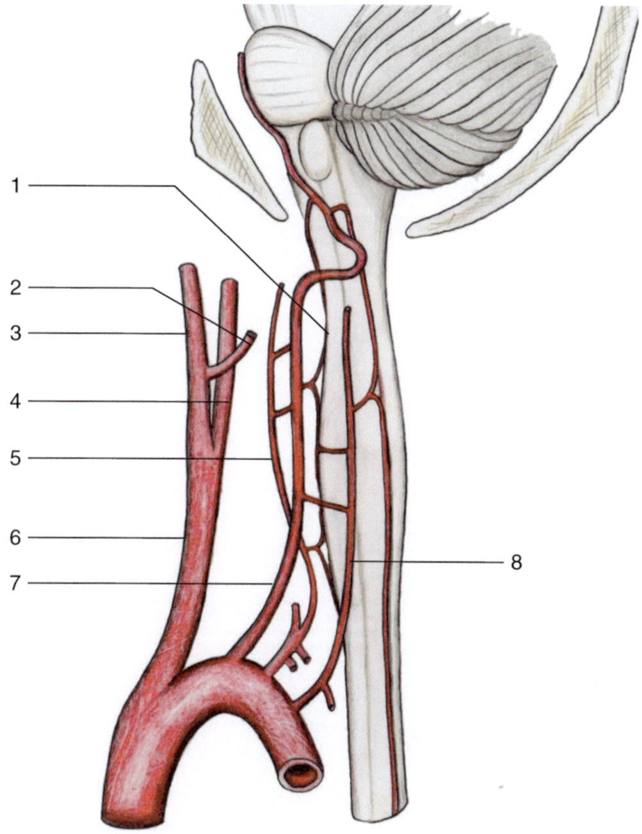

Fig. 3 (1) Ventral spinal artery; (2) occipital artery, (3) external carotid artery, (4) internal carotid artery, (5) ascending cervical artery, (6) common carotid artery, (7) vertebral artery and (8) deep cervical artery

intercostal artery is known as the subcostal artery and accompanies the twelfth rib.

The intercostal arteries differ on the two sides of the aorta. The arteries on the right side, especially the upper vessels, are longer than those on the left because the aorta lies to the left side of the vertebral column.

On the right side, the intercostal arteries course over the right side of the vertebral bodies, crossed by the thoracic duct, esophagus and major vena azygos, and covered by the pleura and lung.

On the left side, the upper two intercostal vessels are crossed by the left superior intercostal vein, and the next two are crossed by the accessory hemiazygos vein. The lower left intercostal arteries are crossed by the hemiazygos vein (minor). The left pleura and lung cover the left-sided arteries.

The intercostal arteries have two branches, ventral and dorsal:

- The ventral branches initially cross the vertebrae somewhat obliquely because of the downward direction of the ribs. They continue towards the angle of the rib. At the costovertebral articulation, they are crossed by the sympathetic chain. The ventral branches are accompanied by a nerve and a vein to their termination between two intercostal muscles.
- The dorsal branches arise from the intercostal arteries opposite the space bounded by the transverse process of the vertebra above, the costal process below and the body of the vertebra medially. The dorsal branches travel towards the intervertebral foramen where they divide into a muscular and a spinal branch. The spinal branch enters the intervertebral foramen where it supplies ligaments, laminae, nerve roots, dura and the spinal cord [6].

Abdominal Aorta (Fig. 4)

The abdominal portion is at the lower border of T12 and usually ends at approximately the level of the fourth lumbar vertebra. At L4 the abdominal aorta divides into the right and left common iliac arteries. Initially the abdominal aorta is located centrally, but as it courses distally it slightly deviates to the left side [5].

The abdominal aortic branches are divided into three types: parietal (right and left phrenic arteries, and the four pairs of right and left lumbar arteries), visceral (celiac, mesenteric,

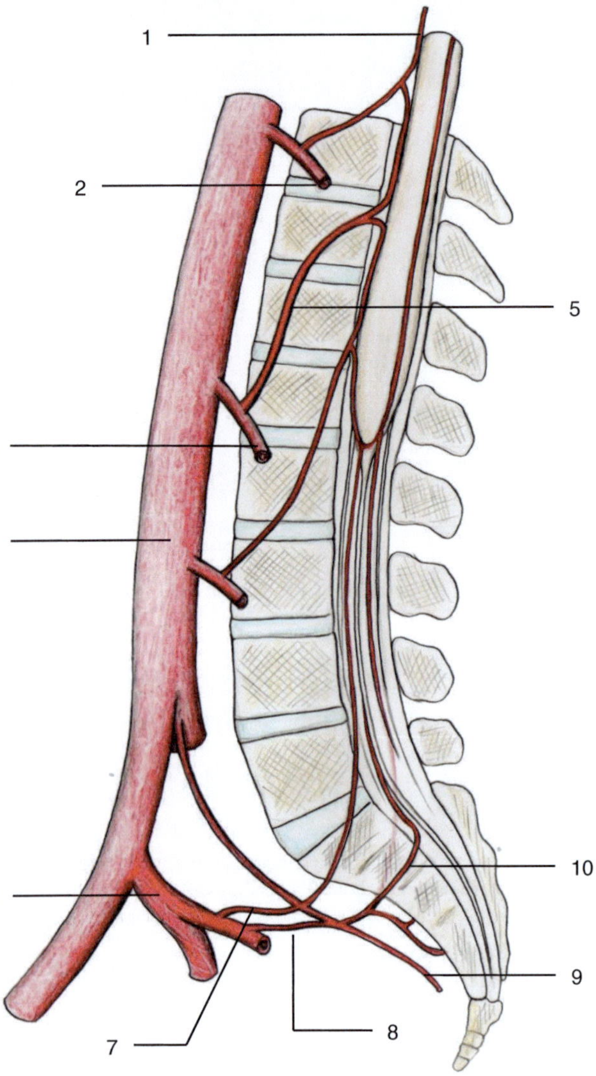

Fig. 4 (1) Ventral spinal artery, (2) intercostal artery, (3) lumbar artery, (4) abdominal aorta, (5) artery of lumbar intumescence (Adamkiewicz), (6) internal iliac artery, (7) Desproges-Gotteron artery, (8) lateral sacral artery, (9) median sacral artery and (10) artery of the filum

renal …arteries) and the terminal branches: the right and left common iliac arteries and the median sacral artery. However, this vascular bifurcation is variable and can occur anywhere from the upper half of L3 to the lower border of L5.

The eight lumbar segmental arteries (four on each side) arise from the dorsal aspect of the abdominal aorta. Because the aorta is situated somewhat to the left of the midline, the right lumbar arteries are longer than are those on the left side. These vessels pass through the middle and around the four upper lumbar vertebrae.

As the arteries curve around the bodies of the vertebrae, they pass beneath the sympathetic trunk. The upper two lumbar arteries course under the crura of the diaphragm. The right lumbar arteries pass beneath the vena cava, and the upper two on the right side are situated under the cisterna chyli. Both the right and left lumbar arteries are under the tendinous arch of the psoas muscles situated along the sides of the vertebral bodies.

The arteries continue under the psoas until they arrive at the interval between the transverse process of the vertebrae and the medial edge of the quadratus lumborum muscle. While the lumbar arteries are coursing under the psoas, they are accompanied by rami of the sympathetic chain and the lumbar veins. Ventral to the transverse process, the lumbar arteries are crossed by branches of the lumbar plexus. A fifth pair of lumbar arteries is often given off from the middle sacral artery opposite the fifth lumbar vertebrae.

Like the intercostal arteries, the lumbar arteries course to the foramen and divide into a dorsal vertebral branch and a ventral muscular branch. The ventral branch travels forward between the abdominal muscles and terminates by anastomosing with other abdominal wall arteries.

The origin of the common iliac arteries usually occurs opposite the left side of the middle of the fourth lumbar vertebra. They terminate opposite the lumbosacral articulation by dividing into the external and internal iliac arteries. The external iliac artery continues to the brim of the pelvis to the lower limb; the internal iliac artery descends medially. The right and left arteries differ in their relations to nearby structures.

Because of the bifurcation of the aorta a little to the left of the midline, the right common iliac artery is approximately 5 cm long and the left one is 4 cm. The right common iliac artery is crossed in front by the ureter and the ovarian artery in the female, sympathetic nerve branches descending to the hypogastric plexus, the inferior mesenteric artery termination, the sigmoid colon and the sigmoid mesocolon. From behind, the right iliac artery lies on the right common iliac vein, the end of the left common iliac vein and the beginning of the vena cava. These venous structures separate it from the fourth and the fifth vertebra and the L4L5 interspace. To the right of the right iliac artery are located the inferior vena cava, the termination of the right iliac vein and the psoas. Along the left border of the right common iliac artery are seated the right common iliac vein, the end of the left common iliac vein, and the superior hypogastric plexus [7].

The shorter left common iliac artery is crossed in front by the ureter, the ovarian artery in the female, branches of the sympathetic nerve and termination of the inferior mesenteric artery, the sigmoid colon and the sigmoid mesocolon. Located behind the left common iliac artery are the lower border of the fifth lumbar vertebra, the L4L5 disc space, the body of L5 and the L5S1 disc interspace. To the left of the left common iliac artery is the psoas muscle. On the right side of the artery are the left common iliac vein, the hypogastric plexus and the middle sacral artery.

The artery of Adamkiewicz, the great radicular artery, usually enters the vertebral canal between T7 and L4. Its greatest sites of location are between T9 and T11 on the left side [8, 9].

Blood Supply of the Vertebral Structures (Figs. 5 and 6)

The Vertebral Body [10, 11]

At the cervical level, the vascularization is provided by the ascending branches of the right and left subclavian arteries: lower thyroid artery, ascending cervical artery, deep cervical artery. They are organized in three axes: prevertebral (thyroid and ascending cervical arteries), latero-vertebral (vertebral artery) and dorsal (deep cervical artery). These three axes are largely anastomosed between each other and ensure vascularization to the vertebrae.

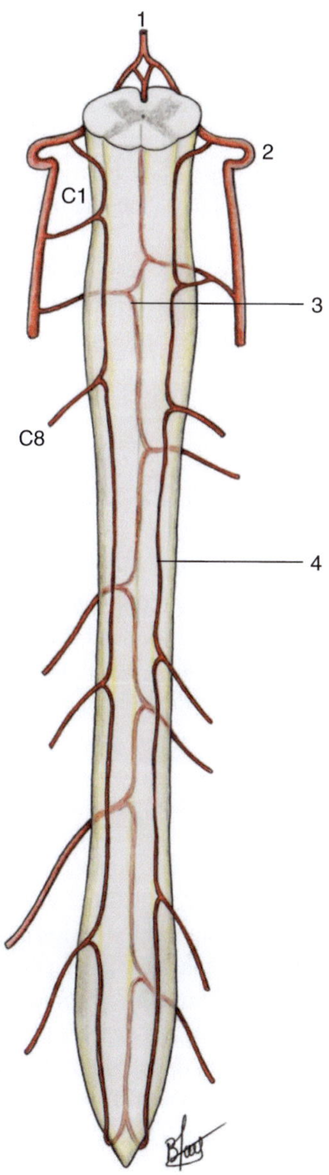

Fig. 5 (Dorsal view) (1) Basilar artery, (2) vertebral artery, (3) ventral spinal artery and (4) dorsal spinal artery

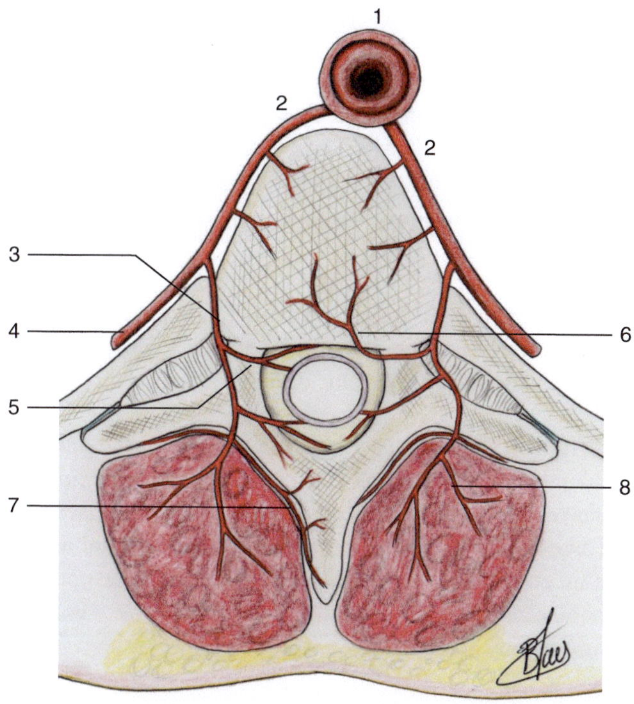

Fig. 6 (1) Thoracic aorta, (2) posterior intercostal arteries, (3) dorsal branch, (4) ventral branch, (5) root artery, (6) retrovertebral artery, (7) medial muscular branch and (8) lateral muscular branch

At the thoracic and lumbar level, the blood supply is derived from the intercostal and lumbar arteries.

The vertebral body is fed by two arterial groups:

- a prevertebral group formed by the artery of the vertebral body and the periosteal branches.
- an intracanalicular group formed by the ventral spinal canal branch.

The Ventral Group

It is formed of multiple small periosteal branches coming from the trunk of the intercostal artery which vascularize the peripheral portion of the ventral and lateral sides of the vertebral body.

The aorta lies laterally on the left side and its particular position accounts for the differences observed according to side and level. These are periosteal branches numbering between two and four per intercostal artery on the right side, and often less numerous on the left side where they arise lateral to the insertion of the ventral longitudinal ligament.

According to the course they take, three types of different vessels may be distinguished:

- ascending vessels arising from the superior surface of the intercostal artery and passing superiorly. They divide into several periosteal branches which supply the superior half of the vertebral body, may give an anastomotic branch to the descending artery of the vertebral body which arises from the suprajacent intercostal artery.

- descending vessels which originate from the inferior surface of the intercostal artery pass downwards and give off periosteal branches to supply the inferior half of the vertebral body.
- recurrent arteries usually arising from the superior surface of the intercostal artery, and which pass superiorly then transversely and medially, and may anastomose with the corresponding artery on the opposite side.

While all three arrangements may be met at the thoracic and lumbar level, such is not the case in the superior thoracic spine where the branches to the vertebral bodies arise from the ascending segment of the trunk of the intercostal artery, and ascend vertically before penetrating the corresponding vertebrae at the level of the ventral intercostal artery without giving off any collaterals.

The Dorsal Group

The dorsal group provides the majority of the vascularization of the vertebral body and comes from the ventral branch of the retrocorporeal artery via two perforating branches which penetrate the vertebral body through its vascular hilum whose branches vascularize the dorsal side of the vertebral body and most of the central corporeal region.

This group is formed by the anastomotic network behind the vertebral body. The ventral spinal canal branch arises from the dorsospinal artery close to its origin, either in isolation or more frequently via a common trunk with the radicular artery. In certain cases, they may originate directly from the trunk of the intercostal artery in front of the origin of the dorsal branch. This anatomical arrangement is a relatively frequent finding at the lumbar and superior dorsal levels.

The ventral spinal canal branch runs a descending and oblique course downwards and medially following the curve of the ventral surface of the spinal nerve as it passes out of the intervertebral foramen at a variable distance on the spinal process. Once it has penetrated the spinal canal, it divides into a large ascending branch and more slender descending branch.

– The ascending branch passes obliquely upwards and medially, on the dorsal surface of the vertebral body, passes beneath the dorsal longitudinal ligament and then divides at the level of the central part of the vertebral column into several branches: an anastomotic branch to the descending branch of the subjacent intercostal artery, another one to the retrovertebral artery on the other side and several intraosseous branches which penetrate the body of the vertebrae via the basivertebral foramen (of Hann).
– Among the several variations which can exist, it is worth pointing out the isolated origin of the descending branch directly from the trunk of the dorsospinal artery or even one of its terminal branches. In this case, this branch passes behind the spinal nerve, crossing its inferior surface to reach the ventral or inferior part of the intervertebral foramen.

The Costovertebral Joint

The costovertebral vascularization is fed by branches coming from the ventral branch of the intercostal artery and the two branches coming from the dorsospinal artery during its passage through the paravertebral space.

There are two distinct vascular sources:

- a transverse branch from the ventral intercostal artery of very slender calibre, it arises from the superior surface of the ventral intercostal artery near to its origin, sometimes from the first perforating branch in its proximal segment. It ascends vertically and then it is just near the inferior border of the rib as far as the medial extremity of the transverse process.
- branches arising from the supra and subjacent dorsal arteries during their course in the paravertebral gutter, providing a blood supply to the posterior surface of the transverse process.

The Dorsal Arch

The dorsal arch receives a double blood supply:

– the intracanalicular portion supplied by an arterial network situated in the epidural space and formed by branches of the dorsal spinal canal branch;
– the dorsal portion supplied by branches of the medial muscular branch of the dorsospinal artery.

Intracanalicular System

It is formed by the dorsal spinal canal artery and its branches. It arises from the trunk of the dorsospinal artery after the radiculomedullary artery, or sometimes via a common trunk with it, but rarely from a branch of division of the dorsospinal artery. It penetrates the spinal canal by passing through the intervertebral foramen, behind the spinal nerve and then runs a variable course in the epidural space and terminates on the median line with respect to the origin of the spinal process in anastomosing with its counterpart from the opposite side.

It gives several branches to the dorsal arch:

- a vertical anastomotic branch with its adjacent neighbour situated above and just medial to the articular process. Its situation is more lateral than that of the retrovertebral anastomoses.
- an osseous branch which is constant and which supplies the lamina.
- a branch penetrating the root of the spinal process in the median line.

Dorsal System

Its blood supply is assured by branches coming from the medial muscular branch of the dorsospinal artery. The latter is easily identified by virtue of its course which is practically identical at all levels: it passes firstly medially, just near the lamina, then on reaching the root of the spinous process, it becomes oblique downwards and dorsally, running the length of the spinous process. At the point of the spinous process, it anastomoses with a branch of its subjacent neighbour.

During its course it gives off several osseous branches:

- periosteal branches assuring the blood supply to the dorsal surface of the lamina and spinal process.
- a branch to the intervertebral joint. It arises from the initial part of the medial muscular branch and its short vertical course behind the articular process is characteristic. This latter branch is bigger at the lumbar level than at the thoracic one.

The Intervertebral Foramen [6]

The intervertebral foramina, regardless of the segment considered, are traversed by nerve roots and also by veins and arteries, some going to the spinal cord. The radicular arteries vary in position, number, calibre and division, some of them feed the spinal cord.

In the cervical intervertebral foramen, the nerve roots are usually located at or below the disc plane, protected from it by the uncus.

The lumbar intervertebral foramen has two parts, one superior and rigid, where nerve components pass and usually the radicular or radiculomedullary arteries; the other inferior part is more mobile and exposed to disc changes. It is difficult to categorize the veins, which can be found in both parts.

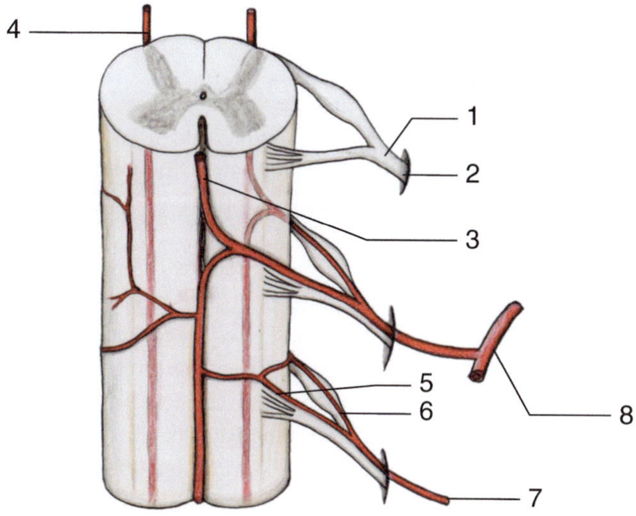

Fig. 7 (Ventral view) (1) spinal nerve, (2) intervertebral foramen and dura mater, (3) ventral spinal artery, (4) dorsal spinal artery, (5) ventral radicular artery, (6) dorsal radicular artery; (7) radicular artery and (8) segmental artery

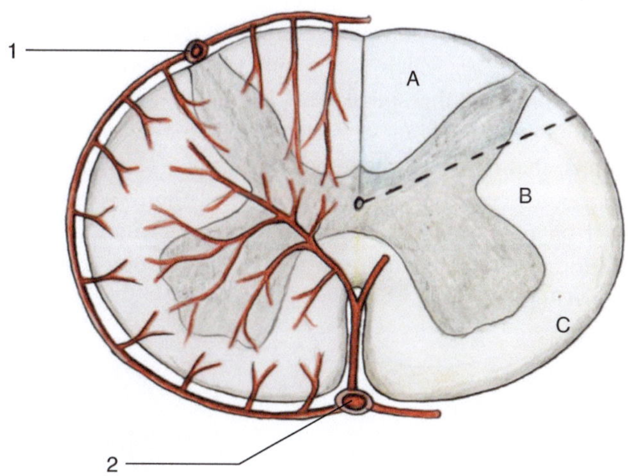

Fig. 8 (1) Dorsal spinal artery and (2) ventral spinal artery

Blood Supply of the Spinal Cord (Figs. 5, 7 and 8)

The Radiculomedullary Arteries

The radiculomedullary arteries supply the spinal cord, the spinal roots, dura and bony wall of the spinal canal. These vessels give off a branch that enters the intervertebral foramen and then divides into a vertebral branch supplying the vertebral body and a radicular branch that pierces the dura and accompanies the spinal nerve root. The radicular branch further divides into ventral and dorsal radicular branches, coursing along the ventral and dorsal nerve roots, respectively.

The longitudinal spinal axes are supplied by segmental vessels at various spinal levels. They are referred to as radiculomedullary arteries in order to distinguish them from radicular arteries that merely supply the nerve roots and do not contribute to the longitudinal spinal axes, and from radiculomeningeal arteries that supply the nerve root as well as the nerve root sleeve and adjacent dura. These arteries are classified depending on their contribution to the spinal cord:

- Radicular arteries only supplying the nerve root and dura.
- Radicular arteries supplying the nerve roots, the dura and the dorsal spinal arteries.
- Radicular arteries following the ventral surface of the spinal cord, bifurcating at the midline into ascending and descending branches, which ultimately form the ventral spinal artery.

There are also intersegmental anastomoses along the ventrolateral aspect of the vertebral body and adjacent to the transverse process. Each segmental artery is connected to the neighbouring segmental artery via these anastomoses. Thus, the anastomotic network around the spine necessitates investigation of the two adjacent vertebral levels above and the two below a tumour to exclude a potential shunt between the segmental arteries.

Of the 62 left and right radicular branches, only a few of these segmental vessels provide a significant contribution to the ventral and dorsal spinal axes. The course of radicular branches at the cervical level is relatively horizontal while their trajectory becomes progressively steeper as one progresses in a caudal direction. The radiculomedullary arteries divide into the ventral and dorsal radiculomedullary arteries which accompany the ventral and dorsal nerve roots. At the spinal cord level, they divide into a prominent descending branch and a smaller ascending branch that both join the longitudinal axis. This results in a prominent cranial loop with the typical "hairpin" appearance on angiography. The cranial loop has a wider angle in anterior radiculomedullary arteries than in the posterior ones (Fig. 9).

- 6–8 ventral radiculomedullary arteries make functional connections to the ventral spinal artery.
- The number of ventral radiculomedullary arteries is extremely variable between individuals and at various spinal cord levels.
- 11–20 dorsal radiculomedullary arteries (also called the radiculopial arteries) supply the dorsal spinal arteries. The junctions between the dorsal radiculomedullary arteries and the dorsal spinal arteries also exhibit a characteristic hairpin configuration, but the dorsal arterial junctions are located off the midline. Dorsal radiculomedullary arteries are more numerous and have a smaller diameter than their ventral counterparts, but their number is variable.

Radiculomedullary arteries are usually asymmetric and reach the cord from either the left or the right side, but generally not from both sides at the same segmental level. In those rare instances in which arteries from both sides join the ventral spinal artery at the same segment, a diamond-shaped pattern may occur. This pattern is most often observed angiographically in children. Similarly, it is either the ventral or the dorsal vessel that reaches the cord but generally not both vessels at the same level.

When ventral and dorsal spinal contributors are provided by the same radicular artery, the variant takes the name of an artery of Lazorthes.

At the Cervical Level

The radiculomedullary arteries arise from the vertebral artery and the ascending and deep cervical arteries. A prominent

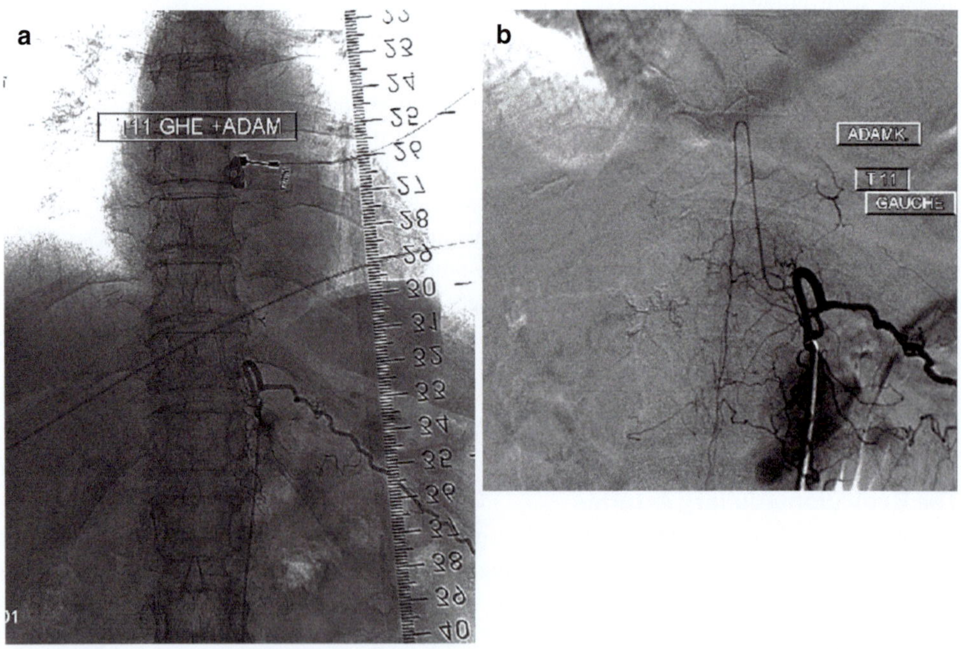

Fig. 9 Radiculomedullary artery and angiography

radiculomedullary artery, called the artery of the cervical enlargement, is present at the level of cervical vertebrae C5 or C6. This artery originates from the vertebral artery. However, as a variant, it can also originate from the branches of the costocervical and thyrocervical trunk. Additional contributions may be present from anastomoses with the external carotid artery via the occipital and ascending pharyngeal arteries.

In the upper cervical region (C1–C3), ventral radiculomedullary arteries are generally rare or absent because blood supply is provided by the two ventral spinal rami from the distal vertebral arteries.

At the Thoracolumbar Level

The radiculomedullary arteries arise from the supreme intercostal, dorsal intercostal and lumbar arteries. The blood supply to the sacrum and the cauda equina is via the lateral sacral and the iliolumbar arteries from the internal iliac artery. The ventral and dorsal spinal arteries are connected through a basket-shaped anastomotic network at the level of the conus medullaris.

From the dorsal intercostal and lumbar arteries, the dorsospinal branch divides at the level of the neural foramen into the radicular artery and the muscular branch. The muscular branch continues dorsally to the neural foramen and supplies the paraspinal musculature. The radicular artery enters the spinal canal and divides into the ventral and dorsal branches, each of which further divides over the surface of the spinal cord into the ascending and descending rami. The radicular artery also provides somatic branches which supply the ventral and dorsal bony walls of the neural canal.

The Great Ventral Radiculomedullary Artery (The Artery of Adamkiewicz)

It is the largest radiculomedullary artery in the thoracolumbar region, and it is the major supplier of blood to the ventral spinal artery at the lower thoracic and upper lumbar levels. This artery characteristically makes a sharp hairpin, turn caudally as it joins the ventral spinal artery. In 75% of individuals, this artery arises at T9–T12 vertebral level most often on the left side. When it arises above the T8 or below L2 level, there is usually a second major radiculomedullary arterial supplying the ventral spinal artery. Half of the patients have a blood supply from two ventral radiculospinal arteries supplying the thoracolumbar region, a little less than half of the patients from a single one, and rarely from three arteries.

Other Variations

Bilateral lower lumbar vessels may arise from a common midline trunk. Another variation, usually seen in the thoracic region, is a common intersegmental trunk in which the ipsilateral segmental arteries serving two adjacent vertebral levels arise from the same trunk.

In a complete intersegmental trunk, each segmental artery provides a dorsospinal branch; however, in an incomplete intersegmental trunk, one of the segmental arteries lacks the dorsospinal branch, which emerges directly from the aorta. Recognition of a dorsospinal branch that emerges directly from the aorta is important because the dorsospinal branch usually provides a radiculomedullary branch to the ventral spinal artery. An intercostal artery providing a radiculomedullary artery may arise from an intercostobronchial trunk together with the bronchial artery. The intercostobronchial trunk is more often on the right side.

The Longitudinal Arterial Axis

The blood supply of the spinal cord can schematically be divided into three longitudinal vascular axes, supplied by segmental vessels at various levels of the spinal cord, which comprise the ventral spinal artery and the two dorsal spinal arteries. At the upper cervical level, an additional paired longitudinal artery called lateral spinal arteries exists.

Ventral Spinal Artery

There are only 6–8 ventral branches of the radicular arteries along the length of the spine. The distribution of these branches enables the distinction of three large arterial areas. The anterior spinal artery is not continuous, for in the midthoracic region there exists a critical narrow zone.

- *The cervicothoracic region* extends from the cervicomedullary junction to the first two or three thoracic segments.
- The vascularization of the superior cervical segments is provided by the ventral artery descending from the intracranial vertebral arteries and rarely going below the 4th cervical segment. This ventral artery results from the junction of two small ventral spinal rami originating from the intracranial portion of each vertebral artery. These rami course ventromedially to form a single descending channel that runs along the ventral sulcus of the spinal cord. There is often an asymmetry in calibre of these two rami and it is not unusual to see the ventral artery as the continuation of a single vertebral artery branch. The newly formed vessel runs in the subpial space of the ventral sulcus, dorsal to the ventral spinal veins, and has a fairly straight course, although deflections towards the junction of the segmental feeding vessels may occur.
- The artery of cervical enlargement that accompanies the C6 nerve root arises from the deep cervical artery.
- The lower segments are supplied by an artery descending from the costocervical trunk. This region has multiple vascular collaterals which originate from the vertebral arteries and from branches of the costocervical or thyrocervical trunks.

The diameter of the ventral spinal artery generally gradually gets narrower down at the upper thoracic level but increases in size immediately below its junction with ventral radiculomedullary arteries.

- *The midthoracic region comprises the vertebral segments from T4 to T8.*

This region has a smaller blood supply and most often, only one radiculomedullary artery supplies the ventral spinal artery in this region, usually arising at the T4 or T5 level. This region is the border zone between the midthoracic and thoracolumbar regions and is particularly vulnerable to ischemia when one of the functional radiculomedullary arteries is occluded.

- *The thoracolumbar region extends from the T8 segment to the conus medullaris.*

A single large vessel usually supplies this region, commonly referred to as the artery of Adamkiewicz. It usually enters from T9 to T12 and is on the left in almost 75% of individuals. In about 10%, the vessel originates at a lower level and accompanies the L1 or L2 nerve roots. In 15% the major artery enters from T5 to T8. In these cases, an additional branch feeds the anterior spinal artery in the region of the conus medullaris.

At the level of the conus, there is a constant anastomosis uniting the ventral spinal and the two dorsal spinal arteries. This "anastomotic loop for the conus medullaris" is constant. Several sacral radicular branches converge on its convexity. Desproges-Gotteron describe a radiculomedullary artery following the L5 root in the L5S1 foramen; in case of compression by herniation, tumour or after foraminal infiltration, we can observe conus medullaris ischemia (Fig. 10) [12].

Dorsal Spinal Arteries

These paired arteries represent the major blood flow located on the dorsal surface of the spinal cord. They run parallel to each other adjacent to the origins of the dorsal nerve roots.

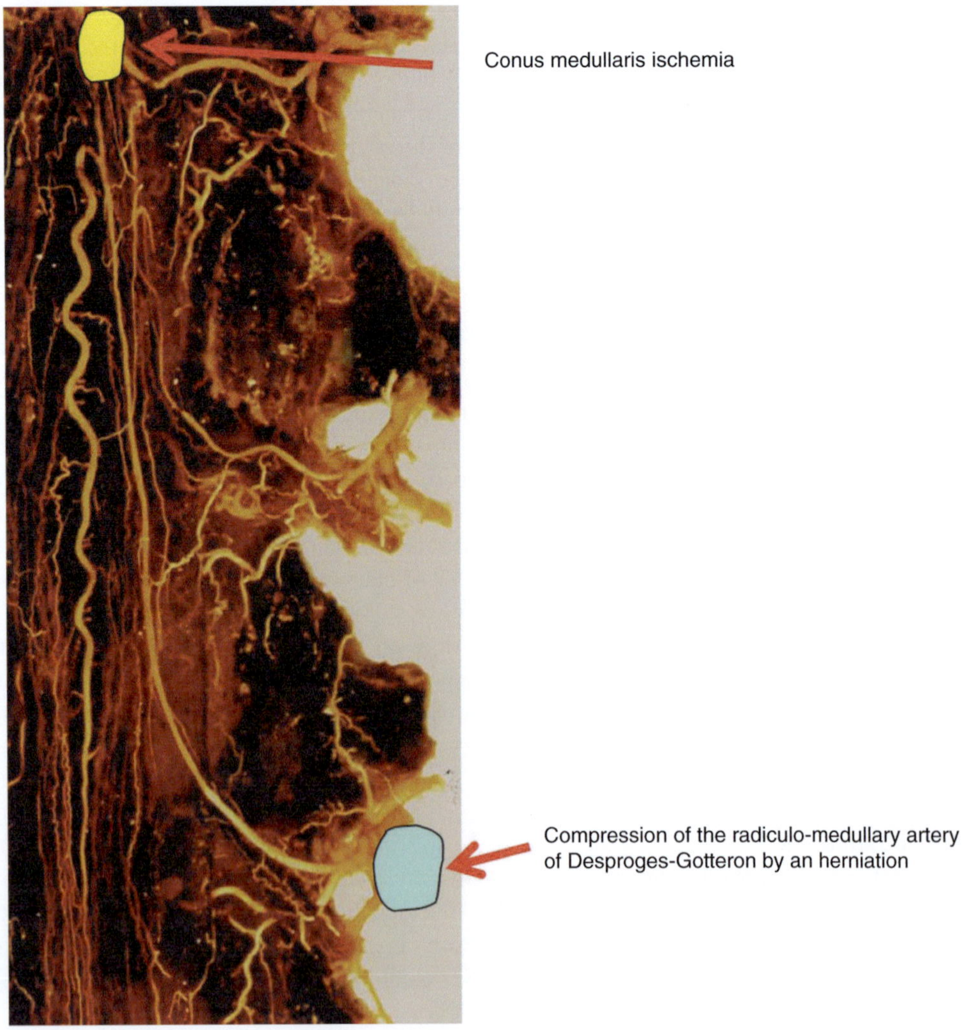

Fig. 10 The radiculomedullary artery of Desproges-Gotteron (Crock)

These two arteries, which are about a third of the size of the ventral spinal artery, generally originate from the inferior or dorsal aspect of the vertebral artery, near but proximal to its point of dural penetration, or alternatively from the posterior inferior cerebellar artery (PICA)

When the dorsal spinal artery originates from the vertebral artery, it takes, with the vertebral artery, a parallel ascending course until they reach the lateral surface of the medulla oblongata. The vertebral artery then passes over the ventral aspect of the pontomedullary junction, while the dorsal spinal artery turns dorsolaterally and, after a sharp curve, courses caudally along the dorsal aspect of the spinal cord. At the apex of the curve, the dorsal spinal artery generally gives off an ascending branch that anastomoses with the PICA at the level of the restiform body.

Ten to twenty feeders contribute to the dorsal spinal artery at various levels throughout the spine. The most cephalad feeding artery originates from the intradural vertebral arteries.

Transverse connections across the dorsal surface of the spinal cord connect the paired dorsal spinal arteries.

In contrast, no significant arterial anastomoses are present over the lateral surface of the spinal cord. Only at the conus medullaris do the dorsal spinal arteries encircle the spinal cord to join the ventral spinal artery.

Lateral Spinal Artery [13]

For a long time, authors have described an artery ventral to the dorsal cervical root and have named it "the lateral spinal artery". But this artery was presented as an anatomical variation.

Lasjaunias et al. have described the so-called lateral spinal artery. It originates lateral to the medulla, from either the PICA or the intradural vertebral artery. It then courses caudally, running parallel to the spinal component of the 11th cranial nerve, dorsal to the dentate ligament, and ventral to the dorsal spinal nerve roots to C4. The collaterals of this artery supply the 11th cranial nerve and the lateral and dorsal surface of the spinal cord via the C1–C4 spinal nerves. The artery terminates at C4 or C5 in the classical dorsolateral arterial axis, dorsal to the dorsal roots of the spinal nerves.

The lateral spinal artery anastomoses rostrally with the PICA branches at the level of the restiform body, with the extradural arteries arising from the vertebral or occipital arteries at each metameric level (particularly C2), and with the contralateral system dorsally.

The normal variations of the lateral spinal artery that have been recorded correspond to a transfer of certain branches of the embryonic lateral spinal artery by a combination of spontaneous regression and persistence of specific arterial channels within the vascular network of the neural tube. The metameric arteries of the region (first, second and third segmental arteries) play an important role in the persistence of either the extradural intersegmental anastomosis for the future vertebral artery (the vertebral artery represents the persistence of six to seven consecutive intersegmental arteries) or the intradural intersegmental anastomosis (future lateral spinal artery).

Intrinsic Spinal Cord Vascularization

The fixed nature of the intramedullary arterial distribution contrasts with the variability of the afferent arterial supplies.

Two groups of arteries arise from the ventral spinal artery and dorsal spinal arteries and directly supply the neural tissue: the central sulcal arteries or sulcocommissural arteries, and peripheral arteries.

Central Arteries

At each segmental level, the ventral spinal artery gives off a central branch which reaches, via the ventral median fissure, the ventral white commissure of the spinal cord, and then turns laterally to one side to enter the grey matter of the ventral horn. These arteries constitute the so-called centrifugal system (of Adamkiewicz). Arteries going to the right generally alternate irregularly with arteries going to the left. Sometimes, a common stem giving rise to a left and a right central artery can be observed, and this most frequently occurs at the lumbar and sacral levels.

On reaching the grey matter, central arteries divide into an ascending and a descending branch that extend upwards and downwards so that there is a considerable overlap at the capillary level.

Central arteries are generally particularly large, numerous and densely packed in the regions of the cervical and lumbar enlargement of the cord.

Peripheral Arteries

The ventral spinal artery and the dorsal spinal arteries each give off small lateral pial branches that run along the circumference of the cord and constitute the "centripetal system" (of Adamkiewicz).

They give off perpendicular branches that penetrate the spinal cord at right angles and supply the outer rim of the spinal cord.

- In the cervicothoracic area, the superficial anastomotic network is rich and the central arteries are large and numerous.
- In the midthoracic area, the superficial anastomotic network is poor. The central arteries are small in diameter, few in number and spaced out.
- In the thoracolumbar area, the superficial anastomotic network is rich. The central arteries are large in diameter and numerous.

The lack of collaterals between the ventral spinal artery and dorsal spinal arteries functionally separates these vascular territories. The perimedullary anastomotic system appears insufficient while intramedullary anastomoses are without functional value. The grey–white junction represents a potential vulnerable zone.

The territories of the central arteries and peripheral arteries overlap in an area consisting of the inner portion of the white matter and the outer edge of the grey matter (except for the dorsal halves of the post horns, which are supplied by peripheral arteries). The widest overlap exists in the dorsal and lateral columns.

Anastomotic Arterial Pathways [14]

The "substitution pathways" of the arterial vascularization of the central axis of the nervous system are laid out on several anastomotic levels.

Anastomoses of the Afferent Arterial Supply

Superior or Cervicothoracic Area

There are not only the two or three arteries issuing from the vertebral arteries and that coming from the costocervical trunk but also the occipital, deep cervical and ascending cervical arteries.

The vertebral artery anastomoses with collaterals of the ascending and deep cervical arteries and collaterals of the occipital artery. These anastomoses constitute a "suboccipital arterial crossroads", and they have a potential value in case of deficiency of one vertebral artery.

Midthoracic Area

The arterial supply comes from one of the midthoracic spinal branches.

- The dorsal spinal branches are united by their different collaterals.
- The artery destined for the vertebral body anastomoses, within the vertebra itself, with its supra and subjacent homologues and also the contralaterals.
- The branch that penetrates the spinal canal through the intervertebral foramen anastomoses within the dorsal longitudinal ligament and vertebral body with the homologous supra and subjacent branches, but particularly with the contralateral homologous branch.
- The terminal branches of the dorsal arteries which spread out within the adjacent muscular mass also anastomose widely with the supra and subjacent homologues.

Throughout the length of the vertebral column, there is a longitudinal substitution pathway situated within these muscular masses from the nuchal to the lumbar region.

Thus, substitution pathways exist between the arterial blood supplies, not only in the midthoracic area of the spinal cord but throughout the length of the vertebral column. It is impossible to estimate their functional value.

Thoracolumbar Area

The artery of the lumbar enlargement may be compensated for by other arteries, probably non-functional in the physiological state.

Outside the vertebral column, there are arterial anastomoses analogous to those found in the cervical and thoracic spinal cord. From occiput to sacrum, horizontal anastomoses unite the vertebral branches of cervical, thoracic and lumbar arteries and vertical anastomoses unite the dorsal muscular branches of these arteries.

Inside the spine, some sacral spinal branches that lead to the communicating branch of the conus medullaris certainly have even greater functional value. There are one or two arteries for each root of the cauda equina. The branches accompanying these roots enter the ventral and dorsal spinal arteries, respectively.

Peri-Axial Anastomoses

The periaxial anastomoses unite the ventral and dorsal spinal arteries. There is no continuous perimedullary longitudinal substitution pathway. The three areas are functionally isolated because there is a poor vascularization in the midthoracic area where anastomoses are more or less present.

Intra-Axial Anastomoses

The central arteries sometimes anastomose with their neighbours by vertical branches situated within the grey matter. Only a few very fine and non-functional anastomoses unite the terminal branches of the central arteries and those of the radial arteries (Fig. 11).

Venous Drainage of the Spinal Structures (Figs. 12 and 13)

Intra-Vertebral Venous Network

Medullary Venous Network

It is made of central veins which present a radiating position and run off, via horizontal perimedullary veins, into two principal veins, the ventral spinal vein and the dorsal spinal vein, whose gauge is very variable.

– *the ventral spinal veins* lead into the ventral median spinal sulcus, accompanying the ventral spinal artery, and drain the anterior quarter of the spinal cord. This ventral drainage consists of three parallel, longitudinal veins, and appears to be continuous from the cephalic to the caudal extremity of the spinal cord.

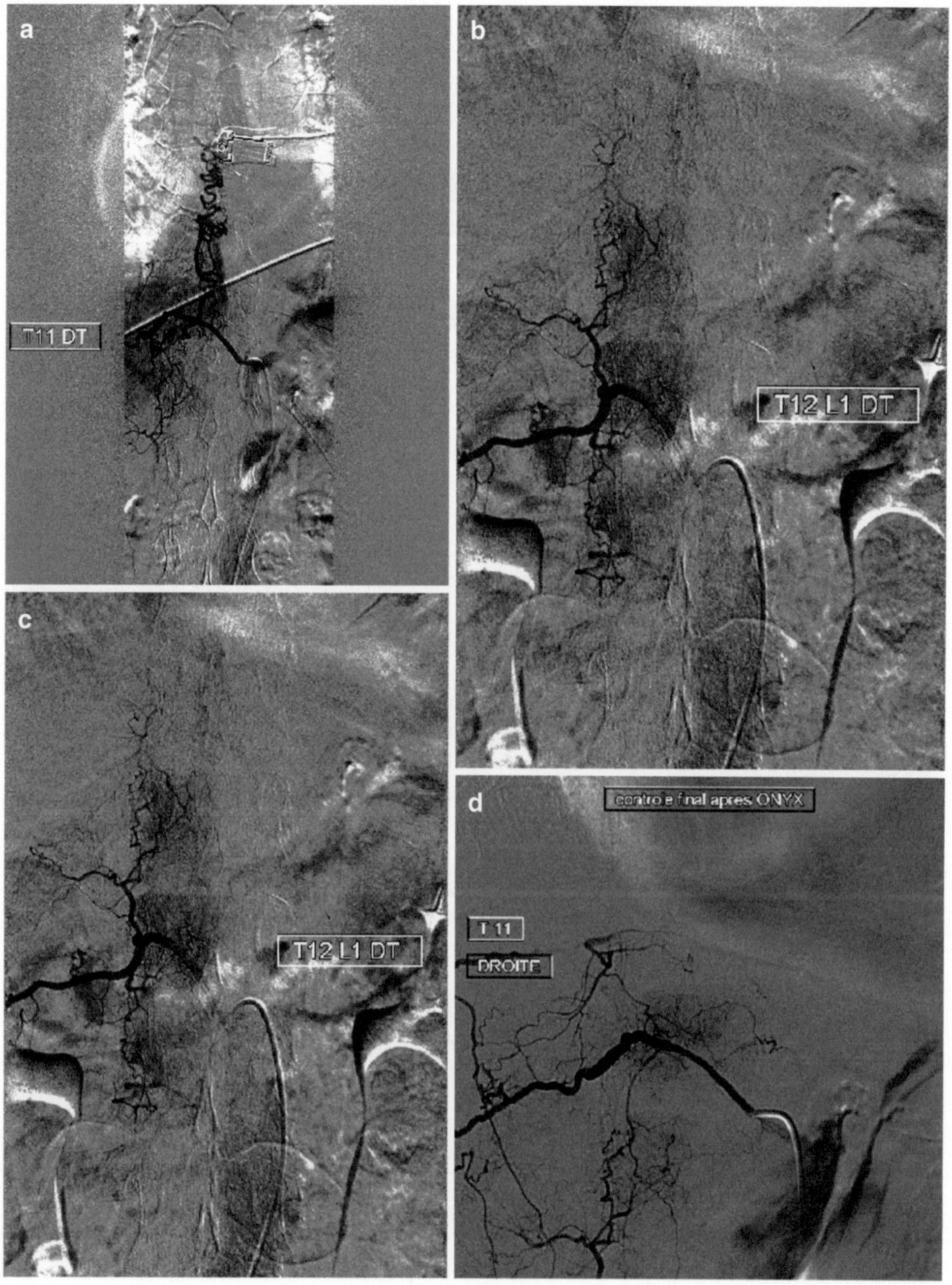

Fig. 11 (**a–c**) Dural fistula at T11 on the right, at the level of the intervertebral foramen, with a very fast filling of the perimedullary veins. It is observed that Adamkiewicz's artery is on the opposite side, at t11 on the left. At the injection at l1, an anastomosis between the foraminal artery in t12 and the fistula is observed, the anastomosis is indirect and there is only one afferent to the fistula. (**d**) Final radiograph after embolization of the fistula (with onyx)

– *the dorsal spinal veins*, with a larger gauge, are often bulkier at the level of the cervical or lumbar spinal enlargement. These veins can be duplicated in the cervical area. They drain the posterior three-quarters of the spinal cord. The dorsal drainage consists of three veins: two travel with the dorsolateral spinal arteries and one courses in the midline in the dorsal median sulcus.

These veins anastomose forming a superficial venous network on the surface of the spinal cord. These superficial veins give rise to the dorsal and ventral radicular veins which accompany the nerve roots as they exit the intervertebral foramen.

Intradural Drainage

There are a varying number of ventral and dorsal radiculomedullary veins. Usually, there are 2 or 3 radiculomedullary veins in the cervical area, one at the upper dorsal level, one at the middle dorsal level, 2 at the level of the conus medullaris and one in the lumbar area (filum vein). These veins run into the intraspinal plexuses.

The ventral and dorsal contributions of the internal venous system form a confluence at the intervertebral foramen. Two veins course along the upper and lower pedicle, completely surrounding the nerve root.

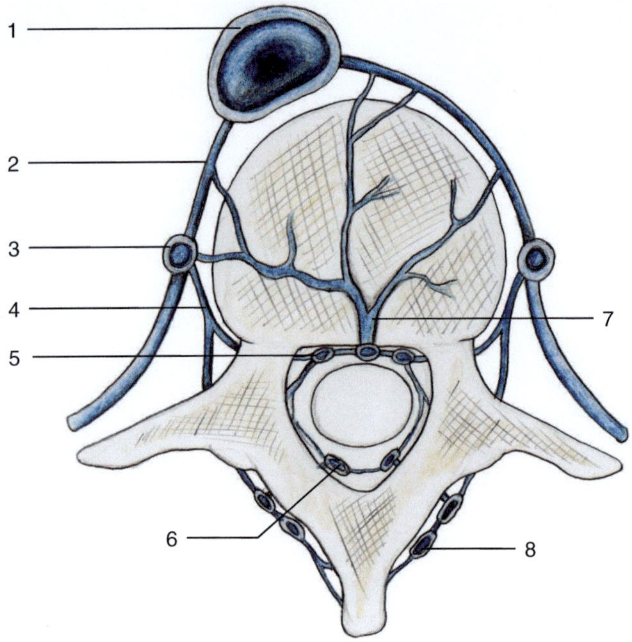

Fig. 12 (1) Inferior vena cava, (2) lumbar vein, (3) ascending lumbar vein, (4) intervertebral vein, (5) transverse retrocorporeal venous plexus (ventral internal venous plexus or ventral epidural venous plexus), (6) epidural dorsal venous plexus, (7) basivertebral vein and (8) external dorsal venous plexus

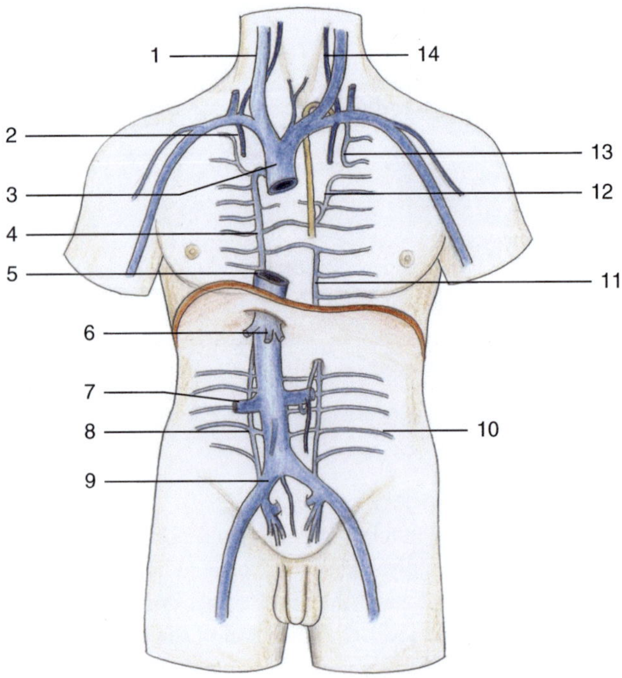

Fig. 13 (1) Right internal jugular vein, (2) right internal thoracic vein, (3) superior vena cava, (4) azygous vein, (5) inferior vena cava, (6) hepatic veins, (7) right renal vein, (8) right ascending lumbar vein, (9) right common iliac vein, (10) lumbar vein, (11) hemi-azygous vein, (12) accessory hemi-azygous vein, (13) superior left intercostal vein and (14) vertebral vein

Extradural Plexuses [15, 16]

This internal venous system forms a "ladder-like" network along the dorsal aspect of the vertebral bodies, which tends to be particularly prominent on the upper cervical and lumbar regions. At sites where the vessels cross-connect, they receive a large feed from the basivertebral sinus. Very little venous drainage occurs around the disk space. The ventral half of the epidural venous plexuses is larger and more regular than the dorsal half.

An extensive network of anastomosing, interconnecting and extradural venous channels extend from the base of the skull to the sacrum. However, the organization or the ventral and dorsal vertebral venous plexuses is different according to the level of the spine.

- *The ventral internal vertebral venous plexus* is found throughout the length of the spine. It consists of two longitudinal veins each located in the lateral part of the spinal canal and joined at the midline by retrocorporeal anastomotic veins. These veins are horizontal and located halfway up behind the vertebral bodies, which they drain through a basivertebral vein, but only from the third cervical vertebra.
  - At the cervical level, the ventral plexus cannot be seen in the medial part of the canal, being located more laterally behind the dorsal longitudinal ligament. Behind C2, the retrocorporeal vein is particularly enlarged and is butterfly-shaped.
  - At the thoracic level, the longitudinal veins are more voluminous and extend laterally and medially. Usually, they are juxtaposed. They remain behind the dorsal longitudinal ligament, but the retrocorporeal veins which join them become more ventral and are located in front of the dorsal longitudinal ligament, just behind the vertebral body.
  - At the lumbar and sacral levels, the ventral plexus is large. The ventral longitudinal veins consist of several sinusoidal venous channels forming wide lakes of venous plexus. So, the dorsal plexus does not display two veins and becomes plexiform.
- *The dorsal internal vertebral venous plexus* is related to the ventral one by anastomotic veins. It cannot be seen at the cervical level. It appears at the thoracic level as narrow channels located in the angle between the laminae and pedicles. At T1 level, an oblique anastomosis joins the dorsal aspect of the ventral plexus, goes backwards and downwards to the dorsal plexus.

A horizontal anastomosis is found between the ventral and dorsal plexuses at each segmental level. Another narrower anastomosis located in front of the superior third of the lamina joined both dorsal plexuses.

These ventral and dorsal internal venous plexuses are joined to the external vertebral venous plexuses by two veins through the intervertebral foramina.

- At the cervical level, there is a wide venous flow made of a voluminous superior vein and a smaller inferior one. The spinal roots are masked by the veins which have a horizontal course to the vertebral vein.
- At the thoracic level, there are two veins, both cross the spinal roots with an upward course.
- At the lumbar level, the intervertebral foramen is wide and the two veins are separate. The superior vein is located in the superior part of the foramen, while the inferior vein is located in its inferior part. Only the inferior vein crosses the spinal nerve root, with an oblique downward course.

Extra-Vertebral Venous Network

Vertebral veins and perivertebral venous plexuses communicate with the internal system through the ligamentum flavum at each spinal level. The dorsal vertebral arches are drained by a central vein of the spinous process and veins of the lamina. These vessels drain towards the pedicles and also anastomose with the internal and external plexuses.

Vertebral Veins

The cervical vertebral vein accompanies the vertebral artery in the transverse process foramen in the upper cervical vertebrae, emerges from the transverse process foramen of the sixth cervical vertebrae, joins the deep cervical vein, descends laterally, then drains into the upper portion of the brachiocephalic vein. Just below the sixth vertebra, the vertebral vein is adjacent to the vertebral artery located ventrolaterally to the musculus longissimus coli.

The bilateral vertebral veins are united with the epidural venous plexus via the intervertebral veins, in which the blood flow may be reversed.

Perivertebral Venous Plexuses

Perivertebral venous plexuses in and around the lower cervical and upper thoracic vertebrae communicate with each other. In addition, anastomoses exist between the vertebral venous system and the azygos and oesophageal veins.

Ventral External Plexuses (Longitudinal Prevertebral Vein)

Two longitudinal prevertebral veins are located medially to the musculus longissimus coli on the anterior surface of the cervical vertebrae and anastomose with the vertebral veins on each side.

There are stepladder-like anastomoses between the bilateral vertebral veins at the ventral aspect of the cervical vertebrae.

Dorsal External Plexuses (Deep Cervical and Dorsal Intercostal Veins)

The deep cervical vein receives tributaries from the deep muscles at the back of the neck, runs forward above the neck of the first rib, and terminates in the lower part of the vertebral vein.

The bilateral deep cervical veins are united with each other via the plexuses around the spinous process of the cervical vertebrae and also anastomose with the dorsal intercostal vein.

Those veins form a venous plexus on the dorsal surface of the laminae and the spinous and transverse processes of vertebrae.

In Fig. 14 we can note the difference between anterior and posterior (more developed) cervical external plexuses.

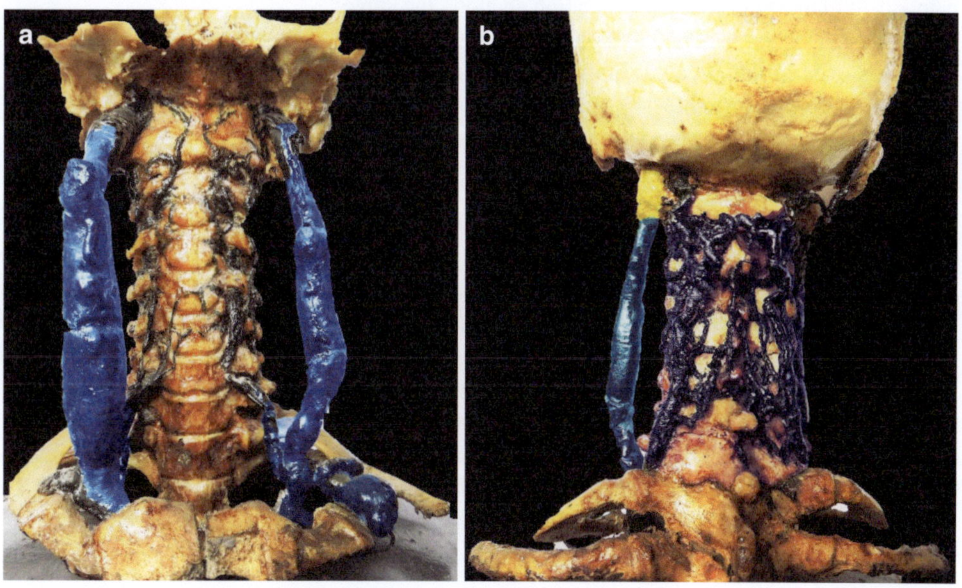

Fig. 14 Difference between anterior (**a**) and posterior (**b**) (more developed) cervical external plexuses. (Courtesy of the Museum of Anatomy, University of Montpellier–Pr. F. Bonnel)

Basivertebral Veins

Basivertebral veins are tortuous vascular channels in the vertebral bodies and unite with the longitudinal prevertebral veins and the ventral epidural venous plexus.

Communications Between the Vertebral Venous System and Systemic Veins

Longitudinal Prevertebral Vein and Azygos System

- In the upper thorax, the epidural venous plexuses are anastomosed with the superior intercostal veins via the intervertebral veins. The blood of the neck and upper extremities can run downward in the epidural venous plexuses, reach the superior intercostal vein and then drain into the azygos vein.
- The lumbar intercostal veins consist of four or five segmental pairs that accompany, in part, the corresponding arteries. Their dorsal branches drain the structures of the back and have free connections with the vertebral plexuses. The lumbar veins may empty separately into the inferior vena cava or common iliac, but generally they are united on each side by a vertical connecting vein, the ascending lumbar vein. Each ascending lumbar vein enters the thorax behind the psoas major and medial arcuate ligament on the corresponding side. The right vein joins the right subcostal veins and forms the azygos vein. The left joins the left subcostal vein and forms the hemiazygos vein. The left upper lumbar veins and ascending lumbar vein are usually connected with the left renal vein.

The vertebral venous system is a valveless plexiform network with a longitudinal pattern. This venous system enables communication of systemic veins and serves an important role as collateral vessels, especially in patients with venous stenosis or obstruction. This intra-canalar longitudinal pattern is involved in the metastatic dissemination all along the spine; it is why the isolated vertebral metastasis is rare (Fig. 15).

Valves exist in the radicular branches, and that is rare in the central nervous system.

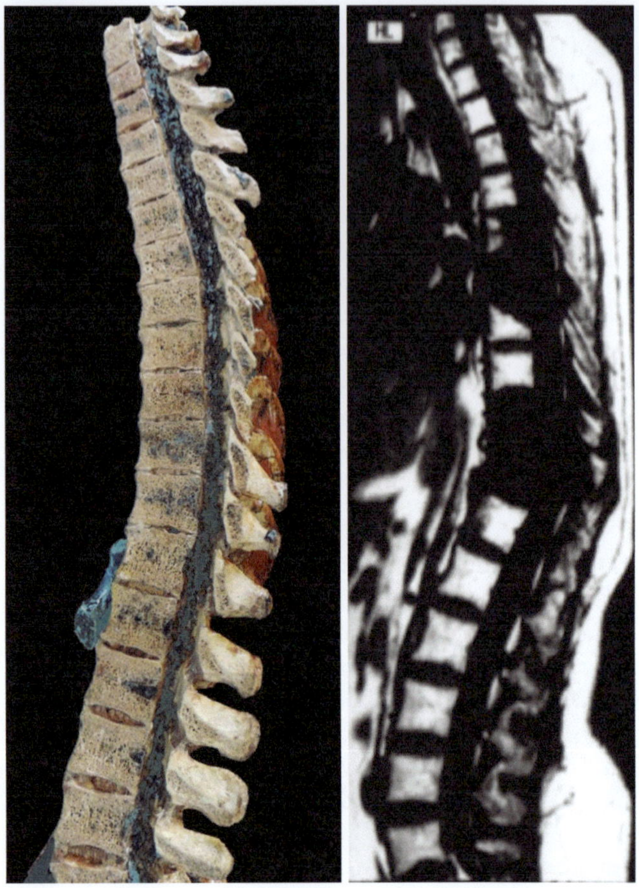

Fig. 15 The intra-canalar longitudinal pattern is involved in the metastatic dissemination all along the spine; it is why the isolated vertebral metastasis is rare. (Courtesy of the Museum of Anatomy, University of Montpellier–Pr. F. Bonnel)

Inferior Vena Cava

The junction of the external and internal iliac veins forms the right and left common iliac veins, respectively. Because of the relative positions of the inferior vena cava and the aorta, the left common iliac vein lies directly below the bifurcation of the aorta.

The inferior vena cava is a large, valveless, venous trunk, and it is formed by the junction of the two common iliac veins, slightly below and to the right of the bifurcation of the aorta, and receives the blood from the lower limbs and much of the blood from the back and from the walls and contents of the abdomen and pelvis. The right renal artery crosses behind the vena cava.

Focus on the Filum Terminale [12]

The distribution of the vascularization of the filum terminale appears constant.

A single artery, the artery of the filum, arises from the termination of the ventral spinal axis, either by trifurcation or from the proximal part of one of the two branches of the anastomotic ansa of the conus medullaris. The artery travels in front of the filum, with rapidly diminishing calibre; rarely, it can be followed into the sacral canal. The artery of the filum is of a calibre proportional to that of the filum and appears to be a nutrient vessel.

The vein of the filum travels in front of that structure, behind the artery; its calibre is uniform, unrelated to that of the filum, it traverses the dura below and is continuous with the ventral spinal vein above. No vessels were found on the dorsal aspect of the filum. The dorsal spinal vein also shares in the drainage.

The vein of the filum is more than a simple vein draining an agenesic neural structure. It represents a true venous axis capable of functioning in two directions: descending towards the sacral venous plexuses and the hypogastric vein, and ascending towards the medullary veins as in the case of sacral dural fistulae or arteriovenous shunts of the filum terminale. In the latter case, the ascending drainage is towards the caval-azygos system and also towards a possible intraspinal venous drainage.

References

1. Ozkan E, Gupta S. Embolization of spinal tumors: vascular anatomy, indications and technique. Tech Vasc Interv Radiol. 2011;14(3):129–40.
2. Pait TG, Elias AJR, Tribell R. Thoracic, lumbar, and sacral spine anatomy for endoscopic surgery. Neurosurgery. 2002;51(suppl. 2):52–67.
3. Siclari F, Burger IM, Fasel JHD, Gailloud P. Developmental anatomy of the distal vertebral artery in relationship to variants of the posterior and lateral spinal arterial systems. Am J Neuroradiol. 2007;28:1185–90.
4. Zawilinski J, Litwin JA, Nowogrodzka-Zagorska M, Gorczyca J, Miodonski AJ. Vascular system of the human spinal cord in the prenatal period: a dye injection and corrosion casting study. Ann Anat. 2001;183:331–40.
5. Chiras J, Morvan G, Merland JJ, Bories J. Blood supply to the thoracic and lumbar spine. Anat Clin. 1982;4:23–31.
6. Demondion X, Lefebvre G, Fisch O, Vandenbussche L, Cepparo J, Balbi V. Radiographic anatomy of the intervertebral cervical and lumbar foramina (vessels and variants). Diagn Interv Imaging. 2012;93:690–7.
7. Tribus CB, Belanger T. The vascular anatomy anterior to the L5S1 disk space. Spine. 2001;26:1205–8.
8. Alleyne CH, Cawley CM, Shengelaia GG, Barrow DL. Microsurgical anatomy of the artery of Adamkiewicz and its segmental artery. J Neurosurg. 1998;89:791–5.
9. Charles YP, Barbe B, Beaujeux R, Boujan F, Steib JP. Relevance of the anatomical location of the Adamkiewicz artery in spine surgery. Surg Radiol Anat. 2011;33:3–9.
10. Groen RJM, Ponssen H. Vascular anatomy of the spinal epidural space. Clin Anat. 1991;4:413–20.
11. Wells-Roth D, Zonenshayn M. Vascular anatomy of the spine. Oper Tech Neurosurg. 2003;6(3):116–21.
12. Djindjian M, Ribeiro A, Ortega E, Gaston A, Poirier J. The normal vascularization of the intradural filum terminale in man. Surg Radiol Anat. 1988;10:201–9.
13. Lasjaunias P, Vallee B, Person H, ter Brugge K, Chiu M. The lateral spinal artery of the upper cervical spinal cord. Anatomy, normal variations and angiographic aspects. J Neurosurg. 1985;63:235–41.
14. Lazorthes G, Gouaze A, Zadeh JO, Santini JJ, Lazorthes Y, Burdin P. Arterial vascularization of the spinal cord. Recent studies of the anastomotic substitution pathways. J Neurosurg. 1971;35:253–62.
15. Chaynes P, Verdie JC, Moscovici J, Zadeh J, Vaysse P, Becue J. Microsurgical anatomy of the internal vertebral venous plexuses. Surg Radiol Anat. 1998;20:47–51.
16. Ibukuro K, Fukuda H, Mori K, Inoue Y. Topographic anatomy of the vertebral venous system in the thoracic inlet. Am J Roentgenol. 2001;176:1059–65.

Part IV

Functional Anatomy

Systemic Approach to the Functioning of the Spine

J. Sénégas

A system is a set of elements in dynamic interaction, organized according to a purpose.
Joel de Rosnay [1].

Introduction

Within the constraints of bipedalism, the result of the spinal functional program may appear, at first glance, to be simple in view of the complexity of the structure that evolution has selected to accomplish it.

It consists, on the one hand, of maintaining postures, with or without loads (states of static equilibrium) and, on the other hand, in performing flexural/straightening and/or rotational movements, with or without loads, according to an optimal trajectory (*states of dynamic equilibrium*).

The control of these states of equilibrium in time and space is an acceptable definition of the concept of vertebral stability, and there are many formulations.

The vertebral structure includes vertebrae, discs, fibrous elements all composed of highly differentiated connective tissues, and muscles. It is also worth mentioning a host of sensory receptors (measurement of acceleration, force, displacements, etc.).

Functionally, the vertebral system presents a complex multi-scale organization that allows to spread over time several responses adapted to the problems of balance of the vertebral column. We can thus distinguish three different control modules:

- a tissue module that immediately responds to the constraints in compression, tension or torsion thanks to the mechanical properties of its connective and muscular constituents (elasticity, rigidity, and contractility) without any latency time.
- a cellular module which, by mechanobiological effect, adapts in a delayed manner to the same constraints by synthesizing new protein constituents (various proteoglycans and collagens) which guarantee the homeostasis of the extracellular matrix. We are talking about adaptive remodeling.
- the third functional control module of the column is a neural module that is both medullary and cerebral.

The motricity (motor function) of the vertebral structure is totally dependent on the spinal and cerebral nervous control centers where intangible instructions are developed for turning, until the action stops, in feedback loops where they undergo incessant adjustments (positive or negative gains) to match the results obtained (outputs) to the task required to control spinal stability. Any state of static or dynamic equilibrium is ultimately dependent on these feedbacks.

The first constituents (the structural elements) are material, and the second (the instructions and the feedbacks) are virtual.

The constitutive elements of any dynamic system are, therefore, interdependent and interact in a circular process of causality [2–7].

The understanding of the nature and functioning of any complex entity, especially in the living, necessarily implies a double cognitive approach:

- one is analytic that can identify its components and their connections, then evaluate their properties.
- the other is synthetic, focused on the dynamic effects of their interactions. This is the systematic approach to the problem. Both methods are completely complementary.

This holistic method of approaching the complexity of the living resonates with any doctor. Medical diagnosis requires, firstly, a detailed and comprehensive assessment of structural and functional unit failures (symptomatology), then a second approach, this time synthetic, which consists of grouping the pathological data in a proper nosological setting and then establish a prognosis as relevant as possible.

J. Sénégas (✉)
Spinal Unit, University Hospital, Bordeaux, France

J. M. Vital, D. T. Cawley (eds.), *Spinal Anatomy*, https://doi.org/10.1007/978-3-030-20925-4_29

The purpose of this work is to enlighten the reader to:

1. complete, for the structural analysis of "mechanical" vertebral pathology, the imaging data, as efficient as it is, by those coming from functional exploration techniques, which are already available, which should be done among the routine preoperative investigations (quantitative functional assessments, kinematic analyzes, numerical simulations);
2. adopt methods of analysis of automation engineers, which have already become essential to progress in the understanding and management of complex pathologies in general. While the collaboration of the mechanics and the spinologist works perfectly, it is critical to develop it with the automation engineers. The analysis of the vertebral system according to the laws of systems engineering should cause an important strategic inflection in the field of spinal pathology.

Organization of a System

(Functional diagram, state variables, complexity, hypercomplexity, …)

The functional diagram of a system is a simplified graphic representation called a functional diagram, describing the hardware components and virtual links that convey information. It can be used in two ways: (1) for a qualitative analysis and (2) for a quantitative analysis if we reliably know the laws of each component and if the tools to do so exist [2, 3].

This is usually the case for common industrial servo systems whose components have well-defined properties and perfectly defined functional parameters: actuators (motors, cylinders), transformation and adaptation devices (drives, reducers), sensors and correctors (control elements for modulating the behavior of the server system). In these cases, the operating state of the system can, in principle, be known at any time thanks to the mathematical formulation of the functional parameters of each component and links (state variables). This is the basic functional scheme of automobiles, planes as well as an industrial chocolate production line [2–7].

In these cases, the functional diagram provides an overall qualitative and quantitative representation of the system concerned.

We speak of linear systems when the effects are proportional to the causes. Basic knowledge of matrix theory and linear algebra is sufficient to understand and quantify them.

Nonlinear systems are more difficult to study. In these systems, the effects are not proportional to the causes. They cannot be described by linear differential equations with constant coefficients. Most physical systems are nonlinear.

Over the last decade, there have been important conceptual changes in the formulation of complex systems. New mathematical techniques have introduced some uncertainty in the modeling of controls with, as a consequence, a multivariable feedback. The integration of this type of uncertainty is seen as a progress, decisive in the treatment of complex systems because the group processing of certain multivariable parameters makes it possible to increase the robustness of these systems (robust control theory) [8, 9].

Living systems are immeasurably more complex than industrial systems. We can speak of hypercomplexity. These are open systems in constant interaction with the environment. They are maintained through variable flows of energy and information. Nonlinearity and variability of controls are the rule. The order does not exist a priori, it is created and maintained by the action (dynamic systems).

Living systems also have five characteristics of their own:

1. The storage of energy material is limited so that their performance periodically collapses (fatigue) until the recovery of reserves after a shorter or longer period (recovery). In living beings, endurance thus becomes an essential parameter for maintaining performance [10, 11].
2. The controls are not only electric but also biochemical.
3. A living organism manufactures, maintains, transforms, and repairs (up to a certain point) its own components through a permanent process of genetically programmed production.
4. Their performances vary spontaneously throughout their life (growth/learning, fullness, aging).
5. Living systems can replicate.

Finally, the only invariant of living systems lies in their organization which ensures the durability of the action parameters (homeostasis) [8, 9].

Qualitative Analysis of the Vertebral System (Fig. 1)

Like all systems, the vertebral system is defined by a boundary that separates all its constituents from the environment. In the case of the vertebral system, it is the body skin that is the frame of the system.

The Entries

Solicitations from the outside environment are not information but physical interactions. They can, without transformation, directly reach the vertebral structure and trigger a passive instant mechanical response.

Another mode of entry follows the path of sensory transducers. It is these signals that trigger the activation of the

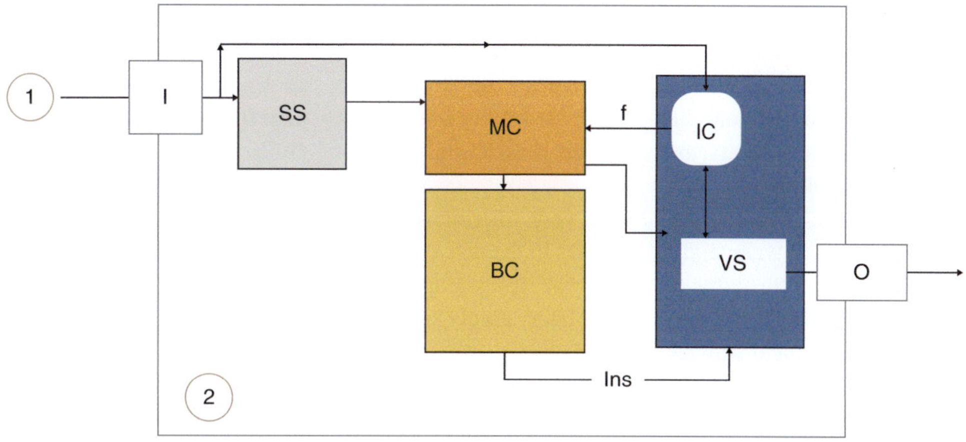

Fig. 1 Simplified diagram of the vertebral system: 1. Environment, 2. Inside the body. *I* inputs, *O* outputs, *SS* sensory sensors, *IC* intrinsic control, *MC* medullary control, *BC* brain control, *Ins* instruction, VS vertebral structure, *f* feedback

system (the task at hand). To be integrated under the form of information that can be used by a living organism, these exogenous signals must be encoded [12] by transducers (sensors).

The task to be accomplished can also be generated within the system itself (endogenous signals). The order then comes directly from a nerve center. In these cases, no conversion is necessary.

Transducers (Receivers or Sensors)

These devices convert a physical or chemical interaction signal into a nerve message (creating a membrane potential variation) [12, 13]. It is an active process that consumes energy.

- Sensorial receptors (visual, vestibular, auditory, olfactory, or cutaneous) encode information from the environment for the brain.
- Sensitive receptors encode endogenous information. They feed the interactions and continuously monitor a host of data including position, velocity, and even some parameters of tissue metabolism. They abound in the vertebral structure (mechanoreceptors, proprioceptors, chemoreceptors). There are intramuscular sensors (neuromuscular spindles) and sensors located in periarticular fibrous structures (free ending fibers, Ruffini and Pacinian corpuscles, Golgi tendinous bodies, etc.) [14]. At least seven types of myelinated afferent nerve fibers (I, II, alpha, gamma, Ib, III, etc.) emerge.

At this stage, the information is already desynchronized because each type of nerve fiber has a different conduction velocity depending on the thickness of the myelin sheath.

Mechanoreceptors combine to construct the kinesthetic sense.

It is of course necessary to add to this flow of circulating information which come from the sensory sensors of the pain.

All transducers and afferent fibers deteriorate progressively with age, but sometimes also because of neurological pathologies (degenerative or specific peripheral neuropathies). These abnormalities often escape the medical examination. They result in a loss of information or a delay in the transmission of signals which, by themselves, can compromise the equilibrium states of the spinal system by altering its performance [12, 13].

Controls

There are three types of controls: tissue-based, cellular, and neurologic.

- Intrinsic or tissue-based, organizes the expression of the mechanical and biological properties of the vertebral connective tissues.
- Neurological, they receive the relative encoded information, integrate them, and develop an action program (motor program or instruction). For the vertebral column, there are two different but interconnected neurological controls: spinal cord control and cerebral control.
- Cellular.

Tissue-Based Control

The mechanical properties of the connective tissue: bone, fibrous, or muscle of the vertebral column allow an instantaneous to mechanical stresses.

The components of the vertebral structure (discs, vertebrae, ligaments, and muscles) resist compressive or stretching forces by deforming. It is the collagen fibers, the elastic fibers, and the extracellular proteins that are responsible for this. Passive stretching of the tendons is used to store potential energy and then return it as kinetic energy, provided that the reaction is almost immediate to avoid dissipation in the form of heat. This phenomenon, called energy restitution storage, leads to a significant metabolic energy saving, for example in humans (up to 50% according to Linsted,

2002). It also intervenes at the spinal column level where it increases endurance in dynamic stabilization efforts. Thanks to their mechanical properties, the connective structures of the column thus participate totally in the control of vertebral stability, as well as the neurological activation of the musculature.

Cyclic mechanical stress plays a very important role in the movement of water and metabolites in the disc and articular cartilages. The hydration of the disc, for example, is by percolation through the epiphyseal plates largely under the effect of mechanical stresses.

Cellular Control

The mechanical constraints, moreover, regulate a good part of the cellular and extracellular metabolism of the components of the vertebral system through a network of macromolecules, a group of surface proteins, the integrins connected to the collagen fibers. They function as real mechanoreceptors. Prolonged mechanical stresses trigger an adaptive remodeling process of bone, fibrous, or muscular components. Genetically programmed, it involves an impressive number of intra and extracellular proteins (hormones), growth factors, enzymatic cascade, cell activity regulating factors such as MAP kinase (mitogen-activated protein), and also mobilizes stromal cells (i.e., strain). This mechanobiological control makes it possible to temporarily adapt the resistance of vertebral materials to the mechanical requirements of vertebral stability.

Neurological Checks

Spinal cord control is an automatic neurological control (reflex). The afferent signals from the sensors converge to the motor neurons located in the anterior horns of the cord at variable speeds depending on the number of synaptic relays (mono or polysynaptic reflexes). The operating time varies on average from 0.5 ms to 20 ms. It gets longer with age.

Pain signals are normally scrambled to a certain threshold by proprioceptive signals at the level of the posterior horns (gate control), but any peripheral demyelination may disturb this protective mechanism by improving nerve conduction gaps.

Cerebral control is more complex and slower (100–1000 ms).

The brain response is developed through neural modules often spatially and temporally remote.

Very schematically, the so-called voluntary cortical response begins with a process of identifying the task. A mental image of the body and its relationship to the environment is progressively elaborated by diffusion of the signals from the perception areas to the associative areas of integration. For vision, for example, information progresses from the primary visual cortex to the posterior parietal area, and then to the prefrontal cortex.

The next step is the motor programming. It obligatorily refers to the memory of sensorial and sensitive information relating to the experience of previous movements of the column (procedural memory). The memory then publishes tangible recipes of governance.

This predictive programming integrates the optimal tension of each muscle involved in the desired balance, corresponding to a specific posture or displacement. It must also determine the type (slow I, fast IIa or IIb) and number of muscle fibers to recruit in each muscle, and decide on the need for coactivation of other peri-vertebral muscle groups or even located at a distance from the column. If it is a question of maintaining a posture, the muscular contractions will be isometric, but most often it is a question of programming displacements which require dynamic contractions [10].

Cerebral control offers a great deal of flexibility in the choice of the most efficient and/or the least expensive energy control strategy (set shifting or task switching). The running of the motor protocol can even be pre-programmed, as for example in certain sports exercises or for any repetitive activity in general [15].

Motor programming is under the permanent control of the basal ganglia. It can, however, be interrupted, delayed, or modified at any moment under the effect of emotions. In this context, the motor response can be both shifted in time (1–2 s) and lose in precision with respect to the reality according to the degree of attention of the subject. The level of psychological "motivation" of the subject is also an important parameter for demanding efforts.

Finally, the decision to execute the motor program (the instruction) is formed at the level of the supplementary motor area, then reaches the actual motor area from which the axons of the pyramidal pathway emerge.

But programming and controlling muscles is not enough. The cortical signals that descend toward the medullary motor neurons are permanently controlled and filtered by the cerebellum which, consistent with the pyramidal pathway, has the peculiarity to represent only 11% of the cerebral volume but to possess by contrast 50% of the neurons of the brain human.

Finally, the action sequences (cerebral function) reach, via the spinal cord, the selected muscles whose finely tuned contractions are supposed to provide an optimal response.

Outputs

A system is essentially a variable transformer. The input variables (task to be accomplished) are transformed into output variables that are supposed to represent the task ideally accomplished.

In fact, the output data are not, in most cases, immediately optimal. In addition, the delay introduced by the process of setting up the motor program necessitates adjustments at the entry level.

Feedback

They ensure the adjustment of output variables to input variables. This device returns to the controls the output data that represents the action of the system on the environment. It is fundamental to the dynamics of change within the system.

This device is referred to feedback loops.

There are two types:

- Positive feedback loops that amplify the behavior of the system to optimize the adjustment of the control.
- Negative feedback loops, on the contrary, tend to stabilize the system when the action appears finalized.

The sensory receptors that are integrated into the vertebral structure continuously send data to the nerve controls which, in turn, regulate the instructions continuously. This refers to positive or negative gains. Gains tend to zero when the error between inputs and outputs approaches zero.

Feedbacks are essential to maintain muscle activation that ensures stability. The functional adjustment of the vertebral system is thus perpetually updated thanks to the information circulating in the feedback loops.

Any diagram of a living system is of course only an extreme simplification of reality. There is no feedback loop but a considerable number of links that convey the feedback data. The performance of the system depends on the accuracy of the signals flowing in these loops. Any degree of uncertainty in the data is a noise generator leading to some approximation in the representation of the system at the controls.

Quantitative Analysis of the Vertebral System

The quantitative analysis of a system can be partial or global.

Partial Analysis

It is a unitary approach, based on structure. This approach is similar to the analysis of symptomatology in medicine.

In practice, for the vertebral system, it is reduced more and more to the analysis of imaging provided by radiology.

The tremendous development of vertebral imaging (CT, MRI, EOS, …) has led, as in many specialties, to a reductionist attitude, especially in the analysis of degenerative pathology. The situation has become caricatural in clinical case discussion meetings. In most cases, therapeutic decisions refer mainly to topological data from imaging and some parsimonious information about the discomfort and pain of the patient. The patient actually disappears from these discussions while interns have never had so many ways to represent him. The use of only their smartphone can capture in video, the patient himself, his history and physical examination. It would thus be easy to contribute to the discussions of clinical cases. The fascination produced by the images seems to inexorably discourage any other attempt to find out more.

It must be restated that modern imagery is a static exam, which cannot rely on functional data. It does not necessarily explain the pain. Most degenerative lesions and the sometimes significant deformities that can result are painless and have an acceptable functional impact [16]. Imagery is naturally indispensable, but it must be contextualized.

The assessment of vertebral system failures cannot be reduced to morphological analysis. It is now possible to perform numerical simulations from imagery, and even to introduce other physical information such as force platform data or surface EMG. A technical and financial effort is of course necessary to trivialize these explorations and also a good dose of voluntarism that is justified by the often uncertain results of complex vertebral surgery.

Analysis of Overall Functional Capacity

The overall analysis is to measure the overall performance of the vertebral system in the process of maintaining the balance of posture or movement along an optimal trajectory.

It is an integrative approach to the functioning of the vertebral system, the counterpart of a stress test with VO_2 Max for a cardiorespiratory assessment device.

The tools of this exploration exist but are not all integrated in the current practice as for the industrial systems.

Oswestry Disability Index (ODI) scales are widely used to assess the impact of physical disability resulting from lumbar degenerative pathology. Other scores take into account the psychological and social impact of the pathology (SF36, SF12, etc.).

These scores are primarily established to quantify surgical performance. The data collected does not make it possible to evaluate the specific functional performance of the vertebral system.

The same goes for tests of evaluation of the capacities with physical effort. These tests, developed in the 1980s (*Pile test, Iserhagen work system, Ergos, etc.*) are primarily intended to assess the level of aptitude of a subject for physical work by subjecting him to work simulation or increasing efforts to lift, using exercises that most often involve the entire body without isolating the spinal system. Ruan [17] has shown that this type of evaluation is unreliable for patients with some degree of disability and is therefore unsuitable for preoperative predictive evaluation [18, 19].

The overall evaluation of the specific performance of the spine for surgical treatment must make it possible to measure the specific performance of the vertebral system alone (strength, endurance) with the objective of assessing whether the patient has a good probability of benefiting from surgery most often involving the fusion of several intervertebral mobile segments. The stiffening of the thoracolumbar spine on several segments inevitably entails an important modification of the kinematics of the column, in particular an increase in the bending moments at the hips when fusion comprises the spinopelvic junction. Therefore, a reliable preoperative assessment of the performance of the vertebral system is a predictive test of the patient's ability to tolerate the side effects of the intervention. We will see later that kinematic simulation allows, as of today, to appreciate these effects with good reliability.

The most used machines since the 1980s are isokinetic devices (Aristokin (Biometrics), Cybex (Medimex), Prothia (Broda), etc.). Their operating principle is to maintain a constant speed in keeping with their resistance. We measure not a force but the torque created by a force and its lever at the level of a dynamometer. It is possible to choose a concentric or eccentric contraction mode. We obtain the following parameters:

- Linear (cm/s) or angular velocity (°/s)
- Moment of maximum force
- Maximum work (Nm)
- Maximum power (J)
- Angle of maximum efficiency.

The reproducibility of the tests is satisfactory for the same subject, for the same device and the same examiner. These devices are widely used in the USA, and in the EU, especially in Germany. Their high price (50,000–90,000 €), their operating and maintenance costs are the main reasons for their limited use. The data obtained make it possible to make an accurate assessment of the level of spinal performance of a subject, but the results are biased because of the isokinetics which impose conditions that do not correspond to the stabilization of the living vertebral column. Moreover, they do not lend themselves to the measurement of controls, gains in feedback and the robustness of the system, a parameter that is nevertheless essential for judging its adaptability [20–23]. Finally, they also lend themselves very poorly to numerical simulation. This is why the future lies rather in methods based on the science of systems.

Methods based on systemic analysis:

Their principle is to treat the system as a black box. The inputs are varied and the variations of the outputs measured.

We can thus study the general properties of the system: *Stability, optimality, robustness* [7].

For the vertebral column, the principle of the method consists of placing the subject to be evaluated on an unstable seat equipped with a platform of force, or standing on a platform of force, and to apply precise dynamic stresses at the level of the pelvis by recording the angular displacements using potentiometers.

The measured data concern the amplitude of the displacements, the velocity, the forces, the delays of establishment of balance, the errors of signal which materializes the difference between the entries and the outputs, the gains of the controls. The robustness of the system is also calculated. These data are materialized by graphs (for more details on the protocols, refer to references [7, 24–27]).

This method makes it especially possible to make a numerical simulation of the state of functioning of the vertebral system as one can obtain with a stress test of the heart. The simulation is to vary the parameters that seem to play an important role. Alternative scenarios with predictive intent can be developed. Other parameters can be coupled to these examinations, including surface EMG for the measurement of reflex responses and proprioception analysis [7, 11, 24, 28–30].

Finally, thanks to this specific method of the system, the state of the vertebral system can be evaluated from measurable experimental data.

It is thus possible to mathematically formulate the overall behavior of the system with respect to a static or dynamic equilibrium reference, and to calculate its performances (height of the set point, speed of establishment of equilibrium, duration of the maintenance of the equilibrium …) it is at their optimality, as well as the robustness of the system which designates the ability to maintain performance despite intrinsic or extrinsic disturbances.

Performances

The analysis of the data obtained by the experimentation (or the simulation) makes it possible to qualify and to quantify the performances of the system:

- Stability,
- Optimality (accuracy, speed, damping),
- Robustness.

Stability Whether maintaining a posture or moving, the process is stable when the output status matches the initial goal of the inputs. For example, maintaining the standing position inclined forwards at approximately 30°, or unsupported lifting of a load of 20 kg.

The notion of stability can thus be recreated with an objective of action [29].

The height of the performance (force) is set by the level of the instruction. The endurance (derived from power over time) corresponds to the time of instruction [11, 31] (Fig. 2).

There is, of course, a relationship between performance and energy cost. The force applied is a function of muscular recruitment and secondarily the coactivation of other muscle groups. An excess of rigidity of the vertebral segments by muscular overactivation is however not a guarantee of better

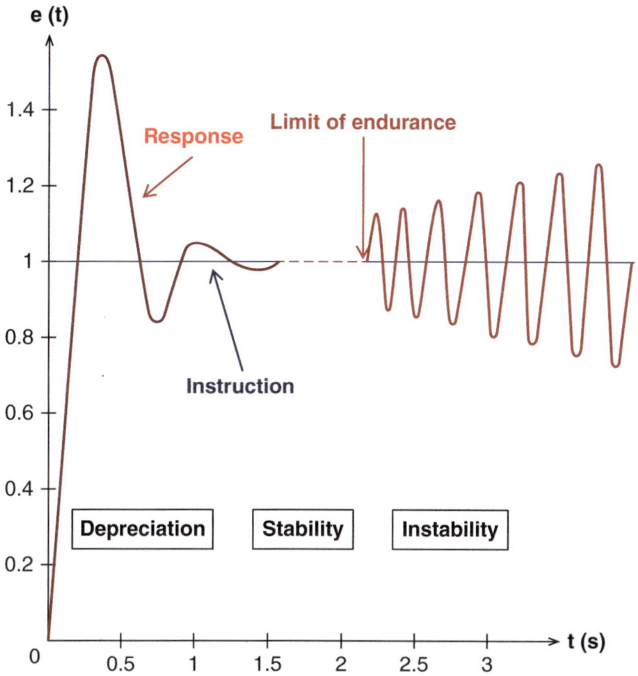

Fig. 2 Representation of the depreciating stabilization of a static equilibrium with respect to an instruction and the instability arising from fatigue

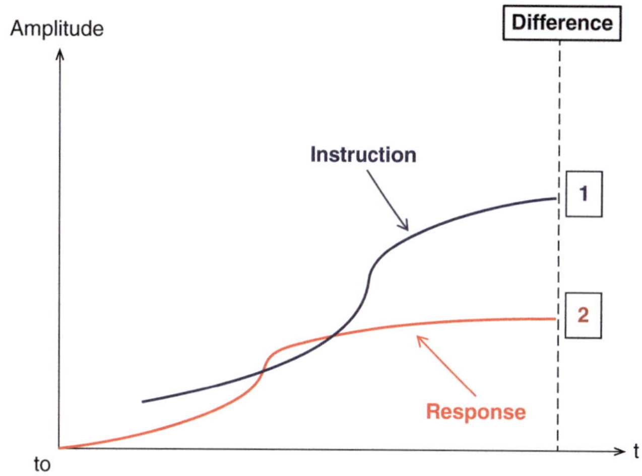

Fig. 3 The precision is expressed by the difference between the instruction and the response. For static equilibrium (left) and dynamic equilibrium (right): 1. nominal trajectory; 2. disturbed trajectory

vertebral stability, especially in dynamic balance [32–34]. This situation of excess muscular coactivation is characteristic of episodes of acute low back pain.

Stability refers to the ability of the system to reach the setpoint accurately and quickly. The error signal represents the difference between the input and output parameters with respect to time.

Speed is the time that the system takes to react to changes in the input signal (response time).

Finally the damping capacity of the oscillations is also an important parameter.

Robtuness is the property that allows the system to maintain its functions despite internal or external disturbances [26, 27, 35], and the uncertainty of representations (Selling 2004). Indeed, despite the magnitude of the flow of information sent back to the controls, the representation of the vertebral system remains an approximation. Robustness allows it to operate however with a certain degree of uncertainty in the data.

One of the foundations of the robustness of living systems is the extreme redundancy of constituents and controls that contributes to stability at all scales.

Robustness is a different concept of stability. The robustness can be increased by lowering the stability conditions [34].

Like the other parameters mentioned, robustness is a measurable parameter in global tests inspired by the systemic (Fig. 3).

Fault Factors of the Vertebral System

Functional failures of the vertebral system can include both structural abnormalities in the column and its "soft envelope," and failures of controls and/or interactions.

Failures Related to the Vertebral Structure

Degenerative lesions of the spine (discs, epiphyseal plates, zygapophyseal joints, and peri-vertebral ligaments) result from a sudden (traumatic) or chronic mechanical overload. The existence of scoliotic or kyphotic deformation is a predisposing factor. Genetic factors and age also play a particularly important role.

Repeated mechanical stresses greater than the resistance and damping capacities of the constituents of the vertebral structure alter the nutrition process of the intervertebral disc. This results in a depressurization which, in turn, lowers the mechanical performance of the elements concerned. At the same time, at the cellular level, an apoptosis process, an inflammatory molecular cascade, and a degradation of the adaptive remodeling phenomenon are triggered. All of these factors interact in a circular causality.

Inadequate thoracopelvic musculature (in strength and endurance) is a major factor in the degeneration of the vertebral system [10, 15, 25, 36], especially in elderly patients (sarcopenia) and may easily be at the origin of degenerative kyphosis. These deformities, reducing the thoracopelvic flexion moments, materialize the mechanical adaptation of the vertebral structure to the weakness of the posterior musculature (extensors of the column, gluteal muscles, and hamstrings). The correction of such deformities, associated with extensive thoracopelvic fusion, inevitably leads to an increase in bending moments which may be insurmountable by some patients.

In motivated patients, however, muscle performance can be substantially improved by preoperative rehabilitation for a few months [37].

Transducer Failures

They result from a degeneration of sensorial and/or sensation receptors most often related to age. The resulting signal degradation leads to an increase in noise and deteriorates system performance at the control level. This results in particular disorders of proprioception that may escape the examination during the surgical consultation as the system is sufficiently robust.

Proprioception disorders can be improved by appropriate preoperative management.

Failures Related to Controls

There is, of course, a host of central injuries that can alter the instructions. Parkinson's disease and other degenerative cerebrospinal pathologies are common and often evaluated in elderly subjects.

The lack of integration of control feedbacks is probably a common cause of dysfunction that can, even for a simple lumbago, induce excessive lumbar stiffness and pain by abnormal muscle coactivation [32–34, 38].

Emotional fragility also disrupts the development and continuation of the motor program. At the time of the operative decision, it certainly deserves more than an intuitive evaluation.

Conclusion

The spine surgeon must anticipate the side effects of the most unpredictable techniques that he plans to apply and take into account of the specificities for each patient. Most often it is to predict the functional consequences of particularly extensive vertebral arthrodesis, such as pedicle subtraction osteotomy. These techniques can have detrimental mechanical effects, especially in weakened patients.

The considerable weight given to conventional radiological imaging in the operative decision seems excessive to us. A major effort should be made to develop digital simulation of the vertebral kinematics and be able to apply it routinely.

It must be admitted, however, that the correction of geometrical anomalies can rightly result in undeniable success in the hands of very experienced surgeons.

The evidence suggests, however, that in many cases these procedures are not always sufficient to achieve pain relief and a substantial improvement in the patient's functional disability despite the rigor of angular corrections and the quality of the arthrodeses. Sometimes even the patient's condition can be aggravated. A worrying uncertainty about the lack of data at the time of the decision-making process hovers over the results of this major surgery. It is still increasing in older patients, often with multiple deficiencies. We now know, often at our expense, that the determinants of scoliosis surgery in childhood, primarily structural and occurring in systems generally endowed with excellent robustness, are obviously not applicable to degenerative deformities of the aging adult.

Systems analysis is likely to open new horizons for the planning of complex surgical procedures on the spine. As in other medical specialties that have integrated it, it can produce a decisive strategic inflection both in the field of surgery and that of the rehabilitation of spinal disorders.

References

1. De Rosnay J. Le macroscope. Paris: Seuil; 1975.
2. Donnadieu G, Quarks M. La systémique: penser et agir dans la complexité. Paris: Liaisons; 2002.
3. Durand D. La systémique. PUF; 2013.
4. Forrester JW. Principles of systems. Cambridge: MIT Press; 1969.
5. Le Moigne JL. La modélisation des systèmes complexes. Paris: Dunod; 1999.
6. Von Bertalanffy L. Théorème général des systèmes. Malakoff: Dunod; 2012.
7. Xu Y, Choi J, Reeves NP, Cholewicki J. Optimal control of the spine system. J Biomech Eng. 2010;132:051004.
8. Carlson JM, Doyle J. Complexity and robustness. Proc Natl Acad Sci U S A. 2002;99(Suppl 1):2538–54.
9. Kitano H. Biological robustness. Nat Rev Genet. 2004a;5:826–37.
10. Granata KP, Slota GP, Bennett BC. Paraspinal muscle reflex dynamics. J Biomech. 2004a;37:241–7.
11. Lariviere C, Bilodeau M, Forget R, Vadeboncoeur R, Mecheri H. Poor back muscle endurance is related to pain catastrophizing in patients with chronic low back pain. Spine. 2010a;35:E1178–86.
12. Corey DP, Roper SD, editors. Sensory transduction: Society of General Physiologists, 45th Annual Symposium. Marine Biological Laboratory, Woods Hole, Massachusetts 1991. New York: Rockefeller University Press; 1992.
13. Swinkels A, Dolan P. Regional assessment of joint position sense in the spine. Spine. 1998;23:590–7.
14. Buxton DF, Peck D. Neuromuscular spindles relative to joint complexities. Clin Anat. 1989;2:211–24.
15. Van Daele U, Hagman F, Truijen S, Vorlat P, Van Gheluwe B, Vaes P. Differences in balance strategies between nonspecific chronic low back pain patients and healthy control subjects during unstable sitting. Spine. 2009;34:1233–8.
16. Panjabi MM. The stabilizing system of the spine. Part I. Function, dysfunction, adaptation, and enhancement. J Spinal Disord. 1992;5:38–9.

17. Ruan CM, Haig AJ, Geisser ME, Yamakawa K, Buchholz RL. Functional capacity evaluations in persons with spinal disorders: predicting poor outcomes on the Functional Assessment Screening Test (FAST). J Occup Rehabil. 2001;11(2):119–32.
18. Brouwer S, Reneman MF, Dijkstra PU, Groo-Thoff JW, Schellekens JMH, Goeken LNH. Test-retest reliability of the Isernhagen work systems functional capacity evaluation in patients with chronic low Back pain. J Occup Rehabil. 2003;13(4):207–18.
19. Hazard RG, Reeves V, Fenwick JW. Lifting capacity. Indices of subject effort. Spine. 1992;17:1065–70.
20. Gremion G, Mahler F, Chantraine A. Mesures isocinétiques de la force musculaire du rachis: influence de l'âge, de l'activité physique et des lombalgies. Ann Readapt Med Phys. 1996;39:439.
21. Luoto S, Hupli M, Alaranta H, Hurri H. Isokinetic performance capacity of trunk muscles. Part II: coefficient of variation in isokinetics in maximal effort and in submaximal effort. Scand J Rehabil Med. 1996;28:207–10.
22. Vézirian T, Voisin P, Vanhee JL. Evaluation isocinétique des fléchisseurs et extenseurs du tronc avec et sans correction de la gravité. Ann Kinesithé. 1996;23:62–7.
23. Timm KE. Clinical applications of a normative database for the Cybex TEF and TORSO spinal isokinetic dynamometers. Isokinet Exerc Sci. 1995;5:43–9.
24. Lariviere C, Kearney R, Mecher H, Ludwig D, Shirazi-Adl A, Gagnon D. Évaluation biomécanique des déterminants de la stabilité lombaire. Rapport IRSST; 2012. R.742.
25. Hoshino Y, Nakamura K, Kariya Y, Saita K, Ito K. Trunk muscle weakness as a risk factor for low back pain. A 5-year prospective study. Spine. 1999;24:54–7.
26. Reeves NP, Popovich JM, Priess MC, Cholewicki J, Choi J, Radcliffe CJ. Reliability of assessing trunk motor control using position and force tracking and stabilization tasks. J Biomech. 2014;47(1):44–9.
27. Reeves NP, Everding VQ, Cholewicki J, Morrisette DC. The effects of trunk stiffness on postural control during unstable seated balance. Exp Brain Res. 2006;174:694–700.
28. Granata KP, Rogers E, Moorhouse K. Effects of static flexion-relaxation on paraspinal reflex behaviour. Clin Biomech. 2005;20:16–24.
29. Jacazinski RJ, Flash JM. Control theory for humans: quantitative approaches to modelling performance. Mahwah: Lawrence Erlbaum Associates; 2003.
30. Van Daele U, Huyvaert S, Hagman F, Duquet W, Van Gheluwe B, Vaes P. Reproducibility of postural control measurement during unstable sitting in low back pain patients. BMC Musculoskelet Disord. 2007;8:44.a.
31. Granata KP, Slota GP, Wilson SE. Influence of fatigue in neuromuscular control of spinal stability. Hum Factors. 2004b;46: 81–91.
32. Moorehouse K, Granata K. Role of reflex dynamics in spinal stability: intrinsic muscle stiffness alone is insufficient for stability. J Biomech. 2007;40:1058–65.
33. Radebold A, Cholewicki J, Polzofer GK, Greene HS. Impaired postural control of the lumbar spine is associated with delayed muscle response times in patients with chronic idiopathic low back pain. Spine. 2001;26:724–30.
34. Reeves NP, Narendra KS, Cholewicki J. Spine stability: the six blind men and the elephant. Clin Biomech. 2007;22: 266–74.
35. Slota GP, Granata KP, Madigan ML. Effects of seated wholebody vibration on postural control of the trunk during unstable seated balance. Clin Biomech. 2008;23:381–6.
36. Cholewicki J, Silfies SP, Shah RA, Greene HS, Reeves NP, Alvi K, Goldberg B. Delayed trunk muscle reflex responses increase the risk of low back injuries. Spine. 2005;30:2614–20.
37. McGill SM. Low back stability: from formal description to issues for performance and rehabilitation. Exerc Sport Sci Rev. 2001;29:26–31.
38. Potvin JR, O'Brien PR. Trunk muscle co-contraction increases during fatiguing, isometric, lateral bend exertions. Possible implications for spine stability. Spine. 1998;23: 774–8.

Kinematics of the Spine

Jean Marc Vital, J. Sénégas, C. Garnier, and H. Bouloussa

The vertebral column, in recognition of the superposition of the intervertebral mobile segments of Junghanns, can be similar to a flexibility that acts along three axes perpendicular to each other: X, Y, and Z. There are translations along these axes which, when they are over-developed, are pathological, and especially rotations defining the three movements of the vertebral column (Fig. 1):

- rotation around the transverse X-axis: flexion–extension
- rotation around the vertical Y-axis: true right and left rotation
- rotation around the anteroposterior Z-axis: right and left lateral inclination.

The intervertebral joint is therefore an articulation with six degrees of freedom (DOF), three DOF in translation, and three DOF in rotation [1].

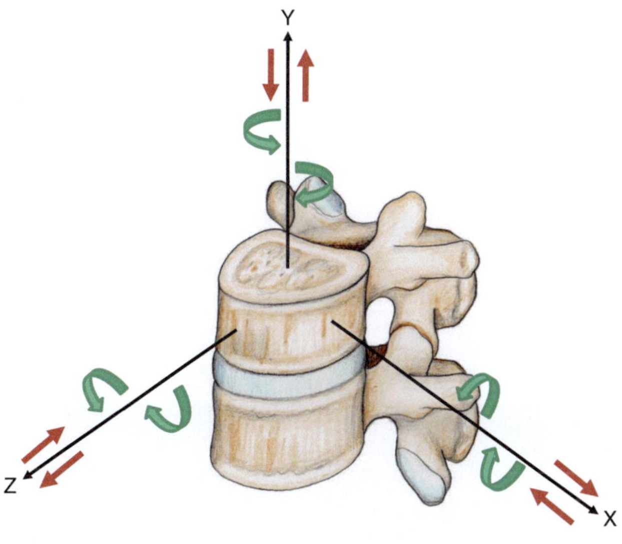

Fig. 1 The three axes of the spinal movements

J. M. Vital (✉) · J. Sénégas · C. Garnier · H. Bouloussa
Spinal Unit, University Hospital, Bordeaux, France

The movements occur in the disc and articular facet joints, assimilated into three coaxial joints which therefore have no locking position (Fig. 2). The tensioning of the ligamentous structures, including the intervertebral disc and the

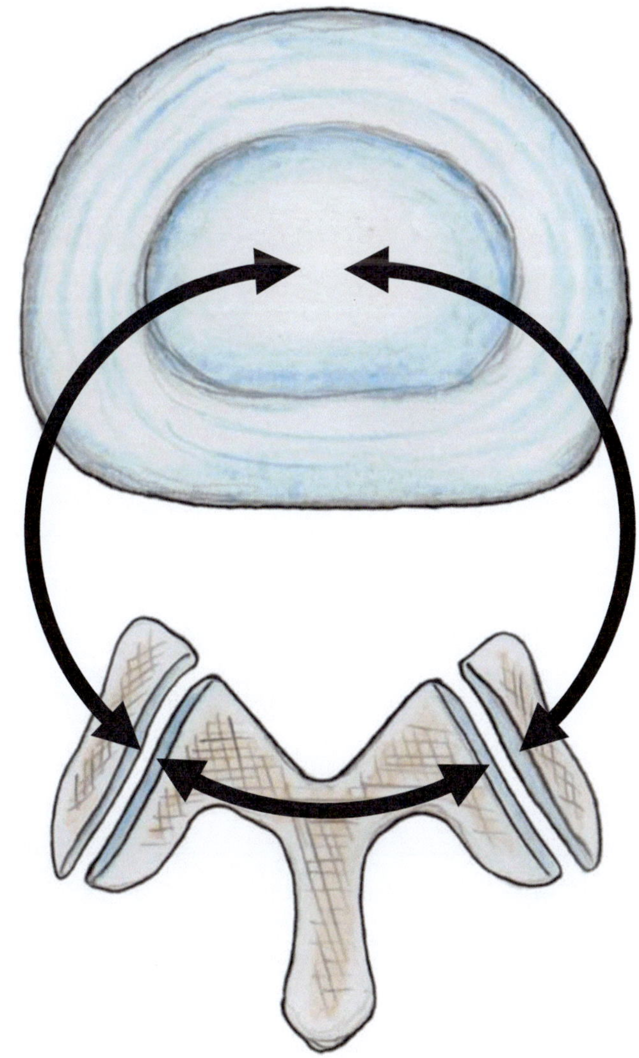

Fig. 2 Coaxiality of the joints of the intervertebral segment

J. M. Vital, D. T. Cawley (eds.), *Spinal Anatomy*, https://doi.org/10.1007/978-3-030-20925-4_30

osseous constraints are stabilizing structures which can be exceeded in extreme situations, especially in micro- or macro-trauma.

According to Panjabi [2], when a load is applied to a spinal functional unit (SFU), the result is a range of motion (ROM), which, before reaching its maximum, passes through a neutral zone and an elastic zone. The neutral zone is the portion of the intervertebral mobility area closest to the rest position, in which the joint has the largest capacity for movement with minimal resistance to intervertebral mobility. The elastic area corresponds to the magnitude of intervertebral mobility located between the end of the neutral zone and the limit of the ROM. It is interesting to note that in the setting of disc degeneration, the neutral zone will increase, as well as translations, which signifies instability (Figs. 3 and 4).

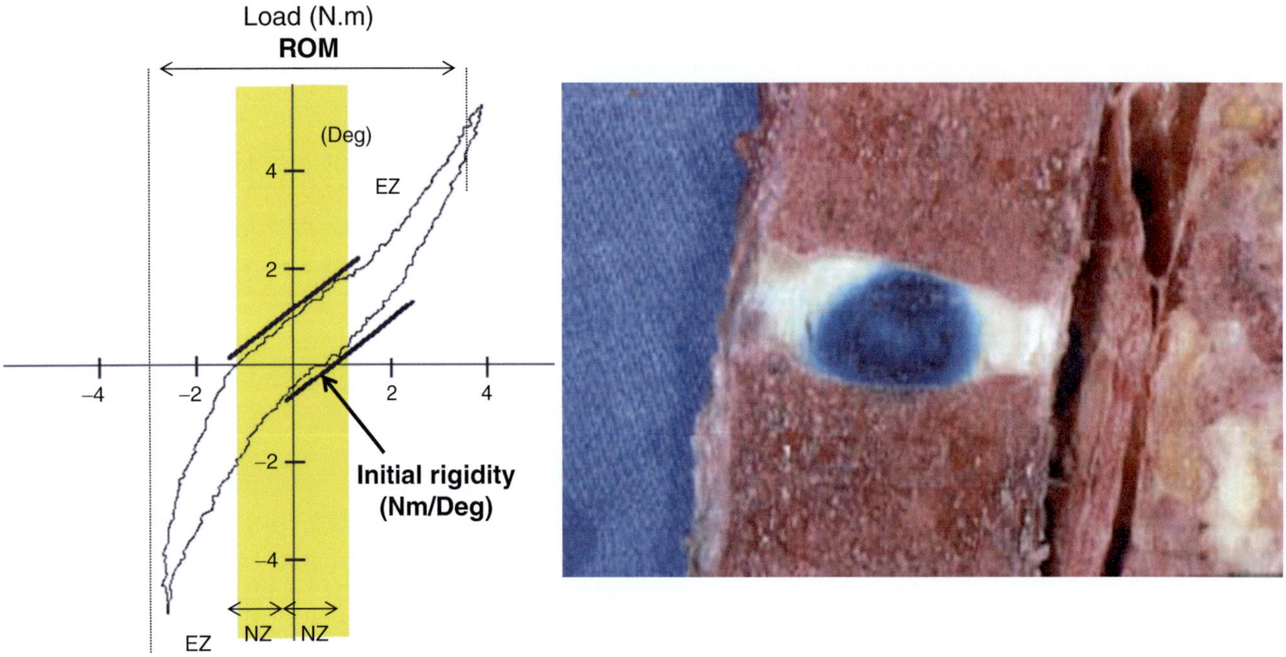

Fig. 3 Neutral (NZ) and elastic (EZ) zones on a normal mobile segment

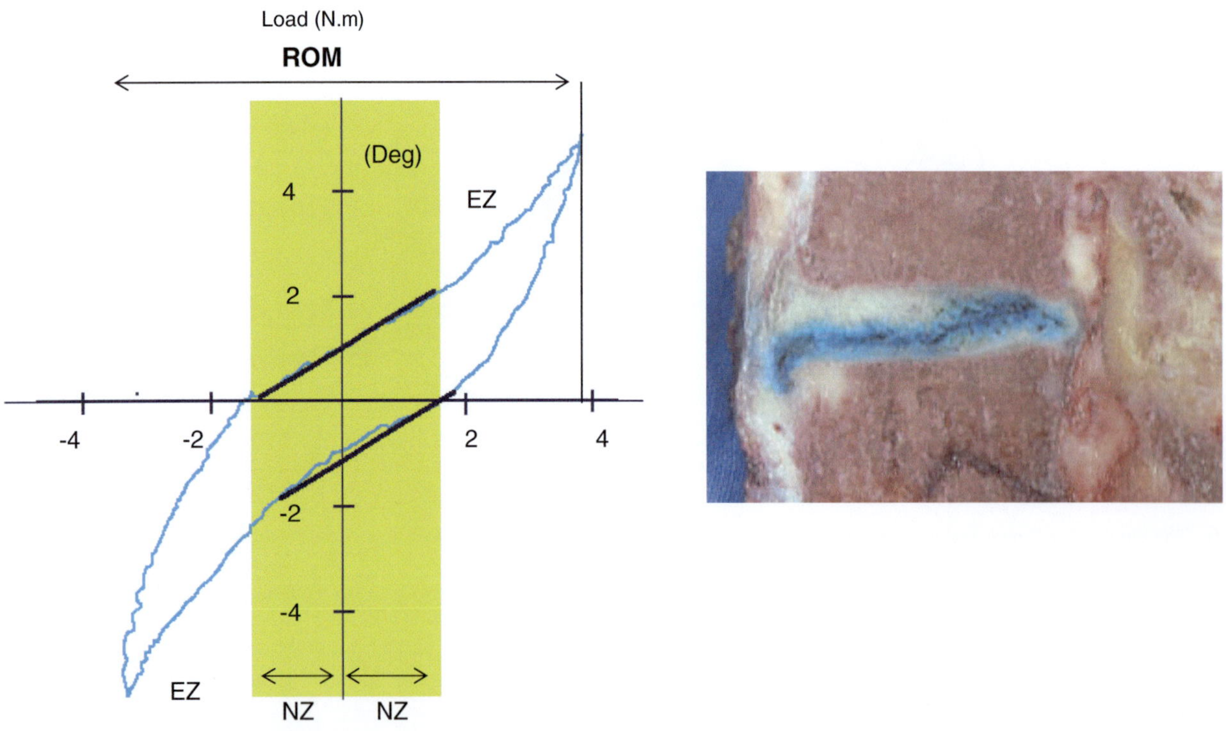

Fig. 4 Neutral (ZN) and elastic (ZE) zones on a degenerate mobile segment

Methods for Measuring Spinal Mobility

This evaluation can be done in vitro and in vivo.

In Vitro Measurements

In vitro measurements are performed on cadaveric subjects, usually of elderly subjects but isolated from any musculoligamentous envelope, which explains why angular values are usually increased compared to those measured on living subjects. The physical measurement means are displacement sensors, ultrasound or X-rays.

In Vivo Measurements

The in vivo measurements are for active movements which seek to assess the overall and intersegmental mobility. Many processes can be used: simple goniometers or inclinometers (liquid or gravity) and especially more accurate electronic (cervical range of motion® or CROM®) [3], electrogoniometers, magnetic devices (e.g., Fastrack® or Isotrack®) [4], ultrasound devices (Zebris®), videofluoroscopy, and finally optoelectronic devices (Vicon®).

Medical imaging includes dynamic X-rays, cineradiography, CT, and MRI.

Dynamic radiographs are performed routinely in the clinical setting, mainly for cervical and lumbar evaluation. On these images, the flexion–extension and less often the right and left lateral inclination can be measured. Rotation is perfectly explored only through computed tomography (CT).

The dynamic flexion–extension lateral cervical radiographs are in a sitting position: the subject is asked, for the exploration of flexion, to try to touch the sternum with the chin and to explore extension by bringing the head as far back as possible. The dynamic lumbar images of flexion–extension can be done according to different techniques. The technique of Putto [5], which is with the patient seated or standing, hyperflexion of the trunk in hyperextension with gluteal support is the most recognized (Fig. 5); the same author showed that he obtained less amplitude by positioning the patient in less flexion and extension. We can also achieve these positions of flexion–extension on a Swedish chair, a method used in the evaluation of spinal fusion [6] (Fig. 6). Wood [7] studied patients with spondylolisthesis and shows that images performed in flexion–extension on the supine subject were more sensitive than those practiced in standing.

Dynamic images for lateral inclination were investigated by Weitz [8] to recognize indirect signs of lumbar disc herniation. Dupuis [9] did a study of dynamic radiographs in lateral inclination to recognize signs of instability.

More conventionally, the intervertebral instability is likely if it exists between extremities of flexion and extension, an angular intervertebral mobility of greater than 10° [9], or even 20° [10], and vertebral translation of more than 3 mm [11], 4 mm [9], or even 5 mm [10].

With the help of image software, one can refine the evaluation of intersegmental mobility and calculate the position of the instantaneous centers of rotation (ICRs) [6]. Gertzbein [12] demonstrated on cadaveric parts that there was dispersion of these ICRs in degenerate and unstable intervertebral segments (Fig. 7).

Finally, the evaluation of dynamic views of lumbosacral mobility is crucial to recognize the patient's ability to correct their pelvic retroversion in the setting of anterior truncal imbalance. We can evaluate the amplitude of anteversion in standing with an image in a single leg lunge position as described by Hovorka in the chapter "The Reserve of Hip Extension and its Relationship with the Spine" and by Lazennec [13] (Fig. 8), in a procubitus position with a cushion positioning the femurs in hyperextension (Fig. 9).

CT is less used in this setting but enhances evaluation of rotation. It was used by Penning [14] at the cervical level, Morita [15] to evaluate flexion–extension in the thoracic region, and Fujimori [16] to evaluate lateral inclination in the thoracic region. Husson [17] describes signs of lumbar instability in the face of abnormal decoaptation (uncoupling) on rotating scanners.

Dynamic MRI is mainly used to evaluate the neurological content of the spinal canal. Vitzhum [18] used it to evaluate thoracic movements.

Finally, intraoperative rigidity measurement was described for the first time by Ebara [19] with intraoperative distraction of the spinous processes surrounding the tested intervertebral segment according to the force (F) and displacement (D); the rigidity is proportional to the ratio: delta F/delta D (Fig. 10). An unstable segment will have low rigidity, characterized by significant displacement for a small applied force. Brown [19] has developed an automated device that can best adjust the intensity of the applied force. Like Hasegawa [21], who has a great deal of experience in this field, Brown maintains that the indication of a flexible or rigid arthrodesis is governed by these results for measurement of rigidity.

Amplitude of Spinal Movements

Figure 11 shows the distribution of movement amplitudes between the cervical, thoracic, and lumbar segments in flexion, extension, rotation, and lateral inclination.

Global amplitudes (Figs. 12, 13, and 14).

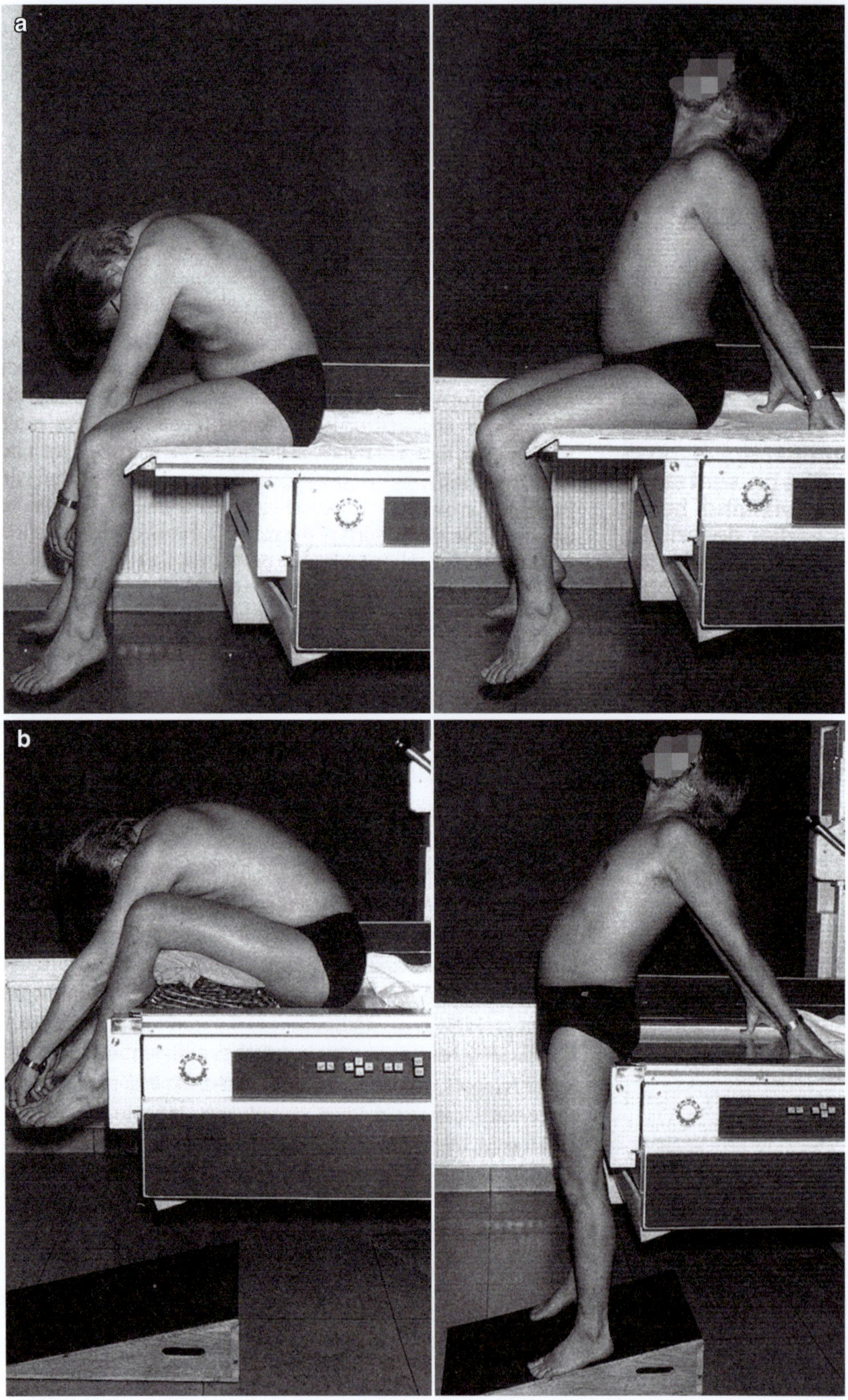

Fig. 5 Dynamic images in lumbar flexion–extension according to Putto [5]; method b is preferable to a

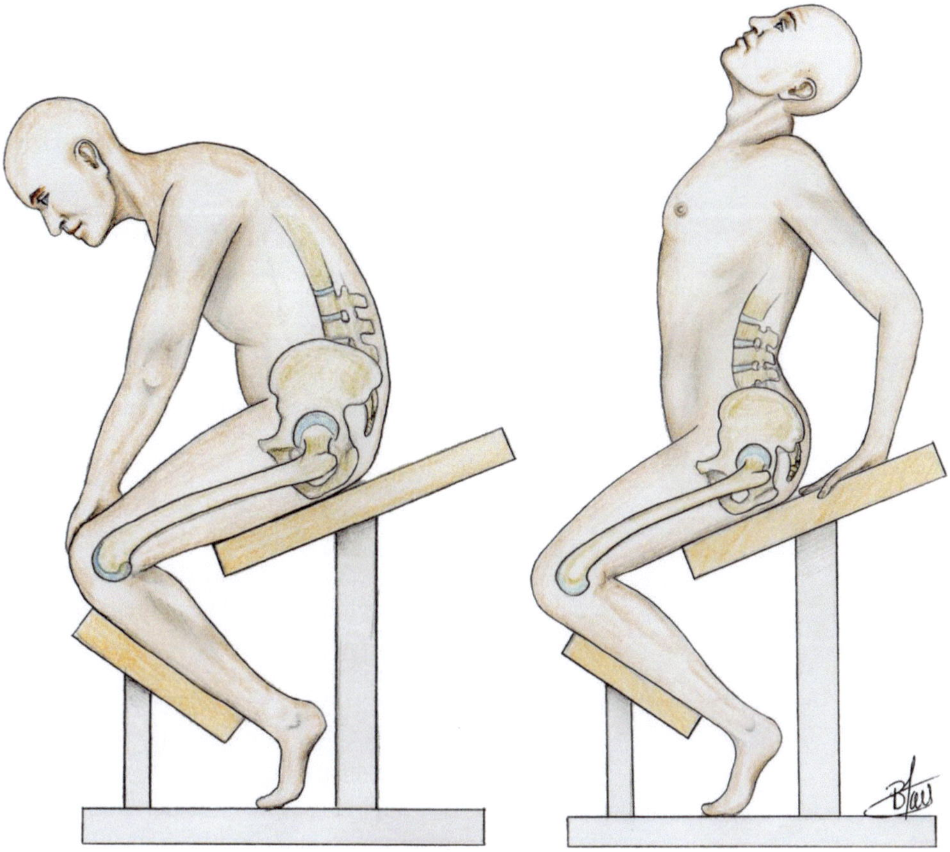

Fig. 6 Dynamic images in lumbar flexion–extension on Swedish seat, according to Templier [6]

Fig. 7 Dispersion of ICR on a degenerate lumbar intervertebral segment, according to Gertzbein [12]

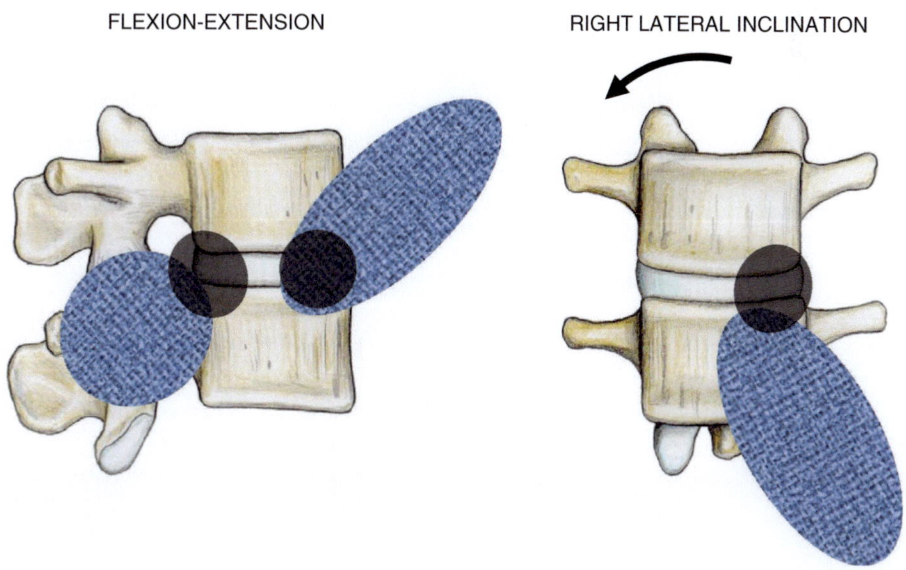

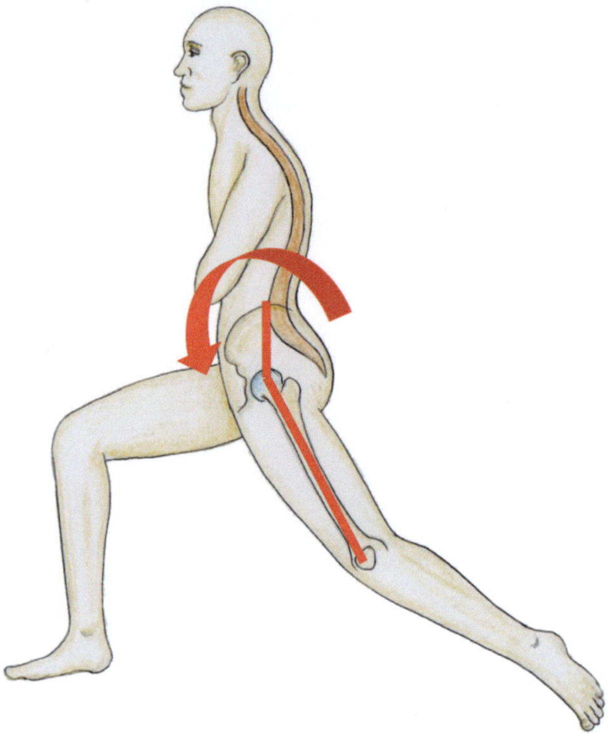

Fig. 8 Diagram of posterior lunge (Hovorka) which allows assessment of the ability of pelvic anteversion and extension of the hip joint

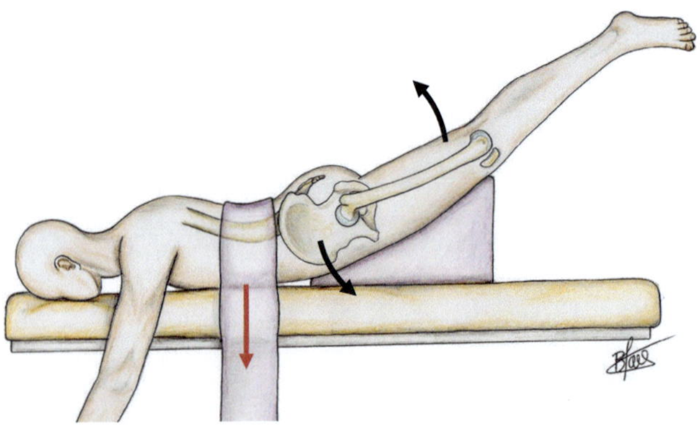

Fig. 9 Image with reduction of pelvic retroversion

Flexion has a total amplitude of 145°–150° with an average cervical flexion of 70°, a thoracic flexion of 30°, and a lumbar flexion of 45°.

Extension has a total amplitude of 165° with an average cervical extension of 80°, a thoracic extension of 40°, and a lumbar extension of 45°.

Lateral inclination has an overall amplitude of 65°–80° with a cervical inclination of 15°–30°, a thoracic inclination of 30°, and a lumbar inclination of 20°.

The rotation has an overall amplitude of 90–95° with a cervical rotation of 50°, a thoracic rotation of 30°, and a lumbar rotation of 10°.

Table 1 shows the total thoracic mobilities according to the different authors.

White and Panjabi [2] have shown, in vitro, that these last two movements of inclination and rotation are reflexively or automatically associated (Fig. 15).

Ishii [22 and 23] has shown more recently, in vivo, that lateral inclination and lateral rotation were in the same direction in the lower cervical spine but that there was an opposite rotation in the upper cervical spine (Fig. 16). This coupling was confirmed by Fujimori [16].

The diagrams of Castaing [24] show the amplitudes of cervical flexion–extension (Fig. 17), cervical lateral inclination (Fig. 18), cervical rotation (Fig. 19), the different movements of the thoracic spine (Fig. 20), and finally the different movements of the lumbar spine (Fig. 21).

At the cervical level, Ordway [26] describes on the dynamic views in flexion–extension of the cervical spine the presence of protraction (or protrusion) and retraction movements. In protraction, there is a flexion of the C3C7 segment and an associated extension of the OC1C2 segment. In retraction, there is an extension of the C3C7 segment and an associated flexion of the OC1C2 segment (Fig. 22).

At the thoracic level, with CT, Morita [15] found a flexion–extension of 31.7° and Fujimori [16] a lateral inclination of 25°.

Fig. 10 Measurement of intraoperative rigidity (R) according to Ebara [20]. R = delta F/delta D

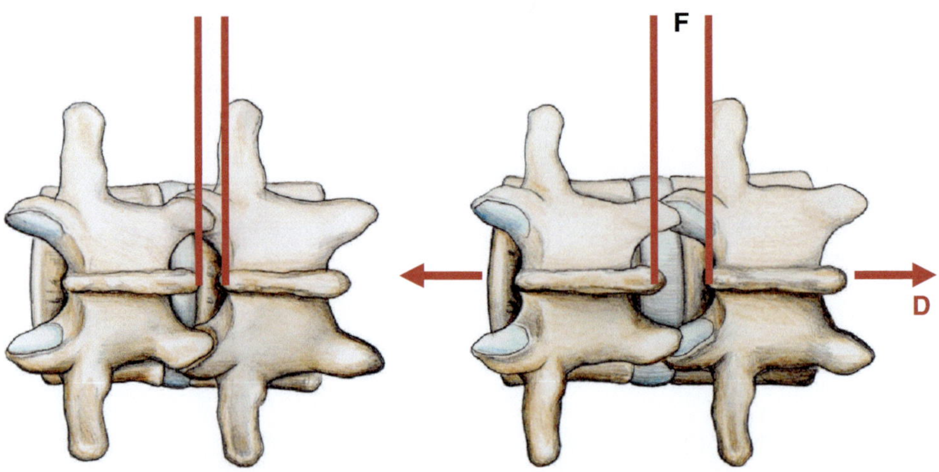

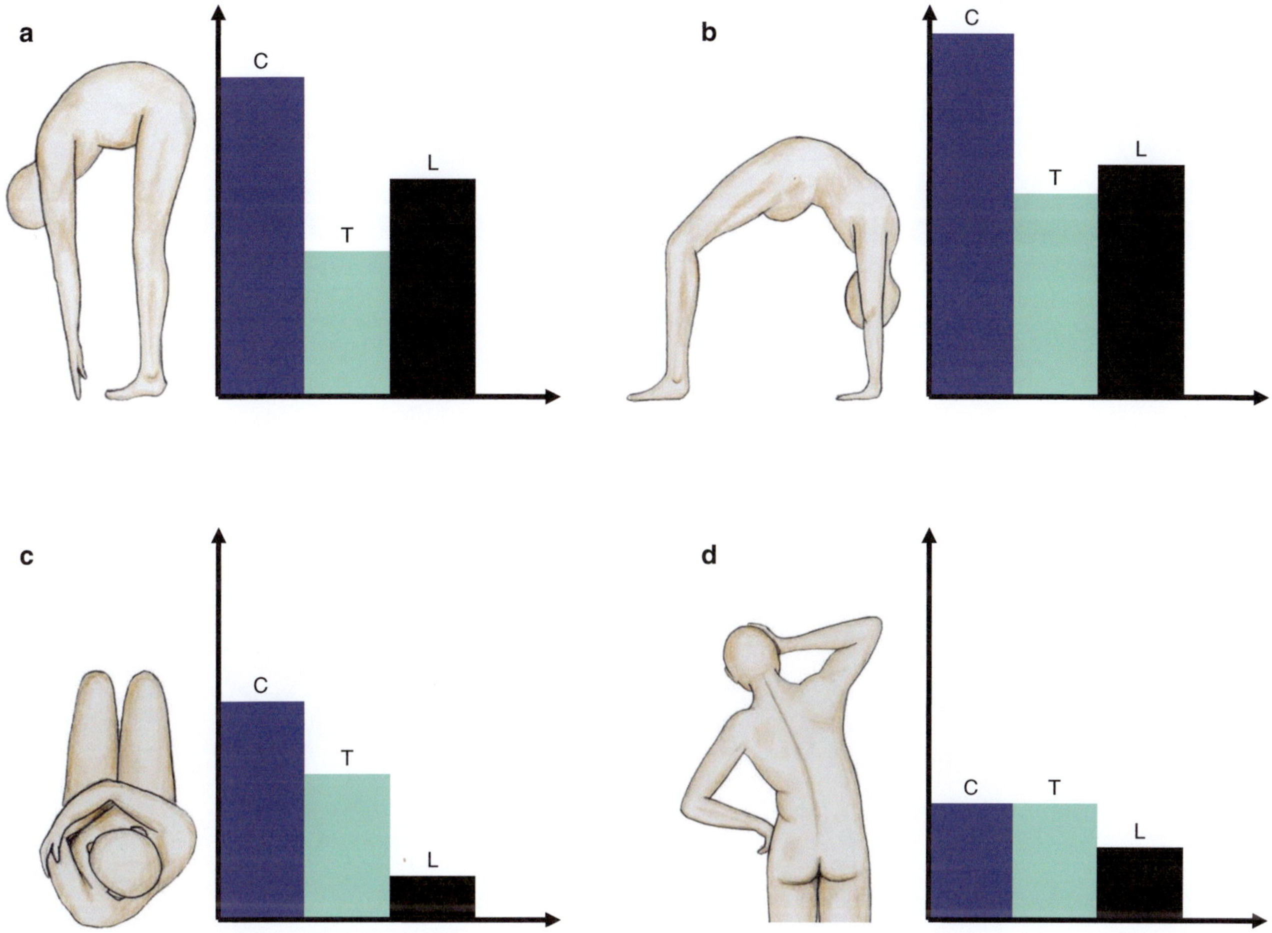

Fig. 11 Respective participation of the different cervical (C), thoracic (T), and lumbar (L) segments in flexion (**a**), extension (**b**), axial (**c**), and lateral (**d**) movements

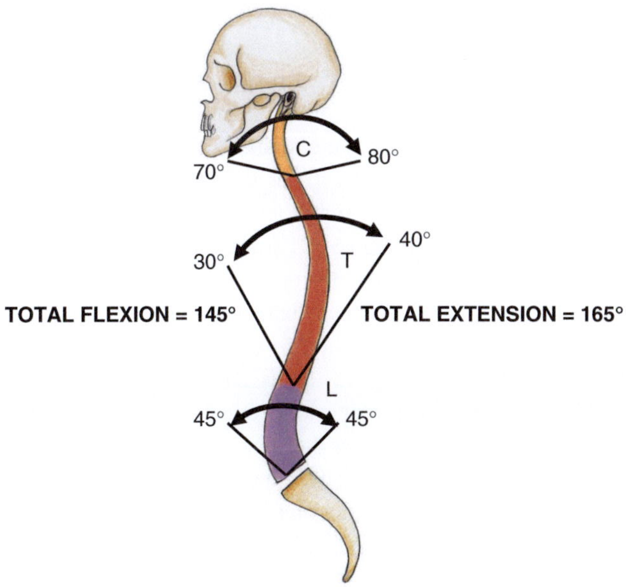

Fig. 12 Overall amplitudes of flexion–extension

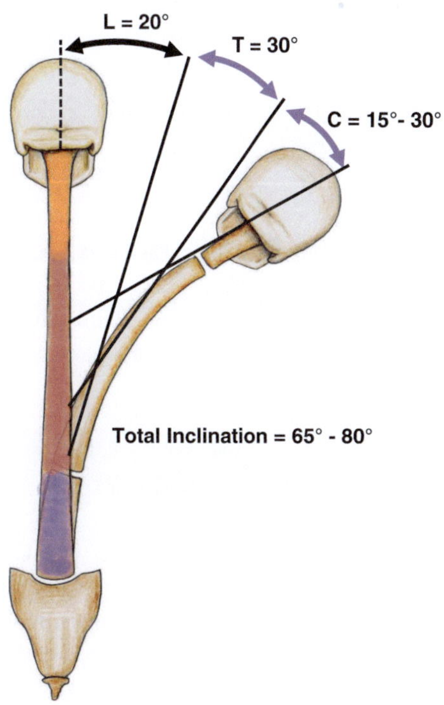

Fig. 13 Overall inclinations of lateral inclination

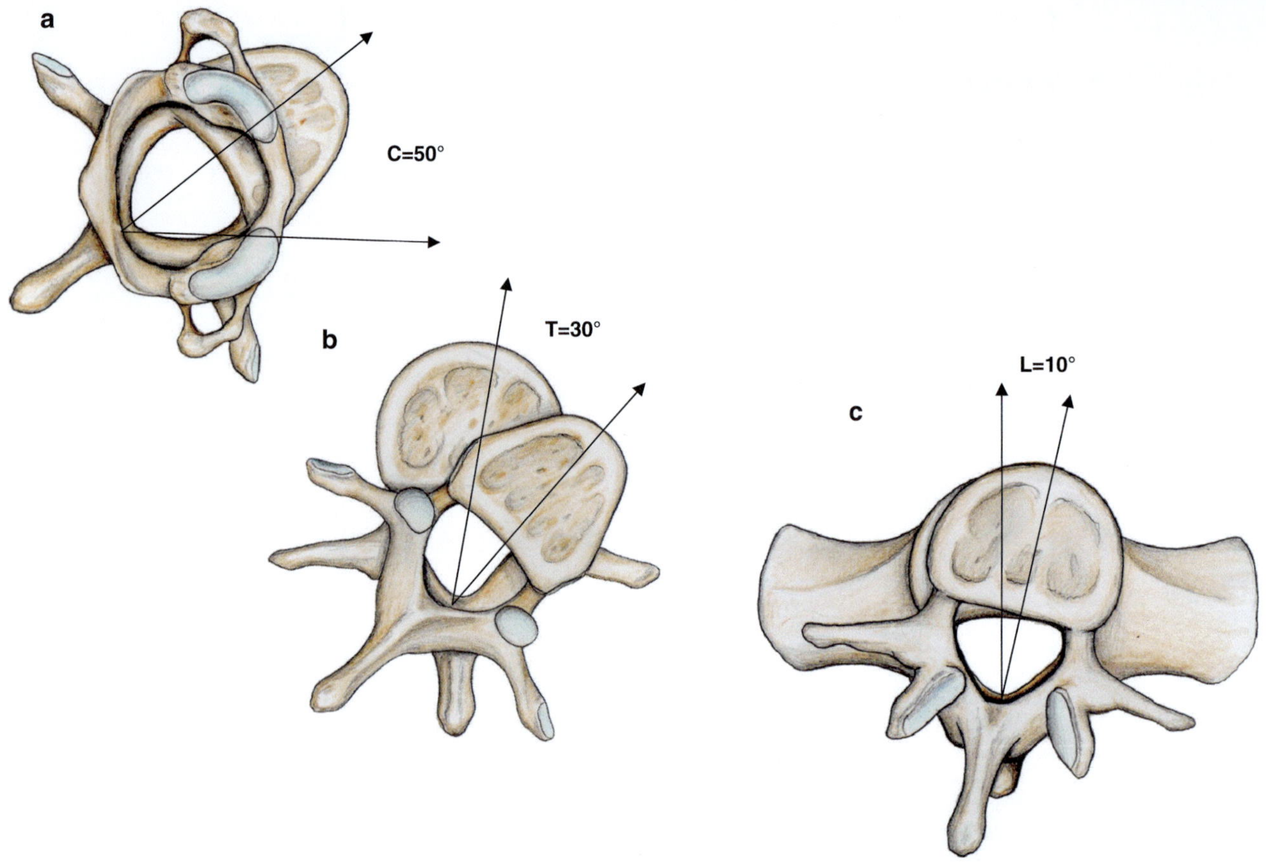

Fig. 14 Overall amplitudes of lateral rotation (views from above): (**a**) cervical, (**b**) thoracic, and (**c**) lumbar

Table 1 Total thoracic mobility

Authors	Flexion–extension	Lateral inclination	Unilateral rotation
Louis [22]	50°	20°	35°
White and Panjabi [2]	62°	36°	32.5°
Vanneuville [45]	64°	35.5°	36°
Castaing [24]	70°	30°	30°
Kapandji [23]	70°	–	37°

Segmental Amplitudes and Motion Analysis

We recall that these movements are mainly in rotation and also in translation which is much smaller and which become pathological if too important.

The Upper Cervical Spine (OC1C2)

At the level of the upper cervical spine (OC1C2), Table 2 summarizes the amplitudes proposed by the different authors. At OC1, despite the spheroidal shape of the surfaces, there is practically only a flexion–extension motion; the occipital condyles recede with respect to the upper articular surfaces of C1 in flexion and advance in extension. The center of the movement is at the occiput (Fig. 23).

At the C1C2 level in flexion, the neural arc of C1 slightly loses its parallelism with that of C2, without C1's nosing forward as in certain high cervical instabilities. In extension, the neural arc tilts backwards. The center of the movement is in the middle of the articular mass of C1 (Fig. 23).

The rotational movement is essential at C1C2 since it has an amplitude of more than 25° for each side, i.e., half of the total amplitude of rotation in the cervical region. In this movement, which mainly affects the atlanto-axial joints, there is a shift toward the front of the lower articulation of C1 on the side opposite to the rotation and a sliding toward the rear of this same lower articulation of C1 from the side of the rotation (Fig. 24). This is reflected in the open-mouth radiograph by an asymmetry of the AO distances between the axis (O) and the lateral masses of C1 (A) (Fig. 25) which is not pathological and does not mean in any way a C1C2 rotary subluxation.

The ICR of the movement is located in the middle of the dens process, at mid-distance from the joints involved in the movements, lateral and anterior atlanto-axial. For Castaing [24], there are two types of rotation: one around the odontoid with symmetrical displacements of the two C1C2 joints and the other around a fixed C1C2 articulation (Fig. 26). It is interesting to note that there are two types of C1C2 rotary subluxation involving these two modes of rotation. Finally, Fig. 27 shows that there is a lateral inclination of 8° at C2C3, 3° at OC1, and virtually no inclination at C1C2.

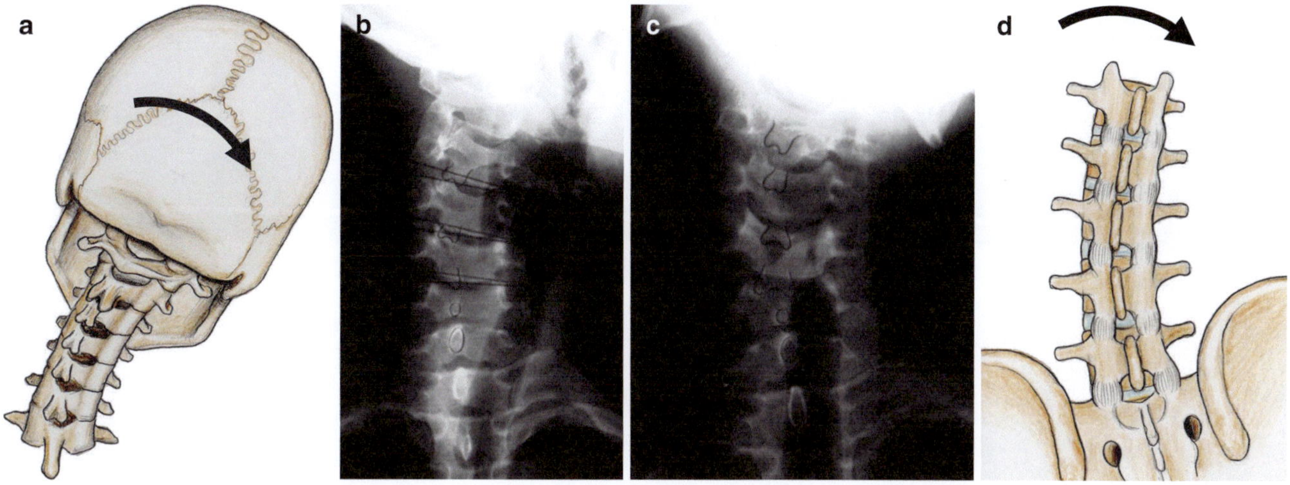

Fig. 15 Automatically associated tilt and rotation movements in cervical (**a**), inclination (**b**), rotation (**c**), and lumbar (**d**)

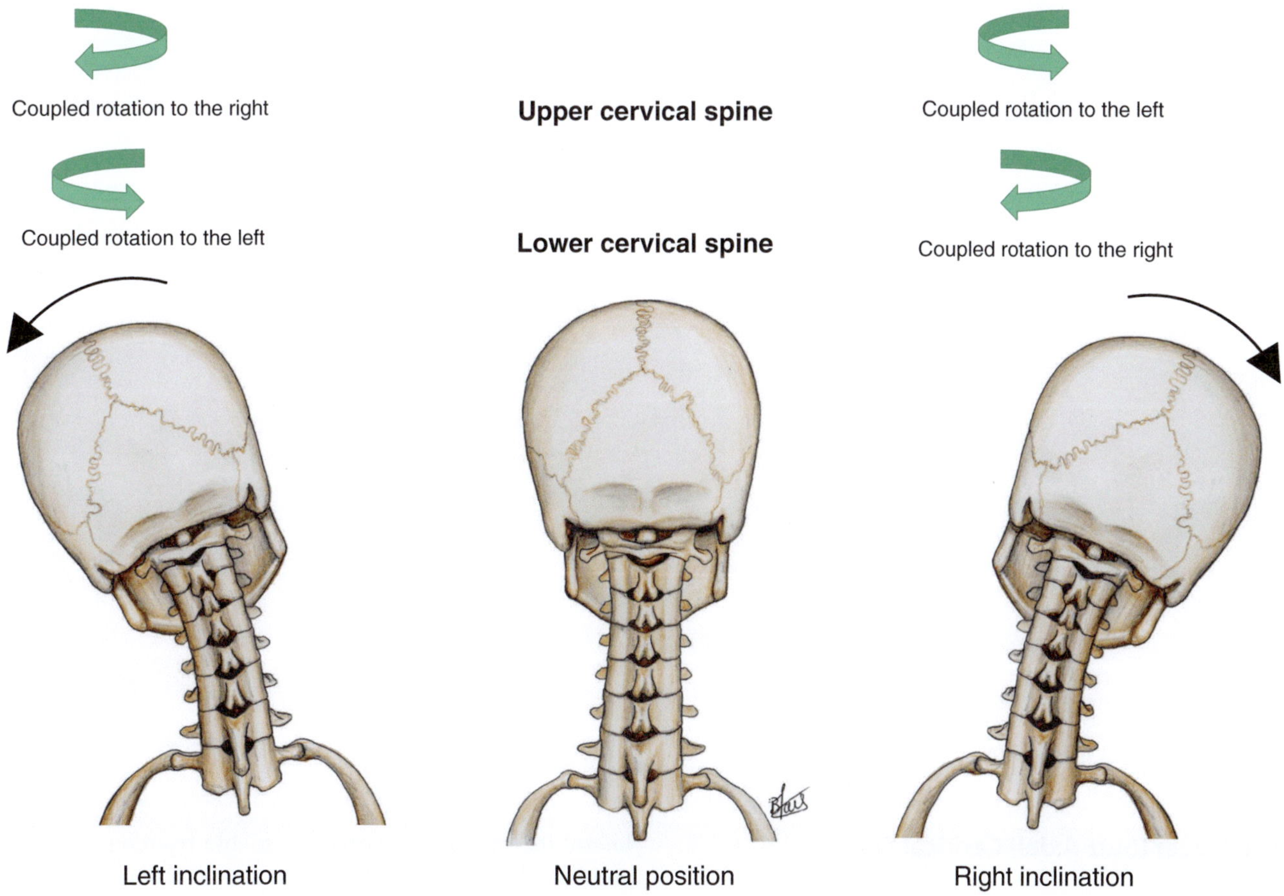

Fig. 16 Coupling rotation inclination at the cervical spine (Ishii [25])

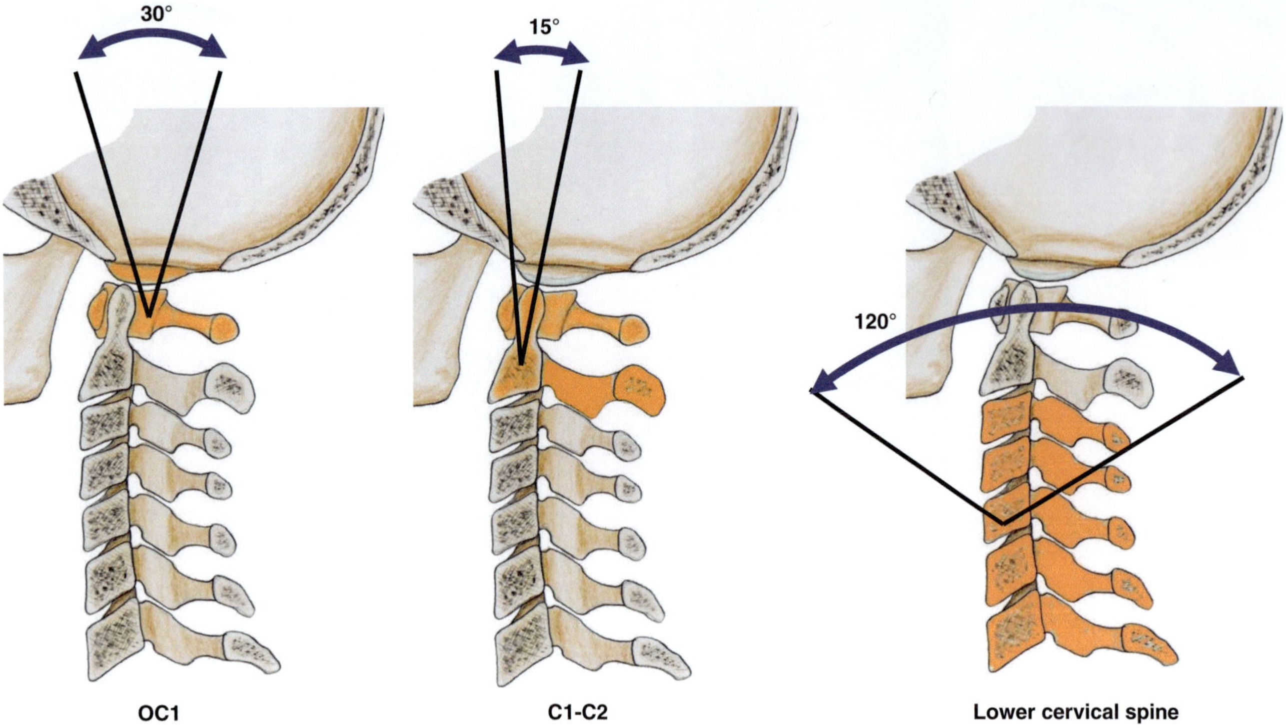

Fig. 17 Cervical flexion–extension amplitudes (Castaing [24])

Fig. 18 Cervical lateral inclination amplitudes (Castaing [24])

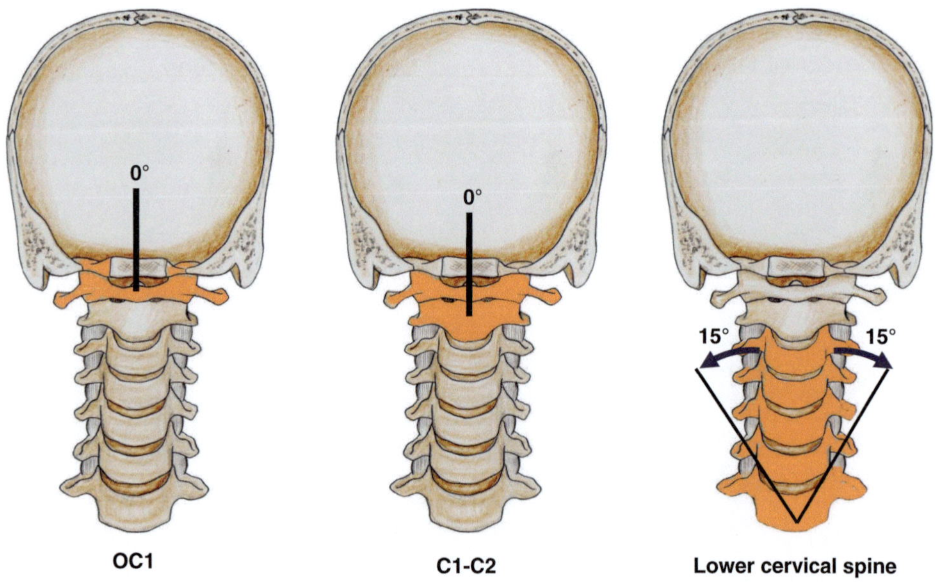

The Lower (Sub-Axial) Cervical Spine

Tables 3, 4, and 5 show different amplitudes reminiscent of intersegmental mobility noted in vitro and in vivo in the literature. The C5C6 segment is the most mobile, especially in flexion–extension and one will recall that the lesions of degenerative instability are most common at this level. The amplitudes of movement in rotation and lateral inclination are slightly variable from one level to another. The C7T1 segment is the least mobile in all movements.

The flexion–extension ICR, for a given intervertebral segment, is located in the middle of the lower part of the lower vertebral body (Fig. 27). Similarly, White and Panjabi [2], showed that ICRs are, for the 3 movements, at the level of the lower vertebral body (Fig. 28).

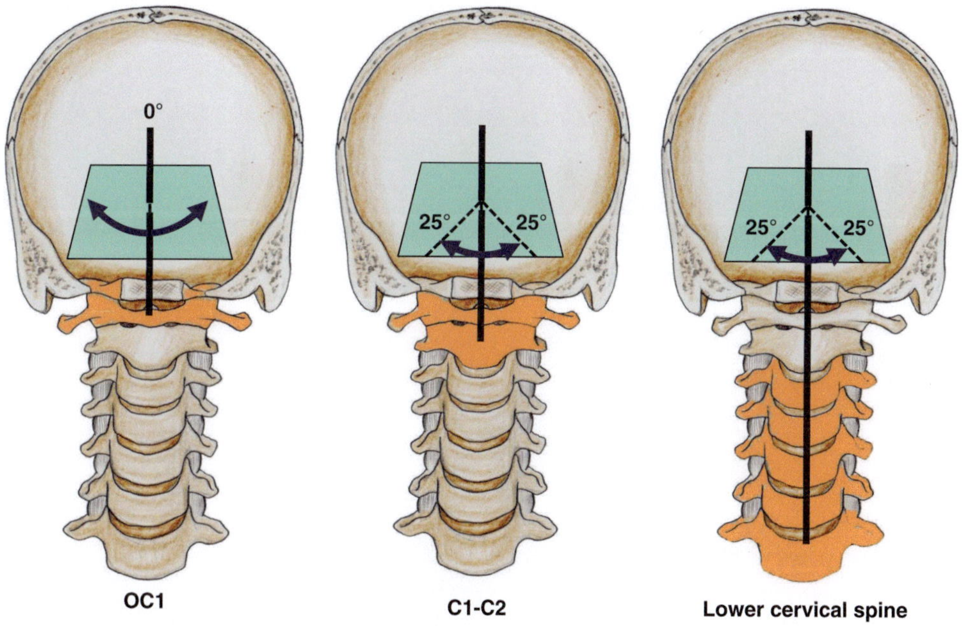

Fig. 19 Amplitudes of cervical rotation (Castaing [24])

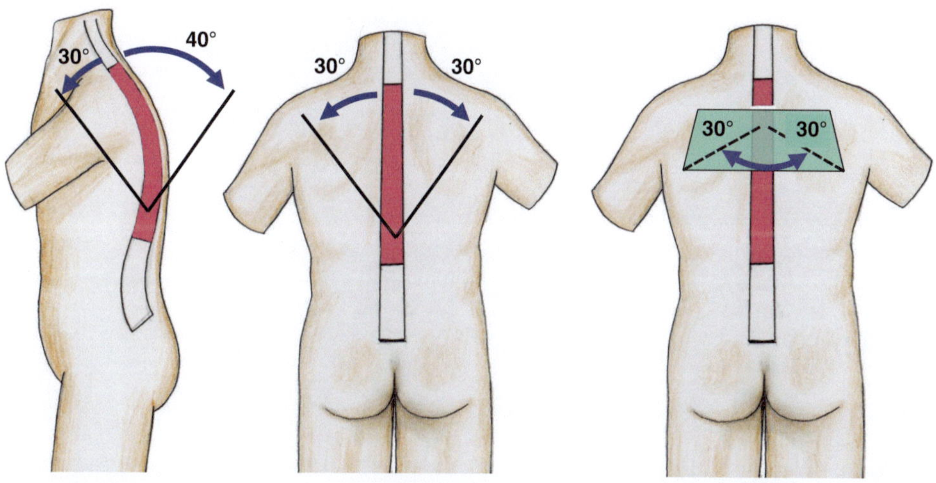

Fig. 20 Amplitudes of thoracic movements (Castaing [24])

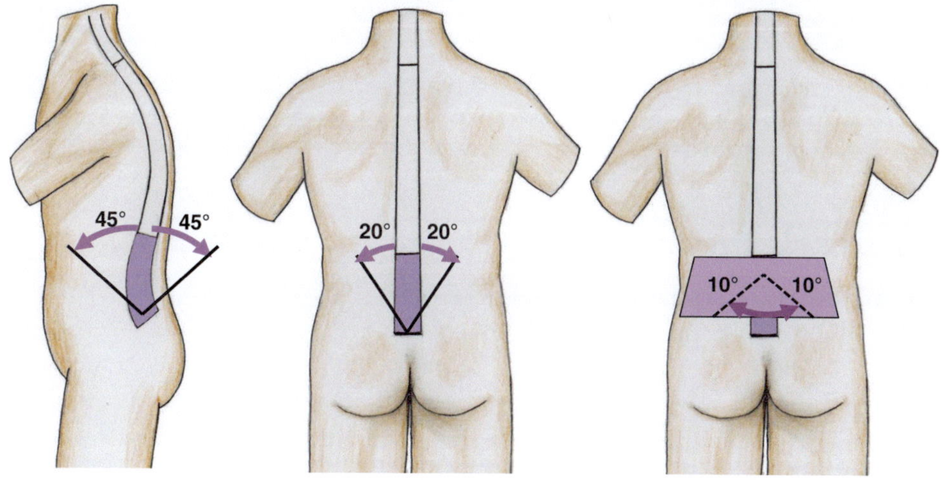

Fig. 21 Amplitudes of lumbar movements (Castaing [24])

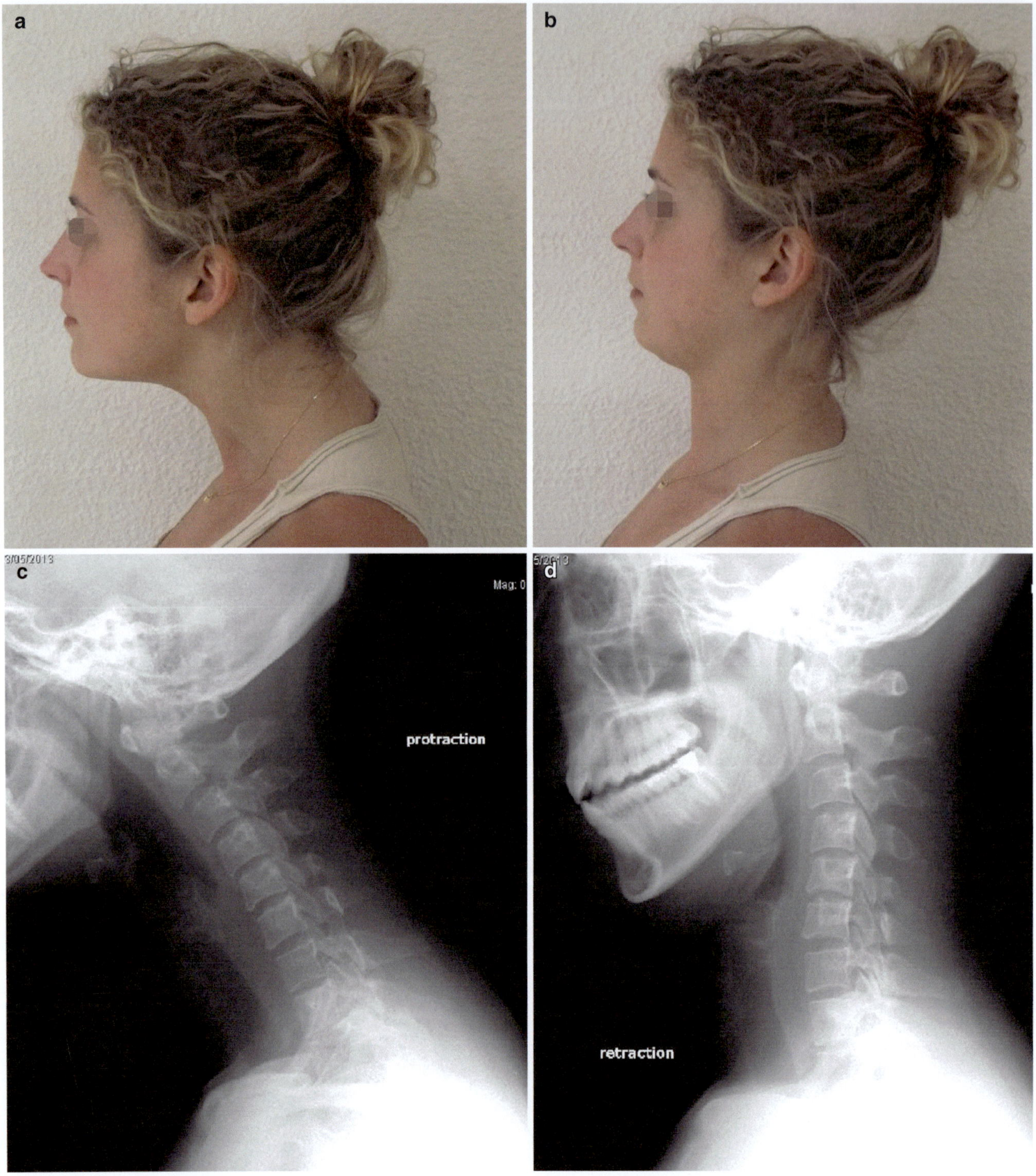

Fig. 22 Protraction (**a**, **c**) and retraction (**b**, **d**) movements

Table 2 Intersegmental motion upper cervical spine

	OC1			C1C2		
Authors	Flexion–extension	Lateral inclination	Axial rotation	Flexion–extension	Lateral inclination	Axial rotation L&R
Roy Camille [27]	50°	15°–20°	0°	10°	5°	40°
Brugger [28]	15°	0°	0°	15°	0°	80°
White and Panjabi [2]	25°	8°	0°	25°	0°	47°
Penning [29]	30°	5°	2°	30°	5°	81°
Louis [22]	20°	8°	8°	0°	0°	48°
Wen [30]	28.5°	8.3°	–	25.5°	9.8°	–
Watier [31]	28.7°	6.7°	11°	22.3°	9.3°	71°

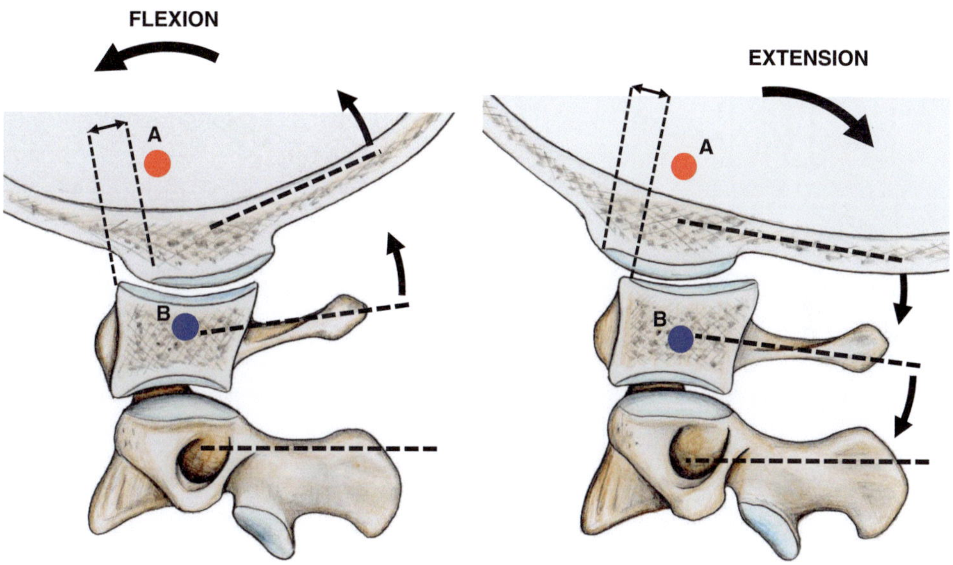

Fig. 23 Flexion–extension movements at OC1C2. A = ICR of the occipitocervical joint and B = ICR of the C1C2 joint

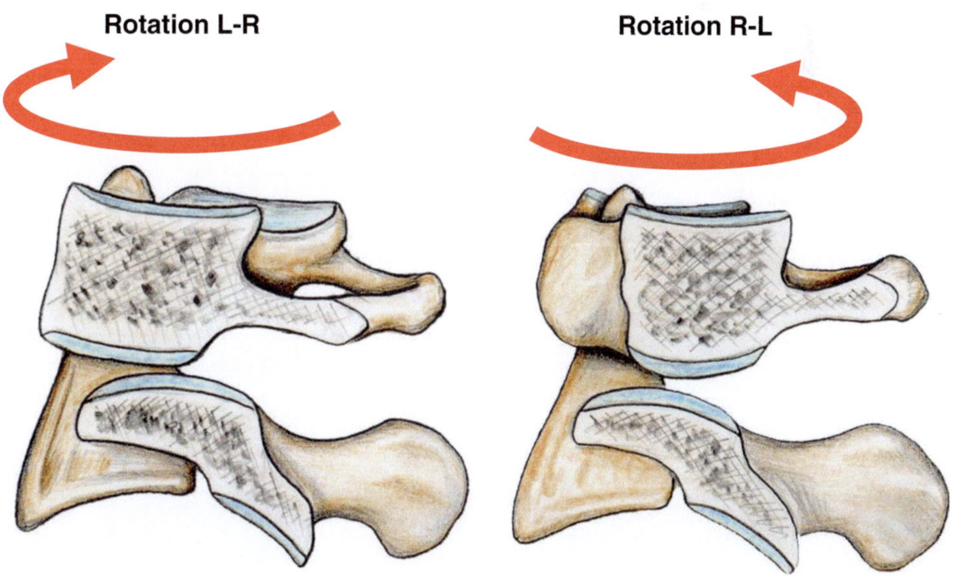

Fig. 24 Rotational movements at C1C2

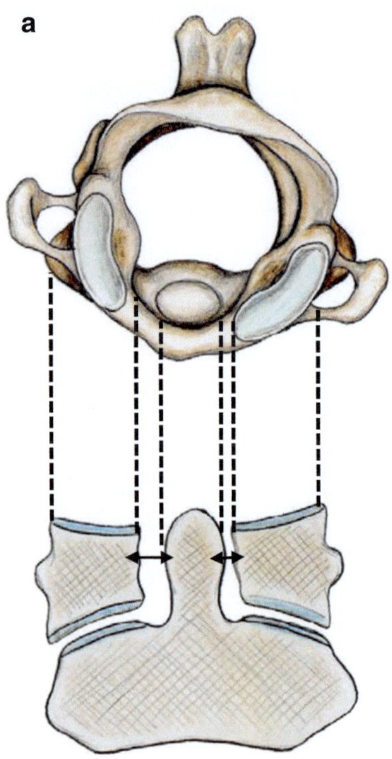

Fig. 25 Coronal projections of C1C2: Symmetrical if there is no rotation (**b**), asymmetrical if there is rotation (**a** and **c**)

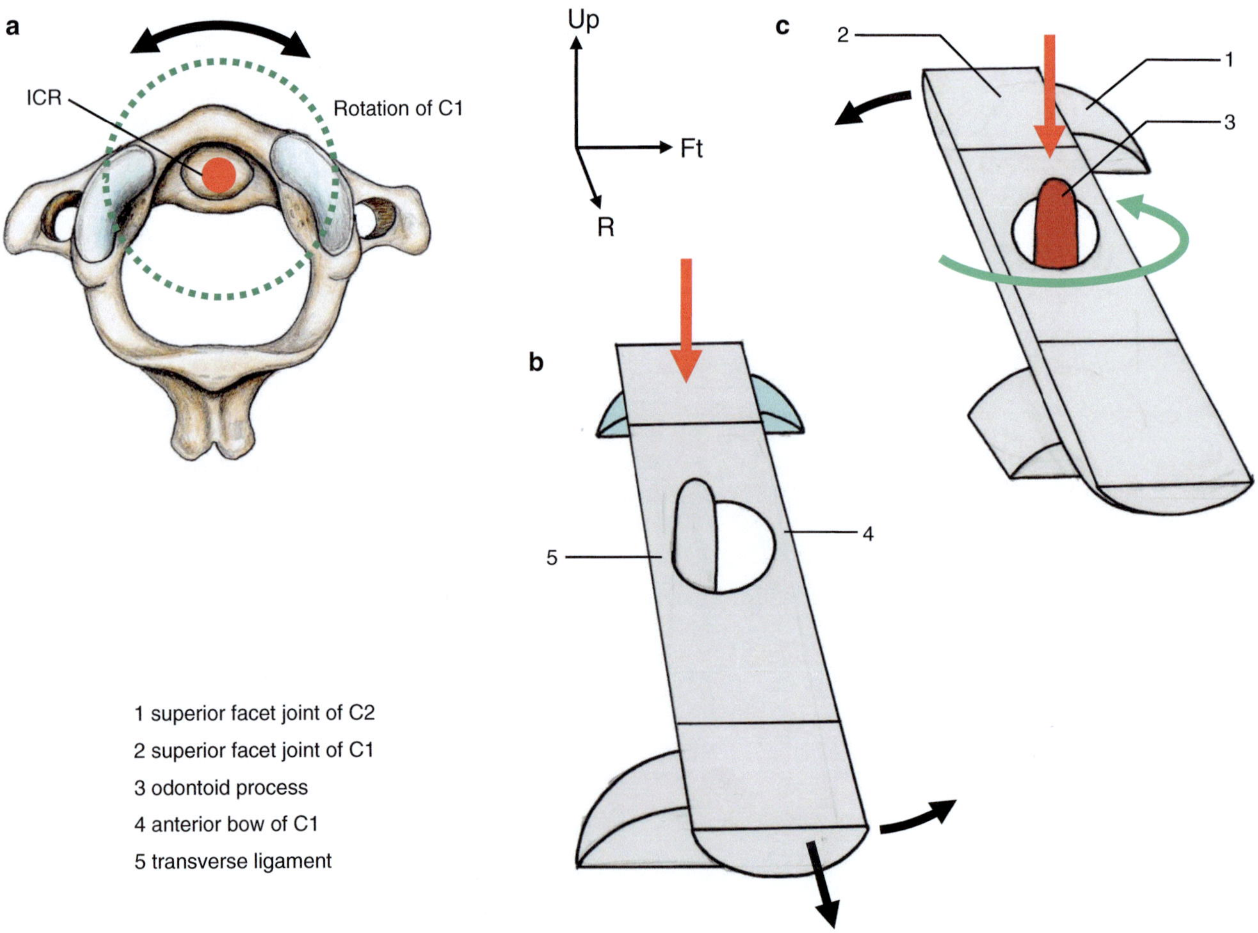

Fig. 26 ICR at the C1C2 rotation movement on a superior view (**a**), rotation around the left C1C2 articular facet joint (red arrow) (**b**), rotation around the odontoid (red arrow) (**c**) 1. Superior facet joint of C2; 2. Superior facet joint of C1; 3. odontoid process; 4. Anterior arc of C1; 5. Transverse ligament

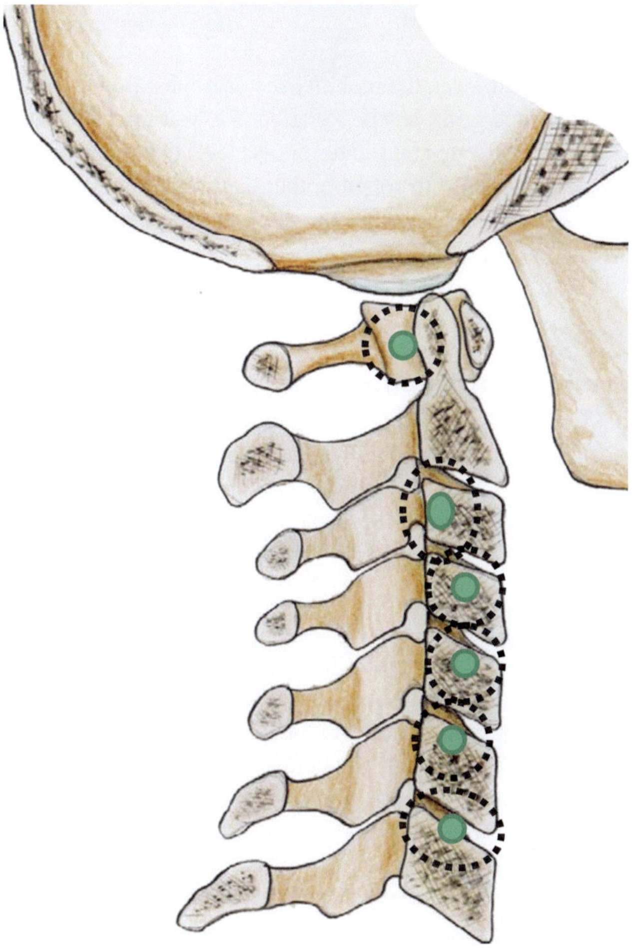

Fig. 27 ICR in flexion–extension according to Dvorak [32]

Table 3 Intersegmental sub-axial cervical flexion–extension motion

Authors	Flexion–extension sub-axial cervical spine					
	C2C3	C3C4	C4C5	C5C6	C6C7	C7T1
White and Panjabi [2]	8°	13°	12°	17°	16°	9°
Penning [29]	12°	18°	20°	20°	15°	–
Louis [22]	15°	15°	20°	22°	18°	10°
Dvorak [32]	12°	17°	21°	23°	21°	–
Wen [30]	11.8°	14.7°	13.3°	13.8°	12.3°	–
Watier [31]	7.3°	10.8°	13.8°	13.4°	10.8°	–
Lansade [33]	9°	16°	17°	17°	14°	–

Table 4 Intersegmental sub-axial cervical lateral inclination motion

Authors	Lateral inclination sub-axial cervical spine					
	C2C3	C3C4	C4C5	C5C6	C6C7	C7T1
White and Panjabi [2]	10°	11°	11°	8°	7°	4°
Penning [29]	6°	6°	6°	6°	6°	–
Louis [22]	10°	12°	12°	8°	9°	10°
Dvorak [32]	12.6°	13.4°	11°	10.6°	9.2°	–
Wen [30]	6.7°	6.7°	10.5°	11.2°	8.6°	–
Watier [31]	4°	3°	3°	4°	6°	–
Lansade [33]	6°	9°	8°	9°	11°	–

Table 5 Intersegmental sub-axial cervical rotation

Authors	Rotation sub-axial cervical spine					
	C2C3	C3C4	C4C5	C5C6	C6C7	C7T1
White and Panjabi [2]	9°	11°	12°	10°	9°	8°
Penning [29]	6°	13°	13.6°	13.8°	10.8°	–
Louis [22]	12°	12°	14°	12°	12°	12°
Watier [31]	9.5°	10.8°	12.3°	9°	10°	–
Ishii [34]	2°	4°	5°	4°	2°	–
Lansade [33]	8°	9°	7°	9°	6°	–

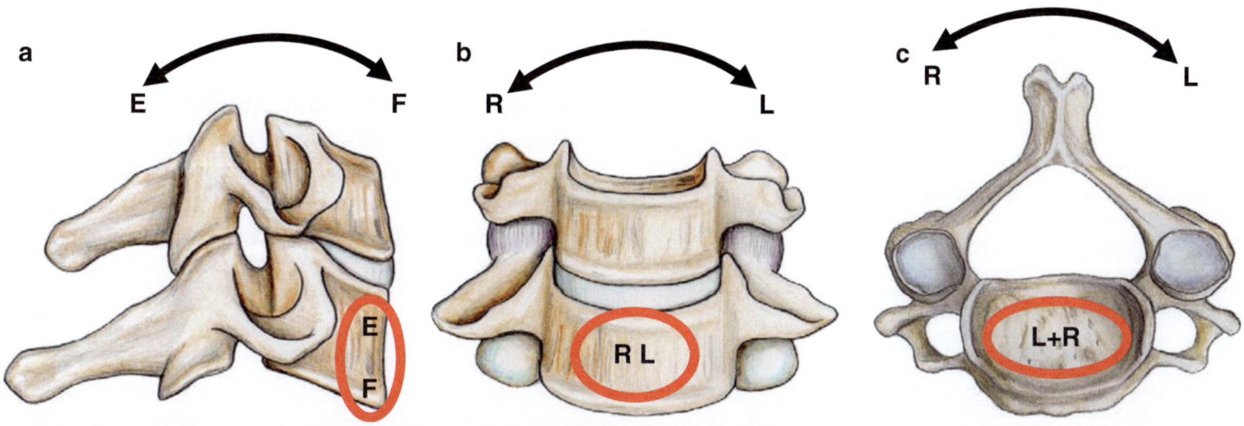

Fig. 28 ICR in flexion–extension (**a**), lateral inclination (**b**), and rotation (**c**) at the sub-axial cervical spine, according to White and Panjabi [2]

The Table 6 of Watier [31] shows the values of normal anteroposterior and lateral translations observed during flexion–extension and lateral inclination movements. These figures may seem high in clinical practice since it is estimated:

- that in C2C3, there can exist in flexion a physiological anterolisthesis of 2.5–3.5 mm (particularly in a child with a flexion hinge at C2C3),
- then from C3 to C7, this anterolisthesis can reach 1.5–2 mm. Beyond these limits, there is instability as in cervical severe sprain where the offset reaches 3 mm.

The Thoracic Spine

At the thoracic spine, the magnitudes are much lower, as the ribcage significantly attenuates the intersegmental mobility. Flexion–extension is three times greater at the lower thoracic level than the upper thoracic level where rotation is almost nil. Lateral inclination is apportioned equally at all levels (Table 7). ICRs are at the lower mid-vertebral body level in flexion, inclination, and rotation (Fig. 29).

Table 6 Cervical translation, according to Watier [31]

Level	Anteroposterior translation (in mm) average (standard deviation)	Level	Lateral inclination translation (in mm) average (standard deviation)
C0C1	−8.1 (2.7)	C0C1	5.7 (3.1)
C1C2	3.4 (1.5)	C1C2	−1.8 (3.2)
C2C3	3.1 (2.3)	C2C3	−1.5 (0.6)
C3C4	3.3 (2.3)	C3C4	−1.7 (0.9)
C4C5	3.6 (1.7)	C4C5	−2.1 (1.3)
C5C6	3.4 (1.8)	C5C6	−2.1 (1.3)
C6C7	2.1 (1.3)	C6C7	−1.9 (0.9)
C7T1	1.3 (1)	C7T1	−0.9 (0.7)

The minus sign (−) signifies a posterior translation in flexion–extension or contralateral in inclination

The Lumbar Spine

At the lumbar level, the mobility sector is most important for the L4L5 and L5S1 levels. Rotation is low at the L5S1 level (Table 8). ICRs are at the anterior disc level in flexion, further back in extension. In rotation, they are in the middle of the disc and toward the side of the disc opposite the side of the inclination (Fig. 30). We recall that Gertzbein [12] demonstrated a dispersion of these ICRs on degenerate discs (Fig. 7).

Evolution of Amplitudes with Age

Numerous authors have shown decreased range of motion at all spinal levels with age.

Arbogast [36] measured the range of motion in 67 children (including 39 girls) for age groups 3–5, 6–8, and 9–12 years, demonstrating how flexion and extension vary little with age, unlike lateral inclination and rotation (Fig. 31).

Wong [37] evaluated the lumbar level in 100 individuals classified into four age groups (20–30 years (group A), 30–40 years (group B), 40–50 years (group C), and more than 50 years (group D)); Fig. 32 shows a decrease in the amplitudes of movement, with a radical change from 50 years. Swinkels [38] did the same study in the cervical region of 400 volunteers for the four same age brackets; with identical results—net reduction of mobility after 50 years, as shown in Table 9.

The study of the influence of aging on mobility has mostly been studied at the level of the cervical spine. Figure 33 by Castaing [24] shows this decrease in mobility. Youdas [3] conducted a study on cervical spine mobility with CROM® by age group and gender on 171 women and 166 men aged between 11 and 97 years old. For this author, there is a linear decrease in mobility over all decades. In a meta-analysis, Chen [39] notes a linear decrease of 4° per decade for each cervical movement. Finally, for Feipel [40], this decrease in mobility is not linear.

Table 7 Intersegmental Thoracic Motion

	Flexion–extension		Lateral inclination (one side)		Axial rotation (one side)	
Authors	Vanneuville [45]	White and Panjabi [2]	Vanneuville [45]	White and Panjabi [2]	Vanneuville [45]	White and Panjabi [2]
T1 T2	4°	4°	3°	3°	4.5°	4°
T2 T3	4°	4°	3°	3°	4°	4°
T3 T4	4°	4°	3°	3°	4°	4°
T4 T5	4°	4°	3°	3°	4°	4°
T5 T6	4°	5°	3°	3°	4°	4°
T6 T7	5°	6°	3°	3°	4°	4°
T7 T8	6°	6°	3°	3°	4°	3.5°
T8 T9	6°	6°	3°	3°	3.5°	2°
T9 T10	6°	9°	3°	2.5°	2°	2°
T10 T11	7°	12°	4°	4.5°	1°	1°
T11 T12	12°	12°	4.5°	4°	1°	1°
Total	63°	72°	35.5°	35°	36°	33.5°

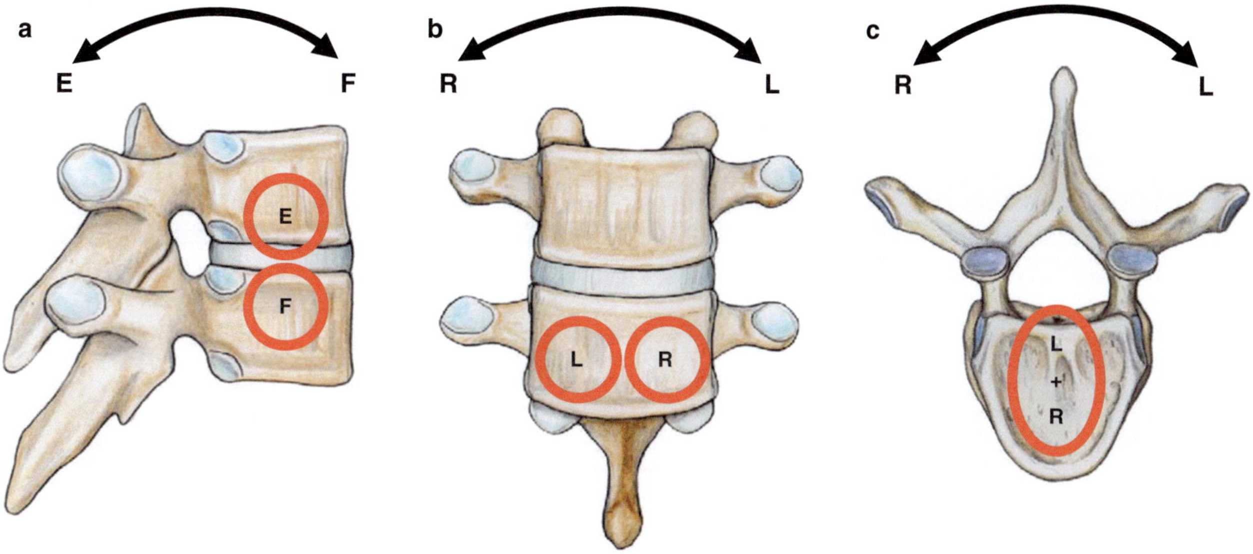

Fig. 29 ICR in flexion–extension (**a**), lateral inclination (**b**), and rotation (**c**) motion at the thoracic level, according to White and Panjabi [2]

Table 8 Inter-segmental Lumbar Motion

	Flexion–extension		Lateral inclination	Axial rotation
Authors	White and Panjabi [2]	Pearcy [35]	White and Panjabi [2]	White and Panjabi [2]
L1 L2	12°	13°	6°	2°
L2 L3	14°	14°	6°	2°
L3 L4	15°	13°	8°	2°
L4 L5	17°	16°	6°	2°
L5S1	20°	14°	3°	5°

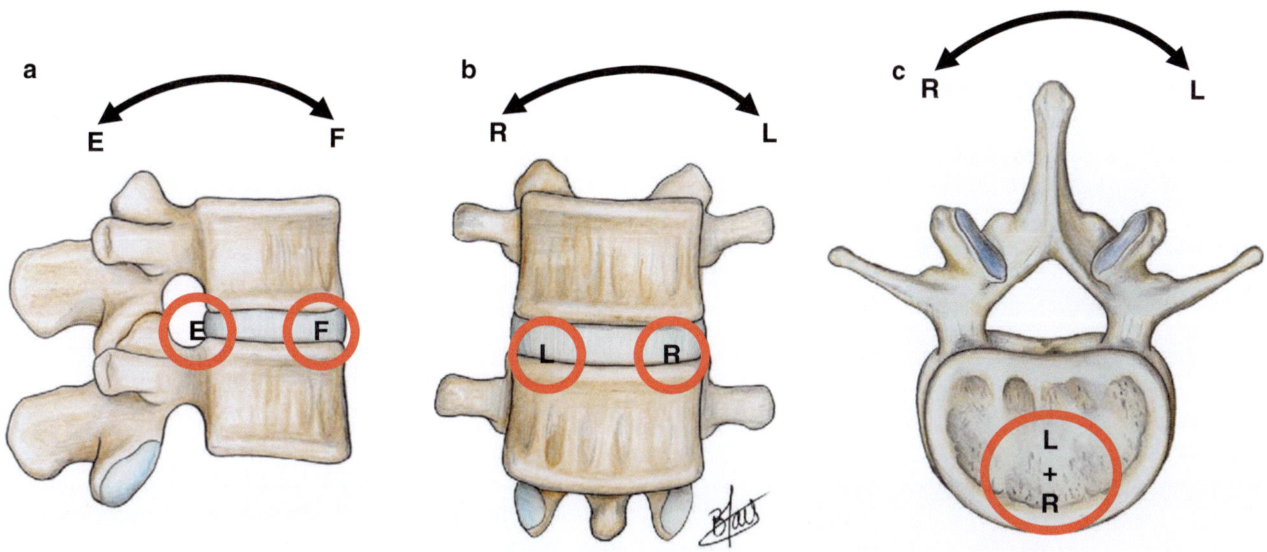

Fig. 30 ICR in flexion–extension (**a**), lateral inclination (**b**), and rotation (**c**) motion at the lumbar level, according to White and Panjabi [2]

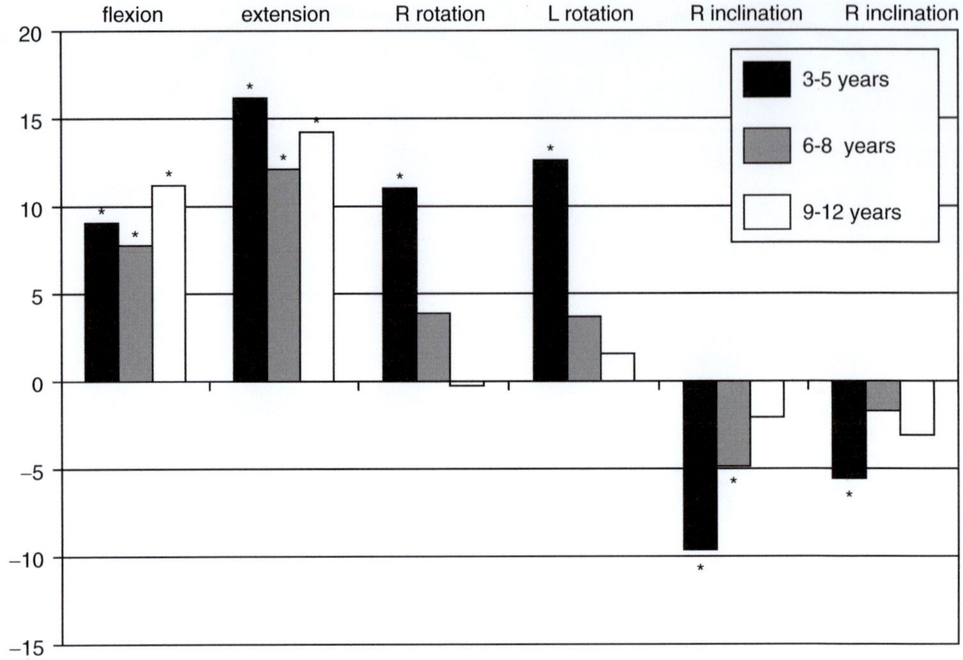

Fig. 31 Evolution of cervical mobility according to three age groups in children (Arbogast [36])

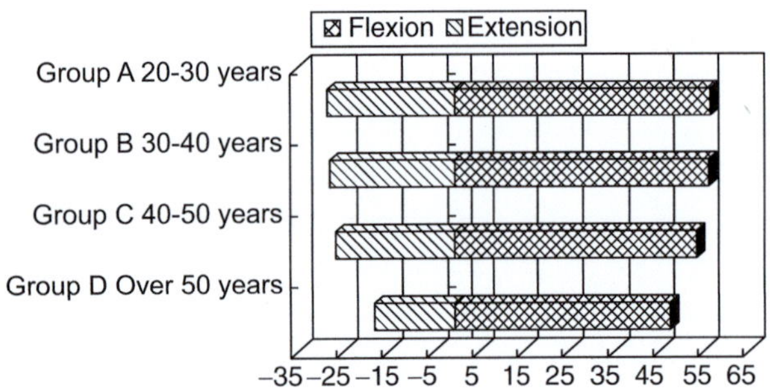

Fig. 32 Diagram showing the mobility reduction in lumbar flexion–extension especially from 50 years (group D) (Wong [37])

Table 9 Evolution of motion by age [38]

Mobility according to age				
Movement	20–29 years N = 100	30–39 years N = 100	40–49 years N = 100	50–59 years N = 100
Flexion	60°	58°	59°	53°
Extension	75°	69°	66°	64°
Right inclination	46°	43°	41°	38°
Left inclination	45°	42°	40°	38°
Right rotation	78°	79°	79°	71°
Left rotation	79°	79°	78°	71°

It is obvious that this loss of mobility due to aging is related to disc narrowing, posterior articular arthrosis, ligament stiffness, and muscular fat degeneration.

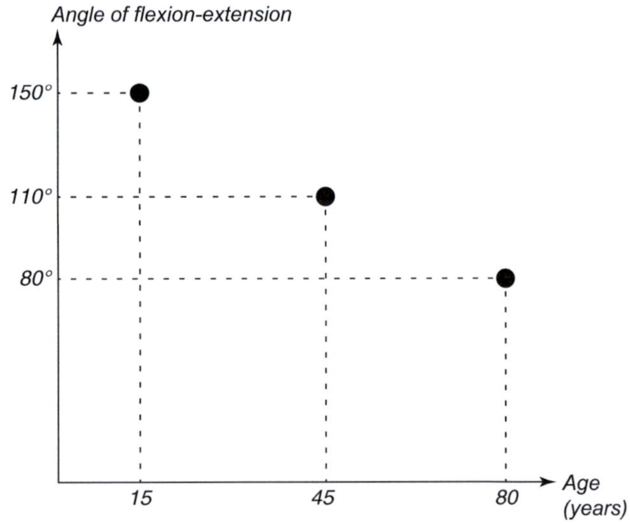

Fig. 33 Diagram showing the reduction of motion of flexion–extension (Castaing [24])

The Movements of the Vertebral Column in Daily Life

Few articles in the literature have focused on the range of motion of the various spinal segments during everyday activities. We will simply quote Bible [41] which describes 15 activities of everyday life that he has evaluated in 30 men and 30 women, ranging in age from 20 to 75 years.

These 16 activities are as follows:

- sitting down
- sitting in a car
- reading with a book on the knees
- cutting meat with knife and fork and bringing it to the mouth
- putting on socks
- tying shoes
- arising from a sitting position
- washing the hands while standing
- to wash the hair in the shower
- shaving the face
- putting on makeup
- picking up an object off the floor with bended knees
- picking up an object off the floor by leaning forward
- walking
- ascending the stairs
- descending the stairs.

All of these activities involve variably different spinal segments and are fully described in Figs. 34, 35, and 36.

The author insists that a small proportion of movements are involved in these daily movements (Table 10).

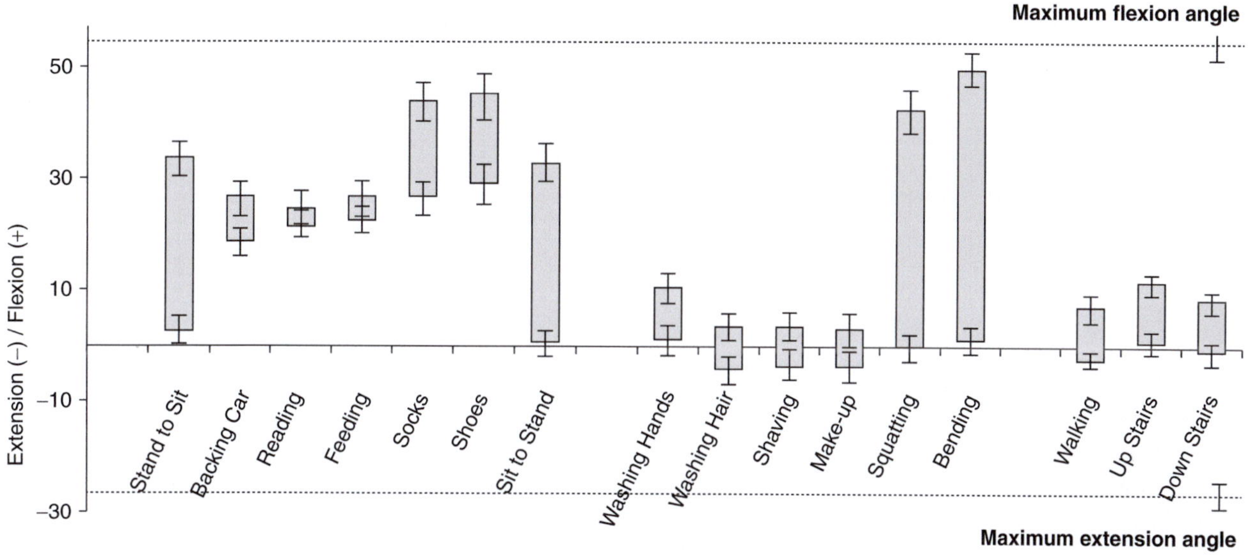

Fig. 34 Percentage of flexion and lumbar extension in the movements of everyday life (Bible [41])

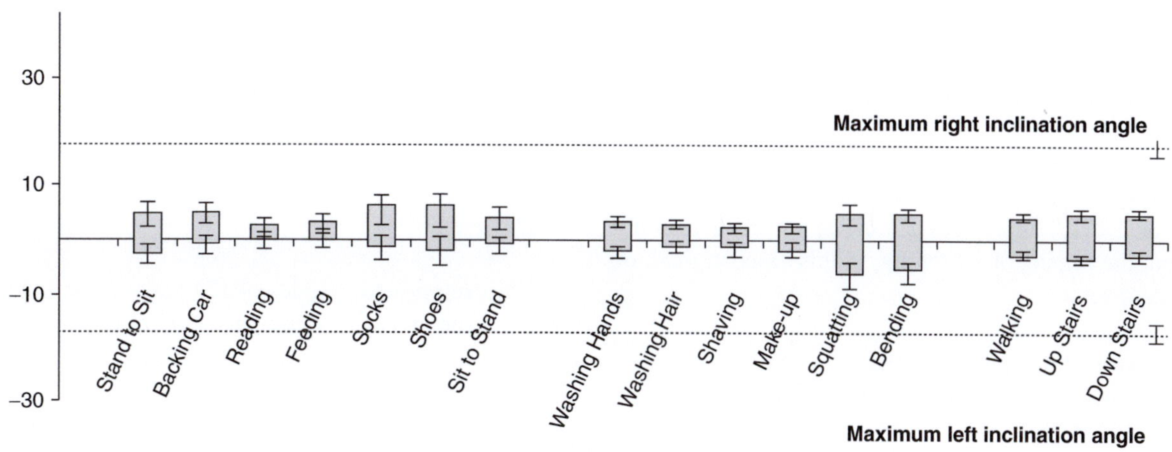

Fig. 35 Percentage of lumbar lateral inclination movement in the movements of everyday life (Bible [41])

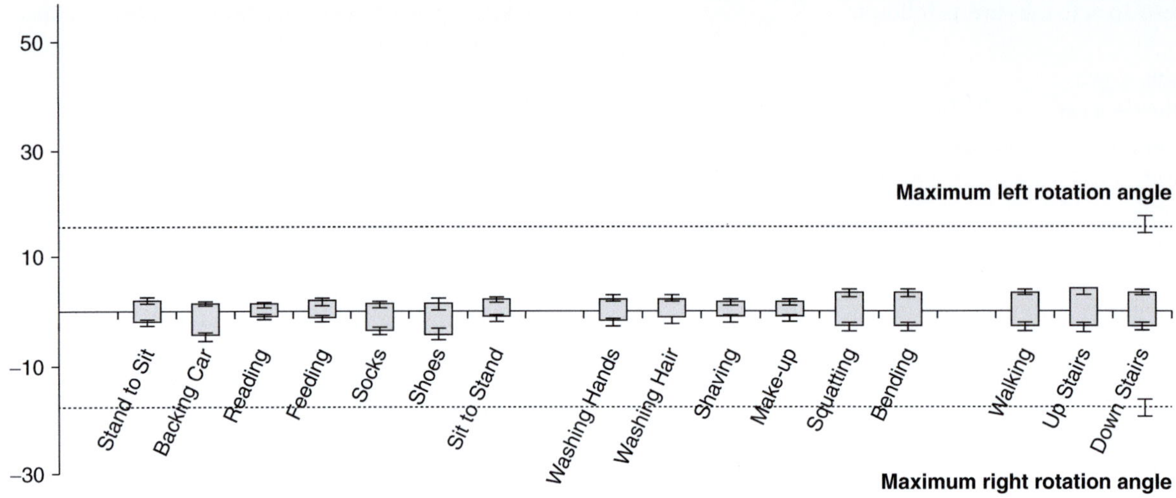

Fig. 36 Percentage of lateral rotation movement in the movements of everyday life (Bible [41])

Table 10 Percentage of flexion–extension, inclination, and rotation in the movements of everyday life [41]

	Percentage of complete movement		
Activities of daily life	Percentage of flexion–extension	Percentage of inclination	Percentage of rotation
Sit	37	20	12
Sit in a car	10	16	18
Read a magazine on the knees	4	6	6
Cut meat with fork and knife and bring to the mouth	5	8	9
Put on socks	22	19	14
To lace shoes	20	20	16
Getting up from a sitting position	39	14	10
Wash the hands while standing	12	15	12
Wash hair in the shower	9	11	12
To shave	8	11	9
Makeup	7	11	8
Pick an object off the ground by bending the knees	52	31	18
Pick an object off the ground by leaning forward	59	29	18
Walk	11	19	19
To go upstairs	13	22	20
Go down the stairs	11	21	18

More recently, Sciubba [42] has evaluated the repercussions of spinal arthrodesis with extension to the pelvis on other movements of daily life with the ten criteria of Hart [43] constituting the "Lumbar Stiffness Disability Index or LSDI " appreciating more appropriately, in our opinion, the impact of stiffening, in this case surgical, on everyday life:

1. Bend forward to put on trousers
2. Lean forward to put on stockings or socks
3. Drive a car
4. Wipe after toileting
5. Lean forward to pick up a small object on the ground
6. Go to bed or get up from bed
7. Sit or stand up from a chair
8. Wash the lower half of the body
9. Enter and exit the car
10. Have sex

In this retrospective series of 134 patients, Sciubba [42] compares the impact of spino-pelvic arthrodesis, with proximal extension to the thoracolumbar or upper thoracic (UT) spine. Both groups had statistically similar scores at 2 years compared to preoperative values with the exception of questions #2 (Bend through your waist to put socks and shoes on) and #8 (bathe lower half of body) in which UT reported increased difficulty. The greatest change from pre-operatively involved dressing or bathing the lower half of the body among patients with upper thoracic fixation. The only domain for which UT had greater impairment was in performing personal hygiene functions after toileting. Finally, some images by Muybridge [44] show the involvement of the various spinal segments in daily life (Figs. 37, 38, 39, 40, 41, 42, 43, 44, 45, 46, 47, 48, and 49).

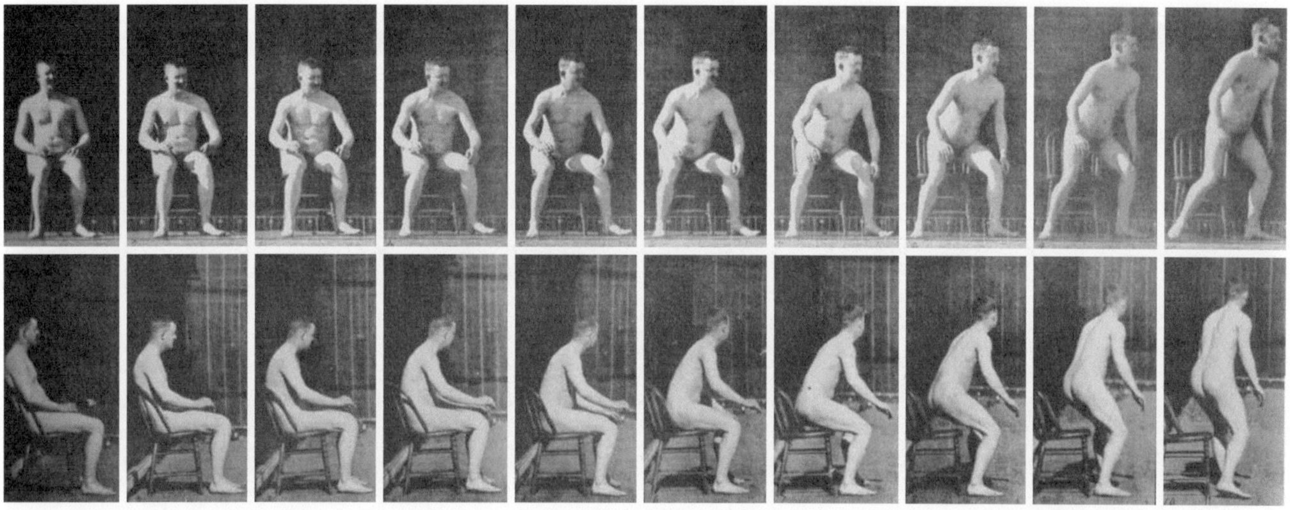

Fig. 37 Action of getting up from a seat; note the extension of the lumbar spine at the end of the movement (Muybridge [44])

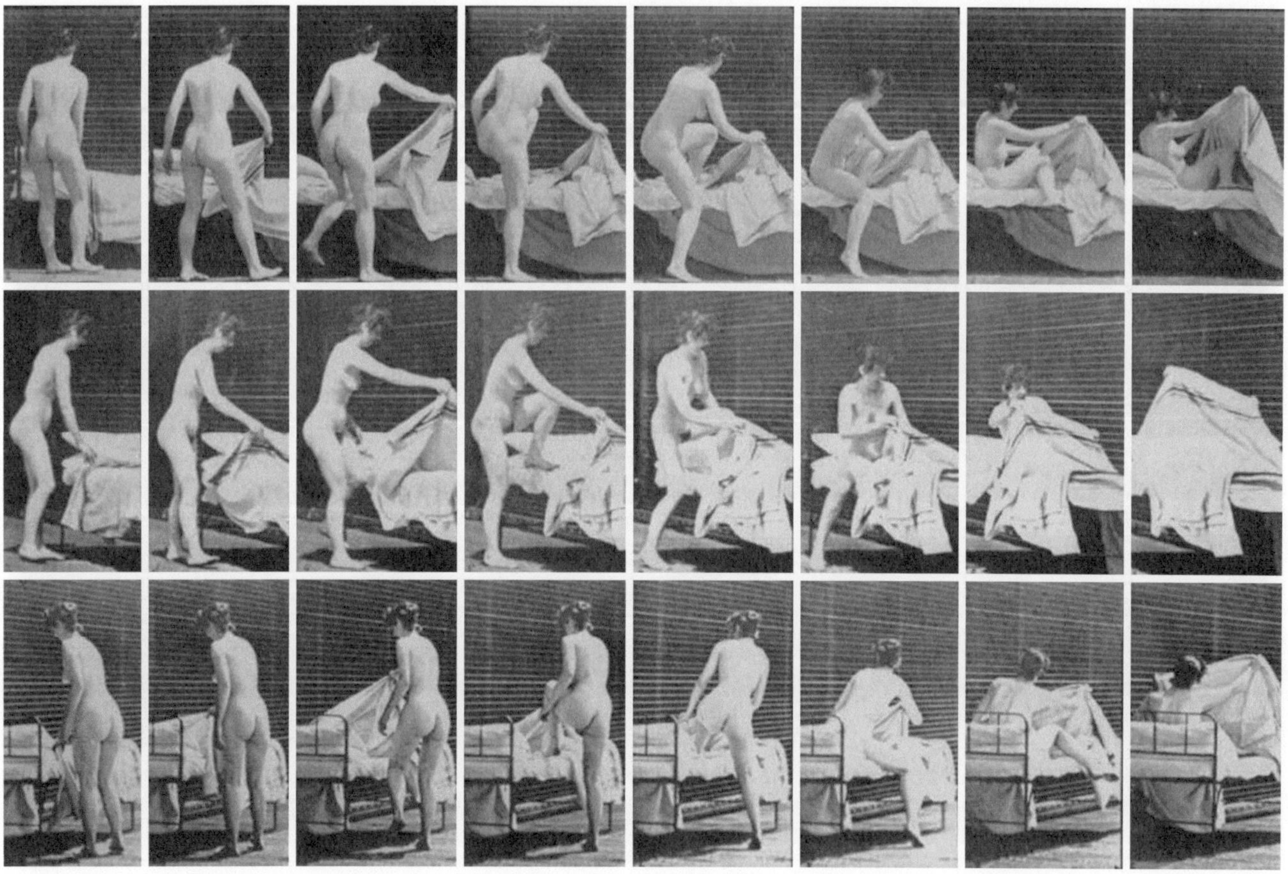

Fig. 38 Action of lying down in bed; flexion and rotation of the lumbar spine exist at the end of the movement (Muybridge [44])

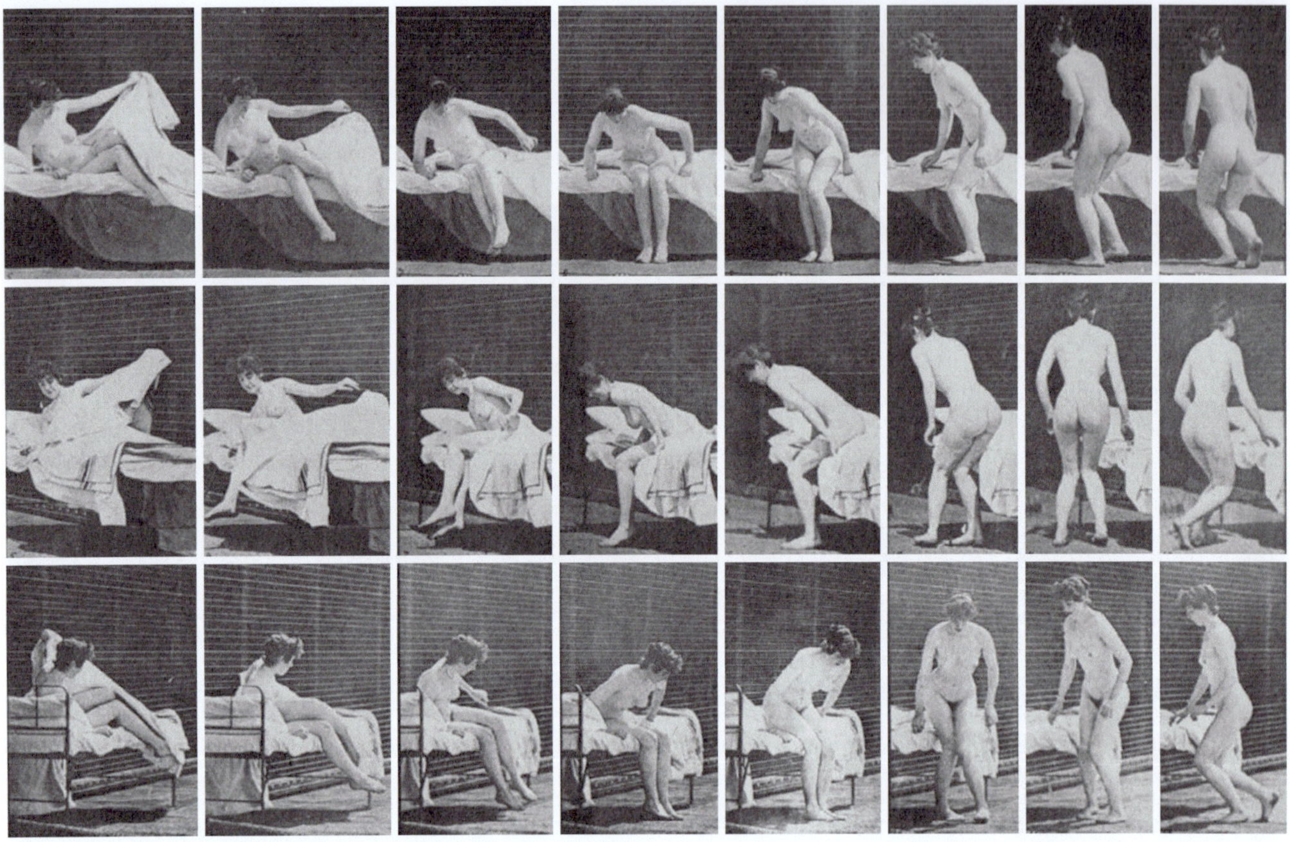

Fig. 39 Action of getting up from bed; extension and rotation of the lumbar spine are well marked at the end of the movement (Muybridge [44])

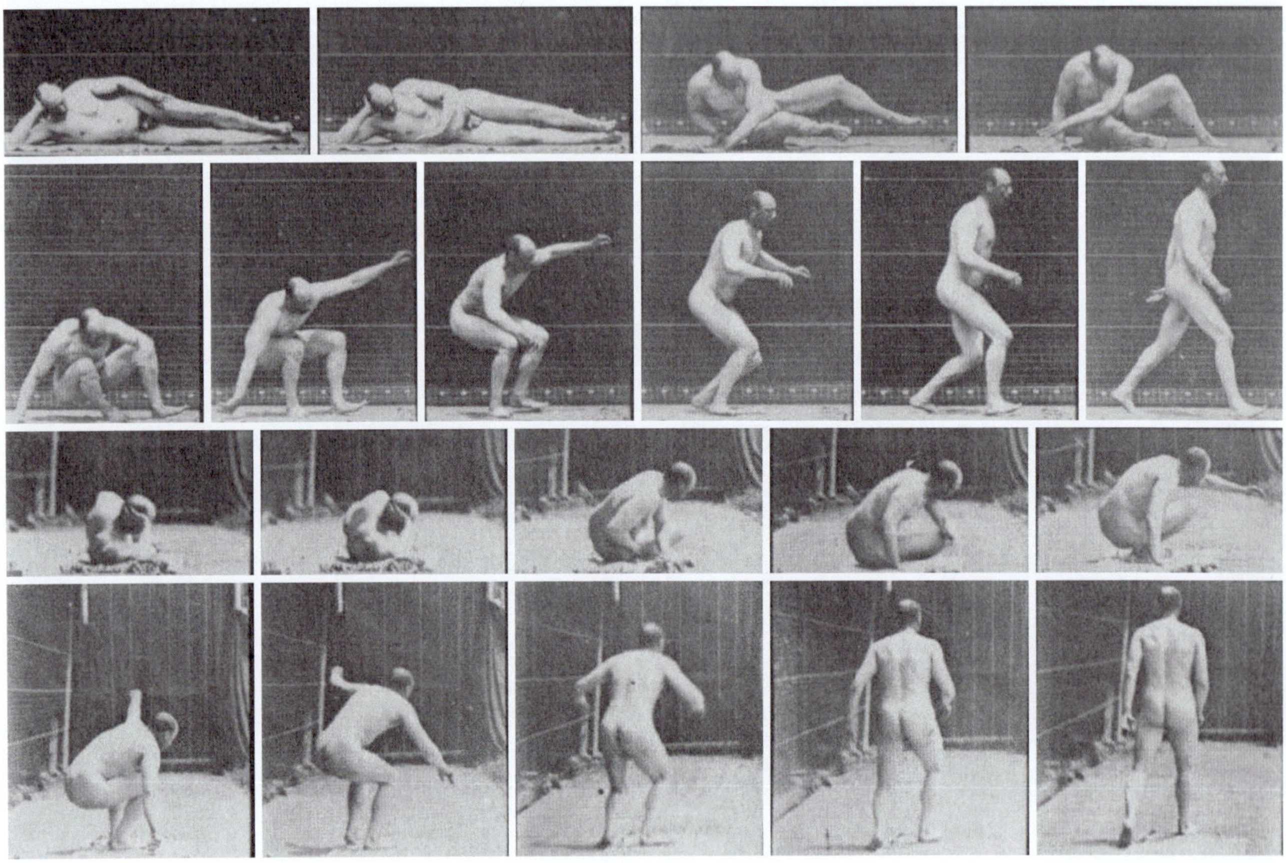

Fig. 40 Action of rising from a lying position on the ground; this difficult movement requires a marked lumbar extension with rotation (Muybridge [44])

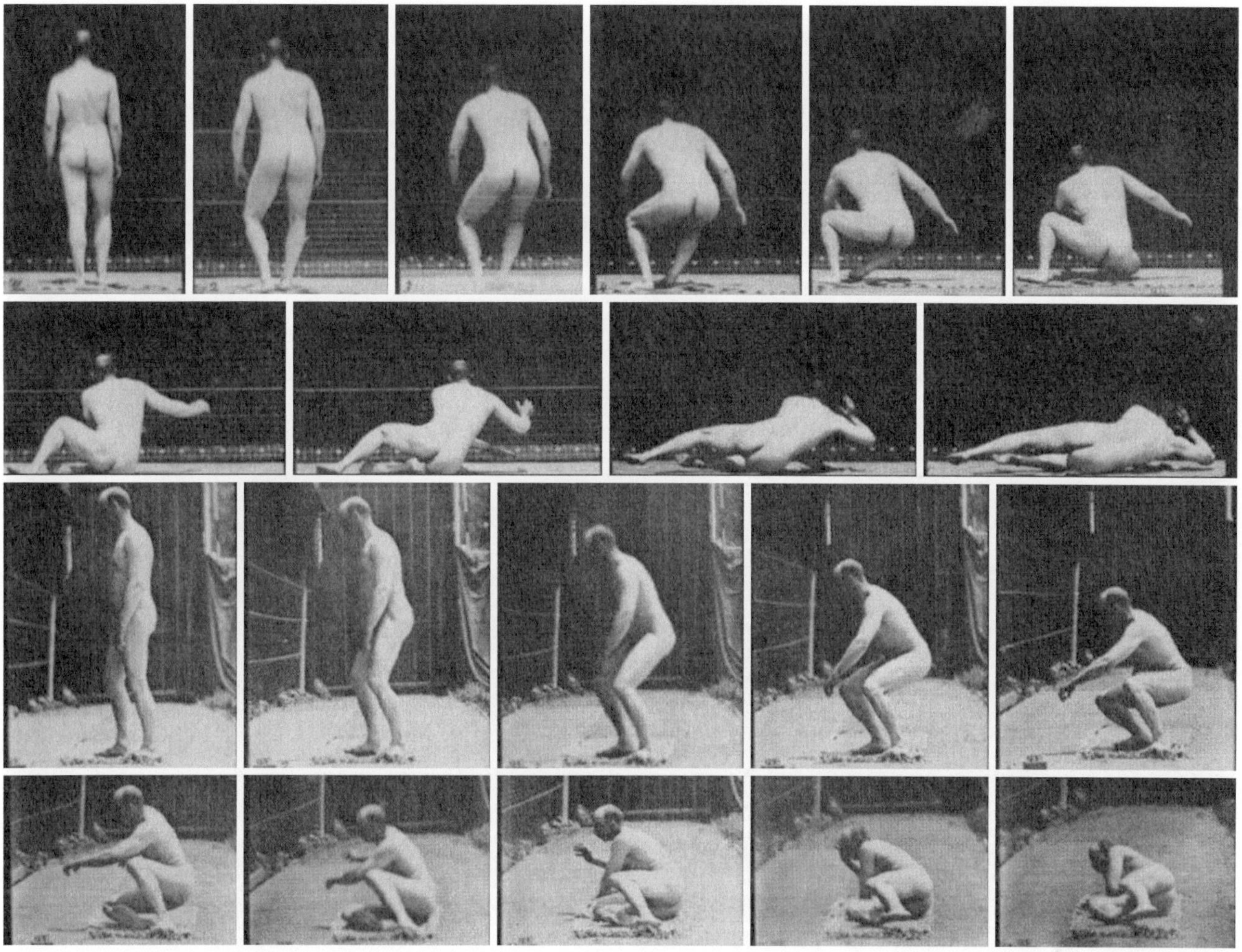

Fig. 41 Action of lying down on the ground; this movement is consistently in lumbar kyphosis but imposes inclination and rotation (Muybridge [44])

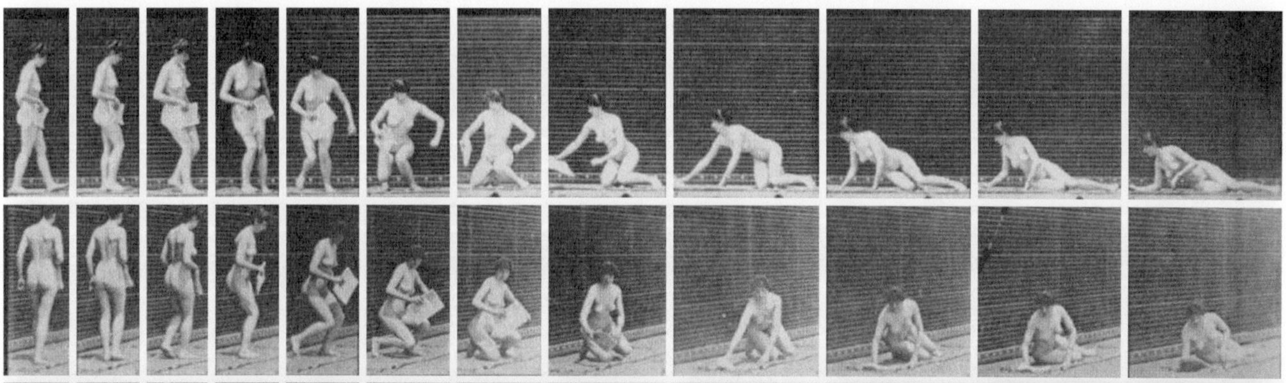

Fig. 42 Action of lying on the floor by bending the knees; flexion of the lumbar spine is reduced to the detriment of rotational tilt movements (Muybridge [44])

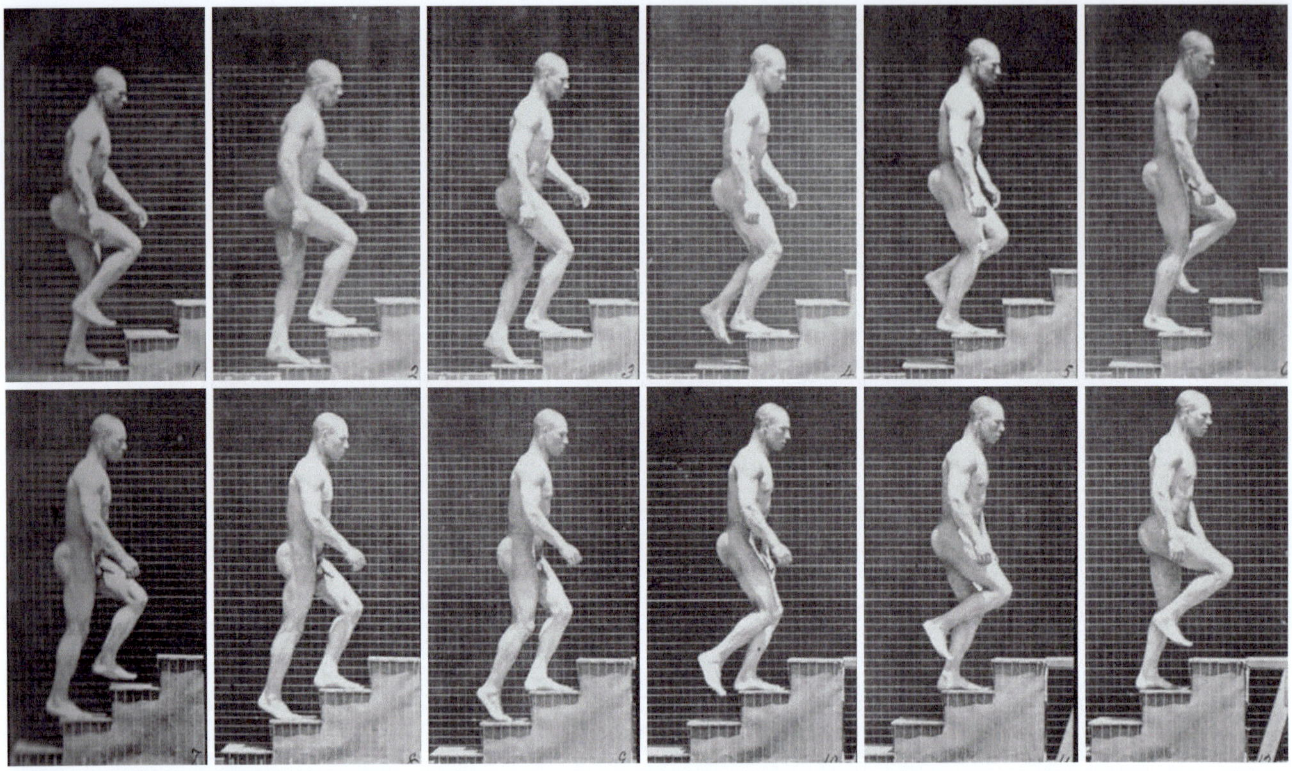

Fig. 43 Action of climbing stairs; note the relative unchanging shape of the entire spine (Muybridge [44])

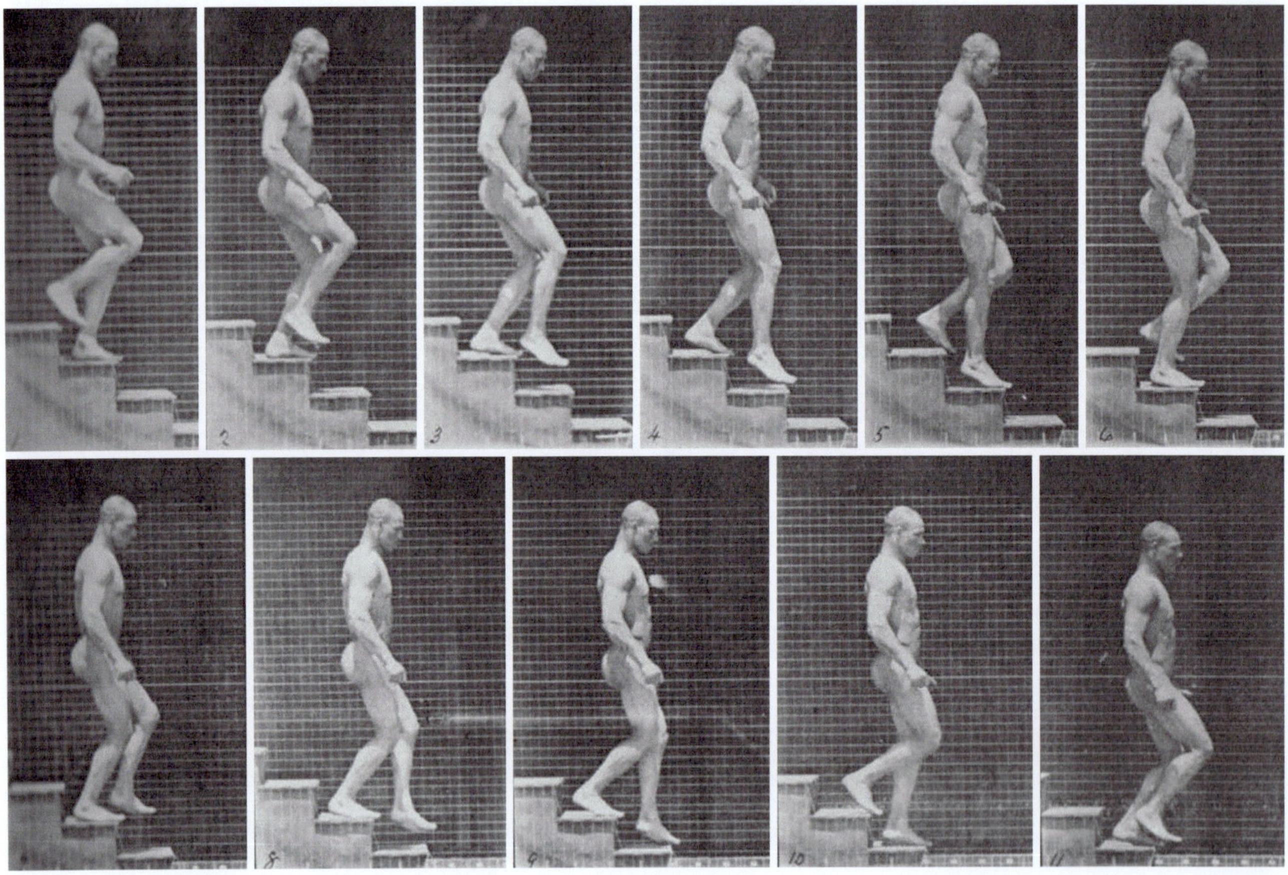

Fig. 44 Descending the stairs; note the largest extension of the lumbar spine (Muybridge [44])

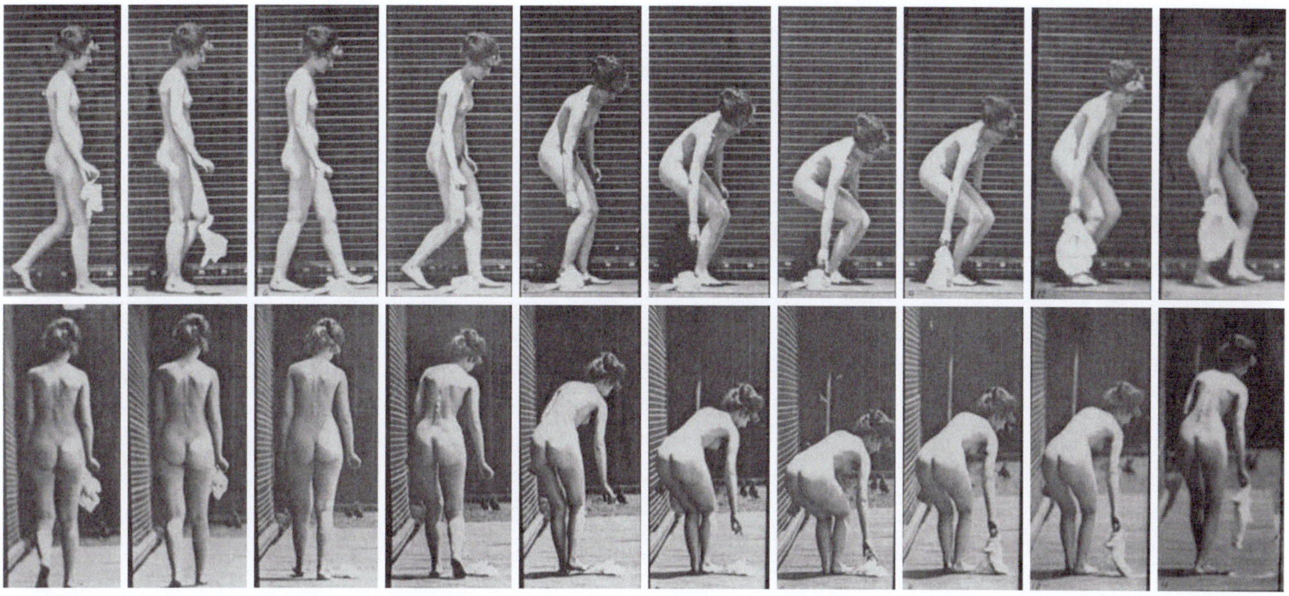

Fig. 45 Action of picking up an object on the ground on the side; this movement involves a rotation to the same side, but the flexion of the knees reduces flexion of the lumbar spine (Muybridge [44])

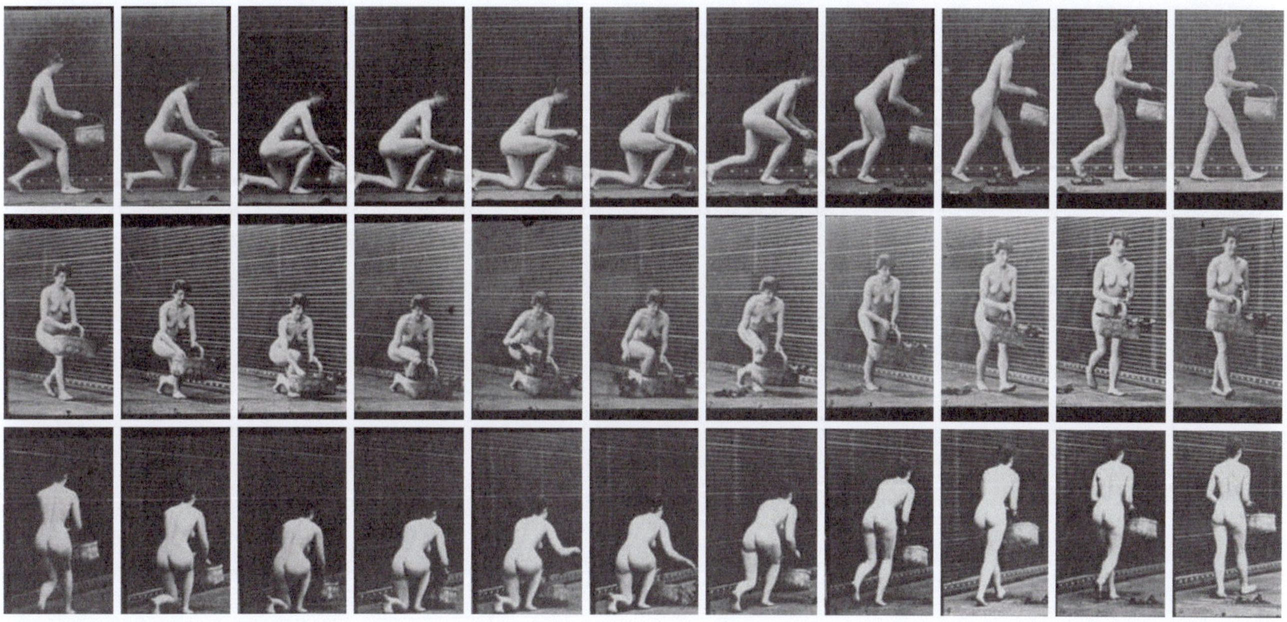

Fig. 46 Action of picking up an object in front by putting one knee on the ground; the flexion of the hips and knees reduces that of the lumbar spine (Muybridge [44])

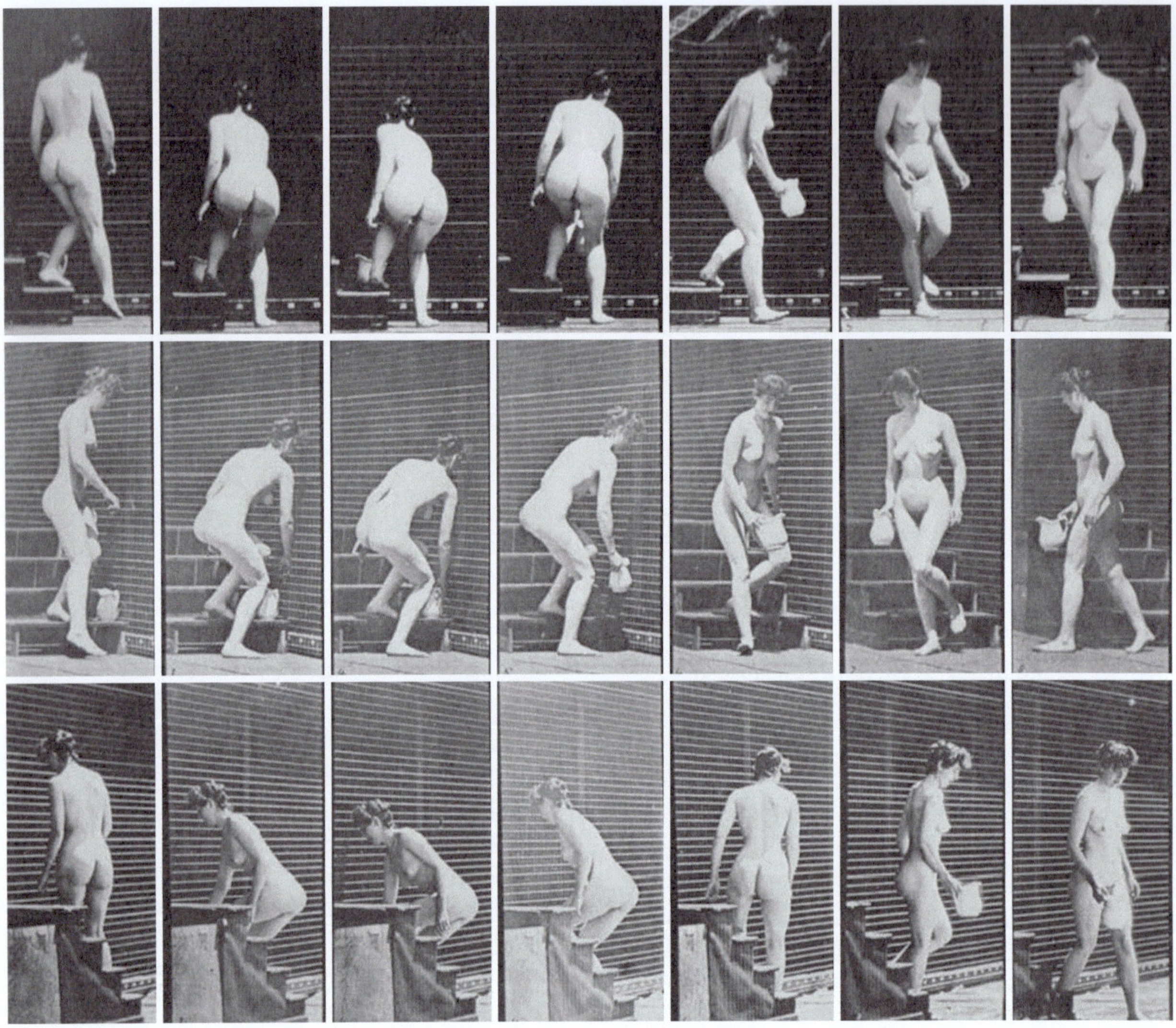

Fig. 47 Action to pick up an object on the ground at the foot of a staircase; this movement involves significant flexion and rotation (Muybridge [44])

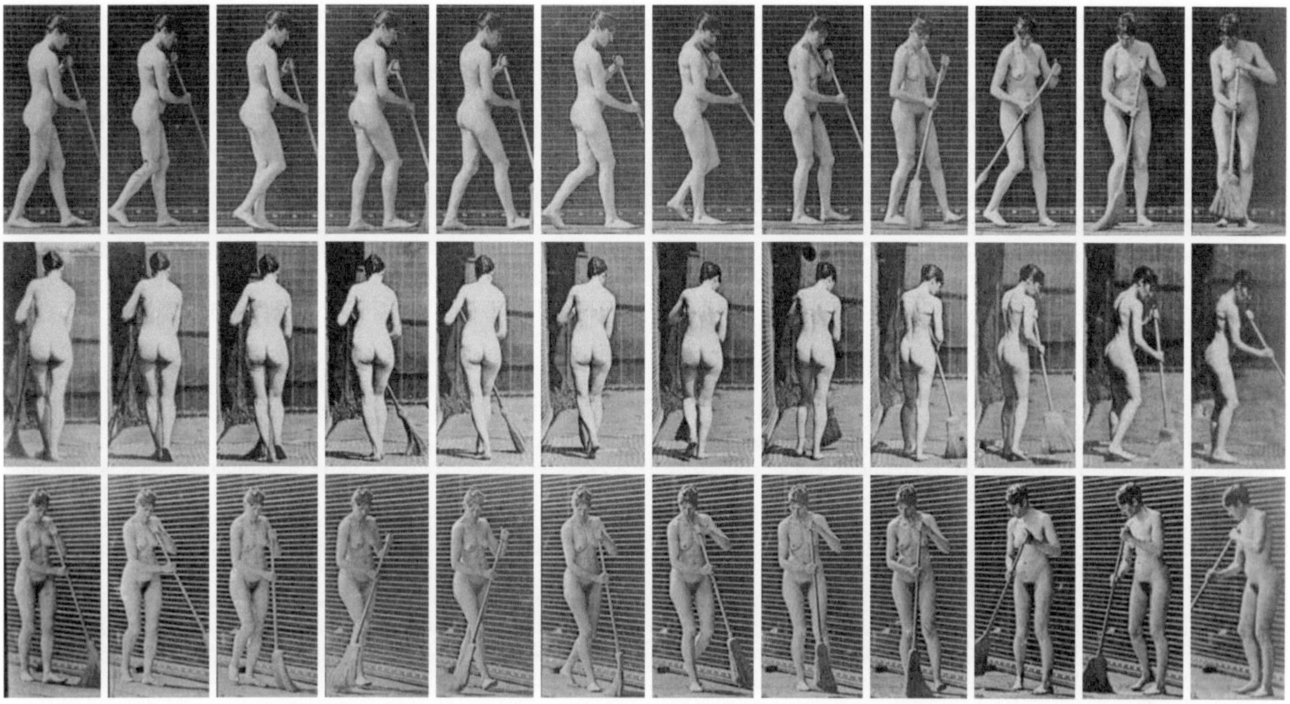

Fig. 48 Sweep action; this involves rotational movements, but the lumbar spine is not stressed in flexion–extension (Muybridge [44])

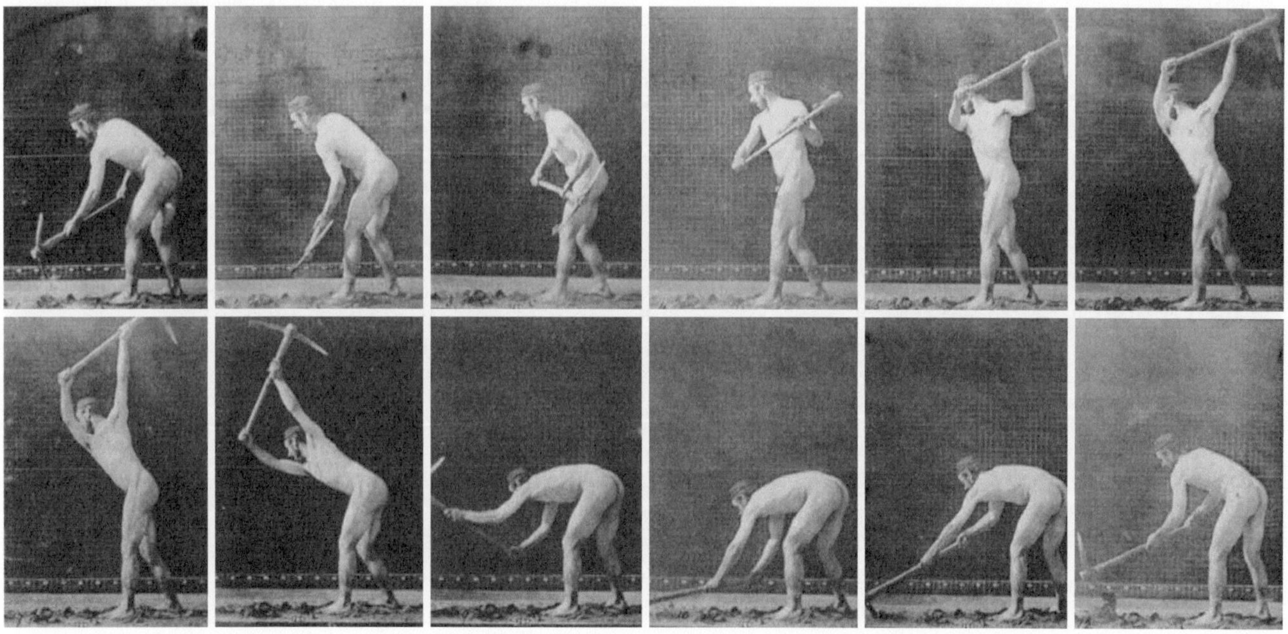

Fig. 49 Picking action; this movement involves large movements of rotation and flexion–extension (Muybridge [44])

References

1. Lavaste F. Biomécanique du rachis. In: Cahiers d'Enseignements de la SOFCOT. Paris: Expansion Scientifique Publications; 1997.
2. White A, Pajabi MM. Clinical biomechanics of the spine. Philadelphia: Lippincott; 1978.
3. Youdas JW, Garrett TR, Suman VJ, Bogard CL, Hallman HO, Carey JR. Normal range of motion of the cervical spine: an initial goniometric study. Phys Ther. 1992;72(11):770–80.
4. Pearson N, Walmsley RP. Trial into the effects of repeated neck retractions in normal subjects. Spine. 1995;20:1245–51.
5. Putto E, Talltoth K. Extension-flexion radiographs for motion studies of the lumbar spine; a comparison of two methods. Spine. 1990;15:107–10.
6. Templier A, Skalli W, Diop A, Vital JM, Mazel C, Saillant G, et al. Evaluation radiographique quantitative des arthrodèses rachidiennes lombaires: protocole et analyse préliminaire d'une série multicentrique de 119 cas. Rachis. 2001;13:23–37.
7. Wood KB, Popp CA, Transfeldt EE, Geissele AE. Radiographic evaluation of instability in spondylolisthesis. Spine. 1994;19:1697–703.
8. Weitz EM. The lateral bending sign. Spine. 1981;6:388–97.
9. Dupuis PR, Yonghing K, Cassidy JD, Kirkaldy-Willis WH. Radiologic diagnosis of degenerative lumbar spinal instability. Spine. 1985;10:262–76.
10. Hayes MA, Howard TC, Gruel CR, et al. Roentgenographic evaluation of lumbar spine flexion-extension in asymptomatic individuals. Spine. 1989;14:327–31.
11. Dvorak J, Panjabi MM, Chang DG, Theiler R, Grob D. Functional radiographic diagnosis of the lumbar spine; flexion-extension and lateral bending. Spine. 1991;16:562–71.
12. Gertzbein SD, Seligman J, Holtby R, et al. Centrode patterns and segment instability in degenerative disc disease. Spine. 1985;10:257–61.
13. Lazennec JY, Brusson A, Folinais D, Zhang A, Pour AE, Rousseau MA. Measuring extension of the lumbar pelvic-femoral complex with the EOS® system. Eur J Ortho Surg Traumatol. 2015;25:1061–8.
14. Penning L, Wilmink JT. Rotation of the cervical spine. A CT study in normal subjects. Spine. 1987;12:732–8.
15. Morita D, Yukawa Y, Nakashima H, Ito K, Yoshida G, Machino M, Kanbara S, Iwase T, Kato F. Range of motion of thoracic spine in sagittal plane. Eur Spine J. 2014;23:673–8.
16. Fujimori T, Iwasaki M, Nagamoto Y, Matsuo Y, Ishii T, Sugiura T, Kashii M, Murase T, Sugamo To K, Yoshikawa H. Kinematics of the thoracic spine in trunk lateral bending: in vivo three-dimensional analysis. Spine J. 2014;14:1991–9.
17. Husson JL, Poncer R, de Korvin B, Meabed J. Apport du scanner en Twist-test dans la mesure de l'instabilité du rachis lombaire. Rev Chir Orth. 1994;79(sup 1):117.
18. Vitzhum HE, Konig A, Seifert V. Dynamic examination of the lumbar spine by using vertical, open magnetic resonance imaging. J Neurosurg Spine. 2000;93(1):58–64.
19. Brown MD, Holmes DC, Heiner AD. WEHMAN KF. Intraoperative measurement of lumbar spine motion segment stiffness. Spine. 2002;27:954.
20. Ebara S, Harada T, Hosono N, Inoue M, Tanaka M, Morimoto Y, et al. Intraoperative measurement of lumbar spinal instability. Spine. 1992;17:S41–50.
21. Hasegawa K, Kitahara K, Hara T, Takano K, Shimoda H, Homma T. Per op evaluation of lumbar segmental instability in degenerative diseases by using a new intraoperative measurement system. J Neurosurg Spine. 2008;8:255–62.
22. Louis R. Chirurgie de rachis. Anatomie chirurgicale et voies d'abord. Heidelberg: Springer; 1982.
23. Kapandji IA. Physiologie articulaire 3, Tronc et Rachis. Paris: Maloine; 1994.
24. Castaing J, Santini JJ. Anatomie fonctionnelle de l'appareil locomoteur: le rachis. Paris: Editions Vigot; 1983.
25. Ishii T, Mukai Y, Hosono N, Sakaura H, Naka Jima Y, Sato Y, Sugamoto K, Yoshikawa H. Kinematics of the upper cervical spine in rotation: in vivo three-dimensional analysis. Spine. 2004;29:E139–44.
26. Ordway NR, Seymour RJ, Donelson RG, Hojnowski LS, Edwrads WT. Cervical flexion, extension, protrusion, and retraction; a radiographic segmental analysis. Spine. 1999;24:240–7.
27. Roy-Camille R. Atlas des coupes anatomiques du tronc. Paris: Masson; 1959.
28. Brugger A. Les syndromes vertébraux radiculaires et pseudoradiculaires. Documenta Geigy. Acta Rhumatol. 1961;18:19.
29. PENNING L. Normal movements of the cervical spine. Am J Roentgenol. 1978;30:317–26.
30. Wen N. Contribution à l'étude expérimentale du comportement mécanique in vitro du rachis cervical. Mémoire Ensam Paris. 1993.
31. Watier B. Comportement mécanique du rachis cervical: une revue de littérature. Mechanical behaviour of cervical spine: literature update. ITBM-RBM. 2006;27:92–106.
32. Dvorak J, Panjabi MM, Novotny JE, Antinnes JA. In vivo flexion/extension of the normal cervical spine. J Orthop Res. 1991;98:28–34.
33. Lansade C. Analyse cinématique tridimensionnelle du rachis cervical sain et pathologique in vivo. Thèse de Doctorat de l'Ecole Nationale Supérieure d'Arts et Métiers, spécialité "Mécanique". Paris. 2009.
34. Ishii T, Mukai Y, Hosono N, Sakaura H, Fujii R, Nakajima Y, Tamura S, Iwasaki M, Yoshikawa H, Sugamoto K. Kinematics of the cervical spine in lateral bending: in vivo three-dimensional analysis. Spine. 2006;31(2):155–60.
35. Pearcy M, Portek I, Sheperd J. Three-dimensional x-ray of normal movement in the lumbar spine. Spine. 1984;9:295–7.
36. Arbogast KB, Gholve PA, Friedman JE, Maltese MR, Tomasello MF, Dormans JP. Normal cervical spine range of motion in children 3-12 years old. Spine. 2007;32:E309–15.
37. Wong KW, Leong JCY, Chan MK, Luk DK, Lu WW. The flexion-extension profile of lumbar spine in 100 healthy volunteers. Spine. 2004;29:1636–41.
38. Swinkels RA, Swinkels Meewisse IE. Normal values for cervical range of motion. Spine. 2014;39:362–7.
39. Chen J, Solinger AB, Pncet JF, Lantz CA. Meta-analysis of normative cervical motion. Spine. 1999;24:1571–8.
40. Feipel V, Salvia P, Klein H, Rooze M. Head repositioning accuracy in patients with whiplash-associated disorders. Spine. 2006;31:E51–8.
41. Bible JE, Biswas D, Miller CP, Whang PG, Grauer JN. Functional range of motion of the lumbar spine during 15 activities of daily living. J Spinal Disord Tech. 2010;23:107–12.
42. Sciubba DM, Scheer JK, Smith JS, Lafage V, Klineberg E, Gupta M, Mundis GM, Protopsaltis S, Kim HJ, Hiratzka JR, Koski T, Shaffrey CI, Bess S, Hart RA, Ames PA. Which daily functions are most affected by stiffness following total lumbar fusion. Spine. 2015;40:1338–44.
43. Hart RA, Gundle KR, Pro SL, et al. Lumbar stiffness disability index: pilot testing of consistency, reliability, and validity. Spine J. 2013;13:157–61.
44. Muybridge E. The human and animal locomotion photographs. Cologne: Taschen; 2010.
45. Vanneuville G, Escande G, Guillot M, Chazal J, Tanguy A, Bourges M, Vergegarnet J, Deubelle A. Eléments de biomécanique du rachis. 63e Congrès de l'Association des Anatomistes. Clermont-Ferrand: Edit Bloc-santé; 1980.

Spinal Balance

J. P. Farcy

The Choice of Words

Balance

It is a French word used everywhere. It means equilibrium and is crucial to ensure that the proper functions of forces are working together. Forces to be balanced must always have flexibility to allow the smallest adjustment. Forces generated by weight and gravity must be evenly applied on each spine segment to adjust to body motion. When the word "Balance" is applied to the spine, its meaning is limited to postural alignment, which is a component, although essential, of the total body balance.

Alignment

Structural modifications of the anatomy over millions of years of evolution have brought us to the upright bipedal posture affecting the entire musculo-skeletal system. Important modifications of the pelvis and the spine have been crucial to ensure the body's stability in the erect position. Alternated segments of the spine, the head, the cervical spine, the thoracic spine, the lumbar spine, and the pelvis have a "center of mass" aligned on a vertical line perpendicular to the ground. Each one of those parts is included in a defined shape, which in the coronal plane, defines the body's axis and in the sagittal plane are organized in curves to insure enough strength to carry the upper body's weight. Details of the sagittal alignment were well defined in Pierre Roussouly's Chap. 6.

J. P. Farcy (✉)
Orthopaedic Surgery NYU University, New York, NY, USA
e-mail: jpfarcy@orthospine.com

Equilibrium

All the structural modifications of the mammal's anatomy to evolve into the bipedal species, consists of a displacement of the body's gravity center on a vertical line, which falls on a point at the center of a small support surface. Combined actions of the musculo-skeletal system controlled by the spine and pelvis structure ensure the body's balance. Balance is even more essential when the center of mass displaced by mobility must be aligned with the center of gravity, to avoid falling while walking, running, or jumping (Fig. 1).

Such a permanent adjustment to motion requires energy which must be controlled for dynamic bipedal harmonious function.

Posture

Upright posture, and by extension sway and destabilizing movement, are specific to the human species. Ideally in the standing position all centers of gravity and centers of body and segment mass are located on the line of gravity which projects at the center of the support surface. This posture of man standing can vary infinitely within the limits of the cone of economy described in Chap. 12 by Jean Dubousset. The variations of posture will then depend on the application of forces, moreover by the perception's modification induced by individual psychological or emotional status.

Stability

Can be defined as a continuity of anatomical structures between the vertebrae which constitute the vertebral column. This continuity of the structures must be rigorously maintained during the very extreme movements of the elements constituting the whole spine. This stability can be interrupted by accidental or degenerative causes. The consequences are a modification of the global spine alignment and thus affect

J. M. Vital, D. T. Cawley (eds.), *Spinal Anatomy*, https://doi.org/10.1007/978-3-030-20925-4_31

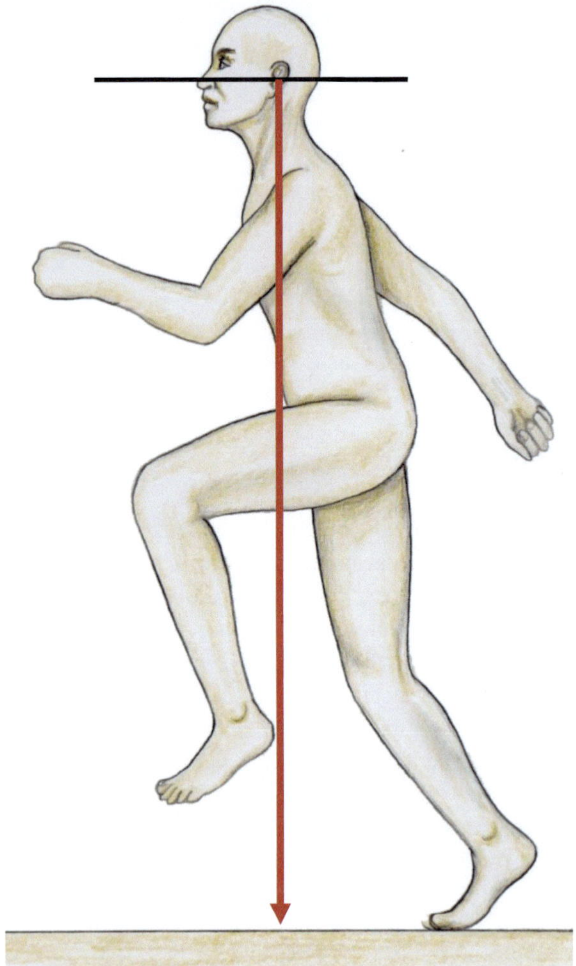

Fig. 1 Man in motion. The line going by inner ear and eye shows the "semi-circular canals" plane which must stay perpendicular to the gravity line during motion

balance. However, the infinite possibilities offered by the flexibility of the spine whilst retaining the role of protecting the nervous system represent its essential function; stability in motion.

From Alignment to Equilibrium

Evaluated and measured, alignment gives an accurate rendition of the ideal structure of the vertebral column obtained in both posteroanterior and lateral radiographs in the standing position. The criteria for this alignment are clearly presented with their morphological and chronological variations in the in-depth study made by Pierre Roussouly and Jean Dubousset (Chaps. 8 and 12). The hip extension criteria are well illustrated by Istvan Hovorka (Chap. 7). These radiological and clinical criteria are complemented by neuro-muscular studies, which are together implied in the concept of spine alignment. It is possible to define the ideal alignment of an individual's spine and pelvis in correlation with body's mass and muscle tone and therefor understand the interactions between the axis of the body and the stays that hold it. Sagittal spine alignment requires full mobility of the hip, including hip extension reserve as a guarantee of functional lumbar lordosis. Pelvis version (pelvic tilt) in correlation with lumbar lordosis induce both thoracic kyphosis and cervical lordosis. As a result, the head's center of mass is maintained on the body's line of gravity. Head and neck segments, with specific powerful stays, control horizontal vision, playing an essential role in balance.

With the brain as control system.

Both static and dynamic balance require a permanent perception of control to select and perform the most appropriate action.

CNS integrity to assimilate all input to transform them in enriched cognition.

↓

Harmony

Importance of Spine Anatomy

The Pelvis

When discs, facet joints, and ligaments degenerate causing lumbar lordosis, the pelvis evolves into retroversion. Pelvis retroversion is visible on a lateral spine radiograph, obtained while standing, where the shadow of the femoral head is seen in front of the body's line of gravity. Such pelvis retroversion combined with maximum hip extension makes the standing upright posture impossible without flexing the knees. Body balance is maintained at the expense of lumbar spine lordosis modification, to the limits imposed by pelvis retroversion. The final result is a cascade of discs, facets, and ligament degeneration, ending up in vertebrae rotatory dislocations and adult spine deformity.

Thoraco-Lumbar Spine

Made up of 17 segments, each individualized, is made up of two zones that operate in a symbiotic mode. The lumbar part, made up of five more voluminous segments presents a sagittal curvature in lordosis. It is also the most mobile while supporting the most important load. Its flexibility, not limited by the rib cage, is much greater than the 12 chest segments with physiological curvature in kyphosis. These two curves compensate each other to such an extent that the increase in the degree of curvature of one corresponds to an increase in the degree of curvature of the other. Let us increase the lumbar lordosis, and we shall see the thoracic kyphosis increase, displacing the head forward increasing stress applied on the cervical spine, affecting the overall spine alignment.

The Cervical Spine

Composed of two complementary segments, it ensures the movement of rotation, lateral flexion, extension, and flexion of the head. The cranial segment is made up of two vertebrae connected to each other, and to the occipital bone, by a complex system of joints constituting three axes of mobility to allow 3 degrees of freedom of the head's movement. The remainder of the five underlying segments is composed of similar vertebrae, whose articular facets allow a combination of rotation and lateral flexion. Such complexity of movement implies difficulty to adapt to conditions of extreme load, stretching the possibilities of resistance and muscle tone to their limits, in order to control the head's position.

Spine and Central Nervous System: (CNS) and (PNS)

It may look obvious that standing upright is a given privilege, however, it requires neurological implication of such complexity redefined every year by neuroscience discoveries. Research conducted by Christine Assaiante [1] demonstrated balance control development over years in synchronicity with CNS development. Body balance for a major part is maintained by the cervical action of all neck muscles, ensuring the inner ear's vestibular stability when acceleration is transmitted to the head by body motion. Head control does not only guarantee good function of the oculo-vestibular reflex, it insures enlarged perception of the environment, and by extension of its specific input at each given moment [2, 3] (Fig. 1). A cervical kyphosis, progressively made permanent by the weakening of the extensors, reduces the visual field and considerably limits the perceptive inputs which are very important to the enrichment of cognition (Fig. 2). Reduction in visual acuity affects not only cognition but also a slowing down of the plasticity of the brain. As a result, other osteo-muscular and tactile perceptions can insidiously compromise the proprioception of the healthy adult. Becoming less engaged, the brain participates less and less in action, and progressive uncertainty creeps in to compromise the feeling of safety. The pattern of behavior is reduced to limit them, and when apprehension becomes fear, the vicious circle is closed.

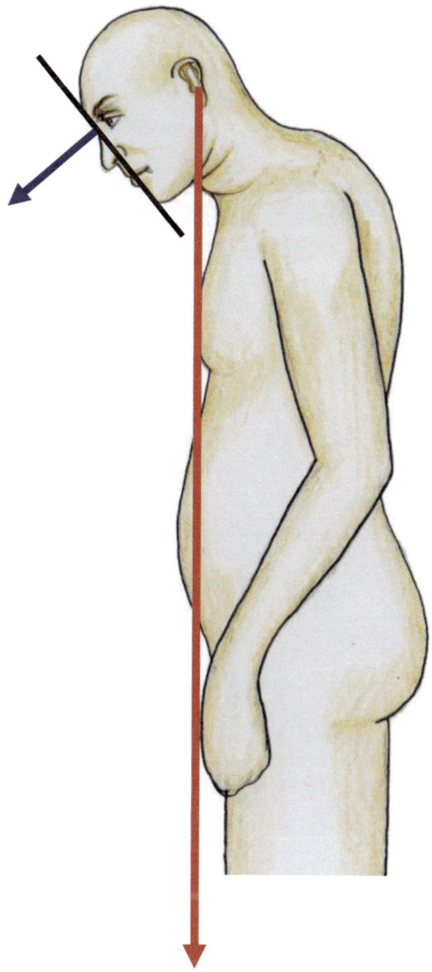

Fig. 2 Man affected by a severe cervical kyphosis. Standing upright; Limited cervical mobility. Limited visual perception. Limited function of the oculo-vestibular reflex

A Word from Neurosciences

Since 1984, with the establishment of centers for cognitive studies, neurosciences have focused mainly on improving learning in the more general framework of education. The cognition that allows the brain to have a keypad that gets richer, constantly needs the continuous input of all perception. Among the perceptions indispensable to permanent enrichment are those that all the senses have to offer, and which are integrated in the form of cognition's repertoire which is continually renewed (Fig. 4). The wide sweep of a gaze of the eye with the multiple degrees of freedom of movement of the head is one of the best guarantees of a continuous enrichment of cognition. Unlimited, permanent capture of the environment is facilitated by an intact oculo-vestibular reflex (Figs. 3 and 4).

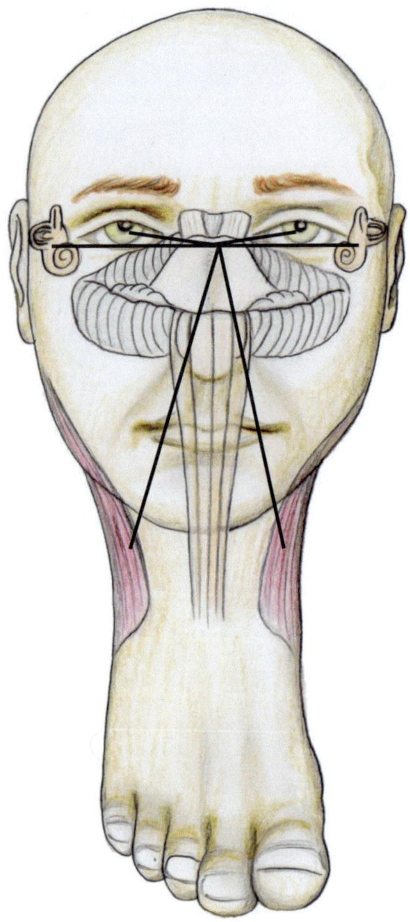

Fig. 3 Balance, a very intricate symbiosis of multiple systems (Tran Ba Hu)

As a corollary, it is necessary to keep posture erect facilitating the important position of the semi-circular canals and eye's gaze on a line perpendicular to the axis of gravity.

Search for Harmony

Anatomists and surgeons need to preserve the alignment of the spine, both in the coronal sagittal and transversal plane so that the head, the seventh cervical vertebra, the third lumbar vertebra, and the center of the pelvis are all on the line of gravity projected at a point between the two internal malleoli in the standing posture. We know that in adults, even without recognized pathology, the muscular tone degenerates, the joints become less mobile, and the spine deforms. This deformation occurs under the influence of the gravitational force as soon as the anatomical structures begin to degenerate.

It is these deformations which cause pain and which we treat by widening the spinal canal, ensuring the stability of the vertebrae and correcting the alignment. But in doing so, the correction is made at the cost of stiffness which leaves no room for adjustment mainly when it is extended to more vertebrae. In search of harmony, could it be possible to find a compromise so that the centers of pressure can be aligned with the center of gravity without the constraint imposed by a large zone of rigidity? It is necessary to preserve both "spinal alignment and dynamic balance." When they fail it has a negative impact on the function of the CNS. Unsuspected possibilities of brain plasticity can be lost without full attention given to spine balance. In light of this evidence the

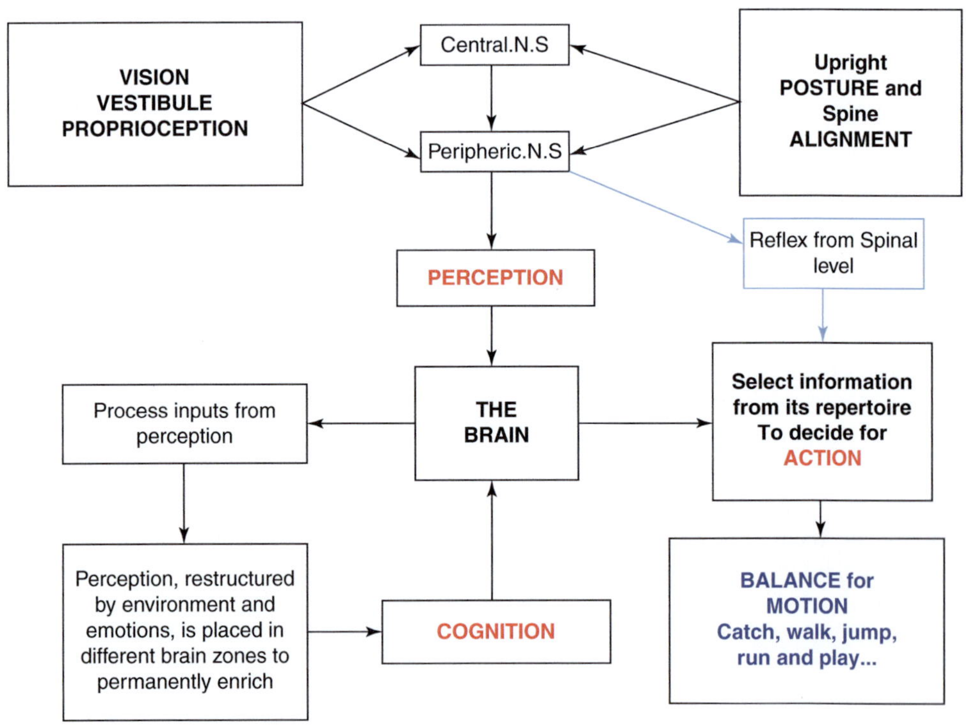

Fig. 4 An algorithm to define balance and alignment

choice of a surgical compromise between the perfect and rigid correction and a relative correction, allowing for enough adjustment must be the main concern [4]. "Spinal balance" needs flexibility to counter a loss of horizontal sight, with the increasingly suboptimal direction of sight then focused downward toward a space restricted to the ground in front of the feet. (Fig. 2).

A Look at the Future

Is it possible to pursue the alignment of the spine while preserving its power of adjustment? Is a preventative minimally invasive intervention feasible to delay the disabling consequences of discs and ligament degeneration?

References

1. Assaiante C. Factors associated with the increased perceptual reliance on the visual reference frame with age. Laboratory of Neuroscience Cognitive. Marseille: University of Aix-Marseille.
2. Roll JP, Roll R. From eye to foot: a proprioceptive chain involved in postural control. Amsterdam: Elsevier; 1988.
3. Amblard B, Berthoz A, Clarac F. Posture and gait: development, adaptation and modulation. Proceedings of the 9th. International Symposium on Posritural and Gait Research. New York: Excerpta Medica; 1988.
4. Berthoz A. The brain's sense of movement. Cambridge: Harvard University Press; 1997.

Biomechanics and Spinal Modelling

W. Skalli, D. Mitton, P. Rouch, and J. Dubousset

Introduction

Among the essential biomechanical functions of the spine are those of maintaining a stable erect position and of allowing movements during walking, activities of daily living or when practicing a sport. An important function is also to effectively protect the spinal cord. These functions involve different interacting systems, mainly the osteoarticular system (bone structures and disco-ligament binding elements) and the muscular system that both stabilizes and mobilizes the skeleton. Motor control for activation of muscular actuators is performed based on information from many proprioceptive sensors.

This neuromusculoskeletal assembly is particularly complex. The goal of the biomechanical engineer is to develop quantitative methods to describe the geometry, to describe the internal architecture on a detailed scale, to propose constitutive equations for the tissues, associated with their mechanical properties. It is also to model this system, at different levels, to better understand the mechanisms that govern its normal or altered operation. To model is to propose a schematic mathematical representation focusing on a particular aspect. This numerical approach is inseparable from the experimental analysis which makes it possible to observe the phenomena for setting relevant models and validating them. The first research in modelling at ENSAM began in the 1980s, under the impetus of F. Lavaste in collaboration with R. Roy Camille. It has continuously evolved since, in close collaboration between engineers and clinicians. This chapter addresses the modelling aspects through geometric modelling, which allows a quantitative description of the morphology, and through biomechanical modelling, which aims to understand how these very specific structures react under the effect of the mechanical loads to which they are subjected, thus shedding further light on the functional anatomy.

The models can be made at different scales, macroscopically (for an extended vertebral segment, for the spine or the body as a whole) or microscopically, for example to study in detail the arrangement between the collagen fibres of an intervertebral disk and elastin fibres that constitute interlamellar bridges [1], or to understand the relationship between bone trabecular architecture and macroscopic mechanical properties [2].

We will remain on a more macroscopic approach and, through some examples, we will illustrate the value of modelling, for a fundamental objective of understanding the basic mechanisms, as well as for clinical issues such as the aid to the diagnosis and the therapeutic management.

Geometric Modelling of the Spine

Geometric Modelling of the Skeleton from Biplane Imagery

The basis for quantitative observation is the shape and pose of each vertebra and trunk as a whole, including the spine, pelvis and ribcage. The development of the EOS® low-dose biplanar X-ray system and the associated 3D reconstruction [3] allowed for the first time quantitative observation of the 3D skeleton in the erect position. The 3D reconstruction method is based on the design of a geometric model of each bone structure. For example, a vertebra of reference, with its vertebral body, its spinous process and its transverse process can be characterized by geometric attributes (dimensions, orientations of the articular facets, etc.). Databases associated with statistical models show that these geometric attributes are

W. Skalli (✉) · P. Rouch
Institut de Biomécanique Humaine Georges Charpak, Arts et Métiers ParisTech, Paris, France
e-mail: wafa.skalli@ensam.eu; Philippe.rouch@ensam.eu

D. Mitton
Univ Lyon, Université Claude Bernard Lyon 1, IFSTTAR, LBMC UMR_T9406, Lyon, France
e-mail: david.mitton@ifsttar.fr

J. Dubousset
National Academy of Medicine, Paris, France
e-mail: jean.dubousset@wanadoo.fr

J. M. Vital, D. T. Cawley (eds.), *Spinal Anatomy*, https://doi.org/10.1007/978-3-030-20925-4_32

correlated for the same vertebra (transversal inferences) and for the vertebrae of the same spine (longitudinal inferences). Therefore only few anatomical landmarks are digitized on X-rays (Fig. 1a) and are used to infer all the geometric attributes of all vertebrae, which allows pre-sizing and positioning of each vertebra in coherence with the digitized information. The theoretical radiographic projections of this initial model are calculated and superimposed with a pair of real radiographs (Fig. 1b). Adjustments are then made, manually or automatically, to bring the simulated radiographic images into coherence with the real radiographic images, and to obtain a realistic model of the object (Fig. 1c, d) [3–6].

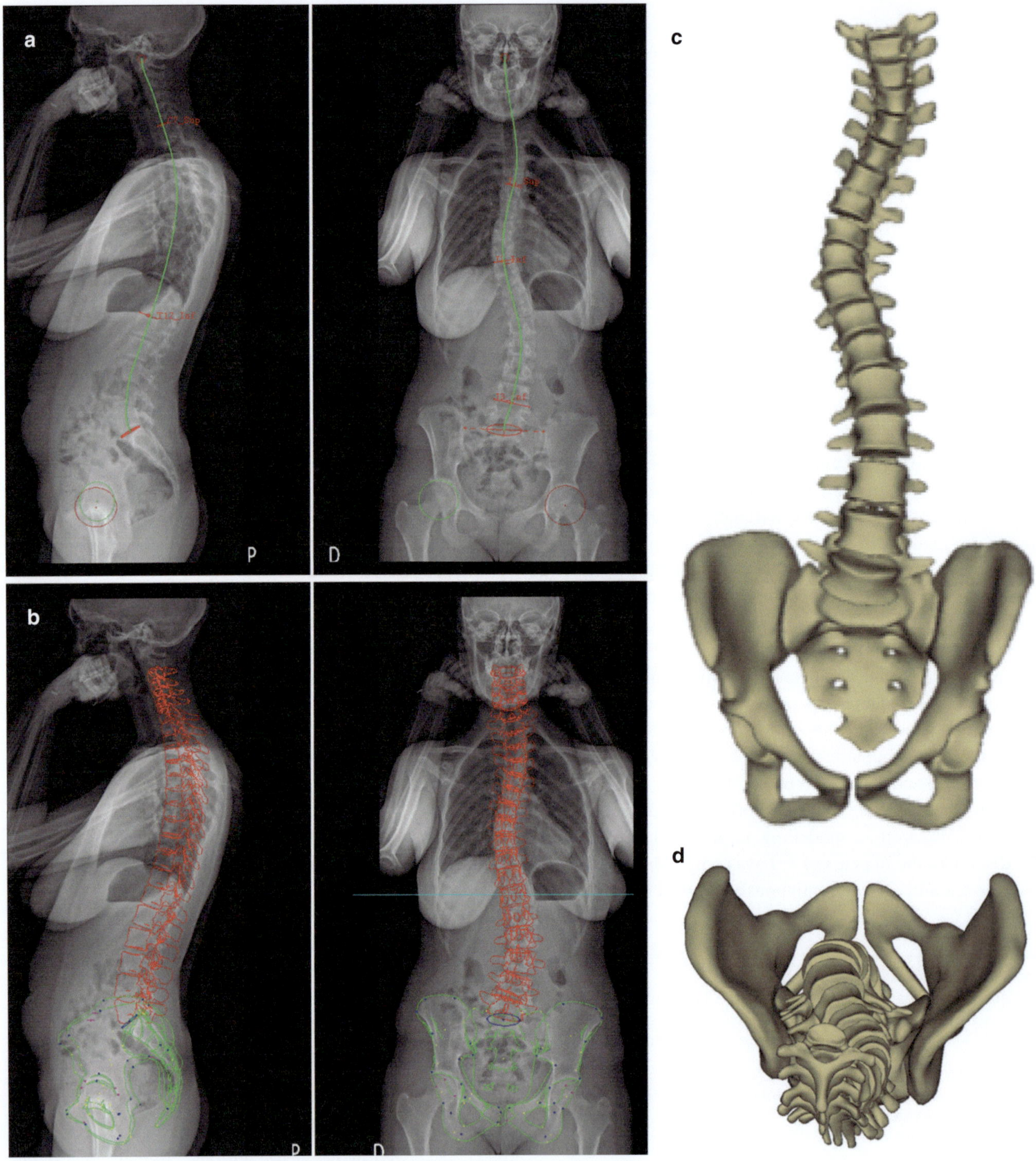

Fig. 1 3D reconstruction process of the spine: (**a**) anatomical landmarks are digitized; (**b**) the initial model is retroprojected on X-rays to allow model adjustments; (**c**) 3D reconstruction in superior view; (**d**) 3D reconstruction in frontal view

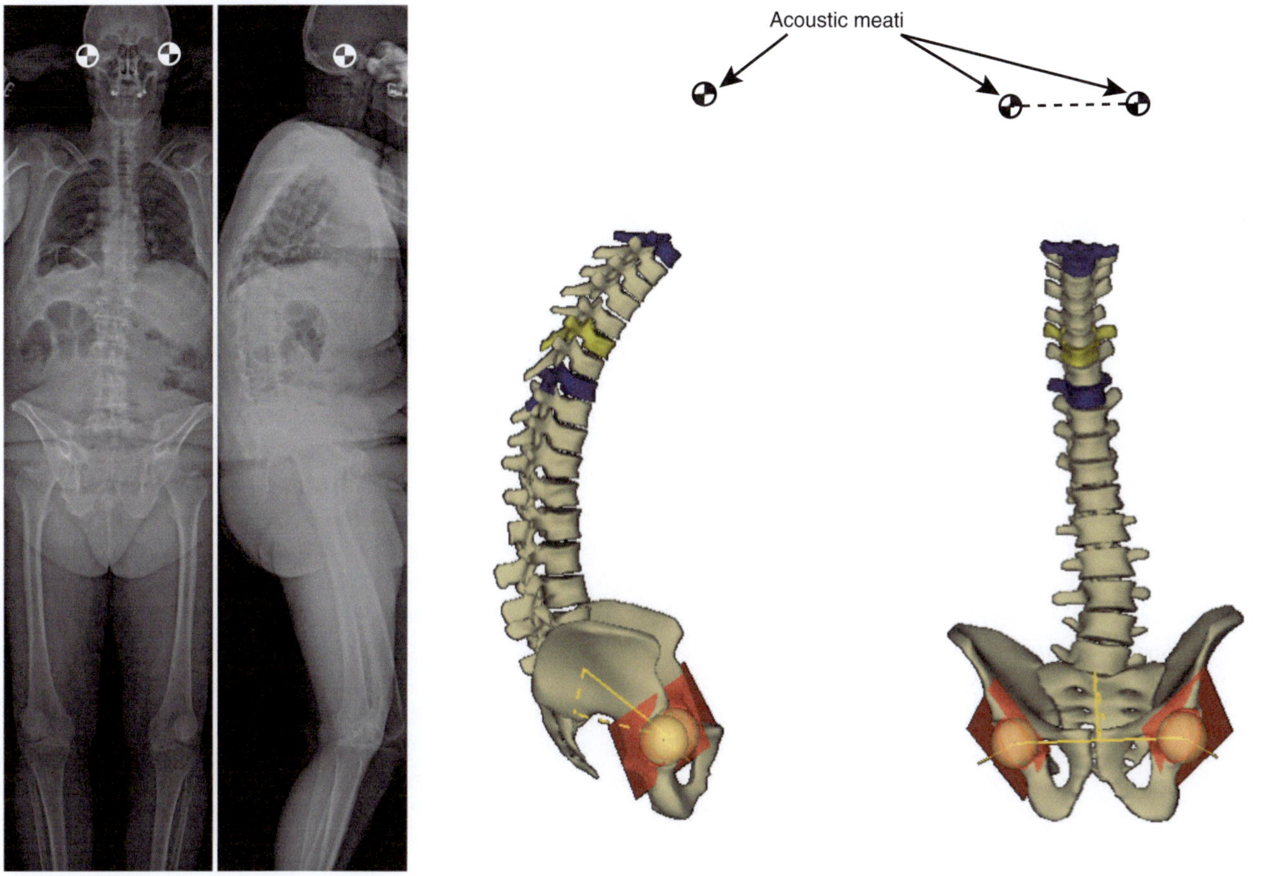

Fig. 2 For this patient, the maximized retroversion of the pelvis is insufficient to avoid tilting forward, bending of the knees is necessary to maintain the erect posture, with the head above the pelvis. The head center of mass is close to the center of acoustic meati (CAMs)

The possibility of viewing in 3D and from different angles is rich in lessons, as highlighted in the chapter on EOS. In particular, head-to-toe analysis has shown how the erect posture is characterized by maintaining the head above the pelvis [7] and how the aging subject or postural disturbance implements a compensation strategy, by retroverting the pelvis, or even flexing the knees, to maintain this erect posture (Fig. 2).

This three-dimensional modelling of the vertebral column provides new insight into the quantitative analysis of scoliotic deformities, described qualitatively by the pioneers René Perdriolle [8], Jean Dubousset, Henri Graf and Ginette Duval Beaupère. Thus it is now established that the main scoliosis curvature has at its extremities, called junctional zones, a limit vertebra which is rotated in the horizontal plane with respect to the adjacent vertebrae (intervertebral axial rotation, IAR—in the inferior and superior zones). The apical vertebra, the most laterally deviated, is also usually the most rotated in the horizontal plane (vertebral axial rotation, VAR). Within the main curvature, each vertebra is rotated relative to the other, from the apex to the lower limit and from the apex to the upper limit, thus describing a torsion phenomenon which is clearly visible in Fig. 1 [9]. Finally, this scoliotic curvature is also characterized by hypokyphosis in the apical region, when observed in the plane of curvature.

Coupled with the modelling of the rib cage, this 3D reconstruction makes it possible to objectify the effect of conservative [10, 11] or surgical [12] treatments. In a study carried out in collaboration with the teams of Saint Etienne University Hospital (Dr Ebermeyer and Courtois) and Trousseau Hospital (Pr Vialle), the analysis of 42 scoliosis patients treated before and after bracing shows that if the brace corrects overall, the angle of Cobb, the lordosis is however decreased in 60% of the cases, and the parameters of the horizontal plane (VAR, torsion, gibbosity) are unchanged in more than 60% of the cases. Vertebral axial rotation is even increased in 14% of cases [13]. Larger scale analyses, linked to the clinical outcome of brace treatment, should lead to a better understanding leading to improved practices and equipment.

Indeed, numerical models make it possible to build large databases in multicentric studies, provided that acquisition protocols are harmonized. The use of data analysis techniques and/or artificial intelligence provides powerful means to classify the data, find the most influential parameters, and ultimately identify useful biomechanical markers for diagnosis and/or development of the therapeutic strategy.

An illustration concerns the identification of a severity index allowing early detection of progressive scoliosis. Screening is important because the treatment is all the more effective when undertaken early. Quantitative observations made on many scoliosis curves lead to establish a "scoliotic deformity signature", that is to say to characterize the pattern of deformity using a few descriptor parameters (Cobb angle, AIR, AVR, hypokyphosis in apical zone, rotation). A normal spine may randomly present one or other of these attributes, but not this structured combination, and its "signature" will be very different. This very specific pattern of deformity may appear in the early phase. Therefore, it is possible, from the first examination, to establish the signature of each spine and, using a mathematical classification method known as factorial discriminant analysis, to compute a severity index that varies from 0 to 1 depending on whether the signature of the studied spine is closer to that of normal spines or that of severe scoliosis. An initial validation was performed on 56 patients, for whom the severity index was established at the first examination and followed until the end of their growth. The results showed that, in more than 80% of cases, scalability or stability can be predicted from this first examination [14]. These promising results have led to the initiation of data collection on a larger scale to consolidate scientific evidence and to reliably use this index in clinical practice. The follow-up time for the validation is long because it is sometimes necessary to wait several years for the future progression of the patient to be proven; we are now at 64 patients with similar conclusive results.

For degenerative scoliosis in adults, such approaches can be considered and have been initiated [15] to look for early warning signals, especially related to intervertebral rotations which could further be translated into true rotational dislocations destabilizing the spine.

These examples illustrate how quantitative three-dimensional analysis is likely to shed new light on spinal pathology. In addition, these geometric models provide a valuable foundation for the biomechanical models that will be presented below.

Biomechanical Modelling of Spine

Biomechanical modelling aims to analyse the response of a mechanical system to forces to which this system is subject. Such modelling consists in schematizing on the one hand the shape of the structure of interest (that is to say, to build a geometric model), and on the other hand the mechanical behaviour of the different components, by describing their constitutive equations. These equations are established by mechanical tests which quantify the internal mechanical stress (force per unit area, in N/mm^2) as a function of the strain (relative variation in length or angulation, in %). The constitutive equations can be very complex and we will provide a simplified vision. By way of example, the stress–strain curve of a sample of cortical bone is shown in Fig. 3a. The equation is linear and the slope of the line corresponds to the modulus of elasticity E (or Young's modulus), which characterizes the stiffness of the considered tissue. Another essential mechanical characteristic is the mechanical strength of the tissue considered, that is to say the maximum stress that can be supported before damage to this material. Soft tissue behaviour is generally nonlinear (Fig. 3b), with stiffness progressively increasing with increasing deformation.

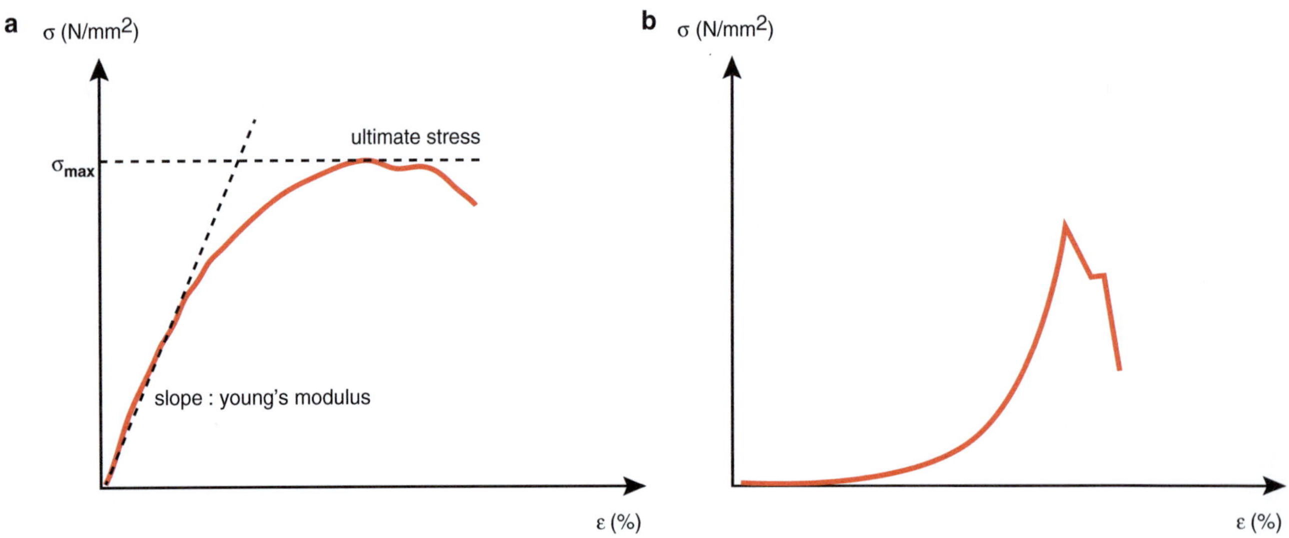

Fig. 3 The stress–strain curves make it possible to characterize the stiffness of the material, expressed by the Young's modulus, as well as its strength, expressed by the maximum admissible stress: (**a**) typical curve for bone tissue, the behaviour of which is linear, (**b**) typical curve for a ligament, the behaviour of which is nonlinear

Biomechanical Modelling and Conceptual Analysis

Mechanical modelling therefore requires the completion of geometric modelling by describing schematically the mechanical characteristics of each material in each region of the model. Internal kinematic links must also be modelled (for example, inter-facet contact). A particularly powerful modelling technique, finite element modelling (FEM), is widely used in mechanics and other areas of physics and developed for the spine since the 1980s.

Figure 4 shows two model examples, for a lumbar segment and for a cervical segment. The models are said in finite elements because the virtual structure is mapped in a finite number of elements, each element having its own characteristics. Such an approach makes it possible to differentiate the mechanical characteristics of the cortical and cancellous bone (and to consider their variability within a given vertebra), to differentiate the annulus of the nucleus, the anterior and posterior fibres of the intervertebral disc, each of the ligaments, etc.

Dedicated software then allows to simulate different types of forces exerted on this structure and to compute the mechanical response, in terms of displacements, local strain and global deformation, and mechanical stresses which, if they are excessive, cause the damage to this system. Of course, because of simplifying assumptions and the resultant schemata, the validation of these models is essential to verify the relevance of the numerical response. Spinal models are generally validated by in vitro mechanical tests, in which vertebral segments are fixed at their base and subjected to controlled mechanical loads (compression, flexion, extension, lateral inflexion, rotation). The movements of one vertebra relative to the other are then measured in the three planes of the space, which makes it possible to obtain the behaviour curves (forces or couples vs. linear or angular displacements). Numerical simulation makes it possible to apply virtually the same forces under the same experimental conditions, and the numerical results are compared with the experimental results (Fig. 5) [16]. This model becomes more refined as knowledge evolves.

Once validated, these models are valuable tools to help thinking: indeed, we can, all things being equal, remove and modify components and analyse their effect. For example, these models allowed to identify the role of geometric parameters in the biomechanical response of the spine [17, 18]. These models are also a powerful means of computer-assisted design of implants: indeed, the simulation of pathology and surgical instrumentation can be realized, and provided that the modelling of the instrumented segment is validated, numerous options can be simulated by varying the different design parameters [19, 20]. Figure 6 shows different examples of implant modelling, and Fig. 7 shows the impact of two posterior implants on the distribution of

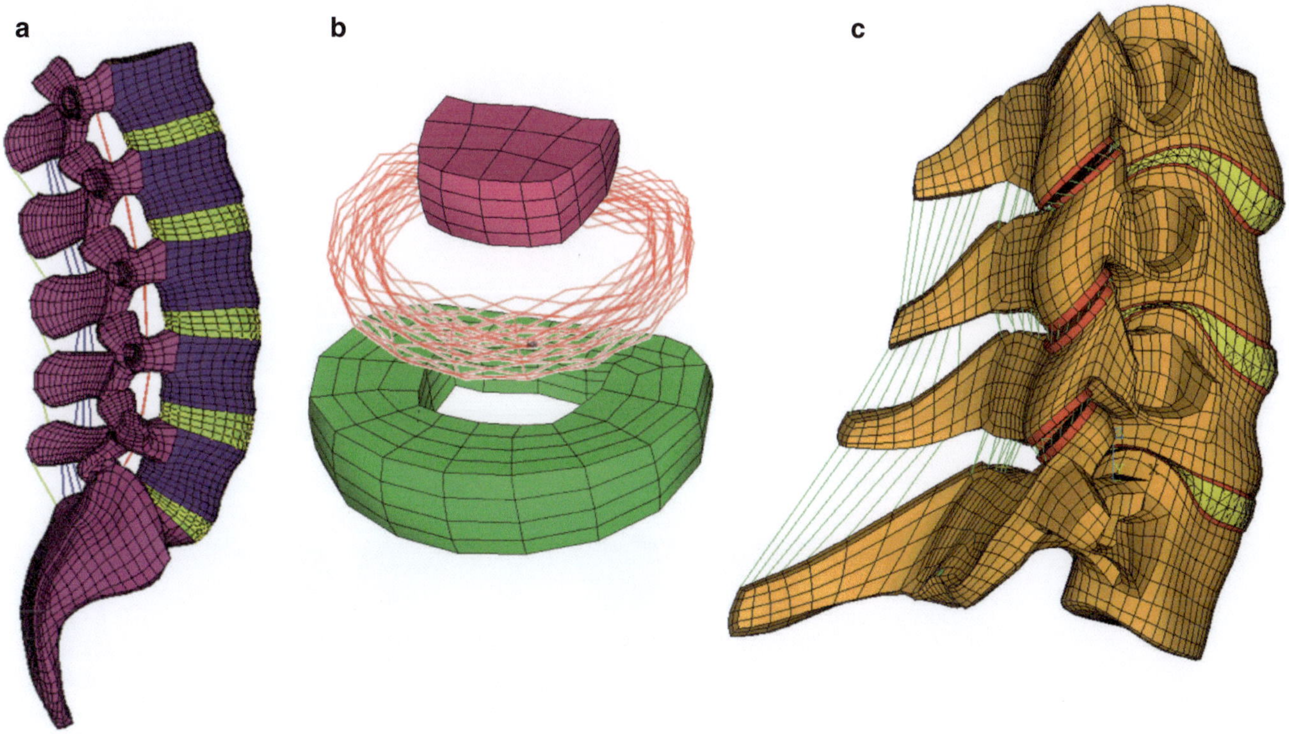

Fig. 4 (**a**) Lumbar vertebral segment model; (**b**) exploded view of the intervertebral disc, highlighting the differentiated modelling between the matrix of the annulus, the collagen fibres included in this matrix and the nucleus; (**c**) model of cervical spine

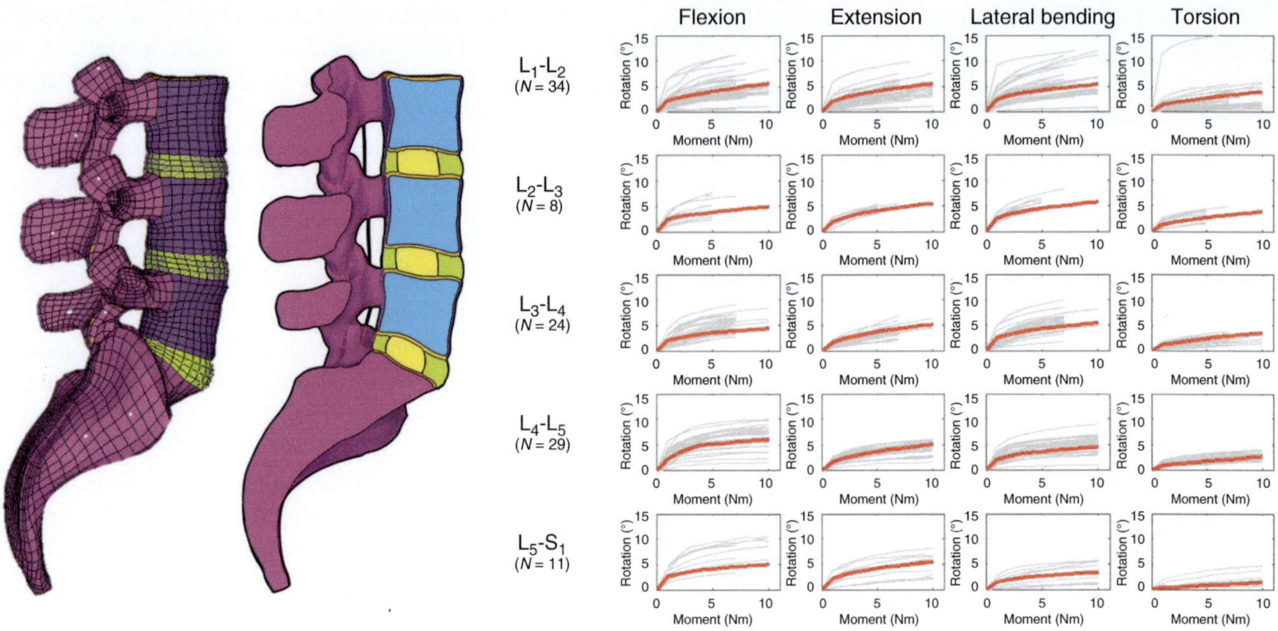

Fig. 5 For each vertebral level and each type of load, flexion extension, extension, lateral bending and rotation, the in vitro experiments make it possible to quantify the curves of rotations as a function of the applied moment (a grey line by specimen). The behaviour of each model is compared to the different experimental results, to verify that the curves are similar and that the numerical results are within the experimental corridor

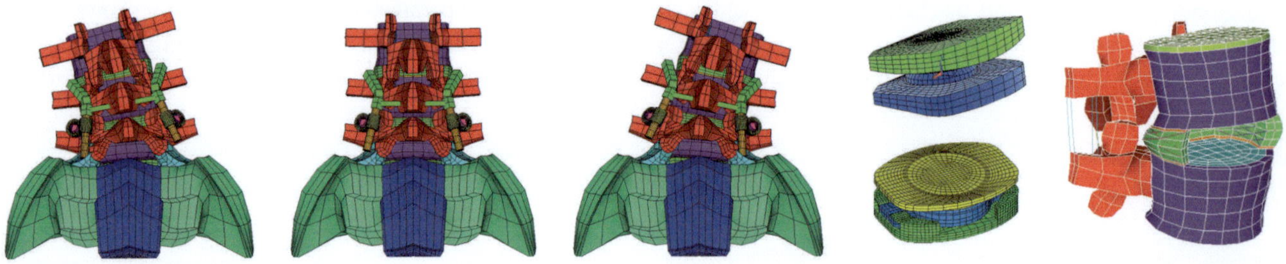

Fig. 6 Simulation of lesions and virtual insertion of different implants

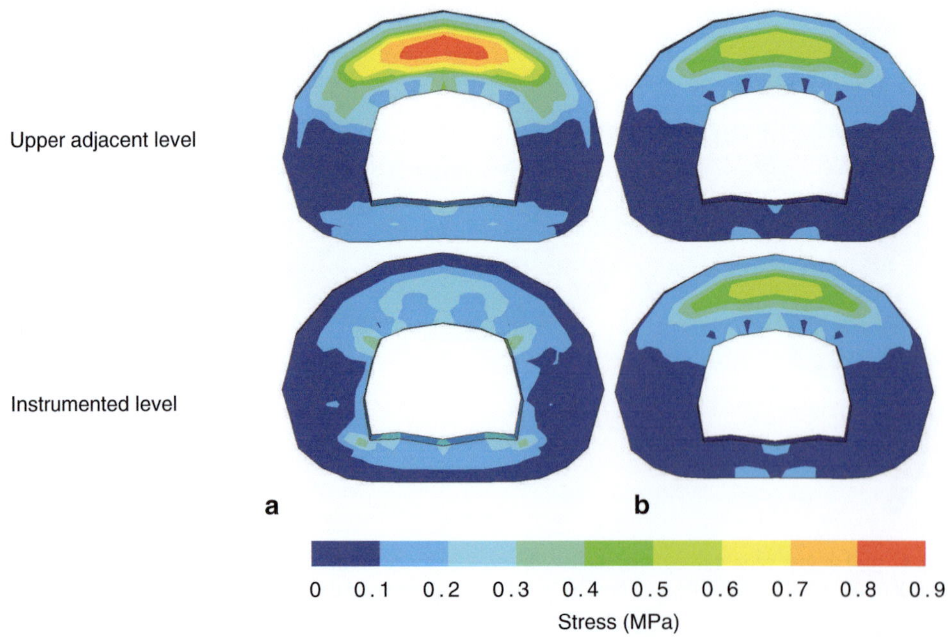

Fig. 7 Example of a numerical result, showing the stress distribution in the intervertebral disc, for two variants—(**a**, **b**) of the same posterior implant

stresses in the intervertebral disc at the instrumented level and at the adjacent level. Some companies now use modelling on a regular basis because such an approach can drastically reduce the design time of an implant.

To illustrate the essential enlightenment that modelling offers, we are interested in dynamic instrumentation using pedicular screws and flexible longitudinal connection elements. "Screw loosening" is a mechanical complication resulting in a deterioration of the bone quality around the screws, impacting the holding of the anchorage. A meta-analysis [21] has shown that the rate of screw loosening varies according to scientific publications of 0–72%. This very large variability can be related to differences in implant concepts. Finite element analysis helps to understand that longitudinal stiffness, along the axis of the connecting elements, is of paramount importance. When bending is performed, the interpedicular distance (at the entry points of the screws) increases in an intact vertebral segment (Fig. 8). If the implant breaks this variation, the movement is altered and local stresses can appear. Modelling allows, all things being equal, variation of the stiffness of the longitudinal element. Results show that when the implant, even if it is flexible, has a high longitudinal stiffness, it yields increased mechanical stresses in the pedicles, which may be responsible for the degradation of the anchorage [16]. Although the clinical outcome of a spinal surgery is really very multifactorial, such a conceptual study allows understanding of a key factor of the variability of results from one type of dynamic implant to another, which is useful to better outline the specifications of such implants.

Subject-Specific Modelling and Treatment Planning

Beyond the conceptual models, it is important to use personalized modelling when the question is, for a given patient, to understand the factors explaining a degenerative process or a mechanical complication because each patient is unique and has his own specificities. A subject-specific geometric model can be obtained from biplanar radiography, or sectional imaging (CT, MRI) or even from ultrasound imaging. However, to build a biomechanical model, it is also essential to document the mechanical properties of the components. There are still technical difficulties, even if great progress has been made in recent years, either by inverse methods for surgery simulation [22, 23] or by direct characterization by ultrasonic elastography, in particular for intervertebral discs [24]. It is also necessary to customize the mechanical loads that may vary depending on the normal or altered postural alignment, and the effectiveness of the muscular actuators. These components will be the subject of paragraph 4.

We will illustrate the interest of these subject-specific models by two very different clinical applications, relating on the one hand to osteoporosis fractures and on the other hand to the simulation of the effect of bracing for scoliosis.

Personalized Simulation to Estimate the Resistance of an Osteoporotic Vertebra

Osteoporosis is a diffuse disease that causes bone fragility, and its prevention is a major issue in public health. Vertebral fractures cause an alteration of the sagittal balance, resulting in severe pain and an increased risk of secondary fractures, impacting the quality of life and independence of the person. Characterization of bone strength is essential to identify at-risk individuals and target preventative therapies. The routine clinical examination is bone osteodensitometry, or DXA (Dual X-Ray Absorptiometry), to estimate bone mineral density (BMD). However, the intrinsic resistance of the vertebra also depends on its shape. Custom finite element models are constructed from QCT (quantitative CT) scanner images, in which the images are previously calibrated for conversion of

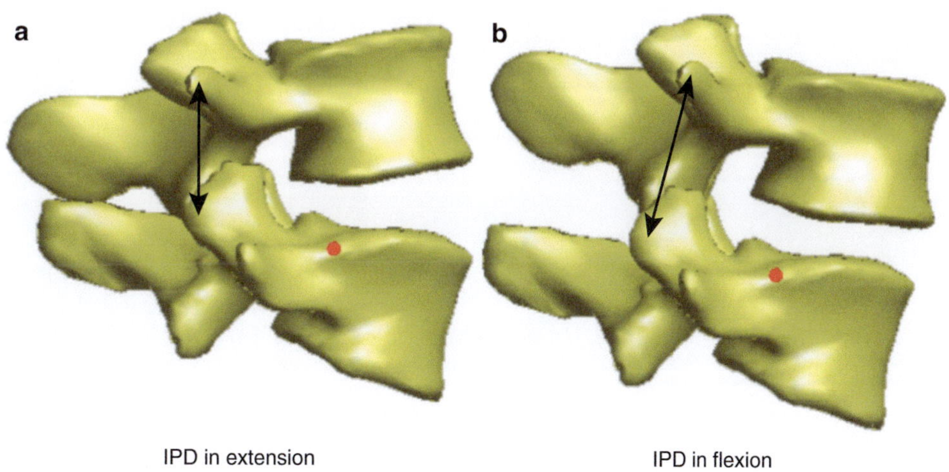

Fig. 8 Between full flexion and full extension, the interpedicular distance (IPD) between the entry points of the pedicle screws varies. When the longitudinal element does not allow any elongation, the modelling shows that it results in increased stress in the pedicles, which may explain a deterioration of the anchorage

Hounsfield units ((HU), associated with the attenuation coefficient of the medium traversed) to BMD. The mechanical properties being correlated with the BMD can be personalized for each "element" which composes the model. The latter is then validated by performing mechanical compression tests in vitro on vertebrae that have been scanned beforehand. Subject-specific models are constructed and test conditions are reproduced to compare the estimated fracture strength by numerical simulation with that measured experimentally. Figure 9 shows the ability of such models to estimate the fracture limit for each of the vertebrae.

Such models have been used, for example, to study the sensitivity of different parameters on bone strength [25]. Other things being equal, it has been shown that the displacement of 1 cm of the lever arm of the load exerted on a vertebra is likely to cause an increase of more than 100% of the mechanical stresses and a decrease of approximately 50% of the strength. This explains the particularly detrimental effect of an alteration of the postural alignment, which results in the increase of the lever arm of the loads exerted on the vertebrae, thus increasing the risk of fracture. This point will be included in paragraph 4.

These models are also used for clinical trials to objectify the effect of drugs on bone reinforcement [26], or to better understand the influence of mechanical properties of bone cement during vertebral restoration [27]. They are not yet used in clinical routine because the systematic realization of scanners for screening is difficult to envisage, but research is very active to build such models from biplane imaging in dual energy. The first proofs of concept in vitro are made [28, 29], with a coefficient of correlation between numerical and experimental strength r^2 of 0.84, between that of the model resulting from the scanner ($r^2 = 0.96$) and the prediction by DXA ($r^2 = 0.74$). Biplane radiography also has the advantage of the standing position, making it possible to also consider the postural alignment of the subject.

Personalized Simulation to Estimate the Effect of a Scoliosis Brace

When a scoliosis has to be corrected by brace, the correction strategy is difficult to establish for each individual, which explains the sometimes insufficient corrections and the fact that the effectiveness of the braces is variable [30]. To move from the geometric model to the biomechanical model, the mechanical properties of the intervertebral discs and the different connecting tissues (ligaments, costovertebral and costotransverse junctions, intercostal muscles) are documented. Although these characteristics can hardly be customized today, the mechanical properties of the ribs, which directly affect the correction transfer from the ribcage to the spine, can be adjusted according to the age of the patient [31, 32]. The numerical simulation consists, at this stage, in simulating the points of support exerted by the brace to account for the biomechanical response of the spine. Validation of such models can only be done with respect to real in vivo data, and a first validation protocol is to compare the numerical results with the results from pre-treatment and post-treatment corset acquisitions. The comparison involves both

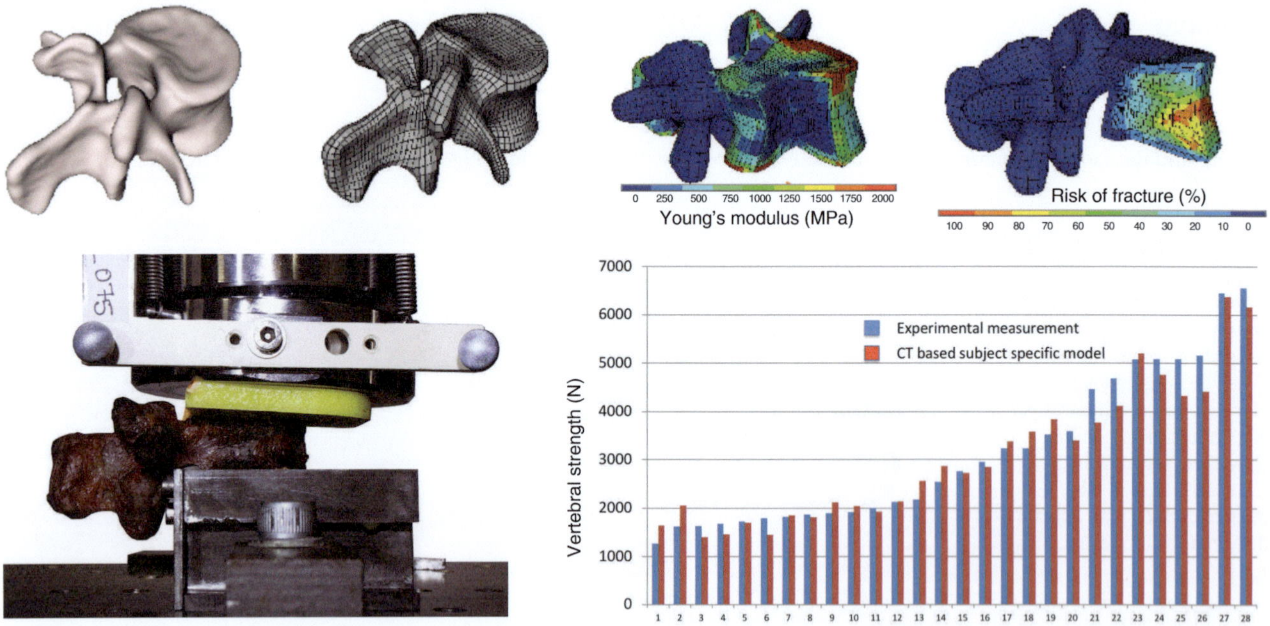

Fig. 9 For 28 vertebrae between L1 and L3, comparison between the experimental fracture force and the estimated rupture force by simulation, for models whose geometry and mechanical properties are customized from scanner imagery

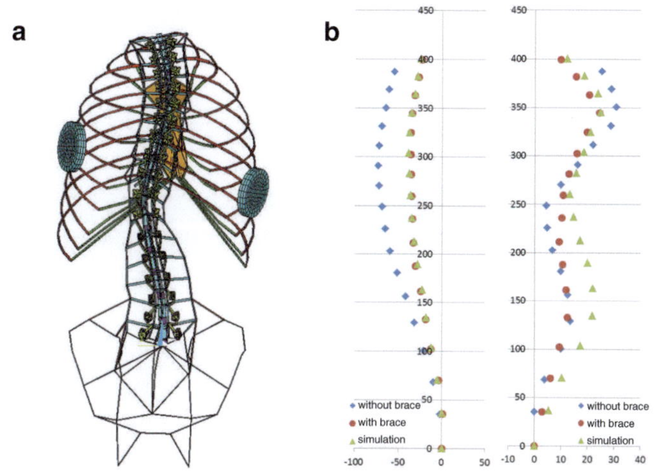

c

	Pre-brace	post brace measured	post-brace: simulation
T4-T12 kyphosis (°)	26	21	18
L1-L5 lordosis (°)	36	31	30
Cobb angle (°)	22	13	12
AVR (°): vertebra axial rotation at the apical level	8	7	5
Torsion (°)	11	8	10
Rib hump (°)	9	7	7

Fig. 10 Example of evaluation of a correction simulation by brace: (**a**) personalized model and simulation of correction pads; (**b**) comparison of the spinal line before, after brace and simulation; (**c**) comparison of the values of clinical parameters obtained by simulation with the parameters measured from post-brace 3D reconstructions

the spinal line and the main clinical parameters of interest: Cobb angle, hump, lordosis, kyphosis, vertebral and intervertebral rotations, and torsion (Fig. 10). Although still preliminary, the results on 42 patients are promising [24] and open the way to the exploitation of modelling as a real tool of reflection to plan the correction considering the specificities of the patient and the results of the predictive simulations.

Postural Alignment, Barycentremetry and Muscle Modelling

The spine is an essential component of the musculoskeletal system, and a gradual evolution has emerged over the last 30 years, from a very local view of the area of direct interest (functional unit or extended vertebral segment) to the global vision considering the longitudinal skeleton as a whole. The chapter on sagittal balance clearly shows the interindividual morphological differences in pelvic incidence and their impact on spinal alignment.

The gravity line, which is the vertical line passing through the subject's centre of gravity, can be localized with regard to the skeleton by associating a force platform with a monoplane [33] or biplane radiograph system [34, 35]. This measurement is important to understand how each individual adjusts his or her posture to maintain this gravity line (GL) within the polygon of support formed by the feet, a condition of balance in the erect position. But it is complex to combine, in clinical routine, radiographic measurements and force platforms, with a relative positioning of the two systems. The modelling approach is useful for estimating the location of LG without an additional platform [36, 37].

3D reconstruction from biplane radiographs of the outer envelope is now fast and accurate (Fig. 11) [38]. It allows computing the volume of each body segment. By estimating the density of each body segment in databases, it is possible to deduce the mass of each segment and the location of its centre of mass. The baricentre of all segments corresponds to the subject's global centre of gravity, which thus can be estimated by modelling. The interest is also to quantify the location of the centre of mass above a given vertebral level (Fig. 12).

To understand why this element is important, we must keep in mind the fundamental research on the biomechanical behaviour of isolated spinal segments: when a centred compression force is exerted on the upper vertebral body of a functional unit, the compression is very high, of the order from 200 to 400 N in the cervical zone and from 4000 to 6000 N in the lumbar zone. When this force Fc is deviated forwards, the lever arm (D) yields a bending moment $Mf = Fc \times D$.

However, the physiologic bending moment is quite low, of the order of 2 Nm in the cervical and 20 Nm in the lumbar spine, which means that if the lever arm is 10 cm (0.1 m), the allowable compression force for a vertebral segment drops to 20 N cervical and 200 N lumbar.

The barycentremetry, by locating the centre of mass of each corporal segment, makes it possible to estimate this lever arm in a realistic way. The work is still preliminary, but by way of example, the external envelope was calculated and the barycentremetry was carried out for 32 asymptomatic subjects in three age groups (12 from 20–40 years, 10 from 41–60 years and 10 from over 61). The centre of mass of the area above L1 moves forward with age, with a lever arm that varies on average from

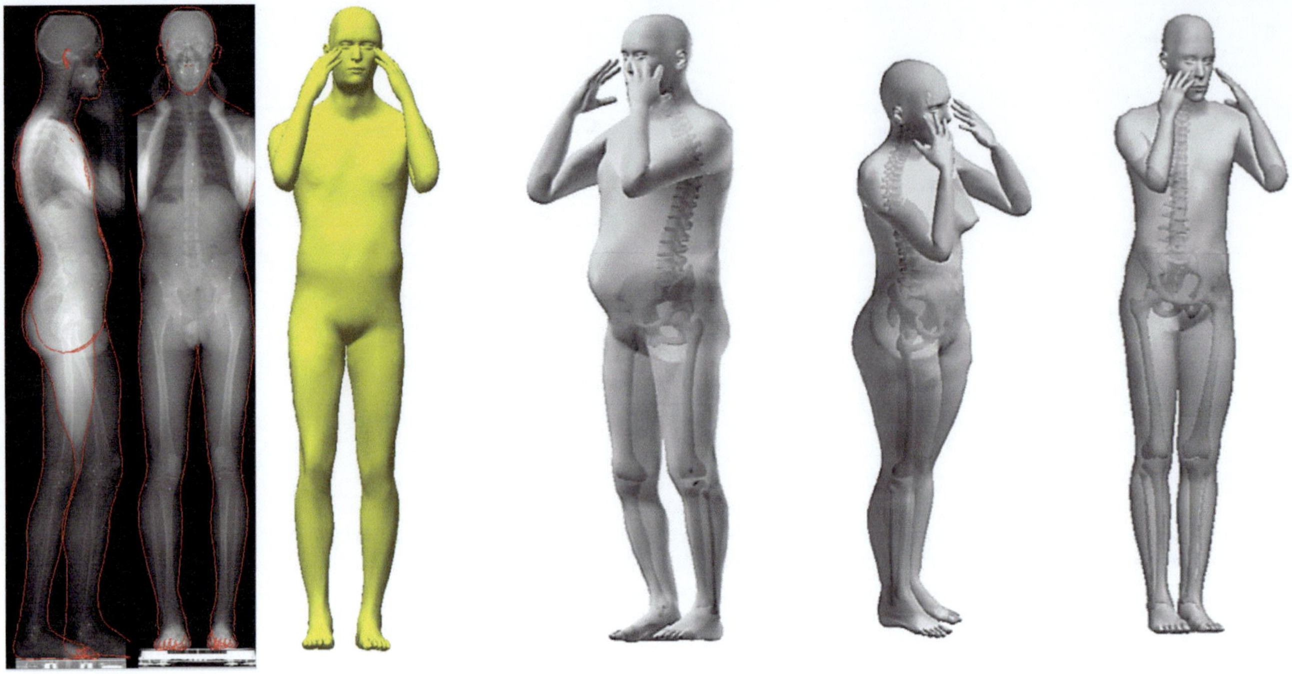

Fig. 11 Reconstruction of the outer envelope from biplanar X-rays, allowing consideration of interindividual variabilities

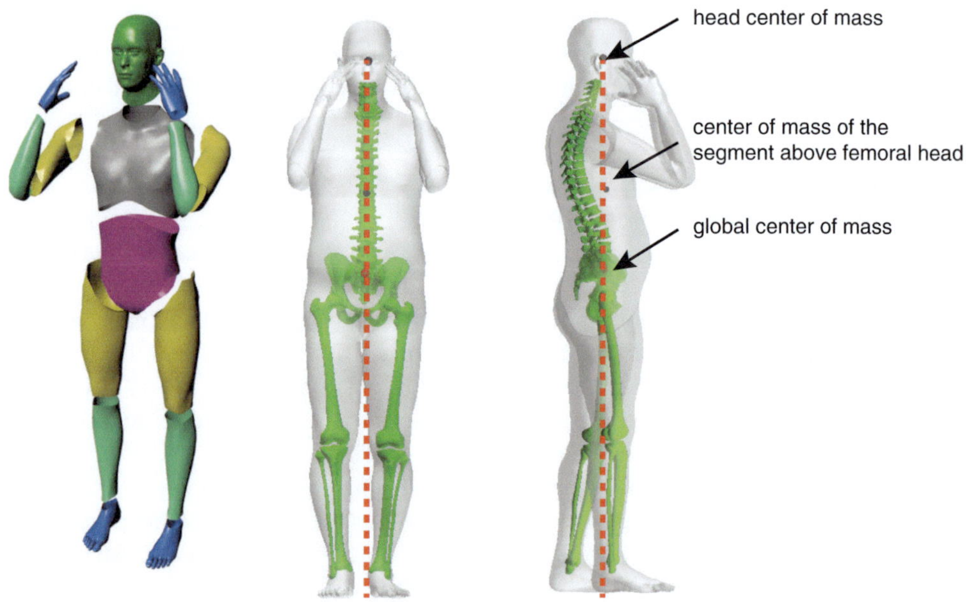

Fig. 12 For each body segment, the mass and the center of mass can be calculated, allowing the calculations of barycentremetry and the estimation of the line of gravity. Center of mass (CoM) head. CoM segment above the femoral heads. Global CoM

13 mm for group 1 to 37 and 44 mm for groups 2 and 3, respectively. With identical bone mineral density, finite element modelling shows that the permissible compressive force drops from 4000 N to 1000 N under the effect of the moment induced by this lever arm. This modelling illustrates the interest of also analysing the postural alignment, and not only the bone mineral density, when one is interested in the risk of fracture of osteoporosis [39]. Another essential parameter to consider is the muscular system; indeed, the muscles are essential components of spinal biomechanics because they allow regulation of the bending moment, and also the shear forces and the moments of lateral inflexion and torsion.

However, the chapter on anatomy shows how complex and subtle this muscular architecture is, with a large number of muscles, to reconcile stability and precise control of posture and movement. For biomechanists, muscular modelling is an active field of research, based on the approach of roboticists who are interested in the control of systems:

- The state of the system is continuously measured with the help of *sensors*;

- A *control system* verifies that this state respects the set-points related for example to the stability and/or to the security of the system;
- A *command system* associated with the control system drives the actuators to regulate the system if necessary and maintain it in the desired state.

For the control of the posture and the movement of the spine, the sensors are numerous at the level of the skin, the eyes, the vestibular system and also at the level of the ligaments, with the proprioceptive sensors which alert in case of abnormal intervertebral displacements. The nervous system provides control and command of muscular actuators to regulate posture and ensure accurate and stable movement.

Alteration of any of the elements can lead to disturbances: the alteration of sensors, control and command can affect the processing of information that can be altered or slowed down. Altered muscle actuators, due to muscle atrophy or fatty infiltration, can affect the ability to regulate posture and movement.

The analysis of these complex mechanisms is all the more difficult because there are still technological blocks because many parameters of interest are hardly accessible to measurement: for example electromyography (EMG), carried out more easily for assessing the superficial muscles, can measure muscle activation but it cannot directly assess muscular effort. Nevertheless, the progress of functional MRI and electroencephalography (EEG) should shed valuable light on the aspects related to muscular control.

The complexity is also linked to the multiplicity of co-activated muscles, to manage the synergy and muscle antagonisms for a permanent control of the stability of the system.

However, in this field too, modelling is making progress: research in muscle modelling makes it possible to exploit MRI data for a quantitative calculation of muscle volumes and fatty infiltration of muscles [40, 41]. The exploitation of ultrasound elastography also appears very promising [42]. As for the modelling of muscular activation, different mathematical approaches are proposed in the literature [43]. Models simulating postural control from proprioceptive information have been proposed [44]. The personalization of the models will allow better understanding of the vicious cascade that occurs when postural alignment and/or the muscular system is altered, in order to progress towards the prevention of aggravation of certain spinal pathologies.

Conclusion

With the development of computer science and numerical simulation tools, modelling brings one of the elements of understanding of the functional anatomy of the spine.

Geometric modelling allows today observation of the skeleton in 3D, in erect position, which helps diagnose and objectify the effect of a therapeutic intervention. Longitudinal studies should reveal a number of degradation mechanisms.

Biomechanical modelling considers both the geometrical and mechanical properties of the components. This is an increasingly useful way to help design implants and functional restoration systems. The evolution towards personalized modelling opens up promising prospects for helping to plan treatments that consider the specificities of each individual. These models are still at the research level, but they are reaching maturity and should in the near future be usable in clinical practice.

The biomechanical analysis of the spine cannot be complete without considering the mechanical loads that are exerted, relative to gravity and the muscular efforts. Advances in barycentremetry analysis, in personalized muscle modelling and in muscular control modelling, should lead to a better understanding of the involved mechanisms.

Thus, modelling provides valuable insights for a better, earlier and more accurate diagnosis, and for a quantitative assessment of the effect of treatments. The better understanding of the mechanisms of degradation with individual specificities should be a source of major progress and breakthrough innovations in prevention and therapeutic management.

Acknowledgements It is difficult to thank everyone involved in the research mentioned in this chapter. Thank you to the team of the ENSAM Biomechanics Laboratory, now the Georges Charpak Institute of Human Biomechanics, as well as the clinical and industrial partners of this research.

This research is benefited from financial support under the ParisTech biomecAM Chair in subject-specific modelling, with the support of the Yves Cotrel Foundation for research in spinal pathology, the Protéor company, Société Générale and the Covéa group. This Chair allows basic research, which is essential to progress. Thanks to the institutional supports and partners of the European VPHOP project, the FUI STEREOS + and DEXEOS projects and the CORSIN project.

Beyond these references and the rich international scientific literature on the subject, the reader will be able to refer to the PhDs on Spine research carried out at ENSAM on various aspects, in order to deepen the aspects addressed in this document of biomechanics and spine modelling, both by engineers and by clinicians: W. Skalli (1983), F. Lavaste (1990 state thesis), S. Robin (1992), N. Maurel (1993), W. Koubaa (1995), JL. Descrimes (1995), S. Veron (1997), P. Leborgne (1998), A. Templier (1998), N. Bertholon (1999), C. Lecire (1999), A. Mitulescu (2001), V. Pomero (2002), R. Dumas (2002), V. Lafage (2002), B. Fréchède (2003), Ph. Dupont (2004), S. Campana (2004), N. Champain (2004), O. Gille (2006), Y. Lafon (2006), MA. Rousseau (2007), S. Champain (2008), T. Mosnier (2008), E. Sapin (2008), A. Laville (2010), C. Barrey (2011), X. Drevelle (2011), J. S. Steffen (2011), A. Courvoisier (2012), B. Ilharreborde (2012), Y. P. Charles (2012), C. Travert (2013), B. Moal (2014), L. Venancio (2014), M. Prud'homme (2014).

References

1. Adam C, Rouch P, Skalli W. Inter-lamellar shear resistance confers compressive stiffness in the intervertebral disc: an image-based modelling study on the bovine caudal disc. J Biomech. 2015;48(16):4303–8.

2. Prot M, Saletti D, Pattofatto S, Bousson V, Laporte S. Links between mechanical behavior of cancellous bone and its microstructural properties under dynamic loading. J Biomech. 2015;48(3):498–503.
3. Dubousset J, Charpak G, Dorion I, Skalli W, Lavaste F, Deguise J, Kalifa G, Ferey S. A new 2D and 3D imaging approach to musculoskeletal physiology and pathology with low-dose radiation and the standing position: the EOS system. Bull Acad Natl Med. 2005;2:287–97.
4. Pomero V, Mitton D, Laporte S, De Guise JA, Skalli W. Fast accurate stereoradiographic 3D-reconstruction of the spine using a combined geometric and statistic model. Clin Biomech. 2004;3:240–7.
5. Humbert L, Guise JA, Aubert B, Godbout B, Skalli W. 3D reconstruction of the spine from biplanar X-rays using parametric models based on transversal and longitudinal inferences. Med Eng Phys. 2009;31:681–7.
6. Skalli W. Stéréoradiographie basse dose EOS: de la recherche à la routine clinique. Resuscitation. 2011;100:241–53.
7. Amabile C, Pillet H, Lafage V, Barrey C, JM V, Skalli W. A new quasi-invariant parameter characterizing the postural alignment of young asymptomatic adults. Eur Spine J. 2016;25(11):3666–74.
8. Perdriolle R. La scoliose, son étude tridimensionnelle. Paris: Maloine éditeur; 1979. 144p.
9. Steib JP, Dumas R, Mitton D, Skalli W. Surgical correction of scoliosis by in situ contouring: a detorsion analysis. Spine. 2004;29(2):193–9.
10. Courvoisier A, Drevelle X, Vialle R, Dubous Set J, Skalli W. 3D analysis of brace treatment in idiopathic scoliosis. Eur Spine J. 2013;22(11):2427–32.
11. Lebel DE, Alaubaidi Z, Shin EJ, Howard A, Zeller R. Three dimensional analysis of brace biomechanical efficacy for patients with AIS. Eur Spine J. 2013;22(11):2445–8.
12. Ilharreborde B, Sebag G, Skalli W, Mazda K. Adolescent idiopathic scoliosis treated with posteromedial translation: radiologic evaluation with a 3D low-dose system. Eur Spine J. 2013;22(10):2335.
13. Vergari C, Courtois I, Ebermeyer E, Boulous SA H, Vialle R, Skalli W. Experimental validation of a patient-specific model of orthotic action in adolescent idiopathic scoliosis. Eur Spine J. 2016;25(10):3049–55.
14. Vergari C, Abelin-Genevois K, Kohler R, Dre Velle X, Ebermeyer E, Courtois I, Dubousset J, Skalli W A preliminary validation of a severity index for early detection of progressive adolescent idiopathic Scoliosis. Scoliosis Research Society 49th annual meeting, 2014; Anchorage, Alaska, USA; 2014.
15. Ferrero E, Lafage R, Challier V, Diebo B, Gui Gui P, Mazda K, Schwab F, Skalli W, Lafage V. Clinical and stereoradiographic analysis of adult spinal deformity with and without rotatory subluxation. Orthop Traumatol Surg Res. 2015;101(5):613–8.
16. Venanciolima L Contribution à la modélisation biomécanique personnalisée du rachis lombaire intact et instrumenté. Thèse de doctorat Ecole nationale supérieure d'arts et métiers ENSAM; 2014.
17. Robin S, Skalli W, Lavaste F. Influence of geometrical factors on the behavior of lumbar spine segments: a finite element analysis. Eur Spine J. 1994;3(2):84–90.
18. Laville A, Laporte S, Skalli W. Parametric and subject-specific finite element modelling of the lower cervical spine. Influence of geometrical parameters on the motion patterns. J Biomech. 2009;42:1409–15.
19. Lafage V, Gangnet N, Sénégas J, Lavaste F, Skalli W. New interspinous implant evaluation using an in vitro biomechanical study combined with a finite-element analysis. Spine. 2007;32:1706–13.
20. Charles YP, Persohn S, Steib JP, Mazel C, Skalli W. Influence of an auxiliary facet system on lumbar spine biomechanics. Spine. 2011;36:690–9.
21. Prud'homme M, Barrios C, Rouch P, Charles YP, Steib JP, Skalli W. Clinical outcomes and complications after pedicle-anchored dynamic or hybrid lumbar spine stabilization: a systematic literature review. J Spinal Disord Tech. 2015;28(8):E439–48.
22. Lafage V, Dubousset J, Lavaste F, Skalli W. 3D finite element simulation of Cotrel-Dubousset correction. Comput Aided Surg. 2004;9(1–2):17–25.
23. Lafon Y, Lafage V, Steib JP, Dubousset J, Skal Li W. In vivo distribution of spinal intervertebral stiffness based on clinical flexibility tests. Spine. 2010;35:186–93.
24. Vergari C, Dubois G, Vialle R, Gennisson JL, Tanter M, Dubousset J, Rouch P, Skalli W. Lumbar annulus fibrosus biomechanical characterization in healthy children by ultrasound shear wave elastography. Eur Radiol. 2016;26(4):1213–7.
25. Travert C, Jolivet E, Sapindebrosses E, Mit Ton D, Skalli W. Sensitivity of patient-specific vertebral finite element model from low dose imaging to material properties and loading conditions. Med Biol Eng Comput. 2011;49:1355–61.
26. Keaveny TM, Mcclung MR, Genant HK, Zan Chetta JR, Kendler D, Brown JP, Goemaere S, Recknor C, Brandi ML, Eastell R, Kopperdahl DL, Engelke K, Fuerst T, Radcliffe HS, Libanati C. Femoral and vertebral strength improvements in postmenopausal women with osteoporosis treated with denosumab. J Bone Miner Res. 2014;29(1):158–65.
27. Kinzl M, Schwiedrzik J, Zysset PK, Pahr DH. An experimentally validated finite element method for augmented vertebral bodies. Clin Biomech (Bristol, Avon). 2013;28(1):15–22 5.
28. Choisne J, Valiadis JM, Travert C, Rouch P, Skalli W. Vertebral strength prediction under anterior compressive force using a finite element model. Comput Methods Biomech Biomed Engin. 2015;18(Suppl 1):1900–1. 21st Congress of the European Society of Biomechanics 2015; Prague, Czech Republic.
29. Travert C. Estimation du risque de fracture ostéoporotique du rachis thoraco-lombaire par un modèle en élément finis personnalisé. Thèse de doctorat. Ecole nationale supérieure d'arts et métiers ENSAM; 2012.
30. Weinstein SL, Dolan LA, Wright JG, Dobbs MB. Effects of bracing in adolescents with idiopathic scoliosis. N Engl J Med. 2013;369:1512–21.
31. Pezowicz C, Glowacki M. The mechanical properties of human ribs in young adult. Acta Bioeng Biomech. 2012;14:53–60.
32. Zhu Y. In vivo study on children of the mechanical behavior of thorax and the mechanical properties of ribs. Biomechanics. Thèse Université Claude Bernard Lyon I; 2014.
33. El Fegoun AB, Schwab F, Gamez L, Champain N, Skalli W, Farcy JP. Center of gravity and radiographic posture analysis: a preliminary review of adult volunteers and adult patients affected by scoliosis. Spine. 2005;30(13):1535–40.
34. Gangnet N, Pomero V, Dumas R, Skalli W, Vital JM. Variability of the spine and pelvis location with respect to the gravity line: a three-dimensional stereoradiographic study using a force platform. Surg Radiol Anat. 2003;25(5–6):424–33.
35. Steffen JS, Obeid I, Aurouer N, Hauger O, Vital JM, Dubousset J, Skalli W. 3D postural balance with regard to gravity line: an evaluation in the transversal plane on 93 patients and 23 asymptomatic volunteers. Eur Spine J. 2010;19:760–7.
36. Pillet H, Bonnet X, Lavaste F, Skalli W. Evaluation of force plateless estimation of the trajectory of the Centre of pressure during gait. Comparison of two anthropometric models. Gait Posture. 2010;31:147–52.
37. Sandoz B, Laporte S, Skalli W, Mitton D. Subject-specific body segment parameters' estimation using biplanar X-rays: a feasibility study. Comput Methods Biomech Biomed Engin. 2010;13:649–54.
38. Nérot A, Choisne J, Amabile C, Travert C, Pil Let H, Wang X, Skalli W. A 3D reconstruction method of the body envelope from biplanar X-rays: evaluation of its accuracy and reliability. J Biomech. 2015;48(16):4322–6.

39. Choisne J, Amabile C, Nérot A, Haschaka T, Travert C, Pillet H, Skalli W. Upper body center of mass location affects the factor of risk for vertebral fractures proceedings of ASBMR (American Society for Bone and Mineral Research) meeting 2015; Seattle, Washington, USA; 2015.
40. Moal B, Bronsard N, Raya JG, Vital JM, Schwab F, Skalli W, Lafage V. Volume and fat infiltration of spino-pelvic musculature in adults with spinal deformity. World J Orthop. 2015;6(9):727–37.
41. Li F, Laville A, Bonneau D, Laporte S, Skalli W. Study on cervical muscle volume by means of three-dimensional reconstruction. J Magn Reson Imaging. 2014;39(6):14116.
42. Dubois G, Kheireddine W, Vergari C, Bonneau D, Thoreux P, Rouch P, Tanter M, Gennisson JL, Skalli W. Reliable protocol for shear wave elastography of lower limb muscles at rest and during passive stretching. Ultrasound Med Biol. 2015;41(9):2284–91.
43. Dreischarf M, Shiraziadl A, Arjmand N, Rohlmann A, Schmidt H. Estimation of loads on human lumbar spine: a review of in vivo and computational model studies. J Biomech. 2016;49(6):833–45.
44. Pomero V, Lavaste F, Imbert G, Skalli W. A proprioception-based regulation model to estimate the trunk muscle forces. Comput Methods Biomech Biomed Engin. 2004;7(6):331–8.

Anatomy Is a Living Language

A. Dimeglio and F. Bonnel

Every generation is called to write a new page in the history of anatomy. Questioning the past is necessary to discover a new world.

Anatomy: Open Thought on Modernity

Anatomy is a living language! It is not fixed. Anatomy books have, for pedagogical convenience, restricted this to a finite world. But from generation to generation, anatomy has been able to overcome this all-too rigid conformity. If the part is immutable, the expressions are multiple. With time, anatomy has been able to renew itself.

Medical imaging has accompanied this change; the three-dimensional scanner has revealed anatomy's intimate nature. Magnetic resonance has pushed the boundaries of the invisible by illuminating muscles, tendons, and ligaments. Ultrasound has uncovered the hidden fetus by delving into the sinuous folds of the spine and the brain. Growth reconciled anatomy with its original identity. Biomechanics has dynamized it by introducing movement. The quantified analysis of walking showed that the flexibility of the spine and the pelvis was a prerequisite for fluid movement of the lower limbs. The EOS, by apprehending the musculoskeletal apparatus in its entirety, has inscribed the spine in the corporal space.

Embryology: The Essence (of Things) of Life

A critical period, a decisive period, everything happens at an exponential speed. Everything is ordinanced to the millimeter and the second. Synchronized, harmonized, hierarchical, this choreographic ballet obeys a ternary rhythm: first, a mesenchymal phase, then cartilaginous, and then ossification. These three successive and superimposed phases do not tolerate the slightest deception at the origin of the malformations. The vessels and the nerves preside over the simultaneous construction of several organs: spine, heart, kidney. Chromosome non-compliance explains Klippel Feil's syndrome: cervical vertebral malformations are accompanied by a constellation of malformations observed in the kidney, heart, cord, and upper limb.

The container and the contents of the vertebral column control each other. The non-closure of the neural plate leads to a loss of the posterior arch at the origin of a myelomeningocele. At 2 months (60 days) of intrauterine life, everything is arranged! The "anonymous" mesenchymal tissue gives way to a miniature model of the body with a well-defined cartilaginous supporting frame and an ossification that spreads over 17 years.

Growth: A Volumetric Revolution, a Morphological Emancipation

At birth, 30% of the skeleton is ossified. Ossification is tenacious, irresistible. It gradually gains ground and seizes the cartilaginous cartilage; the morphology changes. The vertebral body, initially ovoid, takes the form of a parallelepiped (three-dimensional parallelogram). In contrast, the thorax at birth is circular and becomes, over time, ovoid. Growth is a volumetric revolution: chest volume is 8% at birth, 30% at 5 years, and 50% at 10 years.

Growth Is Not Linear

Each growth site has its own pace. Between 5 years and the beginning of puberty, when the lower limb grows, the trunk slows; the reverse occurs at puberty. At 5 years old, the height reaches 70% of its final size and the thoracic area 30%. All

A. Dimeglio (✉)
Department of Pediatric Orthopedic Surgery, Polyclinique Saint Roch, Montpellier, France

F. Bonnel
Orthopedic Surgery, Clinique Beau Soleil, Montpellier, France

J. M. Vital, D. T. Cawley (eds.), *Spinal Anatomy*, https://doi.org/10.1007/978-3-030-20925-4_33

growths are not contemporaneous, but all are synchronized. Strategies must follow these phases of acceleration and deceleration.

The Interdependence of Growths Explains the Domino Effect

Any abnormal growth of the spine induces an abnormal growth of the thorax which leads to an abnormal growth of the heart and lungs. It all starts with scoliosis and everything can end with cardiorespiratory failure. Campbell proposes to treat "chest retraction" first and foremost: it is the parasol effect to give more room for lung growth.

The Vilebrequin Effect Is Omnipresent

Growth cartilages are masters of the game. Controlling a serious infantile scoliosis requires the theoretical neutralization of all the growth cartilages involved in the curvature. No instrumentation is able to control the crankshaft effect. An insurmountable challenge! On the one hand, the temptation is great to neutralize the evolutionary curvature; on the other, everything must be done to save mobility. According to the work of Canavese and Karol, early arthrodesis of the spine has negative consequences for the growth of thorax and lungs. The surgical approach of the growing spine should be as economical as possible. Any extensive dissection creates the conditions for spontaneous arthrosis. Early severe scoliosis, whatever its cause, is initially a true "orthopedic" disease that, over time, changes in nature. It is transformed and becomes a pediatric disease with serious cardio-pulmonary consequences.

Puberty Idiopathic Scoliosis: Indomitable

The technical feats, by pedicle screw fixation which completely corrects the curvature, must not make us forget that the arthrodesis is an incurable anatomical sacrifice. It is never the final solution; it is a statement of failure. The maximum is not necessarily the optimum. Growth leads us to favor mobility and prescribe arthrodesis. In the end, what matters is not the amount of raw material (screw, rod, etc.) but the amount of gray matter. The control of a spinal curvature first involves strategic intelligence.

COBB Angle: A Virtual Value

It does not reflect the real world, the global spatial reality of spinal deformity. What matters is not the Cobb angle but the remaining growth: 20° scoliosis at 5 years is distressing, 20° at 10 years is a concern, whereas 20° at 15 years is reassuring. "What matters is not the angle of Cobb, but the cone of stability" (Dubousset).

Balance: A Priority, an Ardent Obligation

It is necessary to write about balance. Global equilibrium is actually the product of 1000 postures, 1000 matches, 1000 coordinated compensations. In the context of normal and pathological variants, each individual has its morphological specificity and therefore a spinal balance which is part of his personality.

After Growth the Spine Continues Its Destiny

Aging begins very early with, as a priority, the lumbar spine, which is first concerned with the lumbosacral junction. Protecting one's lumbar spine early in life by addressing the correct spinal economy and alignment is important.

The Time Has Come to Review the Hierarchies

For decades, anatomy books have prioritized bone. Experience has shown that ligaments, intervertebral discs, muscles, and fasciae are more important than bone structures. "The soft is more resistant than the hard." The viscoelasticity of the column in severe scoliosis is a parameter to be considered, halo traction retains its flexibility.

The Muscles and Their Fascia Play an Essential Role

The collapse of the spine in paralytic scoliosis is the perfect illustration. Their disposition between long and short are mixed and is on a short scale. The pennation of the fascicles intervenes mechanically in the first degree.

The Curvatures of the Column Promote Mobility, Elasticity, Resistance, and Balance

They are in correspondence and harmonious tension to distribute the constraints. They watch each other, oppose each other, compete with each other … and are finally accomplices. The loss of lumbar lordosis heavily compromises walking. Arthrodesis of thoracic kyphosis has upstream mechanical consequences (cervicalgia) and downstream consequences (lumbago).

Scoliotic Disease Is a Life-Long Illness

Over time, imperceptibly, 10° of lumbar scoliosis become 40° or 50° by 50 years. The aggravation is favored by muscular and disc degeneration, ligament fatigue.

The Surgeon Has a Physical Relationship with the Anatomy

Anatomy is his privileged partner. With experience, the surgeon tames it, feeling it, knowing where the risk is. Screw insertion to the pedicles is more than a technical audacity, it is a reasoned provocation. The surgeon knows that one has to be polite with the anatomy, with muscles and ligaments. But after surgery, nothing will be like before. There is no return to anatomical innocence.

Anatomy is a ruthless justice of the peace. There is no compromise possible. A perfect result supposes a perfect functional restitution.

Anatomy: A Regalian Discipline

It is a universal constitutional discipline.

It sets the rule.

It is essential without concession.

It is available in all languages.

It is timeless.

Its story has been tirelessly repeated since the origin of man.

Research: Positive Insubordination

Under repeated attacks of research, anatomy has been reborn in other forms. Without to denounce its past, it has torn herself away from the "motionless fixity" of schemas and sketches; it has distanced itself from static iconographic conventions. It knew how to renew itself as a living language. It has seized time with the study of growth. It apprehended the space with the EOS. It enriched itself with the study of walking. It has been enlarged by annexing the pelvis and renaming it to be called pelvic vertebrate. It appropriated the thorax as the fourth dimension of the spine. It echoes Schumpeter's quote: "Questioning the past is necessary to discover a new world." From generation to generation, anatomy is never quite the same or quite another.

Tomorrow: Another Day

Yesterday, Professor René Louis's book marked his time. For those starting their career in spinal surgery, one must start by reading this essential book that is still relevant today by its basic precepts. Today, the book edited by Professor Jean-Marc Vital and Derek Cawley is a continuation of that of Prof. Louis. It is the product of many enriching discussions between the authors. *It bears witness to the inexhaustible fecundity of anatomy;* as soon as it is closed, we perceive the necessity of writing another one … but tomorrow is another day.

The 10 stages of puberty.

		Hand	Olecranon	Triradiate cartilage	Risser
11-year-old girl	1	Sesamoid of the thumb	Double ossification	Open	0
13-year-old boy	2	Sesamoid of the thumb	Ovoid	Open	0
	3	Sesamoid of pronounced thumb	Quadrangular	Closed	0
	4	Sesamoid of pronounced thumb	Start of fusion	Closed	0
	5	Distal fusion of the thumb	Fused	Closed	0
13-year-old girl	6	Distal phalanx fusion	Fused	Closed	1
15-year-old boy	7	Metacarpophalangeal fusion	Fused	Closed	2
	8	Interphalangeal fusion	Fused	Closed	3
	9	Fusion ulna	Fused	Closed	4
	10	Fusion radius	Fused	Closed	5

Index

J. M. Vital, D. T. Cawley (eds.), *Spinal Anatomy*, https://doi.org/10.1007/978-3-030-20925-4

W

Z

FSC
www.fsc.org
MIX
Papier aus verantwortungsvollen Quellen
Paper from responsible sources
FSC® C105338

If you have any concerns about our products,
you can contact us on
ProductSafety@springernature.com

In case Publisher is established outside the EU,
the EU authorized representative is:
Springer Nature Customer Service Center GmbH
Europaplatz 3, 69115 Heidelberg, Germany

Printed by Libri Plureos GmbH
in Hamburg, Germany